ULTRASONOGRAPHY
IN
OBSTETRICS
AND GYNECOLOGY

ULTRASONOGRAPHY
IN
OBSTETRICS
AND GYNECOLOGY

Peter W. Callen, M.D.

Professor of Radiology,
Obstetrics, Gynecology and Reproductive Science
University of California, San Francisco
School of Medicine
San Francisco, California

W.B. SAUNDERS COMPANY

A Division of
Harcourt Brace & Company
Philadelphia   London   Toronto   Montreal   Sydney   Tokyo

W.B. SAUNDERS COMPANY
A Division of
Harcourt Brace & Company

The Curtis Center
Independence Square West
Philadelphia, Pennsylvania 19106

Library of Congress Cataloging-in-Publication Data

Ultrasonography in obstetrics and gynecology / [edited by] Peter W. Callen. — 3rd ed.

  p.   cm.

Includes bibliographical references and index.

ISBN 0–7216–6712–0

  1. Ultrasonics in obstetrics.   2. Generative organs, Female—Ultrasonic imaging.   I. Callen, Peter W.

[DNLM: 1. Fetal Diseases—diagnosis.   2. Fetal Monitoring.
3. Genital Diseases, Female—diagnosis.   4. Obstetrics.
5. Ultrasonography.   WQ 100 U47 1994]

RG527.5.U48U47   1994

618′.047543—dc20

DNLM/DLC   93–6621

Ultrasonography in Obstetrics and Gynecology, 3rd edition   ISBN 0–7216–6712–0

Printed in the United States of America.

Last digit is the print number: 9   8   7   6   5   4   3   2

To
Mom and Dad,
Karen, Melanie, Brooke, Andy and Daniel

Contributors

N. SCOTT ADZICK, M.D.
Associate Professor of Surgery and Pediatrics, University of California, San Francisco, School of Medicine, San Francisco, California.
Prenatal Management of the Fetus with a Correctable Defect

GERALDINE BALLARD, R.D.M.S.
Chief Ultrasound Technologist, University of Manitoba Health Sciences Centre, Winnipeg, Manitoba, Canada.
Normal Anatomy of the Female Pelvis

BERYL R. BENACERRAF, M.D.
Clinical Professor of Obstetrics, Gynecology, and Reproductive Biology, Harvard Medical School; Co-Director, Consultative Obstetrical Ultrasound, Brigham & Women's Hospital, Boston, Massachusetts.
Ultrasound Evaluation of the Fetal Face

CAROL B. BENSON, M.D.
Associate Professor of Radiology, Harvard Medical School; Co-Director of Ultrasound, Brigham & Women's Hospital, Boston, Massachusetts.
Ultrasound Evaluation of Amniotic Fluid

GINA M. BROWN, M.D.
Maternal-Fetal Fellow, Columbia University College of Physicians and Surgeons, New York, New York.
Endovaginal Sonographic Evaluation of the Obstetric and Gynecologic Patient

JOSEPH P. BRUNER, M.D.
Assistant Professor of Obstetrics and Gynecology, Vanderbilt University Medical Center, Nashville, Tennessee.
Doppler Ultrasonography in Obstetrics and Gynecology

PETER W. CALLEN, M.D.
Professor of Radiology, Obstetrics, Gynecology, and Reproductive Sciences, University of California, San Francisco, School of Medicine, San Francisco, California.
The Obstetric Ultrasound Examination
α-Fetoprotein Screening Programs: What Every Obstetric Sonologist Should Know
Ultrasound Evaluation of Gestational Trophoblastic Neoplasia
Artifacts, Pitfalls, and Normal Variants

WINSTON A. CAMPBELL, M.D.
Associate Professor of Obstetrics and Gynecology; Associate Director, Maternal-Fetal Medicine, Director, Maternal-Fetal Intensive Care Unit, University of Connecticut Health Center, Farmington, Connecticut.
Antepartum Fetal Assessment by Ultrasonography: The Fetal Biophysical Profile

DARYL H. CHINN, M.D.
Staff Radiologist, Department of Radiology, Hoag Memorial Hospital Presbyterian, Newport Beach, California.
Ultrasound Evaluation of Hydrops Fetalis

JAMES P. CRANE, M.D.
Professor of Obstetrics, Gynecology, and Radiology; Associate Vice Chancellor and Associate Dean for Clinical Affairs, Washington University School of Medicine, St. Louis, Missouri.
Ultrasound Evaluation of Fetal Chromosome Disorders

SYDNEY M. DASHEFSKY, M.D.
Assistant Professor of Radiology, University of Manitoba Health Sciences Centre, Winnipeg, Manitoba, Canada.
Normal Anatomy of the Female Pelvis

PETER M. DOUBILET, M.D., Ph.D.
Associate Professor of Radiology, Harvard Medical School; Co-Director of Ultrasound, Brigham & Women's Hospital, Boston, Massachusetts.
Ultrasound Evaluation of Amniotic Fluid

VICKIE A. FELDSTEIN, M.D.
Assistant Professor of Radiology, University of California, San Francisco, School of Medicine, San Francisco, California.
The Role of Computed Tomography and Magnetic Resonance Imaging in Obstetrics

ROY A. FILLY, M.D.
Professor of Radiology and Obstetrics, Gynecology, and Reproductive Sciences and Vice Chairman, Department of Radiology, Chief, Section of Diagnostic Ultrasound, University of California, San Francisco, School of Medicine; Co-Director, Fetal Treatment Program, University of California, San Francisco Medical Center, San Francisco, California.
α-Fetoprotein Screening Programs: What Every Obstetric Sonologist Should Know
Ultrasound Evaluation During the First Trimester
Ultrasound Evaluation of Normal Fetal Anatomy
Ultrasound Evaluation of the Fetal Neural Axis
Ovarian Masses . . . What to Look for . . . What to Do
Ectopic Pregnancy

HARRIS J. FINBERG, M.D.
Director of Diagnostic Ultrasound, Phoenix Perinatal Associates, Phoenix, Arizona.
Ultrasound Evaluation in Multiple Gestation

ALAN W. FLAKE, M.D.
Assistant Professor of Surgery, University of California, San Francisco, School of Medicine, San Francisco, California.
Prenatal Management of the Fetus with a Correctable Defect

ARTHUR C. FLEISCHER, M.D.
Professor of Radiology, Obstetrics, and Gynecology; Chief of Diagnostic Sonography, Vanderbilt University Medical Center, Nashville, Tennessee.
Doppler Sonography in Obstetrics and Gynecology

JAMES D. GOLDBERG, M.D.
Associate Professor of Obstetrics, Gynecology, and Reproductive Sciences, University of California, San Francisco, School of Medicine; Attending Physician, University of California Hospitals, San Francisco, California.
The Role of Genetic Screening in the Obstetric Patient

RUTH B. GOLDSTEIN, M.D.
Associate Professor of Radiology and Obstetrics, Gynecology, and Reproductive Sciences, University of California, San Francisco, School of Medicine, San Francisco, California.
α-Fetoprotein Screening Programs: What Every Obstetric Sonologist Should Know
Ultrasound Evaluation of the Fetal Thorax
Ultrasound Evaluation of the Fetal Abdomen
Doppler Sonography in Obstetrics and Gynecology

LUÍS FLÁVIO GONÇALVES, M.D.
Research Fellow, Department of Radiology, Vanderbilt University Medical Center, Nashville, Tennessee.
Ultrasound Evaluation of Abdominal Wall Defects

FRANK P. HADLOCK, M.D.
Professor of Radiology, Baylor College of Medicine, Houston, Texas.
Ultrasound Determination of Menstrual Age
Ultrasound Evaluation of Fetal Growth
Sonographic Prediction of Fetal Lung Maturity

DEBORAH A. HALL, M.D.
Assistant Professor of Radiology, Harvard Medical School; Radiologist, Massachusetts General Hospital, Boston, Massachusetts.
Ultrasound Evaluation of the Uterus

MICHAEL R. HARRISON, M.D.
Professor of Surgery and Pediatrics, Chief, Division of Pediatric Surgery; Director, Fetal Treatment Center, University of California, San Francisco, School of Medicine, San Francisco, California.
Prenatal Management of the Fetus with a Correctable Defect

SUSAN C. HOLT, M.D.
Assistant Professor of Radiology, Section of Diagnostic Ultrasound, University of Manitoba Health Sciences Centre, Winnipeg, Manitoba, Canada.
Normal Anatomy of the Female Pelvis

HEDVIG HRICAK, M.D., Ph.D.
Professor of Radiology, Urology, and Radiation Oncology, and Chief,
Uroradiology Section, University of California, San Francisco, School of Medicine,
San Francisco, California
*The Role of Magnetic Resonance Imaging in the Evaluation of Gynecologic
Disease*

PHILIPPE JEANTY, M.D., Ph.D.
Associate Professor of Radiology and Assistant Professor of Obstetrics and
Gynecology, Vanderbilt University Medical Center, Nashville, Tennessee.
Ultrasound Evaluation of Abdominal Wall Defects

CLIFFORD S. LEVI, M.D.
Associate Professor of Radiology and Section Head of Diagnostic Ultrasound,
University of Manitoba Health Sciences Centre, Winnipeg, Manitoba, Canada.
Normal Anatomy of the Female Pelvis

DANIEL J. LINDSAY, M.D.
Assistant Professor of Radiology, University of Manitoba Health Sciences Centre,
Winnipeg, Manitoba, Canada.
Normal Anatomy of the Female Pelvis

EDWARD A. LYONS, M.D.
Professor and Chairman, Department of Radiology, University of Manitoba Health
Sciences Centre, Winnipeg, Manitoba, Canada.
Normal Anatomy of the Female Pelvis

BARRY S. MAHONY, M.D.
Co-Director, Ultrasound Division, Swedish Hospital Medical Center, Seattle,
Washington.
Ultrasound Evaluation of the Fetal Musculoskeletal System
Ultrasound Evaluation of the Fetal Genitourinary System

ANA MONTEAGUDO, M.D.
Assistant Professor of Obstetrics and Gynecology, Columbia University College of
Physicians and Surgeons, New York, New York.
Endovaginal Sonographic Evaluation of the Obstetric and Gynecologic Patient

MARK J. POPOVICH, M.D.
Assistant Clinical Professor of Radiology, University of California, San Francisco,
School of Medicine, San Francisco, California.
*The Role of Computed Tomography and Magnetic Resonance Imaging in
Obstetrics*
*The Role of Magnetic Resonance Imaging in the Evaluation of Gynecologic
Disease*

WILLIAM G. M. RITCHIE, M.D.
Clinical Professor of Radiology, University of Pennsylvania School of Medicine;
Radiologist, Pennsylvania Hospital, Philadelphia, Pennsylvania.
Ultrasound Evaluation of Normal and Induced Ovulation

JOHN F. RODIS, M.D.
Assistant Professor of Obstetrics and Gynecology; Director, Perinatal Genetics,
University of Connecticut Health Center, Farmington, Connecticut.
*Antepartum Fetal Assessment by Ultrasonography: The Fetal Biophysical
Profile*

KLAUS G. SCHMIDT, M.D.
Assistant Professor, Department of Cardiology, Children's University, Heidelberg,
Germany.
Ultrasound Evaluation of the Fetal Heart

NORMAN H. SILVERMAN, M.D.
Professor of Pediatrics and Radiology (Cardiology); Director, Pediatric
Echocardiography Laboratory, University of California, San Francisco, School of
Medicine, San Francisco, California.
Ultrasound Evaluation of the Fetal Heart

ILAN E. TIMOR-TRITSCH, M.D.
Professor of Clinical Obstetrics and Gynecology, Columbia University College of
Physicians and Surgeons; Director, Obstetrical and Gynecological Ultrasound,
Presbyterian Hospital, New York, New York.
Endovaginal Sonographic Evaluation of the Obstetric and Gynecologic Patient

RONALD R. TOWNSEND, M.D.
Associate Professor of Radiology, University of Colorado Health Sciences Center,
Denver, Colorado.
Ultrasound Evaluation of the Placenta and Umbilical Cord

ANTHONY M. VINTZILEOS, M.D.
Professor of Obstetrics, Gynecology, and Pediatrics, and PHS Professor and
Endowed Chair in Maternal-Fetal Medicine; Director, Maternal-Fetal Medicine
and Obstetrics, University of Connecticut Health Center, Farmington, Connecticut.
*Antepartum Fetal Assessment by Ultrasonography: The Fetal Biophysical
Profile*

JOHN A. WORRELL, M.D.
Assistant Professor of Radiology, Vanderbilt University Medical Center, Nashville,
Tennessee.
Doppler Sonography in Obstetrics and Gynecology

ISABEL C. YODER, M.D.
Associate Professor of Radiology, Harvard Medical School; Radiologist,
Massachusetts General Hospital, Boston, Massachusetts.
Ultrasound Evaluation of the Uterus

Preface

It has now been nearly six years since the last edition of this book was published. This long interval has been in keeping with my desire not to write and edit a new edition unless it would involve a major revision with significantly new changes. Likewise, as in the past, I have tried to incorporate the changes that you, the readers, have suggested. As a result, in addition to major revisions of previous chapters, 12 new chapters have been added to reflect areas of either new technologic change or reader interest. In addition, color photographs or illustrations have been added throughout the text. Although it may seem unusual to have a chapter dealing with gynecologic magnetic resonance imaging in a sonographic text, that modality is so frequently interrelated that it was believed to be of sufficient interest to include in this text.

Like the field of diagnostic ultrasonography, this book has grown over the past decade. What was initially a book of 20 chapters and 346 pages is now one of 34 chapters and more than 700 pages. Despite the increase in the size of this book, I have maintained the same objective that I had in previous editions: to produce a text that is not just a reference book but one that a reader would likely read in its entirety.

As the editor, I chose those contributors for this multiauthored text who are leading authorities and whose work is informative and readable. One will undoubtedly encounter differing philosophies or approaches to similar problems in this text. Rather than attempt to make this a homogeneous work, I retained this diversity of opinion, as much as possible. I tried to ensure that the quality of the illustrations and readability of the text were uniformly high.

There are many people to thank for their contributions and help: first, my family, for their patience and understanding; my close friend and associate, Roy Filly, for his major contributions and helpful suggestions; and the sonographers, fellows, and residents with whom I work. I wish to thank my secretary, Peggy Bragg, for her assistance and Lisette Bralow, the Editor-in-Chief, Medical Books, and the production staff at W.B. Saunders for their hard work. I also wish to thank the authors for their hard work and timely contributions and, lastly, you the reader, for your suggestions and continued interest in this text.

PETER W. CALLEN

Contents

CHAPTER *1*

■■■■■■■

The Obstetric Ultrasound Examination

PETER W. CALLEN, M.D.

It has now been more than two decades since ultrasonography was first used to evaluate the obstetric patient. In its infancy the questions that this modality sought to answer were quite basic: Is there a pregnancy? Is the fetus alive? Is there a singleton or a twin gestation? What is the location of the placenta? What is the gestational age? Probably few envisioned that the day would come when ultrasonography would be used to answer questions as to the presence of subtle anatomic defects such as cleft lip or palate or clubfoot abnormality. Likewise, at its inception it was difficult to convince clinicians as to the usefulness of this new diagnostic modality. Now it is unusual for a patient not to have at least one ultrasound examination during her pregnancy.

Although the almost universal enthusiasm for this modality is exciting, it has raised a new series of questions and problems. Is the ultrasound examination safe? How should the obstetric ultrasound examination be performed? Who should perform the ultrasound examination? Should screening ultrasound examinations be performed on every pregnant patient, and if so, how often? How does one avoid the mushrooming medical malpractice crisis as it relates to the diagnostic ultrasound examination? These questions and problems are addressed in the following discussion.

SAFETY OF ULTRASOUND EXAMINATION

It was not long after the inception of ultrasound evaluation that questions were raised as to the safety of this new modality. In an attempt to answer these concerns, studies were initiated to determine if there was an association between diagnostic ultrasound studies in utero and chromosomal abnormalities, altered fetal growth, learning disabilities, or even malignancy.[1-4] Although these studies are ongoing there is little evidence to indict ultrasonography as causing abnormalities in the human fetus.[5]

The major biologic effects of ultrasonography are believed to be thermal (a rise in temperature) and cavitation (production and collapse of gas-filled bubbles).[6, 7] Although it has been shown that a rise in temperature of less than 1°C may occur during diagnostic ultrasound evaluation, this is unlikely to have any clinical impact in humans.[8, 9] Likewise, cavitation (which requires the preexistence of stable gas-filled

nuclei) may occur with in vitro experiments but is also unlikely to occur in humans.[10]

The major difficulties with the studies investigating a possible deleterious effect of diagnostic ultrasound evaluation are threefold: (1) experimental ultrasound exposure levels often far exceeded those that are normally used diagnostically; (2) the systems used to show ultrasound effect (plants, cell culture, laboratory animals) may not be applicable to humans; and (3) many studies that have demonstrated adverse effects in vitro have not been reproducible.[6]

A review of the safety of ultrasound with respect to the fetus has concluded that "current data indicate that there are no confirmed biologic effects on patients and their fetuses from the use of diagnostic ultrasound evaluation and that the benefits to patients exposed to the prudent use of this modality outweigh the risks, if any."[6] Although one may obtain some reassurance of the safety of ultrasound evaluation from the previous statements, until adequate long-term studies are performed, ultrasound evaluation (like any other medical test) should be performed only when there are clear clinical indications.

INDICATIONS FOR OBSTETRIC ULTRASOUND EXAMINATION

It has been estimated, in some countries, that as many as 90% to 100% of women seeking obstetric care will have at least one ultrasound examination during pregnancy.[11, 12] In Glasgow, Scotland, where routine scanning is employed, the average number of scans per pregnancy is 2.8.[13]

If ultrasound evaluation is relatively safe and noninvasive and has the potential for yielding important diagnostic information, then why not use this modality in every pregnant patient? As one might imagine, there is much controversy over this single issue.

In countries where routine prenatal ultrasound examination is practiced, investigators have noted that ultrasound scanning is beneficial in detecting congenital malformations, in diagnosing twins and placenta previa, and in identifying patients at risk for postmaturity and intrauterine growth retardation.[12, 14] Although these observations are clearly important, the major question still unanswered is whether patient outcome is significantly improved by screening ultrasound examinations. In one study in which the routine use of prenatal ultrasound examination was evaluated, researchers found no benefit from the routine use of "office ultrasound."[15] Most important errors of gestational age and most twin pregnancies were suspected clinically and diagnosed by an indicated, as opposed to a screening, ultrasound examination.[15]

Several studies have examined the sensitivity of ultrasound assessment for the detection of congenital anomalies.[16] These studies have demonstrated that in a low-risk population the sensitivity is low, approximately 34%, while the specificity is quite high at 99%.[17, 18] When targeted examinations of a high-risk population are performed the sensitivity is significantly improved, to greater than 90%.[19, 20]

Even if one concludes, based on the previous information, that screening ultrasound examinations are a worthwhile endeavor, two major issues must still be addressed. First, the cost of such an undertaking would be large. With approximately 4 million deliveries in the United States annually, the cost of screening every woman with a conservative estimate of $200 per examination would be $800 million. If one adds the additional cost for multiple examinations the added health care costs would be over $1 billion.

The second issue involves the persons who perform the screening examinations. Many believe the best solution would be to have virtually any examiner do the screening as long as he or she would willingly refer all questions to more experienced persons. Although that might conceivably alleviate the problem with the false-positive examination, it would not address the issues of missing an abnormality due to examiner inexperience and a large number of unnecessary "second look" examinations.

As a result of the explosion in the number of ultrasound examinations, a number of persons and organizations began the process of developing a consensus of indications for the performance of the ultrasound examination. In 1983–1984, a panel from the National Institutes of Health convened and, after obtaining input from a number of experienced sonologists, developed a list of indications for obstetric and gynecologic ultrasound evaluation[21]:

- Estimation of gestational age by ultrasound evaluation for confirmation of clinical dating for patients who are to undergo elective repeat cesarean delivery, induction of labor, or elective termination of pregnancy
- Evaluation of fetal growth (when the patient has an identified etiology for uteroplacental insufficiency, such as severe preeclampsia, chronic hypertension, chronic significant renal disease, or severe diabetes mellitus, or for other medical complications of pregnancy when fetal malnutrition, i.e., intrauterine growth retardation [IUGR] or macrosomia, is suspected)
- Vaginal bleeding of undetermined etiology in pregnancy
- Determination of fetal presentation when the presenting part cannot be adequately assessed in labor

- Suspected multiple gestation
- Adjunct to amniocentesis (chorionic villus sampling)
- Significant uterine size/clinical dates discrepancy
- Pelvic mass detected clinically
- Suspected hydatidiform mole
- Adjunct to cervical cerclage
- Suspected ectopic pregnancy
- Adjunct to special procedures
- Suspected fetal death
- Suspected uterine abnormality
- Intrauterine contraceptive device localization
- Ovarian follicle development surveillance
- Biophysical profile for fetal well-being (after 28 weeks' gestation)
- Observation of intrapartum events (e.g., version/extraction of second twin, manual removal of placenta)
- Suspected polyhydramnios or oligohydramnios
- Suspected abruptio placentae
- Adjunct to external version from breech to vertex presentation
- Estimation of fetal weight and/or presentation in premature rupture of membranes and/or premature labor
- Abnormal serum α-fetoprotein value for clinical gestational age when drawn
- Follow-up observation of identified fetal anomaly
- History of previous congenital anomaly
- Serial evaluation of fetal growth in multiple gestations
- Estimation of gestational age in late registrants for prenatal care

Although there may be some exceptions to this list, it serves as a useful guideline for referral for ultrasound evaluation in the obstetric and gynecologic patient.

WHO SHOULD PERFORM THE ULTRASOUND EXAMINATION AND HOW SHOULD IT BE PERFORMED?

Theoretically, the answer to who should perform the ultrasound examination should be extremely easy. In fact, it is one of the most controversial issues relating to the ultrasound examination. The answer should be that only those persons who have had adequate training (including didactic as well as supervised "hands on" experience) should perform and interpret an ultrasound examination.

More than 10 years ago the Joint Task Group on Training for Diagnosis in Obstetrical and Gynecologic Ultrasound developed guidelines for the postresident physician who completed residency programs in either radiology or obstetrics and gynecology that did not provide formal training in obstetric and gynecologic ultrasound evaluation.[22] These guidelines included a recommendation of a minimum of 3 months' experience in obstetric and gynecologic ultrasound evaluation. In addition, it was recommended that this training include 1 month of supervised and documented training in an established ultrasound facility. Such training should include basic physics, technique, performance, and interpretation. In addition, the physician should obtain 2 months of practical experience (at least 200 examinations) before the offering of services as a physician with competence in diagnostic ultrasound examination.[22] There is no reason to believe that in the subsequent 10 years, with the increased complexity of this field, that these guidelines should be anything but more stringent.

The "turf" battles between radiologists and obstetricians as to who should perform the examination are unfortunate. As long as the examining physician is adequately trained and performs the minimum standard obstetrical ultrasound examination, as per the guidelines of the American College of Radiology (ACR) and American Institute of Ultrasound in Medicine (AIUM) and the American College of Obstetricians and Gynecologists (ACOG), the specialty of the examiner does not matter.[23, 24] I, however, do not believe in the practice of self-referral. Self-referral examinations tend to be performed more frequently[25] and are often less "complete" and of a lower quality than when they are performed by a dedicated ultrasound practitioner. Except in localities where there are no diagnostic ultrasound specialists, patients should be referred to practitioners whose major practice is daily ultrasonography. The potential issues of inconvenience and difficulty in scheduling examinations will undoubtedly always be remedied by practicing sonologists eager for referrals.

Although the previous list of clinical indications addresses the circumstances in which the ultrasound examination should be performed, it does not address the problem of how the examination is performed. In the early 1980s it became clear that obstetric ultrasound studies were being performed by a variety of persons with disparate levels of training and that the examinations were quite different from practitioner to practitioner. There was concern that as the number of examinations was dramatically increasing, their quality was decreasing. In an attempt to address this problem the ACR Commission on Ultrasound, with minor modification by the AIUM, developed guidelines to serve as a standard for the performance of the obstetric ultrasound examination.[26] These guidelines were modified slightly in 1991.[23] Although there may be those sonologists who exceed these guidelines, they serve as a minimum standard for all practitioners of obstetric ultrasonography[27]; and although the ACOG never officially sanctioned the guidelines, an ACOG technical bulletin appeared in 1988 with very similar standards.[24]

The concept of the "level 1" and "level 2" ultrasound examination, while initially useful in the α-fetoprotein (AFP) screening programs, has spread to the routine ultrasound examination and has been dramatically misused. Unfortunately, many examiners have chosen to "hide behind" a *level* of ultrasound or a brand or type of ultrasound scanner to justify a less than adequate examination.[28] It is for this reason that the ACR/AIUM and ACOG developed guidelines as to the minimum standard for an ultrasound examination.

In fact, there are two types of ultrasound examinations, but they do not conform specifically to the concept of the levels described in the AFP screening programs (see Chapter 3). The first is the standard ultrasound examination that is performed on every patient regardless of the request. The second is a "targeted" examination in which a specific abnormality or abnormalities are sought because the patient is at risk or because an abnormality was suggested on an earlier examination.

The actual ACR/AIUM guidelines are presented in Table 1–1. What follows is my own bias as to what constitutes an appropriate ultrasound examination. In some respects, this is an expansion of the guidelines previously mentioned. Because this multiauthored text is essentially a detailed review of the obstetric ultrasound examination, I recognize that my viewpoint in this chapter and those of the authors of the subsequent chapters may differ.

ULTRASOUND EQUIPMENT AND DOCUMENTATION

It seems there will always be differences of opinion as to which ultrasound machines produce the best images. With the present state of ultrasound technology these differences are often quite subjective, particularly among the state-of-the-art machines. Most ultrasound machines utilize phased-array real-time technology. This technology allows for more consistent images and less downtime owing to the absence of moving parts in the transducers.

An often controversial issue is *which* transducer should be used for the ultrasound examination. The answer to this statement is that as many transducers should be used as are necessary to answer the question for which the patient is referred. There is a misconception that the "newest" transducer introduced by a manufacturer may be the only one that is needed. When sector and, ultimately, endovaginal probes were first introduced many practitioners believed that these transducers alone could be used for the entire examination. Many learned the hard way that using only a single transducer restricts the field of view or visualization of detail, making diagnosis more difficult.

The most common transducers, which are the "workhorses" of the ultrasound laboratory, are a linear array and sector transducer (3 to 5 MHz) and an endovaginal probe (5 to 10 MHz). The higher-frequency transducers are most useful to achieve high-resolution scans, and the lower-frequency transducers are useful in those circumstances in which increased penetration of the sound beam is necessary. Variations of transducer technology include convex linear transducers and multifrequency probes. Doppler technology and color Doppler flow imaging are exciting new areas of present investigation. This technology is still investigational and at this time is certainly not part of the standard ultrasound examination.

Whatever technology is used, the examination should be documented as some form of "hard copy." The purpose of documentation is twofold. First, the

Table 1–1. GUIDELINES FOR PERFORMANCE OF THE ANTEPARTUM
OBSTETRIC ULTRASOUND EXAMINATION*

These guidelines have been developed for use by practitioners performing obstetric ultrasound studies. A limited examination may be performed in clinical emergencies or as a follow-up to a complete examination. In some cases, an additional or specialized examination may be necessary. Although it is not possible to detect all structural congenital anomalies with diagnostic ultrasound examination, adherence to the following guidelines will maximize the possibility of detecting many fetal abnormalies.

Equipment

These studies should be conducted with real-time scanners, using an abdominal or vaginal approach, or both. A transducer of appropriate frequency (3 MHz or higher abdominally, 5 MHz or higher vaginally) should be used. A static scanner (3 to 5 MHz) may be used but should not be the sole method of examination. The lowest possible ultrasonic exposure settings should be used to gain the necessary diagnostic information.

Comment: Real-time studies are necessary to reliably confirm the presence of fetal life through observation of cardiac activity, respiration, and active movement. Real-time studies simplify evaluation of fetal anatomy as well as the task of obtaining fetal measurements. The choice of frequency is a tradeoff between beam penetration and resolution. With modern equipment, 3- to 5-MHz abdominal transducers allow sufficient penetration in nearly all patients, while providing adequate resolution. During early pregnancy, a 5-MHz abdominal or a 5- to 7-MHz vaginal transducer may provide adequate penetration and produce superior resolution.

Documentation

Adequate documentation of the study is essential for high-quality patient care. This should include a permanent record of the ultrasound images, incorporating whenever possible the measurement parameters and anatomic findings proposed in the following sections of this document. Images should be appropriately labeled with the examination date, patient identification, and, if appropriate, image orientation. A written report of the ultrasound findings should be included in the patient's medical record regardless of where the study is performed.

Guidelines for First-Trimester Sonography

Overall Comment: Scanning in the first trimester may be performed either abdominally or vaginally. If an abdominal scan is performed and fails to provide definitive information concerning any of the following guidelines, a vaginal scan should be performed whenever possible.

1. The location of the gestational sac should be documented. The embryo should be identified and the crown-rump length recorded.
   Comment: The crown-rump length is an accurate indicator of fetal age. Comparison should be with standard tables. If the embryo is not identified, characteristics of the gestational sac including mean diameter of the anechoic space to determine fetal age and analysis of the hyperechoic rim should be noted. During the late first trimester, biparietal diameter and other fetal measurements may also be used to establish fetal age.
2. Presence or absence of fetal life should be reported.
   Comment: Real-time observation is critical in this diagnosis. It should be noted that fetal cardiac motion may not be visible before 7 weeks abdominally and frequently at least 1 week earlier vaginally as determined by crown-rump length. Thus, confirmation of fetal life may require follow-up evaluation.
3. Fetal number should be documented.
   Comment: Multiple pregnancies should be reported only in those instances when multiple embryos are seen. Because of variability in fusion between the amnion and chorion, the appearance of more than one saclike structure in early pregnancy is often noted and may be confused with multiple gestation or amniotic band.
4. Evaluation of the uterus (including cervix) and adnexal structures should be performed.
   Comment: This will allow recognition of incidental findings of potential clinical significance. The presence, location, and size of myomas and adnexal masses should be recorded.

Guidelines for Second- and Third-Trimester Sonography

1. Fetal life, number, and presentation should be documented.
   Comment: Abnormal heart rate and/or rhythm should be reported. Multiple pregnancies require the reporting of additional information: placenta number, sac number, comparison of fetal size, and, when visualized, fetal genitalia and presence or absence of an interposed membrane.
2. An estimate of the amount of amniotic fluid (increased, decreased, normal) should be reported.
   Comment: Although this evaluation is subjective, there is little difficulty in recognizing the extremes of amniotic fluid volume. Physiologic variation with stage of pregnancy must be taken into account.
3. The placental location and appearance and its relation to the internal cervical os should be recorded.
   Comment: It is recognized that placental position early in pregnancy may not correlate well with its location at the time of delivery.
4. Assessment of gestational age should be accomplished using a combination of biparietal diameter (or head circumference) and femur length. Fetal growth and weight (as opposed to age) should be assessed in the third trimester and requires the addition of abdominal diameters or circumferences. If previous studies have been performed, an estimate of the appropriateness of interval change should be given.
   Comment: Third-trimester measurements may not accurately reflect gestational age. Initial determination of gestational age should therefore be performed before the third trimester whenever possible. If one or more previous studies have been performed, the gestational age at the time of the current examination should be based on the earliest examination that permits measurement of crown-rump length, biparietal diameter, head circumference, and/or femur length by the equation:

$$\text{current fetal age} = \text{initial embryo/fetal age} + \text{number of weeks from first study}$$

The current measurements should be compared with norms for the gestational age based on standard tables. If previous studies have been performed, interval change in the measurements should be assessed.

   a. Biparietal diameter at a standard reference level (which should include the cavum septi pellucidi and the thalamus) should be measured and recorded.
   Comment: If the fetal head is dolichocephalic or brachycephalic, the biparietal diameter alone may be misleading. On occasion, the computation of the cephalic index, a ratio of the biparietal diameter to fronto-occipital diameter, is needed to make this determination. In such situations, the head circumference or corrected biparietal diameter is required.
   b. Head circumference is measured at the same level as the biparietal diameter.
   c. Femur length should be measured routinely and recorded after the 14th week of gestation.
   Comment: As with biparietal diameter, considerable biologic variation is present late in pregnancy.

Table 1–1. GUIDELINES FOR PERFORMANCE OF THE ANTEPARTUM
OBSTETRIC ULTRASOUND EXAMINATION* Continued

d. Abdominal circumference should be determined at the level of the junction of the umbilical vein and portal sinus.
   Comment: Abdominal circumference measurement may allow detection of growth retardation and macrosomia—conditions of the late second and third trimester. Comparison of the abdominal circumference with the head circumference should be made. If the abdominal measurement is below or above that expected for a stated gestation, it is recommended that circumference of the head and body be measured and the head circumference/abdominal circumference ratio be reported. The use of circumferences is also suggested in those instances in which the shape of either the head or body is different from that normally encountered.
5. Evaluation of the uterus and adnexal structures should be performed.
   Comment: This will allow recognition of incidental findings of potential clinical significance. The presence, location, and size of myomas and adnexal masses should be recorded.
6. The study should include, but not necessarily be limited to, the following fetal anatomy: cerebral ventricles, four-chamber view of the heart (including its position within the thorax), spine, stomach, urinary bladder, umbilical cord insertion site on the anterior abdominal wall, and renal region.
   Comment: It is recognized that not all malformations of the previously mentioned organ systems (e.g., the spine) can be detected using ultrasonography. Nevertheless, a careful anatomic survey may allow diagnosis of certain birth defects that would otherwise go unrecognized. Suspected abnormalities may require a specialized evaluation.

*The *comments* are those that appeared in the originally published guidelines.
Modified from Guidelines for performance of the antepartum obstetrical ultrasound examination. J Ultrasound Med 10:577, 1991.

---

identification of normal structures is important so they can be viewed retrospectively and compared with later images if pathologic processes are ultimately demonstrated. Second, if a pathologic problem is identified, it can be shown to referring examiners who will be doing further examinations.

Initially, laboratories used rapid-process film of the Polaroid type for hard copy documentation. The cost and difficulty of mounting these images made this impractical. Many laboratories then turned to multiformat cameras that used radiographic-type film. These cameras added some flexibility but were not without their own problems, including the inconsistency and downtime of these cameras as well as the added complication of processing time and materials. Some have chosen videotape as a means of documentation to obviate some of these difficulties. The difficulty with this methodology is the time it takes to view and compare individual planes of section, particularly when pathologic processes are demonstrated. It is likely that in the next several years most state-of-the-art ultrasound machines will record their images in digital format in computer workstations. These images can then be transferred directly to viewing monitors or cameras.

In addition to the hard copy "film," a written report of the ultrasound examination should be included in the patient's medical record. When significant pathologic processes are present the referring physician should be notified immediately before the patient leaves the examination area. This immediate communication should occur not only in cases of fetal malformations but also in cases of oligohydramnios or diminished fetal movement.

TERMINOLOGY

There are undoubtedly hundreds of terms that are used in obstetrics and ultrasonography that are either incorrect or confusing. Many of these will be addressed later in this chapter and in other chapters in this text.

Two areas in which terminology is often either misused or misunderstood in obstetric ultrasonography are fetal life and age. The term *viability* is defined as the ability to survive in the extrauterine environment. Even in cases of very late third-trimester examinations, this statement cannot be used with 100% certainty. I prefer to state that the embryo or fetus is *living,* if that is the case, and use the term *nonviable* for those embryos or fetuses that either are dead or are not capable of living in the extrauterine environment.

The second often confusing term is *gestational age.* Taken as it sounds, this term would seem to imply the actual age of the fetus from conception to the present. In fact, this term, which is widely used by obstetricians and sonologists alike, is most often meant to be synonymous with *menstrual age. Menstrual age* refers to the length of time calculated from the first day of the last normal menstrual period to the point at which the pregnancy is being assessed. The true age of the embryo or fetus, *fetal age,* is rarely known accurately unless the patient has had assisted fertilization or has extremely regular menstrual periods and the day of conception is known. Some examiners subtract 2 weeks from the menstrual age to arrive at the fetal age.

In this text the terms *gestational age* and *menstrual age* will be used interchangeably. The important point for any examiner to remember is not which term is necessarily preferable but rather that the person interpreting the examination and the physician who ordered the examination both use the same terminology.

THE FIRST-TRIMESTER ULTRASOUND EXAMINATION

Identification of an Intrauterine Pregnancy

Patients referred for first-trimester ultrasound evaluation often have vaginal bleeding, which raises the question of an ectopic pregnancy or a threatened abortion. The primary goal of ultrasound evaluation in the first trimester is to determine whether the pregnancy is intrauterine and whether the embryo is living. With present-day equipment, particularly endovaginal transducers, both of these tasks should be readily accomplished at very early stages of gestation. The same care taken in concluding that a pregnancy in the second or third trimester has a lethal malformation should be applied in deciding that an early pregnancy is nonviable. If there is reasonable doubt about embryonic life, a repeat examination in as few as 7 to 10 days will invariably make the conclusion unequivocal.

Fetal Number

There is no question that, with a careful examination, the true number of embryos can be accurately determined in the first trimester. The literature has emphasized that it is important not to overestimate the number of developing gestations by misinterpreting findings such as a "double sac sign," fluid in the uterine cavity, the yolk sac, or the presence of the amnion as evidence of multiple sacs or embryos and thus multiple gestations. However, the examiner may be just as likely to underestimate the number of developing gestations and embryos if a thorough evaluation of the gestational sac is not made for all embryos. It is my experience that when multiple gestations are missed using ultrasound assessment, it is usually from a less than optimal first-trimester examination. It is for these reasons that some investigators prefer that if one ultrasound examination is to be done concentrating on fetal number, it should be done in the early to middle second trimester of pregnancy.

Estimating Gestational Age

The subject of estimating gestational age is covered in detail in Chapter 7. Some estimate of gestational age should be made when an ultrasound examination is performed in the first trimester. The two most common methods of gestational age estimation are mean gestational sac diameter and crown-rump length. For many years the crown-rump length has been acclaimed as the most reliable method of estimating gestational age in utero. The crown-rump length is a highly accurate method of estimating gestational age using ultrasound evaluation (accuracy ±3–7 days). Other measurements, such as the head circumference or femur length, done in the second trimester are nearly as accurate and have the added benefit of allowing one to assess fetal morphology to a better advantage in a larger fetus. I believe that the first-trimester ultrasound examination should not be done for the sole purpose of obtaining more accurate measurements if there is not a clinical reason why it cannot be done in the second trimester.

Morphologic Abnormalities

Since the advent of endovaginal ultrasound transducers there have appeared numerous reports documenting morphologic abnormalities detected in the embryonic stage in the first trimester. Abnormalities involving virtually every organ system have been reported. In light of these reports, I am frequently asked the question: When is the earliest time that a particular abnormality can be detected? My reply is often that while early detection of a morphologic abnormality is useful, the confident unequivocal detection of an abnormality is even more important. Unless one is extremely confident of the existence of an abnormality in the first trimester, a follow-up examination should be performed.

Certainly, a single screening examination should not occur in the first trimester. One should beware of three potential pitfalls in diagnosis in the first trimester: (1) the normal extra-abdominal position of the embryonic intestine simulating an abdominal wall defect, (2) the prominence of the normal integument simulating soft tissue edema, and (3) the potential false-negative diagnosis of anencephaly.[29–31]

Placenta

In very early pregnancies, it may be difficult to ascertain the site of the developing placenta. If, however, the examiner can confidently identify the site of placentation, either anterior or posterior, this information should be documented. There are a number of cases in which the early first-trimester ultrasound examination is the only examination obtained during pregnancy. Later in pregnancy, if either an amniocentesis or a cesarean section is planned and no ultrasound equipment is available, it would be helpful to know the location of the placental site from an earlier examination.

Uterus and Adnexa

The maternal uterus should be carefully examined for evidence of uterine abnormalities, particularly in high-risk patients. Late in pregnancy, these anomalies may be extremely difficult to detect. If uterine myomas are detected, their size, site, and relationship to the cervix should be recorded. It should be remembered that transient myometrial contractions may simulate myomas.

The adnexa should be carefully searched for the presence of cysts as well as ovarian neoplasms, both benign and malignant. Again, later in pregnancy, as the adnexal areas are displaced superiorly, they may be extremely difficult to evaluate adequately.

THE SECOND- AND THIRD-TRIMESTER ULTRASOUND EXAMINATIONS

Fetal Number and Fetal Life

Although evaluating the number of fetuses may be difficult during early pregnancy, it should be extremely easy and accurate in the second and third trimesters. The increased perinatal morbidity and mortality of multiple gestations make it mandatory that a "surprise twin" at delivery be a rare event in any patient who has had a second- or third-trimester ultrasound examination. The major potential error in determining the number of fetuses is one of underestimation. This mistake, when made, is likely due to either not evaluating the fundal region or not making sure that the fetal head is associated with its body rather than that of a twin. When a multiple gestation is identified, it is important to determine, if possible, the number of placentas and the number of gestational sacs (the chorionicity and amnionicity).

In the ultrasound report, a statement should be made that the fetus was living, if this was the case, by virtue of cardiac motion being identified. Ideally, the diagnosis of fetal death should be confirmed by more than one examiner based on the absence of cardiac motion for at least 3 minutes. The lack of fetal motion should not be interpreted as representing fetal death.

Fetal Position

Once fetal life and number have been identified, then the fetal lie and presenting part must be determined. Fetal lie refers to the relationship of the long axis of the fetus to the long axis of the uterus. Presentation defines the presenting fetal part closest to the cervix. The most common fetal lie is longitudinal, and the most common presenting part is the fetal head. Fetal lies or presentations other than these are referred to as malpresentations. Their significance lies in increased perinatal morbidity during delivery.

The advent of real-time ultrasound evaluation has placed an additional demand on the sonographer. If the sonologist interpreting the scans has not performed the examination he or she must be able to deduce the lie and presentation from several images rather than a single one. This may be done only by understanding the normal fetal anatomy and applying it to the scanning position (Figs. 1–1 and 1–2). Likewise, some congenital anomalies (e.g., dextrocardia, abnormal right-sided abdominal cystic mass) will be recognized only fortuitously if a structure is identified as abnormal by virtue of its abnormal position related to the lie and presentation of the fetus.

As mentioned previously, the most common presenting part is the fetal head—the cephalic presentation. (I prefer the use of the term *cephalic* rather than *vertex* since the latter term may also be used to describe a location on the fetal head.) When the head is adjacent to the lower uterine segment, it is likely that the fetus is in cephalic presentation; however, one must see all images before coming to that conclusion. The fetal body may also be low in the uterus with the fetal head, and thus the fetus would be in a transverse lie rather than in a cephalic presentation.

Fetal malpresentations require that the sonographer extend the examination to answer two additional questions important to the referring obstetrician. First, what specifically is the presenting part (i.e., foot, buttocks in the case of a breech presentation, or shoulder in the case of a fetus in transverse lie) (Figs. 1–3 and 1–4). Second, is there an associated fetal malformation or placental abnormality that may be causally related to the abnormal lie?[32]

Assigning Gestational Age and Weight

The assignment of gestational age and weight is covered in detail in Chapters 7 and 9. It is important to remember several concepts when assigning gestational age using ultrasonography. First, measurements made early in pregnancy, for the most part, are more accurate than those made near term. Second, pathologic states should be taken into consideration when deciding which body parts to use in assigning gestational age or weight. Most ultrasound machines allow the user to select out of the gestational age calculation those body parts that are abnormal. The abdominal circumference measurement is likely to be inaccurate in the presence of fetal ascites, and the femur length measurement is unreliable in fetuses with short-limbed dwarfism. Third, every obstetric ultrasound report should relate the calculated sonographic age to the patient's menstrual age. Because menstrual histories are frequently inaccurate, there is often a tendency to not believe any woman's menstrual history in deference to the calculated sonographic age. In doing so, however, one runs the risk of assigning an earlier gestational age to a fetus that is in fact older but growth retarded. Likewise there is the possibility of assigning an earlier gestational age to a pregnancy that is post term, placing the fetus at risk for fetal postmaturity syndrome or in utero death. Fourth, the calculated fetal weight should be stated not only in grams but also as a percentile based on the patient's menstrual age. Again, if the patient's menstrual dates are inaccurate, the obstetrician can make the decision not to become alarmed at a reported low weight percentile. This is far better than misinterpreting a growth-retarded fetus as normal by relating only the estimated weight to the ultrasound-determined age. Fifth, if there has been a previous ultrasound examination, there should be some statement in the report as to whether the fetal growth has been normal or abnormal. Finally, sonograms attempting to assess normal or abnormal interval growth should have an interval of no less than 2 weeks. It may be difficult to determine whether there has been a growth abnormality versus a measurement error if scans are done with a shorter interval.

Amniotic Fluid Volume

During the past several years, there has been tremendous interest in the role of amniotic fluid in fetal development and well-being. Although there is relatively good agreement on the significance of extremes of amniotic fluid volume, there is controversy over the methodology used to make the diagnosis of either too much or too little amniotic fluid. I believe that the diagnosis of oligohydramnios and polyhydramnios can

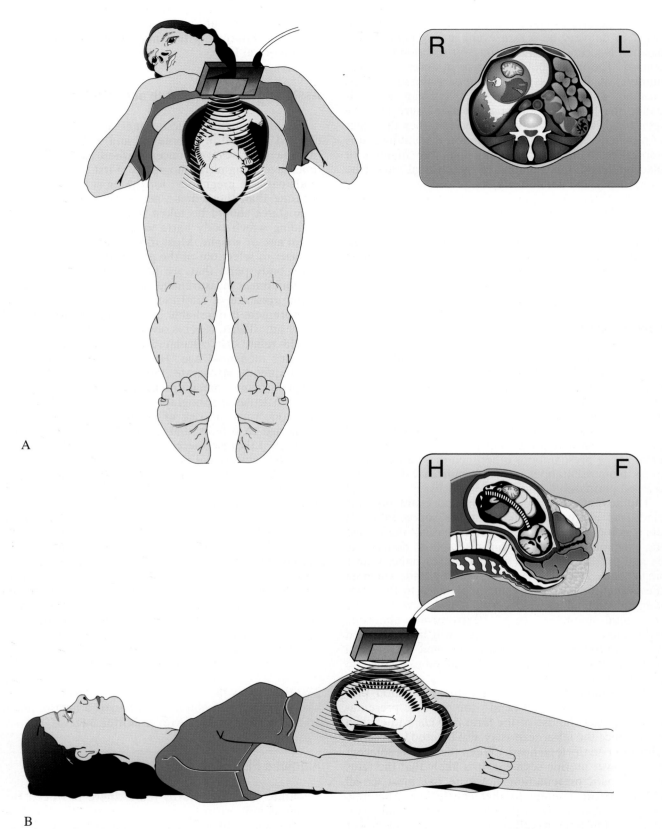

Figure 1–1. *A.* Illustration of a transverse plane of section of the gravid uterus. The fetus is in cephalic presentation so this scan transects the fetal abdomen transversely. *B.* Longitudinal plane of section of the same fetus. These images are viewed with the maternal head to the left of the recorded image.

**A. Longitudinal Lie
Cephalic Presentation**

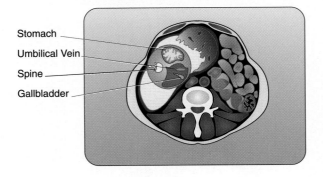

Stomach
Umbilical Vein
Spine
Gallbladder

**B. Longitudinal Lie
Breech Position**

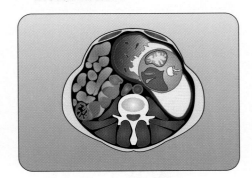

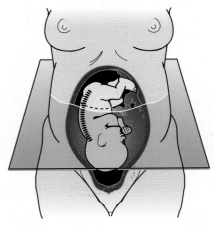

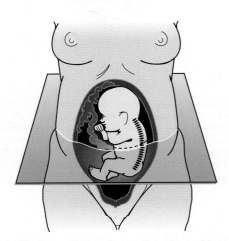

Figure 1–2. Knowledge of the plane of section across the maternal abdomen (longitudinal or transverse) as well as the position of the fetal spine and left-sided (stomach) and right-sided (gallbladder) structures can be used to determine the fetal lie and presenting part. *A.* This transverse scan of the gravid uterus demonstrates the fetal spine on the maternal right with the fetus lying with its right side down (stomach anterior, gallbladder posterior). Because these images are viewed looking up from the patient's feet, the fetus must be in a longitudinal lie and cephalic presentation. *B.* When the gravid uterus is scanned transversely and the fetal spine is on the maternal left, with the right side down, the fetus is in a longitudinal lie and breech presentation.

Illustration continued on following page

C. Transverse Lie
   Head, Maternal Left

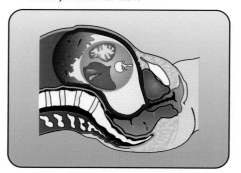

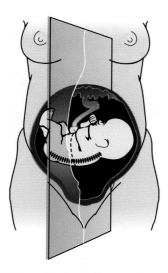

D. Transverse Lie
   Head, Maternal Right

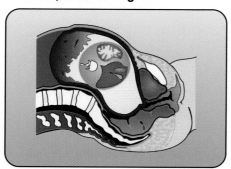

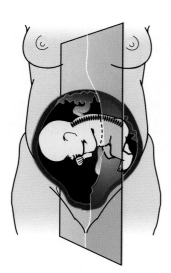

Figure 1–2 *Continued C.* When a longitudinal plane of section demonstrates the fetal body to be transected transversely and the fetal spine is nearest the lower uterine segment, with the fetal right side down, the fetus is in a transverse lie with the fetal head on the maternal left. *D.* When a longitudinal plane of section demonstrates the fetal body to be transected transversely and the fetal spine is nearest the uterine fundus with the fetal right side down, the fetus is in a transverse lie with the fetal head on the maternal right. Although real-time scanning of the gravid uterus quickly allows the observer to determine fetal lie and presentation, this maneuver of identifying specific right- and left-sided structures within the fetal body forces one to determine fetal position accurately and identify normal and pathologic fetal anatomy.

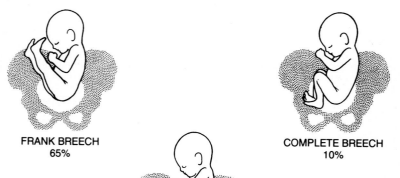

FRANK BREECH
65%

COMPLETE BREECH
10%

FOOTLING BREECH (Single or Double)
25%

Figure 1–3. Illustration of the types of breech presentation. In a frank breech presentation (the most common), the thighs are flexed at the hips with the legs and knees extended. In complete breech (the least common), the thighs are flexed at the hips and there is flexion of the knees as well. One or both hips and knees are extended in the footling breech. The risk of cord prolapse is greatest with a footling breech and least with a frank breech.

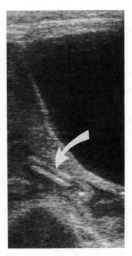

Figure 1–4. Longitudinal scan of a footling breech presentation. In this scan, the leg *(arrow)* and foot extend into the lower uterine segment and cervix.

best be made subjectively. The difficulty with objective measurements is that they are often too stringent and are often not related to gestational age. The ability to assess amniotic fluid volume subjectively at different stages of gestation is readily learned and should not be difficult for most examiners. Two points should be remembered when assessing amniotic fluid volume. First, amniotic fluid volume is large compared with fetal volume at early stages of gestation and should not be misinterpreted as polyhydramnios. Conversely, in term patients the normal volume of amniotic fluid is quite small so that only small pockets may be seen. Second, patients who are obese often appear to have less than normal volumes of amniotic fluid. This may in part be due to scattering of sound with artifactual echoes within the amniotic fluid.

In making the diagnosis of oligohydramnios, one should remember two points. First, because, in most cases, this will imply the likelihood of a fetal renal malformation or severe growth retardation in the absence of ruptured membranes, this diagnosis should only be made when there is essentially no amniotic fluid. The only exception to this is when there is a small amount of fluid in an early or mid second-trimester examination. Second, because of the association of severe diminution of amniotic fluid with fetal death, the obstetrician should be alerted immediately if this diagnosis is made, before the patient leaves the ultrasound evaluation area.

The diagnosis of polyhydramnios, while seeming to be less serious, in many cases may in fact be associated with significant complications to the mother and fetus. In the mother, preterm labor and ruptured membranes may occur; and in the fetus, fetal anomalies may be present. Although many cases of polyhydramnios ultimately result in a normal fetus, the high number of anomalous fetuses with this condition reported in the literature should alert the sonographer to perform a thorough evaluation when this diagnosis is suggested.[33, 34]

Amniotic Fluid Volume in Multiple Gestations

If one looks at a list of causes of polyhydramnios in many obstetric texts, multiple gestations will most likely appear. Although increased amniotic fluid volume may appear in twin gestations, in most cases the cause is some abnormality of pregnancy.[35] Many of these cases are due to the twin transfusion syndrome.[36]

The Placenta

As mentioned earlier, whenever the placenta is identified in pregnancy, its position and relationship to the cervix should be noted in the interpretation. The literature has emphasized the large number of false-positive diagnoses of placenta previa that are made either early in pregnancy or in the presence of an overdistended urinary bladder.[37, 38] Although this is true, one must not be lulled into a sense of security in thinking that all low-lying placentas will "go away" and be clinically unimportant. If after a variety of maneuvers and transducers (Trendelenburg position, emptying the bladder, translabial scanning) one is still unsure about the relationship of the edge of the placenta to the cervical os, the placenta should be interpreted as low lying and a placenta previa cannot be excluded. These patients will therefore be followed more closely clinically.

Abruptio placentae is a diagnosis that is often difficult to make using ultrasonography. One should remember that the myometrium and its vessels, as well as a transient myometrial contraction, may simulate a hematoma and that these potential false-positive diagnoses should be avoided. Because most clinicians are aware that abruptio placentae is a difficult diagnosis, they often refer patients for ultrasound evaluation to exclude a placenta previa rather then to specifically view the abruption.

Fetal Malformations

The subject of fetal malformations is among the most emotionally charged issues that either the parents or diagnostician may have to face. During the past 10 years, ultrasound evaluation has undergone a transformation that has allowed us to answer not only the basic question as to whether the patient is pregnant but also whether a fetal anomaly is present. As smaller and smaller abnormalities are identified, the question now becomes what degree of assurance should a patient expect from a report that no anomaly was seen during a routine ultrasound examination. This is a complex issue. The large number of anatomic structures that can be detected by ultrasound studies have necessitated that anomaly detection, by and large, be a *targeted* examination. To examine every patient for all anomalies would be highly impractical. Fortunately, most *major* anomalies will be detected as part of a routine evaluation with several minor modifications.

Table 1–2. THE ROUTINE ULTRASOUND EXAMINATION

Structure or Measurement	Abnormality
Fetal head (biparietal diameter, head circumference)	Anencephaly, hydrocephalus, encephalocele, cystic hygroma
Fetal heart	Cardiac abnormality, thoracic mass, pleural effusion
Fetal abdomen (abdominal circumference)	Esophageal atresia (absent stomach), small bowel atresias (dilated bowel), ascites, hydronephrosis, gastroschisis, omphalocele
Femur length	Skeletal dysplasias, short-limbed dwarfism
Amniotic fluid	Polyhydramnios due to gastrointestinal obstruction or oligohydramnios from renal disease
Placenta	Placenta previa, abruptio placentae, chorioangioma

As was mentioned in the discussion of the first-trimester ultrasound examination, fetal anomalies have been described in virtually every organ system at almost every gestational age. However, it is my recommendation that if a single ultrasound or a targeted (level 2) examination is performed, it should be done at a gestational age of 20 weeks. The reason for this is that the fetus will be of a sufficient size to exclude most abnormalities and still allow time for a follow-up examination, if necessary. I have frequently noted that abnormalities that were not seen at 18 to 19 weeks' gestational age became apparent at 20 weeks. The slight loss of accuracy in assigning gestational age at this time is well worth the gain in visibility of fetal anatomy and pathology.

A list of the structures or measurements visualized as part of a routine examination and of the corresponding abnormalities that might be detected fortuitously is provided in Table 1–2. The only additional modification to this would be a careful evaluation of the fetal spine and posterior fossa (cisterna magna). Because neural tube defects can be devastating to the fetus and not seen as part of the routine evaluation, it is important to evaluate these areas specifically.

The patient and the referring obstetrician should be made aware that during the standard ultrasound examination, while many abnormalities may be fortuitously detected, more subtle lesions are likely to be detected only when the fetus is known to be at risk for a specific malformation. Anatomic malformations are likely to grow during pregnancy just as the fetus does; a defect seen at birth may have been too small to be detected earlier in pregnancy. Last, it is important for sonologists to know the limits of their expertise. If a malformation is suspected and the examiner has had little experience with the abnormality in question, the case should be referred to a more experienced examiner. Only in this way will patients best be served.

Uterus and Adnexa

Evaluation of the uterus and adnexa becomes more difficult the later in gestation that the examination occurs. The most common abnormalities that are likely to be detected are uterine myomas. As stated earlier, it is important to measure the size, record the location, and define the relationship of the myoma to the cervix. If ovarian abnormalities are suspected and not seen, patients should have a postpartum examination.

MALPRACTICE AND OBSTETRIC ULTRASOUND EXAMINATION

It is likely that each person reading this text has been touched in some way by the present malpractice crisis. For most of us this crisis has resulted in increased costs of goods and services, but for some it has meant being the defendant in a malpractice suit.

Data on the number of claims of malpractice and their settlements are difficult to obtain. In one report, Sanders[39] reported malpractice claims in diagnostic ultrasonography in 228 cases. Obstetric ultrasound examinations represented the majority (78%) of the cases.

Some of the more common reasons for the initiation of malpractice suits (whether legitimate or not) include the following:

- Unreasonable expectations of the ultrasound examination on the part of the patient and the referring physician
- Physician performing the examination has inadequate training or equipment
- Failure to seek consultation in difficult cases
- Inadequate or incomplete study
- Misinterpretation of the ultrasound examination (resulting in the inability to terminate before the legal state limit, wrongful termination, or preterm or postterm delivery)
- Poor communication with referring clinicians (improper wording, lack of timely communication)
- Failure to maintain ultrasound equipment
- Failure to adequately supervise personnel

It is my desire that this text, through the education process of the sonologist, will help alleviate errors in diagnosis and thus reduce the number of these cases. Unfortunately, despite the best medical care some malpractice suits are brought against physicians.

CONCLUSION

The appeal of the ultrasound examination is that it is a noninvasive, safe procedure that has a high degree of patient acceptance and can yield a wealth of information. It is always a delight to examine the obstetric patient and reassure her about her pregnancy, when appropriate.

When a pathologic process is first identified, the role of the sonologist is that of a *detective*, who attempts to piece together all of the information to arrive at the correct diagnosis (Fig. 1–5). While discovering a pathologic process is always disconcerting, the sonologist can be a counselor to the patient and the clinician and help guide them to appropriate management decisions.

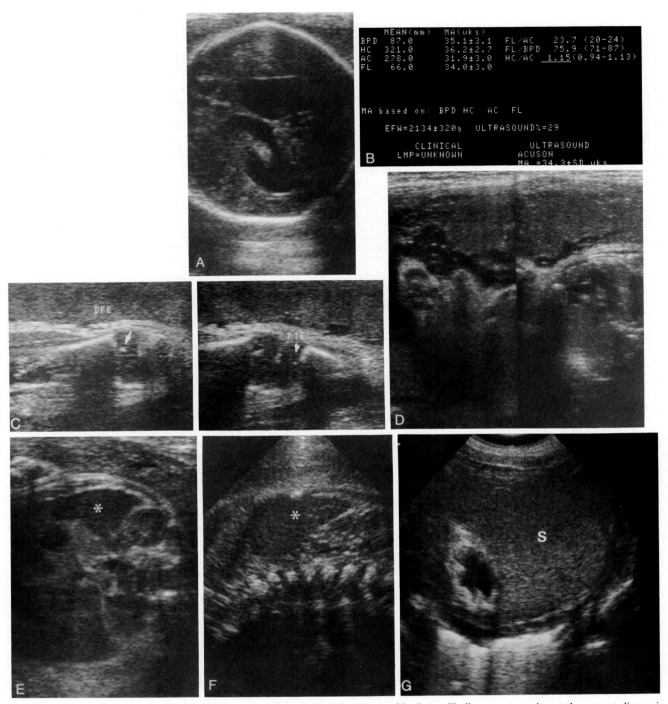

Figure 1–5. This is an excellent example of how observation of all of the sonographic signs will allow one to arrive at the correct diagnosis. The patient was referred because a "cyst" was seen in the fetal head on initial sonographic scanning. *A.* Slightly angled transverse axial scan of the fetal head demonstrates moderate ventriculomegaly. (The dilated ventricles were what were incorrectly interpreted as a fetal intracranial cyst.) *B.* The ultrasound "worksheet" reveals measurements of the fetal head (BPD, HC), abdomen (AC), and femur (FL) that are all different from one another. The main differential at this point is that either the head is enlarged and the femur and abdomen more correctly represent the gestational age or that the head measurements are normal and the fetal abdomen is small from growth retardation. One might assume that the head measurements are abnormally large owing to the ventricular dilatation. In fact, the fetal head does not usually enlarge until the ventricular dilatation is significantly more pronounced.[40] *C.* The next step would be to evaluate the epiphyseal ossification centers. In this fetus both the distal femoral epiphyseal (DFE) and proximal tibial epiphyseal (PTE) centers *(arrows)* show calcification, indicating a fetus with a likely minimum gestational age of 34 to 35 weeks. *D.* These joined dual images of the long axis of the uterus demonstrate little amniotic fluid. The information from images *C* and *D* would seem to indicate that this fetus is likely of 34 to 35 weeks' gestation with a small abdomen (31 weeks' gestation), little amniotic fluid, and probable growth retardation. *E* and *F.* Transverse and coronal planes of section of the fetal abdomen show an enlarged spleen (*). *G.* A post natal sonogram confirms the splenomegaly (S). At birth, the neonate was growth retarded and antibody titers confirmed the diagnosis of cytomegalovirus infection.

There are times, however, when an abnormality is strongly suspected but it may be equivocal or may not fit into a specific category. Under these circumstances, the best pathway for the sonologist to follow is to do a follow-up examination and seek consultation. If time does not allow a follow-up examination, then the sonologist should communicate to the referring physician and the patient that a definitive answer is not possible and decisions will have to be made with less-than-perfect information.

I am hopeful that this text will serve two purposes: to educate and to excite. If those reading this text maintain the same enthusiasm for obstetric and gynecologic sonography that I have, I will have fulfilled my goal.

References

1. Goss SA: Sister chromatid exchange and ultrasound. J Ultrasound Med 3:463, 1984.
2. Stark CR, Orleans M, Haverkamp AD, Murphy J: Short- and long-term risks after exposure to diagnostic ultrasound in utero. Obstet Gynecol 63:194, 1984.
3. Cartensen E, Gates AH: The effects of pulsed ultrasound on the fetus. J Ultrasound Med 3:145, 1984.
4. American Institute of Ultrasound in Medicine: Safety statements. J Ultrasound Med 2:S19, 1983.
5. Merritt CRB: Ultrasound safety: What are the issues? Radiology 173:304, 1989.
6. Reece EA, Assimakopoulos E, Zheng X-Z, et al: The safety of obstetric ultrasonography: Concern for the fetus. Obstet Gynecol 6:139, 1990.
7. Kremkau WF: Biologic effects and possible hazards. Clin Obstet Gynecol 10:395, 1983.
8. American Institute of Ultrasound in Medicine, Bioeffects Committee: Bioeffects consideration for the safety of diagnostic ultrasound. J Ultrasound Med 7(suppl):53, 1988.
9. Wells PNT: The safety of diagnostic ultrasound: Report of a British Institute of Radiology Working Group. Br J Radiol 20 (suppl):1, 1987.
10. Carstensen EL: Acoustic cavitation and the safety of diagnostic ultrasound. Ultrasound Med Biol 13:597, 1987.
11. Report of the Royal College of Obstetricians and Gynaecologists Working Party on Routine Ultrasound Examination in Pregnancy, December 1984.
12. Eik-Nes S, Okland O, Aure J, Ulstein M: Ultrasound screening in pregnancy: A randomized controlled trial. Lancet 1:1347, 1984.
13. Whitfield CR: The routine ultrasound scan in all pregnancies. Presented before the World Society of Perinatal Medicine Meeting. Washington, DC, September 8–12, 1984.
14. Persson PH, Kullander S: Long-term experience of general ultrasound screening. Am J Obstet Gynecol 146:942, 1983.
15. Ewigman B, Le Fevre M, Hesser J: A randomized trial of routine prenatal ultrasound. Obstet Gynecol 76:189, 1990.
16. Pitkin RM: Screening and detection of congenital malformations. Am J Obstet Gynecol 164:1045, 1991.
17. Li TCM, Greenes RA, Weisberg M, Millan D, Flatley M, Goldman L: Data assessing the usefulness of screening obstetrical ultrasonography for detecting fetal and placental abnormalities in uncomplicated pregnancy: Effects of screening a low risk population. Med Decis Making 8:48, 1988.
18. Levi S, Crouzet P, Schaps JP, et al: Ultrasound screening for fetal malformations. (Letter) Lancet 1:678, 1989.
19. Sabbagha RF, Sheikh A, Tamura RK, et al: Predictive value, sensitivity and specificity of ultrasonic targeted imaging for fetal anomalies in gravid women at high risk for birth defects. Am J Obstet Gynecol 152:822, 1985.
20. Manchester DK, Pretorius DH, Avery C, et al: Accuracy of ultrasound diagnoses in pregnancies complicated by suspected fetal anomalies. Prenat Diagn 8:109, 1988.
21. The Use of Diagnostic Ultrasound Imaging in Pregnancy: US Department of Health and Human Services, Public Health Service, National Institutes of Health, NIH publication No. 84-667. Washington, DC, US Government Printing Office, 1984.
22. Joint Task Group on Training for Diagnosis in Obstetrical and Gynecologic Ultrasound, American Institute of Ultrasound in Medicine: Guidelines for minimum post residency training in obstetrical and gynecologic ultrasound. J Ultrasound Med 1:R40, 1982.
23. Guidelines for performance of the antepartum obstetrical ultrasound examination. J Ultrasound Med 10:577, 1991.
24. Hobbins J: Ultrasound in pregnancy. American College of Obstetricians and Gynecologists Technical Bulletin No. 116. Washington, DC, American College of Obstetricians and Gynecologists, 1988.
25. Hillman BJ, Joseph CA, Mabry MR, et al: Frequency and cost of diagnostic imaging in office practice: A comparison of self-referring and radiologist-referring physicians. N Engl J Med 393:1604, 1990.
26. Leopold G: Antepartum obstetrical ultrasound examination guidelines. J Ultrasound Med 5:241, 1986.
27. Leopold G: Responsibilities associated with obstetric sonography. AJR 153:1255, 1989.
28. Filly RA: Level 1, level 2, level 3 obstetric sonography: I'll see your level and raise you one. Radiology 172:312, 1989.
29. Schmidt W, Yarkoni S, Crelin E, Hobbins JC: Sonographic visualization of physiologic anterior abdominal wall hernia in the first trimester. Obstet Gynecol 69:911, 1987.
30. Hertzberg BS, Bowie JD, Carroll BS, et al: Normal sonographic appearance of the fetal neck in the first trimester: The pseudomembrane. Radiology 171:427, 1989.
31. Goldstein RB, Filly RA, Callen PW: Sonography of anencephaly: Pitfalls in early diagnosis. J Clin Ultrasound 17:397, 1989.
32. Neilson DR: Management of the large breech infant. Am J Obstet Gynecol 107:345, 1970.
33. Sivit CJ, Hill MC, Larsen JW, Lande IM: Second-trimester polyhydramnios: Evaluation with US. Radiology 165:467, 1987.
34. Barkin SZ, Pretorius DH, Beckett MK, et al: Severe polyhydramnios: Incidence of anomalies. AJR 148:155, 1987.
35. Hashimoto BE, Callen PW, Filly RA, Laros RK: Ultrasound evaluation of polyhydramnios and twin pregnancy. Am J Obstet Gynecol 154:1069, 1986.
36. Mahony BS, Filly RA, Callen PW: Amnionicity and chorionicity in twin pregnancies: Prediction using ultrasound. Radiology 155:205, 1985.
37. Zemlyn S: The effect of the urinary bladder in obstetrical sonography. Radiology 128:169, 1978.
38. Laing FC: Placenta previa: Avoiding false-negative diagnoses. J Clin Ultrasound 9:109, 1981.
39. Sanders RC: The effect of the malpractice crisis on obstetrical and gynecological ultrasound. In Chervenak F, et al (eds): Textbook of Obstetrical and Gynecological Ultrasound. Boston, Little, Brown & Co, 1993, pp 263–276.
40. Callen PW, Chooljian D: The effect of ventricular dilatation upon biometry of the fetal head. J Ultrasound Med 5:17, 1986.

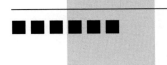

CHAPTER 2

The Role of Genetic Screening in the Obstetric Patient

JAMES D. GOLDBERG, M.D.

The availability of prenatal diagnosis for a wide range of genetic disorders has been a major advance in the area of reproductive genetics. Historically, couples at risk were given information regarding their reproductive chances of producing an affected offspring. These couples then had the option of taking their chances or not reproducing at all. The advent of prenatal diagnosis for many genetic diseases has allowed these couples the option of having unaffected offspring. In addition, progress has also been made in prospective population screening tests both to identify couples at risk for having an offspring affected with a genetic disorder and to screen for abnormal fetuses.

Ultrasound evaluation has played a central role in the development of the various approaches to prenatal diagnosis. In this chapter the focus is on the interface between reproductive genetics and ultrasound evaluation. A brief discussion of the epidemiology of genetic defects and of genetic counseling principles is presented followed by a description of the various prenatal diagnostic procedures and their relationship to ultrasound evaluation. The importance of sonographic guidance will become evident as the various techniques are described.

EPIDEMIOLOGY OF GENETIC DEFECTS

All pregnancies carry a baseline risk of a birth defect. The incidence varies somewhat depending on what defects are included, but most geneticists quote a figure of 3% to 4% for major congenital anomalies. It is important to keep this baseline figure in mind when counseling couples regarding their risk of a specific defect. The etiologies for these birth defects can be broken down into several major categories. These include (1) chromosomal disorders, (2) single-gene or mendelian disorders, (3) polygenic or multifactorial disorders, and (4) teratogenic or environmental effects.

Chromosomal disorders encompass approximately 0.5% of neonatal birth defects. The incidences of the more common chromosomal abnormalities are listed in Table 2–1.

Single-gene or mendelian disorders comprise approximately 1% of congenital defects. A large number of mendelian disorders have been described, although the incidence of any specific disorder is, in general, rare. For example, cystic fibrosis (one of the most common disorders in white, northern European persons) has a carrier frequency of approximately 1 in 20, resulting in a disease frequency of approximately 1 in 1600. The current edition of McKusick's *Mendelian Inheritance in Man* lists 1864 autosomal dominant disorders, 631 autosomal recessive disorders, and 161 X-linked disorders.[1]

Multifactorial or polygenic disorders account for another approximately 1% of birth defects. These disorders are due to the effects of several different genes and/or environmental effects. Examples of these types of disorders are listed in Table 2–2. Multifactorial disorders carry a recurrence risk of 2% to 5% in first-degree relatives. Multiple affected persons in a pedigree would increase this risk. Tables of empiric recurrent risk figures for most of the common multifactorial disorders are available. Another category that falls into this general area is that of multiple congenital abnormalities of unknown etiology. In general, these occurrences are believed to be multifactorial and carry a recurrence risk of 2% to 5%. One exception to this is in the case of parental consanguinity, in which recurrence risks may be as high as 25%.

Teratogens or environmental exposures are thought to cause less than 1% of congenital abnormalities. There are only a limited number of teratogens that have been proven to have a deleterious effect on the fetus. Although the number is small, this area is important because these exposures are potentially preventable.

PRINCIPLES OF GENETIC COUNSELING

Fundamental to the prenatal diagnosis of any disorder is the provision of nondirective genetic counseling. It is essential that the couple at risk be informed of all their reproductive options. If they choose to undergo prenatal diagnostic studies, they must understand the risks and advantages of any procedures they are to undergo. This is particularly important for any new procedure for which the safety and accuracy have not been adequately assessed.

Before attempting the prenatal diagnosis of any inherited disease, it is essential to establish or confirm the specific disorder under consideration. Efforts must be directed toward eliminating the possibility of misdiagnosis due to phenotypic, metabolic, or genetic

Table 2–1. CHROMOSOMAL ABNORMALITIES IN LIVEBORNS

Type of Abnormality	Incidence
Numerical aberrations	
Sex chromosomes	
47,XYY	1/1,000
47,XXY	1/1,000
45,X	1/10,000
47,XXX	1/1,000
Autosomal trisomies	
13–15	1/20,000
16–18	1/8,000
21–22	1/800
Structural abnormalities	
Balanced	
Robertsonian	
t(Dq;Dq)	1/1,500
t(Dq;Gq)	1/5,000
Reciprocal translocations and inversions	1/7,000
Unbalanced	
Robertsonian	1/14,000
Reciprocal translocations and inversions	1/8,000
Inversions	1/10,000
Deletions	1/5,000
Markers	1/8,000

Modified from Hamerton JL, Canning N, Ray M, et al: A cytogenetic survey of 14,069 newborn infants: I. Incidence of chromosome abnormalities. Clin Genet 8:223–245, 1975. © Munksgaard International Publishers Ltd., Copenhagen, Denmark.

heterogeneity. In the case of an enzymatic or molecular diagnosis the precise defect must be demonstrated in the proband or affected relatives. If the proband is deceased, the heterozygosity of both parents (or of the mother for an X-linked disease) must be documented. In the case of a dysmorphic syndrome, all manifestations of the disorder must be known and looked for at the time of evaluation.

INDICATIONS FOR PRENATAL DIAGNOSIS

The most common indications for prenatal diagnostic studies are listed in Table 2–3. By far the most frequent indication is advanced maternal age. Many studies have shown an increased incidence of chromosomal trisomy with advanced maternal age.[2] It is important to realize when quoting risk figures that the incidence at 16 weeks' gestation of fetal aneuploidy is approximately

Table 2–2. POLYGENIC/MULTIFACTORIAL TRAITS

Hydrocephaly (most forms)
Neural tube defects
Cleft lip, with or without cleft palate
Cleft palate
Cardiac abnormalities
Diaphragmatic hernia
Omphalocele
Renal agenesis
Müllerian fusion defects
Limb reduction defects
Pyloric stenosis
Talipes equinovarus

Table 2–3. INDICATIONS FOR PRENATAL DIAGNOSIS

Chromosomal Abnormality
Advanced maternal age
Previous child with a chromosomal disorder
Balanced translocation carrier for a chromosomal disorder
Single-Gene Defects
Previous child with an inherited metabolic disorder
Heterozygous couples detected prospectively by screening programs
Previous child with a disorder detectable by ultrasound evaluation
Multifactorial Disorders
Previous child with a neural tube defect
Previous child with a developmental defect or malformation syndrome detectable by ultrasound evaluation
Environmental Defects
Prenatal exposure to teratogenic drug or infectious agent

double that of neonates, implying a natural spontaneous loss rate of aneuploid fetuses from 16 weeks' gestation to term. Maternal age–specific risk figures for fetal chromosomal abnormalities are listed in Table 2–4. Although initial data suggested a paternal age effect for chromosomal aneuploidy, this has not been confirmed in later studies. It is critical to obtain a complete family history, however, since couples with one indication for prenatal diagnosis frequently will have other risk factors identified. Testing on the basis of maternal age by amniocentesis or chorionic villus sampling (age 35 or older) detects approximately 20% of cases of Down syndrome. Eighty percent of cases of Down syndrome will occur in the nontested group. Maternal serum screening using α-fetoprotein will detect approximately 20% of cases of Down syndrome in the tested group.[3] Preliminary studies using "triple markers" (α-fetoprotein, unconjugated estriol, and human chorionic gonadotropin) have increased this detection rate to approximately 60%.[4]

The family history of a genetic disorder is another common indication for prenatal diagnosis if a specific molecular, enzymatic, or structural defect is diagnosable in the fetus. As mentioned earlier, the precise diagnosis must be known to provide accurate prenatal

Table 2–4. MATERNAL AGE–SPECIFIC ANEUPLOIDY RATES AT TIME OF AMNIOCENTESIS

Maternal Age (yr) at Delivery	Aneuploidy Rate (%)
35	0.78
36	0.97
37	1.2
38	1.5
39	1.9
40	2.4
41	3.1
42	3.9
43	4.9
44	6.3
45	8.0
49	21.1

Modified from Hook EB, Cross PK, Schreinemachers DM: Chromosomal abnormality rates at amniocentesis and in live-born infants. JAMA 249:2034, 1983.

diagnostic studies. The inheritance pattern of the disorder under evaluation must also be known to provide accurate risk figures, keeping in mind that some disorders have differing patterns of inheritance in different families. In addition, the ethnic background of a couple under evaluation must be ascertained, since certain ethnic groups have an increased incidence of specific disorders, such as sickle cell disease in blacks, Tay-Sachs disease in Ashkenazi Jews, and thalassemia in Asians and persons of Mediterranean descent.

Teratogen exposures are becoming an increasing indication for prenatal ultrasound evaluation. This is a particularly difficult area because only a very few teratogens have been confirmed in the literature. Many, if not most, of the reports in the literature of a specific drug causing a birth defect are case reports. These types of reports suggest a possible association only and do not prove cause and effect. In an effort to help the sonologist in this area, many of the reported associations are listed in Table 2–5.

TECHNIQUES FOR PRENATAL DIAGNOSIS

Amniocentesis

The traditional approach to prenatal diagnosis has been transabdominal amniocentesis performed at approximately 16 weeks' gestation. The amniotic fluid obtained contains desquamated fetal cells that can be grown in tissue culture and karyotyped or used for a variety of metabolic assays or DNA extraction. The volume of amniotic fluid at 15 menstrual weeks has been shown to be 125 mL, which increases 50 mL/wk for the next 13 weeks.[5] Initial studies indicated that procedures performed before 15 to 16 weeks' gestation resulted in a significant incidence of "dry taps." With improved ultrasound techniques this can be minimized and procedures can technically be performed much earlier in gestation. This provides the advantage of an earlier, safer termination of pregnancy if an affected fetus is diagnosed and the couple elects to terminate the pregnancy. The safety of performing amniocentesis before 15 to 16 weeks' gestation, however, is not well documented. Preliminary studies suggest an increased fetal loss as compared with the well-established loss-rate at 15 to 16 weeks of 0.5%.[6]

The technique I use for second-trimester amniocentesis is as follows. Sector-array real-time ultrasonography is performed to assess gestational age, fetal life, fetal number, and placental localization. If possible, a placenta-free window is located and the position marked by indenting the maternal abdomen. Increased fetal morbidity has been reported with procedures that traverse the placenta.[7] The abdomen is then prepared with an iodine antiseptic, and the skin and subcutaneous tissues are infiltrated with local anesthetic. The ultrasound transducer is then placed in a polyethylene "sandwich" bag that has been gas sterilized, and sterile gel is placed on the abdomen. The position of the amniotic fluid pocket is reconfirmed and a 22-gauge 3.5-inch spinal needle is inserted under direct ultrasound guidance. The obturator is then removed, a syringe is attached to the needle, and 24 mL of amniotic fluid is withdrawn after discarding the first 0.5 mL to avoid maternal cell and blood contamination. Approximately 1.4% of specimens are discolored, usually reflecting heme pigment.[8]

The usefulness of continuous ultrasound monitoring has been debated. Although no significant decrease in fetal morbidity has been reported, a significant decrease in the incidence of bloody and dry taps of the first needle insertion and in the number of patients who required multiple needle insertions has been reported.[9] In addition, it is extremely reassuring to the patient to know that the fetus is not in the needle's path. Additional information is also provided in instances in which fluid is not immediately obtained owing to tenting of the membranes or a uterine contraction. In most prenatal diagnostic centers this has become the standard of care.

If a twin gestation is identified on ultrasound examination, additional counseling and a change in the amniocentesis technique are necessary. Since one third of twin gestations are monozygotic, the increased risk for a twin gestation would be five-thirds times the maternal age–specific risk. For indications other than advanced maternal age the specific risks for twin gestations have been derived and should be discussed with the couple.[10] Review of amniocentesis for twins done at our institution (330 sets) revealed a loss rate of 3.57%.[11] This was believed not to be greater than the increased baseline loss rate for twins as compared with singletons.

The technique for sampling a twin gestation involves first visualizing the dividing membrane and identifying an amniotic fluid pocket in both sacs. After removal of fluid from the first sac, 0.5 mL of indigo carmine dye is instilled. Methylene blue should not be used owing to reports of fetal hemolysis and bowel atresia when the dye is injected intra-amniotically.[12, 13] Aspiration of clear fluid from the second sac ensures proper placement. A single-puncture technique has been reported.[14] This involves a single puncture of the maternal abdomen and puncture of the dividing membrane to access the second sac. This approach must be viewed with caution, however. Gilbert and colleagues[15] have reported several cases of severe fetal abnormalities in twin gestations following in utero rupture of the dividing membrane. Further large prospective studies are needed in this area.

The finding of a single affected fetus in a twin gestation presents a significant counseling dilemma. The couple has various options open to them. They can choose to do nothing and allow the pregnancy to continue with the birth of one normal infant and one with a potential disability. Another option is to terminate the pregnancy, thus terminating both a normal and an abnormal fetus. A third alternative is selective termination of the affected fetus. In initial reports cardiac puncture with air injection was used to terminate the affected fetus. We have found fetal intracardiac injection of potassium chloride to be safe and effective.[16]

Table 2–5. SELECTED MEDICATIONS AND REPORTED ASSOCIATED MALFORMATIONS*

Drug	Malformation
Acetazolamide	Sacrococcygeal teratoma
Amantadine	Cardiac defects
Aminopterin	Neural tube defects, hydrocephalus, limb shortening, cleft lip/palate, clubfoot
p-Aminosalicylic acid	Ear deformity, limb deformity, hypospadias
Amitriptyline	Limb reduction, micrognathia, hypospadias
Amobarbital	Anencephaly, cardiac defects, limb deformity, cleft lip/palate, polydactyly, genitourinary defects, clubfoot
Amphetamine	Cerebral injury in neonates
Aspirin	Intracranial hemorrhage, intrauterine growth retardation
Bromides	Polydactyly, gastrointestinal anomalies, clubfoot
Busulfan	Intrauterine growth retardation, cleft palate, neural tube defects
Captopril†	Second-trimester hypocalvaria
Carbamazepine†	Neural tube defects, cardiac defects
Chlorambucil	Renal agenesis, cardiac defects
Chlordiazepoxide	Microcephaly, duodenal atresia, cardiac defects
Chloroquine	Wilms tumor, hemihypertrophy, tetralogy of Fallot
Chlorothiazide	Fetal bradycardia
Chlorpheniramine	Polydactyly, gastrointestinal defects, hydrocephalus
Chlorpromazine	Microcephaly, syndactyly
Chlorpropamide	Microcephaly, hand anomalies
Clomiphene	Microcephaly, neural tube defects, cleft lip/palate, cardiac defects, syndactyly, clubfoot
Cocaine	Spontaneous abortion, placental abruption, cardiac defects, urinary tract and limb abnormalities, bowel atresias, intrauterine growth retardation
Coumarin derivatives†	Spontaneous abortion, intrauterine growth retardation, neural tube defects [open and closed] (dorsal midline dysplasia), cardiac defects, scoliosis, limb hypoplasia, cleft palate
Cyclophosphamide	Cleft palate, hand abnormalities, cardiac defects, intrauterine growth retardation
Cytarabine	Hand abnormalities (lobster claw deformity), lower limb defects, neural tube defects, cardiac defects
Daunorubicin	Intrauterine growth retardation
Diphenhydramine	Cleft lip/palate, genitourinary defects, clubfoot, cardiac defects
Disulfiram	Clubfoot, VACTERL syndrome, phocomelia
Ethanol (alcohol)†	Intrauterine growth retardation, microphthalmia, micrognathia, microcephaly, hypoplastic maxilla, cardiac defects, genitourinary defects, radioulnar synostosis, Klippel-Feil anomaly, diaphragmatic hernia
Ethoheptazine	Umbilical hernia, hip dislocation
Ethosuximide	Cleft lip/palate, hydrocephalus, patent ductus arteriosus, spontaneous hemorrhage in the neonate
Etretinate†	Neural tube defects, facial dysmorphia, multiple synostoses, syndactylies, limb reduction
Fluorouracil	Radial aplasia, pulmonary hypoplasia, esophageal and duodenal atresia, cloacal malformation
Fluphenazine	Ocular hypertelorism, cleft lip/palate, imperforate anus
Griseofulvin	Conjoined twins
Haloperidol	Limb reduction, aortic valve defect
Heroin	Intrauterine growth retardation, multiple and varied congenital malformations
Ibuprofen	Oligohydramnios, premature closure of patent ductus arteriosus
Imipramine	Diaphragmatic hernia, cleft palate, excencephaly, renal cystic dysplasia
Indomethacin	Oligohydramnios, premature closure of patent ductus arteriosus, phocomelia, penile agenesis
Isoetharine	Clubfoot
Levothyroxine	Cardiac defects, polydactyly

Table 2–5. SELECTED MEDICATIONS AND REPORTED ASSOCIATED MALFORMATIONS* *Continued*

Drug	Malformation
Lithium†	Cardiac defects (Ebstein anomaly, ventricular septal defect, coarctation, mitral atresia), neural tube defects
Lysergic acid diethylamide	Intrauterine growth retardation, limb reduction, neural tube defects, cardiac defects
Marijuana	Intrauterine growth retardation, facial anomalies
Mechlorethamine	Intrauterine growth retardation, oligodactyly, malformed kidneys
Meclizine	Eye and ear defects, hypoplastic heart, respiratory defects
Melphalan	Intrauterine growth retardation
Meprobamate	Cardiac defects, omphalocele, joint abnormalities
Mercaptopurine	Cleft palate, microphthalmia, intrauterine growth retardation
Methimazole	Patent urachus
Methotrexate	Intrauterine growth retardation, hypertelorism, dextroposition of the heart, absent digits, absence of frontal bone
Methotrimeprazine	Hydrocephalus, cardiac defects
Metronidazole	Spontaneous abortion and limb, cardiac, urinary, and facial abnormalities
Minoxidil	Omphalocele, clinodactyly, cardiac defects (ventricular septal defects and transposition)
Norethindrone	Neural tube defects, hydrocephalus
Norethynodrel	Cardiac defects
Nortriptyline	Limb reduction
Oxazepam	Neural tube defects, intrauterine growth retardation
Paramethadione†	Spontaneous abortions, intrauterine growth retardation, cardiac defects
Penicillamine	Hydrocephalus, flexion deformities, perforated bowel
Phenacetin	Craniosynostosis, anal atresia, musculoskeletal and urinary tract defects
Phensuximide	Ambiguous genitalia
Phenylephrine	Eye and ear abnormalities, syndactyly, clubfoot, musculoskeletal defects
Phenylpropanolamine	Eye and ear abnormalities, polydactyly
Phenytoin†	Microcephaly, hypertelorism, cleft lip/palate, hypoplasia of distal phalanges, short neck, broad nasal ridge
Procarbazine	Intrauterine growth retardation, cardiac defects, oligodactyly, malformed kidneys
Prochlorperazine	Cleft palate/micrognathia, cardiac defects, skeletal defects
Propoxyphene	Limb abnormalities, omphalocele, micrognathia, clubfoot, microcephaly
Quinacrine	Renal agenesis, neural tube defects
Quinine	Neural tube defects, hydrocephalus, limb defects, facial defects, cardiac defects, urogenital abnormalities, vertebral abnormality, gastrointestinal anomaly
Retinoic acid†	Hydrocephalus, neural tube defects, microphthalmia, microcephaly, cardiac defects, limb abnormalities, cleft palate
Sodium iodide†	Ablation of fetal thyroid gland
Sulfasalazine	Cleft lip/palate, hydrocephalus, cardiac defects, urinary tract abnormalities
Sulfonamides	Limb hypoplasia, urinary tract abnormalities
Thioguanine	Absent digits
Tolbutamide	Syndactyly, cardiac defects
Trimethadione†	Intrauterine growth retardation, microcephaly, cleft lip/palate, cardiac defects, malformed hand, clubfoot, ambiguous genitalia, esophageal atresia, tracheoesophageal fistula
Valproic acid†	Neural tube defects, cardiac defects, facial dysmorphism, hypertelorism, protruding eyes, micrognathia, hydrocephalus, cleft lip/palate, microcephaly, limb reduction, scoliosis, renal hypoplasia, duodenal atresia, hand deformity

*Many of the listed associations are based on case reports that have appeared in the medical literature. It is likely that in many cases the reported association was coincidental to, rather than resultant from, the medication. In all cases of suspected teratogenetic effects a reproductive geneticist or teratologist should be consulted.
†Proven teratogens.
Modified from Briggs GG, Freeman RK, Yaffe SJ: Drugs in Pregnancy and Lactation. Baltimore, Williams & Wilkins, 1990.

Chorionic Villus Sampling

As described earlier, amniocentesis at 16 weeks' gestation followed by culture and analysis of the obtained amniocytes frequently results in a prenatal diagnosis being made at 19 to 20 weeks' gestation. If an affected fetus is diagnosed and the couple elects a termination of pregnancy, a second-trimester termination procedure is necessary with its increased medical and psychological risks as compared with a first-trimester termination. Because of this, research efforts have been directed toward developing an early first-trimester diagnostic procedure.

The first attempt to obtain chorionic villus cells was reported by Hahnemann and Mohr in 1968.[17] These and other investigators were able to obtain trophoblast by transcervical hysteroscopy from women undergoing mid second-trimester termination of pregnancy. The yield of tissue, however, was extremely low, and there was difficulty in culturing what little tissue they had. The use of ultrasonography to guide the sampling and improved tissue culture techniques have provided for the development of routine chorionic villus sampling. In addition to providing guidance of the catheter into the trophoblast, ultrasound evaluation provides many other advantages for chorionic villus sampling. One of the most important is in verifying that a fetus is living before sampling is performed. Studies have shown that over 10% of women presenting for chorionic villus sampling have nonviable gestations.[18] Multiple gestations can also be identified in most instances. It must be recognized, however, that a proportion of multiple gestations observed in the first trimester will revert to a lower-order gestation as pregnancy progresses.[19] Ultrasound evaluation also identifies local uterine variations such as fibroids or uterine contractions that can interfere with insertion and placement of the sampling catheter.

There are two commonly used approaches to chorionic villus sampling. One approach uses transcervical insertion of a sampling catheter under direct ultrasound guidance. The other approach is a transabdominal one using a needle under direct ultrasound guidance. The choice of method is dictated by the implantation site and the uterine position. I choose whichever method that I believe would be easiest to obtain a sample. Sampling is most commonly performed at between 10 and 12 menstrual weeks. There have been several reports of an increased incidence of limb reduction defects in procedures performed earlier in gestation.[20]

The technique of transcervical chorionic villus sampling is as follows. With the use of a sector scanner, fetal life is documented, multiple gestations are looked for, the trophoblast is localized, and the sampling path is estimated. Manipulation of bladder volume frequently helps in optimizing the sampling position. The patient is then put in the lithotomy position, a speculum is inserted, and the vagina is prepped with an iodine antiseptic. Under direct ultrasound visualization the sampling catheter, a 16-gauge polyethylene catheter with a malleable stainless steel obturator, is inserted into the area of the trophoblast, as shown in Figure 2–1. A 20-mL syringe is then attached to the catheter, and with 5 to 10 mL of negative pressure the sample

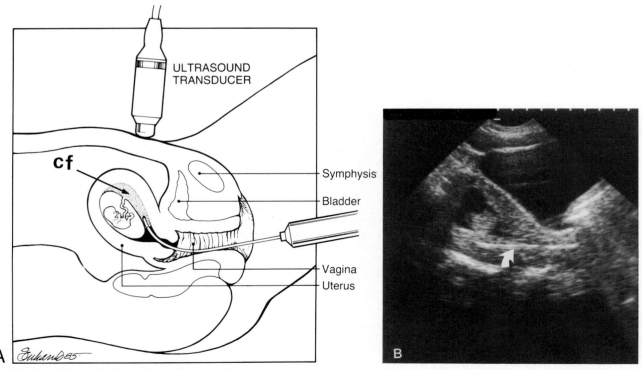

Figure 2–1. *A.* Schematic of chorionic villus sampling procedure. *B.* Sonogram of chorionic villus catheter *(arrow)* in posteriorly implanted trophoblast. (*A,* from Gabbe SG, Niebyl JR, Simpson JL (eds): Obstetrics: Normal and Problem Pregnancies, 2nd ed. New York, Churchill Livingstone, 1991.)

Table 2–6. INDICATIONS FOR FETAL BLOOD SAMPLING

Confirm chromosomal mosaicism found on amniocentesis
Rapid karyotyping
Fetal blood grouping
Assessment of fetal anemia or thrombocytopenia
Hemoglobinopathies
Hemophilia A, hemophilia B, and other clotting disorders
Immunodeficiencies and other white blood cell disorders
Inborn errors of metabolism

is aspirated as the catheter is removed. The sample is immediately examined under a low-power dissecting microscope to determine its adequacy. A tenaculum is occasionally needed to stabilize the cervix. As many as three passes of the catheter are performed, if necessary, with a new catheter used each time. No anesthesia is necessary; however, a cramping sensation is frequently reported by the patient as the catheter passes through the internal os of the cervix.

The transabdominal technique is similar to ultrasound-guided amniocentesis, but a 20-gauge needle is guided into the trophoblast. Negative pressure is applied, and the needle is moved up and down in the area of the trophoblast.

US and Canadian prospective studies of transcervical chorionic villus sampling have demonstrated the safety of the technique.[21, 22] The US collaborative study demonstrated a nonsignificant increase in loss rate compared with 16-week amniocentesis of 0.8%. The Canadian study also reported a nonsignificant increased loss rate of 0.6%. The addition of the transabdominal approach has resulted in a further decrease in loss rate at the University of California-San Francisco. I believe that the risk for procedure-related fetal loss is the same following chorionic villus sampling and mid second-trimester amniocentesis. An interesting observation has been the long learning curve associated with chorionic villus sampling as compared with amniocentesis.[23]

Rhesus Sensitization

The risk of rhesus (Rh) sensitization following amniocentesis or chorionic villus sampling is controversial. Several studies have suggested an increased risk of sensitization based on the finding of fetal red blood cells in the maternal circulation after the procedure or of an increased level of maternal serum α-fetoprotein.[24, 25] Two large retrospective studies, however, found no increase in isoimmunization in women not receiving Rh prophylaxis after amniocentesis.[26, 27] Most centers, however, do administer Rh immune globulin after amniocentesis. There is some suggestion that the administration of Rh immune globulin following chorionic villus sampling may actually increase the fetal loss rate.[28] In addition, it has been suggested that if early prophylaxis is given it should be repeated at regular intervals during the pregnancy to avoid an enhancement phenomenon.[25]

Fetal Blood Sampling

As listed in Table 2–6 there are many indications that require access to the fetal circulation and the sampling of fetal blood. The most common indication is the confirmation of abnormal findings found on amniocentesis or chorionic villus sampling. Another frequent indication is the need for a rapid chromosomal diagnosis. Analysis of fetal blood requires 48 to 72 hours compared with 2 to 3 weeks with amniocentesis. An increasingly common indication is the finding of a structural anomaly on ultrasound evaluation. In a report by Nicolaides and colleagues,[29] summarized in Table 2–7, a significant number of fetuses found to have a structural anomaly on ultrasound examination were aneuploid.

In the past, fetal blood sampling was performed by fetoscopic-guided puncture of the umbilical vessels. The first prenatal diagnosis by fetoscopy was reported in 1974 by Hobbins and associates.[30] The procedure involved transabdominal insertion of a 1.7-mm endoscope through a 3.2-mm trocar. The fetal vessels were then visualized on the placental surface and needled under direct vision for a fetal blood sample. Samples obtained in this way were frequently mixed with maternal blood. A significant advance in the fetoscopic procedure was reported by Rodeck and coworkers,[31] when under direct vision the umbilical cord was punctured near its insertion into the placenta. This resulted in pure fetal samples being obtained in almost all cases. This highly specialized technique was available only at a limited number of centers around the world. A 5% fetal loss rate was reported for patients undergoing fetoscopy at these centers.[32]

The current approach to fetal blood sampling was initially described by Daffos and colleagues.[33] This procedure involves percutaneous umbilical blood sampling under sonographic guidance. These investigators reported over 600 cases of fetal blood sampling with a fetal loss rate of less than 1%. This approach has become the method of choice for fetal blood sampling and fetal intravascular transfusion. Studies suggest that the complication rate following the procedure is dependent on the indication for sampling. Fetuses with intrauterine growth retardation and/or structural

Table 2–7. INCIDENCE OF CHROMOSOMAL ANEUPLOIDY

Disorder (No. Patients)	Incidence
Nonimmune hydrops fetalis (12/37)	32%
Omphalocele (8/12)	67%
Duodenal atresia (1/3)	33%
Obstructive uropathy (9/39)	23%
Unilateral pleural effusion (1/3)	33%
Severe intrauterine growth retardation and oligohydramnios (2/10)	20%
Hydrocephalus (2/9)	22%
Choroid plexus cyst (3/4)	75%

Modified from Nicolaides KH, Rodeck CH, Gosden CM: Rapid karyotyping in nonlethal fetal malformations. Lancet 1:283, 1986.

anomalies are at a significantly increased risk of fetal distress.[34]

The procedure is performed as follows. The area of the umbilical cord insertion into the placenta is visualized by a sector scanner. This is the optimal area for sampling because the cord is fixed at this location. The umbilical cord insertion into the fetus or a free loop of cord may also be used; however, this approach is frequently more difficult owing to cord movement. Other investigators have reported the use of the fetal intrahepatic vein[35] or direct puncture of the fetal heart to obtain blood.[36] The mother is then given parenteral sedation both for maternal comfort and to decrease fetal movements. Intramuscular or intravenous fetal injections of curare or pancuronium bromide (Pavulon) have been reported to be useful in eliminating fetal movement during the longer intravascular transfusion procedures.[37, 38] The long-term effects of temporary fetal paralysis are unknown. The abdomen is then prepped and draped, and the insertion site and subcutaneous tissues are infiltrated with local anesthetic. While the subcutaneous tissue is being infiltrated the angle of the needle insertion can be checked sonographically. Under ultrasound guidance a 22- or 25-gauge 3.5-inch spinal needle is advanced into the umbilical circulation as shown in Figure 2–2. Samples of fetal blood are then aspirated into preheparinized syringes.

The fetal blood sample is immediately analyzed using a Coulter cell sizer to verify fetal origin. The fetal red blood cell size is plotted against a maternal sample and will show a larger size distribution. Kleihauer-Betke staining may also be performed for additional verification. The ability to analyze the sample immediately makes it possible to obtain a second sample if a maternal specimen has been obtained.

Fetal Tissue Sampling

Some inherited diseases are expressed only in a specific tissue, and thus sampling of that tissue is necessary if a prenatal diagnosis is to be made. Fetal liver, fetal skin, and fetal muscle have been obtained by ultrasonically guided biopsy.[39–41] These procedures are performed only at a few referral centers.

DNA Methodology

As progress is made in the elucidation of the specific molecular defect in an ever-increasing number of genetic diseases, prenatal diagnosis will be possible by DNA analysis. Since DNA is present in every nucleated cell, minimally invasive techniques such as amniocentesis or chorionic villus sampling may replace the more invasive procedures such as fetal blood sampling or fetal liver biopsy for the prenatal diagnosis of many diseases. The list of diseases diagnosable by DNA analysis is continually expanding. Thus, before

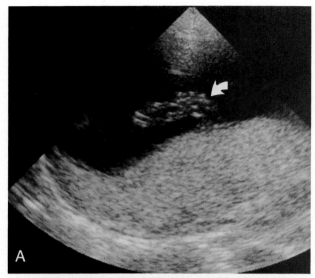
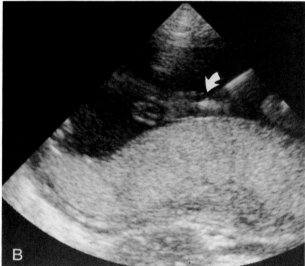

Figure 2–2. *A.* Sonogram of posterior insertion of umbilical cord into placenta *(arrow)*. *B.* Sonogram of sampling needle in umbilical cord at the insertion site *(arrow)*.

attempting a prenatal diagnosis a current compendium or geneticist should be consulted.

FUTURE PROSPECTS

Safe and reliable access to the fetal circulation is opening up a new era in fetal prenatal diagnosis and fetal therapy. Therapy involving fetal intravascular transfusion of red blood cells or platelets for isoimmunization is routinely performed.[42, 43] In addition, the availability of early first-trimester prenatal diagnosis may provide opportunities for prenatal therapy for certain disorders by replacement of missing enzymes or cofactors, by somatic gene replacement, or by stem cell transplantation. Ultrasound evaluation will continue to play a critical role in the development of these new approaches to fetal prenatal diagnosis and therapy.

References

1. McKusick VA: Mendelian Inheritance in Man. Baltimore, Johns Hopkins University Press, 1990.
2. Hook EB, Cross PK, Schreinemachers DM: Chromosomal abnormality rates at amniocentesis and in live-born infants. JAMA 249:2034, 1983.
3. New England Regional Genetics Group: Combining maternal serum alpha-fetoprotein measurements and age to screen for Down syndrome in pregnant women under age 35. New England Regional Genetics Group Prenatal Collaborative Study of Down Syndrome Screening. Am J Obstet Gynecol 160:575, 1989.
4. MacDonald ML, Wagner RM, Slotnick RN: Sensitivity and specificity of screening for Down syndrome with alpha-fetoprotein, hCG, unconjugated estriol, and maternal age. Obstet Gynecol 77:63, 1991.
5. Fuchs F: Volume of amniotic fluid at various stages of pregnancy. Clin Obstet Gynecol 9:449, 1966.
6. Hanson FW, Tennant FR, Hune S, et al: Early amniocentesis: Outcome, risks, and technical problems at ≤ 12.8 weeks. Am J Obstet Gynecol 166:1707, 1992.
7. Kappel B, Nielsen J, Brongaard Hansen K, et al: Spontaneous abortion following mid-trimester amniocentesis: Clinical significance of placental perforation and blood-stained amniotic fluid. Br J Obstet Gynaecol 94:50, 1987.
8. Hess LW, Anderson RL, Golbus MS: Significance of opaque discolored amniotic fluid at second-trimester amniocentesis. Obstet Gynecol 67:44, 1986.
9. Romero R, Jeanty P, Reece EA, et al: Sonographically monitored amniocentesis to decrease intraoperative complications. Obstet Gynecol 65:426, 1985.
10. Hunter AGW, Cox DM: Counselling problems when twins are discovered at genetic amniocentesis. Clin Genet 16:34, 1979.
11. Anderson RL, Goldberg JD, Golbus MS: Prenatal diagnosis in multiple gestation: 20 years' experience with amniocentesis. Prenat Diagn 11:263, 1991.
12. McEnerney JK, McEnerney LN: Unfavorable neonatal outcome after intra-amniotic injection of methylene blue. Obstet Gynecol 61(suppl):35, 1983.
13. van der Pol JG, Wolf H, Boer K, et al: Jejunal atresia related to the use of methylene blue in genetic amniocentesis in twins. Br J Obstet Gynaecol 99:141, 1992.
14. Bahado-Singh R, Schmitt R, Hobbins JC: New technique for genetic amniocentesis in twins. Obstet Gynecol 79:304, 1992.
15. Gilbert WM, Davis SE, Kaplan C, et al: Morbidity associated with prenatal disruption of the dividing membrane in twin gestations. Obstet Gynecol 78:623, 1991.
16. Golbus MS, Cunningham N, Goldberg JD, et al: Selective termination of multiple gestations. Am J Med Genet 31:339, 1988.
17. Hahnemann N, Mohr J: Genetic diagnosis in the embryo by means of biopsy from extraembryonic membranes. Bull Eur Soc Hum Genet 2:23, 1968.
18. Jones S, Dorfmann A, Patton L, et al: Non-viable pregnancy in patients anticipating chorionic villus sampling. Am J Hum Genet 34:A257, 1986.
19. Landy HL, Weiner S, Corson SL, et al: The "vanishing twin": Ultrasonographic assessment of disappearance in the first trimester. Am J Obstet Gynecol 155:14, 1986.
20. Firth HV, Boyd PA, Chamberlain P, et al: Severe limb abnormalities after chorion villus sampling at 56–66 days' gestation. Lancet 1:762, 1991.
21. Rhoads GG, Jackson LG, Schlesselman SE, et al: The safety and efficacy of chorionic villus sampling for early prenatal diagnosis of cytogenetic abnormalities. N Engl J Med 320:609, 1989.
22. Canadian Collaborative CVS-Amniocentesis Clinical Trial Group: Multicenter randomized clinical trial of chorion villus sampling and amniocentesis: First report. Lancet 1:1, 1989.
23. Goldberg JD, Porter AE, Golbus MS: Current assessment of fetal losses as a direct consequence of chorionic villus sampling. Am J Med Genet 35:174, 1990.
24. Blakemore KJ, Baumgarten A, Schoenfeld-Dimaio M, et al: Rise in maternal serum alpha-fetoprotein concentration after chorionic villus sampling and the possibility of isoimmunization. Am J Obstet Gynecol 155:988, 1986.
25. Bowman JM, Pollack JM: Transplacental fetal hemorrhage after amniocentesis. Obstet Gynecol 66:749, 1985.
26. Golbus MS, Stephens JD, Cann HM, et al: Rh isoimmunization following genetic amniocentesis. Prenat Diagn 2:149, 1982.
27. Tabor A, Jerne S, Bock JE: Incidence of rhesus immunisation after genetic amniocentesis. Br Med J 293:533, 1986.
28. Smidt-Jensen S, Philip J: Comparison of transabdominal and transcervical CVS and amniocentesis: Sampling success and risk. Prenat Diagn 11:529, 1991.
29. Nicolaides KH, Rodeck CH, Gosden CM: Rapid karyotyping in nonlethal fetal malformations. Lancet 1:283, 1986.
30. Hobbins JC, Mahoney MJ: In utero diagnosis of hemoglobinopathies: Technique for obtaining fetal blood. N Engl J Med 290:1065, 1974.
31. Rodeck CH, Campbell S: Umbilical-cord insertion as source of pure fetal blood for prenatal diagnosis. Lancet 1:1244, 1979.
32. The status of fetoscopy and fetal tissue sampling: The results of the first meeting of the International Fetoscopy Group. Prenat Diagn 4:79, 1984.
33. Daffos F, Capella-Pavlovsky M, Forestier F: Fetal blood sampling during pregnancy with use of a needle guided by ultrasound: A study of 606 consecutive cases. Am J Obstet Gynecol 153:655, 1985.
34. Maxwell DJ, Johnson P, Hurley P, et al: Fetal blood sampling and pregnancy loss in relation to indication. Br J Obstet Gynaecol 98:892, 1991.
35. Nicolini U, Nicolaidis P, Fisk NM, et al: Fetal blood sampling from the intrahepatic vein: Analysis of safety and clinical experience with 214 procedures. Obstet Gynecol 76:47, 1990.
36. Antsaklis AI, Papantoniou NE, Mesogitis SA, et al: Cardiocentesis: An alternative method of fetal blood sampling for the prenatal diagnosis of hemoglobinopathies. Obstet Gynecol 79:630, 1992.
37. de Crespigny LC, Robinson HP, Quinn M, et al: Ultrasound-guided fetal blood transfusion for severe rhesus isoimmunization. Obstet Gynecol 66:529, 1985.
38. Seeds JW, Bowes WA: Ultrasound-guided fetal intravascular transfusion in severe rhesus isoimmunization. Am J Obstet Gynecol 154:1105, 1986.
39. Holzgreve W, Golbus MS: Prenatal diagnosis of ornithine transcarbamylase deficiency utilizing fetal liver biopsy. Am J Hum Genet 36:320, 1984.
40. Esterly NB, Elias S: Antenatal diagnosis of genodermatoses. J Am Acad Dermatol 8:655, 1983.
41. Evans MI, Greb A, Kunkel LM, et al: In utero fetal muscle biopsy for the diagnosis of Duchenne muscular dystrophy. Am J Obstet Gynecol 165:728, 1991.
42. Berkowitz RL, Chitkara U, Goldberg JD: Intrauterine intravascular transfusions for severe red blood cell isoimmunization: Ultrasound-guided percutaneous approach. Am J Obstet Gynecol 155:574, 1986.
43. Daffos F, Forestier F, Muller JY, et al: Prenatal treatment of alloimmune thrombocytopenia. Lancet 2:632, 1984.

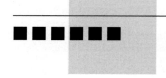

α-**Fetoprotein Screening Programs: What Every Obstetric Sonologist Should Know***

ROY A. FILLY, M.D.
PETER W. CALLEN, M.D.
RUTH B. GOLDSTEIN, M.D.

α-Fetoprotein (AFP) is a glycoprotein that is synthesized predominantly in the normal fetal liver, but also in the yolk sac and gut.[1] It is produced only in very low concentrations by adult liver cells. This protein demonstrates an electrophoretic motion similar to that shown by albumin and is the major circulatory protein of the early fetus.

α-Fetoprotein is found in high concentration in fetal serum. Serum levels peak at 2 to 3 mg/mL at approximately the 14th week of gestation, after which the level progressively decreases.[1] Normally, small quantities of AFP enter the amniotic fluid compartment. The quantity of AFP in amniotic fluid is much more dilute (measured in micrograms per milliliter) than fetal serum concentrations (Table 3–1). The mechanism by which AFP passes from the fetal circulation into the amniotic fluid is not fully understood, although two likely pathways are fetal proteinuria and transudation across immature epithelium (normal events in early pregnancy). The AFP in amniotic fluid demonstrates a unimodal concentration curve, peaking in early second trimester, and then, as with fetal serum AFP, declining as pregnancy progresses.[1] Very small quantities (measured in nanograms per milliliter) of this protein enter the maternal circulation from the amniotic fluid compartment and across the placenta. Maternal serum levels of AFP rise progressively from the 7th week to the 32nd week and then decline.[1] Pregnancies that do not produce fetal tissues (e.g., hydatidiform mole) are characterized by an absence of AFP.

Measurement of AFP in amniotic fluid (AF-AFP) has been successfully employed for many years to detect open neural tube defects in the fetus.[1-4] When an open neural tube defect is present, a portion of the fetus lacks a normal integumentary covering. For example, in anencephaly there is no skin covering the abnormality. Instead the cranial surface is covered by a thick angiomatous stroma (Fig. 3–1). In meningocele, or myelomeningocele (Fig. 3–2), and many cephaloceles (Fig. 3–3), only a membranous covering, or no covering at all, is present. This allows abnormally large quantities of AFP to "leak" into the amniotic fluid, which is reflected as an abnormal increase in the maternal serum level.[5]

Neural tube defects are among the most common congenital anomalies occurring in the United States. The overall prevalence of these malformations has been estimated to be 16 per 10,000 (0.16%) births.[1] However, the prevalence is higher in the eastern United States than in the western United States and higher among whites than blacks. The prevalence is very much higher in children born to families with a history of neural tube defects. In the United States, the risk of recurrence after one child with a neural tube anomaly is 2% to 3%, and after a second abnormal child the risk is approximately 6%.[1] Because the birth of a child with a neural tube defect may cause emotional as well as possible financial hardship, patients at risk for recurrence of neural tube defects in a subsequent pregnancy are routinely screened with measurement of AF-AFP levels. However, if all women who had previously been delivered of a child with an open neural tube defect were screened by amniocentesis for elevation of the AF-AFP, only 10% of all fetuses with an open neural tube defect would be detected; 90% occur as first-time events.[1] The risks of amniocentesis make AF-AFP determination impractical as a screening tool. Maternal serum AFP rather than AF-AFP must be employed for large-scale screening studies of pregnant women.

---

*This chapter is adapted from Filly RA, Callen PW, Goldstein RB: Alpha-fetoprotein screening programs: What every obstetrical sonologist should know. Radiology 188:1–9, 1993, with permission of the publisher.

Table 3–1. COMPARISON OF α-FETOPROTEIN LEVELS

Sample Site	Approximations
Maternal serum	30 ng/mL
Amniotic fluid	20,000 ng/mL
Fetal plasma	3 million ng/mL

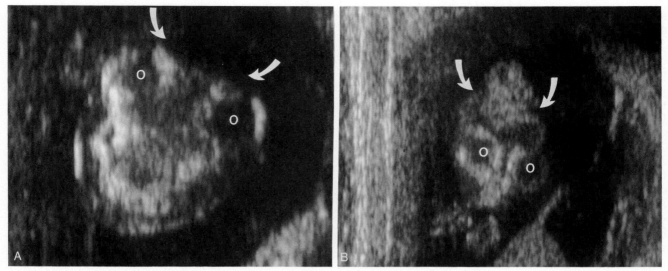

Figure 3–1. Anencephaly. *A.* Note absence of calvarium *(curved arrows)* above the orbits (o). *B.* Presence of angiomatous stroma *(curved arrows)* should not dissuade the examiner from the correct diagnosis of anencephaly.

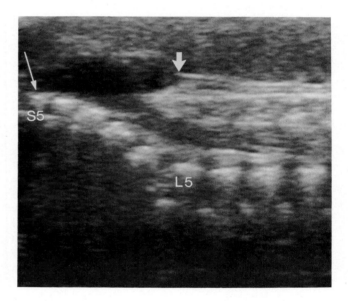

Figure 3–2. Myelomeningocele. The top of the lesion *(short arrow)* is estimated by counting up from the last sacral ossification center *(long arrow)*, assumed to be S4 in the second trimester and S5 in the third trimester. The age of this fetus was 36 menstrual weeks, and the top of the myelomeningocele was at L5.

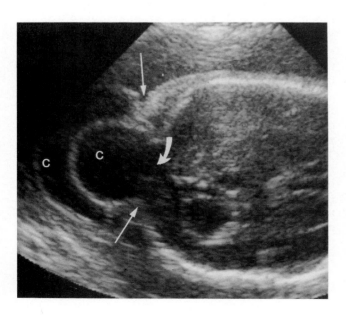

Figure 3–3. Cephalocele. Acute angles with integument *(long arrows)*, calvarial defect *(curved arrow)*, and "cyst within a cyst" (c) appearance (possibly reflect the herniated fourth ventricle into the cephalocele sac) help to distinguish this lesion from a cystic hygroma.

ROUTINE MATERNAL SERUM α-FETOPROTEIN SCREENING

Maternal serum AFP (MS-AFP) screening was first performed in Great Britain.[6] However, in Great Britain, the general population risk for neural tube defect is substantially greater than in the United States.[7] In Great Britain the overall frequency of neural tube defects is 5 to 7 per 1000 pregnancies compared with 1 to 2 per 1000 pregnancies in the United States. Nonetheless, a number of screening programs have been instituted in the United States and demonstrate clear evidence for benefit despite the lower prevalence.[8-11] Table 3–2 demonstrates the probability of an abnormal fetal outcome when the MS-AFP level is elevated for a patient in the United States compared with a patient in Great Britain owing to the lower population prevalence.[6, 7]

To minimize the number of false results, selection of the normal range is critical. Setting the upper limit of normal at a high level reduces false-positive rates, but it also reduces the number of abnormal cases detected. Setting a lower level for the upper limit improves the detection rate but increases the false-positive rate (Table 3–3).[1] The cutoff value for maternal serum levels should be adjusted for the mother's weight. Other factors known to affect the maternal serum levels include diabetes and ethnicity.[12, 13] False-negative results occur because the range of normal values overlaps those of abnormal fetuses.

Significant abnormalities are detected by both abnormally high and abnormally low levels of AFP in the maternal serum. The causes and associations of high MS-AFP levels have been more widely publicized than those that cause low MS-AFP levels.[5, 12-17] Low levels are seen in patients who are not pregnant, have a hydatidiform mole (absence of fetal tissues), have had a fetal death, have a misdated pregnancy, have a trisomic fetus, or have a normal pregnancy.[18-23] It is particularly the category of trisomic fetuses that has generated so much interest. Approximately 20% of fetuses with trisomy 21 are found in women undergoing amniocentesis for a maternal age of more than 35 years. An additional 20% of fetuses with trisomy 21 are found in women whose MS-AFP level is low after adjustment for age.[24] The risk of trisomy when the MS-AFP level is low is significant enough to warrant amniocentesis for karyotyping. In California, 7% of pregnant women are older than the age of 35. Con-

versely, only 3% of pregnant women screened by MS-AFP are judged to have an abnormally low level. Therefore, twice as many fetuses with Down syndrome will be detected per amniocentesis performed for low MS-AFP compared with those performed for advanced maternal age. The potential of finding this additional 20% of fetuses with Down syndrome through MS-AFP testing is highly attractive. This yield may be further increased by also measuring human chorionic gonadotropin levels and serum estriol levels in conjunction with the MS-AFP.[25] These three markers (so-called triple markers) refine the risk for trisomy to a greater degree than MS-AFP alone.

Causes of elevated MS-AFP levels are also numerous. However, the vast majority are encompassed in the following list: twins, fetal death, misdated pregnancies, neural tube defects, other anatomic abnormalities, aberrations in the placenta, and normals.[5, 14-17, 26] Furthermore, there is a growing body of evidence that in the absence of an anatomic abnormality an elevated MS-AFP level may portend obstetric problems later in pregnancy.[27, 28]

Technical errors can occur in the measurement of AFP.[29-31] To eliminate these errors, all abnormal test results should be checked by repeat measurement. False results are more commonly obtained for other reasons.[32] Because false-positive results may lead to termination of a normal pregnancy, the reasons for false-positive results should be carefully excluded. The most common of these is overlap of the upper end of normal with the lower end of the abnormal range. Other common entities are multiple pregnancy and errors in dating. Less common causes of false elevations are concurrent maternal liver disease and collection of MS-AFP samples after amniocentesis (fetal-maternal blood mixing).

There are numerous benefits to a screening program for MS-AFP (Table 3–4). These include identification of early twins and early fetal death. Many misdated pregnancies are reassigned a corrected gestational age. The program finds many structural and chromosomal anomalies and thereby decreases the anxiety of parents of normal fetuses. As noted earlier, it identifies potential obstetric problems and can point the way to identification of patients who harbor a hydatidiform mole or choriocarcinoma or who are not pregnant at all.

Unfortunately, such programs also have significant problems that must be minimized (see Table 3–4). One of the most significant is the anxiety caused by physiologically increased or decreased AFP levels.[33, 34] Im-

Table 3–3. CUTOFF VALUES OF MATERNAL SERUM α-FETOPROTEIN LEVELS TO DETECT ABNORMALITY

	Anencephaly	Spina Bifida	Normal
2.0 MOM	91%	90%	7.2%
2.5 MOM	88%	79%	3.3%
	(97%)*	(80%)*	

MOM, multiples of median.
*Results from California maternal serum α-fetoprotein program, which uses 2.5 MOM as a cutoff value.

Table 3–2. PROBABILITY OF AN ABNORMAL OUTCOME IF THE MATERNAL SERUM α-FETOPROTEIN LEVEL IS ELEVATED AND POPULATION STATISTICS ARE KNOWN

	Maternal Serum α-Fetoprotein	Population Incidence	Probable Abnormal Fetus
Great Britain	2.5 MOM	4.5/1000	1/10
United States	2.5 MOM	2/1000	1/20
California program	2.5 MOM		1/15

MOM, multiples of median.

Table 3–4. BENEFITS AND PROBLEMS IN
α-FETOPROTEIN SCREENING PROGRAMS

Benefits
- Finds many structural and chromosomal anomalies
- Identifies early twins
- Identifies early fetal death
- Redates many misdated pregnancies
- Decreases anxiety for normals
- Identifies potential obstetric problems
- Identifies hydatidiform mole/choriocarcinoma
- Identifies nonpregnant females believed to be pregnant

Problems
- Anxiety caused by physiologically increased α-fetoprotein levels
- Affected children "missed" by the screening program
- Affected children born to late registrants or noncomplying women
- Probable need for 40,000 more amniocenteses per year
- Pregnancy losses of normal fetuses due to complications of amniocentesis
- Mothers who elect to abort solely on finding of abnormal α-fetoprotein levels
- Sonographic false-positive and false-negative results

portantly, affected fetuses will be missed by the screening program and the parents of these children will feel especially "cheated." Similarly, there will be affected children born to late registrants or women who do not comply with the program. Some mothers will lose normal fetuses because of the complications of amniocentesis. Importantly, mothers may elect to abort a fetus solely on the basis of an abnormal AFP level that is falsely positive or may fall victim to a sonographic false-positive or false-negative diagnosis. A national program of this nature would generate approximately 40,000 more amniocenteses per year, which must, in many instances, be followed up with high-level ultrasonography. Developing and maintaining high-quality centers to perform these tasks would be difficult.

Maternal serum AFP testing has had very encouraging results. These results have caused the American College of Obstetricians and Gynecologists to recommend that pregnant women at the appropriate gestational age be offered this test.[35] As large numbers of women are screened, virtually all sonologists doing obstetric diagnosis will encounter patients in whom abnormal MS-AFP levels have been recorded. Familiarity with guidelines for the appropriate sonographic evaluation of a pregnancy in which an abnormal MS-AFP result has been obtained is becoming increasingly important.

THE CALIFORNIA MS-AFP SCREENING PROGRAM

The California MS-AFP Screening Program has already tested well over 1 million women. In this chapter we will concentrate on patients with elevated MS-AFP levels because sonography plays a greater role in this group.[11, 36] Californian physicians are required to offer MS-AFP testing to all patients of appropriate gestational age. The patient may decline the program. If the patient accepts entry into the program, a fee of $53 is charged. This fee covers the cost of the MS-AFP test and any subsequent genetic counseling, sonography, amniocentesis, or other pertinent tests engendered by an abnormal result, including the right to seek a second opinion if desired.

General programmatic considerations in a large-scale MS-AFP screened population are outlined in Figure 3–4. Within the California program, a limited number of prenatal diagnostic centers are permitted to provide counseling for patients, amniocenteses, and targeted sonograms. All practitioners must meet specified guidelines. However, prenatal diagnostic centers are permitted latitude in following some aspects of the program. A major one revolves around when the patient undergoes a level 2 sonogram. Some centers recommend the level 2 sonogram for those patients with elevated AF-AFP levels, as illustrated in Figure 3–4. However, at other centers a level 2 examination is performed before the amniocentesis in an effort to decrease the number of amniocenteses performed. At the University of California San Francisco (UCSF), level 2 examinations are performed on patients with elevated AF-AFP levels (predominant group) or women who have an elevated MS-AFP level but decline amniocentesis. Therefore, the data presented here should be viewed with this information in mind.

There are considerable differences, from the sonographic perspective, in these two philosophies. If a center elects to do level 2 sonograms before the amniocentesis there are major consequences. First, there will be a need to do approximately 10 times more level 2 sonograms. A more important consequence is that the prevalence of disease in the sonographic test population will decrease 10-fold, thereby placing a greater emphasis on the "normal" result. Unfortunately, the normal result is the less reliable sonographic conclusion. Importantly, these examinations would be performed earlier in gestation than those that are done following the amniocentesis. All sonologists recognize the benefits of 1 or 2 weeks of growth in early pregnancy in terms of visualization of fetal structures. As noted earlier, we have followed the more "traditional" philosophy of performing level 2 examinations when the AF-AFP level is elevated. This gives the additional advantage of knowing the result of acetylcholinesterase testing. Therefore, our results would serve as a useful comparison for institutions electing to perform level 2 examinations in advance of the amniocentesis.

Very tight control is exercised at the laboratory testing level, and the number of laboratories performing the assay is extremely limited. Each is licensed by the state government. As noted earlier, all abnormally elevated samples are retested and a second specimen is drawn from the patient for comparative analysis if the value is high and was drawn at 16 menstrual weeks. If, however, the degree of elevation is substantial (greater than 3 multiples of the median [MOM]) or the gestational age is greater than 17 menstrual weeks, the latter steps are deleted. Among the first 1.1 million women tested in the California program, approximately 5% tested positive and approximately 2% had

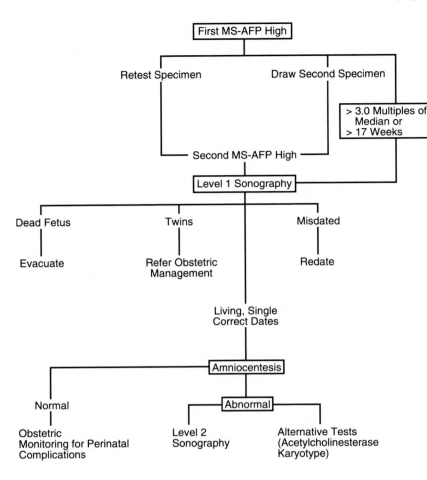

Figure 3–4. Programmatic considerations in a large-scale MS-AFP–screened population. MOM, multiples of median.

elevated MS-AFP levels. Among the positive high results, 16% were readjusted to normal when retested. The remaining 84% were referred to prenatal diagnostic centers for level 1 sonography. As in the laboratories that perform MS-AFP testing, the prenatal diagnostic centers also must meet stringent state requirements and periodic reviews.

This, by the way, is the context in which the term *level 1* was introduced into the sonologic lexicon, and some clarification of this term is appropriate. A level 1 sonogram is, for all intents and purposes, a standard obstetric sonogram as described in the American Institute of Ultrasound in Medicine and American College of Radiology guidelines published in 1986 and modified in 1991.[37] Its goals are determination of fetal number, gathering of fetal biometric data (and the subsequent calculations that can be made from these), estimation of amniotic fluid volume, localization of the placenta, and detection of uterine and adnexal masses. Although not specifically done to detect fetal anomalies, there is a reasonable probability during the course of the data gathering that anomalies will be detected, and a prudent effort should be made to do so. This "prudent" effort is further defined by a number of sonographic views specified in the guidelines as useful for detecting anomalies. The indication for a level 1 sonogram is not defined by pregnancy risk (i.e., low-risk pregnancies get level 1 sonograms while high-risk pregnancies get level 2 sonograms). The performance

of a level 1 sonogram is also not defined by the technical capability or intellectual prowess of the examiner or the cost of the sonographic machine employed. Rather, the definition is related to the intent of the examination. Level 2 examinations are "directed" or "targeted" to answer specific questions, far and away the most common of which is, "Does the fetus have a morphologic abnormality?" Indeed, unless there is a reason not to do so, a patient should get a level 1 examination every time a sonogram is performed during the second or third trimester. That the examination performed was a level 1 sonogram is neither an excuse for failing to make observations that should be made during the course of the sonogram nor an excuse to inadequately document that the information was carefully obtained.

Level 1 Sonography

The major purpose for level 1 sonography is to identify misdated pregnancies (18%), multiple gestations (10%), and unsuspected fetal death (5%) among women who have abnormal MS-AFP levels. At present, the biparietal diameter only is employed to estimate age in the California MS-AFP program. Although composite ages from multiple biometric parameters are more accurate for dating, the rationale in this instance is to increase detection of myelomeningoceles. This anomaly is associated with smaller than average biparietal diameter measurements.[38] A small biparietal diameter makes any MS-AFP level "appear" higher. Therefore, relying on the probability that myelomeningocele fetuses, as a group, have smaller than average biparietal diameter measurements, these fetuses will be more conspicuous in the test population.

Although the intent of the level 1 examination is not to search out all potentially diagnosable anomalies that might generate an elevation of the MS-AFP, a number of the anomalous fetuses in the group are recognized during the course of this examination. Virtually all cases of anencephaly are detected. Some of the other more conspicuous neural tube defects are noted as well, including cephaloceles and myelomeningoceles. The same is true of ventral wall defects. Because anencephaly is readily diagnosed and uniformly fatal, no further referral is required unless the patient wishes a second opinion. However, the other lesions have varying prognoses. Further diagnostic testing can disclose features that affect the prognosis. This information is valuable in counseling parents and in case management. Therefore, such cases should go on to level 2 sonography.

Amniocentesis After Abnormal Result of MS-AFP Test

Following readjustment by results of the level 1 sonogram, approximately 65% of women will remain in the abnormal zone. The major risk with a low MS-AFP level is a chromosomal abnormality, which can be most reliably diagnosed by amniocentesis and karyotyping of fetal cells. Therefore, more women (75%) offered amniocentesis when the MS-AFP level is low elect to proceed with this test than when the MS-AFP level is high (66%). This is in large part because sonography can more accurately identify anomalies in the high MS-AFP group than in the low MS-AFP group. Other factors influence women's choices, including the type of abnormality likely to be diagnosed and the potential risks of the procedure.

Of the first 1.1 million women screened in the California MS-AFP program, 38,500 (3.5%) had either an abnormally low or high MS-AFP level.[36] Of these, 37,000 (96%) reported for genetic counseling and sonography at prenatal diagnostic centers. Of these, 20,000 underwent amniocentesis. This filtration process is, of course, designed to extract from the patient pool at large those who have an extremely high risk of abnormality. This process is highly successful. Among the 1.1 million patients screened, 1390 anomalies (morphologic and chromosomal) were detected (prevalence of 1.3/1000). Of those patients who went to prenatal diagnostic centers, the prevalence increased to 38/1000. If the patient underwent amniocentesis, the risk of an anomalous fetus further increased to 70/1000.

The anomalies detected by the California program between 1987 and 1990 were as follows:

Neural Tube Defects		Non–Neural Tube Defect Abnormalities	
Anencephaly	417	Ventral wall defects	286
Spina bifida	247	Down syndrome	163
Encephalocele	46	Other chromosomal abnormalities	231
Total	710	Total	680

Level 2 Sonography

Conceptually, patients whose amniocentesis shows an elevated level of AFP are referred for detailed or targeted (level 2) sonograms. Simply stated, level 2 sonographic examination of a patient whose AF-AFP level is significantly increased should be conducted in a fashion designed to detect a fetal anomaly that might explain the noted elevation.

Common Causes
1. Open neural tube defects
   a. Anencephaly (and its variants)
   b. Encephalocele
   c. Open spina bifida
   d. Amniotic band syndrome resulting in non–embryologically positioned neural tube defects
2. Abdominal wall defects
   a. Omphalocele
   b. Gastroschisis
   c. Gastropleuroschisis from amniotic band syndrome
3. Cystic hygromas
4. Neural axis anomalies (not associated with open neural tube defects, e.g., hydrocephalus, Dandy-Walker malformation)

Other Causes
1. Teratomas that contact the amniotic fluid
   a. Sacrococcygeal
   b. Lingual
   c. Retropharyngeal
2. Renal abnormalities
3. Esophageal atresia with or without tracheoesophageal fistula
4. Duodenal obstruction

A general obstetric examination should be obtained that includes documentation of biometric data, including biparietal diameter, head circumference, abdominal circumference, and femur length. These parameters can then be used to calculate a composite sonographic age and body proportionality ratios. It is also important to quantitate the amount of amniotic fluid, which will be a secondary sign of some of the previously described disorders. Composite images should be obtained to survey the entire uterine cavity to exclude a previously missed fetus papyraceus.

After these standard features have been evaluated, specific fetal morphologic structures should be demonstrated. The additional studies include multiple transverse axial sonograms of the head to exclude an encephalocele and to document the size of the lateral ventricles and the presence of the cisterna magna.

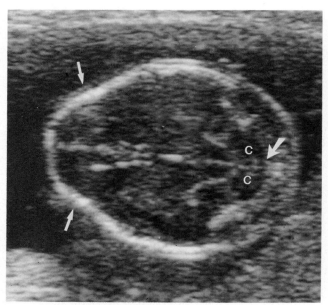

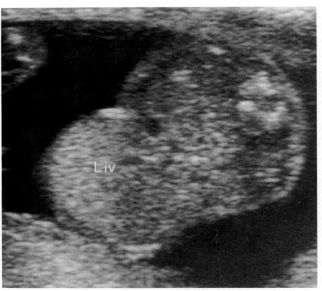

Figure 3–7. Omphalocele. Exteriorized liver (Liv) is seen within the omphalocele sac.

Figure 3–5. Cranial findings associated with open spina bifida and the Chiari II malformation include inward scalloping of the frontal bones *(straight arrows)*, known as the "lemon sign," and "banana" configuration of the cerebellum (c) and effaced cisterna magna *(curved arrow)*.

Because open spina bifida lesions are nearly always associated with Chiari II malformations, there is an effacement of the cisterna magna in virtually all such fetuses[39] (Fig. 3–5) and an increase in ventricular size in 80% to 85% of cases. Obtaining such images assumes, of course, that all anencephalic fetuses have been previously detected.

Transverse axial sonograms of the neck are obtained to exclude cystic hygroma (Fig. 3–6). These sonograms should also demonstrate a midline position of the hypopharynx and/or the trachea to exclude retropharyngeal teratoma. Transverse axial and coronal sono-

grams of the face of the fetus will exclude exophytic cranial (lingual) teratomas. Transverse axial sonograms of the abdomen are then obtained to document the size of the fetal stomach and the absence of a dilated duodenum as well as the demonstration of one or both kidneys and the umbilical cord insertion. A normal cord insertion and adjacent abdominal wall excludes nearly all omphaloceles (Fig. 3–7) and gastroschises. However, in small hernias of the cord (essentially small omphaloceles) (Fig. 3–8) it is possible for the cord insertion to be nearly normal in appearance. Similarly, in a fetus with gastroschisis, the defect in the abdominal wall may be obscured and the anomaly only recognized by visualization of bowel loops floating freely in the amniotic fluid. The stomach is documented to exclude those cases of esophageal atresia without tracheoesophageal fistula and of duodenal obstruction. A useful secondary finding in this regard is the quantity of amniotic fluid, which is virtually always increased in upper gastrointestinal obstructions. Unfortunately, it is now known that polyhydramnios is not always manifest in early cases of tracheoesophageal fistula.

The examination is then directed toward the spine. Open spina bifida lesions without a sac are likely to be the most difficult abnormalities to detect. Thus, careful scrutiny of the spine in both longitudinal and transverse axial sections is recommended. Longitudinal views of the sacrum, while somewhat insensitive for open spina bifida, are excellent for the detection of sacrococcygeal teratoma (Fig. 3–9) and sacral agenesis. Transverse axial sonograms of the spine must cover from the cranial cervical junction to the ischial ossification centers. However, it is not necessary to record an image at every level, although every level should be examined more than one time. Any patient with a fetus that maintains a persistently supine position must be scheduled for reexamination.

A few final points should be considered. If destructive procedures will be used to evacuate the fetus, and an encephalocele is demonstrated, special note of the

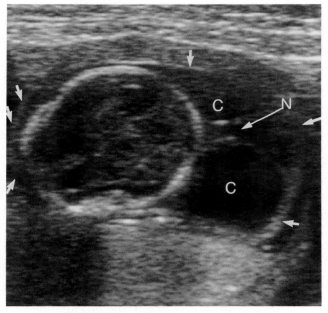

Figure 3–6. Cystic hygroma. Integumentary edema is circumferential around the head and neck *(small arrows)*. Posterior cystic mass (C) appears continuous with skin. N, nuchal ligament.

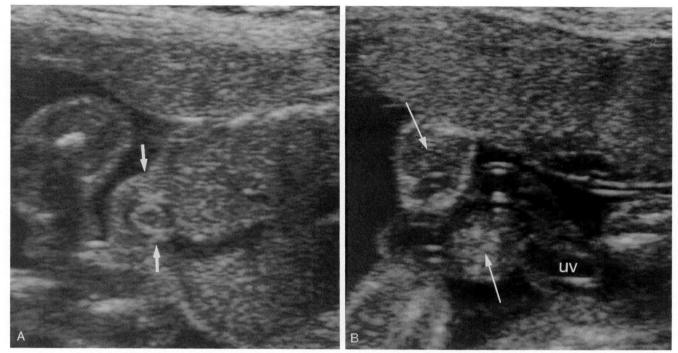

Figure 3–8. "Bowel only" omphalocele. *A.* Very small defect of the abdominal wall *(arrows)* is a subtle observation. *B.* Collapsed bowel loops *(arrows)* are observed within the umbilical cord a few centimeters from the fetal abdominal wall. uv, umbilical vein.

kidneys and an image of the fetal hand are warranted to exclude Meckel syndrome (encephalocele, polydactyly, cystic dysplastic kidneys, microcephaly) because the recurrence risk for this autosomal recessive syndrome is very much greater than for an encephalocele alone. When cystic dysplasia of the kidneys is present in Meckel syndrome, oligohydramnios will virtually always be present. Some examiners look for a clubfoot deformity as a secondary sign of a neural axis abnormality; however, primary demonstration of an open neural tube defect should always be the major goal of an examination. Some examiners may wish to perform a more comprehensive examination than is outlined earlier. Finally, consideration should be given to a later repeat examination when the initial study is negative (especially if the MS-AFP or AF-AFP level was very high).

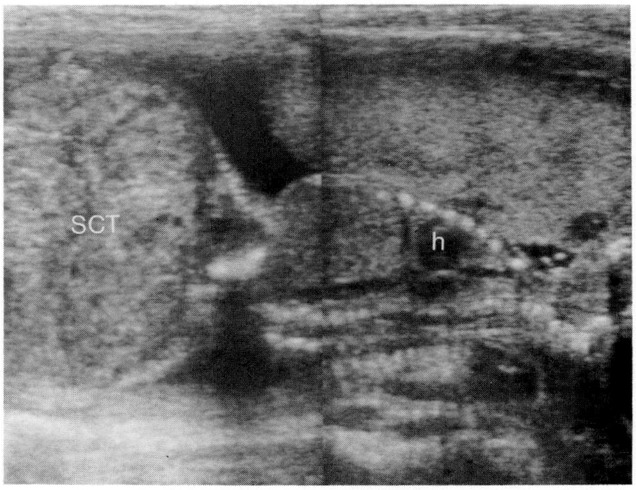

Obviously, a rather broad array of anomalies are encompassed in the list of lesions that may be encountered. The prognosis varies widely in this group. Even among single categories of malformations the prognosis will vary substantially.

Myelomeningocele is an excellent example of a serious malformation that, nonetheless, has a broad spectrum of prognosis (Table 3–5). The prognosis is affected by the location[40] and size of the defect (see Fig. 3–2), the presence of spinal deformity (e.g., kyphosis, scoliosis), associated clubfoot deformity, associated hydrocephalus, and concomitant central nervous system or extra–central nervous system malformations or chromosomal anomalies. Virtually all of these features can be assessed in utero, thereby allowing parents to make a more informed decision. Indeed, in our experience, the level 2 examination is used more to further characterize anomalies than to detect them because a relatively high percentage of abnormal fetuses are recognized on the sonogram preceding the amniocentesis.

After an elevated AF-AFP level is detected, sonog-

Figure 3–9. Large sacrococcygeal teratoma. h, heart; SCT, sacrococcygeal teratoma.

Table 3–5. PROGNOSTIC FACTORS WITH MYELOMENINGOCELE

Location and size of defect
Open versus closed lesion
Associated hydrocephalus
Clubfoot formation
Other associated malformations
Postnatal complications (e.g., shunt infections)

Table 3–6. DETECTION OF ALL ANOMALIES: DATA FROM UNIVERSITY OF CALIFORNIA SAN FRANCISCO, 1978–1990

	Anomaly Present	Anomaly Absent
Positive sonogram	84	0
Negative sonogram	5	174

Sensitivity, 94%; specificity, 100; positive predictive value, 100%; negative predictive value, 97%; prevalence, 34%.

raphy can accurately assess the presence and type of anomaly. The experience at the UCSF prenatal diagnostic center in all cases where the AF-AFP level was elevated from January 1978 through June 1990 is detailed in Tables 3–6 and 3–7.[41–43] Obviously, these data include a longer time span than the California AFP program has existed. Patients with an elevated AF-AFP level discovered during an amniocentesis done for maternal age are also included. Two hundred and sixty-three cases in which the AF-AFP level was elevated were obtained from a total of 22,355 amniocenteses.

In our experience, sonography has been an excellent test to identify the normal pregnancies that have an elevated AF-AFP concentration and segregate them from the pathologic pregnancies. Only 5 of 263 fetuses seen at UCSF between 1978 and 1990 with an elevated AF-AFP concentration had anomalies undetected by sonography (see Table 3–6) and 3 of these are developing normally following corrective surgeries.[43] The remaining two anomalous fetuses, although they exhibited normal sonograms, were prospectively identified as cases of congenital nephrosis because of their extremely high levels of AF-AFP. The rule that "normal is the most difficult diagnosis to make" clearly applies in this situation. Although sonographic performance was weakest in this area, the negative predictive value of sonography alone was 97% (see Table 3–6), which is a still highly accurate result.

Furthermore, sonography detects neural tube defects with an extraordinarily high degree of sensitivity and specificity. When results of the AF-AFP testing were known, as well as the results of acetylcholinesterase testing, no neural tube defects were missed (see Table 3–7). Additionally, sonography can accurately diagnose other congenital anomalies that may cause an elevated AF-AFP concentration (Table 3–8). Many of these anomalies have remarkably different prognoses. One of the major benefits of sonography is its ability to gather valuable information and separate fetuses

Table 3–7. DETECTION OF OPEN NEURAL TUBE DEFECTS: DATA FROM UNIVERSITY OF CALIFORNIA SAN FRANCISCO, 1978–1990

	Defect Present	Defect Absent
Positive sonogram	32	0
Negative sonogram	0	231

Sensitivity, 100%; specificity, 100%; positive predictive value, 100%; negative predictive value, 100%; prevalence, 12%.

Table 3–8. FINAL DIAGNOSIS IN 263 FETUSES WITH ELEVATED AMNIOTIC FLUID α-FETOPROTEIN LEVELS BETWEEN JANUARY 1978 THROUGH DECEMBER 1990 AT THE UNIVERSITY OF CALIFORNIA SAN FRANCISCO

	Amniotic Fluid α-Fetoprotein	
	2–2.5MOM	>2.5MOM
Neural axis abnormalities:		
Myelomeningocele	2	18
Anencephaly	0	8
Encephalocele	0	4
Hydrocephalus (not associated with myelomeningocele)	3	2
Dandy-Walker malformation	2	0
Other anomalies:		
Gastroschisis	1	10
Cystic hygroma	2	9
Genitourinary disease	4	5
Omphalocele	3	2
Amniotic band syndrome	1	3
Tracheoesophageal fistula	1	0
Pharyngeal teratoma	0	1
Skeletal abnormalities	1	1
Hydrops (without cystic hygroma)	1	0
Fetal death	1	4
Total anomalies	22	67
Normal	135	39
Totals	157	106

MOM, multiples of median.

into their proper prognostic groups. For example, a fetus with an isolated omphalocele has a far better prognosis than a fetus with an omphalocele and other associated anomalies (Fig. 3–10).[44] Even among fetuses with isolated lesions, sonography can help to stratify

Table 3–9. RESULTS OF AMNIOTIC FLUID α-FETOPROTEIN (AFP) SCREENING: UNIVERSITY OF CALIFORNIA SAN FRANCISCO, 1984–1990 (14,737 AMNIOCENTESES)

Result	%
Amniotic fluid AFP level exceeding 2.0 MOM	1.5
Neural tube defect present with amniotic fluid AFP >2.0 MOM	12
Anomalous fetuses with amniotic fluid AFP >2.0 MOM	33
Anomalous fetuses with amniotic fluid AFP between 2.0 and 2.5 MOM	14
Anomalous fetuses with amniotic fluid AFP >2.5 MOM	58
Anomalous fetuses with amniotic fluid AFP >10.6 MOM	100
Probability of anomalous fetus when acetylcholinesterase level was positive (including trace positive)	81
Probability of anomalous fetus when the acetylcholinesterase level was positive (excluding trace positive)	100
Probability of a normal outcome when acetylcholinesterase level was negative	87
Anomalous fetuses detected sonographically	94
Percent of cases in which a combination of sonography and amniotic fluid AFP level allowed a confident diagnosis of an anomalous fetus	97
Probability of a correct programmatic distinction of normal versus anomalous fetus	>99
Percent of open neural tube defects detected sonographically	100

MOM, multiples of median.

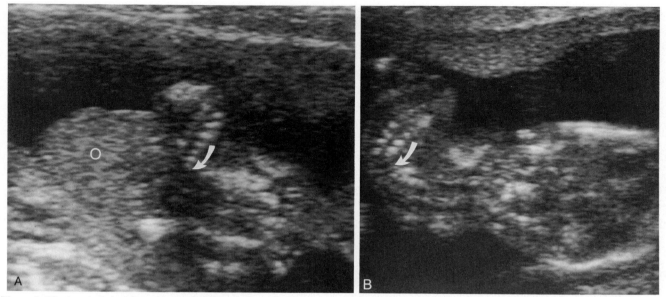

Figure 3–10. Amniotic band syndrome and limb–body wall complex. *A.* Omphalocele (o) and acute angulation of the spine *(curved arrow).* *B.* Characteristic acute angulation of the spine *(curved arrow)* suggests this is not a simple omphalocele.

the fetuses into prognostic categories. For example, a fetus with a sacral myelomeningocele has a significantly different prognosis than a fetus with a thoracic myelomeningocele.[45]

Our data suggest that open neural tube defects are generally not present with AF-AFP concentrations less than 2.5 MOM (see Table 3–8). Open neural tube defects were found in only two cases over the past 12 years when the AF-AFP concentration was less than 2.5 MOM. One case was not pathologically confirmed, but the sonographic features were virtually pathognomonic for a myelomeningocele. All other open neural tube defects studied before 20 weeks' gestation had AF-AFP concentrations greater than 2.5 MOM. This observation is consistent with previously presented data.[3]

In summary, our experience documents that MS-AFP screening leading to testing of the AF-AFP and subsequent sonography is an excellent method to diagnose numerous defects in high-risk patients (Table 3–9). Pregnancies with an elevated AF-AFP concentration clearly fall into this category. More recently, it has been suggested that mothers with elevated MS-AFP levels could be screened with sonography better than with amniocentesis to confirm or deny the presence of a fetal anomaly.[46–58] It is clear that sonography has the capacity to detect neural tube defects and other causes of elevation of AFP when relatively small numbers of examinations are performed with a great deal of care in a population with a relatively high prevalence of fetal anomalies.[59] Whether this can be achieved with the higher numbers of examinations required and the lower prevalence rate when screening all patients with elevations of MS-AFP levels remains to be seen.

References

1. Main DM, Mennuti MT: Neural tube defects: Issues in prenatal diagnosis and counseling. Obstet Gynecol 67:1, 1986.

2. Goldberg MF, Oakley GP: Interpreting elevated amniotic fluid alpha-fetoprotein levels in clinical practice: Use of the positive predictive value concept. Am J Obstet Gynecol 133:126, 1979.

3. Crandall BF, Matumota M: Risk associated with an elevated amniotic fluid alpha-fetoprotein level. Am J Med Genet 39:64, 1991.

4. Sheffield LJ, Sackett DL, Goldsmith CH, et al: A clinical approach to the use of predictive values in the prenatal diagnosis of neural tube defects. Am J Obstet Gynecol 145:319, 1983.

5. Brock DJH, Barron L, Duncan P, et al: Significance of elevated mid-trimester maternal plasma alpha-fetoprotein values. Lancet 1:1281, 1979.

6. UK Collaborative Study on Alpha-fetoprotein in Relation to Neural-Tube Defects: Maternal serum alpha-fetoprotein measurement in antenatal screening for anencephaly and spina bifida in early pregnancy. Lancet 1:1323, 1977.

7. Greenberg F, James LM, Oakley GP: Estimates of birth prevalence rates of spina bifida in the United States from computer-generated maps. Am J Obstet Gynecol 145:570, 1983.

8. Milunsky A, Jick SS, Bruell CL, et al: Predictive values, relative risks, and overall benefits of high and low maternal serum α-fetoprotein screening in singleton pregnancies: New epidemiologic data. Am J Obstet Gynecol 161:291, 1989.

9. Haddow JE, Kloza EM, Smith DW, Knight GJ: Data from an alpha-fetoprotein pilot screening program in Maine. Obstet Gynecol 62:556, 1983.

10. Burton BK, Sowers SG, Nelson LH: Maternal serum α-fetoprotein screening in North Carolina: Experience with more than twelve thousand pregnancies. Am J Obstet Gynecol 146:439, 1983.

11. Cowan LS, Phelps-Sandall B, Hanson FW, et al: A prenatal diagnostic center's first-year experience with the California α-fetoprotein screening program. Am J Obstet Gynecol 160:1496, 1989.

12. Milunsky A, Alpert E, Kitzmiller IL, et al: Neural tube defects, diabetes, and serum α-fetoprotein screening. Am J Obstet Gynecol 142:1030, 1982.

13. Macri JN, Kasturi RV, Hu MG, et al: Maternal serum α-fetoprotein screening: III. Pitfalls in evaluating black gravid women. Am J Obstet Gynecol 157:820, 1987.

14. Crandall BF, Robinson L, Grau P: Risk associated with an elevated amniotic fluid alpha-fetoprotein level. Am J Med Genet 165:581, 1991.

15. Warner AA, Pettenati MJ, Burton BK: Risk of fetal chromosomal anomalies in patients with elevated maternal serum alpha-fetoprotein. Obstet Gynecol 75:64, 1990.

16. Petrikovsky BM, Nardi DA, Rodis JF, Hoegsberg B: Elevated maternal serum alpha-fetoprotein and mild fetal uropathy. Obstet Gynecol 78:262, 1991.

17. Killam WP, Miller RC, Seeds JW: Extremely high maternal serum alpha-fetoprotein levels at second-trimester screening. Obstet Gynecol 78:257, 1991.

18. Davenport DM, Macri JN: The clinical significance of low maternal serum α-fetoprotein. Am J Obstet Gynecol 146:657, 1983.

19. Palomaki GE, Knight GJ, Holman MS, Haddow JE: Maternal serum α-fetoprotein screening for fetal Down syndrome in the United States: Results of a survey. Am J Obstet Gynecol 162:317, 1990.

20. Palomaki GE, Haddow JE: Maternal serum α-fetoprotein, age, and Down syndrome risk. Am J Obstet Gynecol 156:460, 1987.

21. Hershey DW, Crandall BF, Perdue S: Combining maternal age and serum α-fetoprotein to predict the risk of Down syndrome. Obstet Gynecol 68:177, 1986.

22. Simpson JL, Baum LD, Depp R, et al: Low maternal serum α-fetoprotein and perinatal outcome. Am J Obstet Gynecol 156:852, 1987.

23. Drugan A, Dvorin E, Koppitchm FC III, et al: Counseling for low maternal serum alpha-fetoprotein should emphasize all chromosome anomalies, not just Down syndrome! Obstet Gynecol 73:271, 1989.

24. New England Regional Genetics Group Prenatal Collaborative Study of Down Syndrome Screening: Combining maternal serum α-fetoprotein measurements and age to screen for Down syndrome in pregnant women under age 35. Am J Obstet Gynecol 160:575, 1989.

25. MacDonald ML, Wagner RM, Slotnick RN: Sensitivity and specificity of screening for Down syndrome with alpha-fetoprotein, hCG, unconjugated estriol, and maternal age. Obstet Gynecol 77:63, 1991.

26. Thomas RL, Blakemore KJ: Evaluation of elevations in maternal serum alpha-fetoprotein: A review. Obstet Gynecol Surv 45:269, 1990.

27. Robinson L, Grau P, Crandall BF: Pregnancy outcomes after increasing maternal serum alpha-fetoprotein levels. Obstet Gynecol 74:17, 1989.

28. Hamilton MPR, Abdalla HI, Whitfield CR: Significance of raised maternal serum α-fetoprotein in singleton pregnancies with normally formed fetuses. Obstet Gynecol 65:465, 1985.

29. Evans MI, Belsky R, Greb A, et al: Wide variation in maternal serum alpha-fetoprotein reports in one metropolitan area: Concerns for the quality of prenatal testing. Obstet Gynecol 72:342, 1988.

30. Milunsky A, Alpert E: Prenatal diagnosis of neural tube defects: II. Analysis of false-positive and false-negative alpha-fetoprotein results. Obstet Gynecol 48:6, 1976.

31. Macri JN, Kasturi BE, Krantz DA, Hu MG: Maternal serum α-fetoprotein screening: II. Pitfalls in low-volume decentralized laboratory performance. Am J Obstet Gynecol 156:533, 1987.

32. Platt LD, Golde SH, Artal R, et al: False-negative maternal serum alpha-fetoprotein determinations in myelodysplasia: The role of ultrasound. Am J Obstet Gynecol 144:352, 1982.

33. Burton BK, Dillard RG, Clark EN: The psychological impact of false-positive elevations of maternal serum α-fetoprotein. Am J Obstet Gynecol 151:77, 1985.

34. Burton BK, Dillard RG, Clark EN: Maternal serum α-fetoprotein screening: The effect of participation on anxiety and attitude toward pregnancy in women with normal results. Am J Obstet Gynecol 152:540, 1985.

35. Alpha-Fetoprotein. American College of Obstetricians and Gynecologists Technical Bulletin No. 154. Washington, DC, American College of Obstetricians and Gynecologists, 1992.

36. Platt L, Feuchtbaum L, Filly RA, et al: The California maternal serum α-fetoprotein screening program: The role of ultrasonography in the detection of spina bifida. Am J Obstet Gynecol 166:1328, 1992.

37. Leopold G: Antepartum obstetrical ultrasound examination guidelines. J Ultrasound Med 5:241, 1986.

38. Wald N, Cuckle H, Boreham J, et al: Small biparietal diameter of fetuses with spina bifida: Implications for antenatal screening. Br J Obstet Gynaecol 87:219, 1980.

39. Goldstein RB, Podrasky AE, Filly RA, Callen PW: Effacement of the fetal cisterna magna in association with myelomeningocele. Radiology 172:409, 1989.

40. Kollias SS, Goldstein RB, Cogen PH, Filly RA: Estimation of the spinal level of prenatally detected myelomeningoceles: Sonographic accuracy. Radiology 185:109, 1992.

41. Slotnick N, Filly RA, Callen PW, Golbus M: Sonography as a procedure complementary to α-fetoprotein testing for neural tube defects. J Ultrasound Med 1:319, 1982.

42. Hashimoto BE, Mahony BS, Filly RA, et al: Sonography, a complementary examination to alpha-fetoprotein testing for fetal neural tube defects. J Ultrasound Med 4:307, 1985.

43. Robbin M, Filly RA, Fell S, et al: Elevation of the amniotic fluid alpha-fetoprotein: Sonographic evaluation. Radiology 188:165, 1993.

44. Hughes MD, Nyberg DA, Mack LA, Pretorius DH: Fetal omphalocele: Prenatal US detection of concurrent anomalies and other predictors of outcome. Radiology 173:371, 1989.

45. Eldon FL: Myelomeningocele: Selection for treatment. In O'Brien MS (ed): Pediatric Neurological Surgery. New York, Raven Press, 1978.

46. Hogge WA, Thiagarajah S, Fergusson JE II, et al: The role of ultrasonography and amniocentesis in the evaluation of pregnancies at risk for neural tube defects. Am J Obstet Gynecol 161:520, 1989.

47. Lindfors KK, McGahan JP, Tennant FP, et al: Mid-trimester screening for open neural tube defects: Correlation of sonography with amniocentesis results. AJR 149:141, 1987.

48. Richards DS, Seeds JW, Katz VL, et al: Elevated maternal serum alpha-fetoprotein with normal ultrasound: Is amniocentesis always appropriate? A review of 26,069 screened patients. Obstet Gynecol 71:203, 1988.

49. Drugan A, Zador IE, Syner FN, et al: A normal ultrasound does not obviate the need for amniocentesis in patients with elevated serum alpha-fetoprotein. Obstet Gynecol 72:627, 1988.

50. Nadel AS, Green JK, Holmes LB, et al: Absence of need for amniocentesis in patients with elevated levels of maternal serum alpha-fetoprotein and normal ultrasonographic examinations. N Engl J Med 323:557, 1990.

51. Schell DL, Drugan A, Brindley BA, et al: Combined ultrasonography and amniocentesis for pregnant women with elevated serum α-fetoprotein: Revising the risk estimate. J Reprod Med 35:543, 1990.

52. Thornton JG, Lilford RJ, Newcombe RG: Tables for estimation of individual risk of fetal neural tube and ventral wall defects, incorporating prior probability, maternal serum α-fetoprotein levels, and ultrasonographic examination results. Am J Obstet Gynecol 164:154, 1990.

53. Watson WJ, Chesceir NC, Katz VL, Seeds JW: The role of ultrasound in evaluation of patients with elevated maternal serum alpha-fetoprotein: A review. Obstet Gynecol 78:123, 1991.

54. Katz VL, Seeds JW, Albright SG, et al: Role of ultrasound and informed consent in the evaluation of elevated maternal serum alpha-fetoprotein. Am J Perinatol 8:73, 1991.

55. Linfors KK, Gorczyca DP, Hanson FW, et al: The roles of ultrasonography and amniocentesis in evaluation of elevated maternal serum α-fetoprotein. Am J Obstet Gynecol 164:1571, 1991.

56. Tyrrell S, Howel D, Bark M, et al: Should maternal α-fetoprotein estimation be carried out in centers where ultrasound screening is routine? Am J Obstet Gynecol 158:1092, 1988.

57. Laurence KM, Elder G, Evans KT, et al: Should women at high risk of neural tube defect have an amniocentesis? J Med Genet 22:457, 1985.

58. Morrow RJ, McNay MB, Whittle MJ: Ultrasound detection of neural tube defects in patients with elevated maternal serum alpha-fetoprotein. Obstet Gynecol 78:1055, 1991.

59. Steinhaus KA, Bernstein R, Bocain ME: Importance of accurate diagnosis in counseling for neural tube defects diagnosed prenatally. Clin Genet 39:355, 1991.

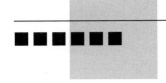

CHAPTER *4*

Ultrasound Evaluation of Fetal Chromosome Disorders

JAMES P. CRANE, M.D.

Cytogenetic abnormalities affect 1 in every 200 children, with autosomal aneuploidy, sex chromosome abnormalities, and structural rearrangements occurring with approximately equal frequency.[1] At present, genetic amniocentesis is typically offered only to women known to be at increased risk for chromosome abnormalities on the basis of maternal age, family history of a cytogenetic abnormality, or low maternal serum α-fetoprotein (MS-AFP) levels. This policy results in detection of fewer than one third of all chromosomally abnormal fetuses.

Many cytogenetic abnormalities are associated with structural birth defects capable of being diagnosed at second-trimester ultrasound evaluation. This diagnostic capability coupled with the fact that the majority of pregnant women undergo ultrasound examination during pregnancy provides a powerful noninvasive tool for prenatal diagnosis of cytogenetic abnormalities in low-risk pregnant women.

In this chapter the focus is on the current status of sonographic biometry as a means of screening for fetal chromosome abnormalities and specific patterns of malformation associated with common cytogenetic disorders, including trisomies 13, 18, and 21, Turner syndrome, and fetal triploidy syndrome.

SONOGRAPHIC BIOMETRY AS A SCREENING TOOL FOR CYTOGENETIC ABNORMALITIES

Essential Characteristics of Screening Tests

The potential value of sonographic biometry depends on the sensitivity, positive screening rate, and positive predictive value of the measured parameter. Ideally, a screening test should have a high sensitivity combined with a low positive screening rate and high predictive value. For example, if sensitivity is too low, the screening tool will have little impact on the overall prevalence of chromosome abnormalities. An inordinately high positive screening rate is also undesirable, resulting in unwarranted anxiety for many women carrying normal fetuses and exposing them unnecessarily to the risks of genetic amniocentesis.

The positive predictive value of an abnormal sonographic finding can be used to determine the appropriateness of amniotic fluid chromosome studies. For example, let us assume that 1 in every 100 fetuses with a given sonographic finding has Down syndrome. This can be compared with the risk of a procedure-related pregnancy loss secondary to second-trimester amniocentesis (approximately 1 in 200 chances).[2] Invasive testing would be reasonable in this situation since the odds of detecting a chromosome abnormality by amniocentesis would outweigh the risk of losing a normal pregnancy secondary to the procedure. In contrast, the wisdom of amniocentesis must be questioned for sonographic parameters with predictive values greater than 1 in 200 since more normal fetuses will be lost by invasive testing than abnormal fetuses detected.

Maternal age of 35 years and older and low MS-AFP levels are widely accepted indications for genetic amniocentesis.[3, 4] The sensitivity, positive screen rates, and positive predictive values for these screening criteria are illustrated in Table 4–1 and can be used as a benchmark with which to compare sonographic biometry.

Persons with Down syndrome often exhibit short stature and redundant skin folds at the nape of the neck. These dysmorphic features can, on occasion, be recognized sonographically during the second trimester of pregnancy. This knowledge has led to the investigation of sonographic biometry as a noninvasive screening tool for Down syndrome.

Nuchal Skin Fold Thickness

Redundant nuchal skin folds are present in 80% of newborns with Down syndrome.[5] Sonographic assessment of fetal nuchal skin fold thickness was first proposed by Benacerraf and colleagues in 1985.[6]

Measurements are typically performed at between 15 and 21 weeks' menstrual age using a transverse axial image that is directed in a suboccipital-bregmatic plane (Fig. 4–1). Critical internal landmarks include the cavum septi pellucidi, cerebral peduncles, cerebellar hemispheres, and cisterna magna. Nuchal skin fold thickness is measured with electronic calipers from the outer skull table to the outer skin surface, with values of greater than or equal to 6 mm considered abnormal. The mean intraobserver and interobserver errors for this measurement are only 0.63 mm and 0.53 mm, respectively, assuming care is taken to achieve the correct plane.[7]

The effectiveness of nuchal skin fold thickness as a

Table 4–1. CURRENTLY EMPLOYED SCREENING TOOLS FOR DETECTION OF DOWN SYNDROME

Screening Criteria	Sensitivity	Positive Screening Rate	Positive Predictive Value
Maternal age ≥35 years[3]	20%	5%	1/110
Low MS-AFP levels (general population)[4]	33%	5%	1/169

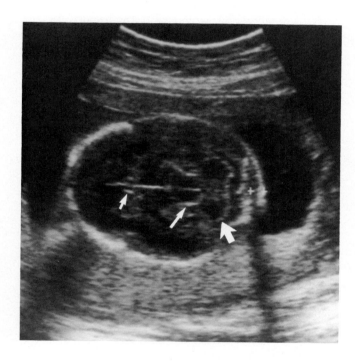

Figure 4–1. Correct plane for measuring nuchal skin fold thickness. Critical landmarks include the cavum septi pellucidi *(short arrow)*, cerebral peduncles *(long arrow)*, and cerebellar hemispheres *(broad arrow)*. Calipers (+) are placed from the outer skull table to the outer skin surface.

Table 4–2. NUCHAL SKIN FOLD THICKNESS FOR DOWN SYNDROME DETECTION

Study	No. of Patients		Sensitivity	Positive Screening Rate	Positive Predictive Value*
	Total Population	Trisomy 21			
Benacerraf et al[8]	3825	21	43%	0.1%	1/3.6
Crane and Gray[7]	6567	26	42%	1.3%	1/8

*Positive predictive value is based on a 1 in 710 prevalence of trisomy 21 in the general population.

Table 4–3. BIPARIETAL DIAMETER/FEMUR LENGTH RATIO FOR DETECTION OF DOWN SYNDROME

Study	No. of Patients with Trisomy 21	Sensitivity	Positive Screening Rate	Positive Predictive Value*
Benacerraf et al[8]	20	70%	5%	1/47
Lockwood et al[10]	35	51%	7%	1/103
Dicke et al[11]	33	18%	4%	1/169
Hill et al[12]	22	36%	7%	1/172
Brumfeld et al[13]	15	40%	2%	1/277
Hadlock et al[14]	16	19%	12%	1/469
Perella et al[9]	19	26%	23%	1/628

*Positive predictive value is based on a 1 in 710 prevalence of trisomy 21 in the general population.

screening tool for Down syndrome has been independently confirmed by two large prospective clinical trials (Table 4–2).[7, 8] The sensitivity and positive screen rates in both studies were superior to those associated with either advanced maternal age or low MS-AFP levels. The predictive value of nuchal skin fold thickness for Down syndrome was also quite high (1/4 to 1/13), even after adjustment for the prevalence of Down syndrome in the general population (1/710 births). Given these findings, genetic amniocentesis should be offered when a nuchal skin fold thickness of 6 mm or greater is observed. Perella and associates[9] were unable to confirm the value of sonographically measured nuchal skin fold thickness; however, this study was retrospective and used images that were not specifically taken for the purpose of nuchal skin fold measurement.

Femur Length

Femur length is an indirect measure of stature. It is therefore not surprising that fetuses with Down syndrome have slightly shorter femurs than do chromosomally normal fetuses. The appropriateness of the femur length can be assessed at between 15 and 23 weeks' menstrual age using either the biparietal diameter/femur length ratio or the observed-to-expected femur length ratio.[8, 10] The latter is based on a formula that takes into account the normal relationship between the biparietal diameter and the femur length. Any fetus with a biparietal diameter/femur length ratio above 1.5 standard deviations for menstrual age is considered as having a positive screening test. When the observed-to-expected femur length ratio is used, values below 0.92 standard deviation indicate disproportionate shortening of the femur.[8]

The efficacy of the biparietal diameter/femur length ratio and the observed-to-expected femur length ratio for Down syndrome detection is illustrated in Tables 4–3 and 4–4.[8-17] As noted, some investigators have found sensitivities, positive screening rates, and predictive values that support the use of these ratios as indications for genetic amniocentesis. Other studies, however, have failed to confirm a strong enough association between femur length and Down syndrome to warrant invasive testing. Accordingly, it is important for prenatal diagnostic centers to assess the usefulness of these approaches in their own institutions before deciding what action, if any, is appropriate in the event of a positive screening result. It is also imperative that each center establish its own normal reference curve since mean values and standard deviations may vary significantly from one institution to another (Fig. 4–2). These steps will ensure that optimal sensitivity and specificity are achieved.

Humeral Length

In 1989, Fitzsimmons and coworkers[18] reported that humeral lengths are also shorter than expected in trisomy 21. This observation was based on postmortem measurements in 37 fetuses with Down syndrome compared with 174 chromosomally normal subjects. The results of two subsequent sonographic studies of humeral length and Down syndrome are summarized in Table 4–5. Both groups of investigators confirmed that humeral length is shortened in trisomy 21, although conflicting results were reported with respect to the usefulness of humeral length as a predictor of Down syndrome.[19, 20]

Table 4–4. OBSERVED-TO-EXPECTED FEMUR LENGTH RATIO FOR DETECTION OF DOWN SYNDROME

Study	No. of Patients with Trisomy 21	Sensitivity	Positive Screening Rate	Positive Predictive Value*
Benacerraf et al[8]	28	68%	2%	1/22
Grist et al[15]	6	50%	6%	1/105
Dicke et al[11]	33	15%	10%	1/455
LaFollette et al[16]	30	12%	13%	1/619
Hill et al[12]	22	50%	15%	1/249
Nyberg et al[17]	49	14%	6%	1/303

*Positive predictive value is based on a 1 in 710 prevalence of trisomy 21 in the general population.

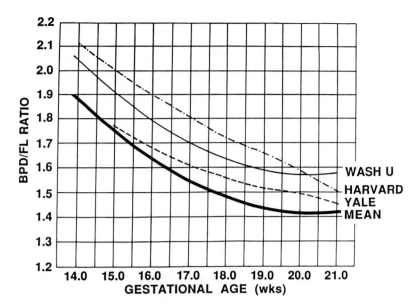

Figure 4–2. Nomogram of biparietal diameter (BPD)/femur length (FL) comparing 1.5-SD thresholds at Washington, Harvard, and Yale Universities. Solid bold line represents the Washington University mean.

Summary

Sonographic biometry offers a noninvasive means of identifying some pregnancies at increased risk for Down syndrome in otherwise "low-risk" populations. It should be remembered, however, that at least 50% of fetuses with Down syndrome will have no recognizable sonographic abnormality. Ultrasound evaluation should therefore not be used as a substitute for genetic amniocentesis when other valid risk factors such as advanced maternal age or low MS-AFP levels are present.

A potential area for future exploration is the combined use of sonographic, biochemical, and historical parameters to develop patient-specific risks for Down syndrome. Although the biparietal diameter/femur length ratio, nuchal skin fold thickness, serum estriol level, serum human chorionic gonadotropin concentration, and maternal age may not be entirely independent of one another, mathematic models can be applied to take this into account and enhance both sensitivity and specificity.

SONOGRAPHIC MALFORMATIONS ASSOCIATED WITH THE COMMON CHROMOSOME DISORDERS

Chromosome abnormalities are often associated with a characteristic constellation of malformations and dysmorphic features, many of which can be recognized sonographically. In this section, the fetal phenotypes associated with trisomies 13, 18, and 21, Turner syndrome, and triploidy syndrome are presented.

Trisomy 21

Down syndrome is the single most common cytogenetic abnormality among liveborn infants, occurring in 1 in every 710 births. Children with Down syndrome are moderately retarded with an average IQ score of approximately 50, although milder or more severe degrees of intellectual handicap can also be observed.[21] Fortunately, social performance exceeds mental age by several years. As a result, children with Down syndrome typically interact well within society. Fifteen to 20% of infants with Down syndrome will die during the first year of life, usually of congestive heart failure or leukemia. Children who survive the first year commonly live to adulthood, although mortality rates exceed those for normal persons at any given age.[22]

Sonographic abnormalities associated with Down syndrome are illustrated in Figures 4–3 through 4–6 and listed in Table 4–6. Certain of these malformations deserve special comment. Duodenal atresia occurs in 8% of fetuses with Down syndrome and is characterized sonographically by the "double bubble" sign (see Fig. 4–4), which results from distention of the stomach and duodenum proximal to the level of obstruction. Polyhydramnios is often present owing to impaired reabsorption of amniotic fluid by the intestines. These

Table 4–5. OBSERVED-TO-EXPECTED HUMERAL LENGTH FOR DETECTION OF DOWN SYNDROME

Study	No. of Patients with Trisomy 21	Sensitivity	Positive Screening Rate	Positive Predictive Value
Benacerraf et al[19]	24	50%	6%	1/33
Rotmensch et al[20]	43	28%	9%	1/244

Positive screen defined as an observed-to-expected humeral length ratio of <0.91.

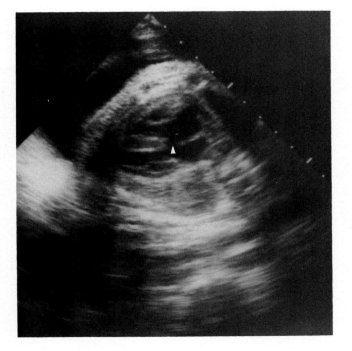

Figure 4–3. Four-chamber view of heart in a fetus with Down syndrome and atrioventricular canal. The septal leaflets of the atrioventricular valves cannot be identified and a ventricular septal defect and primum atrial septal defect are apparent *(arrowhead).*

findings may occasionally be apparent during the second trimester of pregnancy but are typically not seen until after 22 to 24 weeks of menstrual age. The sonographic finding of duodenal atresia carries a 30% risk for associated Down syndrome. Fetal karyotyping is therefore appropriate.

Nonimmune hydrops is a common second-trimester presentation of many chromosome abnormalities, including trisomies 13, 18, and 21 as well as Turner syndrome. Overall, 14% to 18% of hydropic fetuses will have an underlying cytogenetic disorder. Fetal karyotyping should therefore be included as a part of the diagnostic evaluation of this pregnancy complication. Other potential etiologies for nonimmune hydrops and appropriate diagnostic studies are presented in Table 4–7.

More recently, Benacerraf and colleagues reported an association between mildly dilated renal pelves and Down syndrome.[23] With the use of the criteria shown in Table 4–8, 25% of fetuses with Down syndrome had pyelectasis as compared with only 2.8% of normal subjects. Corteville and colleagues[24] confirmed an increased frequency of trisomy 21 among fetuses with pyelectasis but noted that other sonographic abnor-

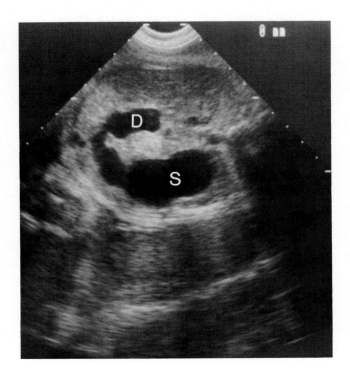

Figure 4–4. Transverse axial view through fetal abdomen showing dilated stomach (S) and proximal duodenum (D) (double-bubble sign) secondary to duodenal atresia.

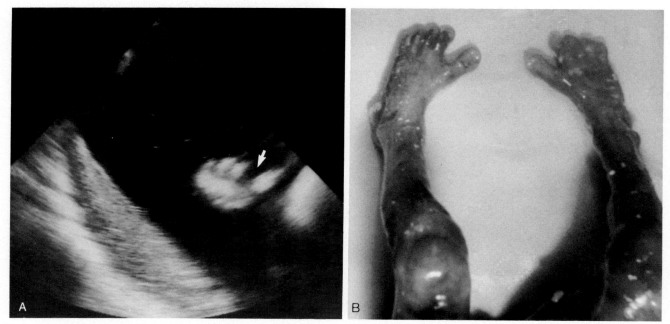

Figure 4–5. Sonogram *(A)* and gross photograph *(B)* of fetus with Down syndrome with widely spaced first and second toes *(arrow)*, a common dysmorphic feature in trisomy 21.

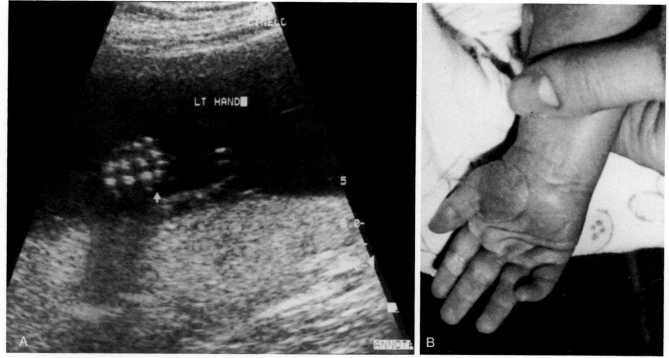

Figure 4–6. Sonogram *(A)* and gross photograph *(B)* showing clinodactyly with hypoplastic middle phalanx of fifth digit. This dysmorphic finding is observed in nearly 50% of infants with Down syndrome.

Table 4–6. SONOGRAPHIC FINDINGS IN
DOWN SYNDROME

Thickened nuchal skin fold
Cystic hygroma
Mildly dilated cerebral ventricles
Congenital heart disease (40%)
  Ventricular and atrial septal defects
  Atrioventricular canal
Esophageal atresia
Duodenal atresia (8%)
Diaphragmatic hernia
Nonimmune hydrops
Renal pyelectasis (17% to 25%)
Short femur and humerus
Clinodactyly of fifth digits
Widely spaced first and second toes

malities were also commonly observed. The sensitivity (4%) and predictive value (1 in 340) of isolated pyelectasis would not appear to warrant invasive testing.

Trisomy 13

Trisomy 13, or Patau syndrome, occurs with a frequency of 1 in 5000 births. Affected children are profoundly mentally retarded and may experience a variety of neonatal problems, including seizures, hypotonia or hypertonia, apneic episodes, feeding difficulties, and generalized failure to thrive.[25] Early death is typical, with 50% of infants with trisomy 13 dying within 1 month and only 18% surviving more than 1 year.

Sonographic abnormalities commonly associated with trisomy 13 are listed in Table 4–9. Second-trimester fetal growth retardation is observed in 43% of cases, while polyhydramnios and hypotonia may become apparent during the third trimester.[26] Congenital heart disease occurs in over 80% of fetuses with trisomy 13, with ventricular septal defects, atrial septal defects, and dextrocardia being most common.[25]

Table 4–7. NONIMMUNE HYDROPS: ETIOLOGY AND
EVALUATION

Potential Causes
Chromosome abnormality (14%–18%)
Congenital infection (cytomegalovirus, parvovirus, syphilis, toxoplasmosis)
Structural heart defects
Cardiac arrhythmias
Fetal-to-maternal hemorrhage
Twin-transfusion syndrome
α-Thalassemia (Southeast Asian or Mediterranean ethnic origin)

Diagnostic Evaluation
Indirect Coombs' test
Kleihauer-Betke test
Rapid plasma reagin, cytomegalovirus, parvovirus, and toxoplasmosis titers
Amniotic fluid viral cultures
Amniotic fluid cytogenetic studies
Fetal echocardiography including M-mode
Mean corpuscular volume, hemoglobin electrophoresis, and serum iron concentration

Central nervous system anomalies are present in nearly 70% of fetuses with trisomy 13 and may include holoprosencephaly, agenesis of the corpus callosum, and deafness secondary to malformation of the organ of Corti.[27] Holoprosencephaly is characterized by incomplete division of the cerebral hemispheres and can be recognized sonographically using the criteria listed in Table 4–10 and illustrated in Figure 4–7. Sonographic findings in agenesis of the corpus callosum include absence of the cavum septi pellucidi and colpocephaly with dilatation of the occipital horns of the lateral ventricles (Fig. 4–8).

Craniofacial malformations are also common in trisomy 13 and may include micrognathia, sloping forehead, cleft lip and/or palate (60% incidence), and microphthalmia (Fig. 4–9).

Sonographic assessment of the hands and feet may increase the index of suspicion for trisomy 13 when other major malformations are apparent. Specific anomalies may include postaxial polydactyly, camptodactyly, and overlapping digits (Fig. 4–10).

Finally, trisomy 13 can be associated with a variety of gastrointestinal and renal malformations, including omphalocele, renal cortical cysts, hydronephrosis, and horseshoe kidney.[25] Fetal karyotyping should be performed in all cases of sonographically detected omphalocele since 30% to 40% of these fetuses will have either trisomy 13 or trisomy 18.[28–30] Amniocentesis is not essential in fetuses with isolated renal malformations unless other risk factors (advanced maternal age, low MS-AFP screening test result, family history of chromosome abnormalities) are present.

Trisomy 18

Trisomy 18, or Edward syndrome, is the second most common autosomal trisomy, occurring with a frequency of 1 in 3000 births. Neonatal complications are similar to those observed in trisomy 13 and may include initial hypotonia followed by hypertonia, apnea, and poor sucking ability necessitating nasogastric tube feedings. Affected children are severely retarded, fail to thrive, and have reduced survival, with 30% dying within 1 month and 90% dying within 1 year.[25]

Table 4–11 is a summary of recognizable sonographic abnormalities in trisomy 18. General features may include second-trimester fetal growth retardation (59%), polyhydramnios, and diminished fetal activity.[26] Congenital heart disease is present in more than 90% of affected fetuses, with ventricular and atrial septal defects being most common.[25]

Other anomalies in trisomy 18 amenable to sonographic diagnosis include diaphragmatic hernia, hydronephrosis, horseshoe kidney, esophageal atresia with or without tracheoesophageal fistula, and omphalocele. Small omphaloceles containing only bowel (Fig. 4–11) are more commonly associated with a chromosomal etiology[31, 32]; however, fetal karyotyping is recommended regardless of omphalocele content and size.

Trisomy 18 can be associated with a variety of limb malformations, including clubfoot deformity, general-

Table 4–8. RENAL PYELECTASIS AND DOWN SYNDROME

Investigator	Sensitivity	Positive Screening Rate	Positive Predictive Value
Benacerraf et al[23]*	25%	2.8%	Not stated
Corteville et al[24]†			
All cases	17%	2.2%	1/90
Isolated pyelectasis	4%	2.2%	1/340

*Pyelectasis defined as an anteroposterior pelvic diameter of ≥4 mm from 15 to 20 weeks, ≥5 mm from 20 to 30 weeks, ≥7 mm from 30 to 40 weeks.
†Pyelectasis defined as an anteroposterior pelvic diameter of ≥4 mm from 14 to 32 weeks and ≥ 7 mm after 32 weeks.

ized arthrogryposis, and clenched hands with overlapping digits (Fig. 4–12).[33–35] Careful sonographic assessment of the extremities can therefore yield helpful clues when other major structural anomalies are apparent.

Fetuses with trisomy 18 often have a characteristic facial profile, with micrognathia, dolichocephaly, and a prominent occiput (Fig. 4–13A). When viewed in a transverse axial plane, the fetal skull may have an unusual strawberry-shaped configuration (see Fig. 4–13B). A common intracranial finding in trisomy 18 is enlargement of the cisterna magna (≥10 mm anteroposterior diameter) (Fig. 4–14).[36–38] Although usually not apparent during the early second trimester, this sonographic clue can be noted in approximately 44% of fetuses with trisomy 18 after 24 weeks' gestation.

Choroid plexus cysts (Fig. 4–15) are common in trisomy 18, occurring in nearly 30% of cases.[39] Most of these fetuses will have other sonographically detected anomalies that prompt fetal karyotyping.[39–43] The appropriateness of genetic amniocentesis for isolated choroid plexus cysts remains controversial since choroid plexus cysts are also observed in 0.7% to 3.6% of normal second-trimester fetuses.[44–48] Benacerraf and associates[39] estimated that 477 amniocenteses would be required to identify each fetus with trisomy 18 if isolated choroid plexus cysts were considered an indication for invasive testing. Amniocentesis would seem ill advised from a risk–benefit perspective given these

odds. It has been suggested that large, complex, or bilateral choroid plexus cysts carry a greater risk for trisomy 18 than do small, unilateral simple cysts.[49, 50] These reports are largely anecdotal, however, and without appropriate controls. In summary, sonographic detection of choroid plexus cysts should prompt a careful fetal anatomic survey, including echocardiography. Other risk factors, including maternal age, MS-AFP levels, and family history, should also be taken into account. Genetic amniocentesis is appropriate in those instances in which other anomalies, fetal growth retardation, or historical risk factors are identified.

Turner Syndrome

Most cases of Turner syndrome are caused by a missing X chromosome (45,X karyotype). Other karyotypic abnormalities resulting in a Turner phenotype may include isochromosome Xq, Xp deletions, and ring X chromosomes.[27] Mosaicism with a concomitant normal cell line occurs in 15% of cases.

The vast majority of 45,X conceptions result in first- or second-trimester miscarriage. The incidence of Turner syndrome among liveborn females is 1 in 2500. Physical stigmata typically include short stature, low hairline, webbed neck, cubitus valgus, shield chest with widely spaced nipples, hearing loss (50%), renal malformations (especially horseshoe kidney), and congenital heart disease (15% to 20%). Affected females are also infertile and fail to develop menses and secondary sexual characteristics owing to ovarian dysgenesis. Mental retardation is rare, although motor IQ scores tend to be slightly lower than those of chromosomally normal siblings.[51] Sonographic findings in Turner syndrome may include cystic hygromas, nonimmune hydrops, renal anomalies, and cardiac malformations. Coarctation of the aorta accounts for nearly 70% of the cardiac defects associated with Turner syndrome and is usually not detectable during the second trimes-

Text continued on page 47

Table 4–9. SONOGRAPHIC FINDINGS IN TRISOMY 13

Second-trimester–onset intrauterine growth retardation (43%)
Third-trimester hydramnios
Congenital heart disease (>80%)
  Ventricular septal defect, atrial septal defect
  Dextrocardia
Central nervous system malformations (>70%)
  Holoprosencephaly
  Agenesis of corpus callosum
Craniofacial malformations
  Micrognathia
  Sloping forehead
  Cleft lip and/or palate
  Microphthalmia
Extremity abnormalities
  Postaxial polydactyly
  Camptodactyly
  Overlapping digits
Renal malformations
  Renal cortical cysts
  Hydronephrosis
  Horseshoe kidney
Omphalocele

Table 4–10. SONOGRAPHIC FINDINGS IN HOLOPROSENCEPHALY

Fused lateral ventricles with or without dorsal cyst
Variable presence of falx
Cavum septi pellucidi absent
Thalami fused, third ventricle absent
Microcephaly/trigonencephaly
Hypotelorism/cyclopia
Single nostril, proboscis

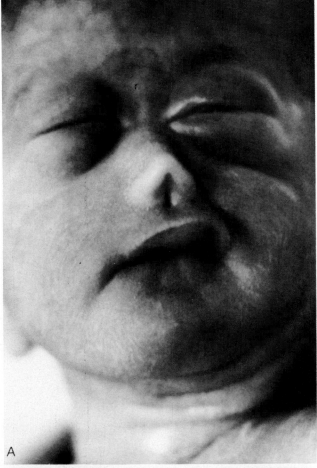

Figure 4–7. *A.* Fetus with trisomy 13 and holoprosencephaly, hypotelorism, and a single nostril. *B.* Sonogram shows common ventricle with large dorsal cyst.

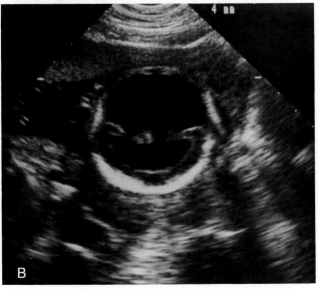

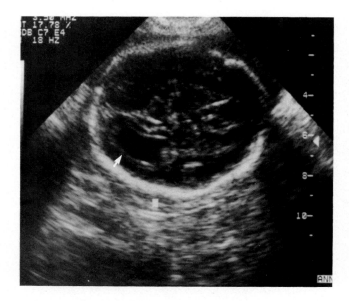

Figure 4–8. Agenesis of the corpus callosum. Note absence of cavum septi pellucidi and prominent occipital horn of lateral ventricle *(arrow).*

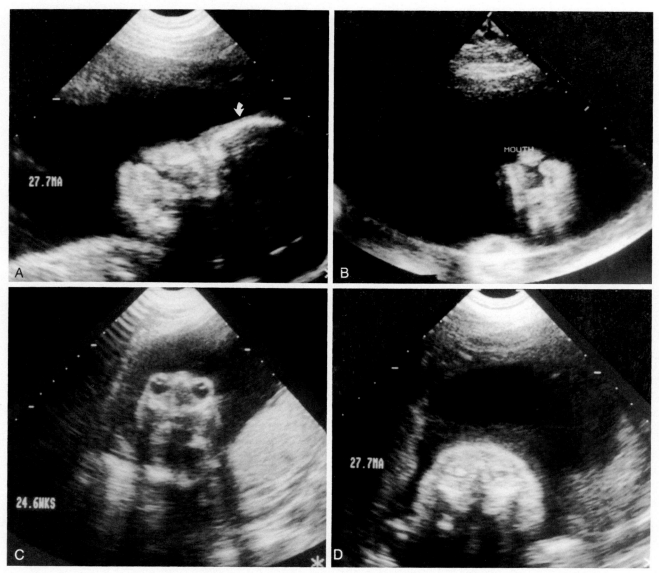

Figure 4–9. Craniofacial malformations in trisomy 13. *A.* Abnormal facial profile with micrognathia and sloping forehead *(arrow). B.* Cleft lip and palate. *C.* Transverse axial view of orbits in a normal fetus. *D.* Transverse axial view of orbits in a fetus with trisomy 13 and microphthalmia.

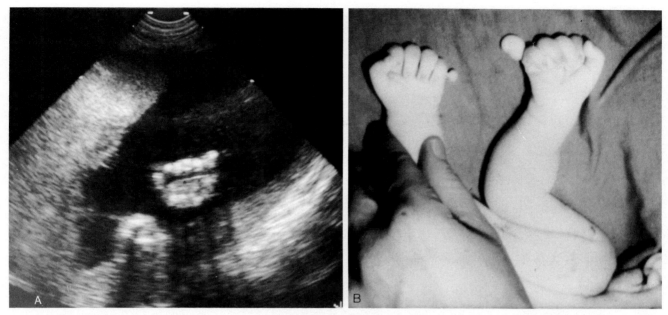

Figure 4–10. Sonogram *(A)* and gross photograph *(B)* demonstrating postaxial polydactyly of the hands in trisomy 13.

Table 4–11. SONOGRAPHIC FINDINGS IN TRISOMY 18

Second-trimester–onset intrauterine growth retardation (59%)	Craniofacial malformations
Third-trimester polyhydramnios	Micrognathia
Congenital heart disease (90%)	Dolichocephaly
Diaphragmatic hernia	Prominent occiput
Omphalocele	Strawberry-shaped skull
Esophageal atresia with or without tracheoesophageal fistula	Intracranial malformations
Hydronephrosis, horseshoe kidney	Large cisterna magna
Limb malformations	Choroid plexus cysts
Clubfoot deformity	
Generalized arthrogryposis	
Clenched hands	

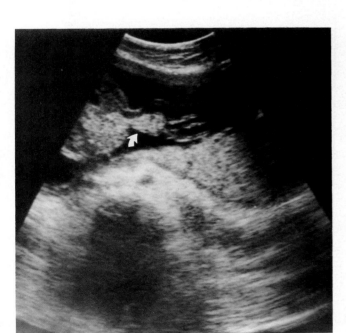

Figure 4–11. Fetus with trisomy 18 and small omphalocele filled with bowel *(arrow)*.

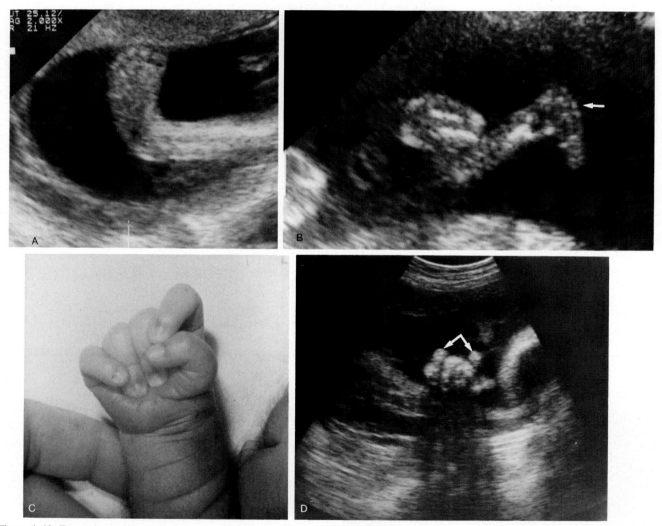

Figure 4–12. Extremity malformations associated with trisomy 18. *A.* Clubfoot deformity. *B.* Rocker-bottom feet *(arrow).* *C* and *D.* Clenched hands with overlapping digits *(arrows).*

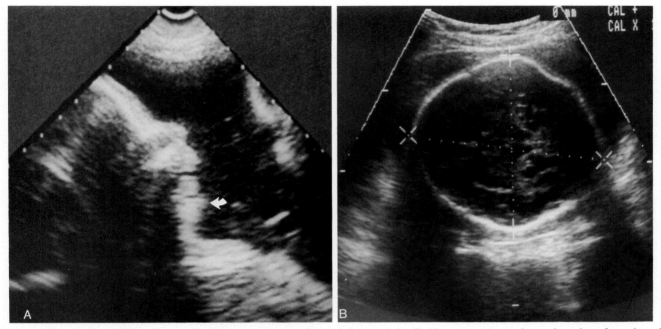

Figure 4–13. *A.* Fetus with trisomy 18 and micrognathia *(arrow)* and dolichocephaly. *B.* Note unusual strawberry-shaped configuration of the skull.

ter. Fetuses with coarctation may, however, exhibit right ventricular enlargement during late pregnancy owing to increased shunting across the ductus arteriosus to the descending aorta.

Fetuses with Turner syndrome commonly exhibit cystic hygromas, nuchal edema, or pterygium colli. These abnormalities all result from jugular lymphatic obstruction. Embryologically, the jugular lymphatic sacs should develop communications with the internal jugular veins at approximately 40 days after conception.[25] Failed or delayed communication results in enlargement of the jugular lymphatics. Specific sonographic findings are dependent on gestational age. For example, first-trimester fetuses may exhibit only mild edema in the posterior cervical region (Fig. 4–16),

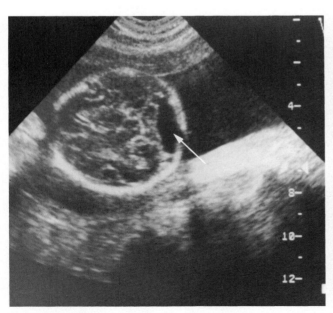

Figure 4–14. Fetus with trisomy 18 and large cisterna magna *(arrow).*

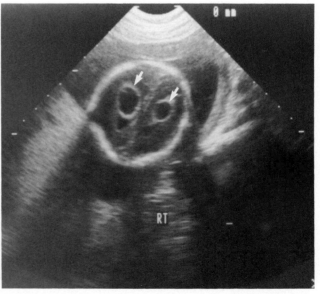

Figure 4–15. Choroid plexus cysts *(arrows)* are observed in 30% of fetuses with trisomy 18.

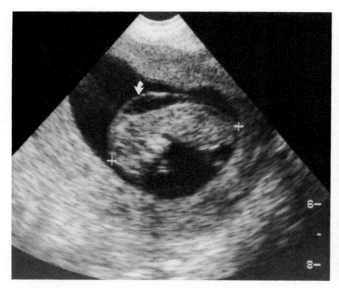

Figure 4–16. Posterior cervical edema *(arrow)* in an 11-week embryo. Chorionic villus sampling confirmed a 45,X karyotype.

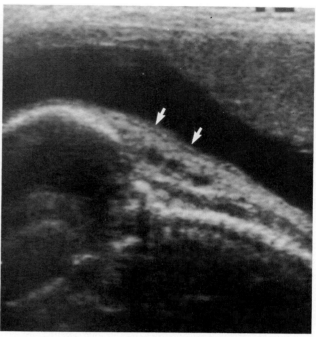

Figure 4–18. Coronal view showing residual webbing of the neck *(arrows)* in a 19-week fetus with spontaneously resolving cystic hygromas.

whereas older fetuses typically present with large multiloculated cysts and generalized hydrops (Fig. 4–17). Survival is rare once hydrops has developed, although spontaneous resolution has been reported.[52–61] This suggests that delayed communication between the lymphatic and jugular venous systems can ultimately be established in some instances and likely explains the webbed appearance of the neck in liveborn infants with Turner syndrome (Fig. 4–18).

Finally, it should be emphasized that sonographic detection of cystic hygromas or nuchal edema should prompt fetal karyotyping. Overall, a cytogenetic abnormality will be found in 47% to 73% of these cases.[56, 61] Second-trimester fetuses with cystic hygromas are more likely to have Turner syndrome, while nuchal edema during the first trimester is commonly associated with other aneuploid states, including trisomies 13, 18, and 21.[60, 61]

Triploidy Syndrome

Triploidy is characterized by a complete extra set of chromosomes. This phenomenon most commonly results from fertilization of an egg by two different sperm,

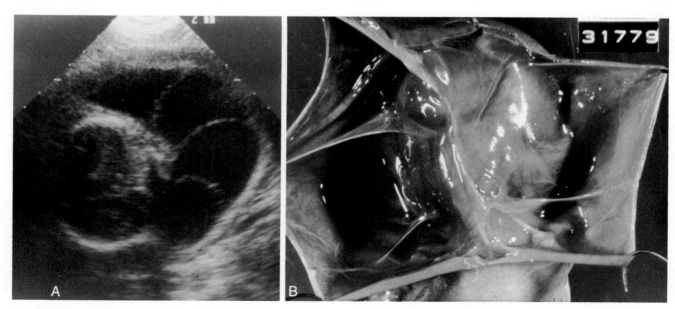

Figure 4–17. *A.* Transverse axial view through cranium and posterior cervical region showing large multiloculated cystic hygromas with thinwalled septations. *B.* Gross photograph of cystic hygroma opened at autopsy.

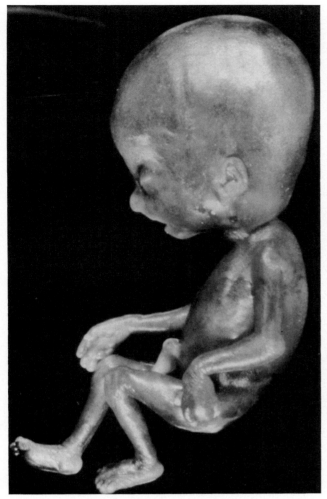

Figure 4–19. Mid-trimester triploid fetus illustrating severe head-to-body disproportion.

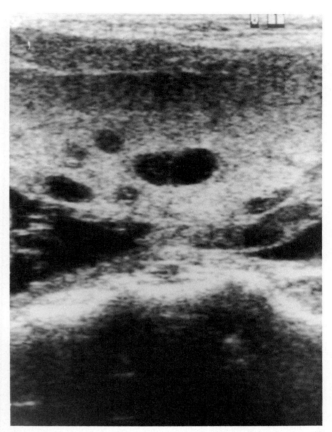

Figure 4–20. Large hydropic placenta and oligohydramnios in a 22-week triploid fetus.

CONCLUSION

Sonographic identification of any structural birth defect mandates a detailed and complete fetal anatomic survey, including echocardiography. Fetal karyotyping should be offered whenever more than one malformation or other risk factors (e.g., maternal age, low MS-AFP level, family history of birth defects) are apparent. Even when isolated, certain fetal anomalies (Table 4–12) carry a sufficiently high risk for cytogenetic abnormalities to warrant chromosome studies. This information can be crucial in ensuring that parents

although diandry and digyny are responsible for some cases. Triploid conceptions account for nearly 20% of chromosomally abnormal miscarriages; however, live-birth is rare, occurring in fewer than 1 in 2500 pregnancies.[62]

Second-trimester fetuses with triploidy syndrome have severe intrauterine growth retardation with a disproportionately small trunk (Fig. 4–19). Other fetal anomalies may include multicystic renal dysplasia, hydronephrosis, ambiguous genitalia, congenital heart disease, omphalocele, cleft lip and/or palate, ocular hypertelorism, microphthalmia, and central nervous system malformations such as holoprosencephaly, agenesis of the corpus callosum, hydrocephalus, and meningocele.[63–66]

Aberrations in amniotic fluid volume are common in triploidy syndrome with both oligohydramnios and polyhydramnios being described. A unique sonographic finding in triploidy is enlargement and molar degeneration of the placenta (Fig. 4–20), although this feature is observed only in those cases in which the extra set of chromosomes is paternal in origin.[63–66]

Table 4–12. ISOLATED FETAL ANOMALIES WARRANTING AMNIOCENTESIS

Holoprosencephaly
Ventriculomegaly
Agenesis of the corpus callosum
Thickened nuchal skin fold or nuchal edema
Cystic hygroma
Congenital heart disease
Esophageal atresia
Duodenal atresia
Diaphragmatic hernia
Omphalocele
Nonimmune hydrops
Generalized arthrogryposis

are fully informed and in allowing an appropriate plan of obstetric management to be established.

References

1. Adams MM, Erickson JD, Layde PM, et al: Down's syndrome: Recent trends in the United States. JAMA 246:758, 1981.
2. Tabor A, Philip J, Madsen M, et al: Randomised controlled trial of genetic amniocentesis in 4606 low-risk women. Lancet 1:1287, 1986.
3. Schreinemachers DM, Cross PK, Hook EB: Rates of trisomies 21, 18, 13, and other chromosome abnormalities in about 20,000 prenatal studies compared with estimated rates in live births. Hum Genet 61:318, 1982.
4. DiMaio MS, Baumgarten A, Greenstein RM, et al: Screening for Down's syndrome in pregnancy by measuring maternal serum alpha-fetoprotein levels. N Engl J Med 317:342, 1987.
5. Hall B: Mongolism in newborn infants. Clin Pediatr 5:4, 1966.
6. Benacerraf BR, Barss VA, Laboda LA: A sonographic sign for the detection in the second trimester of the fetus with Down's syndrome. Am J Obstet Gynecol 151:1078, 1985.
7. Crane JP, Gray DL: Midtrimester sonographically measured nuchal skin fold thickness as a screening tool for Down syndrome. Obstet Gynecol 77:553, 1991.
8. Benacerraf BR, Gelman R, Frigoletto FD: Sonographic identification of second-trimester fetuses with Down's syndrome. N Engl J Med 317:1371, 1987.
9. Perrella R, Duerinckx AJ, Grant EG, et al: Second-trimester sonographic diagnosis of Down syndrome: Role of femur-length shortening and nuchal fold thickening. AJR 151:981, 1988.
10. Lockwood C, Benacerraf B, Krinsky A, et al: A sonographic screening method for Down syndrome. Am J Obstet Gynecol 157:803, 1987.
11. Dicke JM, Gray DL, Songster GS, Crane JP: Fetal biometry as a screening tool for the detection of chromosomally abnormal pregnancies. Obstet Gynecol 74:726, 1989.
12. Hill LM, Guzick D, Belfar HL, et al: The current role of sonography in the detection of Down syndrome. Obstet Gynecol 74:620, 1989.
13. Brumfield CG, Hauth JC, Cloud GA, et al: Sonographic measurements and ratios in fetuses with Down syndrome. Obstet Gynecol 73:644, 1989.
14. Hadlock FP, Harrist RB, Martinez-Poyer J: Fetal body ratios in second trimester: A useful tool for identifying chromosomal abnormalities. J Ultrasound Med 11:81, 1992.
15. Grist TM, Fuller RW, Albiez KL, Bowie JD: Femur length in the US prediction of trisomy 21 and other chromosomal abnormalities. Radiology 174:837, 1990.
16. LaFollette L, Filly RA, Anderson R, Golbus MS: Fetal femur length to detect trisomy 21: A reappraisal. J Ultrasound Med 8:657, 1989.
17. Nyberg DA, Resta RG, Hickok DE, et al: Femur length shortening in the detection of Down syndrome: Is prenatal screening feasible? Am J Obstet Gynecol 162:1247, 1990.
18. FitzSimmons J, Droste S, Shepard TH, et al: Long-bone growth in fetuses with Down syndrome. Am J Obstet Gynecol 161:1174, 1989.
19. Benacerraf BR, Neuberg D, Frigoletto FD: Humeral shortening in second-trimester fetuses with Down syndrome. Obstet Gynecol 77:223, 1991.
20. Rotmensch S, Luo J, Liberati M, et al: Fetal humeral length to detect Down syndrome. Am J Obstet Gynecol 166:1330, 1992.
21. Selikowitz M: Down Syndrome: The Facts. New York, Oxford University Press, 1990.
22. Baird PA, Sadovnick AD: Life expectancy in Down syndrome adults. Lancet 2:1354, 1988.
23. Benacerraf BR, Mandell J, Estroff JA, et al: Fetal pyelectasis: A possible association with Down syndrome. Obstet Gynecol 76:58, 1990.
24. Corteville JE, Dicke JM, Crane JP: Fetal pyelectasis and Down syndrome: Is genetic amniocentesis warranted? Obstet Gynecol 79:770, 1992.
25. Jones KL: Smith's Recognizable Patterns of Human Malformation, 4th ed. Philadelphia, WB Saunders, 1988.
26. Dicke JM, Crane JP: Sonographic recognition of major malformations and aberrant fetal growth in trisomic fetuses. J Ultrasound Med 10:433, 1991.
27. de Grouchy J, Turleau C: Clinical Atlas of Human Chromosomes, 2nd ed. New York, John Wiley & Sons, 1984.
28. Choiset PA, Porrier NL, Thepot F, et al: Chromosomal prenatal diagnosis: Study of 936 cases of intrauterine abnormalities after ultrasound assessment. Prenat Diagn 9:255, 1989.
29. Crawford DC, Chapman MG, Allan LD: Echocardiography in the investigation of anterior abdominal wall defects in the fetus. Br J Obstet Gynecol 92:1034, 1985.
30. Gilbert WM, Nicolaides KH: Fetal omphalocele: Associated malformations and chromosomal defects. Obstet Gynecol 70:633, 1987.
31. Nyberg DA, Fitzsimmons J, Mack LA, et al: Chromosomal abnormalities in fetuses with omphalocele: Significance of omphalocele contents. J Ultrasound Med 8:299, 1989.
32. Benacerraf BR, Saltzman DH, Estroff JA, Frigoletto FD: Abnormal karyotype of fetuses with omphalocele: Prediction based on omphalocele contents. Obstet Gynecol 75:317, 1990.
33. Bundy AL, Saltzman DH, Pober B, et al: Antenatal sonographic findings in trisomy 18. J Ultrasound Med 5:316, 1986.
34. Benacerraf BR, Miller WA, Frigoletto FD: Sonographic detection of fetuses with trisomies 13 and 18: Accuracy and limitations. Am J Obstet Gynecol 158:404, 1988.
35. Benacerraf BR, Frigoletto FD, Greene MF: Abnormal facial features and extremities in human trisomy syndromes: Prenatal US appearance. Radiology 159:243, 1986.
36. Comstock CH, Boal DB: Enlarged fetal cisterna magna: Appearance and significance. Obstet Gynecol 66:25S, 1985.
37. Thurmond AS, Nelson DW, Lowensohn RI, et al: Enlarged cisterna magna in trisomy 18: Prenatal ultrasonographic diagnosis. Am J Obstet Gynecol 161:83, 1989.
38. Nyberg DA, Mahony BS, Hegge FN, et al: Enlarged cisterna magna and the Dandy-Walker malformation: Factors associated with chromosome abnormalities. Obstet Gynecol 77:436, 1991.
39. Benacerraf BR, Harlow B, Frigoletto FD: Are choroid plexus cysts an indication for second-trimester amniocentesis? Am J Obstet Gynecol 162:1001, 1990.
40. Nicolaides KH, Rodeck CH, Gosden CM: Rapid karyotyping in non-lethal fetal malformations. Lancet 1:283, 1986.
41. Gabrielli S, Reece EA, Pilu G, et al: The clinical significance of prenatally diagnosed choroid plexus cysts. Am J Obstet Gynecol 160:1207, 1989.
42. Ostlere SJ, Irving HC, Lilford RJ: Fetal choroid plexus cysts: A report of 100 cases. Radiology 175:753, 1990.
43. Fitzsimmons J, Wilson D, Pascoe-Mason J, et al: Choroid plexus cysts in fetuses with trisomy 18. Obstet Gynecol 73:257, 1989.
44. Clark SL, DeVore GR, Sabey PL: Prenatal diagnosis of cysts of the fetal choroid plexus. Obstet Gynecol 72:585, 1988.
45. Chitkara U, Cogswell C, Norton K, et al: Choroid plexus cysts in the fetus: A benign anatomic variant or pathologic entity? Report of 41 cases and review of the literature. Obstet Gynecol 72:185, 1988.
46. Chan L, Hixson JL, Laifer SA, et al: A sonographic and karyotypic study of second-trimester fetal choroid plexus cysts. Obstet Gynecol 73:703, 1989.
47. Chinn DH, Miller EI, Worthy LM, Towers CV: Sonographically detected fetal choroid plexus cysts: Frequency and association with aneuploidy. J Ultrasound Med 10:255, 1991.
48. Perpignano MC, Cohen HL, Klein VR, et al: Fetal choroid plexus cysts: Beware the smaller cyst. Radiology 182:715, 1992.
49. Furness ME: Choroid plexus cysts and trisomy 18. Lancet 2:693, 1987.
50. Hertzberg BS, Kay HH, Bowie JD: Fetal choroid plexus lesions: Relationship of antenatal sonographic appearance to clinical outcome. J Ultrasound Med 8:77, 1989.
51. Robinson A, Bender BG, Borelli JB, et al: Sex chromosomal aneuploidy: Prospective and longitudinal studies. In Ratcliff SG, Paul N (eds): Prospective Studies on Children With Sex Chromosome Aneuploidy, p 23. New York, Alan R. Liss, 1986.
52. Bernstein HS, Filly RA, Goldberg JD, Golbus MS: Prognosis of fetuses with a cystic hygroma. Prenat Diagn 11:349, 1991.
53. Pijpers L, Reuss A, Stewart PA, et al: Fetal cystic hygroma: Prenatal diagnosis and management. Obstet Gynecol 72:223–224, 1988.

54. Rodis JF, Vintzileos AM, Campbell WA, Nochimson DJ: Spontaneous resolution of fetal cystic hygroma in Down's syndrome. Obstet Gynecol 71:976, 1988.
55. Bronshtein M, Rottem S, Yoffe N, Blumenfeld Z: First-trimester and early second-trimester diagnosis of nuchal cystic hygroma by transvaginal sonography: Diverse prognosis of the septated from the nonseptated lesion. Am J Obstet Gynecol 161:78, 1989.
56. Chervenak FA, Isaacson G, Blakemore KJ, et al: Fetal cystic hygroma: Cause and natural history. N Engl J Med 309:822, 1983.
57. Mostello DJ, Bofinger MK, Siddiqi TA: Spontaneous resolution of fetal cystic hygroma and hydrops in Turner syndrome. Obstet Gynecol 73:862, 1989.
58. Chodirker BN, Harman CR, Greenberg CR: Spontaneous resolution of a cystic hygroma in a fetus with Turner syndrome. Prenat Diagn 8:291, 1988.
59. Macken MB, Grantmyre EB, Vincer MJ: Regression of nuchal cystic hygroma in utero. J Ultrasound Med 8:101, 1989.
60. Pircon RA, Porto M, Towers CV, et al: Ultrasound findings in pregnancies complicated by fetal triploidy. J Ultrasound Med 8:507, 1989.
61. Shulman LP, Emerson DS, Felker RE, et al: High frequency of cytogenetic abnormalities in fetuses with cystic hygroma diagnosed in the first trimester. Obstet Gynecol 80:80, 1992.
62. Boue J, Boue A, Laza P: Retrospective and prospective epidemiological studies of 1500 karyotyped spontaneous human abortions. Teratology 12:11, 1975.
63. Crane JP, Beaver HA, Cheung SW: Antenatal ultrasound findings in fetal triploidy syndrome. J Ultrasound Med 4:519, 1985.
64. Lockwood C, Scioscia A, Stiller R, et al: Sonographic features of the triploid fetus. Am J Obstet Gynecol 157:285, 1987.
65. Edwards MT, Smith WL, Hanson J, et al: Prenatal sonographic diagnosis of triploidy. J Ultrasound Med 5:279, 1986.
66. Shulman LP, Emerson DS, Felker RE, et al: High frequency of cytogenetic abnormalities in fetuses with cystic hygroma diagnosed in the first trimester. Obstet Gynecol 80:80, 1992.

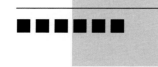

CHAPTER 5

Endovaginal Sonographic Evaluation of the Obstetric and Gynecologic Patient

ILAN E. TIMOR-TRITSCH, M.D.
ANA MONTEAGUDO, M.D.
GINA M. BROWN, M.D.

Most sonologists would undoubtedly agree that the introduction of endovaginal sonography nearly a decade ago has dramatically advanced our ability to evaluate the gynecologic and obstetric patient. Although the most common application of this technology has been in the imaging of ovarian pathology, its utility in early pregnancy evaluation has been quite dramatic.[1-15]

In this chapter the utilization of endovaginal sonography in obstetrics and gynecology is described. Although specific clinical applications are briefly discussed, the major focus is on the technology and actual examination itself. The use of endovaginal sonography in specific clinical situations is described in other chapters in this text.

EQUIPMENT

The technology of the endovaginal probe has undergone dramatic change since its introduction nearly 10 years ago.[11-15] As with the rest of sonography, single-element mechanical sector transducers have been replaced by electronically focused multielement transducers. It is of interest that the actual shaft of the transducer has also changed significantly. The original endovaginal transducers had a sharp anteroposterior angulation ("broken handle").[8, 10] The purpose of this configuration was to allow easy needle puncture above the handle in patients undergoing ovum retrieval. The angulation of the ultrasound probe created a number of problems. The orientation was awkward compared with the standard straight forward-looking palpation that is done during clinical examinations. Likewise, with this design, lateral motion of the transducer was restricted by the patient's thighs. In correcting these difficulties biomedical engineers compounded the problem by changing the in-line, in-axis scanning "fan" to an off-axis, off-line scanning angle. To adequately evaluate the adnexa the examiner needed to image one side and then rotate the probe 180° to image the contralateral side. The image orientation would then need to be reversed (left to right) to display the image in its customary orientation. It took manufacturers nearly 6 years to respond to sonologists' desire to develop a straight, in-line endovaginal probe.

Two additional engineering advances improved the use of straight probes: a variable scanning field of view in which wider angles (120° to 160°) allowed a panoramic view of the pelvis and a steered field of view enabling a 90° to 110° fan to move from one side to the other. This allowed off-axis scanning without actually moving or angling the probe.

As was mentioned earlier, transducer element technology improved from single-element transducers to annular array probes then to electronic and dynamic focusing using solid-state phased-array transducers. The basic physical principles that apply to conventional transabdominal transducers are applicable to endovaginal transducers as well. The higher the frequency of sound, the higher the resolution but lower depth of penetration (Fig. 5-1). Undoubtedly, the greatest asset of endovaginal probes is the ability to use high-frequency probes (≥5 MHz) adjacent to the organ of interest (Fig. 5-2).

TECHNIQUE

The Examination Table

Virtually any examination table or bed can be used for the performance of an endovaginal examination. Ideally, the patient should be examined on a gynecologic examination table in which there is adequate leg support allowing the patient to elevate her pelvis. It is counterproductive to place the patient in a Trendelenburg position, although a slight anti-Trendelenburg position may be beneficial because it "drains" all of the existing fluid in the abdominal cavity into the pelvic area, resulting in enhanced tissue interfaces, which are advantageous for endovaginal scanning.

Status of the Urinary Bladder

In most cases an empty bladder is necessary to obtain the best results using endovaginal sonography. Partially filled bladders become important in cases in which the anterior cervical lip has to be emphasized on a sagittal scan, in cases of suspected placenta previa, or when cervical anatomy needs to be delineated. A distended urinary bladder may distort pelvic anatomy.

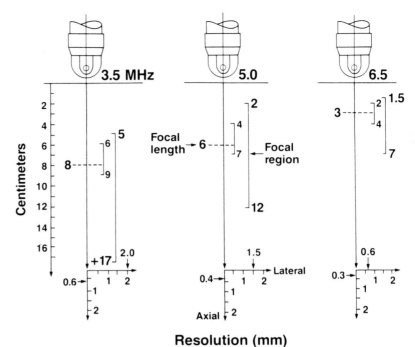

Figure 5–1. Drawing showing the focal region, focal length, as well as the lateral and axial resolution of the 3.5-, 5.0-, and 6.5-MHz probes (From Timor-Tritsch IE, Rottem S, Thaler I: Review of transvaginal ultrasonography: A description with clinical application. Ultrasound Q 6:1, 1988.)

In many cases requiring pelvic sonography it will be necessary to do a transabdominal examination as well as an endovaginal one. In such cases, if the patient presents with a distended urinary bladder, she should first be examined transabdominally then, after voiding, endovaginally.

Pelvic Examination

A thorough manual pelvic examination preceding the ultrasound examination usually provides the gynecologist with preliminary information that will prove important when a subsequent endovaginal scan is done. Some endovaginal probes enable the introduction of one finger alongside the transducer, so that palpation and visualization can occur at the same time.

Patient Information

If an endovaginal examination is to be performed, the procedure should first be explained to the patient. One should mention the similarity between the endovaginal examination and the routinely performed speculum examination, a procedure that the patient has

Figure 5–2. The relationship between the tip of the transvaginal probe inserted into the vagina and the pelvic organs is illustrated. Note the large distance between the abdominal wall and the pelvic organs, which is almost twice the distance of that measured from the tip of the transvaginal probe to the same organs. (Reprinted by permission of the publisher from Timor-Tritsch IE, Rottem S, Elgal S: How transvaginal sonography is done. In Timor-Tritsch IE, Rottem S (eds): Transvaginal Sonography, 2nd ed, pp 15–25. New York, Elsevier Publishing, 1991.)

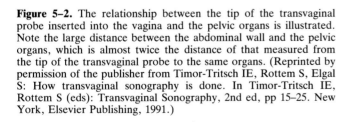

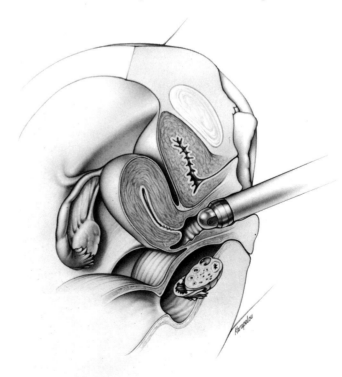

probably experienced previously. If there are any questions regarding the safety of the examination (e.g., ruptured membranes, placenta previa), the referring obstetrician should be contacted before the examination. There have been no documented reports of untoward effects of endovaginal sonography. Most examiners believe that an informed consent is not necessary. If a male examiner is to perform the examination, it is advisable to have a female aide, nurse, or sonographer present.

Preparing the Equipment and the Transducer

The ultrasound scanner, as well as the recording equipment, should be prepared for the examination before the endovaginal probe is inserted into the vagina. All data such as last menstrual period, history, and referring physician should be recorded. It is advantageous to have a foot pedal for freezing the image or activating the equipment to produce hard copy images. In many cases the examiner may have to use his or her other hand to enhance the quality of the picture.

The tip of the transducer is covered with coupling gel and introduced into a condom or protective rubber sheath or into the digit of a sterile rubber glove. A small amount of coupling gel is then applied on top of the probe, easing its vaginal insertion. Infertility patients close to midcycle should be scanned using saline or water to avoid exposure of the sperm to the noxious effects of coupling gels.

After completion of the examination and removal of the probe, the probe is gently cleaned with a paper towel and a disinfectant. A variety of disinfectant solutions are available in spray or other forms, and some work within as little as 10 minutes.[16] It is wise to contact the manufacturer to find out its choices to keep the probes clean. As in all ultrasound examinations the examiner should wear gloves during the examination.

Scanning Technique

To obtain images in different planes, directions, and depths and to obtain a larger field of view, the following maneuvers can be employed:

1. Maneuvering the probe itself
   a. Rotating the handle along the probe's longitudinal axis to change the scanning plane along a 360° range (Fig. 5–3A).
   b. Tilting or angling the probe to point in different directions in the pelvis (see Fig. 5–3B).
   c. Pushing and pulling the probe to align the focal region of interest in the pelvis (see Fig. 5–3C).
2. Manipulating the field of view. This can be done with both mechanical and solid-state electronic probes.
   a. If a variable field of view is available on the equipment, one should always start out with the

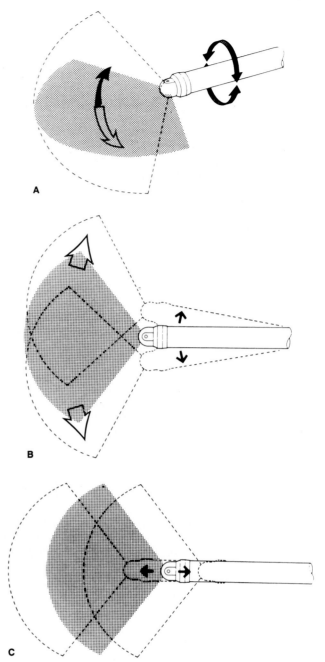

Figure 5–3. Basic scanning directions, planes, and depth achieved by moving the probe or by moving the scanning plane. Any combination of the following can be used to obtain the best image: *A.* The probe can be rotated along its longitudinal axis. Some scanners have the ability to mechanically or electronically move the scanning plane itself up or down *(black and open arrows)* to achieve a larger mobility of the scanning plane. *B.* By angling the shaft, the probe can be pointed in any desired direction; some probes have the ability to move the scanning plane to the left or to the right electronically or mechanically *(open arrows).* *C.* Pushing or pulling the probe aligns the targeted organs within the focal range of the transducer. (Reprinted by permission of the publisher from Timor-Tritsch IE, Rottem S, Elgal S: How transvaginal sonography is done. In Timor-Tritsch IE, Rottem S (eds): Transvaginal Sonography, 2nd ed, pp 15–25. New York, Elsevier Publishing, 1991.)

widest panoramic view and then gradually narrow it down to examine the region of interest.
   b. Steering the field of view has lately been made possible by using electronic or mechanical sector

probes (see Fig. 5–3A and B). Special controls are used to move the field of view from side to side. This enables imaging of the adnexa in coronal or transverse scanning planes. Examining anteriorly or posteriorly situated structures is thus made possible if the probe is rotated to the sagittal plane.

3. Focusing
   a. Electronically, if a solid-state phased array or curvilinear vaginal probe is used.
   b. In mechanical probes, the focusing is achieved in two ways: by electronically filtering and selectively enhancing different frequencies of the emitting crystal and by using an annular array configuration of crystals that are individually focused at different depths; however, the combination of these focusing techniques results in a wider focal range.

Some probes offer electronic or mechanical steering of the scanning plane itself, not only to the two lateral positions but also anteriorly and posteriorly, thus enabling complete scanning of the pelvis without moving the shaft of the probe.

Dynamic Use of the Endovaginal Probe

Significant enhancement of scanning can be achieved by using the maneuvers listed below[3, 4]:

1. The examiner can enhance the ultrasound examination by placing his or her hands on the lower abdomen to keep pelvic structures within "sight" of the probe, much like a regular bimanual examination.

2. Localization of the point of maximal intensity of pain can be ascertained by touching structures with the tip of the transducer probe and observing directly the localization of the pain indicated by the patient.

3. Dense pelvic adhesions can be diagnosed by using the "sliding organs sign": the transducer tip is pointed at the structures in question, and a gentle push–pull movement of several centimeters is started. If no adhesions are present, the organs will move freely past each other and sometimes past the static pelvic wall. This displacement of organs is perceived on the screen as a sliding movement. In case of dense adhesions, such as tubo-ovarian complex, the conglomerate of the uterus, tube, and ovary will not change position with the pushing motion on the probe.[3]

4. Combined examination by using a "fingertip" probe on the index finger can be done so that an examination combining pelvic bimanual examination and endovaginal scanning can be performed. Another way to achieve a combined ultrasound and pelvic examination is to slide in one finger, usually the index finger, alongside a regular endovaginal probe and simultaneously touch and see the structure in question.

The Scanning Routine

A rigid and relatively strict scanning routine should be followed.

1. The probe should scan the cervix while it is introduced into the vagina. A quick examination of the bladder can also be performed at this time.

2. The uterus should then be localized and evaluated in the longitudinal and the transverse planes. When sagittal scanning of the uterus is performed, the cervix should also be included by gently pulling out the probe and directing it toward the cervix.

3. If a pregnancy is present, the gestation should be scanned.

4. The adnexa should next be evaluated. The ovaries and fallopian tubes should be identified as well as any pathologic process related to these structures.

5. The cul-de-sac should be evaluated by tilting the probe posteriorly toward the back of the patient.

6. The probe should be extracted under continuous ultrasound observation and by tilting the probe upward at the time of its complete withdrawal. The urethra and the insertion of the ureters into the bladder can be evaluated. The urinary bladder in the transverse and sagittal planes, as well as the posterior bladder neck and its angle, can also be observed. At the completion of the endovaginal examination it may become evident that a complementary transabdominal examination is required. At this time the formerly empty bladder may be sufficiently filled for the abdominal approach.

Orientation and Image Planes

Endovaginal scanning, since its inception, has been readily accepted as a technique offering superb resolution. What has been difficult for many is an understanding of the orientation and display of pelvic structures using this technique.[17–19] Although this is often difficult to learn initially, once mastered, the steepest part of the learning curve of this technique will be conquered. The remainder of one's learning occurs after scanning a large number of patients with both normal and abnormal findings and gaining the necessary experience.

On-screen orientation is critical to perform this technique adequately. This means the operator is aware at all times of the scanning plane that is displayed on the screen and most importantly which are the true right, left, cephalic, caudal, anterior, and posterior orientations of the displayed image.

The Scanning Planes

Image planes are fixed coordinates used in communication between health care professionals. The conventional imaging planes are sagittal, coronal, and transverse. Longitudinal applies to one dimensional direction along the longest axis of the body. In endovaginal scanning "longitudinal" may also be used to describe a scanning plane imaged using the longest dimension of an organ.

Two planes can be applied to the longitudinal axis of the body: the *sagittal* and the *coronal planes*. In contrast to this, only one plane, the *transverse* or cross-sectional plane, can be applied to the two short axes of the body (i.e., *anteroposterior* and *laterolateral*). For example, the uterus, ovary, and fallopian tube can be imaged in a cross-sectional fashion. Because of the restricted motion of the probe in the vagina only a midsagittal and a midcoronal (or more correctly a transverse) plane can be obtained. As opposed to transabdominal scanning in which the plane of the linear probe can be successively moved laterally in a parallel fashion, with endovaginal scanning one will be able to move the scanning plane only in a radial, fanlike fashion. The apex of this fan is the tip of the transducer.

The uterus, ovaries, and fallopian tubes usually assume different, composite oblique positions within the pelvis. Because of this, their longest dimensions point to different directions that are difficult to describe using classic scanning planes.

Display of Images

As has been mentioned earlier, orientation and display of image planes are critical to adequately perform and interpret endovaginal scans. Traditionally, transabdominal ultrasound images are displayed with the apex of the image at the top of the screen. This represents the anterior aspect of the patient. The posterior aspect is at the bottom of the image. On longitudinal scans the patient's head is at the left of the image and on transverse scans the patient's right side is on the left of the screen.

Endovaginal sonographic scans, owing to the confusion created by the diversity of on-screen display modalities, are shown in various orientations. Roughly 60% of sonologists in the United States display endovaginal images with the apex of the wedge pointing toward the top of the screen. The remainder of sonologists in the United States and approximately 63% in Europe favor placing the apex of the scan at the bottom of the image. The logic behind displaying an image with the apex pointing downward is that it clearly distinguishes the image generated by endovaginal ultrasound from that obtained by transabdominal ultrasound.[20]

Until such standardization of images is reached, it is important to properly label and annotate the pictures created by endovaginal ultrasound so that the orientation and the structures it represents are fully understood.[17]

If the footprint of the transducer (i.e., the apex of the wedge) is on the top of the screen, then

1. On a sagittal, longitudinal plane the filling bladder will be seen on the upper left side of the screen. The fundus of an anteverted uterus will appear pointing to the left of the screen (to the same side where the bladder is displayed), and the cervix will point toward the upper right side of the picture.

2. On cross-sectional, horizontal, or coronal planes of section the patient's right ovary will be seen on the left and her left ovary will be seen on the right side of

the screen. If the same image display is used and the transducer tip is aimed toward the patient's sacrum, the cross section of the rectum will appear on the bottom of the screen.

Virtually all machines offer "left-right" as well as "apex invert" switches. These can be activated as desired. It is of utmost importance that the operator be fully aware of the actual mode of the switch at all times. This avoids misdiagnoses as far as the actual side that a pathologic process is found and subsequently reported. Persons operating vaginal transducers (with angled handles) requiring a left-right switching at the time of transducer rotation of 180° to scan the opposite adnexa (to keep traditional on-screen orientation correct) are particularly susceptible to this error. Labeling the image anew, each time a print is generated, is a prerequisite for avoiding this problem. Some authors have suggested the terms "trans" and "AP" as a reference to the direction of the sound beam in the pelvis.[19]

DOCUMENTATION

Last but not least, the question of documentation has to be addressed. There is a basic difference between the requirements of documentation following an endovaginal sonographic enhanced bimanual examination in the office setting of a gynecologist/obstetrician and that of a laboratory in which imaging is the only service provided.*

Adequate documentation of a endovaginal pelvic examination performed in an office setting to complement the bimanual examination consists of several coherent sentences describing the detected pathology in conjunction with appropriate prints properly annotated. The *lack* of findings does not require taking pictures of *normal* organs. A simple sentence stating that "no apparent pelvic pathology was seen by endovaginal ultrasound evaluation" is all that is required. Imaging specialists or laboratories must document their findings in a much more detailed fashion.*

CLINICAL APPLICATIONS

The applications in which endovaginal sonography are used are wide and increasing each day. Endovaginal sonography is now considered the gold standard in the workup of patients suspected of ectopic pregnancy and in evaluation of first- and early second-trimester pregnancies as well as the infertile patient. The diagnosis of gynecologic diseases such as ovarian, uterine, and

---

*It is the *Editor's* belief that any time that an imaging study is performed there should be documentation of images and a written report in both *normal and abnormal* cases. This is not purely medicolegally driven. Documentation serves as a basis for comparison if the patient subsequently returns with a problem for which a pathologic condition is demonstrated. The editor has seen too many examples in which the "normal" of one examiner, particularly in gynecology, is abnormal to another.

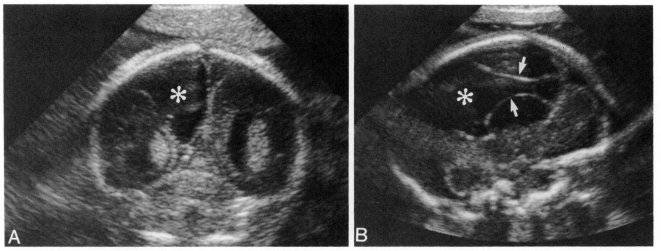

Figure 5–4. *A.* Endovaginal scan of a fetus with an interhemispheric cyst *(asterisk)* and agenesis of the corpus callosum. *B.* Multiple loculations are seen within the cyst *(arrows).*

inflammatory processes within the pelvis cannot be performed without the endovaginal probe. In spite of the unfounded opposition of several clinicians, it is rapidly gaining ground as the primary diagnostic modality for placenta previa and placenta accreta.

New uses or applications using endovaginal sonography have been reported in urologic gynecology and in evaluation of the fetal brain and subtle fetal morphologic abnormalities (Fig. 5–4).[5, 21–23] Finally, color Doppler ultrasound interrogation utilizing the endovaginal probe is the newest and probably not the last of unique applications of endovaginal sonography.[24–32]

In spite of the many advantages of endovaginal sonography, it is only fair to list its few limitations. The only two *absolute* contraindications to performing endovaginal sonography are imperforate hymen and patient refusal. *Relative* contraindications include the fear of introducing infection in a pregnant patient with premature rupture of the membranes and its use in a patient with a virginal introitus.

Since manufacturers constantly reduce the size of transducers, even patients with a virginal or relatively strictured introitus may have an endovaginal ultrasound examination with proper counseling. In an extremely obese patient, one may not be able to obtain as clear a picture of the pelvis as is desirable. This may be due to the large amount of fatty tissue in the pelvis causing significant sound attenuation. Virginal patients or patients with imperforate hymen, as well as postmenopausal patients with extremely advanced age, may not be able to accommodate the vaginal probe.

There is not enough space in this chapter to list all those areas in which the impact of endovaginal sonography has been felt. The reader is referred to individual chapters for in-depth discussions of specific clinical problems. The following are areas in which endovaginal sonography has proved to be invaluable:

Obstetrics

- Early diagnosis of intrauterine pregnancy (Fig. 5–5)
- Early and reliable diagnosis of early pregnancy failure (Fig. 5–6)
- Detection of malformations in the first trimester (Fig. 5–7)
- Comprehensive malformation workup in the early second trimester
- Scanning for fetal central nervous system malformations throughout the entire pregnancy (see Figs. 5–4 through 5–7)
- Diagnosis of placenta previa and placenta accreta
- Color flow studies of fetal blood vessels and the fetal heart

Figure 5–5. Endovaginal scan of a normal 10-week pregnancy. The amnion (A), embryo (E), and yolk sac (Y) can be readily seen in this patient.

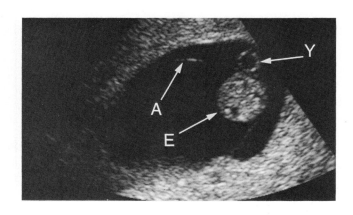

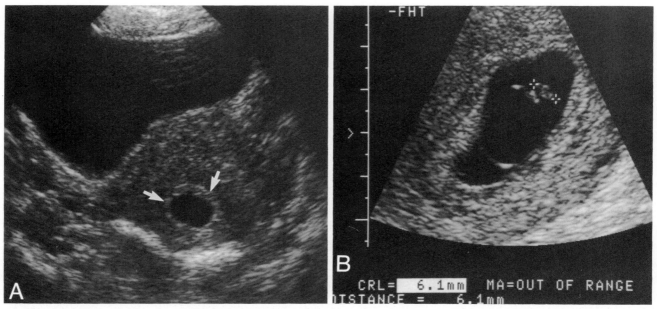

Figure 5–6. A patient presented with vaginal bleeding and an unknown last menstrual period. *A.* Transabdominal scan demonstrates an intrauterine gestational sac *(arrows)* with a mean sac diameter of 14 mm. With this measurement, the absence of an embryo or yolk sac would make this examination equivocal. *B.* Endovaginal scan of the same patient demonstrates an embryo measuring 6.1 mm *(cursors)*. The absence of cardiac activity allows one to diagnose a nonviable gestation.

Gynecology

- Accurate scanning of the uterus and ovaries and fallopian tubes (normal and abnormal) (Figs. 5–8 through 5–10)
- Diagnosis and management of ectopic pregnancies
- Diagnosis and management support for infertility
- Early detection of ovarian and endometrial cancer

including morphologic and color Doppler flow studies (Figs. 5–11 and 5–12)

Interventional Uses

- Aspiration of ova for in vitro fertilization or embryo transfer

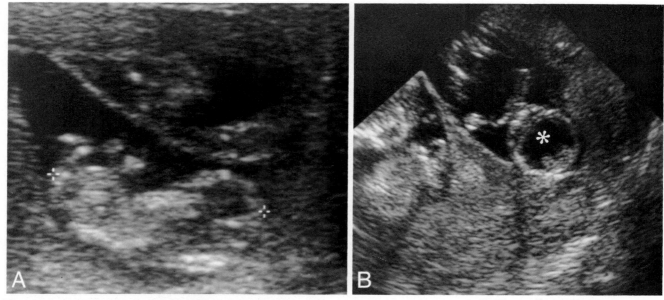

Figure 5–7. *A.* Transabdominal scan done before chorionic villus sampling demonstrates a normal-appearing first-trimester embryo *(cursors)*. *B.* Endovaginal scan of the same patient reveals a large fluid-filled sac within the cranium *(asterisk)* consistent with alobar holoprosencephaly.

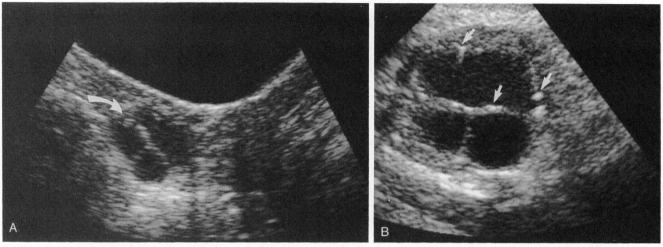

Figure 5–8. *A*. Transabdominal scan of the left ovary demonstrates a cyst *(arrow)* with low-level internal echoes. *B*. Endovaginal scan of the same patient demonstrates the cyst with multiple loculations and reflections likely due to cholesterol crystals within the wall *(arrows)*. These findings are usually seen in endometriosis, which was confirmed at laparoscopy.

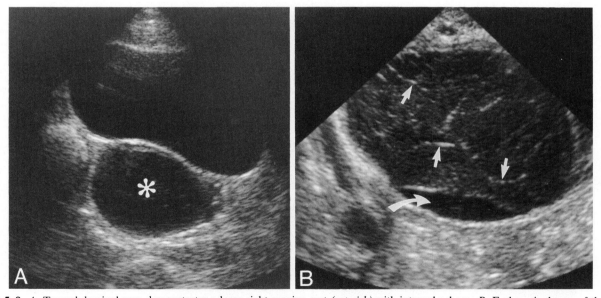

Figure 5–9. *A*. Transabdominal scan demonstrates a large right ovarian cyst *(asterisk)* with internal echoes. *B*. Endovaginal scan of the same patient clearly demonstrates solid tissue (thrombus) within the cyst with lacelike strands *(arrows)* (fibrinous strands) and clot retraction *(curved arrow)*. These findings indicate a benign hemorrhagic cyst.

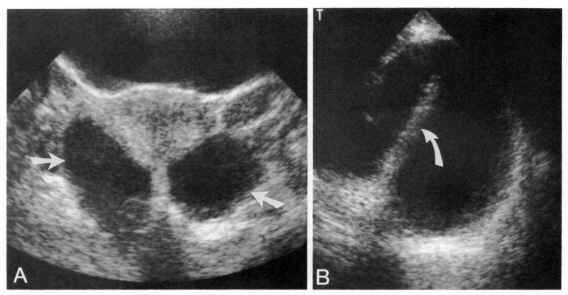

Figure 5–10. *A*. Transverse transabdominal scan demonstrates two cystlike structures *(arrows)* on either side of the uterus. *B*. Endovaginal scan of the left adnexa demonstrates that this fluid-filled structure is a dilated fallopian tube. The linear structure *(arrow)* is secondary to the dilated tube's folding on itself and should not be mistaken for a thick septation.

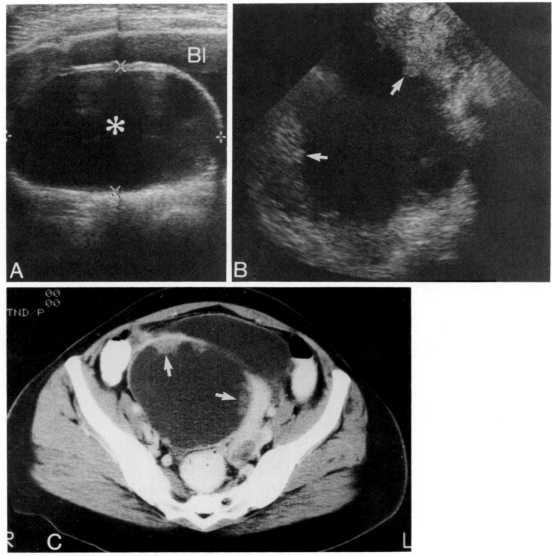

Figure 5–11. *A*. Transabdominal scan demonstrates a large ovarian cyst *(asterisk)* pressing on the urinary bladder (Bl). *B*. Endovaginal scan additionally shows mural nodularity *(arrows)* suggestive of neoplasm. *C*. Computed tomogram of the same patient also demonstrates the nodularity of the cyst wall *(arrows)*. An ovarian carcinoma was found at surgery.

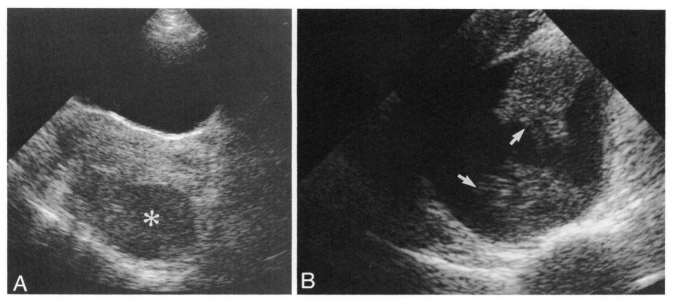

Figure 5–12. *A*. Transabdominal sonogram in a premenopausal patient demonstrates a large cyst *(asterisk)* in the cul-de-sac with low-level internal echoes. *B*. Endovaginal scan of the same patient demonstrates intramural and intraluminal soft tissue *(arrows)*. At surgery a clear cell carcinoma of the ovary was detected.

- Aspiration of ovarian cysts
- Aspiration and drainage of pelvic fluid collections
- Multifetal pregnancy reduction
- Treatment of ectopic pregnancies by injection of potassium chloride, methotrexate, and so on
- Early amniocentesis
- Chorionic villus sampling

References

1. Editorial. Contemp Obstet Gynecol May 1984.
2. Timor-Tritsch IE, Bar-Yam Y, Elgali S, Rottem S: The technique of transvaginal sonography with the use of a 6.5 MHz probe. Am J Obstet Gynecol 158:1019, 1988.
3. Timor-Tritsch IE, Rottem S, Thaler I: Review of transvaginal ultrasonography: A description with clinical application. Ultrasound Q 6:1, 1988.
4. Zimmer EZ, Timor-Tritsch IE, Rottem S: The technique of transvaginal sonography. In Timor-Tritsch IE, Rottem S (eds): Transvaginal Sonography, 2nd ed, pp 61–76. New York, Elsevier, 1991.
5. Timor-Tritsch IE, Rottem S (eds): Transvaginal Sonography, 2nd ed. New York, Elsevier, 1991.
6. Goldstein SR: Endovaginal Ultrasound, 2nd ed. New York, Alan R. Liss, 1991.
7. Fleischer AC, Kepple DM: Transvaginal Sonography: A Clinical Atlas. Philadelphia, JB Lippincott, 1992.
8. Peisner DB: Transvaginal sonography: Equipment. In Timor-Tritsch IE, Rottem S (eds): Transvaginal Sonography, 2nd ed, pp 29–60. New York, Elsevier, 1991.
9. Chervenak FA, Isaacson GC, Campbell S: Ultrasound in Obstetrics and Gynecology. Boston, Little, Brown & Co, 1993.
10. Nyberg DA, Hill LM, Bohm-Velez M, Mendelson EB: Transvaginal Ultrasound. St. Louis, Mosby–Year Book Medical Publishers, 1992.
11. Goldstein SR: Incorporating endovaginal ultrasonography into the overall gynecological examination. Am J Obstet Gynecol 162:625, 1990.
12. Timor-Tritsch IE: Is office use of vaginal sonography feasible? Am J Obstet Gynecol 162:983, 1990.
13. Goldstein SR: How ultrasound enhances the bimanual exam. Contemp Ob/Gyn 37:102, 1992.
14. Timor-Tritsch IE: Office and emergency room use of transvaginal sonography. In Timor-Tritsch IE, Rottem S (eds): Transvaginal Sonography, 2nd ed, pp 493–506. New York, Elsevier, 1991.
15. Frederick JL, Paulson RJ, Sauer JV: Routine use of vaginal ultrasonography in the preoperative evaluation of gynecologic patients: An adjunct to resident education. J Reprod Med 36:779, 1991.
16. Odwin CS, Fleischer AC, Kepple DM, Chiang DT: Probe covers and disinfectants for transvaginal transducers. J Diagn Med Sonograph 6:130, 1990.
17. Timor-Tritsch IE: Standardization of ultrasonographic images: Let's all talk the same language! Ultrasound Obstet Gynecol 2:311, 1992.
18. Rottem S, Thaler I, Goldstein SR, et al: Transvaginal sonographic technique: Targeted organ scanning without resorting to "planes." J Clin Ultrasound 18:243, 1990.
19. Dodson MG, Deter RL: Definition of anatomical planes for use in transvaginal sonography. J Clin Ultrasound 18:239, 1990.
20. Bernaschek G, Deutinger J: Current status of vaginosonography: A worldwide inquiry. Ultrasound Obstet Gynecol 2:352, 1990.
21. Quinn MJ, Beynon J, Mortensen NM, Smith PJB: Transvaginal endosonography in the assessment of urinary stress incontinence. Br J Urol 62:414, 1988.
22. Monteagudo A, Reuss ML, Timor-Tritsch IE: Imaging the fetal brain in the second and third trimester using transvaginal sonography. Obstet Gynecol 77:27, 1991.
23. Benacerraf BR, Estroff JA: Transvaginal sonographic imaging of the low fetal head in the second trimester. J Ultrasound Med 8:325, 1989.
24. Zalud I, Kurjak A: The assessment of luteal blood flow in pregnant and non-pregnant women by transvaginal color Doppler. J Perinatol Med 18:215, 1990.
25. Kurjak A, Zalud I, Jorkovic D, et al: Transvaginal color Doppler for the assessment of pelvic circulation. Acta Obstet Gynecol Scand 68:131, 1989.
26. Kurjak A, Jurkovic D, Alfirevic Z, Zalud I: Transvaginal color Doppler. J Clin Ultrasound 18:227, 1990.

27. Fleischer AC, Rao BK, Kepple DM: Transvaginal color Doppler sonography: Preliminary experiences. Dynamic Cardiovasc Imaging 3:52, 1990.
28. Hata T, Hata K, Senoh D, et al: Transvaginal Doppler color flow mapping. Gynecol Obstet Invest 27:217, 1989.
29. Bourne T, Campbell S, Steer C, et al: Transvaginal colour flow imaging: A possible new screening technique for ovarian cancer. Br Med J 299:1367, 1989.
30. Fleischer AC, Rodgers WH, Rao BK, et al: Transvaginal color Doppler sonography of ovarian masses. J Ultrasound Med 10:563, 1991.
31. Kurjak A, Zalud I, Schulman H: Ectopic pregnancy: Transvaginal color Doppler identifies trophoblastic flow in suspicious adnexa. J Ultrasound Med 10:685, 1991.
32. Jaffe R, Warsof SL (eds): Color Doppler Imaging in Obstetrics and Gynecology. New York, McGraw-Hill Book Company, 1992.

CHAPTER 6

Ultrasound Evaluation During the First Trimester

ROY A. FILLY, M.D.

In the past decade a wealth of new information has become available regarding the first trimester of pregnancy, particularly its earliest beginnings. Programs of in vitro fertilization have caused physicians to look at the first trimester in a new light. This perception has been greatly augmented by powerful newer tools such as radioimmunoassays to detect extremely small quantities of human chorionic gonadotropin (hCG) and high-resolution real-time sonographic systems equipped with endovaginal transducers. Newer sonographic systems enable visualization of early pregnancies before the fifth week after the last normal menstrual period (LNMP) and to identify an implanted pregnancy by 2.5 weeks after conception. Another relatively new program, chorionic villus sampling, is capable of gathering a great deal of sonographic and chromosomal information from pregnancies at 8 to 10 menstrual weeks.

Sonologists have long recognized their potential contribution to the evaluation of early pregnancy. Ian Donald, the early pioneer of obstetric sonography, stated in his Gold Medal address: "We are particularly interested in studying the first twelve weeks of uterine development which are even more interesting than the last twelve weeks. It is surely the most crucial period in any being's existence. . . ."[1]

From the perspective of the sonologist, we are gathering a large amount of new information from intracorporeal transducers. Very high frequency transducers, painlessly introduced into the vagina, yield a view of early pregnancy previously unavailable. These transducers are variously termed *transvaginal* or *endovaginal sonographic transducers,* the latter term being preferable. Endovaginal scanning also serves as an "equalizer"; those sonologists with practices too small to offset the cost of selectably focused, phased-array ultrasound systems will be able to substantially improve their ability to image early pregnancies by availing themselves of this powerful "add on" to existing lower resolution systems.

The sonographic approach recommended in this chapter is one of pragmatism. There is a widely held belief that the way to proceed in sonographically suspected abnormal first-trimester pregnancies is to subject the patient to a seemingly endless sequence of follow-up examinations. Although all diagnosticians recognize the value of adding the dimension of time and serial observation to particularly difficult cases, this philosophy should not become so pervasive that one virtually abdicates diagnostic responsibility. A number of extremely reliable indicators of a nonviable pregnancy have been described; once these have been observed, nothing is gained by prolonging the pregnancy.

WHAT IS A PREGNANCY?

With the advent of in vitro fertilization programs and in view of both moral and ethical questions surrounding legal therapeutic abortion, gynecologists are reexamining the fundamental concept of pregnancy. Is a fertilized ovum (zygote) a pregnancy? Is an implanted blastocyst a pregnancy? What should in vitro fertilization programs, charging women thousands of dollars per attempt, claim as their "pregnancy rate"?[2]

Clinicians and researchers now can detect the presence of a recently implanted pregnancy at a very early age. hCG is first elaborated after implantation of the blastocyst into the decidualized endometrium of the uterus. The hormone is produced by the trophoblastic cells of the developing chorionic villi. Extraordinarily low levels of this hormone (<1 ng/mL) can be detected by radioimmunoassay techniques, making it possible for investigators to confidently detect a pregnancy before a woman misses her first menstrual period.

Numerous studies have addressed the issue of early pregnancy identification and have recorded a surprisingly high loss rate.[2–4] Of 100 ova exposed to fertilization, 16 ova will fail to be fertilized (Fig. 6–1).[3] Of the 84 that become zygotes, a further 15 will fail to implant. Thus 69 blastocysts implant in the uterus and result in detectable levels of hCG *(chemical pregnancy).* However, 27 of these (39%) will abort very near to the expected onset of the ensuing menstruation. In this manner, the developing gestation is lost *(menstrual abortion)* before the woman recognizes even the possibility that she is pregnant. It is not until a woman has missed a menstrual period and a positive pregnancy test is confirmed that an entity exists that can be termed a *clinical pregnancy.* By this point only 42 of the original 100 exposed ova have survived to become a recognized pregnancy even though 84 became embryos. Simply put, half of the embryos are lost before they are recognized by the mother or clinician.

Even among clinically recognized pregnancies the difficult journey is far from complete. Within this group, one fourth will threaten to abort and fully half of these will indeed be lost *(recognized abortion).* Up to this point, the obstetrician has yet to have an opportunity to influence the final outcome. It is only among the remaining 30 potentially viable fetuses that

What is a Pregnancy ?

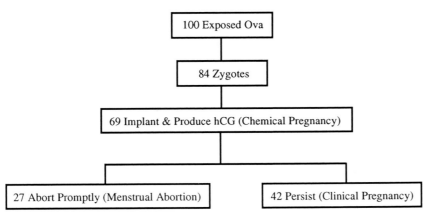

Figure 6–1. Background loss rate in early human pregnancies.

modern obstetrics can begin to make an impact, and even then a further small percentage will be lost, and some viable outcomes will be less than desirable.

These figures become somewhat less depressing when one realizes that the bulk of these losses are not random "bad luck" but rather "nature's way" of eliminating anomalous fetuses. The frequency of chromosomal anomalies in abortuses up to 6 weeks is very high, approximately 70%.[5] Over 99% of chromosomally anomalous fetuses are eliminated during the course of pregnancy. It is a difficult to accept that the unfortunate newborns we sometimes encounter with chromosomal anomalies are, in fact, the "cream of the chromosomally abnormal crop." Their counterparts could not survive the arduous process of development and birth.

NORMAL EARLY EMBRYONIC DEVELOPMENT*

A zygote is formed when an oocyte unites with a sperm cell. Development begins at that moment. Cleavage occurs in the fallopian tube and begins approximately 1 day after fertilization (Fig. 6–2). Subsequent divisions occur rapidly, such that after 3 days a small solid ball of cells (approximately 16) is produced. This entity is called a *morula,* the structure that enters the uterine cavity.

Fluid promptly passes into the morula from the endometrial cavity. This fluid separates the embryonic cells (blastomeres) into two layers. The outer layer or trophoblast eventually becomes the chorionic membrane and the fetal contribution to the placenta, while the inner cell mass gives rise to the embryo, amnion, cord, and secondary yolk sac. This cystic structure is called the *blastocyst* (see Fig. 6–2).

The blastocyst remains within the endometrial cavity approximately 2 days and then attaches to the deci-

dualized endometrial wall. It is the trophoblast immediately adjacent to the inner cell mass that attaches to and begins to invade the endometrial epithelium. By the end of the first week of development, some 3 weeks after the onset of LNMP, the blastocyst is implanted. As further invasion of the endometrium occurs, early chorionic villi develop. These cells elaborate hCG, a substance that can now be measured in a minute quantity; that is, the "pregnancy test" becomes positive.

The blastocyst continues to invade the endometrium until it is virtually submerged, and, indeed, the breeched surface heals over (Fig. 6–3A and B).[7] As the blastocyst cavity expands, a layer of cells separates from the blastocyst wall, forming Heuser's membrane, the exocoelomic membrane, thus creating the primitive or primary yolk sac that occupies the bulk of the early blastocyst cavity. Simultaneously, the smaller amniotic cavity begins to form. Lying between the amniotic cavity and the primary yolk sac is the embryonic disk.

The primitive yolk sac shrinks as the secondary yolk sac takes shape. The embryonic disk now lies between the forming amniotic cavity and the secondary yolk sac (Fig. 6–4A). At the end of the second week of development (4 weeks since the beginning of the LNMP), the blastocyst cavity has attained a size of only 1 mm. Within a few days, the blastocyst cavity has attained a mean diameter of 2 to 3 mm; thereafter, high-resolution sonography can begin to detect the presence of a gestation.

By the end of the third week (5 LNMP weeks), the chorionic cavity is well developed and contains the bulk of the fluid that sonographers call the gestational sac (see Figs. 6–3C and 6–4A and B). The amniotic sac, at this stage, is much smaller than the chorionic cavity. The edges of the amnion are fused with the embryonic disk (see Fig. 6–4A). Folding of the embryo causes it to come to lie within the amniotic cavity (see Fig. 6–4B). As the embryo folds, the dorsal curvature bows into the amniotic sac. The attachment of the amnion to the embryo thus comes to be along its ventral aspect; in fact, the amnion envelops the umbilical cord (see Figs. 6–4C and D and 6–5). The yolk sac's communication with the embryo is progressively "pinched" off, and it comes to lie within the chorionic

---

*The following section was largely excerpted from Dr. Keith Moore's excellent embryologic textbook *The Developing Human: Clinically Oriented Embryology,* 4th ed. Philadelphia, WB Saunders Co, 1988.[6–8]

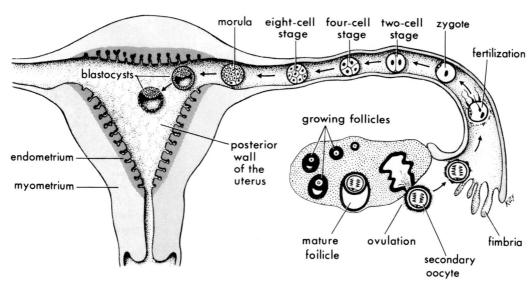

Figure 6–2. Diagram demonstrating the sequence of ovulation, fertilization, and early development of the embryo. The morula is the structure that enters the endometrial cavity. Fluid rapidly enters the morula, creating the blastocyst. The blastocyst is the embryonic structure that implants into the decidualized endometrium. (From Moore KL: The Developing Human: Clinically Oriented Embryology, 4th ed. Philadelphia, WB Saunders, 1988.)

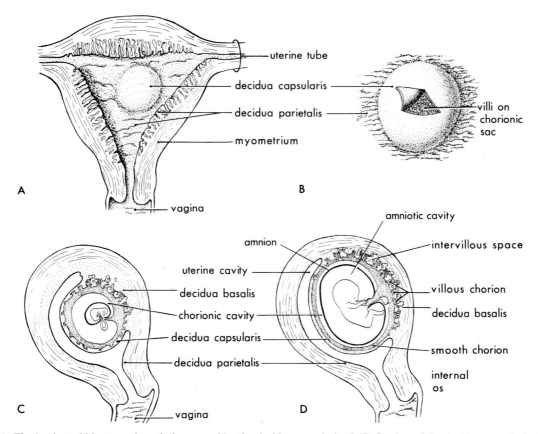

Figure 6–3. *A.* The implanted blastocyst is entirely covered by the decidua capsularis. *B.* Reflection of the decidua capsularis shows multiple chorionic villi covering the chorionic sac. *C* and *D.* Progressive growth brings the decidua capsularis in contact with the decidua parietalis. (From Moore KL: The Developing Human: Clinically Oriented Embryology, 4th ed. Philadelphia, WB Saunders, 1988.)

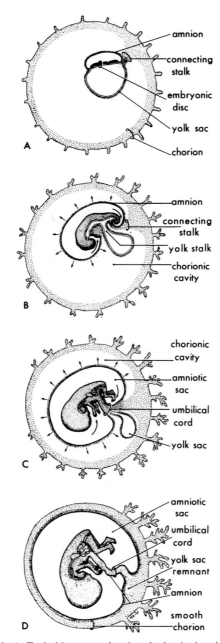

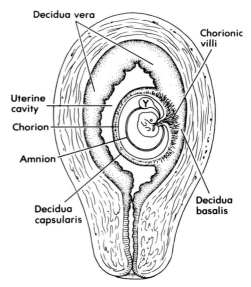

the embryo "officially" becomes a fetus. Thus, the sonographically favored term of "fetal pole" is inappropriate because it usually is employed to refer to an embryo.

An equally vital structure, the placenta, is developing in parallel with the early embryo. Recall that the developing blastocyst is entirely embedded in the endometrial surface, and the decidualized endometrium has healed over it by the end of the second week (4 LNMP weeks) (see Fig. 6–3A and B). The decidua that heals over and covers the surface of the blastocyst is termed the *decidua capsularis*. At 3 weeks of development (5 LNMP weeks), chorionic villi (tertiary type) developing from the trophoblastic layer have proliferated extensively and cover the surface of the blastocyst entirely and equally (see Figs. 6–3B and 6–4A and B). However, as the sac grows and expands into the endometrial cavity, the villi adjacent to the decidua capsularis become compressed and begin to degenerate, producing a bare area of chorion, the chorion laeve (see Figs. 6–3C, and D, 6–4C, and 6–5). This structure eventually becomes the chorionic membrane. As growth continues, the enlarging gestational sac fills the endometrial cavity, bringing the decidual capsularis, which covers the chorion laeve, into intimate and full contact with the decidua lining the remainder of the uterine cavity (the decidua parietalis). The decidua capsularis is now greatly attenuated and eventually fuses with the decidua parietalis, obliterating the endometrial cavity. The decidual capsularis then degenerates and disappears. After the disappearance of the decidua capsularis, the chorionic membrane (from the chorion laeve) in turn fuses with the decidua parietalis. This fusion can be separated and usually is when bleeding occurs. The blood pushes the chorionic membrane away from

Figure 6–4. *A*. Early blastocyst showing the beginning development of the amnion and the secondary yolk sac. The embryonic disk lies between. This structure is attached to the chorion by the connecting stalk. Note that villi are equally distributed around the periphery of the chorion. *B*. The dorsal aspect of the embryo begins to fold into the amnion. This infolding begins to constrict the attachment of the yolk sac to the embryo, forming the yolk stalk. The chorionic villi at the base of the yolk stalk are more prolific than those along the opposite pole of the blastocyst. *C*. The amnion now is enfolding the developing umbilical cord, pushing the yolk sac into the chorionic cavity. A smooth area of chorion is easily seen. *D*. The smooth chorion is now well developed. The amnion is fused to the smooth chorion, and the early placenta is well established. (From Moore KL: The Developing Human: Clinically Oriented Embryology, 4th ed. Philadelphia, WB Saunders, 1988.)

Figure 6–5. Diagram of an early gestation. The embryo lies entirely within the amnion. The amnion has not yet fused with the chorion. Chorionic villi (the chorion frondosum) are intermingled with the decidua basalis. The decidua capsularis covers the smooth chorion. The decidua capsularis is not yet in apposition with the decidua vera. The decidua capsularis covers the smooth chorion. The decidua capsularis is not drawn in apposition with the decidua vera although it is.

cavity. The yolk stalk maintains a connection between the yolk sac and the embryo.

The amniotic cavity progressively enlarges until it obliterates the chorionic cavity toward the end of the first trimester. At the end of the eighth embryonic week (10 weeks since the beginning of the LNMP), the decidua parietalis, reestablishing the potential space of the endometrial cavity.

Conversely, the portion of the trophoblast known as the chorion frondosum demonstrates progressive villus formation and forms the fetal component of the placenta. The chorion frondosum develops around the most deeply imbedded portion of the blastocyst, that portion immediately adjacent to the inner cell mass (early embryo). The maternal component of the placenta arises from the decidua basalis (the decidua adjacent to the chorion frondosum). So-called anchoring villi cause firm adherence of the fetal component to the maternal components. Therefore, by inference, the center of the early placenta marks the site of implantation; the center of the fluid in the gestational sac does not necessarily mark the relative position of implantation (see Figs. 6–3A and C). Because the chorionic membrane (from the chorion laeve) and the fetal placenta (from the chorion frondosum) develop from the same layer of cells, they are firmly attached at the edges.

NORMAL SONOGRAPHIC ANATOMY IN THE FIRST TRIMESTER

There is a natural tendency to relate sonographically observed landmarks in the first trimester of pregnancy to menstrual age. However, from the perspective of a clinical sonologist, it is more practical to relate observations seen on early pregnancy sonograms to the size of the gestational sac rather than to the menstrual or embryonic age of the pregnancy. This is particularly true because an abnormal gestational sac may be discordant (usually smaller) with dates, or the dates may be inaccurate. Because the early gestational sac is elliptical and may be distorted by pressure from focal myometrial contractions or myomas, it is best to judge sac size by estimating a mean sac diameter (MSD).[9–13] The MSD equals the length (craniocaudal dimension), width (transverse dimension), and height (anteroposterior dimension) of the gestational sac, divided by three. These measurements are obtained from the chorionic tissue–fluid interface (Fig. 6–6). Only the width is measured on transverse scans. Longitudinal scans are required to obtain the craniocaudal and anteroposterior dimensions.

With modern sonographic instruments equipped with endovaginal transducers, one can detect a gestational sac when it is only 2 to 3 mm MSD (approximately 4 weeks and 3 days since the LNMP) (Fig. 6–7).[14]* With most high-resolution scanners, even employing a transabdominal approach, one can usually detect gestational sacs as an intrauterine gestational sac when the MSD equals approximately 5 mm (35 days; 5 menstrual weeks).[10] With either technique, the earliest gestational sacs appear as tiny fluid collections surrounded by a uniform thickness rim of moderate amplitude echoes (arising from the developing chorionic villi). At the stage of gestation, when the gestational sac can consistently be detected by endovaginal sonography, hCG levels vary from 500 to 1500 IU/L (Second International Standard). In early pregnancy, hCG levels increase rapidly, doubling approximately every 2 days.[15–17] Therefore, the seemingly large range of 500 to 1500 IU/L actually constitutes only a 3-day difference in reported sonographic appearance times of early gestations. Unfortunately, a variety of other conditions may result in intrauterine fluid collections that may have a similar appearance to early gestational sacs. These include bleeding, endometritis, endometrial cysts, cervical stenosis, and the pseudogestational sac of ectopic pregnancy, to name the most common.[18] However, only the pseudogestational sac of ectopic pregnancy is also associated with detectable circulating levels of hCG.[19–22]

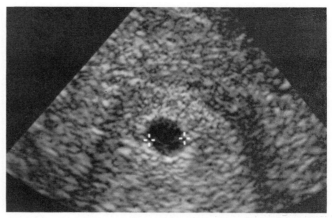

Figure 6–6. Transverse endovaginal sonogram of an early gestation sac (before visualization of a yolk sac). Mean sac diameter is being measured. This image depicts the transverse diameter *(cursors)* measured from the chorionic tissue–fluid interfaces.

Sonographic visualization of early pregnancies has progressively improved since the first observations were made.[1, 9, 17–26] One can begin observations of pregnancies within 10 to 14 days of implantation. Occasionally, sacs smaller than 5 mm MSD are observed by the classic transabdominal methods of uterine visualization through the distended urinary bladder. This method results in a distance of 10 to 15 cm from the transducer surface to the gestational sac. Endovaginal transducers shorten this distance by a factor of 5, thus enabling one to employ higher-frequency transducers and to image in an area of the beam much easier to focus (see Figs. 6–6 and 6–7).[14] Thus, one may reasonably anticipate that the trend to obtain

---

*There is some controversy in the literature regarding the precise age at which ultrasound examination can first detect a gestational sac, with estimates ranging from 3.5 to 5 weeks.[9, 10, 14–23] There is less controversy regarding the size of the gestational sac when it is first observed.[14] This is now thought to be 2 to 3 mm MSD. Similarly, most observers agree that the MSD increases about 1 mm/d in early gestation.[9, 10, 12, 24] Controversy returns when one looks at age estimates of MSD by various authors.[9, 10, 23] Embryologic data and data gathered by de Crispigny and colleagues leave little doubt that MSD is 2 to 3 mm at 4 weeks and 3 to 4 days.[6, 14] It is reasonably safe to assume that a gestational sac reaches 5 mm at 5 weeks.[10] Thus (until an MSD of 25 mm is reached), gestational age in days can be calculated by adding 30 to the MSD (i.e., MSD at 5 weeks = 5 mm).[10, 24]

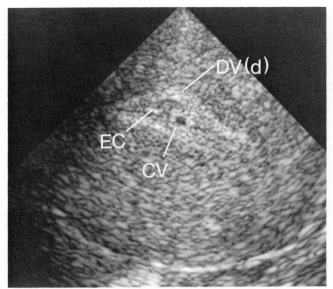

Figure 6–7. Transverse endovaginal sonogram of a very early gestational sac (about the limits of resolution of modern sonography). The complex of echoes is greater than would be estimated from mean sac diameter alone because the surrounding chorionic villi (CV) are also part of the complex. This figure also demonstrates the true origin of the double "decidual" sac sign. The two bright rings of the double sac are actually composed of the ring of chorionic villi (CV) and the deeper layer of the decidua vera [DV(d)]. The superficial layer is less echogenic. EC, endometrial cavity.

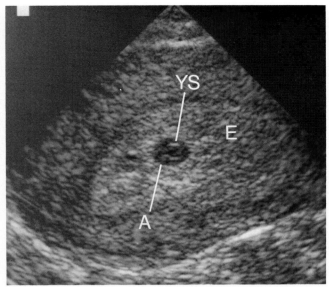

Figure 6–8. Endovaginal sonogram demonstrating the uncommonly observed "double bleb" sign composed of the yolk sac (YS) and amnion (A) lying side by side. Although this early embryonic complex can be resolved, it is likely that the window of opportunity to visualize this structure is very short. E, endometrium.

clearer and clearer images of early embryos will continue.

The early normal gestational sac is filled predominantly with chorionic fluid.[6] Since the surrounding rim of trophoblastic tissue is not included in the measurement of the MSD, the actual complex of echoes identified in early pregnancy is, in fact, more prominent and thus easier to see than suggested by the MSD (see Fig. 6–7).

The earliest embryonic structures are not usually seen with transabdominal sonography until the gestational sac reaches approximately 10 mm MSD and are not consistently seen until the sac reaches a mean diameter of 15 mm (40 to 45 days since the LNMP).[11, 26] The first such structure to be seen is a combination of the yolk sac and the developing amniotic sac.[26] This "double bleb" makes a distinctive pattern within the chorionic cavity, although it is visible for only a brief period and therefore uncommonly seen (Fig. 6–8). The primitive embryonic disk is the line of echoes dividing these minute fluid-containing sacs. The entire echo complex is only a few millimeters in diameter, but the surrounding chorionic fluid provides the background contrast against which the beginnings of human life are observed with high-resolution real-time sonography.

The yolk sac grows slowly (Fig. 6–9), and its wall appears to thicken (Fig. 6–10). At this point, the yolk sac dominates the interior of the gestational sac (see Fig. 6–9).[25, 26] The embryo, lying in close contiguity with the yolk sac, measures only 2 to 3 mm in length and, as such, is less readily visible than the yolk sac itself. Interestingly, in the era when only transabdom-

inal transducers were available, an embryonic marker was more clearly seen at this stage of development than the corpus of the embryo.[11] This marker is the tiny pulsation of the forming embryonic heart, so unmistakable on the screen of the sonographic device. It is, of course, artificial to segregate "the embryo" from the yolk sac, the amnion, or certainly its own heartbeat. These distinctions are drawn only to properly sequence early sonographic observations. With endovaginal transducers it is usually possible to see the

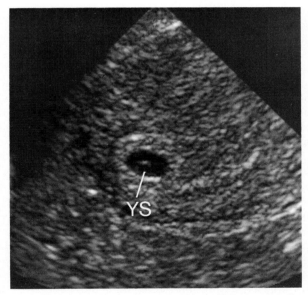

Figure 6–9. Endovaginal sonogram demonstrating an early yolk sac (YS). At this stage of development the yolk sac dominates sonographic observations (i.e., the stage at which the mean sac diameter ranges from 7 to 15 mm). Again, the echogenic reflectors that contribute to the double "decidual" sac sign are visible, as in Figure 6–7.

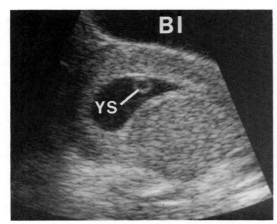

Figure 6–10. High-resolution real-time transabdominal sonogram of an 8-week gestation, demonstrating the yolk sac (YS). The yolk sac wall has considerably thickened by this stage of development. Thus, it has higher subject contrast and is more readily seen. Bl, bladder.

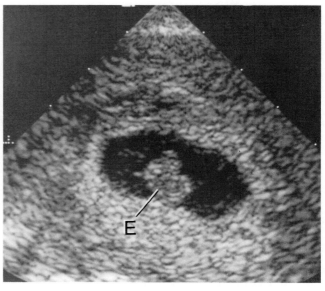

Figure 6–12. Endovaginal sonogram of a normally formed but dead embryo (E). Note the curvature of the embryo enabling discrimination of the "crown" from the "rump." The distinction is less obvious without the presence of a heartbeat to identify the torso.

tiny asymmetric thickening along the yolk sac wall representing the early embryo in which the heartbeat is identified.[27]

Endovaginal transducers have enabled observers to document living embryos in which no visible heartbeat can be recorded. Tiny embryos with crown-rump lengths (CRL) of 2 to 3.9 mm correspond to menstrual ages of 34 to 40 days.[27, 28] Embryologic texts suggest that cardiac activity begins approximately at the 22nd day past conception. This equates to approximately 36 menstrual days or a CRL of 1.5 to 3 mm (i.e., living human embryos can be sonographically visualized before the onset of cardiac pulsations).

When the embryo achieves a CRL of 5 mm it can be consistently seen as a discrete structure separable from the wall of the yolk sac and within which one or several echoes pulsate (all embryos of this size should have visible cardiac pulsations if alive) (Fig. 6–11).[27] At this point, the MSD is usually 15 to 18 mm and the menstrual age is approximately 6.5 weeks. It is not

possible even to discriminate which end of the embryo is its crown and which is its rump, but the unmistakable cardiac pulsations confirm without doubt that this small "clump" of echoes is a living human embryo. From this point forward visualization of the embryo itself dominates the sonologic observations. Intraembryonic structures become progressively clearer. When an embryo reaches approximately 12 mm in CRL the head can be discriminated from the torso (Figs. 6–12 and 6–13). The embryo's head will constitute fully half of its total volume. Progressively, one visualizes limb buds, the umbilical cord (Fig. 6–14), and then the primary ossification centers of the maxilla, mandible, and clavicle (Fig. 6–15).[17, 29] Thereafter, the gamut of visible anatomy rapidly unfolds, especially as viewed by endovaginal techniques as the embryo (through the eighth week of development; 10 menstrual weeks) becomes

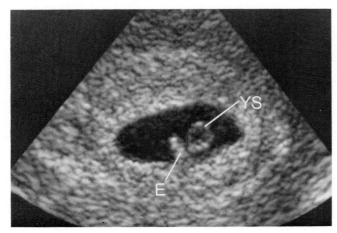

Figure 6–11. Endovaginal sonogram of an early embryo (E) (crown-rump length = 4 to 5 mm). Note that at this stage the embryo lies in close proximity to the yolk sac (YS) because the yolk stalk has not yet developed to any significant degree. Nearly all embryos of this size can be resolved by endovaginal sonography.

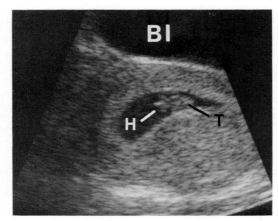

Figure 6–13. Longitudinal transabdominal sonogram of an early pregnancy. A 13-mm embryo is seen within the gestational sac. Note that the head (H) and torso (T) can be discriminated in embryos of this size. Bl, bladder.

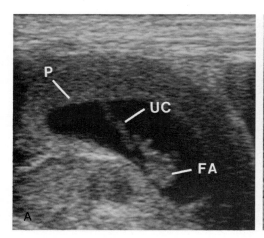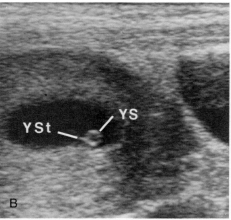

Figure 6–14. Sequential longitudinal transabdominal sonograms of a late first-trimester pregnancy. *A.* The umbilical cord (UC) is seen coursing from the placenta (P) to the fetal abdomen (FA). *B.* The yolk sac (YS) is noted, and a short segment of the terminal yolk stalk (YSt) is seen leading to the yolk sac

the fetus (beginning of the ninth week of development; 11 menstrual weeks). This transition occurs when the CRL reaches approximately 30 to 35 mm.

AMNIOTIC AND CHORIONIC MEMBRANES

Recall that the amnion was among the earliest visible embryonic structures (see Figs. 6–4*A* and 6–8).[26] As it develops it passes through a stage of relative "invisibility." Presumably this period of invisibility relates to the thinness of the amniotic membrane and its proximity to the embryo, both of which would tend to obscure the membrane to the sonographic beam. During this brief period sonographic observations center next on the yolk sac and promptly thereafter on the embryo. However, the amnion quickly "reappears" as a much larger sac with an extremely thin wall (Fig. 6–16).[30, 39] This tends to occur when the embryo reaches a CRL of 8 to 12 mm. Still its thinness is no match for the resolving capacity of modern instruments, once amniotic fluid has separated the membrane from the embryo. Commonly only those portions of the amnion lying perpendicular to the acoustic beam are resolved. The embryo lies entirely within the confines of the amniotic membrane; the yolk sac is excluded and lies within the chorionic cavity (see Fig. 6–16), usually between the amniotic membrane and the fetal surface of the developing placenta. The bulk of the fluid within the gestational sac rapidly changes from the chorionic cavity to the amniotic cavity. Indeed, the chorionic cavity diminishes progressively until ultimately the amnion "fuses" to the chorion to obliterate this cavity.*

One can usually continue to observe the yolk sac well into the late stages of the first trimester. A bright curvilinear echo is commonly observed extending toward the yolk sac.[26] Unlike the amnion, this structure is not a sheet and is usually a brighter reflector. Logically, this reflector represents the yolk stalk (see Figs. 6–14 and 6–16).

An understanding of the points of attachment of the chorionic membrane and amnion is important to characterize accurately the location of various pathologic fluid collections that occur during early pregnancy.[31] Recall that the placenta and chorionic membrane had identical origins and are inseparably fused (see Figs. 6–3 and 6–4). The chorionic membrane always leads to the edge of the placenta. By contrast, the amnion surrounds the fetus and is continuous with and covers the umbilical cord where it joins the placenta (see Fig. 6–4*D*). Thus, the amnion can be separated from the fetal surface of the placenta (unlike the chorionic membrane) but cannot be separated from its junction point with the cord insertion site into the placenta.

Although the chorionic membrane cannot be separated from the placental edge, it is easily separated

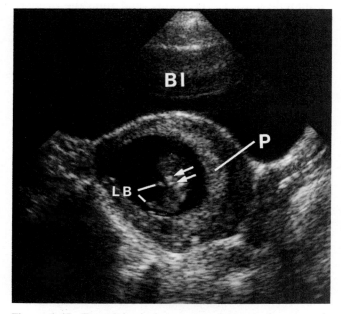

Figure 6–15. Transabdominal sonogram demonstrating an early fetus. Limb buds (LB) can be seen. However, within the head and torso the only visible discrete structures are the primary ossification centers of the maxilla and mandible *(arrows)*. Bl, bladder; P, placenta.

---

*In fact, in the second trimester, puncture of these membranes during amniocentesis commonly allows quantities of amniotic fluid to leak into the chorionic cavity and reestablish this potential space: a so-called chorioamniotic separation. In and of itself a chorioamniotic separation has no proven deleterious effect on a pregnancy and should not be considered evidence for the presence of the amniotic band sequence.

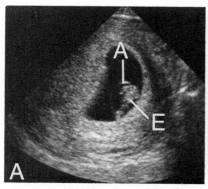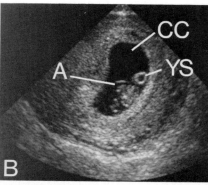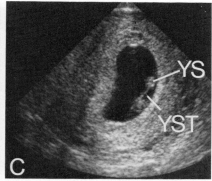

Figure 6–16. *A* through *C.* Sequence of endovaginal sonograms demonstrating the anatomy of an early pregnancy (crown-rump length = 12 mm). The amnion "reappears" at this stage of development. The embryo (E) is confined by the amnion (A). Sufficient amniotic fluid is present to separate the amnion from the embryo. The chorionic cavity (CC) still contains more fluid than the amniotic cavity, but this will rapidly change. The yolk sac (YS) is contained in the chorionic cavity. YST, yolk stalk.

from the endometrial lining (decidua parietalis) to which it is supposedly "fused" by *any* intraendometrial cavity fluid collection. Physicians may inject saline into the endometrial cavity during chorion villus sampling to separate the chorion laeve from the decidua parietalis to locate precisely the junction of the developing chorion frondosum.[32] The only commonly occurring natural (albeit pathologic) fluid collection within the endometrial cavity during early pregnancy is blood, which is seen in women who are in danger of aborting. This is a so-called subchorionic hematoma (Figs. 6–17 through 6–21). It would be preferable to abandon this confusing term in favor of the term *intraendometrial cavity collection,* which accurately describes the anatomic location of the fluid.

Similarly a *chorioamniotic accumulation* is a somewhat confusing term. This simply refers to fluid in the chorionic cavity, a normal and universal finding before "fusion" of the chorion and amnion. Such a collection can be accurately localized because the fluid lies between the fetal surface of the placenta and the membrane (amnion), forming its contralateral boundary (an impossibility for fluid contained in the endometrial cavity [subchorionic collection]).[31] After "fusion," fluid

may reappear in this space following needle puncture that allows amniotic fluid to leak into the chorionic cavity and reestablish this potential space by "stripping away" the amniotic membrane. The "trauma" of second-trimester amniocentesis commonly causes small inconsequential chorioamniotic separations. However, amniocentesis may result in true hemorrhagic complications. The hemorrhage may be either fetal blood (usually devastating) or more commonly maternal blood and may accumulate behind the placenta (abruption) (Figs. 6–22 and 6–23), in the endometrial cavity (subchorionic), in the chorionic cavity (chorioamniotic), or in the amniotic cavity itself. Although all such occurrences are best avoided, an intra-amniotic or chorioamniotic accumulation of blood is not specifically harmful to a fetus.

EVALUATION OF GESTATIONAL AGE

The first trimester is an opportune time to employ the sonographic parameters of pregnancy dating in patients with an uncertain menstrual history. In the first trimester, as throughout the remainder of preg-

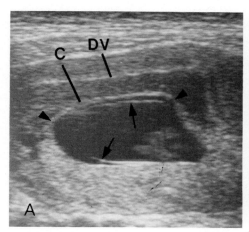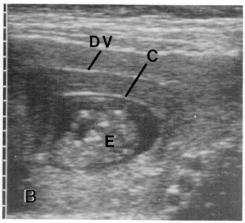

Figure 6–17. Longitudinal *(A)* and transverse *(B)* transabdominal sonograms of a patient experiencing bleeding in the first trimester. A so-called subchorionic hemorrhage has accumulated between the chorion (C) and the decidua vera (DV). Note that the chorion extends circumferentially to meet the edges of the developing placenta *(arrowheads)*. Note as well that the margins of the placenta are separated from the uterine wall (i.e., marginal abruption). The embryo (E) demonstrated an active heartbeat, indicating that this pregnancy should be observed expectantly. Arrows indicate amniotic membrane nearly opposed to the chorion.

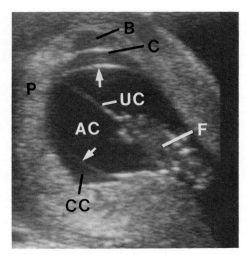

Figure 6–18. Longitudinal transabdominal sonogram through the uterus of a patient experiencing first-trimester bleeding. The fetus (F) is readily identified dangling from its umbilical cord (UC). No fetal heartbeat was identified, confirming nonviability. All of the potential spaces are noted in this case. The amnion *(arrows)* defines the amniotic cavity (AC). Note that the amnion extends to the base of the umbilical cord. The chorionic cavity (CC) lies between the amnion and the chorion (C). The chorion extends to the edge of the placenta (P). Blood (B) has accumulated in the endometrial cavity (i.e., external to the chorion). The blood represents a so-called subchorionic hemorrhage.

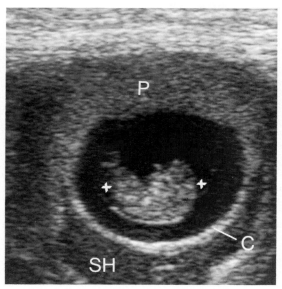

Figure 6–20. Transabdominal sonogram demonstrating a subchorionic hematoma (H) separating the chorionic membrane (C) from the decidua vera. The crown-rump length is measured by the cursor marks. P, developing placenta.

nancy, menstrual age is estimated by measuring the size of a structure. Before embryonic visualization, one can measure the size of the gestational sac (see Fig. 6).[9, 10, 24] After embryonic visualization, the embryo itself can be measured at first in toto (the so-called CRL) (see Figs. 6–20 and 6–23).[33–37] Later, as specific fetal parts become visible, individual fetal parameters can be measured. These are the same in the first trimester as during the remainder of pregnancy (i.e., biparietal diameter [BPD], head circumference, femur length, and abdominal circumference).

From a philosophical perspective, estimation of menstrual age by any biometric measurement is a tradeoff between two competing problems. The first is the measurement's accuracy, and the second is the meas-

urement's predictive validity for age. The feature that most influences the latter is biologic variation. Inexorably, as pregnancy advances, biologic size variation increases. Thus, without question, an individual measurement is more likely to predict the gestational age accurately the earlier in pregnancy it is measured. The opposing feature is ease and accuracy of measurement. Obviously, measurements that result in large interobserver or intraobserver variations manifest significant predictive inaccuracy even though they can be measured at a gestational stage when biologic variation is small.

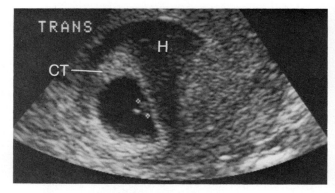

Figure 6–19. Endovaginal sonogram demonstrating a proportionately large subchorionic hematoma (H). The hematoma is partially separating the chorionic tissue (CT) (chorion frondosum) from the uterine wall (i.e., abruption). The embryo (marked by cursors) had a heartbeat.

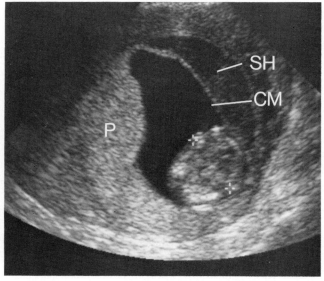

Figure 6–21. Endovaginal sonogram of a large subchorionic hematoma (SH). The fetus survived. CM, chorionic membrane; P, placenta.

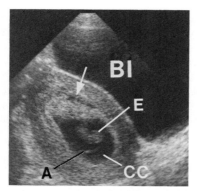

Figure 6–22. Longitudinal transabdominal sonogram through the uterus of a patient experiencing first-trimester bleeding. An embryo (E) is clearly identified. However, no heartbeat was identified, confirming nonviability. A small accumulation of blood *(arrow)* is seen lying between the chorion frondosum and the uterine wall; this indicates an abrupting early placenta. Bl, bladder; A, amnion; CC, chorionic cavity.

One might therefore reason that the most accurate prediction of menstrual age would be obtained by measuring the gestational sac (the earliest sonographically visible structure in pregnancy) between 5 and 6.5 weeks (see Figs. 6–7 through 6–9). It is easily and accurately measured and biologic variation should be quite small. Although no one has ever tested this notion, it is likely true. The fallacy of this concept, of course, is that there is such a narrow window in which to apply it. Furthermore, if the pregnancy dates were known with sufficient accuracy to schedule the examination within this narrow time window, it is unlikely that a mechanism to further improve the dating would be necessary. After 6.5 weeks, the gestational sac can still be measured, but now there is an alternative measurement, the CRL.[33–37] The embryo is as yet too small to have its individual parts measured, but its length can be estimated (see Figs. 6–11, 6–20, and 6–23). There are, unfortunately, some pitfalls in the estimation of the CRL. Since no anatomic marker exists at the tip of the crown or the rump, one must always assume that the "longest" CRL is the most accurate. This, however, can be influenced by beam divergence, beam splitting, side lobe artifacts, the erroneous inclusion of extraneous structures (most notably the yolk sac) (Fig. 6–24), or a change in the resting position of the embryo. The embryo normally rests with a kyphotic curvature, but within a few weeks of its visualization the embryo can begin to extend and straighten itself, "altering" its CRL.

Indeed, Robinson, in his original description of CRL measurement, noted the potential for some of the previously described inaccuracies.[34] The literature is now replete with reports that document beyond any reasonable doubt that early CRL measurement (between 6.5 and 10 menstrual weeks) is the single most accurate method of pregnancy dating.[34–37] The size of the gestational sac, of course, can still be measured accurately during the same time frame; however, available evidence strongly indicates that measurement of a fetal parameter (CRL) is more accurate than the measurement of any general feature of a pregnancy (sac or uterine size).[9] After the 10th week, it is possible to measure specific fetal parts. These specific structures are more accurately measurable than the CRL; however, the CRL can still be measured through the end of the first trimester and is accurate for pregnancy dating. Once visible for measurement, the head and femur become the preferred biometric parameters for estimating gestational age.

The methods used in research experiments conducted by highly motivated examiners may not translate into equivalent predictive accuracies when practiced in the general community or even at other research centers. Campbell and associates investigated this problem, and the results were enlightening.[38] These authors reviewed more than 4500 consecutive pregnancy sonograms and compared the accuracy of a CRL prediction of the estimated date of confinement (EDC)

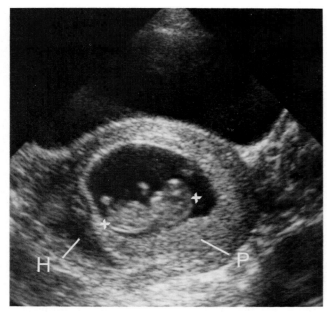

Figure 6–23. Transabdominal sonogram demonstrates a small hematoma (H) that undercuts a modest portion of the placental (P) edge. Cursors mark the crown-rump length measurement.

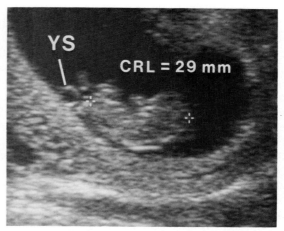

Figure 6–24. Transabdominal sonogram demonstrating an embryo with a crown-rump length (CRL) of 29 mm. It is important not to include the yolk sac (YS) in this measurement.

with that of a BPD obtained before the 18th week. The CRL correctly predicted the EDC (± 14 days) in 85% of cases. Interestingly, the BPD predicted the EDC (± 14 days) in 89% of cases. Even a BPD between 18 to 22 weeks matched the prediction by the CRL. Of further interest, the LNMP predicted EDC (± 14 days) in 85% of cases if an optimal history could be obtained. An optimal history was defined as certainty of the first day of the LNMP, regular cycles, no exposure to birth control pills for at least 2 months, and no unusual bleeding. Unfortunately, such a history was only available in 55% of the patient group.

Despite Campbell's study,[38] the weight of evidence suggests that pregnancies are most accurately dated by sonographic parameters measured in the first trimester.[34–37] The CRL is the most accurate measurement, but an early MSD is also highly accurate. Still, even among those studies documenting improved accuracy of the CRL over a BPD performed at about 18 weeks, the demonstrated improvement in predictive accuracy is only slightly greater than one-half week. *Simply because a pregnancy can be more accurately dated in the first than in the early second trimester does not mean that it should.* Too high a price is paid to gain a small advantage in age estimation. At 18 weeks, one can characterize a large number of important pregnancy parameters that cannot be judged at all in early pregnancy. The placental position can be accurately judged, amniotic fluid volume can be estimated, early shortening of the cervix can be recognized, and numerous fetal anomalies can be detected. Despite the somewhat improved accuracy of pregnancy dating in the first trimester, one is ill advised to pursue pregnancy dating early unless there are other mitigating circumstances besides an uncertain menstrual history. Furthermore, when the menstrual history is optimal, as it is in most pregnant women, ultrasound evaluation is not likely to offer any significant clinical benefit in defining gestational age, even if performed in the first trimester.[38]

THREATENED ABORTION

One could not begin to write about the sonographic diagnosis of abnormal first-trimester pregnancies without recognizing the pioneering work of Dr. Hugh Robinson.[1, 33, 34, 36, 37] Robinson not only set the stage and defined the goals, it is equally clear that in the ensuing decade following his original papers subsequent investigators simply validated his original observations.[38–44] "The primary objective," wrote Robinson, "is to formulate criteria for the sonar (identification) of abnormal pregnancies such that these diagnoses (can) be applied prospectively and with complete reliability in the active management of established early pregnancy failures."[1]

Robinson's objective has largely been achieved, and sonographic diagnosis can now be appropriately applied in threatened abortion, the major indication for sonography in the first trimester. *Threatened abortion* is a clinically descriptive term that applies to women who have vaginal spotting or bleeding, mild uterine cramping, and a closed cervical os during the first 20 weeks of pregnancy. The current discussion will involve women in the first 13 weeks of pregnancy.

Threatened abortion is a common complication that occurs in approximately 25% of clinically apparent pregnancies.[45–47] Despite efforts to alter the outcome, about one half of these pregnancies ultimately abort. In such cases the embryo is most often already dead and usually has been dead for some time. Thus, the administration of progestational drugs is ineffective and only prolongs the natural course of abortion. Although the embryo is dead, chorionic tissue may still be functional, resulting in a persistently positive pregnancy test.

Although nearly all nonviable gestations will eventually abort, spontaneous expulsion is frequently delayed for weeks after the onset of clinical symptoms.[45, 47] This may lead to prolonged vaginal bleeding, infection, and patient anxiety. Although none of these are life threatening, their seriousness should not be underestimated. Clinical management depends on whether the embryo is living. Therefore, the reliable identification of nonviable gestations is important for determining which patients merit uterine evacuation; potentially viable, living embryos, on the other hand, are observed expectantly.

Methods to assess embryonic life include hormonal assays (hCG, estrogen, progesterone, human placental lactogen, pregnancy-specific β-glycoprotein and α-fetoprotein), and sonography.[37, 45, 48–52] Among the hormonal studies, progesterone and hCG levels are more accurate than the others. Falling hCG levels predict pregnancy failure quite accurately.[45] Unfortunately, serial hCG determinations are not uncommonly equivocal. Anembryonic pregnancies and pregnancies complicated by embryonic death may demonstrate normal hCG levels even when villi appear abnormal by gross and microscopic evaluation. It is an attractive hypothesis to assume that low hCG levels are related to abnormal histology of chorionic villi. Unfortunately, this is not necessarily so.[49]

Although such determinations are useful, sonography is the pivotal examination in this clinical setting. Recall that when the patient presents, she has about a 50/50 chance of the pregnancy ending in abortion. However, numerous studies now document that sonographic demonstration of a living embryo alters these statistics dramatically and favorably. Unfortunately, as earlier embryonic identification becomes more common, the fate of these tiny embryos becomes less favorable (see Fig. 6–11).[27, 53] When a living embryo is identified by transabdominal sonography 90% to 97% of cases continue (see Figs. 6–13 and 6–15).[49, 54–57] However, embryonic visualization with transabdominal sonography begins with CRL of 5 mm and becomes universal at 10 mm. Embryos of 2 to 4 mm CRL seen on endovaginal sonography appear not to have as favorable an outcome (Fig. 6–25).[53] The research of Levi and associates[27] would indicate that such embryos will be lost nearly 30% of the time when the mother is bleeding. May and Sturtevant studied 50 embryos seen between 4.5 and 7.5 menstrual weeks.[58] Embryos

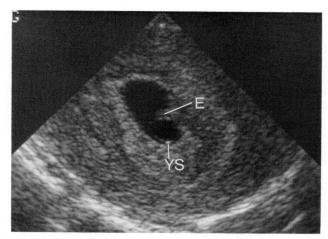

Figure 6–25. Endovaginal sonogram demonstrates a tiny embryo (E) (< 3 mm) located along the margin of an abnormally large and thin-walled yolk sac (YS). No heartbeat was seen. For embryos this small a follow-up examination is required to prove nonviability, which was the case in this pregnancy.

are only uncommonly detected earlier than 6 menstrual weeks; thus one can assume that the bulk of the embryos studied were visualized at between 6 and 7.5 menstrual weeks. Eleven embryos (22%) aborted despite a visible heartbeat. Howe and coworkers[59] closely followed 63 precisely dated early clinically normal pregnancies in which an embryo with a heartbeat was observed. Ten of these pregnancies (15%) aborted (Table 6–1).

These studies and others demonstrate that the background loss rate of very early pregnancies is quite high.[27, 53, 58, 59] There are, of course, further losses in all subsequent stages of pregnancy, but the loss rate falls progressively throughout the remainder of gestation. As noted earlier, endovaginal sonography enables visualization of living embryos that will have a relatively high background loss rate. Considerable interest also exists in better establishing the background loss rate of living embryos in the range of 8 to 12 menstrual weeks since this figure impacts quite directly on the reported procedure-related pregnancy loss rate from chorionic villus sampling.

There are several studies addressing the issue of loss rate in the 8 to 12-menstrual week pregnancy.[54, 55] A comprehensive evaluation had the following results.[54] Among living embryos from 8 to 12 menstrual weeks

Table 6–1. FOLLOW-UP OF PRECISELY DATED EARLY CLINICAL PREGNANCIES

Pregnancies	71 (100%)
Continuing	63 (75%)
Spontaneous abortion	18 (25%)
Embryo	10 (14%)
No embryo	8 (11%)
Heartbeat identified	63 (100%)
Continuing	53 (84%)
Spontaneous abortion	10 (16%)

From Howe RS, Isaacson KJ, Albert JL, Coutifaris CB: Embryonic heart rate in human pregnancy. J Ultrasound Med 10:367, 1991.

Table 6–2. ESTIMATION OF EARLY PREGNANCY FAILURE RATES

Embryo With Heartbeat	Clinical Finding	
	Bleeding	**No Bleeding**
<6 weeks	33%	16%
7–9 weeks	10%	5%
9–11 weeks	4%	1%–2%

Data from references 27, 53, 54, 58, and 59.

the overall abortion rate was 2.3%. The risk decreased following the 10th week (i.e., abortion rate from 7 to 9 weeks was 5% but dropped to 1% to 2% between 10 and 12 weeks). Further subdivision of patients showed a loss rate of 1.3% if the mother was not spotting. However, if spotting was present, 5.4% aborted. Furthermore, risk of abortion increased with maternal age, presumably related to the increased risk of chromosomal anomalies in older mothers. As noted earlier, chromosomal anomalies account for the majority of early pregnancy losses. Similar factors will likely also affect loss rates of earlier embryos identified with endovaginal sonography.

Recall that estimates as high as 50% of early fertilized ova were lost before clinical recognition of a pregnancy.[3, 4] It is not reasonable to assume that sonographic visualization of an embryo with a heartbeat would miraculously cut this loss rate to 5% as was generally quoted in the era when only transabdominal sonography was available. Since we now have the capacity to visualize very tiny embryos in the 5.5- to 6-week age range, evidence suggests that as many as 30% will be lost in women who are threatening to abort and about 15% will abort in women who are clinically normal. The background loss rate falls precipitously to a level of 1% to 2% for clinically normal women as the end of the first trimester is reached and to approximately twice that level in women who are bleeding (Table 6–2).

We may never know or agree on the precise loss rates of "normal" and "threatening" pregnancies at every stage of the first trimester, but some truths and trends are apparent. First, loss rates are high and possibly very high in the 5- to 6-week range, even in women who appear clinically normal. Furthermore, current data indicate that women who are threatening to abort are approximately twice as likely to lose their pregnancy as clinically normal women once sonography has demonstrated a heartbeat (see Table 6–2). Because clinical sonologists have lost confidence that the visualization of an embryonic heartbeat strongly suggests that the pregnancy would continue, efforts have been made to predict pregnancy failure remote from the event in living pregnancies. These efforts have centered on ancillary observations such as intrauterine blood accumulations (subchorionic hematomas) (see Figs. 6–17 through 6–21),[60–62] slow embryonic heartbeats (embryonic bradycardia),[58, 63] disproportionalities in sac size, particularly when the sac appears too small for the size of the embryo present within it (early oligohydramnios),[64, 65] and abnormalities of the yolk sac, particularly yolk sacs that are too large for the stage of early development (see Fig. 6–25).[66, 67]

Some researchers have observed that in the presence of an intrauterine hematoma (appromately one fourth of those women who are threatening to abort) pregnancy loss rates were double the loss rate when no hematoma was present.[60] Others refute this.[61] Partly, the difference in opinions may reside in the precise location, rather than the size of the hematoma (compare Figs. 6–20 and 6–21 with Figs. 6–22 and 6–23). Even small hematomas under the placenta (abruptions) are likely to be more significant than larger collections in the endometrial cavity.

Some observers have suggested that embryos with heart rates less than 85 beats per minute are universally lost.[58, 63] I have personal experience with embryos that have survived despite having exhibited early bradycardia, and Howe and colleagues have published that normal embryos start life with heart rates of less than 85 beats per minute.[59]

Abnormal yolk sac size has been observed in early gestations that subsequently aborted although the gestation otherwise appeared normal.[67] Others have not found this finding to be helpful,[66] and no one considers abnormal size of the yolk sac to be universally predictive of pregnancy failure. Similarly, when the MSD minus the CRL equals 5 or less (i.e., the sac is too small for the size of the embryo), then 80% of the pregnancies ultimately abort.[64, 65, 68] This feature, however, was seen in only 2% of pregnancies.[68]

Although it is reasonable that investigators search out relationships that predict pregnancy failure despite the presence of an embryonic heartbeat, from a personal perspective such observations have little practical value. Once an embryonic heartbeat is observed sonographically, the clear course of action is to observe the patient expectantly. So important is the observation of the embryonic heartbeat that it overrides any simultaneous finding that suggests impending pregnancy loss. That is not to say that observation of "bradycardia" or a sac that is "too small" will not influence outcome, but these features are insufficiently predictive of pregnancy failure to alter management. Some use these features to "prepare" the mother for the worst possible outcome, a practice that adds nothing to management but does add measurably to parental anxiety.

Maternal factors also may influence a women's propensity to lose a pregnancy with a living embryo. These would include most commonly women with numerous or submucous myomas, women with uterine anomalies (didelphic or bicornuate uteri), and women whose mothers were exposed to diethylstilbestrol during pregnancy (DES daughters). However, lethal genetic mutations dwarf maternal causes of early pregnancy loss.

Sonographic demonstration of an embryo that lacks cardiac motion is the most specific evidence of embryonic death (see Figs. 6–12 and 6–22).[49, 57, 69] However, observations with endovaginal sonography have significantly altered the safe utilization of this concept.[27]

Recall that with high-resolution endovaginal sonography it is possible to detect the early embryonic corpus (CRL = 2 to 4 mm) before the onset of cardiac pulsation. Therefore, a cutoff value of 5 mm CRL is recommended for failure to identify cardiac activity in a visualized embryo before diagnosing embryonic death. Embryos of CRL greater than 5 mm who fail to demonstrate a heartbeat may safely be judged as nonviable. Those patients with embryos of CRL less than 5 mm without a visible heartbeat should return for a follow-up examination in 4 days (see Fig. 6–25).

Experienced imaging specialists know that negative observations (no heartbeat observed) are fraught with more problems than positive observations (heartbeat observed), and caution is certainly appropriate when evaluating a patient who is threatening to abort. There are three precautions that should be taken. The first of these is by far the most important. Be sure you are looking at the embryo before you search the entity for a heartbeat. This is a trivially simple exercise when the embryo exceeds 10 mm CRL since it has a discernible head and torso by that time. However, between 2 to 10 mm CRL the embryo has no morphologically recognizable structure other than its heartbeat (which, of course, will not be available for inspection if it is dead). The 2- to 10-mm embryo is seen only as a globular collection of echoes (see Fig. 6–11). Still there are reasonable criteria of observation that can be applied. A recognizable early embryo is at least 2 to 5 mm long and has a reasonable and proportional width with respect to its length (Fig. 6–26). It lies near the yolk sac (see Fig. 6–11), and it may be seen to be surrounded by amnion. Recall, however, that a tiny embryo (2 to 4 mm CRL) may be alive when no sonographic heartbeat can be recorded.

Once one is certain that the structure being interrogated for the presence of a heartbeat is indeed the

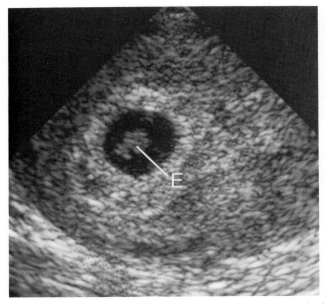

Figure 6–26. An en face view of an early embryo (E) on endovaginal sonography. Note that the embryo is somewhat discoid at this early stage, a feature that helps to reliably identify early embryos.

embryo and that the CRL is greater than 5 mm, the second precaution loses significance, although at first glance it appears to be the pivotal point. This precaution is simply to *observe the embryo thoroughly for evidence of a heartbeat.* No one fears this problem when looking at larger embryos, but confidence wanes when looking at smaller embryos. In fact, simple logic tells us that the smaller the volume that must be interrogated for a heartbeat the less likely one is to overlook it. Missing the heartbeat in a tiny living embryo is not the problem, unless the embryo is so tiny that cardiac contractility has not yet begun, but searching a structure that is not an embryo for a heartbeat is. Still, for many years I have imposed the following rule: before an embryo is judged to be dead, it should be viewed by two independent examiners (usually a sonographer and a physician) each for a 3-minute period. To the inexperienced sonologist 6 minutes may seem a treacherously short period of time to make such a weighty decision, but the experienced examiner knows that 6 minutes is a painfully long time to view a dead embryo with a real-time sonographic device.

The final precaution cannot be simply taught, but all sonologists recognize its importance not only in the situation under consideration but in all scanning situations. We must judge the technical adequacy of the examination. If the technical quality is significantly and adversely affected by either a maternal factor or an instrument factor, extraordinary caution must be applied. With the advent of endovaginal transducers, adverse maternal factors such as obesity or uterine retroflexion can be readily overcome.

When an embryo is identified, the sonologist's task is relatively straightforward; if no heartbeat is seen and the CRL measures more than 5 mm, the pregnancy can be safely evacuated without concern that a potentially viable gestation may be interrupted, whereas the presence of an embryonic heartbeat or visualization of an embryo with a CRL of less than 5 mm and no heartbeat are clear indications for expectant observation. Unfortunately, many abnormal gestations cease development before a recognizable embryo is formed, in which case sonographic assessment is considerably more difficult.[59, 70] Difficulty arises from the fact that normal gestational sacs can be identified sonographically before the detection of the embryo. It then becomes incumbent on the examiner to discriminate a normal early pregnancy from an abnormal anembryonic pregnancy.

Despite the frequency with which "empty" gestational sacs are encountered (see Table 6–1), the literature is sparse regarding the sonographic features that can be said to discriminate normal from abnormal gestations on a single examination. One method that has been suggested is to demonstrate that the gestational sac is small for dates.[1, 40, 48, 50] This approach, however, relies on an accurate menstrual history, which is often lacking.

Sonologists are constantly asked to examine women with "poor dates." What are "good dates" and what deficiencies change dates to "poor" ones? This analysis will be confined to those situations in which a sonologist, seeing a patient for the first time and performing the examination in the first trimester, must judge whether to employ the patient's dates when judging the normalcy of the pregnancy.

As a general rule, one is always better off excluding the patient's dates from considerations about potential viability of an early pregnancy. Throughout the discussion of the sonographic features of threatened abortion the patient's dates were never considered. Only independently judged sonographic parameters are employed. However, some patients have unambiguously reliable dates and in such circumstances the addition of this factor to the analysis can be pivotal in determining that a gestation is no longer viable.

Patients undergoing ovulation induction, artificial insemination, or in vitro fertilization know precisely the date of conception. Indeed, in this small group, one would be ill advised to ignore the patient's dates. In many patients a "minimum" length of gestation can be calculated. This can be done by knowing the date that the pregnancy test became positive and the type and sensitivity of the test employed. For example, if a patient had a "serum" pregnancy test that was positive 4 weeks ago, one can very safely assume that she is at least 7.5 menstrual weeks into the pregnancy (4 weeks since the test and a minimum of 3.5 weeks for the test to become positive). The probabilities, of course, favor that she is even farther along.

Other than these circumstances one imposes an element of risk when "factoring in" a patient's dates in the analysis of the sonographic findings in threatened abortion. This is not to say that most pregnant women are unreliable historians: it is strictly a safety feature. The following features positively influence the validity of dates: infrequent exposure to intercourse, recording the basal body temperature, noting the first day of the LNMP on a calendar, a history of regular periods, an absence of recent exposure to birth control pills, and absence of unusual episodes of bleeding.[38]

A second method used to identify abnormal pregnancies is to evaluate the appearance of the gestational sac. An anomalous sonographic appearance of the gestational sac, when present, has been found to be reliable evidence of an abnormal pregnancy by some observers.[40, 48, 70–72] Others have concluded that, in the absence of an embryo, serial examinations are required to confirm abnormal growth and development before definitive treatment.[13] Anomalous morphologic features that suggest nonviability include a bizarre or irregular sac shape (Figs. 6–27 and 6–28), an unacceptably large sac size that lacks an embryo (see Figs. 6–28 and 6–29), an incompletely or poorly formed decidual reaction, absence of a double decidual sac finding, or the presence of a fluid level within the sac.[1, 40, 48, 50, 72]

Sonography can frequently distinguish abnormal from normal "empty" gestational sacs on a single examination, independent of the menstrual history.[72–75] Among the potential abnormal features listed earlier, one might well expect that some are more predictive than others (Table 6–3).[72] Certain sonographic criteria

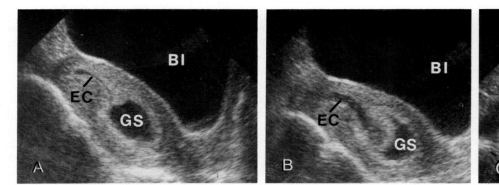

Figure 6–27. Sequential longitudinal transabdominal sonograms (*A* and *B*) with the urinary bladder (BI) distended. Longitudinal sonogram (*C*) with the urinary bladder empty. This sequence of images demonstrates a markedly distorted gestational sac (GS), which is low lying in the endometrial cavity (EC). Additionally, an endometrial accumulation of blood (H) surrounds a substantial percentage of the gestational sac (i.e., subchorionic hemorrhage). Such a gestation is clearly being evacuated by normal processes and can be judged as nonviable with certainty.

are virtually 100% specific and uniformly predict an abnormal outcome. One such criterion is an unacceptably large sac that lacks an embryo. Also, a grossly distorted sac shape invariably predicts an abnormal outcome. Since such features are reliably documented and uniformly predict an abnormal outcome, they should be considered *major criteria* for diagnosing a nonviable gestation.

The cutoff levels for visualization of embryonic parts in a gestational sac visualized by transabdominal sonography are well established and have a wide safety margin (see Table 6–3). These criteria are (1) failure to identify an embryo in a gestational sac with an MSD of 25 mm or more and (2) failure to identify a yolk sac in a gestational sac with an MSD of 20 mm or more.[72] Controversy exists in the literature regarding cutoff levels for endovaginal sonography. Criteria for the MSD at which embryonic visualization consistently occurs range from 10 to 17 mm, and for the MSD at which yolk sac visualization consistently occurs they range from 6 to 8 mm (Table 6–4).[73–75] The safety of absence of yolk sac visualization has recently been challenged.[76] As long as controversy exists, a highly conservative set of criteria for diagnosing nonviability with endovaginal sonography should be chosen by sonologic practitioners. When choosing the limits that are comfortably reliable, one can reasonably assume that endovaginal sonography enables consistent visualization of embryonic structures 1 week earlier than by transabdominal techniques. Therefore, embryos should be visualized in all gestational sacs of 18 mm or more and yolk sacs should be visualized in all gestational sacs of 13 mm or more. More stringent limits may be employed if a given examiner's experience warrants such a selection (see Table 6–4).[73–75]

Pathologic correlation suggests that large gestational sacs that lack an embryo are always abnormal and are usually due to a blighted ovum (anembryonic pregnancy) (see Figs. 6–27 through 6–29).[44, 45, 48, 49, 70] Blighted ova are common in first-trimester abortion and often demonstrate chromosomal anomalies. In the experience of Howe and associates, approximately 45% of failed first-trimester gestations demonstrate anembryonic pregnancies (see Table 6–1).[59] In these patients, trophoblastic activity may continue despite the absence of a developing embryo.[45] The trophoblastic cells continue to elaborate pregnancy hormone, although usually at a much reduced rate, thus attempting to perpetuate this already lost gestation.

Embryos can be consistently detected with endovaginal sonography when they achieve a CRL of 5 mm or more and with transabdominal sonography when they achieve a CRL of 10 mm or more. Within a 25-mm sac one expects to encounter an embryo that has a CRL of 12 mm. Volumetrically a 12-mm embryo is substantially larger than a 5-mm embryo. Even relatively inexperienced examiners are unlikely to fail to identify an embryo of this size. A similar computation may be used for endovaginal sonography. A gestational sac with an MSD of 18 mm is approximately 7 weeks menstrual age. This gives a cushion of approximately

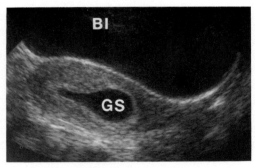

Figure 6–28. Longitudinal transabdominal sonogram of the uterus in a patient who has a threatened abortion and is also considered at risk for ectopic pregnancy. A large, distorted gestational sac (GS) is identified. The choriodecidual reaction surrounding the gestational sac is poorly echogenic compared with the bladder (BI) and myometrial interface reflection, and there is no double decidual sac finding. The mean sac diameter exceeds 25 mm, and no embryo is identified. In the absence of definitive criteria for an intrauterine pregnancy, such a patient must be considered at risk for ectopic gestation. However, if this intraendometrial fluid collection is indeed a gestational sac, one can be confident that it is nonviable (i.e., fulfills a major criterion). Therefore, the initial management decision is straightforward: evacuate the uterus and search for chorionic villi. If these villi are identified, the suspected nonviable gestation has been adequately treated and the ectopic pregnancy has been excluded.

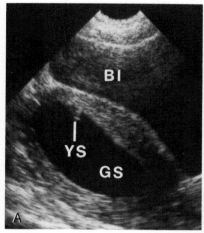
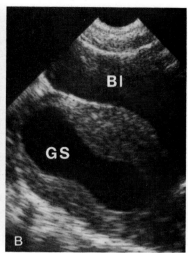

Figure 6–29. *A* and *B.* Sequential longitudinal transabdominal sonograms through the uterus of a patient who has a threatened abortion. A typical abnormal gestational sac of a so-called blighted ovum is seen. The gestational sac (GS) is quite large. An embryo should be clearly identified, yet none is seen. The yolk sac (YS) is readily noted. The margins of the gestational sac are nearly devoid of chorionic and decidual tissues. There can be no question, based on single examination, that this pregnancy is nonviable. Bl, bladder.

1 week over the age one generally detects embryos by endovaginal sonography. Thus, one may confidently employ the stated criterion to establish nonviability. Remember that this criterion is independent of the patient's dates.

That a yolk sac should normally be visible before one can demonstrate an embryo is consistent with normal embryologic development and sonographic observations of normal pregnancies (see earlier).[13, 72–75] The early yolk sac is a more conspicuous structure than the small adjacent embryo and thus detectable at an earlier stage of pregnancy. Its greater conspicuousness is related to two features. First, it is volumetrically larger than the early embryo. Second, it is a fluid-containing sac, thus possessing a relatively high subject contrast. Application of this criterion requires more experience than the identification of an embryo. With endovaginal ultrasound transducers becoming more widely available, even relatively inexperienced observers will likely adopt this criterion (Fig. 6–30). Still, the greatest value of the above criteria is that they are not subjective. The MSD is easily measured, and the yolk sac and embryo are either observed or they are not. However, again it is worthy to mention that not all

investigators agree that yolk sac nonvisualization should be used as a criterion to establish nonviability.[76]

The third major criterion that is uniformly reliable for predicting an abnormal outcome is a distorted sac shape.[72] Although the shape of a normal gestational sac may vary somewhat depending predominantly on the degree of bladder distention, grossly aberrant shapes are readily recognized by experienced sonologists and reliably predict an abnormal outcome. Unfortunately, only about 10% of abnormal gestations meet this criterion. Thus, this criterion, while useful, suffers from two problems. It is somewhat subjective and relatively insensitive.

Currently, I believe a fourth criterion is uniformly and reliably predictive of a nonviable gestation. Remember that the amnion has a period of invisibility. It can be seen clearly when an embryo reaches 13 mm CRL and occasionally is seen when the CRL is 8 mm. Therefore, visualization of the amnion (Figs. 6–31 through 6–33) without concomitent embryonic visualization would be virtually impossible in a normal gestation and would universally predict an anembryonic pregnancy.

The remaining criteria are more subjective, are less

Table 6–3. SENSITIVITY, SPECIFICITY, AND PREDICTIVE VALUES FOR SONOGRAPHIC CRITERIA OF ABNORMAL GESTATIONAL SACS (TRANSABDOMINAL TECHNIQUE)

Sonographic Criterion of Abnormal Sac	Sensitivity (%)*	Specificity (%)†	Positive Predictive Value (%)
Major			
≥ 25 mm without embryo	29	100	100
≥ 20 mm without yolk sac	41	100	100
Minor			
Thin decidual reaction (<2 mm)	28	99	96
Weak decidual amplitude	53	99	98
Irregular contour	37	99	97
Absent double decidual sac	37	98	94
Low position	20	99	94

*Abnormal outcome, n = 83.
†Normal outcome, n = 85.
Specificity and positive prediction of an abnormal outcome increase to 100% when three or more minor criteria are identified.
From Nyberg DA, Laing FC, Filly RA: Threatened abortion: Sonographic distinction of normal and abnormal gestation sacs. Radiology 158:387, 1986.

Table 6–4. SAC SIZE TO DIAGNOSE NONVIABLE EARLY INTRAUTERINE PREGNANCY BY ENDOVAGINAL SONOGRAPHY

Author	Absent Yolk Sac	Absent Embryo
Levi et al[74]	> 8 mm	> 16 mm
Bree et al[75]	> 6 mm	> 10 mm
Jain et al[73]	> 8 mm	> 17 mm
Howe et al[59]	> 13 mm	> 16 mm
University of California, San Francisco		> 18 mm

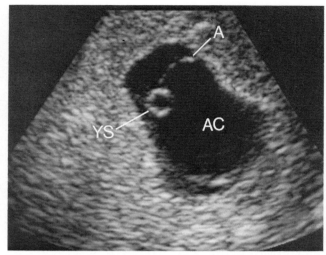

Figure 6–31. Endovaginal sonogram demonstrating a large amniotic cavity (AC) without a visible embryo. One may assume an anembryonic pregnancy exists when this observation is made. YS, yolk sac; A, amnion.

than 100% specific for diagnosing abnormal gestations, and should be considered *minor criteria.*[72] Minor criteria include a thin, weakly echogenic or irregular choriodecidual reaction (see Figs. 6–28 and 6–29), absence of a double decidual sac, and a low position of the gestational sac (see Fig. 6–27). Although diagnostic accuracy employing these criteria will undoubtedly vary with the experience of the interpreter, each minor criterion has a relatively high specificity (98% or greater) and positive predictive accuracy (94% to 98%) for diagnosing an abnormal outcome. Importantly, specificity and predictive accuracy for an abnormal outcome increase to 100% when three or more minor criteria are present.

Of the previously described five minor criteria for identification of abnormal gestations, four relate to the appearance of the "choriodecidual" tissue surrounding the sac fluid. As a rule, normal small sacs have less surrounding chorionic and decidual tissue than larger sacs. This should be kept in mind as an increasing percentage of patients are examined with endovaginal sonography. Although choriodecidual tissue is normally somewhat variable in appearance, clearly deficient choriodecidual tissue is easily noted (see Fig.

6–29). Abnormally thin and/or weakly echogenic choriodecidual tissues reliably correlate with abnormal gestational development (see Fig. 6–28). However, special note should be made that some first-trimester nonviable pregnancies instead show dramatic thickening of the chorionic tissue secondary to hydropic degeneration of villi (Fig. 6–34). Absence of a double decidual sac suggests nonviability of an early pregnancy. The double decidual sac probably disappears when decidual necrosis occurs. Importantly, the presence of a double decidual sac was originally described to discriminate early intrauterine pregnancies from other intrauterine fluid collections not representing true pregnancies. Use of this sign for distinguishing normal from abnormal early pregnancies is a secondary feature and must be judged in concert with other

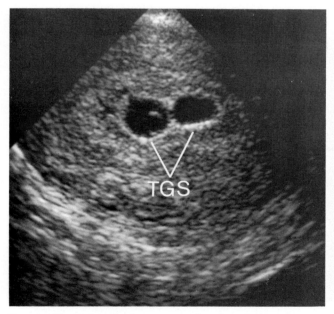

Figure 6–30. Endovaginal sonogram of early twin gestation sacs (TGS). The sac on the left contains a yolk sac while the right sac did not. Only one sac progressed.

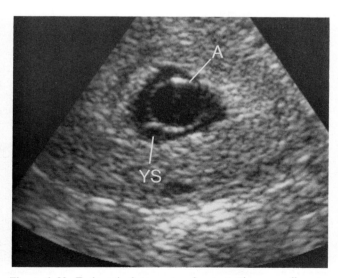

Figure 6–32. Endovaginal sonogram demonstrating a small gestational sac but a large amniotic cavity. Again, a nonviable pregnancy many be inferred from the absence of an embryo when the amnion (A) is clearly seen. YS, yolk sac.

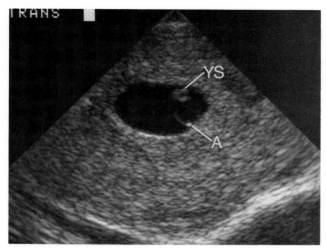

Figure 6–33. A tiny yolk sac (YS) and amnion (A) are seen on this endovaginal sonogram. Amnions like this may have been mistaken for large yolk sacs in the past.

findings of abnormal gestational sac development. Occasionally, a double decidual sac is not visible for small (less than 10 mm) normal gestational sacs.

The fifth, and final, minor criterion used to identify an abnormal gestation is a low position of the gestational sac. This feature has been previously reported as useful by some observers. Low position of the gestational sac is a stage rather than a cause of abortion (see Fig. 6–27). Thus, one would expect this feature to be highly reliable for prediction of subsequent pregnancy loss. Unfortunately, this observation is again a relatively subjective and insensitive one. A low position of the gestational sac, situated in whole or in part within the lower uterine segment, is seen in only 20% of abnormal pregnancies and predicts an abnormal outcome in 94% of cases (see Table 6–3).

CORRELATION OF GESTATIONAL SAC SIZE AND hCG LEVEL

Since "minor criteria" are relatively subjective judgments, it would be helpful to have a less subjective criterion to employ when evaluating small gestational sacs that lack embryonic structures. Sonographic examination of intrauterine contents correlated with si-multaneous serum hCG determinations has been found to be a useful method for evaluating early normal intrauterine pregnancies.[12, 75] A close relationship between sonographic findings and quantitative serum hCG levels normally exists during early pregnancy. Gestational sac size and hCG levels increase proportionately until 8 menstrual weeks, at which time the gestational sac is approximately 25 mm MSD and an embryo should be easily detected by either transabdominal or endovaginal sonography.[10, 61, 62] After 8 weeks, hCG levels plateau and subsequently decline while the gestational sac continues to grow.

As noted earlier, quantitative hCG levels strongly correlate with gestational sac size in normal pregnancies. This enables one to employ a quantitative serum hCG level as an additional, less subjective feature to assist in the establishment of normalcy or abnormalcy of pregnancies without a visible living embryo. Remember that the small gestational sac is the most difficult to evaluate for potentially abnormal features. Evidence indicates that a normal gestational sac can be consistently demonstrated when the hCG level is 1800 mIu/mL (Second International Standard) or greater when using transabdominal sonography. This detection threshold is significantly reduced by endovaginal sonography and may be as low as 500 mIu/mL.[10, 15–17, 75, 77] However, I use the more conservative estimate of 1000 mIu/mL. The relationship between quantitative serum hCG levels and sac size is not unexpected since both sac development and hCG production are a function of trophoblastic activity. A normal gestational sac grows approximately 1.1 mm/d while hCG levels rise exponentially, doubling every 2 to 3 days.[17] The expected relationship between sonographic findings and simultaneous hCG levels is not observed in many abnormal gestations.[77] This augments reliable identification of abnormal gestations on the basis of a single examination despite the absence of a detectable embryo. Again, correlation with the menstrual history is not required and women with an uncertain LNMP and women with irregular vaginal bleeding can be evaluated by this method.

Almost without exception, abnormal pregnancies demonstrate a low hCG level relative to gestational sac development.[12, 51, 77] Comparison of the hCG levels with the gestational sac size demonstrated disproportionately low levels for 65% of abnormal gestational sacs in an evaluation performed with transabdominal

Figure 6–34. Longitudinal (A) and transverse (B) transabdominal sonograms of the uterus in a patient who has a threatened abortion. Unlike the situation in Figure 6–29, the chorionic tissue is markedly thickened (arrow) and demonstrates hydropic villi (HV). This pattern is a less common manifestation in early embryonic demise, associated with villus hydrops rather than atrophy. Bl, bladder.

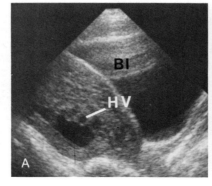
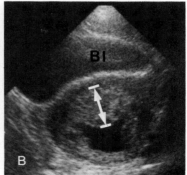

sonography.[77] These data support prior results indicating that hCG levels frequently fall before spontaneous expulsion of nonviable gestations.[12, 78] As expected, similar data are applicable to endovaginal sonography and smaller gestational sacs. However, application of this concept for diagnosis of nonviability in very small sacs is likely to be less helpful than when sac size is larger. Furthermore, simultaneous hCG levels are unlikely to be useful for diagnosing abnormal pregnancies when the sonographic examination fails to detect a gestational sac. In this situation the major competing pathologic diagnosis is ectopic pregnancy.

There is bound to be some overlap between purely sonographic findings of an abnormal sac and correlation of sac size with quantitative hCG levels. Indeed, some data suggest that these two methods identify similar groups of patients.[70] When hCG levels are disproportionately low, the gestation usually demonstrates abnormal sonographic features, including a weak or irregular choriodecidual reaction. This is not unexpected since the chorionic tissue elaborates hCG. However, these sonographic criteria are subjective and require an experienced sonologist for their correct interpretation. Quantitative hCG levels and measurement of the mean sac size are more easily assessed and may be objectively compared with normal data. When the sonographic findings alone are uncertain or when confirmation is desired, a disproportionately low hCG is supportive evidence for an abnormal pregnancy.

This section appropriately began with a quote from Robinson regarding goals and objectives in the evaluation of pregnancy failure and can appropriately end with an admonition from Robinson: "Any other worker wishing to provide (this service) must be prepared to establish these techniques in his own hands with a period of nonintervention and with good lines of communication (with referring clinicians)."[1]

EVALUATION OF MASSES IN EARLY PREGNANCY

There are two relatively common pathologic masses seen in early pregnancy and one very common "physiologic" mass. The pathologic masses are uterine myomas and ovarian corpus luteum cysts; the physiologic mass is the so-called focal myometrial contraction. The myomas must be distinguished from focal myometrial contractions, a sometimes difficult task, and the corpus luteum cysts must be distinguished from ovarian neoplastic cysts (e.g., cystadenomas, cystadenocarcinomas, and cystic teratomas), always an important task.

Distinguishing between a myoma and a focal myometrial contraction (Fig. 6–35) is occasionally difficult, but the following rules usually result in an accurate discrimination. Remember that the following are tendencies, and both overlap and variations exist.

1. A myoma tends to be hypoechoic relative to the adjacent myometrium, but a focal myometrial contraction tends to be isoechoic with the adjacent myometrium.

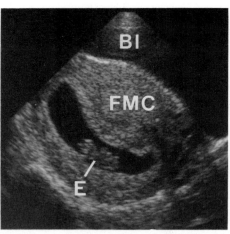

Figure 6–35. Transverse transabdominal sonogram demonstrating a typical focal myometrial contraction (FMC). E, embryo; Bl, bladder.

2. A myoma attenuates the acoustic beam, but a focal myometrial contraction does not.

3. The mass effect of a myoma tends to distort both the serosal and endometrial contours of the uterus, but that from a focal myometrial contraction tends to distort only the endometrial surface.

4. A focal myometrial contraction is virtually always homogeneous; a myoma is sometimes heterogeneous in echo texture.

5. On color Doppler studies a focal myometrial contraction tends to show multiple vessels while a myoma tends to be hypovascular.

If necessary, a patient always can be reexamined after a short interval to distinguish between a contraction and a myoma. It is rarely necessary to delay a patient for this purpose since segregating these two entities is hardly a critical distinction. Occasionally, an exophytic area of myometrial tissue is neither a focal myometrial contraction nor a myoma but a nongravid horn of a bicornuate uterus. This is usually readily recognized since there is decidualized endometrium centrally positioned within the observed tissue.

The major problem caused by myomas in early pregnancy is related to the spontaneous abortion of otherwise normal embryos.[64] This is particularly true of submucous myomas and numerous myomas that distort the uterus. Although myomas may grow to a very large size during pregnancy, undergo necrosis, precipitate preterm labor, or interfere with vaginal delivery, none of these situations pertain to the first trimester.[79]

The life cycle of the corpus luteum begins with rupture of the graafian follicle. The follicle wall collapses, and the cells lining the follicle undergo proliferation and alteration to lutein cells.[80] These cells elaborate progesterone to support any possible pregnancy. Morphologically, a corpus luteum is a thick-walled, noncystic structure that may attain a size up to 2 cm (Fig. 6–36). The corpus luteum continues to enlarge if pregnancy occurs. This structure may now occupy as much as half of the ovary. Normally, the

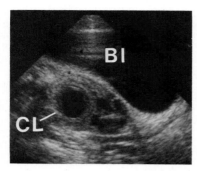

Figure 6–36. Longitudinal transabdominal sonogram of the left ovary in a patient with a normal, ongoing first-trimester pregnancy. A typical corpus luteum cyst (CL) is identified. Note the thick wall and echolucent center. Bl, bladder.

corpus luteum of pregnancy begins to regress after 10 weeks; its function is gradually taken over by the developing placenta. From a practical pathologic perspective, the corpus luteum is called "cystic" when it exceeds 3 cm.[81] It is the central zone that organizes into a cyst; the gelatinous liquid contained therein is fibrin. Occasionally, these cysts become quite large, at times exceeding 10 cm.

Although any type of ovarian tumor may complicate early pregnancy, unilocular cysts, even those with somewhat thickened walls, that are discovered in the first trimester should be assumed to represent corpus luteum cysts and should be observed. These lesions are so common during this stage of pregnancy that it would be impractical to proceed with invasive diagnostic procedures, such as laparoscopy, or to elect to excise the lesion before sufficient time has been allotted to examine the mass serially. Corpus luteum cysts, like the corpus luteum of pregnancy, tend to regress as the end of the first trimester nears.

Follow-up evaluation at the beginning of the second trimester (14 menstrual weeks) usually shows the lesion to be regressing or gone.[79–81] Furthermore, laparotomy for ovarian masses is usually not conducted until the mid second trimester (after the 18th week), provided, of course, that the operation can be postponed until then.[79] This is a period of quiescence of the uterine muscle; thus laparotomy is unlikely to precipitate abortion. This additional time can be used to advantage for further follow-up since, occasionally, these lesions do not regress until later than ordinarily expected. Despite all these precautions and the long period available to follow these masses for regression, corpus luteum cysts occasionally disobey all the rules and continue to expand, and thus become suspect as true ovarian neoplasms.

The decision to remove an asymptomatic ovarian mass is a clinical one.[79] Malignant tumors of the ovary are exceedingly rare complications of pregnancy. Even though ultrasound evaluation may be unable to exclude a malignancy on the basis of observed morphology of the lesion, one should not employ this deficiency as evidence that the mass must be excised.

Glossary

Abortion. The premature expulsion from the uterus of embryonic products of conception or a nonviable fetus.

Blighted ovum. A fertilized ovum in which development has become arrested.

Complete abortion. Abortion in which all the products of conception have been expelled from the uterus and identified.

Fetus. The developing young in the human uterus after the end of the 11th menstrual week. Before this, it is called an embryo; it becomes a neonate when it is completely outside the body of the mother, even before the cord is out.

Imminent abortion. Impending abortion in which the bleeding is profuse, the cervix softened and dilated, and the cramps approach the character of labor pains.

Inevitable abortion. Abortion in progress.

Missed abortion. Retention of a dead pregnancy for at least 2 months.

Viable. Capable of living, especially as it refers to a fetus that has reached such a stage of development that it can live outside the uterus.

References

1. Robinson HP: The diagnosis of early pregnancy failure by sonar. Br J Obstet Gynaecol 82:849, 1975.
2. Soules MR: The in vitro fertilization pregnancy rate: Let's be honest with one another. (Editorial) Fertil Steril 43:511, 1985.
3. Jones HW, Acosta AA, Andrews MC, et al: What is a pregnancy? A question for programs of in vitro fertilization. Fertil Steril 40:728, 1983.
4. Edmonds DK, Linday KS, Miller JR, et al: Early embryonic mortality in women. Fertil Steril 38:447, 1982.
5. Schlesselman JJ: How does one assess the risk of abnormalities from human in vitro fertilization? Am J Obstet Gynecol 135:135, 1979.
6. Moore KL: The beginning of development: The first week. In Moore KL (ed): The Developing Human, 3rd ed, p 14. Philadelphia, WB Saunders, 1982.
7. Moore KL: Formation of the bilaminar embryo. In Moore KL (ed): The Developing Human, 3rd ed, p 40. Philadelphia, WB Saunders, 1982.
8. Moore KL: The fetal membranes and placenta. In Moore KL (ed): The Developing Human, 3rd ed, p 111. Philadelphia, WB Saunders, 1982.
9. Hellman LM, Kobayashi M, Fillisti L, et al: Growth and development of the human fetus prior to the twentieth week of gestation. Am J Obstet Gynecol 103:789, 1969.
10. Nyberg DA, Filly RA, Mahony BS, et al: Early gestation: Correlation of hCG levels and sonographic identification. AJR 144:951, 1985.
11. Cadkin AV, McAlpin J: Detection of fetal cardiac activity between 41 and 43 days of gestation. J Ultrasound Med 3:499, 1984.
12. Batzer FR, Weiner S, Corson SL, et al: Landmarks during the first forty-two days of gestation demonstrated by the β-subunit of human chorionic gonadotropin and ultrasound. Am J Obstet Gynecol 146:973, 1983.
13. Bernard KG, Cooperberg PL: Sonographic differentiation between blighted ovum and early viable pregnancy. AJR 144:597, 1985.

14. de Crispigny LC, Cooper D, McKenna M: Early detection of intrauterine pregnancy with ultrasound. J Ultrasound Med 7:7, 1988.

15. Goldstein SR, Synder JR, Watson C, et al: Very early pregnancy detection with endovaginal ultrasound. Obstet Gynecol 72:200, 1988.

16. Daya S, Woods S, Ward S, et al: Transvaginal ultrasound scanning in early pregnancy and correlation with human chorionic gonadotropin levels. J Clin Ultrasound 19:139, 1991.

17. Timor-Tritsch IE, Farine D, Rosen MG: A close look at early embryonic development with the high-frequency transvaginal transducer. Am J Obstet Gynecol 159:676, 1988.

18. Laing FC, Filly RA, Marks W, et al: Ultrasonic demonstration of endometrial fluid collections unassociated with pregnancy. Radiology 137:471, 1980.

19. Nyberg DA, Laing FC, Filly RA, et al: Ultrasonographic differentiation of the gestational sac of early intrauterine pregnancy from the pseudogestational sac of ectopic pregnancy. Radiology 146:755, 1983.

20. Cadkin AV, McAlpin J: The decidua-chorionic sac: A reliable sonographic indicator of intrauterine pregnancy prior to detection of a fetal pole. J Ultrasound Med 3:539, 1984.

21. Marks WM, Filly RA, Callen PW, et al: The decidual cast of ectopic pregnancy: A confusing ultrasonographic appearance. Radiology 133:451, 1979.

22. Bradley WG, Fiske CE, Filly RA: The double sac sign of early intrauterine pregnancy: Use in exclusion of ectopic pregnancy. Radiology 143:223, 1983.

23. Yeh HC, Goodman JD, Carr L, Rabinowitz JG: Intradecidual sign: A US criterion of early intrauterine pregnancy. Radiology 161:463, 1986.

24. Nyberg DA, Mack LA, Laing FC, Patten RM. Distinguishing normal from abnormal gestational sac growth in early pregnancy. J Ultrasound Med 6:23, 1987.

25. Warren WB, Timor-Tritsch I, Peisner OB, et al: Dating the early pregnancy by sequential appearance of embryonic structures. Am J Obstet Gynecol 161:747, 1989.

26. Yeh HC, Rabinowitz JG: Amniotic sac development: Ultrasound features of early pregnancy—the double bleb sign. Radiology 166:97, 1988.

27. Levi CS, Lyons EA, Zheng XH, et al: Endovaginal US: Demonstration of cardiac activity in embryos of less than 5.0 mm in crown-rump length. Radiology 176:71, 1990.

28. Brown DL, Emerson DS, Felker RE, et al: Diagnosis of early embryonic demise by endovaginal sonography. J Ultrasound Med 9:631, 1990.

29. Mahony BS, Filly RA: High resolution sonographic assessment of the fetal extremities. J Ultrasound Med 3:489, 1984.

30. Jeanty P, Renoy P, Van Kerkem J, et al: Ultrasonic demonstration of the amnion. J Ultrasound Med 1:243, 1982.

31. Burrows PE, Lyons EA, Phillips HJ, Oates I: Intrauterine membranes: Sonographic findings and clinical significance. J Clin Ultrasound 10:1, 1982.

32. Lofberg L, Iosif CS, Edvall H, Gustavii B: Direct vision sampling of chorionic villi during extra-amniotic instillation of physiologic saline. Am J Obstet Gynecol 152:591, 1985.

33. Robinson HP, Fleming JEE: A critical evaluation of sonar crown-rump length measurements. Br J Obstet Gynaecol 82:702, 1975.

34. Robinson HP: Sonar measurement of the fetal crown-rump length as a means of assessing maturity in the first trimester of pregnancy. Br Med J 4:28, 1973.

35. Kurjak A, Cecuk S, Breyer B: Prediction of maturity in the first trimester of pregnancy by ultrasonic measurement of fetal crown-rump length. J Clin Ultrasound 4:83, 1976.

36. Drumm JE: The prediction of delivery date by ultrasonic measurement of fetal crown-rump length. Br J Obstet Gynaecol 84:1, 1977.

37. Chervenak FA, Brightman RC, Thornton T, et al: Crown-rump length and serum human chorionic gonadotropin as predictors of gestational age. Obstet Gynecol 67:21, 1986.

38. Campbell S, Warsof SL, Little D, Cooper DJ: Routine ultrasound screening for the prediction of gestational age. Obstet Gynecol 65:613, 1985.

39. Kohorn E, Kaufman M: Sonar in the first trimester of pregnancy. Obstet Gynecol 44:473, 1974.

40. Duff GB: The prognosis in threatened abortion: A comparison between predictions made by sonar, urinary hormone assays and clinical judgement. Br J Obstet Gynaecol 82:858, 1975.

41. Drumm J, Clinch J: Ultrasound in management of clinically diagnosed threatened abortion. Br Med J 2:424, 1975.

42. Jouppila P: Diagnostics in threatened abortion: A study by ultrasonic, clinical, hormonal and histopathological methods. Ultrasound Med 3A:595, 1976.

43. Smith C, Gregori C, Breen J: Ultrasonography in threatened abortion. Obstet Gynecol 51:173, 1978.

44. Young GB, McDicken WN: Signs of fetal death in early pregnancy. J Clin Ultrasound 6:244, 1978.

45. Hertz JB: Diagnostic procedures in threatened abortion. Obstet Gynecol 66:223, 1984.

46. Fantel AG, Shepard TH: Basic aspects of early (first trimester) abortion. In Iffy L, Kaminetsky HA (eds): Principle and Practice of Obstetrics and Perinatology, vol 1, New York, John Wiley & Sons, 1981, p 553.

47. Cavanagh D, Comas MR: Spontaneous abortion. In Danforth DN (ed): Obstetrics and Gynecology, p 378. Philadelphia, Harper & Row, 1982.

48. Donald I, Morley P, Barnett E: The diagnosis of blighted ovum by sonar. Br J Obstet Gynecol 79:304, 1972.

49. Jouppila P, Huhtaniemi I, Tapanainen J: Early pregnancy failure: Study by ultrasonic and hormonal methods. Obstet Gynecol 55:42, 1980.

50. Anderson SG: Management of threatened abortion with real-time sonography. Obstet Gynecol 55:259, 1980.

51. Braunstein GD, Karow WG, Gentry WC, et al: First trimester chorionic gonadotropin measurements as an aid in the diagnosis of early pregnancy disorders. Am J Obstet Gynecol 131:25, 1978.

52. Ericksen PS, Philipsen T: Prognosis in threatened abortion evaluated by hormone assays and ultrasound scanning. Obstet Gynecol 55:435, 1980.

53. Goldstein RB: Endovaginal sonography in very early pregnancy: New observations. Radiology 176:7, 1990.

54. Wilson RD, Kendrick V, Wittman BK, McGillivray B: Spontaneous abortion and pregnancy outcome after normal first trimester ultrasound examination. Obstet Gynecol 67:352, 1986.

55. Christiaens GC, Stoutenbeek P: Spontaneous abortions in proven intact pregnancies. Lancet 2:57, 1984.

56. Mantoni M: Ultrasound signs of threatened abortion and their significance. Obstet Gynecol 65:471, 1985.

57. Goldstein SR, Subramanyan BR, Raghavendra BN, et al: Subchorionic bleeding in threatened abortion: Sonographic findings and significance. AJR 141:975, 1983.

58. May DA, Sturtevant NV: Embryonal heart rate as a predictor of pregnancy outcome: A prospective analysis. J Ultrasound Med 10:591, 1991.

59. Howe RS, Isaacson KJ, Albert JL, Coutifaris CB: Embryonic heart rate in human pregnancy. J Ultrasound Med 10:367, 1991.

60. Borlum KG, Thomsen A, Clausen I, Eriksen G: Long-term prognosis of pregnancies in women with intrauterine hematomas. Obstet Gynecol 74:231, 1989.

61. Stabile I, Campbell S, Grudzinskas JG: Threatened miscarriage and intrauterine hematomas. J Ultrasound Med 8:289, 1989.

62. Pedersen JF, Mantoni M: Prevalence and significance of subchorionic hemorrhage in threatened abortion: A sonographic study. AJR 154:535, 1990.

63. Laboda LA, Estroff JA, Benacerraf BR: First trimester bradycardia: A sign of impending fetal loss. J Ultrasound Med 8:561, 1989.

64. Nazari A, Check JH, Epstein RH, et al: Relationship of small-for-dates sac size to crown-rump length and spontaneous abortion in patients with a known date of ovulation. Obstet Gynecol 78:369, 1991.

65. Bromley B, Harlow BL, Laboda LA, Benacerraf BR: Small sac size in the first trimester: A predictor of poor fetal outcome. Radiology 178:375, 1991.

66. Reece EA, Scioscia AL, Pinter E, et al: Prognostic significance of the human yolk sac assessed by ultrasonography. Am J Obstet Gyncol 159:1191, 1988.

67. Ferrazzi E, Brambati B, Lanzani A, et al: The yolk sac in early pregnancy failure. Am J Obstet Gynecol 158:137, 1988.

68. Dickey RP, Olar TT, Taylor SN, et al: Relation of small

gestation sac–crown-rump length differences to abortion and abortus karyotypes. Obstet Gynecol 79:554, 1992.

69. Ghorashi B, Gottesfeld KR: The gray scale appearance of the normal pregnancy from 4 to 16 weeks of gestation. J Clin Ultrasound 5:195, 1977.

70. Jouppila P, Herva T: Study of blighted ovum by ultrasonic and histopathologic methods. Obstet Gynecol 55:574, 1980.

71. Young GB, McDicken WN: Signs of fetal death in early pregnancy. J Clin Ultrasound 6:1244, 1978.

72. Nyberg DA, Laing FC, Filly RA: Threatened abortion: Sonographic distinction of normal and abnormal gestation sacs. Radiology 158:397, 1986.

73. Jain KA, Hamper UM, Sanders RC: Comparison of transvaginal and transabdominal sonography in detection of early pregnancy and it complications. AJR 151:1139, 1988.

74. Levi CS, Lyons EA, Lindsay DJ: Early diagnosis of nonviable pregnancy with endovaginal US. Radiology 167:383, 1988.

75. Bree RL, Edwards M, Bohm-Velez M, et al: Transvaginal sonography in the evaluation of normal early pregnancy: Correlation with hCG levels. AJR 153:75, 1989.

76. Kurtz AB, Needleman L, Pennell RG, et al: Can detection of the yolk sac in the first trimester be used to predict the outcome of pregnancy? A prospective sonographic study. AJR 158:843, 1992.

77. Nyberg DA, Filly RA, Filho DLD, et al: Abnormal pregnancy: Early diagnosis by US and serum chorionic gonadotropin levels. Radiology 158:393, 1986.

78. Yuen BH, Livingston JE, Poland BJ, et al: Human chorionic gonadotropin, estradiol, progesterone, prolactin, and B-scan ultrasound monitoring of complications in early pregnancy. Obstet Gynecol 57:207, 1981.

79. Nesbitt REL, Abdul-Karim RW: Coincidental disorders complicating pregnancy. In Danforth DN (ed): Obstetrics and Gynecology. 4th ed, p 542. Philadelphia, Harper & Row, 1982.

80. Blaustein A: Anatomy and histology of the human ovary. In Blaustein A (ed): Pathology of the Female Genital Tract, p 378. New York, Springer Verlag, 1977.

81. Kraus FT: Female genitalia. In Anderson WAD, Kissane JM (eds): Pathology, 7th ed, p 1731. St. Louis, CV Mosby, 1977.

CHAPTER 7

Ultrasound Determination of Menstrual Age

FRANK P. HADLOCK, M.D.

It is important from the outset to establish what is meant by the term *menstrual age* and why it is so important in clinical obstetrics. *Fetal age* actually begins at conception, and an equivalent term is *conceptional age*. By convention, however, obstetricians date pregnancies in menstrual weeks, beginning from the first day of the last normal menstrual period. The appropriate term for this method of fetal dating is *menstrual age,* and this term is used exclusively in this chapter in reference to the duration of a pregnancy using ultrasound evaluation.[1] Many obstetricians also use the term *gestational age*. Although *gestational age* should be equivalent to *conceptual age*, in practice, *gestational age* is used interchangably with *menstrual age*. The term *conceptional age* will only be used to describe pregnancies in which the actual date of conception is known; this is uncommon and is usually restricted to patients who have undergone in vitro fertilization or artificial insemination. If conceptual age is known, the menstrual age should be standardized to reflect conceptual age, based on the assumption of mid-cycle ovulation (menstrual age = conceptual age + 14 days). Once this has been done, the menstrual age is established and should never be changed later in pregnancy. Subsequent fetal measurements then become an index of fetal growth rather than menstrual age.

Knowledge of menstrual age is important to the obstetrician because it affects clinical management in a number of important ways. First, knowledge of menstrual age is used in early pregnancy for the scheduling of invasive procedures such as chorionic villus sampling and genetic amniocentesis and in the interpretation of biochemical tests such as maternal serum α-fetoprotein screening, in which the normal range of values changes over time. Second, knowledge of menstrual age allows the obstetrician to anticipate normal spontaneous delivery, or to plan elective delivery, within the time frame of a term pregnancy (38 to 42 weeks); this also allows the physician to institute measures that will optimize fetal outcome in cases in which labor ensues before 38 weeks or fails to ensue after 42 weeks. Third, knowledge of menstrual age is important in evaluating fetal growth, because the normal range for the size of any fetal parameter changes with advancing age.[1] Thus, a fetal weight of 2000 g would be normal at 33 weeks but would indicate severe growth retardation at 40 weeks. To base important clinical decisions such as these on knowledge of menstrual age, menstrual age should ideally be established or corroborated early in pregnancy.

Before the advent of ultrasound evaluation, the determination of menstrual age was established prenatally by menstrual history, corroborated during pregnancy by physical examination of the fundal height, and confirmed in the postnatal period by physical examination of the neonate.[2, 3] All three of these parameters were notoriously inaccurate (Table 7–1), but the menstrual history could be especially misleading for a number of reasons. First, many women may not accurately recall the first day of the last normal menstrual period, particularly if they are not trying to conceive. Moreover, in those who do remember the last normal menstrual period, it may be unreliable or misleading because of oligomenorrhea, implantation bleeding, the use of oral contraceptives, becoming pregnant in the first ovulatory cycle following a recent delivery, or ovulating very early (<day 11) or very late (>day 21) in the menstrual cycle. The latter point may be particularly important, since Matsumoto and coworkers[4] reported that early or late ovulation occurs in approximately 20% of the population (Fig. 7–1). It is not surprising, then, that both Campbell and colleagues[5] and Waldenström and coworkers[6] found that in patients with optimal menstrual histories (certain last normal menstrual period, regular menses, no exposure to oral contraceptives, and no unusual bleeding), a single second-trimester biparietal diameter (BPD) measurement was more predictive of the estimated date of confinement than an optimal menstrual history. It is for these reasons that the use of ultrasonography as a tool for determining menstrual dates has been so readily accepted into the practice of clinical obstetrics.

Ultrasound studies designed to evaluate the duration of pregnancy are based on measurements of the fetus, using size as an indirect indicator of menstrual age.[5–68] The parameter(s) are chosen for study based on their ease of measurement and the degree to which they can reflect menstrual age. These studies have usually relied on cross-sectional evaluation of large numbers of patients with known dates of the beginning of the last normal menstrual period and no compounding variables in the menstrual history to question its validity. Rossavik and Fishburne have demonstrated that such populations are equivalent to populations with known conception dates for studies of this type.[30] Most studies also eliminate patients with multiple gestation and those with a history that might adversely affect fetal growth. In a properly designed cross-sectional analysis of any fetal parameter, measurements are made in a

Table 7–1. METHODS FOR DETERMINING MENSTRUAL AGE

Clinical or Sonographic Parameter	Variability Estimate (+2 SD)
In vitro fertilization*	±1 day
Ovulation induction*	±3 days
Artificial insemination*	±3 days
Single intercourse record*	±3 days
Basal body temperature record*	±4 days
First-trimester physical examination	±2 weeks
Second-trimester physical examination	±4 weeks
Third-trimester physical examination	±6 weeks
First-trimester sonographic examination (crown-rump length)	±8 % of the estimate
Second-trimester sonographic examination (head circumference, femur length)	±8 % of the estimate
Third-trimester sonographic examination (head circumference, femur length)	±8 % of the estimate

*These are indicators of conceptual age (menstrual age = conceptual age + 14 days).
Adapted from James D. Bowie, M.D.

large number of fetuses evenly distributed over the entire range of menstrual ages, with each fetus being measured only once in gestation; the latter point is important in avoiding bias in variability estimates. The data are then analyzed using regression analysis, with menstrual age as the dependent variable, and equations are generated that will predict menstrual age for any given measurement or set of measurements. Most of the published tables that provide predictions of menstrual age from ultrasound measurements have been generated in this way.[1]

Regardless of the number of sonographic measurements that we employ in predicting menstrual age, it is very important to remember that we are simply inferring age from size and to understand the variability that can be associated with that estimate. The variability, usually the result of measurement error or actual biologic variability in size, is expressed as plus or minus 2 standard deviations (±2SD), which should be applicable to 95% of the fetuses in a normal population. One must always keep in mind, however, that 5% of the time our estimates will be outside this range;

inspection of the magnitude of the maximum errors observed in the original regression data will give a general idea about the largest mistake one could make in predicting menstrual age in a prospective population. Reporting a menstrual age estimate to one or two decimal places for a given fetal measurement or set of measurements, without providing the variability estimate, gives an unrealistic idea about the accuracy of the method. In this chapter, the measurement or set of measurements of the fetus described in the literature that are preferable for determination of menstrual age and the magnitude of the variability associated with their use are determined.

FIRST TRIMESTER OF PREGNANCY (0 TO 13 WEEKS)

The earliest unequivocal sign of pregnancy using ultrasound evaluation is the demonstration of the early gestational sac.[7-13] With the use of the original static image equipment and early transabdominal real-time equipment, the gestational sac could not be visualized until approximately 6 menstrual weeks, but with the new high-resolution real-time equipment, particularly the vaginal probes, the gestational sac can usually be seen by 5 menstrual weeks. The early embryonic pole cannot be seen at this time, but there are two features that differentiate the gestational sac from the pseudo-gestational sac of an ectopic gestation. One is the double decidual sac sign, which is created by apposition of the decidua parietalis and the decidua capsularis.[10] A more reliable sign is the visualization of the yolk sac within the gestational sac; this can be seen using high-resolution vaginal probes during the fifth menstrual week (Fig. 7–2). At this early stage in gestation, the average internal diameter of the gestational sac, calculated as the mean of the anteroposterior diameter, the transverse diameter, and the longitudinal diameter, can provide an adequate estimation of menstrual age in a normally developing pregnancy (Table 7–2). However, the mean sac diameter becomes progressively less reliable as pregnancy advances and the measurement of choice for estimation of menstrual age in the first trimester is the fetal crown-rump length (CRL).

Figure 7–1. Length of the follicular phase of the menstrual cycle in a large number of patients studied by Matsumoto and coworkers.[4] Note that the distribution is skewed to the right, with a higher number of patients ovulating late in the cycle (> day 21) than earlier in the cycle (< day 11). This corresponds to the findings in the study by Waldenstrom and colleagues,[6] in which an early mid-trimester ultrasound study agreed with the menstrual history in only about 80% of the cases. In 3% the age by ultrasound evaluation was greater than expected from the optimal menstrual history (corresponding to early ovulation) and in about 17% the age by ultrasound evaluation was less than expected from the optimal menstrual history (indicating late ovulation). (Adapted from Matsumoto S, Nogami Y, Ohkuri S: Statistical studies on menstruation: A criticism on the definition of normal menstruation. Gumma J Med Sci 11:294, 1962).

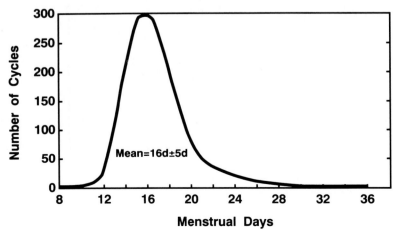

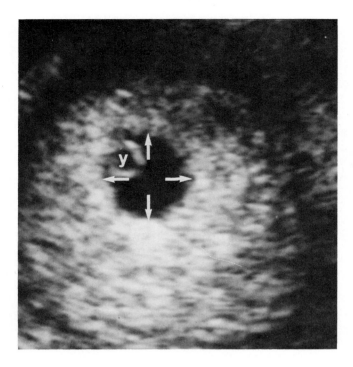

Figure 7–2. This high-resolution endovaginal real-time image demonstrates the appearance of the normal gestational sac at approximately 5 menstrual weeks. At this time the yolk sac (y) is identifiable and confirms that the sac is a pregnancy sac and not the pseudo sac of an ectopic gestation. The arrows indicate the appropriate method of measuring the internal diameters of the sac. The mean sac diameter is calculated as the average of the three internal diameters of the sac (anteroposterior, transverse, and longitudinal). At this stage in gestation, the early embryonic pole is not visible in most cases.

By the sixth menstrual week, one can usually identify the early embryonic pole and definite cardiac activity in normally developing pregnancies (Fig. 7–3A). However, better visualization of the early embryo can be made between 7 and 13 menstrual weeks (Fig. 7–3B). Warren and coworkers[13] have demonstrated the developmental landmarks of the embryo during this time frame (Fig. 7–4). Although these anatomic features can provide clues to the age of the fetus, better estimates of menstrual age can be made by measurement of the fetal CRL.[11, 14–26] When using the CRL to predict menstrual age, one should use the average CRL measurement from three satisfactory images and then refer to published tables or equations for estimation of menstrual age (Table 7–3).

In general, there has been extreme uniformity in the CRL data from various centers dating back to the original studies of Robinson,[14, 15] and it has been demonstrated that measurements made with static image equipment, transabdominal real-time equipment, and endovaginal real-time equipment demonstrate no significant differences. Additionally, Silva and co-

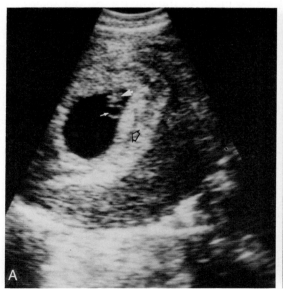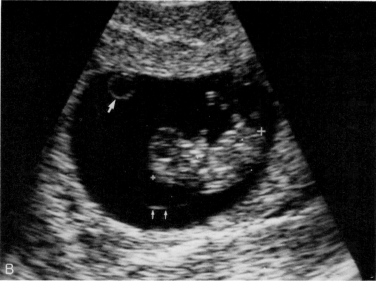

Figure 7–3. *A.* This high-resolution endovaginal real-time image demonstrates the early embryonic pole *(large arrow),* which measures approximately 3 mm in this case, corresponding to a menstrual age of approximately 6 weeks ±8% (±3 days). The yolk sac *(small arrow)* is again identified. The open arrow identifies the double-decidual sac sign. *B.* This high-resolution endovaginal real-time image demonstrates the typical appearance of the crown-rump length. In this case, the crown-rump length measurement is 2.3 cm, corresponding to a menstrual age of approximately 9 weeks. The variability of the mestimate is ±8% (±0.72 weeks). The yolk sac *(arrow)* is again identified, and the unfused amnion *(small arrows)* is also seen.

PERCENT OF EMBRYONIC STRUCTURES PRESENT OR ABSENT

☐ STRUCTURE PRESENT   ■ STRUCTURE ABSENT

WEEKS OF GESTATION	4	5	6	7	8	9	10	11	12
GESTATIONAL SAC ONLY	100	→							
YOLK SAC	0	91	100	→					
FETAL POLE WITH HEART MOTION	0	0	86	100	→				
SINGLE VENTRICLE	0	0	6	82	70	25	0	0	0
FALX	0	0	0	0	30	75	100	100	100
MIDGUT HERNIATION	0	0	0	0	100	100	100	50	0
TOTAL CASES	6	11	15	17	10	13	15	11	6

Figure 7–4. Sequential appearance of significant findings in the first trimester of pregnancy. Note that the gestational sac was identified in 100% of cases beginning at 5 menstrual weeks. (From Warren WB, Timor-Tritsch I, Peisner DB, Raju S, Rosen MG: Dating the early pregnancy by sequential appearance of embryonic structures. Am J Obstet Gynecol 161:747, 1989.)

Table 7–2. RELATION BETWEEN MEAN SAC DIAMETER, MENSTRUAL AGE, AND HUMAN CHORIONIC GONADOTROPIN (hCG) LEVEL

Mean Gestational Sac Diameter (mm)	Predicted Age (wk) Range = 95% CI*	Predicted hCG (mIU/mL) Range = 95% CI†
2	5.0 (4.5–5.5)	1164 (629–2188)
3	5.1 (4.6–5.6)	1377 (771–2589)
4	5.2 (4.8–5.7)	1629 (863–3036)
5	5.4 (4.9–5.8)	1932 (1026–3636)
6	5.5 (5.0–6.0)	2165 (1226–4256)
7	5.6 (5.1–6.1)	2704 (1465–4990)
8	5.7 (5.3–6.2)	3199 (1749–5852)
9	5.9 (5.4–6.3)	3785 (2085–6870)
10	6.0 (5.5–6.5)	4478 (2483–8075)
11	6.1 (5.6–6.6)	5297 (2952–9508)
12	6.2 (5.8–6.7)	6267 (3502–11,218)
13	6.4 (5.9–6.8)	7415 (4145–13,266)
14	6.5 (6.0–7.0)	8773 (4894–15,726)
15	6.6 (6.2–7.1)	10,379 (5766–18,682)
16	6.7 (6.3–7.2)	12,270 (6776–22,235)
17	6.9 (6.4–7.3)	14,528 (7964–26,501)
18	7.0 (6.5–7.5)	17,188 (9343–31,621)
19	7.1 (6.6–7.6)	20,337 (10,951–37,761)
20	7.3 (6.8–7.7)	24,060 (12,820–45,130)
21	7.4 (6.9–7.8)	28,464 (15,020–53,970)
22	7.5 (7.0–8.0)	33,675 (17,560–64,570)
23	7.6 (7.2–8.1)	39,843 (20,573–77,164)
24	7.8 (7.3–8.2)	47,138 (24,067–93,325)

*Predicted age from mean sac diameter is from Daya, S., Wood S, Ward S, et al: Early pregnancy assessment with transvaginal ultrasound scanning. Can Med Assoc J. Reprinted from, by permission of the publisher, CMAJ Vol. 144, 1991.

†Predicted hCG from mean sac diameter is from Nyberg DA, Filly RA, Filho DLD, et al: Abnormal pregnancy: Early diagnosis by US and serum chorionic gonadotropin levels. Radiology 158:393–396, 1986 (hCG calibrated against the Second International Standard).

workers[24] have evaluated patients with known dates of conception using high-resolution vaginal probes, and their data correspond quite nicely with those of the early investigators. The only difficulty with the older studies is that they do not provide data below 7 weeks, and this has posed a problem until very recently for those identifying the early embryo at 6 menstrual weeks using endovaginal real-time equipment. In a comprehensive study of CRL, my colleagues and I[26] have developed measurement tables for establishing menstrual age from CRL as small as 2 mm, and we have extended the range of CRL data up to measurements as large as 12 cm (see Table 7–3). More importantly, perhaps, we have also reevaluated the accuracy of the method and demonstrated that the variability in estimating menstrual age from CRL decreases as pregnancy advances.

The majority of the early studies on the subject of CRL demonstrated that the accuracy of the method in predicting menstrual age was: 3 to 5 days (± 2 SD).[14–16] In the study by MacGregor and associates,[20] however, the accuracy of the technique was demonstrated to decrease as pregnancy advanced into the late first trimester.

Because their study population had known states of conception, this increase in variability with advancing pregnancy was believed to represent early biologic variability in actual fetal size.[20] More recently, my colleagues and I[26] evaluated the accuracy of the method and confirmed that, indeed, the variability in estimating menstrual age from CRL increases as pregnancy advances. In an effort to simplify the reporting of varia-

Table 7-3. PREDICTED MENSTRUAL AGE (MA) (WEEKS) FROM CROWN-RUMP LENGTH (CRL) MEASUREMENTS (CM)*

CRL	MA	CRL	MA	CRL	MA	CRL	MA	CRL	MA	CRL	MA
0.2	5.7	2.2	8.9	4.2	11.1	6.2	12.6	8.2	14.2	10.2	16.1
0.3	5.9	2.3	9.0	4.3	11.2	6.3	12.7	8.3	14.2	10.3	16.2
0.4	6.1	2.4	9.1	4.4	11.2	6.4	12.8	8.4	14.3	10.4	16.3
0.5	6.2	2.5	9.2	4.5	11.3	6.5	12.8	8.5	14.4	10.5	16.4
0.6	6.4	2.6	9.4	4.6	11.4	6.6	12.9	8.6	14.5	10.6	16.5
0.7	6.6	2.7	9.5	4.7	11.5	6.7	13.0	8.7	14.6	10.7	16.6
0.8	6.7	2.8	9.6	4.8	11.6	6.8	13.1	8.8	14.7	10.8	16.7
0.9	6.9	2.9	9.7	4.9	11.7	6.9	13.1	8.9	14.8	10.9	16.8
1.0	7.2	3.0	9.9	5.0	11.7	7.0	13.2	9.0	14.9	11.0	16.9
1.1	7.2	3.1	10.0	5.1	11.8	7.1	13.3	9.1	15.0	11.1	17.0
1.2	7.4	3.2	10.1	5.2	11.9	7.2	13.4	9.2	15.1	11.2	17.1
1.3	7.5	3.3	10.2	5.3	12.0	7.3	13.4	9.3	15.2	11.3	17.2
1.4	7.7	3.4	10.3	5.4	12.0	7.4	13.5	9.4	15.3	11.4	17.3
1.5	7.9	3.5	10.4	5.5	12.1	7.5	13.6	9.5	15.3	11.5	17.4
1.6	8.0	3.6	10.5	5.6	12.2	7.6	13.7	9.6	15.4	11.6	17.5
1.7	8.1	3.7	10.6	5.7	12.3	7.7	13.8	9.7	15.5	11.7	17.6
1.8	8.3	3.8	10.7	5.8	12.3	7.8	13.8	9.8	15.6	11.8	17.7
1.9	8.4	3.9	10.8	5.9	12.4	7.9	13.9	9.9	15.7	11.9	17.8
2.0	8.6	4.0	10.9	6.0	12.5	8.0	14.0	10.0	15.9	12.0	17.9
2.1	8.7	4.1	11.0	6.1	12.6	8.1	14.1	10.1	16.0	12.1	18.0

*The 95% confidence interval is ±8% of the predicted age.

From Hadlock FP, Shah YP, Kanon DJ, Lindsey JV: Fetal crown-rump length: Reevaluation of relation to menstrual age (5–18 weeks) with high-resolution real-time US. Radiology 182:501–505, 1992.

bility estimates, we evaluated the variability as a percentage of the predicted value and demonstrated that the variability is relatively uniform at ±8% for CRL measurements between 2 mm and 12 cm. Thus, for a CRL menstrual age prediction of 8 weeks, the 95% confidence interval is 8 weeks ±8% = 8 weeks ± 0.64 week. Similarly, for a CRL age estimation of 15 weeks, the variability would be 15 weeks ±8% = 15 weeks ±1.2 weeks. We believe that the optimal time for prediction of menstrual age from CRL measurements is between 7 and 9 weeks using high-resolution vaginal probes.

Other measurements of the fetus can also be made in the first trimester of pregnancy. For example, Bovicelli and associates[18] in 1981 evaluated the fetal biparietal diameter in comparison with the first-trimester CRL for predicting menstrual age between 7 and 13 weeks, and in 1982 Selbing[11] reported a similar study. Both groups demonstrated that the first-trimester BPD is a relatively good predictor of menstrual age in this time frame, but in general it is not more accurate than the fetal CRL and adds little, if anything, to the age estimate based on the CRL. Reece and coworkers[21] demonstrated similar results using early fetal abdominal (trunk) circumference in the first trimester of pregnancy. In my practice, the use of high-resolution vaginal probes allows very acceptable images of the head, abdomen, and femur for measurements of head circumference, BPD, abdominal circumference, and femur length from 10 weeks on.[1] But evaluation of the accuracy of these measurements in predicting menstrual age demonstrated that they are not more accurate than the CRL length in predicting age during this time and that their use in conjunction with the CRL does not add sufficient information to justify their use.

Moreover, they are technically more difficult to obtain than the CRL measurement, and I do not believe that their routine use is warranted in the first trimester at this time.

In summary, the accuracy of first-trimester fetal measurements in predicting menstrual age is well documented and is believed to be because there is very little actual biologic variability in fetal size during this time. This is in contrast to the third trimester of pregnancy, in which individual genetic expressions in fetal size can result in a very heterogeneous population. It is also well established that once menstrual age has been determined or corroborated by fetal CRL in the first trimester of pregnancy, the menstrual age of the pregnancy is established and should never be changed based on measurements made later in pregnancy.[1]

SECOND AND THIRD TRIMESTERS OF PREGNANCY (14 TO 42 WEEKS)

Fetal Measurements

In the second trimester of pregnancy, the fetus has grown sufficiently in size so that extreme anatomic detail is visualized, and most major fetal anomalies can be detected using high-resolution real-time ultrasound. There are a number of structures that can be identified and measured during this time,[26–30] but the basic fetal measurements used to estimate age are the BPD, head circumference, abdominal circumference, and femur length (or humerus length).[1] Although obtaining these measurements may seem a difficult task, in fact they can be obtained from six linear measurements of the fetus, as seen in Figures 7–5 through 7–8.

FETAL HEAD MEASUREMENTS (BPD, HC)

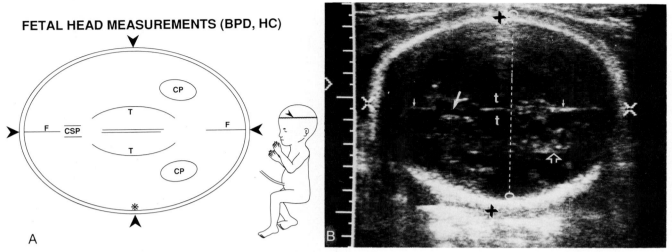

Figure 7–5. *A.* Appropriate transverse axial plane of section for measurement of the fetal biparietal diameter and head circumference. Critical landmarks are the falx (F) anteriorly and posteriorly, the cavum septi pellucidi (CSP) in the midline anteriorly, the thalamic nuclei (T) in the midline, and the choroid plexus (CP) in the atria of the lateral ventricles. The biparietal diameter is measured from the outer to the inner margin of the skull *(top arrowhead to asterisk).* The biparietal diameter and the occipital frontal diameter measured from outer to outer margins *(arrowheads)* are used for calculation of the cephalic index, which is important in assessing fetal head shape. The cephalic index equals the biparietal diameter ÷ occipital frontal diameter × 100. The normal range for this measurement is 78.4 ±4.3. *B.* This high-resolution linear real-time image of the fetal head demonstrates the corresponding anatomy outlined in *A.* The 0---0 line represents the appropriate plane of section for the biparietal diameter. The black cursors (x) mark the outer-to-outer biparietal dimension, and the white cursors (x) indicate the outer-to-outer occipital frontal dimension. These two diameters are used to calculate the cephalic index. In this case, the cephalic index was 9/12 × 100 = 75, which is within the normal range, indicating that the biparietal diameter is an acceptable measure of fetal age in this case.

One must always remember, however, that these images and their measurements must be made with great care in every case, and one must be certain to duplicate the technique of the investigator whose data one is using. Using measurements from poor images, or images that depict fetal anomalies, should be avoided.

BIPARIETAL DIAMETER

The BPD has received the greatest amount of attention in the literature as a means of establishing menstrual age.[26–33] In making this measurement, the fetal head should be imaged in a transverse axial section, preferably with the fetus in a direct occiput transverse position (see Fig. 7–5). The instrument should be set at medium gain so that the parietal bones measure approximately 3 mm in thickness. Intracranial landmarks should include the falx cerebri anteriorly and posteriorly, the cavum septi pellucidi anteriorly in the midline, and the choroid plexus in the atrium of each lateral ventricle; depending on the age of the fetus, one may also visualize the thalamic nuclei and the middle cerebral artery pulsations in the sylvian fissure. The BPD is measured from the outer surface of the

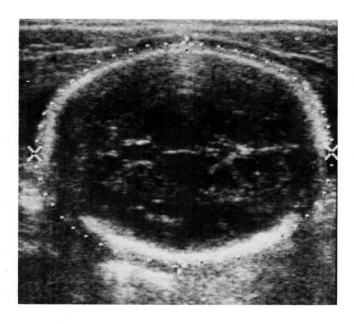

Figure 7–6. This high-resolution real-time image is from the same fetus in Figure 7–5 and demonstrates the ellipse approximation method of measuring head circumference. Although, in general, the head circumference can be calculated using the formula for the circumference of a circle (D1 + D2 × 1.57), in cases of abnormal head shape it is appropriate to use the ellipse formula or to trace the circumference directly.

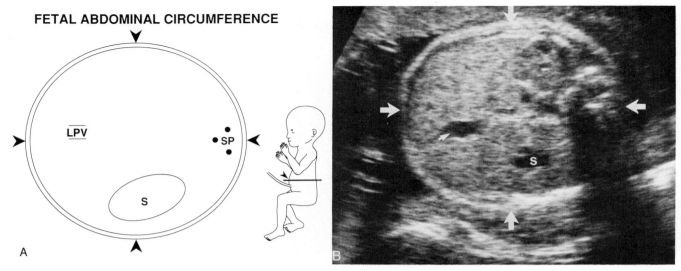

Figure 7–7. *A.* Appropriate transverse axial plane for measurement of the abdominal circumference. The landmarks are the left portal vein (LPV) deep in the liver and, in some cases, the fetal stomach (S). Note the alignment of the three ossification centers of the spine (SP). The abdominal circumference is calculated from the anteroposterior and transverse diameters as indicated by the arrowheads. These measurements are made along the outer-to-outer margin of the fetal abdomen. The circumference can be calculated using the formula for the circumference of a circle (D1 + D2 × 1.57). In cases in which the shape is distorted, the circumference should be calculated based on the formula for an ellipse or traced directly using a map measurer. *B.* This high-resolution linear array real-time image demonstrates the anatomic landmarks and appropriate measurement points *(arrows)* as indicated in *A.* Small arrow indicates the left portal vein. S, stomach.

skull table nearest the transducer to the inner margin of the opposite skull table (outer to inner). The menstrual age can be determined by using a standard reference table (Table 7–4).

All reports on the BPD have demonstrated it to be an accurate predictor of menstrual age before 20 weeks. For example, my colleagues and I[27] demonstrated the variability to be ±1 week (2 SD) in a population of 1771 patients with optional menstrual histories seen between 14 and 20 weeks (Table 7–5). Similar results have been reported by Persson and Weldner[29] and Rossavik and Fishburne[30] in patients with known dates of conception and by de Crespigny and Speirs[33] in a large series of patients whose dates were confirmed by CRL in the first trimester of pregnancy. In addition, Campbell and colleagues[5] and Waldenström and coworkers,[6] in independent studies, have demonstrated that a BPD obtained between 14 and 20 menstrual weeks is a better predictor of the estimated date of confinement than an optimal menstrual history. Virtually all studies have demonstrated a progressive increase in variability from 20 weeks to term, but the degree to which the variability increases in the late third trimester of pregnancy has been a subject of some disagreement in the literature.[31–33, 67] Most early authors concluded that the variability during

FETAL FEMUR LENGTH

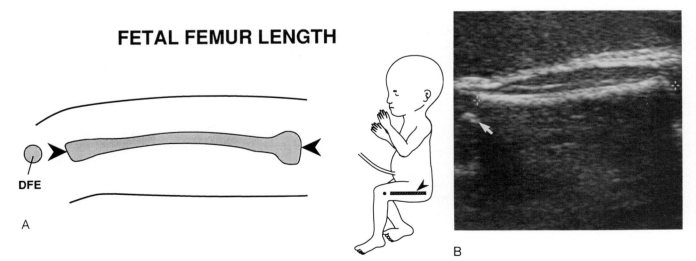

Figure 7–8. *A.* Appropriate plane of section for measurement of the fetal femur length. Ideally, the ultrasound beam should be perpendicular to the bone. The measurement is made along the femur diaphysis *(arrowheads)* and should exclude the distal femoral epiphysis (DFE). *B.* This high-resolution linear array real-time image demonstrates the femur as depicted in *A.* The caliper markers are properly placed for measurement of the bone length of the femur. The small arrow indicates the femoral epiphyseal ossification center, which should never be included in the measurement.

Table 7–4. PREDICTED MENSTRUAL AGE FOR BIPARIETAL DIAMETER (BPD) MEASUREMENTS (2.6 cm–9.7 cm)

BPD (cm)	Menstrual Age (wk)	BPD (cm)	Menstrual Age (wk)
2.6	13.9	6.2	25.3
2.7	14.2	6.3	25.7
2.8	14.5	6.4	26.1
2.9	14.7	6.5	26.4
3.0	15.0	6.6	26.8
3.1	15.3	6.7	27.2
3.2	15.6	6.8	27.6
3.3	15.9	6.9	28.0
3.4	16.2	7.0	28.3
3.5	16.5	7.1	28.7
3.6	16.8	7.2	29.1
3.7	17.1	7.3	29.5
3.8	17.4	7.4	29.9
3.9	17.7	7.5	30.4
4.0	18.0	7.6	30.8
4.1	18.3	7.7	31.2
4.2	18.6	7.8	31.6
4.3	18.9	7.9	32.0
4.4	19.2	8.0	32.5
4.5	19.5	8.1	32.9
4.6	19.9	8.3	33.3
4.7	20.2	8.3	33.8
4.8	20.5	8.4	34.2
4.9	20.8	8.5	34.7
5.0	21.2	8.6	35.1
5.1	21.5	8.7	35.6
5.2	21.8	8.8	36.1
5.3	22.2	8.9	36.5
5.4	22.5	9.0	37.0
5.5	22.8	9.1	37.5
5.6	23.2	9.2	38.0
5.7	23.5	9.3	38.5
5.8	23.9	9.4	38.9
5.9	24.2	9.5	39.4
6.0	24.6	9.6	39.9
6.1	25.0	9.7	40.5

Variability Estimates (±2 SD) (wk)

12–18	±1.2
18–24	±1.7
24–30	±2.2
30–36	±3.1
36–42	±3.2

From Hadlock FP, Deter RL, Harrist RB, et al: Fetal biparietal diameter: A critical reevaluation of the relation to menstrual age by means of real-time ultrasound. J Ultrasound Med 1:97, 1982; and Hadlock FP, Deter LR, Harrist RB, et al: Estimating fetal age: Computer-assisted analysis of multiple fetal growth parameters. Radiology 152:497–501, 1984.

this time frame is approximately ±3½ weeks (2 SD), but Kurtz and coworkers[31] have reported the variability to be ±2 weeks during this time. My colleagues and I believe that this is a statistical phenomenon, since the mathematical evaluation by Kurtz and coworkers[31] was performed on mean values from a number of different centers and does not directly include any of the raw data from the more than 25,000 patients that form the basis of their report. The variability they report, then, represents the confidence interval of the mean and should not be comparable to the standard deviation reported by others.[32] In our studies of patients with optimal menstrual histories, we have consistently demonstrated the variability of late third-trimester BPD age predictions to be approximately ±3½ weeks, and this has been confirmed in a large series of patients in Australia in whom the menstrual ages were confirmed in early pregnancy by CRL.[33] Both of the later studies, however, eliminated patients with head shape abnormalities, multiple gestation, or diseases likely to adversely affect fetal growth. The large variability associated with third-trimester use of the BPD has been confirmed in a study by Benson and Doubilet[46] of patients whose menstrual histories had been established early in pregnancy by CRL; in this study, however, no attempt was made to eliminate multiple gestations or patients with potential growth disturbances. These authors found that the variability in predicting menstrual age using BPD reached a peak at approximately ±4.1 weeks (2 SD) in the late third trimester of pregnancy (Table 7–6).

In certain circumstances (e.g., ruptured membranes, breech presentations, multiple gestations) shape changes in the fetal head may lead to even greater errors than those mentioned here. To recognize the shape changes, one should always measure the cephalic index of the head to assess head shape (see Fig. 7–5). The cephalic index is calculated from the BPD and the fronto-occipital diameter (FOD) measured outer to outer

$$\text{cephalic index} = \text{BPD/FOD} \times 100$$

In the first in utero study on this subject, my colleagues and I[41] evaluated 316 patients at between 14 and 40 menstrual weeks and demonstrated that the cephalic index was essentially age independent over time, with

Table 7–5. VARIABILITY IN PREDICTING MENSTRUAL AGE FROM SONOGRAPHIC MEASUREMENTS (14–20 WEEKS)

Parameter	Variability (2 SD) (Wk)			
	Hadlock et al[27]	Rossavik and Fishburne[30]	Persson and Weldner[29]	Benson and Doubilet[46]
Biparietal diameter	0.94	1.02	0.92	1.40
Head circumference	0.84	0.92	ND	1.20
Abdominal circumference	1.04	1.12	ND	2.10
Femur length	0.96	ND	0.98	1.40
Biparietal diameter, femur length	0.80	ND	0.78	ND
Head circumference, femur length	0.76	ND	ND	ND

ND, no data.

Table 7–6. VARIABILITY IN PREDICTING MENSTRUAL AGE IN THE SECOND HALF OF PREGNANCY (20–42 WEEKS)

Parameter	Variability (±2 SD) (wk)		
	20–26 Weeks	26–32 Weeks	32–42 Weeks
Biparietal diameter	2.1	3.8	4.1
Corrected biparietal diameter	1.9	3.3	3.8
Head circumference	1.9	3.4	3.8
Abdominal circumference	3.7	3.0	4.5
Femur length	2.5	3.1	3.5

Adapted from Benson CB, Doubilet PM: Sonographic prediction of gestational age: Accuracy of second and third trimester fetal measurements. AJR 157:1275, 1991.

a mean value of 78.3 and an SD of 4.4. We concluded that a cephalic index greater than 1 SD above or below the mean (less than 74, greater than 83) may be associated with a significant alteration in the BPD measurement expected for a given menstrual age and that the head circumference can be used effectively as an alternative means of establishing age in such cases. Gray and coworkers[42] found minimal changes in the mean value of cephalic index with advancing age and also concluded that the BPD should be viewed with suspicion as an age indicator when the cephalic index is more than 1 SD above or below the mean for age. An alternative approach to potential head shape variations has been reported by Doubilet and Greenes,[43] who recommend routinely calculating a shape-corrected BPD based on an idealized cephalic index of 78:

$$\text{this shape-corrected BPD} = (\text{BPD} \times \text{FOD})/1.265$$

As expected, when this shape correction is performed, the BPD is equivalent to the head circumference as a predictor of menstrual age because it has been rendered shape independent.[43, 46]

HEAD CIRCUMFERENCE

The neonatal head circumference is an important measurement of neonatal head growth and has gained importance as an in utero ultrasound measurement because it is more shape independent than the BPD. The measurement is made from the same axial image used to measure the BPD (see Fig. 7–5). We have found that reliable estimates of head circumference can be calculated by using the shortest and longest axes of the fetal head measured outer to outer (the same measurements used to calculate the cephalic index). Although ideally one should use the formula for the circumference of an ellipse for this calculation, adequate measurements can usually be made using the formula (D1 + D2) × 1.57. In cases in which the cephalic index indicates extreme dolichocephaly (value <70), the head circumference should ideally be traced

along the outer perimeter of the calvarium using a map measurer or electronic digitizer (see Fig. 7–6). The menstrual age can then be determined by using a standard reference table (Table 7–7).

Several authors have demonstrated that head circumference is one of the most reliable individual parameters for estimation of menstrual age.[34, 35] This is due to its shape independence and the fact that it represents a balance between ease of measurement (and therefore measurement accuracy) and predictive validity for age. For example, in 1982, Law and MacRae[35] demonstrated in a series of 594 patients that the head circumference was superior to the BPD as a predictor of menstrual age. This has been a consistent finding in our studies,[27, 39, 40] and it has also been reported in independent studies by Hill and coworkers[47] and Benson and colleagues.[46] As with the other individual parameters, however, the variability in age prediction from head circumference increases with advancing menstrual age (see Table 7–7). For example, my colleagues and I[27] and Rossavik and Fishburne[30] have demonstrated that this parameter can predict menstrual age to within ±1 week (2 SD) before

Table 7–7. PREDICTED MENSTRUAL AGE FOR HEAD CIRCUMFERENCE MEASUREMENTS (8.5–36.0 cm)

Head Circumference (cm)	Menstrual Age (wk)	Head Circumference (cm)	Menstrual Age (wk)
8.5	13.7	22.5	24.4
9.0	14.0	23.0	24.9
9.5	14.3	23.5	25.4
10.0	14.6	24.0	25.9
10.5	15.0	24.5	26.4
11.0	15.3	25.0	26.9
11.5	15.6	25.5	27.5
12.0	15.9	26.0	28.0
12.5	16.3	26.5	28.6
13.0	16.6	27.0	29.2
13.5	17.0	27.5	29.8
14.0	17.3	28.0	30.3
14.5	17.7	28.5	31.0
15.0	18.1	29.0	31.6
15.5	18.4	29.5	32.2
16.0	18.8	30.0	32.8
16.5	19.2	30.5	33.5
17.0	19.6	31.0	34.2
17.5	20.0	31.5	34.9
18.0	20.4	32.0	35.5
18.5	20.8	32.5	36.3
19.0	21.2	33.0	37.0
19.5	21.6	33.5	37.7
20.0	22.1	34.0	38.5
20.5	22.5	34.5	39.2
21.0	23.0	35.0	40.0
21.5	23.4	35.5	40.8
22.0	23.9	36.0	41.6

Variability Estimates (± 2 SD) (wk)	
12–18	±1.3
18–24	±1.6
24–30	±2.3
30–36	±2.7
34–42	±3.4

From Hadlock FP, Deter RL, Harrist RB, Park SK: Fetal head circumference: Relation to menstrual age. AJR 138:649, 1982. Copyright 1982, American Roentgen Ray Society.

20 weeks' gestation, while Benson and colleagues[46] have demonstrated that the variability in predicting age from head circumference reaches a peak of approximately ±3.8 weeks (2 SD) in the late third trimester of pregnancy (see Tables 7–5 and 7–6).

ABDOMINAL CIRCUMFERENCE

The measurement of the fetal abdominal circumference is made from a transverse axial image of the fetal abdomen at the level of the liver (see Fig. 7–7).[1] A major landmark in this section is the umbilical portion of the left portal vein deep in the liver, with the fetal stomach representing a secondary landmark.[1] This circumference can be traced along its outer margin with a map measurer or electronic digitizer, but we prefer to calculate the circumference using the anteroposterior and transverse diameters measured outer to outer; the circumference then equals $(D1 + D2) \times 1.57$. Great care must be taken when obtaining this measurement to be certain that the image is not inclined side to side or front to back. The image should be as round as possible, and excessive pressure with the transducer should be avoided because it distorts the shape of the abdomen. In some cases, the shape of the abdomen will be distorted because of uterine factors (e.g., decreased amniotic fluid volume, narrow maternal anteroposterior diameter, myometrial contraction), and in such cases the circumference should be traced directly with a map measurer or electronic digitizer. The menstrual age can then be determined by using a standard reference table (Table 7–8).

Of the four basic ultrasound measurements, abdominal circumference has generally had the largest reported variability,[39, 40, 46, 47] and this has been attributed to the fact that abdominal circumference is more acutely affected by growth disturbances than the other basic parameters (see Tables 7–5 and 7–6). I believe, however, that this is probably due more to measurement errors rather than biologic variability, since most authors have gone to extremes to exclude patients with growth disturbances from their study populations. For example, the greatest differences in accuracy between abdominal circumference and the other parameters in the study by Benson and Doubilet[46] were observed in the second trimester of pregnancy, a point in pregnancy in which growth variations would be expected to be minimal. Moreover, during the early third trimester (26 to 32 weeks), a point at which early growth disturbances usually become manifest, Benson and Doubilet[46] demonstrated that the abdominal circumference was more accurate than all of the other basic ultrasound measurements (BPD, head circumference, femur length) in predicting menstrual age (see Table 7–6).

In our own laboratory, the abdominal circumference is only slightly less accurate on average than the other basic measurements, probably because of rigorous attention to measurement technique and elimination of any fetuses at risk for growth abnormalities. Similar results have been reported by Hill and coworkers,[47] who demonstrated that the variability in predicting

Table 7–8. PREDICTED MENSTRUAL AGE FOR ABDOMINAL CIRCUMFERENCE MEASUREMENTS (10–36 cm)

Abdominal Circumfernce (cm)	Menstrual Age (wk)	Abdominal Circumference (cm)	Menstrual Age (wk)
10.0	15.6	23.5	27.7
10.5	16.1	24.0	28.2
11.0	16.5	24.5	28.7
11.5	16.9	25.0	29.2
12.0	17.3	25.5	29.7
12.5	17.8	26.0	30.1
13.0	18.2	26.5	30.6
13.5	18.6	27.0	31.1
14.0	19.1	27.5	31.6
14.5	19.5	28.0	32.1
15.0	20.0	28.5	32.6
15.5	20.4	29.0	33.1
16.0	20.8	29.5	33.6
16.5	21.3	30.0	34.1
17.0	21.7	30.5	34.6
17.5	22.2	31.0	35.1
18.0	22.6	31.5	35.6
18.5	23.1	32.0	36.1
19.0	23.6	32.5	36.6
19.5	24.0	33.0	37.1
20.0	24.5	33.5	37.6
20.5	24.9	34.0	38.1
21.0	25.4	34.5	38.7
21.5	25.9	35.0	39.2
22.0	26.3	35.5	39.7
22.5	26.8	36.0	40.2
23.0	27.3		

Variability Estimates (±2 SD) (wk)

12–18	±1.9
18–24	±2.0
24–30	±2.2
30–36	±3.0
36–42	±2.5

From Hadlock FP, Deter RL, Harrist RB, Park SK: Fetal abdominal circumference as a predictor of menstrual age. AJR 139:367, 1982. Copyright 1982, American Roentgen Ray Society.

menstrual age (14 to 43 weeks) from abdominal circumference in 265 normal-weight fetuses was slightly less than that associated with the BPD. As with all other parameters, however, the variability in predicting menstrual age based on abdominal circumference increases as pregnancy advances. For example, in a retrospective study of patients with menstrual dates corroborated by early CRL, Benson and Doubilet[46] reported a variability of ±4.5 weeks (2 SD) in the late third trimester of pregnancy (see Table 7–6).

FEMUR LENGTH

Because of its size and ease of measurement, the femur length is generally preferred over the other long bones as a means of predicting menstrual age. The femur length measurement is made with the transducer aligned along the long axis of the bone, ideally with the beam exactly perpendicular to the shaft (see Fig. 7–8). The measured ends of the bone should be blunt rather than pointed. After 32 menstrual weeks, one should visualize the distal femoral epiphysis but not include it in the measurement of the femoral shaft. Although virtually all of the early work in femur biometry was done on white populations, it has been demonstrated that these measurements are not altered in any predictable way in other races.[40] It should be noted, however, that pathologic processes (e.g., osteogenesis imperfecta, dwarfism, hypophosphatasia) may result in excessive bowing, hypomineralization, and/or fractures and that the femur should not be used in age predictions in such cases. Once a good measurement has been made, estimates of menstrual age can be obtained from standard reference tables (Table 7–9).

Most studies suggest that the femur length is an accurate predictor of menstrual age in the early second trimester (2 SD = ±1 week), but the variability reported throughout the remainder of pregnancy from several laboratories has been inconsistent (see Tables 7–5 and 7–6).[37, 38, 48, 49] For example, Jeanty and associates[48] reported a uniform variability for the femur length age estimate of ±2.1 weeks throughout the second and third trimesters of pregnancy, suggesting that the femur length is just as accurate at 40 weeks as it is at 14 weeks in predicting age. We and others[55] believe that this is a statistical phenomenon resulting from the use of the wrong test of the variability estimate. Furthermore, although Hill and coworkers[47] found the femur length to be the most accurate of all the individual parameters in predicting menstrual age, Ott[44] found it to be the least accurate. My colleagues and I[39] and Benson and Doubilet[46] have found the femur length to be roughly equivalent in accuracy to the other parameters in estimating menstrual age, reaching a peak variability of approximately ±3.5 weeks in the late third trimester of pregnancy.

OTHER BIOMETRIC PARAMETERS

There are a number of other fetal structures that can be imaged and measured with current high-resolution real-time ultrasound equipment. In the fetal head, these measurements may play a role when the transverse axial image necessary for measurement of the BPD and head circumference is not obtainable. For example, when the head is in a direct occiput-posterior position, the orbits are easily imaged, and several authors have published normal data for both the binocular distance and the interorbital and intraorbital diameters (see Table A–21 in Appendix A).[51, 52] When the fetus is in a direct occiput-anterior position, the posterior fossa is closer to the transducer and the cerebellum can be seen to advantage. Hill and coworkers[54] have published normal data for the transverse diameter of the cerebellum, and some authors believe that it is preferable to other head measurements for age prediction in cases in which fetal growth may be altered (Table 7–10). Other notable measurements that may be used as substitute variables for predicting menstrual age include virtually all of the long bones of the arms and legs (see Appendix A). In addition, normal data have been published for use of the fetal foot length and fetal clavicle length measurements as predictors of menstrual age. The variability associated with age predictions based on these additional biometric parameters is outlined in Table 7–11. It is our belief that these measurements might be useful in certain circumstances but that in general the basic fetal measurements previously mentioned serve as adequate indicators of menstrual age in most cases.

CALCULATION OF MENSTRUAL AGE

The literature is replete with articles that focus on predicting menstrual age using ultrasound measurements of the fetus.[5-68] A common theme among these articles is that the variability in predicting menstrual age increases as pregnancy advances for all fetal parameters (see Tables 7–5 and 7–6). The increase in variability is undoubtedly due for the most part to

Table 7–9. PREDICTED MENSTRUAL AGE FOR FEMUR LENGTHS (1.0–7.9 cm)

Femur Length (cm)	Menstrual Age (wk)	Femur Length (cm)	Menstrual Age (wk)
1.0	12.8	4.5	24.5
1.1	13.1	4.6	24.9
1.2	13.4	4.7	25.3
1.3	13.6	4.8	25.7
1.4	13.9	4.9	26.1
1.5	14.2	5.0	26.5
1.6	14.5	5.1	27.0
1.7	14.8	5.2	27.4
1.8	15.1	5.3	27.8
1.9	15.4	5.4	28.2
2.0	15.7	5.5	28.7
2.1	16.0	5.6	29.1
2.2	16.3	5.7	29.6
2.3	16.6	5.8	30.0
2.4	16.9	5.9	30.5
2.5	17.2	6.0	30.9
2.6	17.6	6.1	31.4
2.7	17.9	6.2	31.9
2.8	18.2	6.3	32.3
2.9	18.6	6.4	32.8
3.0	18.9	6.5	33.3
3.1	19.2	6.6	33.8
3.2	19.6	6.7	34.2
3.3	19.9	6.8	34.7
3.4	20.3	6.9	35.2
3.5	20.7	7.0	35.7
3.6	21.0	7.1	36.2
3.7	21.4	7.2	36.7
3.8	21.8	7.3	37.2
3.9	22.1	7.4	37.7
4.0	22.5	7.5	38.3
4.1	22.9	7.6	38.8
4.2	23.3	7.7	39.3
4.3	23.7	7.8	39.8
4.4	24.1	7.9	40.4

Variability Estimates (±2 SD) (wk)

12–18	±1.0
18–24	±1.8
24–30	±2.0
30–36	±2.4
36–42	±3.2

From Hadlock FP, Deter RL, Harrist RB, Park SK: Fetal femur length as a predictor of menstrual age: Sonographically measured. AJR 138:875, 1982.

Table 7–10. PREDICTED MENSTRUAL AGES FOR TRANSVERSE CEREBELLAR DIAMETERS OF 14 TO 56 mm

Cerebellum (mm)	Menstrual Age (wk)	Cerebellum (mm)	Menstrual Age (wk)
14	15.2	35	29.4
15	15.8	36	30.0
16	16.5	37	30.6
17	17.2	38	31.2
18	17.9	39	31.8
19	18.6	40	32.3
20	19.3	41	32.8
21	20.0	42	33.4
22	20.7	43	33.9
23	21.4	44	34.4
24	22.1	45	34.8
25	22.8	46	35.3
26	23.5	47	35.7
27	24.2	48	36.1
28	24.9	49	36.5
29	25.5	50	36.8
30	26.2	51	37.2
31	26.9	52	37.5
32	27.5	54	38.0
33	28.1	55	38.3
34	28.8	56	38.5

Variability Estimates (+ 2 SD) (wk)

12–8	±1.0
18–24	±1.8
24–30	±2.0
30–36	±2.4
36–42	±3.2

From Hill LM, et al: Transverse cerebellar diameter as a predictor of menstrual age. Obstet Gynecol 75:983, 1990. Reprinted with permission from The American College of Obstetricians and Gynecologists (Obstetrics and Gynecology, 1990, vol. 75, p. 983.)

actual differences in fetal size, since it has been demonstrated consistently in populations with optimal menstrual histories, with known dates of conception, and in whom age was established early in pregnancy by use of the CRL measurement. For example, my colleagues and I[27] studied 1771 patients with perfect menstrual histories and demonstrated that any of the individual parameters can provide accurate estimates of menstrual age (2 SD = ±1 week) between 14 and 20 weeks; Persson and Weldner[29] and Rossavik and Fishburne[30] have demonstrated similar results in patients with known dates of conception (see Table 7–5). In a large study of patients whose dates were confirmed by the "gold standard" of early CRL dating, Benson and Doubilet[46] demonstrated that age estimates from indi-

Table 7–11. VARIABILITY ESTIMATES FOR SECONDARY BIOMETRIC PARAMETERS

Parameter	Variability in Weeks (± 2 SD)				
	12–18	18–24	24–30	30–36	36–42
Binocular distance[52]	1.8	2.4	3.0	4.0	4.0
Cerebellar diameter[54]	1.0	1.8	2.0	2.4	3.2
Clavicle length[56]	6.5	6.5	6.5	6.5	6.5
Radius length[55]	1.8	2.2	2.9	3.5	4.1
Ulna length[48]	3.6	3.6	3.6	3.6	3.6
Tibia length[48]	3.5	3.5	3.5	3.5	3.5
Foot length[53]	1.2	1.7	2.2	2.6	3.1

vidual parameters reach a maximum variability of approximately ±4 weeks in the late third trimester of pregnancy (see Table 7–6). Thus, one should try to establish menstrual age as early in pregnancy as possible. But which measurement(s) should one use to predict age in a given case?

My colleagues and I believe one should avoid the tendency to place excessive emphasis arbitrarily on any one measurement because it has been demonstrated that in a given case any of these measurements could be providing the best estimate of age.[39] With this idea in mind, we postulated, in 1982, that multiple fetal measurements should be used in some combination to provide a composite age estimate.[39] We believed that the use of multiple measurements is especially important when one considers the following: (1) If one is using only one parameter and makes an imaging or measurement error, the magnitude of the error in age prediction could be significantly greater than the reported variability for that parameter. (2) It has been noted by several investigators that normal fetuses may have measurements that are above or below the expected mean value at a given age and that these differences are not always in the same direction, for example, the fetus with a 75 percentile head size and a 25 percentile abdominal size. (3) The process of plane selection of the fetal head, abdomen, and femur allows a detailed look at important anatomic structures and therefore facilitates detection of abnormalities in these areas, including hydrocephalus, encephalocele, bowel obstruction, ascites, renal abnormalities, and dwarfism.

Our initial approach was to use a simple averaging technique in which the estimates of age are simply added and divided by the number of estimates made. For example, consider the measurements obtained in early second trimester in the fetus in Figure 7–9:

Biparietal diameter	3.3 cm = 15.9 weeks
Head circumference	12.4 cm = 16.2 weeks
Abdominal circumference	10.0 cm = 15.6 weeks
Femur length	2.2 cm = 16.3 weeks
Composite age	16.0 weeks ± 1 week

We have subsequently developed regression equations for use in predicting age from any single measurement or combination of measurements,[39] and these equations have been validated prospectively in our own laboratory.[40] We have also demonstrated that the simple averaging technique and the complex regression equations give equivalent results.

The development of this multiple parameter dating approach raises two questions immediately. The first and most obvious question is how many measurements of the fetus must one make to obtain the best estimate of menstrual age. Our studies have examined this issue over the entire 14- to 42-week age range, and we have demonstrated that the use of the four basic measurements results in the greatest accuracy (lack of systematic bias), greatest precision (lowest range of variability), and smallest maximum observed errors.[39]

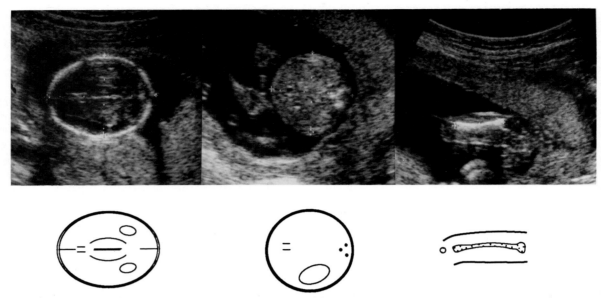

Figure 7–9. These high-resolution real-time images demonstrate the fetal head on the left, the abdomen in the middle, and the femur on the right. Note that the images in this 16-week fetus show some but not all of the anatomic landmarks depicted graphically. Nonetheless, the images are of high quality and very adequate measurements can be made at this stage in gestation.

Although some authors have questioned the validity of the method,[67] our models have now been validated in an independent study by Hill and coworkers in Pittsburgh.[47] Moreover, Hill and coworkers[47] demonstrated that the addition of a fifth parameter (radius length) does not add to the accuracy of the method. From a purely statistical point of view, both my colleagues and I[38] and Hill and coworkers[47] have not been able to demonstrate significant improvement beyond the two-parameter model based on head circumference and femur length. Similar results have been reported in a large study by Persson and Weldner[29] between 14 and 20 weeks (see Table 7–5). While the variability of the two parameter (head circumference, femur length) model will increase as pregnancy advances, we have found that it is relatively constant at ±8% when expressed as a percentage of the estimate. For example, if the composite age estimate based on these two parameters is 20 weeks, then the variability associated with that estimate is 20 weeks ± 1.6 weeks. In the late third trimester, a composite age estimate of 40 weeks would have a corresponding variability of 40 weeks ±3.2 weeks. Because the four-parameter method results in variability estimates of ±7%, we continue to use it in our daily practice.

The second important question that comes to mind using the multiple parameter dating technique is how disparate the individual measurements can be and still be acceptable for incorporation into the composite age estimate. For example, if measurement of the fetal head (BPD or head circumference) gave an age estimate of 20 weeks and measurement of the femur length or humerus length gave an age estimate of 14 weeks, one would know empirically that one of the two measurements is not increasing properly and that the two cannot be averaged to provide a composite age. We have relied heavily on normal fetal body ratio data to deal with this issue (Tables 7–12 and 7–13). For example, if the BPD is to be used in the age estimate, one should first examine the cephalic index, and if it indicates an abnormal head shape, the BPD should either be eliminated in favor of the head circumference or corrected for head shape.[41–43] One can then measure the relationship between femur length and head circumference; and if this is normal, then both measurements can be used for the prediction of age.[63] If the

Table 7–12. NORMAL BODY RATIO DATA (14–21 WEEKS)

Menstrual Week	Cephalic Index (SD = 3.7)[42]	Femur/BPD × 100 (SD = 4.0)[65]	Femur/HC × 100 (SD = 1.0)[65]	Femur/AC × 100 (SD = 1.3)[65]
14	81.5	58.0	15.0	19.0
15	81.0	59.0	15.7	19.3
16	80.5	61.0	16.4	19.8
17	80.1	63.0	16.9	20.3
18	79.7	65.0	17.5	20.8
19	79.4	67.0	18.1	21.0
20	79.1	69.0	18.4	21.3
21	78.8	70.0	18.6	21.5

BPD, biparietal diameter; HC, head circumference; AC, abdominal circumference.

Table 7–13. NORMAL FETAL BODY RATIOS (22–40 WEEKS)

Menstrual Week	Cephalic Index (SD = 4.4)[41]	Femur/BPD × 100 (SD = 5.0)[64]	Femur/HC × 100 (SD = 1.1)[63]	Femur/AC × 100 (SD = 1.3)[62]
22	78.3	77.4	18.6	21.6
23	78.3	77.6	18.8	21.7
24	78.3	77.8	19.0	21.7
25	78.3	78.0	19.2	21.8
26	78.3	78.2	19.4	21.8
27	78.3	78.4	19.6	21.9
28	78.3	78.6	19.8	21.9
29	78.3	78.8	20.0	21.9
30	78.3	79.0	20.3	22.0
31	78.3	79.2	20.5	22.0
32	78.3	79.4	20.7	22.1
33	78.3	79.6	20.9	22.1
34	78.3	79.8	21.1	22.2
35	78.3	80.0	21.4	22.2
36	78.3	80.2	21.6	22.2
37	78.3	80.4	21.8	22.3
38	78.3	80.6	22.0	22.3
39	78.3	80.8	22.2	22.3
40	78.3	81.0	22.4	22.4

BPD, biparietal diameter; HC, head circumference; AC, abdominal circumference.

femur length–head circumference ratio is high, the head measurement should be deleted because of possible microcephaly; if this ratio is low, the femur length age estimate should be deleted because of possible dwarfism.[63] These decisions are based on the assumption of normal anatomy of the head and long bones.

If abdominal circumference is to be included in the age estimate, one must examine the relationship between femur length and abdominal circumference (femur length/abdominal circumference × 100). If this ratio is low, one should avoid using the abdominal circumference because of possible macrosomia; and if it is high, one should avoid avoid using the abdominal circumference because of possible intrauterine growth retardation.[62] Because the abdominal circumference may be affected by abnormal fetal growth, one can make a strong case for eliminating it from the age estimation procedure altogether, particularly in the third trimester of pregnancy.[46] This case is even stronger in view of the fact that my colleagues and I were not able to demonstrate a statistically significant improvement in the age estimation procedure by adding additional parameters to the combination of head circumference and femur length.[27, 39]

We believe that the limiting factor in menstrual age estimates from fetal biometry is the genetic variation in actual fetal size as pregnancy advances, and to some extent the measurement errors associated with their use. We therefore believe that it is unlikely that additional biometric parameters will add to the accuracy of the dating procedure using ultrasound evaluation. It is possible, and even likely, that certain nonbiometric observations may prove helpful in narrowing the variability associated with ultrasound age estimates.[1] These observations include the degree of placental maturation,[59] the amniotic fluid volume,[58] and the maturation of the fetal bowel pattern.[59, 60] The presence of a grade 3 placenta, low amniotic fluid volume (in the absence of ruptured membranes or renal disease), and a mature fetal bowel pattern would make us favor the higher end of the age estimate based on fetal biometry. For example, if our biometric age estimate based on femur length and head size was 34 weeks ±2.7 weeks, we would favor the high end of the estimate (36.7 weeks) in view of these findings. Additionally, the presence or absence of certain epiphyseal ossification centers may play a role in increasing the accuracy of our biometric age estimates.[57] It has been observed that the distal femoral epiphysis is initially seen at 32 to 33 weeks, the proximal tibia epiphysis at 35 to 36 weeks, and the proximal humeral epiphysis at 37 to 38 weeks. Thus, in the case just described, the presence of the distal femoral and proximal tibial epiphyseal ossification centers would again make us favor the higher end of the age estimate, that is, 36.7 weeks.

CONCLUSIONS

In conclusion, I would like to reemphasize the following points:

1. Biometric estimates of age infer age from size and are therefore less accurate as pregnancy progresses because of biologic variability in fetal size and associated measurement errors.

2. If age is known unequivocally by conceptual data, the age is established (menstrual age = conceptual age + 14 days) and should not be changed based on ultrasound measurements. In such cases, ultrasound measurements become an index of growth rather than of age.

3. If a patient's menstrual dates are in question or not known, the patient should be seen for biometric dating as early in pregnancy as possible, preferably in the first trimester by CRL (2 SD = ±8% of the estimate).

4. Beyond the first trimester of pregnancy, age estimates should be based on the multiple parameter technique, preferably before 20 weeks. The optimal combination of parameters is that based on head circumference and femur length. Estimates based on these two parameters in combination should be accurate to within ±8% of the estimate in 95% of normally growing fetuses.

5. The dates should never be changed late in pregnancy based on ultrasound measurements if they have been established early in pregnancy. A classic example of such a case would be the patient who presents in the third trimester at 36 weeks based on accurate menstrual history and early CRL measurement and all fetal measurements indicate an age of 40 weeks. One must understand in such a case that while the size is that of a 40-week fetus, the age has been established at 36 weeks and should not be changed. Misinterpretation of information such as this can lead to iatrogenic prematurity in patients who are candidates for elective cesarean delivery.

References

1. Hadlock FP: Sonographic estimation of fetal age and weight. Radiol Clin North Am 28(1):39, 1990.
2. Beazley JM, Underhill RA: Fallacy of the fundal height. Br Med J 4:408, 1970.
3. Alexander GR, deCaunes F, Hulsey TC, et al: Validity of postnatal assessments of gestational age: A comparison of the method of Ballard et al and early ultrasonography. Am J Obstet Gynecol 66:891, 1992.
4. Matsumoto S, Nogami Y, Ohkuri S: Statistical studies on menstruation: A criticism on the definition of normal menstruation. Gumma J Med Science 11:294, 1962.
5. Campbell S, Warsof SL, Little D, Cooper DJ: Routine ultrasound screening for the prediction of gestational age. Obstet Gynecol 65:613, 1985.
6. Waldenström U, Axelsson O, Nilsson S: A comparison of the ability of a sonographically measured biparietal diameter and the last menstrual period to predict the spontaneous onset of labor. Obstet Gynecol 76:336, 1990.
7. Bernaschek G, Rudelstorfer R, Csaicsich P: Vaginal sonography versus serum human chorionic gonadotropin in early detection of pregnancy. Am J Obstet Gynecol 158:608, 1988.
8. Nyberg DA, Filly RA, Filho DLD, et al: Abnormal pregnancy: Early diagnosis by US and serum chorionic gonadotropin levels. Radiology 158:393, 1986.
9. Daya S, Woods S, Ward S, et al: Early pregnancy assessment with transvaginal ultrasound scanning. Can Med Assoc J 144:441, 1991.
10. Yeh HC, Rabinowitz JG: Amniotic sac development: Ultrasound features of early pregnancy—the double bleb sign. Radiology 166:97, 1988.
11. Selbing A: Gestational age and ultrasonic measurement of gestational sac, crown-rump length and biparietal diameter during first weeks of pregnancy. Acta Obstet Gynecol Scand 61:233, 1982.
12. Goldstein I, Zimmer EA, Tamir A, et al: Evaluation of normal gestational sac growth: Appearance of embryonic heartbeat and embryo body movements using the transvaginal technique. Obstet Gynecol 77:885, 1991.
13. Warren WB, Timor-Tritsch I, Peisner DB, et al: Dating the early pregnancy by sequential appearance of embryonic structures. Am J Obstet Gynecol 161:747, 1989.
14. Robinson HP: Sonar measurement of fetal crown-rump length as means of assessing maturity in first trimester of pregnancy. Br Med J 4:28, 1973.
15. Robinson HP, Fleming JEE: A critical evaluation of sonar "crown-rump length" measurements. Br J Obstet Gynaecol 82:702, 1975.
16. Drumm JE, Clinch J, MacKenzie G: The ultrasonic measurement of fetal crown-rump length as a method of assessing gestational age. Br J Obstet Gynaecol 83:417, 1976.
17. Pedersen JF: Fetal crown-rump length measurement by ultrasound in normal pregnancy. Br J Obstet Gynaecol 89:926, 1982.
18. Bovicelli L, Orsini LF, Rizzo N, et al: Estimation of gestational age during the first trimester by realtime measurement of fetal crown-rump length and biparietal diameter. J Clin Ultrasound 9:71, 1981.
19. Nelson LH: Comparison of methods for determining crown-rump measurement by realtime ultrasound. J Clin Ultrasound 9:67, 1981.
20. MacGregor SN, Tamura RK, Sabbagha RE, et al: Underestimation of gestational age by conventional crown-rump length dating curves. Obstet Gynecol 70:344, 1987.
21. Reece EA, Scioscia AL, Green J, et al: Embryonic trunk circumference: A new biometric parameter for estimation of gestational age. Am J Obstet Gynecol 156:713, 1987.
22. Vollebergh JHA, Jongsma HW, van Dongen PWJ: The accuracy of ultrasonic measurement of fetal crown-rump length. Eur J Obstet Gynecol Reprod Biol 30:253, 1989.
23. Koornstra G, Wattel E, Exalto N: Crown-rump length measurements revisited. Eur J Obstet Gynecol Reprod Biol 35:131, 1990.
24. Silva PD, Mahairas G, Schaper AM, Schauberger CW: Early crown-rump length: A good predictor of gestational age. J Reprod Med 35:641, 1990.
25. Evans J: Fetal crown-rump length values in the first trimester based upon ovulation timing using the luteinizing hormone surge. Br J Obstet Gynaecol 98:48, 1991.
26. Hadlock FP, Shah YP, Kanon DJ, Lindsey JV: Fetal crown-rump length: Reevaluation of relation to menstrual age (5–18 weeks) with high-resolution realtime US. Radiology 182:501, 1992.
27. Hadlock FP, Harrist RB, Martinez-Poyer J: How accurate is second trimester fetal dating? J Ultrasound Med 10:557, 1992.
28. Kopta MM, May RR, Crane JP: A comparison of the reliability of the estimated date of confinement predicted by crown-rump length and biparietal diameter. Am J Obstet Gynecol 145:562, 1983.
29. Persson PH, Weldner BM: Reliability of ultrasound fetometry in estimating gestational age in the second trimester. Acta Obstet Gynecol Scand 65:481, 1986.
30. Rossavik IK, Fishburne JI: Conceptional age, menstrual age, and ultrasound age: A second trimester comparison of pregnancies of known conception date with pregnancies dated from the last menstrual period. Obstet Gynecol 73:243, 1989.
31. Kurtz AB, Wapner RJ, Kurtz RJ, et al: Analysis of biparietal diameter as an accurate indicator of gestational age. J Clin Ultrasound 8:319, 1980.
32. Hadlock FP, Deter RL, Harrist RB, et al: Fetal biparietal diameter: A critical reevaluation of the relation to menstrual age by means of realtime ultrasound. J Ultrasound Med 1:97, 1982.
33. de Crespigny LC, Speirs AL: A new look at biparietal diameter. Aust NZ J Obstet Gynaecol 29:26, 1989.
34. Hadlock FP, Deter RL, Harrist RB, et al: Fetal head circumference: Relation to menstrual age. AJR 138:649, 1982.
35. Law RG, MacRae KDDD: Head circumference as an index of fetal age. J Ultrasound Med 1:281, 1982.
36. Hadlock FP, Deter RL, Harrist RB, et al: Fetal abdominal circumference as a predictor of menstrual age. AJR 139:367, 1982.
37. Hadlock FP, Harrist RB, Deter RL, et al: Fetal femur length as a predictor of menstrual age: Sonographically measured. AJR 138:875, 1982.
38. Hadlock FP, Harrist RB, Deter RL, Park SK: A prospective evaluation of fetal femur length as a predictor of gestational age. J Ultrasound Med 2:111, 1983.
39. Hadlock FP, Deter LR, Harrist RB, et al: Estimating fetal age: Computer-assisted analysis of multiple fetal growth parameters. Radiology 152:497, 1984.
40. Hadlock FP, Harrist RB, Shah YP, et al: Estimating fetal age using multiple parameters: A prospective evaluation in a racially mixed population. Am J Obstet Gynecol 156:955, 1987.

41. Hadlock FP, Deter RL, Carpenter RL, et al: The effect of head shape on the accuracy of BPD in estimating fetal gestational age. AJR 137:83, 1981.

42. Gray DL, Songster GS, Parvin CA, Crane JP: Cephalic index: A gestational age-dependent biometric parameter. Obstet Gynecol 74:600, 1989.

43. Doubilet PM, Greenes RA: Improved prediction of gestational age from fetal head measurements. AJR 142:797, 1984.

44. Ott WJ: Accurate gestational dating. Obstet Gynecol 66:311, 1985.

45. Yagel S, Adoni A, Oman S, et al: A statistical examination of the accuracy of combining femoral length and biparietal diameter as an index of fetal gestational age. Br J Obstet Gynaecol 93:109, 1986.

46. Benson CB, Doubilet PM: Sonographic prediction of gestational age: Accuracy of second and third trimester fetal measurements. AJR 157:1275, 1991.

47. Hill LM, Guzick D, Hixson J, et al: Composite assessment of gestational age: A comparison of institutionally derived and published regression equations. Am J Obstet Gynecol 166:551, 1992.

48. Jeanty P, Rodesch F, Delbeke D: Estimation of fetal age by long bone measurements. J Ultrasound Med 3:75, 1984.

49. Warda AH, Deter RL, Rossavik IK, et al: Fetal femur length: A critical reevaluation of the relationship to menstrual age. Obstet Gynecol 66:69, 1985.

50. Hadlock FP, Deter RL, Roecker E, et al: Relation of fetal femur length to neonatal crown-heel length. J Ultrasound Med 3:1, 1984.

51. Mayden KL, Tortora M, Berkowitz RL: Orbital diameters: A new parameter for prenatal diagnosis and dating. Am J Obstet Gynecol 144:289, 1982.

52. Jeanty P, Cantraine F, Cousaert E, et al: The binocular distance: A new way to estimate fetal age. J Ultrasound Med 3:241, 1984.

53. Mercer BM, Sklar S, Shariatmadar A, et al: Fetal foot length as a predictor of gestational age. Am J Obstet Gynecol 15:350, 1987.

54. Hill LM, et al: Transverse cerebellar diameter as a predictor of menstrual age. Obstet Gynecol 75:983, 1990.

55. Hill LM, Guzick D, Thomas ML, Fries JK: Fetal radius length: A critical evaluation of race as a factor in gestational age assessment. Am J Obstet Gynecol 161:193, 1989.

56. Yarkoni S, Schmidt W, Jeanty P, et al: Clavicular measurement: A biometric parameter for fetal evaluation. J Ultrasound Med 4:467, 1985.

57. Mahony B, Callen P, Filly R: The distal femoral epiphyseal ossification centers in the assessment of third trimester menstrual age: Sonographic identification and measurement. Radiology 155:201, 1984.

58. Rutherford SE, Phelan JP, Smith CV, Jacobs N: The four-quadrant assessment of amniotic fluid volume: An adjunct to antepartum fetal heart rate testing. Obstet Gynecol 70:353, 1987.

59. Petrucha RA, Platt LD: Relationship of placental grade to gestational age. Am J Obstet Gynecol 144:733, 1982.

60. Zilianti M, Fernandez S: Correlation of ultrasonic images of fetal intestine with gestational age and fetal maturity. Obstet Gynecol 62:569, 1982.

61. Goldstein I, Lockwood CJ, Hobbins JC: Ultrasound assessment of fetal intestinal development in the evaluation of gestational age. Obstet Gynecol 70:682, 1987.

62. Hadlock FP, Deter RL, Harrist RB, et al: A date-independent predictor of intrauterine growth retardation: Femur length/abdominal circumference ratio. AJR 141:979, 1983.

63. Hadlock FP, Harrist RB, Shah YP, et al: The use of femur length/head circumference relation in obstetrical sonography. J Ultrasound Med 3:439, 1984.

64. Hohler CW, Quetel TA: The relationship between fetal femur length and biparietal diameter in the last half of pregnancy. Am J Obstet Gynecol 141:759, 1981.

65. Hadlock FP, Harrist RB, Martinez-Poyer J: Fetal body ratios in second trimester: A useful tool for identifying chromosomal abnormalities? J Ultrasound Med 11:81, 1992.

66. Goldstein I, Reece EA, O'Connor T, Hobbins JC: Estimating gestational age in the term pregnancy with a model based on multiple indices of fetal maturity. Am J Obstet Gynecol 161:1235, 1989.

67. Kurtz AB, Needleman L: Ultrasound assessment of fetal age. In Callen PW (ed): Ultrasonography in Obstetrics and Gynecology, 2nd ed. Philadelphia, WB Saunders, 1988.

68. Rose BI, Lamb EJ: Multiple simultaneous predictors of gestational age: An application of Bayer's theorem. Am J Perinatol 5:44, 1988.

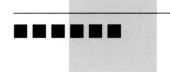

CHAPTER 8

Ultrasound Evaluation in Multiple Gestation

HARRIS J. FINBERG, M.D.

All multiple gestations have substantially higher risks of fetal morbidity and mortality than singleton pregnancies do. The risks become progressively greater as the number of fetuses increases. Among twin pregnancies, there is greater danger of adverse outcome when the twins share a single placenta (monochorionic) than if each has a separate placenta (dichorionic). A still greater danger exists when monochorionic twins also share a single amniotic sac.

Sonography plays an essential role in the diagnosis and management of multiple gestations. It can provide early detection of multifetal pregnancy and accurate determination of the number of placentas and amniotic compartments. Ultrasound evaluation is necessary to identify a variety of specific pathologic conditions that can complicate monochorionic twinning. Intrauterine growth retardation, fetal distress, and premature labor are frequent complications of multiple gestation, and interval sonographic assessment of fetal growth and well-being are reasonably performed in all multifetal gestations.

For the sake of simplicity, the focus in this chapter is on twin pregnancies. All of the general risks of twinning occur and are exaggerated in triplet and higher-order multiple gestations. Similarly, all risks that apply to monochorionic twins also apply to twin pairs or larger groups of fetuses sharing a single placenta within a higher-order multiple gestation.

EMBRYOLOGY AND INCIDENCE OF TYPES OF TWINNING

Twinning occurs either by fertilization of two separate ova (dizygotic) or by fertilization of a single ovum that subsequently divides, yielding two genetically identical embryos (monozygotic).

Dizygotic twinning occurs at significantly different rates among various world populations. The Yoruba people of Nigeria have an incidence of 1 in 20 to 25 pregnancies, a fourfold greater rate than white populations have. The rate in Japan is only 1 in 150 pregnancies.[1] Genetic differences, perhaps related to gonadotropin secretion rates, have been implicated as a predominant cause, but other influences including increasing maternal age, seasonality, and even local environmental and nutritional factors have also been noted to affect dizygotic twinning rates.[2]

The frequency of monozygotic twinning is constant throughout the world at 3.5 per 1000, appearing to be independent of genetic, age, or environmental influences.[2] In the United States twins have occurred in about 1:85 pregnancies, with approximately 70% dizygotic and 30% monozygotic. Therapies for infertile couples including ovulation induction, in vitro fertilization, and intrafallopian gamete transfer all have high rates of twin and higher-order multiple pregnancy, significantly greater than spontaneous rates, reaching 25% for intrafallopian gamete transfer.[3] Nearly all such pregnancies are multizygotic, increasing both the overall incidence of twins and the proportion of dizygotic twins.

All dizygotic twins start as two fertilized ova, each of which becomes a blastocyst that will have a separate implantation site. Therefore, all dizygotic twin pregnancies are dichorionic: each of the embryos has its own placenta and chorionic membrane. Since the amnion forms within the chorionic space and develops subsequent to the chorion, all dichorionic twin pregnancies are necessarily diamniotic also.[2]

In monozygotic twins, the pattern of chorionicity and amnionicity is dependent on the stage at which the single fertilized ovum splits (Fig. 8–1). If the cleavage occurs by the third day, two separate blastocysts develop and a dichorionic diamniotic pregnancy results, just as in all dizygotic cases. This occurs in about 25% of monozygotic twins.

In the other 75% of monozygotic twins, cleavage occurs after day 3, when the single fertilized ovum has reached the blastocyst stage, thus producing a monochorionic twin pregnancy with the single placenta shared by both twins. In nearly all monochorionic twin pregnancies, the splitting occurs between day 4 and 8, before the development of the amnion, with each embryo subsequently forming its own amnion: monochorionic diamniotic twinning.[2]

Monozygotic cleavage occurring between days 8 and 13 produces twins within a single amniotic sac: monochorionic monoamniotic twinning. This very high risk form of twinning is uncommon, accounting for only 2% of monozygotic twin pregnancies. In the rare case when the twinning event happens beyond day 13, embryonic fission is incomplete, resulting in conjoined twins. These are always monochorionic monoamniotic.[2] Two rare variations of dizygotic twinning have been described. Superfetation is defined as the successful fertilization of a second ovum released during an ongoing pregnancy, resulting in twins of unequal age. Soudre and colleagues have reported a convincing example of unequal sized twins, each with normal

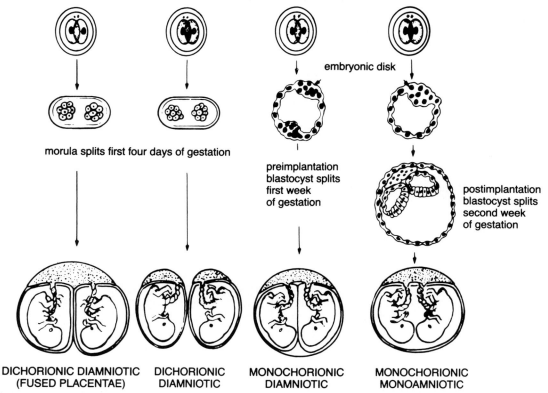

embryonic disk

morula splits first four days of gestation

preimplantation blastocyst splits first week of gestation

postimplantation blastocyst splits second week of gestation

| DICHORIONIC DIAMNIOTIC (FUSED PLACENTAE) | DICHORIONIC DIAMNIOTIC | MONOCHORIONIC DIAMNIOTIC | MONOCHORIONIC MONOAMNIOTIC |

Figure 8–1. Diagram of the development and placentation of monozygotic twins. (From Fox H: Pathology of the Placenta. London, WB Saunders Co., Ltd., 1978.)

growth rates as followed by ultrasound evaluation from 16 weeks' gestation to delivery at 37 weeks. At birth the twins were 1 month different in physical and neurologic maturity by standard developmental criteria.[4] Superfecundation is the fertilization of two ova within a short interval by separate acts of coitus. Such cases are not detectable by sonography but may be proved by detailed genetics if the twins have different fathers.

The type of placentation in twin pregnancies has important prognostic significance. Most, if not nearly all, monochorionic twin placentas have vascular anastomoses between the circulations of the two fetuses. These are most frequently arterial to arterial but may be venous to venous, arterial to venous, or a combination of these types. These circulatory communications provide the pathologic basis for a group of syndromes that specifically affect only monochorionic twin pregnancies and that account, in large measure, for the greater morbidity and mortality of monochorionic as compared with dichorionic twins. These conditions include the twin transfusion syndrome, the twin embolization syndrome, and the acardiac parabiotic twin syndrome.[2]

Dichorionic placentas, whether from dizygotic or monozygotic twinning, may implant in geographically separate regions of the endometrial cavity and develop as distinct individual organs.

They may, alternatively, implant close together and, with growth, coalesce into a single inseparable structure. Fused dichorionic placentas do *not*, with ex-

tremely rare documented exceptions, develop vascular anastomoses between the circulations of the two twins. Dichorionic twins, even with a fused placenta, are therefore not at risk for the syndromes that may afflict monochorionic twins.[5]

MORBIDITY AND MORTALITY IN MULTIPLE GESTATIONS

All multiple gestations have remarkably higher rates of mortality than occur in singleton pregnancies,[6] and for triplets that rate is more than twice as high for twins.[7] Morbidity is similarly two to three times more prevalent in twins than singletons, reported by Ghai and Vidyasagar[6] at 47% versus 27% and by Kovacs and coworkers[8] at 83% versus 32%.

The major causes of adverse outcome are prematurity and intrauterine growth retardation.[6, 8–11] Ghai and Vidyasagar found that birth weight less than 1500 g occurs in 10.1% of twins but in only 1.2% of singletons.[6] Severe prematurity (less than 32 weeks at delivery) accounts for most of the smallest infants, with weights about appropriate for gestational stage in most cases. It would appear that the uteroplacental system can support unrestricted fetal growth up to 3000 g combined fetal weight, but beyond this weight there is a progressive risk of growth retardation. Although specific growth curves have been generated for twin pregnancies, McCulloch suggests that it is more reasonable to use standard singleton growth charts since those designed for twins will incorporate the high incidence of third-trimester growth retardation into the norms.[12]

There is an additional peak in perinatal mortality in the group of twins delivered after 38 weeks' gestation, occurring as a consequence of placental insufficiency, representing, in effect, the postmaturity sequence seen in single pregnancies after 41 to 42 weeks.[6, 10]

The risks of prematurity, growth retardation, and accelerated onset of postmature placental insufficiency affect all multiple gestations. It is clear, however, that monochorionic twins suffer disproportionately more than dichorionic twins from these problems. They are also at specific additional risk from twin transfusion syndrome, twin embolization syndrome, and acardiac parabiotic twin syndrome. Benirschke, in 1964, found the mortality risk for dichorionic twins to be 10%, that for monochorionic diamniotic twins to be 25%, and that for monochorionic monoamniotic twins to be 50%.[13]

There have been important innovations in the diagnosis, assessment and management of multiple gestation over the past 3 decades. A study by Saari-Kemppainen and coworkers[14] studied 9310 pregnant women in Finland who were randomly assigned to routine screening by sonography at 16 to 20 weeks or to scanning for routine indications only, with other aspects of antenatal care otherwise similar. Overall perinatal mortality for all pregnancies was halved for the screened group relative to controls. All twins were detected by the 21st week in the screened group versus 76.3% only in the controls, and perinatal mortality in the small series of twins was 27.8/1000 for screened pregnancies versus 65.8/1000 in controls.

Recent care improvements have reduced the overall loss of twins by about half,[11, 15] but the perinatal mortality of monochorionic twins remains two to three times greater than that of dichorionic pairs, and monoamniotic twins still have a 30% to 50% risk of death.[6, 12, 16] For essentially every category of morbidity, monochorionic twins experience greater occurrence rates and/or severity than do the dichorionic twins. These include degree of growth retardation,[6, 12] presence of congenital malformations,[17] and incidence of spontaneous abortions.[9]

Statistics on perinatal mortality are generally reported on pregnancies in which the fetuses are at least 500 g or beyond 22 weeks' gestational age. Multiple gestations are at greater risk than singleton pregnancies for one or multiple losses in the first half of pregnancy as well. This phenomenon was carefully evaluated by Dickey and colleagues[18] in a population of 4517 patients who became pregnant through infertility treatment. Sonography revealed 227 twin, 43 triplet, and 5 quadruplet pregnancies, all of which had multiple gestational sacs (and were presumably multizygotic). Dickey and colleagues found a loss rate of up to 49% for at least one twin when twinning was initially documented by presence of two gestational sacs and a loss rate of up to 16% when two live fetuses had been seen. With triplets documented by three gestational sacs, the loss rate was up to 82%, with a disappearance rate up to 56% when three live fetuses had been imaged. The patients younger than age 30 experienced lower loss rates than those aged 30 and older (Table 8–1). From a prognostic standpoint for infertility patients, Dickey and colleagues did observe that the chance of getting at least one live infant improved with more gestational sacs: 78% for single sac, 89% for two, and 93% for three. Corroboration of these statistics has been provided by Sampson and de Crespigny studying a group of 59 twin pregnancies conceived by in vitro fertilization and 67 twin pregnancies not from in vitro fertilization, with similar results in both groups. Of live twin pairs detected by 7 weeks, live twin neonates occurred in only 71%. Each twin, if live before 7 weeks, has a 19% risk of in utero death, and, if live between 7 and 10 weeks, had an 11% risk of in utero death.[19]

Twinning in spontaneous pregnancy also occurs at greater rates than are recognized by second- and third-trimester ultrasound evaluation or in birth statistics. Landy and colleagues[20] evaluated 1000 first-trimester pregnancies. Of 54 patients with early sonographic evidence of multiple gestations, 35 were spontaneous and 19 had undergone ovarian stimulation. They found a 3.3% incidence of twins recognized by the presence of two live fetuses, and a 5.4% presumptive total incidence of twinning by including cases with a live fetus and an additional sac that was empty or abnormal. Of these cases with initial documentation of two live

Table 8–1. PERCENTAGE OF LIVE BIRTHS AFTER DOCUMENTATION OF MULTIPLE GESTATIONS BEFORE 9 WEEKS' MENSTRUAL AGE*

Findings	Maternal Age (yr)	Three Live Births (%)	Two Live Births (%)	One Live Birth (%)	No Live Births (%)
Two gestational sacs	<30		63	30	7
	≥30		51	34	15
Two live embryos	<30		91	7	2
	≥30		84	13	3
Three gestational sacs	<30	45	40	5	10
	≥30	17	61	17	4
Three live embryos	<30	90	10		
	≥30	45	33	11	11

*Based on 227 twin and 43 triple pregnancies.
Modified from Dickey RP, et al: The probability of multiple births when multiple gestational sacs or viable embryos are diagnosed at first trimester ultrasound. Hum Reprod 5:881, 1990; by permission of Oxford University Press.

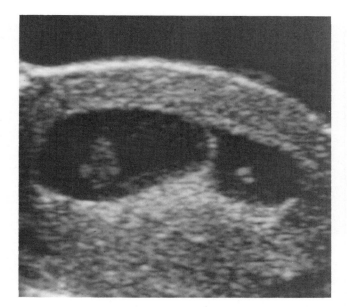

Figure 8–2. Gestational sac too small for size of fetus is a sign of impending death. A scan at 8 weeks (menstrual age) shows live dichorionic twins of similar crown-rump length and with similar heart rates. The sac of the twin to the right of the image has a much smaller volume than the sac of the twin to the left. A scan 2 weeks later showed interval fetal growth but persistent small sac volume and a new finding of bradycardia at 68 beats per minute. One week later, a scan showed death of this fetus.

fetuses, 21% had a subsequent scan that showed only a singleton gestation. Sonographic observations that suggest the risk of impending death of a twin include either one gestational sac smaller than the other, appearing "too small" for the fetus (Fig. 8–2), or one fetus visually smaller than the other.

The criteria of twinning in all of these studies included identification of two separate gestational sacs. Thus these pregnancies were dichorionic and almost certainly predominantly dizygotic. Monochorionic twins are diagnosed in early pregnancy by finding two fetal structures, each with a heartbeat, contained in one gestational sac. These pregnancies have a remarkably high rate of loss. Wenstrom and Gall reported that the ratio of monozygotic to dizygotic twins is 17.5 to 1 in abortuses.[9] In triplet and higher-order multiple gestations, monochorionic twin pairs may occur, and

Table 8–2. COMPARISONS OF MORBIDITY MEASURES IN 15 SETS OF LIVEBORN TRIPLETS AND 15 MATCHED SETS OF TWINS

Measure	Triplets	Twins
Preterm labor	80%	40%
Preterm delivery	87%	26.7%
Mean birthweight	1720 g	2475 g
Gestational age at delivery	33 weeks	36.6 weeks
Growth retardation of one or more neonates	53.3%	6.7%
Size discordancy	66.7%	13.3%
Average neonatal hospital stay	29 days	8.5 days
Ratio of neonates requiring intensive care		5:1

From Sassoon DA, et al: Perinatal outcome in triplet versus twin gestations. Reprinted with permission from The American College of Obstetricians and Gynecologists (Obstetrics and Gynecology, 1990, 75:817).

it is possible to see combined patterns of vanishing fetuses (Fig. 8–3). The disappearance of a twin may be clinically silent but may be accompanied by first-trimester bleeding. The occurrence of bleeding does not appear to reduce the prognosis for successfully carrying the residual twin.[21]

The morbidity and mortality in triplet and quadruplet pregnancies is even greater than in twins.[7, 22, 23] Sassoon and coworkers compared perinatal outcome in 15 triplet pregnancies (all live births) with 15 twin pregnancies carefully matched for age, background, and risk factors. All measures of morbidity were more severe for the triplets except respiratory distress syndrome and intraventricular hemorrhage (Table 8–2).[23] Most early spontaneous twin deaths reabsorb or shrink to nondetectable size over a short time interval. Remnants of a fetus that dies later, particularly after the first trimester, may persist either as an amorphous structure along the placenta or uterine margin (Fig. 8–4) or as a compressed, flattened fetal structure in which

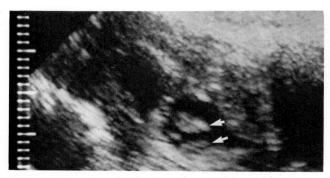

Figure 8–3. Early pregnancy failure with adjacent live monochorionic twins. A 7-week scan shows two live fetuses in the caudal intrauterine sac (second twin along posterior wall of sac). The sac higher within the uterus was empty. At 10 weeks, the empty sac was no longer seen and the twins were alive and thought to be monoamniotic. The patient was delivered of a single healthy infant near term with no detected remnant of a twin.

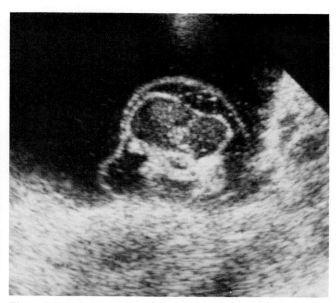

Figure 8–4. Twin remnant in a 36-week pregnancy. A high-resolution view along the chorionic surface of the placenta shows an amorphous, complex structure about 2 cm in diameter in an uneventful pregnancy with late access to care. At delivery of a normal infant, pathologic evaluation confirmed this to be a hyalinized remnant of a twin pregnancy.

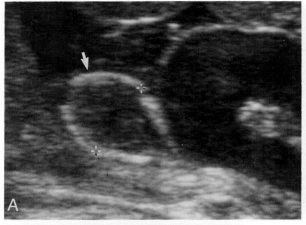

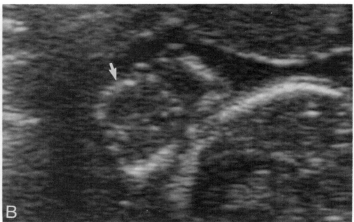

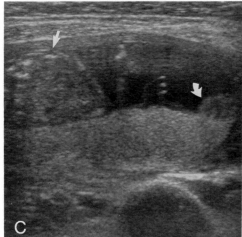

Figure 8–5. Development of a fetus papyraceous in two patients with twins. *A* and *B*. The well-formed torso and head *(arrows)* of a small fetus without heartbeat (average size for 13 weeks by the femur length) is seen adjacent to a live, normal 24-week fetus. *C*. A scan of this patient demonstrated a twin, monochorionic gestation. A repeat scan done in the second trimester demonstrated a normal living fetus on the left of the image *(arrow)* and the small remnant of the dead twin on the right *(curved arrow)*.

bones may still be visualized. This latter condition is referred to by the term *fetus papyraceous* (Fig. 8–5).

Maternal morbidity is also increased in multiple gestations. The risk of proteinuric preeclampsia is five times greater in twins compared with singletons.[9] Lopez-Llera and coworkers[24] reported that the incidence of frank eclampsia in twin pregnancies is three times that in single gestations, and the risk that a patient will develop eclampsia is increased with male-male twin pairs. Five of six maternal deaths in their series occurred in cases of male twins, and the male-male twin pairs themselves also had higher perinatal mortality.

SONOGRAPHIC DETERMINATION OF CHORIONICITY AND AMNIONICITY

One of the primary tasks in evaluating a twin pregnancy is to identify the chorionic and amniotic status, since this will help establish the relative risk of morbidity and mortality in the pregnancy. A decision cascade of imaging criteria provides a logical sequence of observations to seek to make this determination.[25]

1. In pregnancies up to about the 10-weeks stage, count the number of gestational sacs and the number of embryonic heartbeats. Each gestational sac forms its own placenta and chorion. Thus, two gestational sacs imply a dichorionic (and, therefore, also diamniotic) pregnancy, while a single gestational sac must

be monochorionic. There is a high rate of vanishing twin, particularly when twins are diagnosed by recognition of two sacs rather than two live fetuses, each with heartbeat. Until live twins are confirmed, the diagnosis of twinning must be tempered with caution (Fig. 8–6).

2. When monochorionic twins are found up to about 10 weeks, carefully seek the presence of one or two separate amniotic sacs within the chorionic cavity. The amnion grows outward from the embryonic disk, and before 10 weeks the separate amnions of a diamniotic pregnancy will not have enlarged sufficiently to contact each other to create the intertwin septum. Each single amnion is extremely thin and delicate, and it may be very difficult to see on transabdominal scanning. Endovaginal imaging is often more successful (Fig. 8–7). If both twins are present within a single amnion, monoamniotic pregnancy is proven.

Recognition of each embryo and heartbeat is particularly difficult before 8 weeks. A potential pitfall in the diagnosis of multiple gestation is the failure to identify a second embryo in a single gestational sac, whether that is the only sac or one of several. This risk is heightened by uterine myometrial contractions that are frequently present, distorting the shape of the pregnancy sac. An embryo can easily be obscured in an angular corner of such an indented sac. Careful scrutiny of every early pregnancy and liberal use of vaginal sonography are important in avoiding this problem.

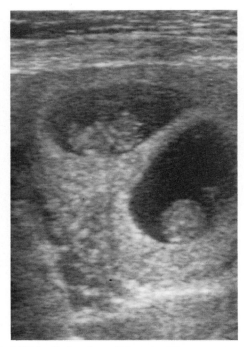

Figure 8–6. Dichorionic twins at 7.7 weeks. Two separate gestational sacs, each containing a live embryo, are seen.

Beyond 10 weeks, gestational sacs are no longer distinctly separable. With their coalescence, the inter-twin membrane is formed and a variety of different criteria related to the fetal gender, placentas, and membranes are used to determine chorionicity and amnionicity. The following order provides a logical sequence for applying these tests. Once a specific step in this decision cascade defines the chorionic and amniotic status of the pregnancy, subsequent steps need not be evaluated. The next three criteria either prove the pregnancy to be dichorionic or they are indeterminate.

3. Determine the gender of the twins. If the twins are a male-female pair, they are necessarily dizygotic and therefore also dichorionic and diamniotic. Like-sex twins and those with unidentified gender are indeterminate by this criterion.

4. Determine the number of placentas. If two separate placentas are present, the pregnancy is dichorionic and must also be diamniotic (Figs. 8–8 and 8–9). A single placental region may occur either in a monochorionic twin pregnancy or with fusion of the two placentas of a dichorionic pregnancy. It is not sufficient to show an anterior and posterior placenta

Figure 8–7. Diamniotic and monoamniotic forms of monochorionic twinning in the first trimester. *A.* Monochorionic diamniotic twins at 7.5 weeks. An endovaginal scan shows a single shared chorionic space surrounded by decidua. Each live twin in this sac is contained within its own very thin amniotic membrane *(arrows)*. These amnions were not detected on transabdominal scans. *B.* Monochorionic mono-amniotic twins at 11.7 weeks. The twins are seen adjacent to one another within the same amniotic sac *(arrows)* C. These monoamniotic twins both have cystic hygromas and generalized body edema. (*B*, Courtesy of B. Kleiner, M.D.)

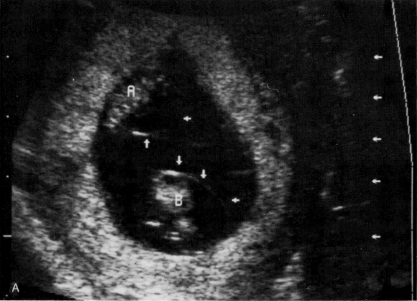

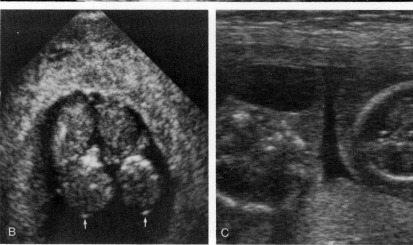

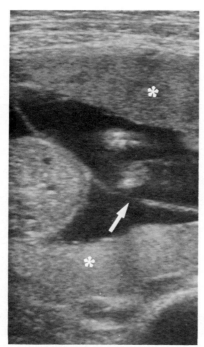

Figure 8–8. Dichorionic twins. Separate placentas (∗) are present along the anterior and posterior walls in this 15-week twin pregnancy. Note also the thick intertwin membrane *(arrow).*

to fulfill this criterion since the placental tissue may be in continuity along a lateral aspect of the uterus. (A rare pitfall could occur if a single shared placenta had a large succenturiate lobe. If that possibility is questioned, application of the next diagnostic steps and identification of the two cord origins from the placenta are likely to resolve this issue.)

5. If there is a single placental region, search for a "chorionic peak." A chorionic peak, also called the twin peak sign, is defined as the presence of a projecting zone of tissue of similar echotexture to the placenta, triangular in cross section and wider at the chorionic surface of the placenta, extending into and tapering to

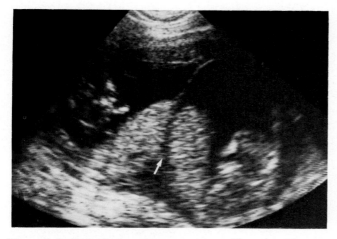

Figure 8–9. Dichorionic twin pregnancy at 12 weeks. The two placentas have formed adjacent to each other, but they have a hypoechoic zone demarcating them as separate *(arrow).* This is accentuated by a myometrial contraction. On scans later in the pregnancy the placentas appeared fused.

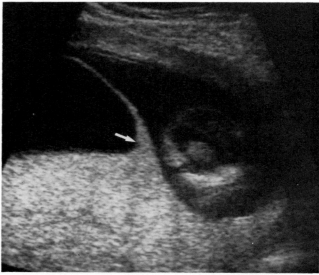

Figure 8–10. Chorionic peak, indicating dichorionic twinning. Placental tissue is present extending into the intertwin membrane at its junction with the chorionic surface, creating a peak with triangular cross section. This finding confirms this 13-week pregnancy to be dichorionic with fused posterior placentas. The membrane is thick and well defined, another finding predictive of dichorionicity.

a point within the intertwin membrane (Fig. 8–10). This phenomenon can occur only in a dichorionic pregnancy because there is a potential interchorionic space between the layers of the twin membrane that is in continuity with the chorionic villi of the placenta (Fig. 8–11A). In a monochorionic pregnancy, the single chorion serves as an intact barrier to the chorionic villi, excluding them from the potential space within the diamniotic membrane (see Fig. 8–11B). Of 15 twin pregnancies in which Finberg identified this twin peak sign, all were dichorionic.[25] The chorionic peak tends to be focal, occurring in one or several sites along the junction of the membrane with the placenta, rather than as a uniform ridge (Fig. 8–12). Absence of this finding neither excludes dichorionicity nor implies monochorionicity. The incidence of identification of the twin peak sign in dichorionic twinning has not yet been established, but with careful evaluation it almost certainly exceeds 50%, in my experience. This observation can be applied between each pair of fetuses of a triplet pregnancy, but it is important to recognize that the placenta of one triplet may contact both, one, or neither of the other placentas (if trichorionic), and the analysis is complex.

6. If the previous criteria are indeterminate, evaluate the presence and thickness of the intertwin membrane. The membrane of a dichorionic pregnancy consists of two layers of amnion and two layers of chorion. It is thicker and more reflective than the monochorionic diamniotic membrane. The latter is composed of two layers of amnion only and is thin, wispy, less reflective, and often hard to image except where it is close to orthogonal to the incident sonographic beam (Figs. 8–13 and 8–14).[26–29]

There are shortcomings to the use of the membrane thickness criterion. There is not an accepted strict

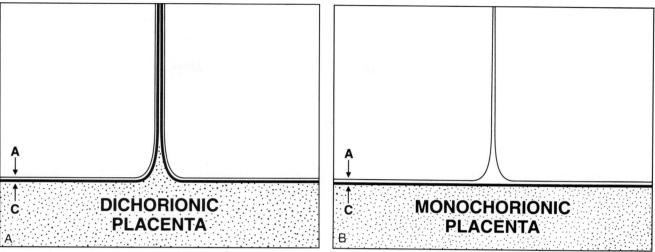

Figure 8–11. *A.* Diagram of the "chorionic peak" sign. The separate chorion and amnion for each twin reflect away from the fused placentas to form the intertwin membrane, consisting of four layers. The proliferating placental villi can grow into the potential interchorionic space of the membrane since there is no physical barrier to their extension into this space. *B.* With a monochorionic diamniotic pregnancy, the intertwin membrane is composed of the two amnions only. The single intact chorion provides an impenetrable barrier to extension of villi into the membrane, and the chorionic peak sign cannot occur. (From Finberg HJ: The "twin peak" sign: Reliable evidence of dichorionic twinning. J Ultrasound Med 11:571–577, 1992.)

definition of what constitutes a thick or thin membrane. The dichorionic membrane thins progressively in the third trimester and becomes less predictive. Townsend and coworkers[26] retrospectively studied 75 twin pregnancies and found a qualitatively thick membrane to have a positive predictive value for dichorionicity of 83%. Detectability of a thick membrane was 89% on first sonograms, falling to only 52% on third-trimester sonograms. Membranes considered thin also had a positive predictive value of 83% but could be recognized as thin in only 54% of monochorionic diamniotic twin pregnancies. Winn and colleagues[27] used a 2-mm thickness to define a thick versus a thin membrane. They achieved a positive predictive rate of 95% for dichorionic and of 82% for monochorionic twinning among 32 twin pregnancies.

The monochorionic diamniotic membrane may ap-

pear artifactually thicker owing to specular reflection when it is exactly orthogonal to the sonographic beam. Filly and colleagues[30] have pointed out that the sonographer's desire to photograph the membrane where it is most prominent increases the risk that evaluation of membrane thickness from hard copy images may be misleading. Real-time assessment allows appreciation of the filmy, wispy quality of a monochorionic diamniotic membrane.

D'Alton and Dudley[31] have reported that sonographically counting the layers of the intertwin membrane

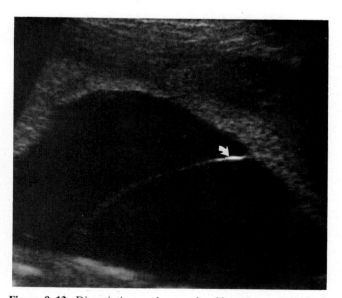

Figure 8–13. Diamniotic membrane of a 22-week monochorionic twin pregnancy. The membrane is thin and, over much of its length, poorly reflective. It appears more echogenic, and artifactually may seem thicker, near the junction with the uterine wall *(arrow)* because the membrane happens to be orthogonal to the incident sonographic beam in this area.

Figure 8–12. Focal regions of chorionic tissue *(arrows)* extension into the intertwin membrane are easily seen in this fused dichorionic placental specimen. These are responsible for the sonographic chorionic peak sign.

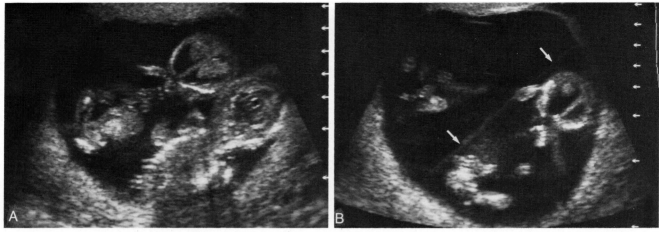

Figure 8–14. Monochorionic diamniotic 12-week twin pregnancy, with thin membrane seen only in some views even on endovaginal images with 7.5-MHz transducer. *A.* Twins are seen in the same chorionic sac, with the membrane not apparent. *B.* With a slight shift in the transducer plane, the diamniotic membrane *(arrows)* is now seen.

accurately predicted chorionicity in 68 of 69 pregnancies: two layers—monochorionic; three or four layers—dichorionic. There have been no confirming studies, and we have been unable to reproduce these observations in our own practice.

7. If no membrane is detected, carefully evaluate the pregnancy conclusively to diagnose or exclude the possibility of monochorionic monoamniotic twinning. When an intertwin membrane is not visualized, possibilities include monoamniotic twinning, presence of a twin with complete oligohydramnios (referred to as a "stuck twin") in which the membrane is closely applied to this twin, and finally a normal twin pregnancy (usually monochorionic diamniotic) in which the membrane is present but not seen owing to its thinness and orientation.[32]

A stuck twin can be suspected when one twin is persistently positioned close to a portion of the uterine wall, often despite polyhydramnios about the other twin. Rolling the pregnant patient into a decubitus lie, so that the questioned stuck twin is nondependent, and demonstrating that this fetus does not shift downward with gravity proves the presence of a restricting membrane (Fig. 8–15). Detailed sonographic inspection of this twin can usually permit visualization of a segment of the membrane, especially between a limb and the torso or between head and shoulder, at least transiently as the fetus attempts to stretch or move (Fig. 8–16).

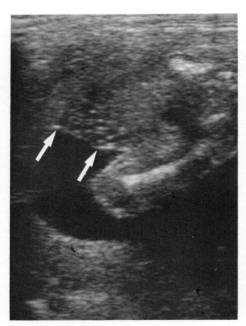

Figure 8–15. Diamniotic twin pregnancy with a "stuck" oligohydramniotic twin due to twin transfusion syndrome. The amniotic membrane is visible *(arrow)*. Normally in these cases the amniotic membrane is not seen but its presence can be inferred because the smaller nonhydropic donor twin does not fall dependently with the patient placed in the lateral decubitus position.

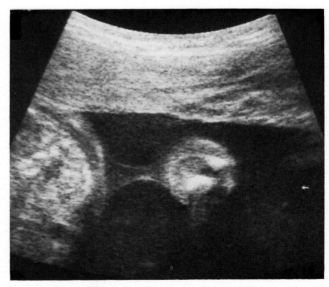

Figure 8–16. A diamniotic twin membrane is seen between the arm and torso of a donor twin with oligohydramnios due to twin transfusion syndrome. The membrane wraps around the body and limbs and becomes stretched and visible as the fetus attempts to abduct the arm. (From Finberg HJ, Clewell WH: Definitive diagnosis of monoamniotic twins. J Ultrasound Med 10:515, 1991.)

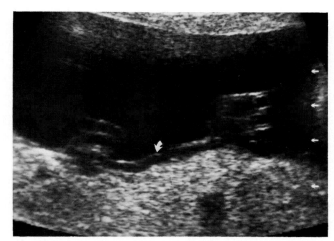

Figure 8–17. Monoamniotic twin pregnancy. Both cord origins from the posterior placenta are seen adjacent to each other, and there is no detectable membrane between them. Note the chorionic surface vessel *(arrow)* running between the two cords. Such vessels provide vascular communications between the circulatory systems of the twins. These can be responsible for monochorionic twin conditions including twin transfusion syndrome, twin embolization syndrome, and acardius.

The management of monoamniotic twins is frequently aggressive, with elective significantly premature cesarean delivery. Diagnosis must, therefore, be certain. The most definite sonographic finding is to follow the umbilical cord of each twin into a common tangle of umbilical cord loops either from the umbilicus of each twin or from the placental origin of each cord (but not from one umbilicus and one placental origin).[33] However, cords need not be intertwined or may be obscured by overlying fetal parts, so this finding may

not be detected in some monoamniotic twin pregnancies.

When both cord origins from a single placenta are seen, the space between them is a prime location to search for the membrane, since it must lie between the cords if it is present. Failure to find the membrane here provides strong support for monoamniotic twinning (Fig. 8–17).

If the sonographic study is not clearly diagnostic, it is reasonable and appropriate to use radiographic confirmation of monoamnionicity before electing early preterm delivery. The most clear-cut, definitive method of proving a pregnancy to be monoamniotic is to demonstrate radiographic contrast material in the intestinal tract of each twin on sonographically selected computed tomographic images performed about 4 hours after the instillation of water-soluble iodinated radiographic contrast agent into one amniotic fluid space by a single amniocentesis.[34] We have used the CT technique three times, twice confirming monoamniotic twins (Fig. 8–18) and once proving the twins to be diamniotic, instead (Fig. 8–19).

MONITORING OF FETAL WELL-BEING AND GROWTH IN MULTIPLE GESTATION

All multiple gestations have high risks of fetal compromise and growth retardation. Standard monitoring tests of fetal well-being, including fetal movement counting and nonstress testing, have limited use in multiple gestation since the pregnant mother may not be able to distinguish the movements of her separate fetuses and there may easily be ambiguity in the source

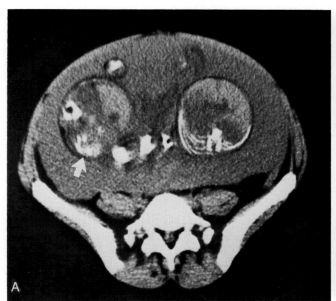
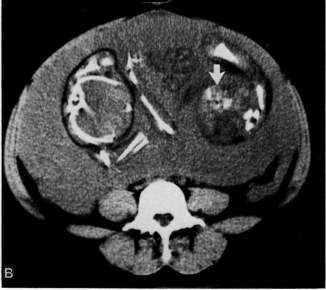

Figure 8–18. Monoamniotic twins proven by demonstrating iodinated contrast agent in the intestinal tract of both twins 4 hours after a single intra-amniotic injection. The two computed tomographic image planes were individually selected by sonography. Contrast agent has largely been cleared from the amniotic space and has concentrated in the fetal gut. *A.* Contrast agent is present in the intestine of the twin toward maternal right *(arrow)*. The intestinal area of the second twin is not in this image plane. *B.* A second selected scan confirms intestinal contrast agent in the left twin *(arrow)*. (From Finberg HJ, Clewell WH: Definitive diagnosis of monoamniotic twins. J Ultrasound Med 10:515, 1991.)

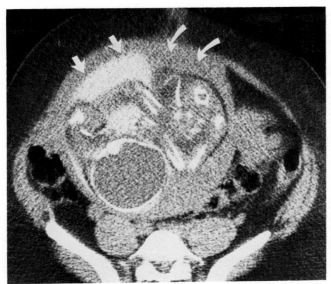

Figure 8–19. Computed tomographic amniogram proves a suspected monoamniotic twin pregnancy to be diamniotic. The patient was difficult to scan owing to obesity. Multiple sonograms at between 16 and 30 weeks' gestation failed to identify an intertwin membrane. The CT scan, with image planes selected using ultrasound, was done at 2 hours after amniotic instillation of an iodinated contrast agent. A sharp demarcation between contrast-enhanced amniotic fluid *(straight arrows)* and nonopacified fluid *(curved arrows)* indicates the plane of a diamniotic membrane.

of heart rate tracings obtained without concurrent imaging. Very heavy reliance is, therefore, placed on sonography to provide early warning signs of fetal distress and of compromise of fetal growth.

Monitoring for fetal well-being is best accomplished by use of the sonographic portions of the biophysical profile, applied separately to each fetus in the pregnancy.[35] The parameters evaluated include fetal movement, tone, breathing activity, and adequacy of amniotic fluid volume. A widely accepted standard of fluid volume, most easily applicable to each gestational sac of a multiple gestation, is identification of a single pocket of fluid with anteroposterior dimension of at least 2 cm, not encroached on by fetal parts or umbilical cord. One cannot apply a four-quadrant amniotic fluid index, since a given gestational space may not occupy all quadrants, and individual fluid pockets may not be unambiguously assignable to a specific fetus.

There is wide agreement that twice-weekly biophysical testing should be performed, beyond the state of viability, in any twin pregnancy showing growth discordancy or below normal amniotic fluid volume in either compartment, as well as in all triplet and higher-order multiple gestations. Reasonable arguments may be made for extending the routine of twice-weekly biophysical profile testing to all twin pregnancies from week 26 on.

Umbilical artery Doppler velocimetry has been suggested as a worthwhile adjunctive study of well-being in twins[36] and triplets,[37, 38] although it is not uniformly recognized as helpful.[39] Giles and coworkers[36] studied 272 twin pregnancies by continuous-wave Doppler study. After the first 100 cases, which were studied but

not reported to clinicians, the subsequent cases were all examined at between 28 and 32 weeks' gestation with results made available for potential influence on clinical management. Between these two groups they found a decrease in corrected perinatal mortality (which excludes anomalous fetuses) from 42.1 to 8.9 per 1000, with fetal deaths reduced from 6 to 1 ($P < .05$). Fewer infants in the study group required neonatal intensive care, 24% versus 38%, and these results were achieved without significant change in gestational age at delivery or cesarean section rate.

Growth discordancy and the consequent risk of compromise of the growth restricted fetus is a major source of morbidity in multiple gestation. An early report by Crane and coworkers[40] found that an intertwin difference of 5 mm in biparietal diameter or of 5% in head circumference, if seen in the second trimester, was associated with high perinatal mortality, much of it secondary to twin transfusion syndrome. Head discordancy after 30 weeks' gestation had a better prognosis.

Most subsequent studies on discordancy have focused on differences in abdominal circumference or estimated fetal weight.[41–46] A difference in abdominal circumference of 20 mm or greater on a scan within 2 weeks of delivery predicted a birthweight discrepancy of 20% or greater with 62% positive predictive value and 93% negative predictive value according to Storlazzi and coworkers.[41] They also found 80% positive predictive value and 93% negative predictive value for estimated fetal weights of 20% difference. Groups headed by O'Brien and associates[43] and Blickstein and Shoham-Schwartz[44] both recommended a weight estimate discordancy of 15% as a safety limit for concern for birthweight disparity at risk of association with increased morbidity (positive predictive value 34%, negative predictive value 95%[43]). Divon and colleagues[46] used either a 15% difference in estimated fetal weight or a 15% difference in umbilical artery systolic-to-diastolic ratio to identify correctly 14 of 18 discordant twin pairs while including only 5 of 40 concordant pairs (Table 8–3).

A report by Secher and associates,[47] reviewing 80 consecutive twin pregnancies, found growth retardation affecting one fetus in 22 cases and affecting both twins in 4 other cases. This helps to point out the concern for using separately generated growth charts for twins or triplets, since these will incorporate the intrinsically higher occurrence of below ideal growth

---

Table 8–3. INDICATORS OF INTERTWIN BIRTHWEIGHT DISCORDANCY THAT MAY BE ASSOCIATED WITH AN INCREASED RISK OF PERINATAL MORBIDITY

Difference in abdominal circumference ≥20 mm
Difference in estimated fetal weight ≥15%
Difference in umbilical artery Doppler A/B ratio ≥15%
Difference in biparietal diameter ≥5 mm*
Difference in head circumference ≥5%*

*Predictive in second but not third trimester and noted to be associated with discordancy as part of twin transfusion syndrome.

of fetuses in multiple gestations, even when they are not overtly compromised.

An additional important source of morbidity and mortality in multiple pregnancies is the occurrence of preterm labor and cervical incompetency. Sonographic assessment of the cervix may play a role in reducing these risks. Michaels and coworkers[48] studied 51 consecutive twin pregnancies prospectively, from initial observation at 14 to 20 weeks until at least 32 weeks, with weekly to biweekly scans of the cervix performed transabdominally using differential bladder filling and emptying. Patients served as their own controls and were evaluated for cervical shortening, dilatation, and protrusion of membranes. Seven study-group patients underwent cerclage as a result of sonographic findings. All twins in the study group survived, while 9 patients among 153 concurrent controls delivered at a mean gestational age of 22.7 weeks with a loss of 17 of 18 of these twins. By 31 weeks, only 1 of the study group had delivered compared with 18 among the controls. The control patients were cared for by their individual obstetricians instead of Michaels and coworkers, and differences in management may have contributed to the improved outcome, but the authors believe that the sonographic cervical assessment was the key factor.

AMNIOCENTESIS IN MULTIPLE GESTATIONS

As with singleton pregnancies, amniocentesis may be used to provide important information for management of multiple gestations, especially with respect to fetal karyotyping, evaluation of maternal serum α-fetoprotein abnormalities, and lung maturity studies. Procedures must be modified to ensure accuracy of sample acquisition and safety to the pregnancy.

In general, information sought should be obtained from each gestational sac. This is most safely performed by sequential individual amniocenteses. To confirm that a subsequent needle placement samples a different sac, 1 to 2 mL of a vital dye, usually indigo carmine, is injected through the first amniocentesis needle after the sample is obtained and before the needle is withdrawn. A subsequent amniocentesis that yields unstained fluid proves the sample to be from a different sac. A single color of dye is sufficient no matter how many amniotic sacs are present: stained fluid has already been sampled while unstained fluid has not.

Two notes of caution should be mentioned. Care must be taken to avoid injection of the dye into the fetal skin. This could produce a permanent tattoo. Methylene blue should not be used as an intra-amniotic dye marker. Its use has been shown to be associated with a 17.0% incidence of jejunal atresia (21 of 123 exposed fetuses), requiring postnatal surgical correction.[49]

Jeanty and coworkers[50] have reported a single-needle technique in twin amniocentesis. They sample one gestational sac and then, under continuous sonographic monitoring, pass the same needle through the interamniotic membrane. An initial aliquot of several milliliters from the second sac is discarded to avoid contamination, and the second sample is then obtained. The procedure was successful in 17 of 18 attempted cases, and no adverse affects were detected.

A potential cause for concern with this single-needle technique is raised by Gilbert and colleagues,[51] who reported eight cases of rupture of a previously documented interamniotic membrane during pregnancy. This resulted in pregnancies that were effectively monoamniotic and in which a 44% mortality rate occurred. Seven of the eight were monochorionic and diamniotic and the other was dichorionic by placental and membrane histology. Although none of these patients had undergone an amniocentesis, one had undergone a laser procedure to ablate placental vascular communications for a twin transfusion syndrome, and a small rent in the intra-amniotic membrane had been created during the procedure. The knowledge that an intertwin membrane, especially a thin, diamniotic membrane, may rupture spontaneously, and the presence of a case in which an iatrogenic hole in a membrane subsequently extended should at least raise caution before one considers adopting the single-needle twin amniocentesis technique.

It is clear that for genetic karyotyping it is necessary to sample fluid from the sac of each fetus present. Any twin pregnancy that appears by sonography to be dichorionic may well be dizygotic. Although there are findings that prove a pregnancy to be dichorionic, there is no sonographic sign after the first trimester that unequivocally shows a pregnancy to be monochorionic (unless it is clearly monoamniotic, in which case there is only one sac to tap). The thin membrane criterion is only 83% accurate, and prudence dictates that karyotyping be separately performed on each twin.

There is a widespread belief that the stress of intrauterine growth retardation has a maturing influence on fetal lungs. If fluid from a larger twin shows mature lung indices, then the smaller, more stressed twin should also have mature lungs. Similarly, presenting twins are considered usually to be less stressed than second twins, so that amniocentesis from the sac of the presenting twin should be predictive of the pulmonary maturity status of both twins. Preliminary experience from our practice suggests that these patterns may be variable. When it is possible to sample amniotic fluid from each sac safely, it remains most reasonable to attempt to do so.

Twin pregnancy is recognized as one of the common causes of elevated maternal serum α-fetoprotein levels, but if serum elevations are greater than four multiples of the singleton median level, there are significantly increased incidences of neural tube defect, fetal and neonatal death, premature delivery, and twin-to-twin birth discordance.[52–54] Caution must be used in the interpretation of amniotic fluid α-fetoprotein and acetylcholinesterase when searching for neural tube defects. α-Fetoprotein can diffuse across dichorionic, diamniotic membranes, and both α-fetoprotein and acetylcholinesterase can diffuse across the diamniotic membrane of a monochorionic twin pregnancy.[55, 56]

CONGENITAL ANOMALIES IN TWINS

Congenital anomalies occur with an increased incidence per fetus in twins and higher-order multiple gestations as compared with singletons. The defects may be concordant or discordant between twins, regardless of whether the pregnancy is monozygotic or dizygotic, but both the incidence of all anomalies and the concordance of anomalies is increased by a factor of as much as four to five times among monozygotic pairs.[9, 57–59] Genetic homogeneity of monozygotic twins is no doubt responsible for much of this concordance, but another factor has also been suggested.

Unlike dizygotic twinning, which occurs at different rates among various genetic populations throughout the world, monozygotic twinning has a constant occurrence rate throughout the world. This has been attributed, by Bulmer as referenced by Benirschke and Kim,[2] to a teratogenic effect on the single fertilized ovum. If this theory is correct, the teratogens that predispose to the twinning event could, if persistent, affect embryologic development and contribute both to the higher overall anomaly rate and the increased frequency of similar abnormalities among monozygotic twins. The fact that concordancy of congenital defects can also occur in dizygotic pairs adds further support for environmental or local teratogenic influences on fetal malformations.

Any abnormality that can affect a singleton pregnancy can occur in either or both members of a twin pregnancy (Fig. 8–20). Some particular categories of congenital anomalies occur more frequently in multiple gestations. These include neural tube defects, hydrocephalus, congenital heart disease, urogenital sinus malformations, chromosomal abnormalities, and single artery umbilical cords.[6] Berg and colleagues[58] performed a statistical analysis on a registry of congenital heart disease compared with a set of controls and found nearly twice as many infants with heart disease to be products of a multiple gestation as in a matched probability set of normal controls. Looping defects occurred in four monozygotic twin pairs but only in one dizygotic twin pair, again implicating some genetic factors. Keusch and coworkers[59] did a similar analysis

on craniofacial abnormalities found in 35 sets of twins (21 monozygotic and 14 dizygotic) among a registry of 1114 patients. The concordance rate was 33% for the monozygotic twins and only 7% for the dizygotic pairs.

A surprising observation was made by Lockwood and colleagues,[60] who reported a case of amniotic band syndrome in a twin pregnancy and reviewed 13 additional case reports. All 12 cases for which zygocity was reported were monozygotic, and all 11 cases for which chorionicity was reported were monochorionic. Of 8 cases that were diamniotic, both twins were separately affected by deformities attributed to bands in 3 cases. In only 1 of 3 monoamniotic cases were both twins affected. Based on these findings, Lockwood and colleagues question the usual "exogenous" theory of amniotic band syndrome and offer a hypothesis of a "primary, perhaps vascular, pathogenesis" for this phenomenon.

In addition to congenital malformations, fetuses within multiple gestations are also at risk for deformations secondary to crowding. These may include clubfoot deformity, other arm and leg distortions, as well as asymmetries to the craniofacial structures or torso. Risks of mechanical deformations rise with increasing numbers of fetuses in the pregnancy.

SYNDROMES SPECIFICALLY ASSOCIATED WITH MONOCHORIONIC TWINS

Nearly all monochorionic twin placentas have vascular communications that interconnect the circulations of both twins. Such connections are extremely rare between dichorionic twins, even when the two placentas grow adjacent to each other and fuse. Twins who share a placenta may, in certain circumstances, transfer blood cells, circulating blood volume, or embolic material through these anastomotic channels. The direction, volume, and significance of these shifts may change dramatically when the clinical status of one or both fetuses deteriorates.

Consider for example, monochorionic twins with a single small chorionic vein-to-vein communication between them. Although both twins are healthy, venous

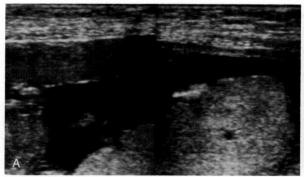 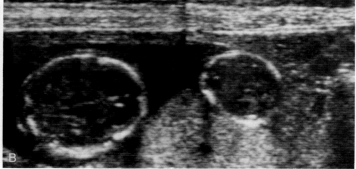

Figure 8–20. Dizygotic twin pregnancy with partial mole and an anomalous fetus due to triploidy in the left-sided gestation. The patient presented at 17.5 weeks with hypertension, acute renal failure, and pulmonary edema. Uterine evacuation was required for maternal indications. *A.* The posterior placenta of the gestation on the right of the image is markedly thickened. The twin on the left with an anterior placenta appeared normal. *B.* The left twin had symmetric growth retardation with all parameters averaging 14 weeks.

pressures are about balanced and no significant shunting of blood volume occurs. If, for whatever reason, one twin dies, the blood pressure in the circulatory system of that twin falls to zero and the normal venous pressure of the remaining twin provides a gradient shunting blood into the vascular bed of the dead twin. The circulatory volume of a fetus is markedly increased by the vascular space available in the placenta, and this factor increases the amount of blood that may be accepted through the shunt. It is common, in this situation of one fetal death, for the live twin to shunt away a sufficient portion of blood volume so that circulatory collapse and death of this second fetus ensues, often within minutes of the death of the first fetus.

The substantial risk of the second twin dying after the death of one monochorionic twin must be figured into the obstetric management plans and the intensity and frequency of fetal monitoring studies performed when even one twin exhibits fetal distress. It should also be noted that this phenomenon provides a nearly absolute contraindication for the selective termination of an anomalous fetus of a monochorionic twin pair.

Three separate syndromes are described that occur as consequences of various vascular communications between monochorionic twins. Twin transfusion syndrome, twin embolization syndrome, and acardiac parabiotic twin syndrome are each associated with grave risks of severe morbidity and mortality.

Twin Transfusion Syndrome

The twin transfusion syndrome is the result of an arteriovenous communication between the circulatory systems of monochorionic twins, usually arising in a shared cotyledon of the common placenta. The syndrome was classically described in neonates, one of whom was growth retarded and anemic while the other was normal to large, plethoric, and sometimes hydropic. Specific criteria of birthweight differences of 15% or more and hemoglobin differences of 5 g/dL or more were considered diagnostic.

This pattern is now recognized as the mild or chronic end of a spectrum of severity, the natural history of which ranges to nearly uniform lethality in utero for both twins with the severe, acute form of twin transfusion syndrome. Anemia/plethora may not, in fact, be a feature of the acute condition. Fisk and colleagues[61] performed umbilical blood samplings on nine twins clinically considered to be suffering from twin transfusion syndrome because of discordant growth and discordant amniotic fluid volumes with monochorionic placentation present. Only one twin pair near term had a hemoglobin difference of 5 g/dL. In acute cases, shifts of circulating blood volume may be more important. Although the syndrome requires only that the twins be monochorionic, the great majority of cases are diamniotic. When the condition is full blown, and the twins are monochorionic and diamniotic, the following findings are seen.

The twin on the arterial side of the communication, referred to as the donor, shunts blood to the other twin, the recipient. The donor twin becomes hypovolemic, leading to severe, generally symmetric growth retardation and to fetal compromise with sluggish or absent movement. The hypovolemia also results in poor renal perfusion, anuria, usually with fetal bladder undetectable, and to severe, often total oligohydramnios of this twin's amniotic sac. As a consequence, the donor twin is held in a fixed position against the wall of the uterus, a phenomenon called the "stuck twin" sign. This twin is at risk of in utero death, but even with survival to delivery there may be pulmonary hypoplasia secondary to oligohydramnios.

The recipient twin becomes hypervolemic. Typically, this twin is normally grown, initially vigorous, and unusually active. The recipient is in a state of constant maximal diuresis and produces copious urine leading to rapidly progressive polyhydramnios. If left unchecked, the polyhydramnios becomes extreme, leading to very premature labor and loss of the pregnancy. If the course is somewhat slower, the circulatory hypervolemia may cause congestive heart failure, hydrops, and death. If either fetus dies in utero, there is a high risk of rapid death of the other twin as well.

The prognosis for both fetuses in the acute twin transfusion syndrome is dismal. Patten and coworkers[62] reported on 25 cases, finding perinatal morbidity in 10% of all twin pairs. Perinatal mortality was 88% for the recipient twin and 96% for the donor twin. The only sonographic finding that seems to correlate with severity (short of fetal hydrops) is the degree of oligohydramnios/polyhydramnios. Complete oligohydramnios of the donor should be taken as strongly prognostic of lethality unless therapy is attempted (see Figs. 8–15 and 8–16). Severe and progressive polyhydramnios of the recipient is strongly indicative of inevitable development of premature labor and delivery unless intervention is initiated. Umbilical artery Doppler studies have shown a difference in systolic-diastolic ratio between the twins of greater than 0.4 in all eight cases studied by Pretorius and coworkers,[63] but they could not differentiate donor from recipient or predict prognosis. Cases in my practice have most frequently shown very slow to absent, or even reversal of, diastolic flow in the umbilical artery of the donor, but also without useful prognostic discrimination of severity (Fig. 8–21).

The grave outlook for twin transfusion syndrome has provided the impetus for some radical interventional therapies. Selective feticide runs the risk of death or embolization syndrome to the remaining twin. Successful removal of one twin and ligation of the cord at open hysterotomy has been performed.[64] Laser ablation of surface chorionic vessels has been attempted through a fetoscope but can only approach posterior and lateral placentas and cannot interrupt communications deep within the placental cotyledon.[65] These methods are too invasive and dangerous to have wide applicability.

An alternative procedure, aggressive volume reduction amniocentesis, appears promising and has been reported by several groups.[66, 67] Elliott and coworkers[66]

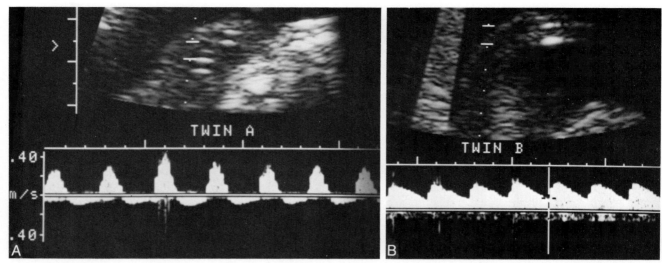

Figure 8–21. Umbilical artery Doppler waveforms in twin transfusion syndrome at 22 weeks' gestation. *A.* There is a very sharp downslope to the systolic pulse with reversal of diastolic flow in the umbilical artery of the donor twin. *B.* The recipient twin has a normal umbilical artery waveform.

performed from 1 to 10 amniocenteses of large volumes of fluid, ranging from 225 to 5000 mL, drained by hand using an 18-gauge needle, from the polyhydramniotic sac of the recipient twin in 17 cases with a "stuck" donor twin. The endpoint of the drainage was the subjective sonographic assessment that the volume of remaining fluid was near lower limits of normal. The patients were scanned twice weekly, and amniocentesis was repeated whenever polyhydramnios reaccumulated. All of the pregnancies achieved a normal amniotic fluid volume and were extended by a mean of

80 days (range, 31 to 119 days.) Twenty-seven of 34 twins survived (a 79% survival rate), and delivery occurred at an average stage of 32.3 weeks (Fig. 8–22). Saunders and coworkers[67] reported the similar use of therapeutic amniocentesis in 19 cases of twin transfusion syndrome with a 37% survival rate. The physiologic basis for the therapeutic benefit to the donor twin is hypothesized to be a reduction in hydrostatic pressure within the overly distended pregnant uterus. This pressure may depress the already compromised circulation of the donor twin below a critical level,

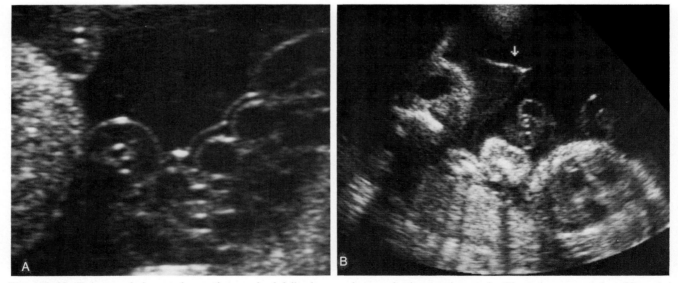

Figure 8–22. Twin transfusion syndrome that resolved following a volume reduction amniocentesis. The twins presented at 25 weeks' gestation. There was severe polyhydramnios about the larger twin, who had ascites. The smaller twin was stuck. *A.* Typical of many twin transfusion syndrome pregnancies, there was gross disparity in the size of the umbilical cords, with the recipient cord being larger. *B.* Following a single volume-reduction amniocentesis, amniotic fluid began to reaccumulate about the stuck twin. The diamniotic membrane *(arrow)* became visible, and urine was seen for the first time in the bladder of the formerly stuck twin (at left of image). Amniotic fluid volumes equilibrated. The smaller twin had a growth spurt. The hydrops of the larger twin resolved, and both twins were healthy at delivery at 37 weeks.

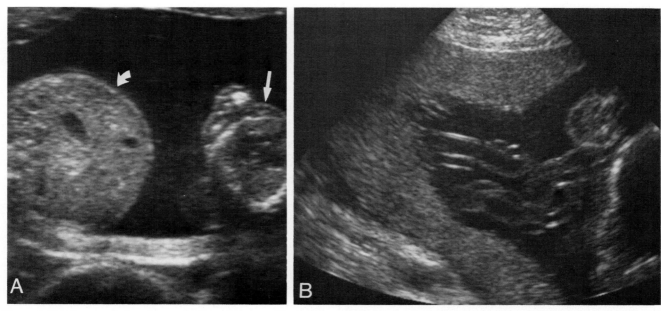

Figure 8–23. Monoamniotic twin transfusion syndrome at 22 weeks' gestation. *A.* There is a smaller donor twin *(straight arrow)* and a larger recipient twin (curved arrow). No membrane was visualized, and no restriction to the movement of either twin was seen as the mother was rolled into different positions. There was polyhydramnios. *B.* Both cord origins at the fundal placenta are seen, and the cords fold around each, confirming the pregnancy to be monoamniotic.

which leads to anuria and complete oligohydramnios. Relief of this pressure appears to improve circulation sufficiently to reinitiate urine production, while improving fetal oxygenation and nutrition.

Twin transfusion syndrome may occur in a monoamniotic pregnancy. Since the donor twin shares the amniotic space with the recipient, it does not become "stuck." The pregnancy will still develop polyhydramnios as in a diamniotic twin transfusion case (Fig. 8–23). It should be noted that oligohydramnios or fetal hydrops may also occur in a dichorionic pregnancy, but etiologies other than twin transfusion syndrome would have to be postulated in that circumstance.

Twin Embolization Syndrome

The in utero death of a monochorionic twin may be followed by the development in the remaining twin of neurologic damage or injury to other organs including the small intestine and kidneys.[30, 68–70] The cause of these abnormalities is theorized to be due to passage of thromboplastic material or of blood clot and detritus from the dead twin, through intraplacental vascular communications into the circulation of the live twin, resulting in thrombotic or embolic events and is referred to as the twin embolization syndrome.

Patten and coworkers[68] found ventriculomegaly, porencephaly, or microcephaly in surviving fetuses of six multiple gestations, five of which were pathologically proven to be monochorionic diamniotic. One of these fetuses also had small bowel atresia requiring surgery. A second had intraperitoneal calcifications without specific clinical correlation. A third had enlarged echogenic kidneys with postnatal clinical evidence of renal

cortical necrosis. Yoshida and Matayoshi[69] found 33 cases with the death of one twin during pregnancy among 133 sets of monochorionic twins. Of these, eight surviving twins (25%) suffered porencephaly, cerebral palsy, and other abnormalities. These researchers found the outcome prognosis to be worse when the co-twin died in the second half of the pregnancy.

Bejar and colleagues[71] studied the risks of antenatal neurologic damage among 89 twins and 12 triplets live born at less than 36 weeks' gestation by evaluating encephalosonograms performed by the third day of postnatal life. Evidence of prenatal cerebral white matter necrosis (brain atrophy or white matter cavitation) was detected in 30% of monochorionic infants and 3.3% of dichorionic infants. Bejar and colleagues demonstrated, by univariate analysis, significant association with polyhydramnios, intrauterine death of the co-twin, hydrops, and pathologic confirmation of placental vascular communications (artery to artery, vein to vein, and artery to vein). The strongest predictor of cerebral damage was vein-to-vein anastomosis, occurring in six of seven infants, followed by artery-to-artery connection and by fetal death of the co-twin. This study indicates that a risk of prenatal neurologic damage, although lower than in monochorionic twins, does still exist for dichorionic twins. Periventricular leukomalacia has been reported on a 27-week in utero scan of a subsequently proven dichorionic fetus with normal growth and normal amniotic fluid volume whose co-twin had complete oligohydramnios secondary to renal agenesis (Fig. 8–24). Postnatal studies confirmed the prenatal diagnosis.

The dangers of neurologic and other organ damage as well as the risk of in utero death of the remaining

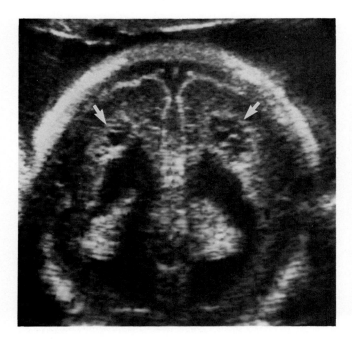

Figure 8–24. In utero identification of periventricular leukomalacia in a twin of a dichorionic pregnancy at 27 weeks' gestation. Multiple small irregular cystic spaces are seen in the parietal periventricular white matter *(arrows)*. The ventricles are mildly enlarged. The subarachnoid spaces are prominent, suggesting the presence of cortical atrophy. There was no known antecedent event. This twin was otherwise normal. The other twin had complete oligohydramnios, diagnosed as due to renal agenesis. All findings were confirmed at birth, including the dichorionicity.

twin following the death of a monochorionic co-twin have implications for management decisions in twin pregnancies in which one or both twins are recognized to be in distress and at risk of death. Very close monitoring and urgent delivery of a surviving twin is an option that requires weighing the uncertain incidence of damage or death to that twin if left in utero against the substantial risks of significantly premature delivery.

One additional potential complication following the death of a twin is the development of maternal disseminated intravascular coagulation. This occurrence has been well documented in singleton pregnancies, when a dead fetus has not been promptly delivered. A case report by Skelly and colleagues[72] described consumptive coagulopathy following one fetal death in an ongoing triplet pregnancy. Romero and coworkers[73] reported successful treatment of this condition after death of a twin. A study of Cherouny and coworkers[74] suggested that this is a rare problem in multiple gestations, failing to find evidence of this condition among 20 cases with death of a fetus after 20 weeks. They recommended conservative management rather than urgent preterm birth, an approach echoed in a study by Goldberger and coworkers.[75]

Acardiac Parabiotic Twin

The acardiac parabiotic twin is a rare and bizarre phenomenon with an incidence of 1 in 35,000 pregnancies. It occurs only in monochorionic twin pregnancy. In this condition, a severely malformed fetus, most often with no formed heart, although occasionally with an inadequate micro two-chambered heart, continues to grow progressively throughout pregnancy. Perfusion of the tissues of this nonviable fetus is accomplished by the presence of paired vein-to-vein and artery-to-artery communications through the placenta to the

circulatory system of the other twin, referred to as the pump twin. Were these not present, this twin would simply be a first-trimester twin death.

Typically the acardiac twin has extremely limited development of the upper half of the body. The head is most often completely absent or occasionally small with holoprosencephaly or other severe brain malformation. Cervical spine, arms, and ribs are absent or hypoplastic. Heart, lungs, and abdominal viscera may all be absent, hypoplastic, or severely malformed. The pelvis and lower extremities are usually much more fully formed. A large dorsal multiloculated cystic hygroma is generally present (Fig. 8–25).

The pattern of development of the acardius is explained by the mechanism of perfusion of this twin. The used, deoxygenated blood of the pump twin travels from the heart to the placenta through the umbilical cord arteries. An artery-to-artery anastomosis in the placenta sends this poorly saturated blood in a retrograde direction through the umbilical arteries of the acardius where it enters the body through the hypogastric arteries. The minimal residual available oxygen is extracted by the tissues of the lower portion of the body of this twin allowing some development and growth. The blood, now fully desaturated, continues to flow in a retrograde direction through the upper body and head, which form poorly if at all, and then flows back to the placenta via the umbilical vein. A vein-to-vein placental anastomosis completes the circulation back into the pump twin. This circulatory pattern gives rise to an alternative name for the acardius phenomenon: twin reversed arterial perfusion (TRAP) sequence. Sherer and coworkers[76] documented the retrograde direction of circulation using Doppler velocimetry of the umbilical cord vessels of both twins in one case of acardius. A case seen in my practice similarly confirms the reversal of blood flow direction (Fig. 8–26).

The added perfusion burden on the cardiovascular

system of the pump twin is the chief cause of morbidity and mortality for this twin, who is the only potentially viable member of the pregnancy. This twin is in a state of persistent high cardiac output, leading to abnormally high renal perfusion and increased urine production. The resultant polyhydramnios may lead to preterm labor. The pump twin is also at risk for high-output congestive heart failure, which may progress to hydrops and death.

Moore and coworkers[77] studied the perinatal outcome in 49 twin pregnancies with an acardiac parabiotic twin. The overall perinatal mortality of the pump twin was 55%. The occurrence of preterm delivery, polyhydramnios, and congestive heart failure were all strongly associated with the ratio of the weights of the acardiac to the pump twin. If the weight of the acardiac twin was greater than 70% that of the pump twin, preterm labor occurred in 90%, polyhydramnios in 40%, and congestive failure in 30%. With acardiac twin weight less than 70%, these rates were preterm delivery in 75%, polyhydramnios in 30%, and congestive heart failure in 10%.

Management strategies for the pump twin may include tocolytic agents and volume reduction amniocentesis to treat preterm labor and frequent interval monitoring studies for signs of congestive failure. If evidence of fetal distress develops at a previable stage, one could consider some form of invasive procedure to ligate the cord of the acardiac twin or otherwise interrupt the circulatory anastomosis.

MORBIDITY AND MORTALITY IN MONOAMNIOTIC TWINNING

Monoamniotic twins are subject to all etiologies of morbidity and mortality that may affect any monochorionic diamniotic twin pregnancy, but they suffer the substantial additional risk of cord entanglement and knotting. The insidious nature of cord accidents is that they may cause death to one or both twins suddenly and without preliminary warning signs that might be detectable by biophysical monitoring studies. The timing of delivery of monoamniotic twins must balance the ongoing risk of unpredictable death with the morbidity and mortality of premature delivery. Cesarean delivery is strongly advocated because of the concern for intrapartum cord accidents. Lumme and Saarikoski[78] in a 20-year review of 23 sets of monoamniotic twins provide support for cesarean delivery. In addition to 4 cases with cord entanglement, they found prolapse of the cord in 3 cases delivered vaginally.

Based on these concerns, coupled with the improving neonatal management of significantly premature infants, Rodis and coworkers[79] have advocated elective cesarean delivery, without proving lung maturity, at or

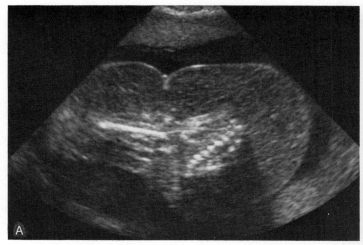

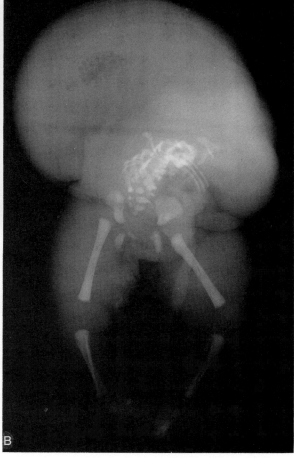

Figure 8–25. Acardiac parabiotic twin at 33 weeks' gestation. There was a normal, nonhydropic twin with moderate polyhydramnios, and in an oligohydramniotic second sac there was an acardius. The normal twin was healthy at a 35-week delivery. *A.* The bony torso of the acardius is small and severely malformed. No organs are recognized. There is gross soft tissue swelling. No head was present. *B.* A specimen radiograph confirms the anatomic features of the acardius.

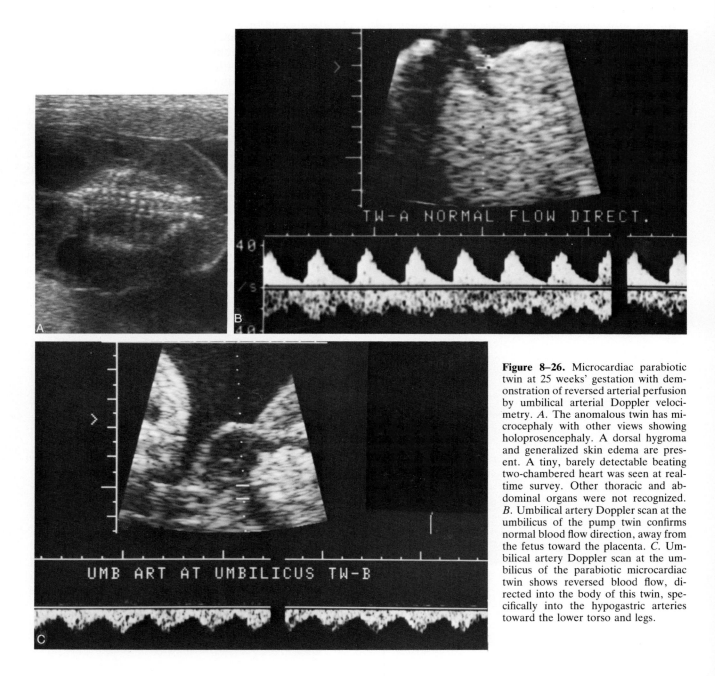

Figure 8–26. Microcardiac parabiotic twin at 25 weeks' gestation with demonstration of reversed arterial perfusion by umbilical arterial Doppler velocimetry. *A.* The anomalous twin has microcephaly with other views showing holoprosencephaly. A dorsal hygroma and generalized skin edema are present. A tiny, barely detectable beating two-chambered heart was seen at real-time survey. Other thoracic and abdominal organs were not recognized. *B.* Umbilical artery Doppler scan at the umbilicus of the pump twin confirms normal blood flow direction, away from the fetus toward the placenta. *C.* Umbilical artery Doppler scan at the umbilicus of the parabiotic microcardiac twin shows reversed blood flow, directed into the body of this twin, specifically into the hypogastric arteries toward the lower torso and legs.

about 32 weeks' gestation. Two retrospective studies of survival rates in monoamniotic twins question the indication for early delivery. Carr and colleagues[80] reviewed hospital records from 1967 to 1988, identifying 24 sets of pathologically proven monoamniotic twins. There were 15 sets with both twins live and 2 sets with one live twin at 30 weeks' gestation, and there were no further deaths beyond that time. Tessen and Zlatnik[81] found 20 sets of monoamniotic twins of at least 20 weeks' gestation over the years 1961 to 1989. They reported 11 deaths through 32nd weeks and none subsequently.

The report by Tessen and Zlatnik, despite arguing against early delivery, presents disturbing data that might well support early elective delivery. Three of their reported 11 fetal deaths occurred in the 32nd week of pregnancy. They have, in addition, annexed an addendum that reports a double fetal death in a 35-week monoamniotic pregnancy, which came to their attention after submission of the manuscript. Lyndrop and Schouenborg[82] reported a monoamniotic double death found at 36 weeks. I also have experienced the death of one twin of a monoamniotic pregnancy at 35 weeks. Based on the dramatic recent improvements in the care and outcome of even very small premature neonates and the more accurate diagnosis of monoamnionicity by current imaging techniques, these several reports of late pregnancy losses suggest that elective cesarean delivery of proven monoamniotic twins at or about 32 weeks may be the most prudent course.

Identification of an intertwin dividing membrane on any sonogram is generally acceptable as proof that these twins are not monoamniotic. Two separate reports have described cases in which rupture of the membrane occurred spontaneously during pregnancy and in which cord entanglement led to morbidity and mortality.[51, 83] It becomes progressively more difficult to visualize the dividing membranes and to trace the course of the umbilical cords in advanced twin pregnancies because of crowding. Nonetheless, one should attempt to document the membrane on each sonogram performed on twins. If the membrane cannot be identified, then one should try to observe the cords. If intertwining of the cords is suggested on the scan, further imaging studies to prove or disprove a ruptured membrane and effective monoamnionicity may be indicated.

CONJOINED TWINS

Conjoined twins result from late and incomplete division of the monozygotic embryonic disk, generally occurring after the 13th day after fertilization. This is a rare sporadic event with prevalence of 1 in 50,000 to 100,000 births and necessarily occurs only in monochorionic monoamniotic pregnancy. Mortality rates are markedly high, and only a very few cases have sufficiently favorable anatomy to permit surgical separation with sustained viability.

The pattern of fusion of conjoined twins is highly variable and has been reviewed by Barth and cowork-

ers.[84] Most cases have symmetry of joined regions. Two forms of nomenclature are used. For those joined regionally, the anatomic site of fusion is named, followed by the suffix *pagus*, from the Greek for fastened. Typical fusions are named thoraco- (chest), omphalo- (umbilical-abdominal), pygo- (sacral), ischio- (pelvic), and cranio- (head). Very extensive zones of fusion may be named by the prefix di- (meaning two), followed by the portion of the twins that is unfused. Examples include dicephalus (two heads on one body), diprosopus (two faces on one head and body), and dipygus (single head and torso with separated pelves and four legs). Asymmetric forms, termed *heteropagus* are exceedingly rare and have a parasitic attachment of a variably sized portion of anatomy appended to or even within any region of the body. Of the various forms of conjoined twins, anterior fusion of some extent from mid chest to umbilicus is most frequent, accounting for up to 75% of cases, and involves some degree of fusion of hearts, liver, and upper gastrointestinal tracts (Fig. 8–27).

Barth and coworkers[84] studied the role of prenatal sonography in diagnosing and assessing 14 cases of conjoined twins. They point out that the diagnosis is usually clear but that several pitfalls should be avoided. Inseparable skin contact sites must be persistent, and at symmetric body zones, to avoid a false-positive diagnosis. A relatively small zone of fusion may be pliable and permit the twins to rotate as much as 180°, so that a vertex-breech presentation does not necessarily exclude conjoined twinning. With a vertex-vertex presentation, engagement of one head within the pelvis may alter the apparent symmetry, thwarting diagnosis. With extreme degrees of fusion, the twins may be mistaken for a singleton (Fig. 8–28).

Barth and coworkers[84] point out that a major role for sonography is to analyze the extent to which organs are shared so that a reasonable assessment of surgical separability can be made. Sharing of a heart or brain virtually excludes successful separation. Even if the hearts are separate, there is a substantial incidence of abnormal cardiac anatomy. If, based on sonographic evaluation, surgical separation and viability appear possible, cesarean section is indicated, since dystocia is likely during vaginal delivery. Even if vaginal delivery is possible, it may cause fetal or maternal injury.

Of the 14 sets of conjoined twins reported by Barth, the mother elected termination in nine cases, 1 set was stillborn, and 3 sets died after birth. The remaining case, omphalopagus, was delivered by cesarean section at 37½ weeks. Following separation one twin was alive and well at 4 months but the other died of cardiac and head malformations. O'Neill and colleagues[85] reported a 30-year experience of surgery in 10 of 13 sets of liveborn conjoined twins. Best results were obtained in twins separated after 4 months of age. There were 16 of 20 initially surviving infants, but 6 of these died up to 10 years following surgery of serious associated congenital anomalies, predominantly cardiac.

Conjoined twins may occur as part of a triplet pregnancy.[86] The separate triplet may have a good prognosis for viability, but as in other forms of multiple

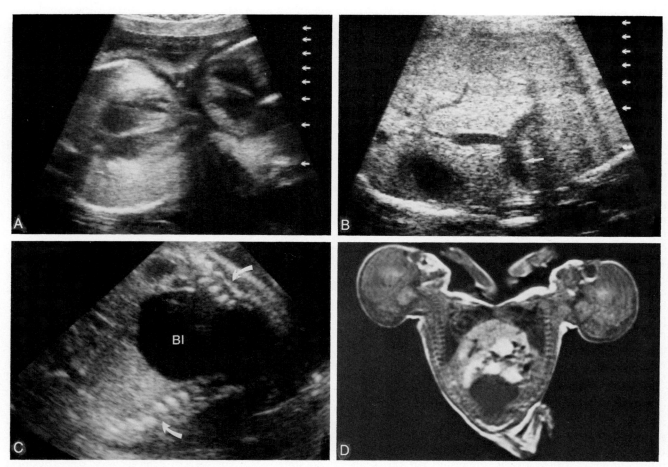

Figure 8–27. Omphaloischiopagus conjoined twins at 25 weeks' gestation. The twins were joined from the xiphoid process of the sternum through the pelvis. There were two normally formed legs and a third hypoplastic leg. There were two normal and two nonfunctional kidneys. Portions of the intestinal tract were shared. The twins were successfully separated at about 1 year of age. *A.* Thoracic level. The hearts were both normal and separate, but a portion of the pericardium was shared. *B.* Upper abdomen. There was broad fusion of the livers. A single umbilical vein *(arrows)* bifurcates into two portal veins. *C.* Coronal view of the pelvis shows an enlarged bladder (Bl) framed by both lumbosacral spines *(arrows)*. A second hypoplastic bladder was present. *D.* Postnatal magnetic resonance image demonstrates the extensive degree of conjunction of the twins.

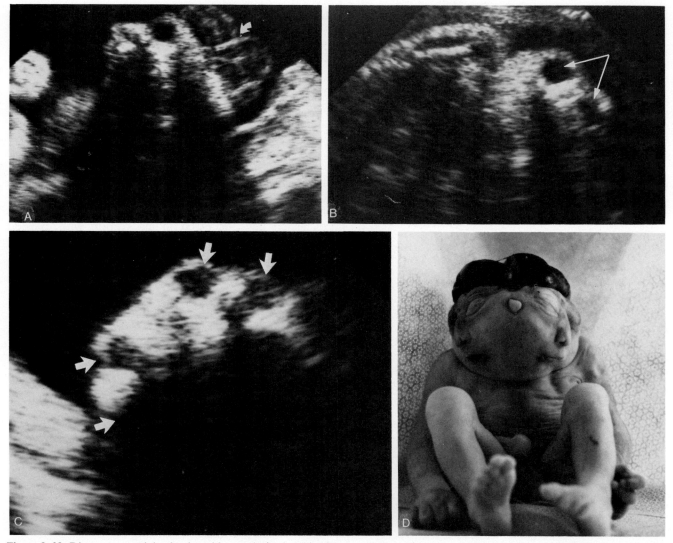

Figure 8–28. Diprosopus conjoined twins with acrania (and rachischisis, not illustrated). The patient first presented for medical care in labor at term. Initial sonograms appeared to show a single fetus with acrania. *A.* The first clue to the presence of conjoined twinning was the orientation of the cleft *(arrow)* in the brain in this image, which shows a profile of the face. If the cleft represents the interhemispheric fissure, it should parallel the profile and not be seen in this view. *B.* A straight-on view of the face seen in profile in the first image shows typical features of the face of an anencephalic/acrania fetus, including the presence of two orbits. *C.* An image plane axial to these two orbits shows a third orbit. A fourth is obscured by the nasal bones. Arrows indicate each orbit. *D.* The features of the stillborn infant confirm the sonographic findings.

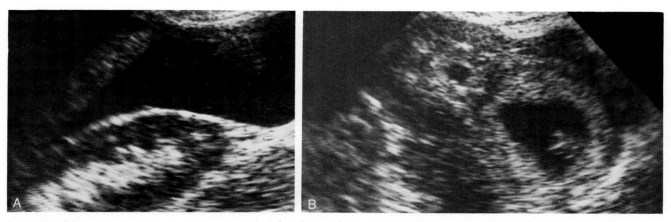

Figure 8–29. Heterotopic pregnancy at 7.5 weeks' gestation. The patient presented with dizziness, abdominal and shoulder pain, but no vaginal bleeding. *A.* A scan of the right upper quadrant shows a very large amount of free fluid, found to be a hemoperitoneum at surgical exploration. *B.* A transverse transabdominal scan of the pelvis shows a live 7.5-week intrauterine pregnancy and, in the right juxtacorneal area, a second smaller ectopic pregnancy. At surgery this was confirmed to be a ruptured and actively bleeding tubal pregnancy, which was successfully resected. The remainder of the pregnancy was uneventful, with successful outcome. (From Laband ST, Cherney WB, Finberg HJ: Heterotopic pregnancy. Am J Obstet Gynecol 158:438, 1988.)

gestation this twin is at risk of complication if there is a shared monochorionic placenta.

HETEROTOPIC MULTIPLE GESTATION

Heterotopic pregnancy, that is, the coexistence of an intrauterine pregnancy and an ectopic pregnancy, has been a rare event, with an estimated incidence of 1 in 30,000 pregnancies. The frequency has increased considerably with the expanding use of assisted fertility techniques. Molloy and coworkers[87] performed 6204 cycles of in vitro fertilization, gamete intrafallopian transfer, or pronuclear stage transfer, achieving 640, 355, and 6 clinical pregnancies, respectively, by each of these techniques. They found 10 surgically proven heterotopic pregnancies in this group for a frequency of about 1% among assisted reproduction pregnancies. My colleagues and I have seen 6 such pregnancies, 4 of which have occurred in association with assisted reproduction (Fig. 8–29).[88] The most recent of these was a chronic tubal pregnancy together with successfully carried in utero dizygotic twins (Fig. 8–30). Rowland and associates[89] reported a case of live tubal ectopic pregnancy together with an intrauterine dichorionic set of triplets (one pair of monochorionic twins and a single fetus in a second sac.)

In this era of assisted reproduction, the sonographer must remain highly vigilant for heterotopic pregnancies. Visualization of a true intrauterine pregnancy cannot be considered as reliably excluding ectopic pregnancy. Coexisting adnexal abnormalities should be

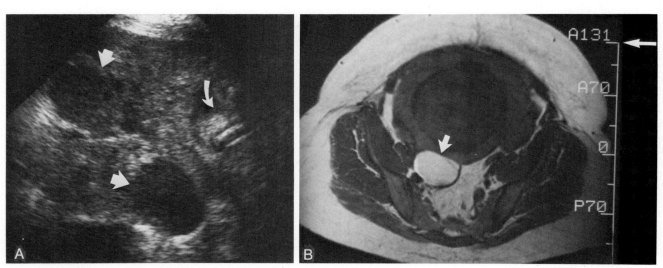

Figure 8–30. Heterotopic chronic right ectopic pregnancy with intrauterine twins. The patient was given clomiphene citrate (Clomid) for pregnancy induction. She presented at 19 weeks with right pelvic pain, severe enough to evaluate extensively. She was scheduled for surgery, but the pain subsided and she remained clinically stable. At a 36-week elective cesarean section the right adnexal process was found to be a chronic ectopic pregnancy. *A.* Sonographic imaging was limited due to maternal obesity, but sonograms showed two right adnexal fluid locules with complex fluid in them *(straight arrows).* Fetal parts are seen in the adjacent uterus *(curved arrow).* *B.* Magnetic resonance image shows a mass (bilobed in other views) with signal characteristics compatible with blood *(arrow).*

critically scrutinized for patterns suggestive of an extrauterine gestational sac.

SELECTIVE REDUCTION OF MULTIFETAL GESTATIONS

Requests for selective abortion while preserving one or more additional fetuses arise in several circumstances. Assisted fertility techniques have led to increasing numbers of twins, triplets, and higher-order multiple gestations. The risk of complete pregnancy loss or the devastating consequences of severe permanent damage to multiple surviving extremely prematurely delivered neonates rises progressively with the number of fetuses present. When a severely anomalous twin coexists with a normal twin, it may jeopardize the healthy twin (e.g., by polyhydramnios leading to preterm labor). Alternatively, a mother may find that she cannot, in conscience, carry the anomalous fetus and will elect complete termination of the pregnancy if elective abortion of the abnormal fetus is not performed.

Selective reduction is most often performed in the first trimester by intracardiac or adjacent intrathoracic injection of potassium chloride. Sonography is used both to guide the needle placement and to confirm cardiac asystole. Some selection criteria can be used to choose the fetus to be aborted or to be preserved.[90]

1. An anomalous fetus, if present, would be selected. Although most anomalies are not detectable in the first trimester, anencephaly and other gross distortions of fetal contours may be recognized.

2. If a gestational sac or a fetus is noticeably smaller than the others present, there is a higher likelihood of

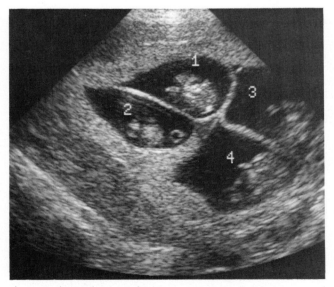

Figure 8–31. Quadruplet pregnancy selectively reduced to twins at 10 weeks' gestation. Fetus No. 2 was smaller than the others and was in a gestational sac also visibly the smallest. This fetus, along with fetus No. 1, was aborted by sonographically guided intracardiac injection of potassium chloride. The remaining twin pregnancy progressed normally.

spontaneous abortion or of aneuploidy of that fetus (Fig. 8–31).

3. If there is a monochorionic twin pair within a higher-order multiple gestation, these should both be selected. They, as a pair, have all the risks of monochorionic twins, including twin transfusion syndrome and higher incidence of spontaneous death.

4. One member of a monochorionic twin pair should not be selectively aborted. Just as in the spontaneous death of one such fetus, the second twin may die quickly from hypovolemia by blood transfusion into the circulatory space of the aborted twin. There is also the risk of twin embolization syndrome, which could produce brain damage or other deficit to the surviving twin. These considerations are clearly important in the case of a monochorionic twin pregnancy with one anomalous twin.

5. Before the selective abortion of an anomalous twin of a dichorionic pregnancy, consider karyotyping both twins (unless they are of different genders). In the presence of most anomalies, the probability of aneuploidy increases above background maternal-age risk. Approximately 25% of spontaneous dichorionic twins (lower percentage with assisted fertility techniques) will be monozygotic, even if they are discordant for anomaly. If the twins are concordant for aneuploidy, selective reduction may be inappropriate.

6. Avoid selective abortion of the presenting fetus. Although the concern is theoretical, potentially the death of the fetus closest to the cervix could lead to transcervical expulsion with increased danger of total abortion of the multiple gestation.

7. If none of these considerations helps determine the appropriate fetus(es) to select, then those that are most accessible, high, and anterior in the uterus should be chosen. The appropriate number of fetuses in a pregnancy at which to consider selective reduction and the appropriate number to which the pregnancy should be reduced, as well as appropriateness of selective reduction in general, are contentious issues. Arguments relative to safety and morality can be advanced on both sides of each of these questions.

Essentially all groups performing selective reductions will offer the procedure in quadruplet and higher grand multiple gestations, and the majority will reduce triplets.[91–96] These groups generally reduce the pregnancy to twins, recognizing that the morbidity and mortality rates for dichorionic twins are higher than for singletons. They express the opinion that the risk of losing the sole remaining fetus and the general social concerns for reducing more than a "necessary" number of fetuses to permit relative pregnancy safety is unacceptable to them. Wapner and Chervenak and their coworkers[97, 98] have taken the stance that there are situations in which reduction from twins or more to singletons may be appropriate and that there are cogent ethical arguments to justify this. My colleagues and I have been faced with the opposite situation on four occasions in which patients wished to salvage as many infants as possible. They elected reduction of one set of sextuplets and three of quintuplets each to quadruplets. Three sets have been delivered with all live born and healthy infants. The fourth set is ongoing, doing well.

The safety and emotional consequences must be carefully reviewed with patients before undertaking selective reduction. Lynch and coworkers[92] reported loss of all fetuses in 8 of 53 completed reduced pregnancies. Tabsh[93] reported only one intrauterine death and one neonatal death among 38 completed pregnancies, with no pregnancy completely lost. Porreco and colleagues[96] specifically compared 13 women with triplets who elected reduction to twins and 11 women with triplets who declined reduction. There was no significant difference in birth weight of infants or age at delivery between the two groups or in neonatal hospital days and maternal complications. The continuing triplet group did have more occurrences and need for treatment of premature labor. Porecco and colleagues have also lectured on an ongoing sense of loss and guilt among many women who have undergone pregnancy reductions with successful outcomes.

At this time, it appears that there are circumstances in which selective reduction of multiple gestation may be an appropriate means of improving pregnancy outcome. There are ongoing controversies as to the specific situations in which to apply the technique and the number of remaining fetuses that should be left. There is general agreement that an individual practitioner is not medically obligated to participate in a pregnancy reduction if the circumstances of the case are contrary to his or her ethical perspective.

References

1. MacGillivray I: Twins and other multiple deliveries. Clin Obstet Gynecol 7:581, 1980.
2. Benirschke K, Kim CK: Multiple pregnancy (first of two parts). N Engl J Med 288:1276, 1973.
3. Jansen RP, Anderson JC, Birrell WS, et al: Outpatient gamete intrafallopian transfer: A clinical analysis of 710 cases. Med J Aust 153:182, 1990.
4. Soudre G, Guettier X, Marpeau L, et al: In utero early suspicion of superfetation by ultrasound examination: A case report. Ultrasound Obstet Gynecol 2:51, 1992.
5. Bardawil WA, Reddy RL, Bardawil LW: Placental considerations in multiple pregnancy. Clin Perinatal 15:13, 1988.
6. Ghai V, Vidyasagar D: Morbidity and mortality factors in twins: An epidemiologic approach. Clin Perinatal 15:123, 1988.
7. Borlum KG: Third-trimester fetal death in triplet pregnancies. Obstet Gynecol 77:6, 1991.
8. Kovacs BW, Kirschbaum TH, Paul RH: Twin gestations: I. Antenatal care and complications. Obstet Gynecol 74:313, 1989.
9. Wenstrom K, Gall SA: Incidence, morbidity and mortality, and diagnosis of twin gestations. Clin Perinatol 15:1, 1988.
10. Fliegner JRH: When do perinatal deaths in multiple pregnancies occur? Aust NZ J Obstet Gynecol 29:371, 1989.
11. Meehan FP, Magani IM, Mortimer G: Perinatal mortality in multiple pregnancy patients. Acta Genet Med Gemellol 37:331, 1988.
12. McCulloch K: Neonatal problems in twins. Clin Perinatol 15:141, 1988.
13. Benirschke K: Twin placenta in perinatal mortality. NY State J Med 61:1499, 1961.
14. Saari-Kemppainen A, Karjalainen D, Ylostalo P, et al: Ultra-

15. Lumme RH, Saarikoski SV: Perinatal deaths in twin pregnancy: A 22-year review. Acta Genet Med Gemellol 37:47, 1988.
16. Nylander PPS: Perinatal mortality in twins. Acta Genet Med Gemellol 28:363, 1979.
17. Coleman BG, Grumbach K, Arger PH, et al: Twin gestations: Monitoring of complications and anomalies with US. Radiology 165:449, 1987.
18. Dickey RP, Olar TT, Curole DN, et al: The probability of multiple births when multiple gestational sacs or viable embryos are diagnosed at first trimester ultrasound. Hum Reprod 5:880, 1990.
19. Sampson A, de Crespigny LC: Vanishing twins: The frequency of spontaneous fetal reduction of a twin pregnancy. Ultrasound Obstet Gynecol 2:107, 1992.
20. Landy HJ, Weiner S, Carson SL, et al: The "vanishing twin": Ultrasonographic assessment of fetal disappearance in the first trimester. Am J Obstet Gynecol 155:14, 1986.
21. Finberg HJ, Birnholz JC: Ultrasound observations in multiple gestation with first trimester bleeding: The blighted twin. Radiology 132:137, 1979.
22. Gonen R, Heyman E, Asztalos EV, et al: The outcome of triplet, quadruplet and quintuplet pregnancies managed in a perinatal unit: Obstetric, neonatal, and follow-up data. Am J Obstet Gynecol 162:454, 1990.
23. Sassoon DA, Castro LC, Davis JL, et al: Perinatal outcome in triplet versus twin gestations. Obstet Gynecol 75:817, 1990.
24. Lopez-Llera M, De la Luna Olsen E, Niz Ramos J: Eclampsia in twin pregnancy. J Reprod Med 34:802, 1989.
25. Finberg HJ: The "twin peak" sign: Reliable evidence of dichorionic twinning. J Ultrasound Med 11:571–577, 1992.
26. Townsend RR, Simpson GF, Filly RA: Membrane thickness in ultrasound prediction of chorionicity of twin gestations. J Ultrasound Med 7:327, 1988.
27. Winn HN, Gabrielli S, Reece EA, et al: Ultrasonographic criteria for the prenatal diagnosis of placental chorionicity in twin gestations. Am J Obstet Gynecol 161:1540, 1989.
28. Hertzberg BS, Kurtz AB, Choi HY, et al: Significance of membrane thickness in the sonographic evaluation of twin gestations. AJR 148:151, 1987.
29. Barss VA, Benacerraf BR, Frigoletto FD: Ultrasonographic determination of chorion type in twin gestation. Obstet Gynecol 66:779, 1985.
30. Filly RA, Goldstein RB, Callen PW: Monochorionic twinning: Sonographic assessment. AJR 154:459, 1990.
31. D'Alton ME, Dudley DK: The ultrasonographic prediction of chorionicity in twin gestation. Am J Obstet Gynecol 160:557, 1989.
32. Mahony BS, Filly RA, Callen PW: Amnionicity and chorionicity in twin pregnancies: Prediction using ultrasound. Radiology 155:205, 1985.
33. Townsend RR, Filly RA: Sonography of non-conjoined monoamniotic twin pregnancies. J Ultrasound Med 7:665, 1988.
34. Finberg HJ, Clewell WH: Definitive prenatal diagnosis of monoamniotic twins: Swallowed amniotic contrast agent detected in both twins on sonographically selected CT images. J Ultrasound Med 10:513, 1991.
35. Finberg HJ, Kurtz AB, Johnson RL, et al: The biophysical profile: A literature review and reassessment of its usefulness in the evaluation of fetal well-being. J Ultrasound Med 9:583, 1990.
36. Giles WB, Trudinger BJ, Cook CM, et al: Umbilical artery flow velocity waveforms and twin pregnancy outcome. Obstet Gynecol 72:894, 1988.
37. Giles WB, Trudinger BJ, Cook CM, et al: Umbilical artery waveforms in triplet pregnancy. Obstet Gynecol 75:813, 1990.
38. Gaziano EP, Knox GE, Bendel RP, et al: Is pulsed Doppler velocimetry useful in the management of multiple gestation pregnancies? Am J Obstet Gynecol 164:1426, 1991.
39. Hastie SJ, Danskin F, Neilson JP, et al: Prediction of the small for gestational age twin fetus by Doppler umbilical artery waveform analysis. Obstet Gynecol 74:730, 1989.

40. Crane JP, Tomich PG, Kopta M: Ultrasonic growth patterns in normal and discordant twins. Obstet Gynecol 55:678, 1980.

41. Storlazzi E, Vintzileos AM, Campbell WA, et al: Ultrasonic diagnosis of discordant fetal growth in twin gestations. Obstet Gynecol 69:363, 1987.

42. Brown CEL, Guzick DS, Leveno KJ, et al: Prediction of discordant twins using ultrasound measurements of biparietal diameter and abdominal perimeter. Obstet Gynecol 70:677, 1987.

43. O'Brien WF, Knuppel RA, Scerbo JC, et al: Birth weight in twins: An analysis of discordancy and growth retardation. Obstet Gynecol 67:483, 1986.

44. Blickstein I, Shoham-Schwartz Z: Characterization of the growth discordant twin. Obstet Gynecol 70:11, 1987.

45. MacLean M, Mathers A, Walker JJ, et al: The ultrasonic assessment of discordant growth in twin pregnancies. Ultrasound Obstet Gynecol 2:30, 1992.

46. Divon MY, Girz BA, Sklar A, et al: Discordant twins: A prospective study of the diagnostic value of real-time ultrasonography combined with umbilical artery velocimetry. Am J Obstet Gynecol 161:757, 1989.

47. Secher NJ, Kaern J, Hansen PK: Intrauterine growth in twin pregnancies: Prediction of fetal growth retardation. Obstet Gynecol 66:63, 1985.

48. Michaels WH, Schreiber FR, Padgett RJ, et al: Ultrasound surveillance of the cervix in twin gestations: Management of cervical incompetency. Obstet Gynecol 78:739, 1991.

49. Pruggmayer MRK, Jahoda MGJ, Van der Pol JG, et al: Genetic amniocentesis in twin pregnancies: Results of a multicenter study of 529 cases. Ultrasound Obstet Gynecol 2:6, 1992.

50. Jeanty P, Shah D, Roussis P: Single-needle insertion in twin amniocentesis. J Ultrasound Med 9:511, 1990.

51. Gilbert WM, Davis SE, Kaplan C, et al: Morbidity associated with prenatal disruption of the dividing membrane in twin gestations. Obstet Gynecol 78:623, 1991.

52. Katz VL, Chescheir NC, Cefalo RC: Unexplained elevations of maternal serum alpha-fetoprotein. Obstet Gynecol Survey 45:719, 1990.

53. Johnson JM, Harman CR, Evans JA, et al: Maternal serum alpha-fetoprotein in twin pregnancy. Am J Obstet Gynecol 162:1020, 1990.

54. Redford DHA, Whitfield CR: Maternal serum alpha-fetoprotein in twin pregnancies uncomplicated by neural tube defect. Am J Obstet Gynecol 152:550, 1985.

55. Johnson VP, Vidgoff J, Wilson N, et al: Alpha fetoprotein and acetylcholinesterase in twins discordant for neural tube defect. Prenat Diagn 9:831, 1989.

56. Stiller RJ, Lockwood CJ, Belanger K, et al: Amniotic fluid alpha-fetoprotein concentrations in twin gestations: Dependence on placental membrane anatomy. Am J Obstet Gynecol 158:1088, 1988.

57. Imaizumi Y, Asaka A, Inouye E: Fetal deaths with birth defects among Japanese multiples, 1974. Acta Genet Med Gemellol 39:345, 1990.

58. Berg KA, Astemborski JA, Boughman JA, et al: Congenital cardiovascular malformations in twins and triplets from a population-based study. Am J Dis Child 143:1461, 1989.

59. Keusch CF, Mulliken JB, Kaplan LC: Craniofacial anomalies in twins. Plast Reconstr Surg 87:16, 1991.

60. Lockwood C, Ghidini A, Romero R: Amniotic band syndrome in monozygotic twins: Prenatal diagnosis and pathogenesis. Obstet Gynecol 71:1012, 1988.

61. Fisk NM, Borrell A, Hubinout C, et al: Fetofetal transfusion syndrome: Do the neonatal criteria apply in utero? Arch Dis Child 65:657, 1990.

62. Patten RM, Mack LA, Harvey D, et al: Disparity of amniotic fluid volume and fetal size: Problem of the stuck twin: US studies. Radiology 172:153, 1989.

63. Pretorius DH, Manchester D, Barkin S, et al: Doppler ultrasound of twin transfusion syndrome. J Ultrasound Med 7:117, 1988.

64. Urig MA, Simpson GF, Elliott JP, et al: Mid-trimester surgical removal of one twin to treat twin-twin transfusion syndrome. Fetal Ther 3:185, 1988.

65. DeLia JE, Cruickshank DP, Keye WR: Fetoscopic neodymium:YAG laser occlusion of placental vessels in severe twin-twin transfusion syndrome. Obstet Gynecol 75:1046, 1990.

66. Elliott JP, Urig MA, Clewell WH: Aggressive therapeutic amniocentesis for treatment of twin-twin transfusion syndrome. Obstet Gynecol 77:537, 1991.

67. Saunders NJ, Snijders RJM, Nicholaides KH: Therapeutic amniocentesis in twin-twin transfusion syndrome appearing in the second trimester of pregnancy. Am J Obstet Gynecol 166:820, 1992.

68. Patten RM, Mack LA, Nyberg DA, et al: Twin embolization syndrome: Prenatal sonographic detection and significance. Radiology 173:685, 1989.

69. Yoshida K, Matayoshi K: A study on prognosis of surviving cotwin. Acta Genet Med Gemellol 39:383, 1990.

70. Fusi L, Gordon H: Twin pregnancy complicated by single intrauterine death: Problems and outcome with conservative management. Br J Obstet Gynecol 97:511, 1990.

71. Bejar R, Vigliocco B, Gramajo H, et al: Antenatal origin of neurologic damage in newborn infants: II. Multiple gestations. Am J Obstet Gynecol 162:1230, 1990.

72. Skelly H, Marivate M, Norman R, et al: Consumptive coagulopathy following fetal death in a triplet pregnancy. Am J Obstet Gynecol 142:595, 1982.

73. Romero R, Duffy TP, Berkowitz RL, et al: Prolongation of a preterm pregnancy complicated by death of a single twin in utero and disseminated intravascular coagulation. N Engl J Med 310:772, 1984.

74. Cherouny PH, Hoskins IA, Johnson TR, et al: Multiple pregnancy with late death of one fetus. Obstet Gynecol 74:318, 1989.

75. Goldberger SB, Rosen DJ, Shulman A, et al: Conservative approach to multiple pregnancy with intrauterine death of one or more fetuses. Int J Gynaecol Obstet 34:367, 1991.

76. Sherer DM, Armstrong B, Shah YG, et al: Prenatal sonographic diagnosis, Doppler velocimetric umbilical cord studies, and subsequent management of an acardiac twin pregnancy. Obstet Gynecol 74:472, 1989.

77. Moore TR, Gale S, Benirschke K: Perinatal outcome of forty-nine pregnancies complicated by acardiac twinning. Am J Obstet Gynecol 163:907, 1990.

78. Lumme RH, Saarikoski SV: Monoamniotic twin pregnancy. Acta Genet Med Gemellol 35:99, 1986.

79. Rodis JF, Vintzileos AM, Campbell WA, et al: Antenatal diagnosis and management of monoamniotic twins. Am J Obstet Gynecol 157:1255, 1987.

80. Carr SR, Aronson MP, Coustan DR: Survival rates of monoamniotic twins do not decrease after 30 weeks' gestation. Am J Obstet Gynecol 163:719, 1990.

81. Tessen JA, Zlatnik FJ: Monoamniotic twins: A retrospective study. Obstet Gynecol 77:832, 1991.

82. Lyndrup J, Schouenborg L: Cord entanglement in monoamniotic twin pregnancies. Eur J Obstet Gynecol Reprod Biol 26:275, 1987.

83. D'Alton ME, Newton ER, Cetrulo CL: Intrauterine fetal demise in multiple gestation. Acta Genet Med Gemellol 33:43, 1984.

84. Barth RA, Filly RA, Goldberg JD, et al: Conjoined twins: Prenatal diagnosis and assessment of associated malformations. Radiology 177:201, 1990.

85. O'Neill JA Jr, Holcomb GW III, Schnauffer L, et al: Surgical experience with thirteen conjoined twins. Ann Surg 208:299, 1988.

86. Apuzzio JJ, Ganesh VV, Chervenak J, et al: Prenatal diagnosis of dicephalous conjoined twins in a triplet pregnancy. Am J Obstet Gynecol 159:1214, 1988.

87. Molloy D, Deambrosis W, Keeping D, et al: Multiple-sited (heterotopic) pregnancy after in vitro fertilization and gamete intrafallopian transfer. Fertil Steril 53:1068, 1990.

88. Laband SJ, Cherney WB, Finberg HJ: Heterotopic pregnancy: Report of four cases. Am J Obstet Gynecol 158:437, 1988.

89. Rowland DM, Geagan MB, Paul DA: Sonographic demonstration of combined quadruplet gestation with viable ectopic and concomitant intrauterine triplet pregnancies. J Ultrasound Med 6:89, 1987.

90. Finberg HJ, Clewell WH: Ultrasound-guided interventions in pregnancy. Ultrasound Q 8:197, 1990.
91. Gonen Y, Blankier J, Casper RF: Transvaginal ultrasound in selective embryo reduction for multiple pregnancy. Obstet Gynecol 75:720, 1990.
92. Lynch L, Berkowitz RL, Chitkara U, et al: First-trimester transabdominal multifetal pregnancy reduction: A report of 85 cases. Obstet Gynecol 75:735, 1990.
93. Tabsh KM: Transabdominal multifetal pregnancy reduction: Report of 40 cases. Obstet Gynecol 75:739, 1990.
94. Evans MI, May M, Drugan A, et al: Selective termination: Clinical experience and residual risks. Am J Obstet Gynecol 162:1568, 1990.
95. Boulot P, Hedon B, Pelliccia G, et al: Obstetrical results after embryonic reductions performed on 34 multiple pregnancies. Hum Reprod 5:1009, 1990.
96. Porrecco RP, Burke MS, Hendrix ML: Multifetal reduction of triplets and pregnancy outcome. Obstet Gynecol 78:335, 1991.
97. Wapner RJ, Davis GH, Johnson A, et al: Selective reduction of multifetal pregnancies. Lancet 335:90, 1990.
98. Chervenak FA, McCullough LB, Wapner RJ: Selective termination to a singleton pregnancy is ethically justified. Ultrasound Obstet Gynecol 2:84, 1992.

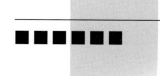

CHAPTER 9

Ultrasound Evaluation of Fetal Growth

FRANK P. HADLOCK, M.D.

The growth of the human fetus, a complex process resulting in an increase in size over time, has been the subject of extensive study.[1-139] Before the advent of ultrasound evaluation, physicians interested in the growth process of the fetus could only look at the infant at delivery and infer what had happened in utero. Based on these observations, clinicians were able to categorize fetuses in very general terms on the basis of their age and size. For example, fetuses were classified as preterm if they were born before 38 menstrual weeks, term if they were born between 38 and 42 menstrual weeks, and post term if they were born beyond 42 menstrual weeks. Similarly, fetuses could be classified by birthweight as small for gestational age, appropriate for gestational age, and large for gestational age. These categories allowed clinicians to recognize that there was a considerable increase in perinatal mobidity and mortality for preterm or post-term fetuses and for fetuses born too small or too large for menstrual age.[1-11]

The use of ultrasound evaluation in obstetrics provides the potential for improvement in prenatal care by allowing recognition of abnormalities of dates and size in utero. As outlined in Chapter 7 on fetal dating, early ultrasound examinations before 20 menstrual weeks provide very accurate characterization of the menstrual age of the fetus (2 SD = ± 1 week). This allows the obstetrician to aggressively and confidently deal with preterm labor when it occurs and to avoid the possibility of post-term delivery. More recently ultrasound evaluation has been applied to fetal size in utero, so that fetuses that are small for gestational age or large for gestational age can be recognized and managed appropriately. In this chapter, the focus is on the proper use of ultrasound evaluation for recognizing these abnormalities of fetal growth.

INTRAUTERINE GROWTH RETARDATION

Clinical Considerations

The *definition* of intrauterine growth retardation (IUGR) is a problematic one, since in a given case we do not know the inherent growth potential of the fetus.[13, 15] For this reason, population standards have been developed and fetuses whose weight falls below the 10th percentile for age are classified as small for gestational age. Although some authors have used the terms *small for gestational age* and *IUGR* synonymously, they should in fact be considered separate

entities. For example, a fetus born at the 5th percentile for weight that has reached its genetic potential may be small in relation to the reference population, but it is not actually growth retarded. On the other hand, a full-term fetus whose weight is at the 50th percentile for age but whose genetic potential was for the 90th percentile could be considered growth retarded. As a practical matter, most authors use the 10th percentile weight for age as a cutoff below which fetuses must be considered small for gestational age. It is the job of the sonologist to help the clinician determine which fetuses are small because of IUGR, so that appropriate management may optimize fetal outcome.

To help the clinician recognize fetuses that are growth retarded, it is important for us to understand the *incidence* of this condition and its associated *etiologies*. The incidence of IUGR in a general low-risk population is only about 5%, reaching a level of approximately 10% in patients who can be considered at risk. Because the low-risk population is a substantially larger group than the high-risk population, approximately one half of all fetuses with IUGR will come from the low-risk population. The at-risk population would comprise all patients subject to the many risk factors associated with IUGR outlined in Table 9–1. In my experience, the most significant maternal factors for IUGR are the history of a previous fetus with IUGR, significant maternal hypertension and/or smoking, the presence of a uterine anomaly (bicornuate uterus or large fibroids), and significant placental hemorrhage.

Historically, the *classification* of IUGR has been based on the morphologic characteristics of the fetuses studied.[29-33] Symmetric IUGR, usually the result of a first-trimester insult (chromosomal abnormality, infection), results in a fetus that is proportionately small throughout pregnancy (Fig. 9–1). Unfortunately, while this group can often be identified in utero, there is very little we can do to impact fetal outcome. Asymmetric IUGR is usually thought to be a process that begins in the late second or early third trimester, resulting from placental insufficiency (Fig. 9–2). The asymmetric IUGR fetus generally exhibits relative head sparing at the expense of abdominal and soft tissue growth, with varying degrees of compromise in fetal length. Doppler studies have demonstrated that this pattern results from preferential blood flow to the fetal brain at the expense of other organ systems. If this process continues unabated to term, the head sparing is usually compromised, and the result is a fetus that is more symmetrically growth retarded. Al-

Table 9–1. CLINICAL PARAMETERS IN ESTIMATION OF GESTATIONAL AGE*

Priority for Estimating Gestational Age	"Estimated" Range for 95% of Cases
1. In vitro fertilization	Less than 1 day
2. Ovulation induction	3–4 days
3. Recorded basal body temperature	4–5 days
4. Ultrasound crown-rump length	± .7 weeks
5. First-trimester physical examination (normal uterus)	± 1 week
6. Ultrasound BPD prior to 20 weeks	+ 1 week
7. Ultrasound gestational sac volume	± 1.5 weeks
8. Ultrasound BPD from 20 to 26 weeks	± 1.6 weeks
9. LNMP from recorded dates (good history)†	± 2–3 weeks
10. Ultrasound BPD 26 to 30 weeks	+ 2–3 weeks
11. LNMP from memory (good history)	3–4 weeks
12. Ultrasound BPD after 30 weeks	3–4 weeks
13. Fundal height measurement	4–6 weeks
14. LNMP from memory (not good history)	4–6 weeks
15. Fetal heart tones first heard	4–6 weeks
16. Quickening	4–6 weeks

Adapted from James D. Bowie, M.D.
BPD, biparietal diameter; LNMP, last normal menstrual period.
*Rule is to always use a more reliable indicator in preference to a less reliable one.
†A "good" history requires knowledge of both LNMP and previous period with regular periods and no use of birth control pills for at least 6 months before the LNMP.

though some authors have disputed the validity of this classification, in my experience it has proven to be a workable one, with approximately one third of growth-retarded fetuses I have seen falling into the symmetric category and approximately two thirds falling into the asymmetric IUGR category.

Finally, and most importantly, the clinical *significance* of IUGR should be considered. The literature has consistently indicated that fetuses suffering from IUGR are at high risk for perinatal morbidity and mortality in comparison with the normal weight peer population.[14–22] For example, in one study of 66 fetuses with IUGR, Hill and associates reported a perinatal mortality rate corrected for severe congenital anoma-

lies of 91 per 1000 deliveries.[83] This compares with a corrected perinatal mortality rate of approximately 4.4 per 1000 deliveries in a large high-risk population closely monitored by antepartum testing, including ultrasound evaluation.[110] Other authors have emphasized that fetuses with IUGR suffer long-term neurologic and intellectual impairment when delivered at term, probably because of chronic hypoxia and severe acidemia in utero.[16–20] However, it has been recognized more recently that early recognition and delivery of growth-retarded fetuses from the hostile intrauterine environment (preferably at approximately 34 to 35 weeks) results in infants whose growth and intellectual development is equivalent to the appropriately grown

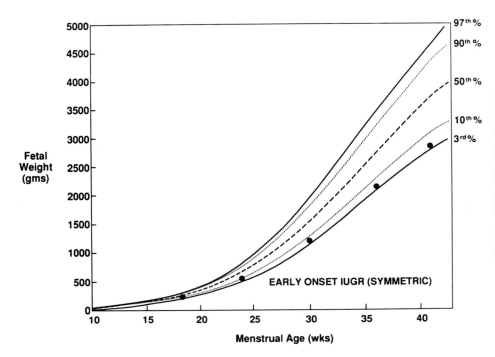

Figure 9–1. Hadlock fetal weight curve demonstrates estimated fetal weight in a case of symmetric intrauterine growth retardation. Note that the weight approximates the third percentile throughout pregnancy. Other sonographic parameters of fetal growth (head size, abdominal circumference, femur length) would show a similar growth pattern throughout pregnancy. This type of growth pattern may be seen in otherwise normal fetuses that are constitutionally small, but it is seen more commonly in fetuses that suffer a first-trimester insult.

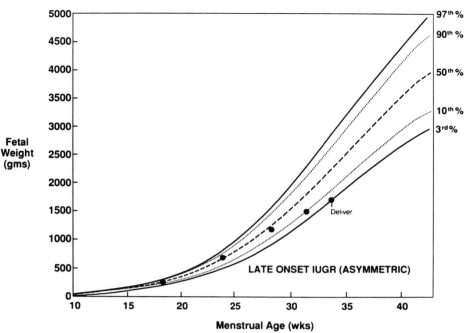

Figure 9–2. Hadlock fetal weight curve demonstrates estimated fetal weight in a case of late-onset asymmetric growth retardation. In these cases, varying degrees of compromise in head size and body length usually occur but abdominal circumference is compromised early. These cases are frequently the result of placental insufficiency. Early delivery at 34 to 35 weeks may keep these fetuses from suffering the increased perinatal morbidity and mortality frequently seen in fetuses with intrauterine growth retardation at term.

peer group at 24 months of age. It is for this reason that those using ultrasound evaluation as a prenatal diagnostic tool must examine every fetus, regardless of the indication of the scan, for evidence of IUGR.

Sonographic Detection

As indicated in Chapter 7 on fetal dating, accurate knowledge of menstrual age is critically important in establishing a diagnosis of IUGR.[36, 37] This is because the normal range values for most fetal growth parameters change over time. Although effective fetal dating can be done in normally growing fetuses as late as 20

menstrual weeks,[42] it is important in fetuses at risk for growth disturbances to establish age as early as possible, since some forms of IUGR may affect crown-rump length growth in the first trimester of pregnancy. For example, Benacerraf was able to detect early IUGR due to aneupoidy at 11 weeks in a patient whose dates were confirmed by crown-rump length at 8 menstrual weeks.[25] The diagnosis of altered growth in the first trimester requires precise knowledge of menstrual age and appropriate population standards for fetal crown-rump length growth.[40] The diagnosis should always be confirmed by follow-up studies, since crown-rump length measurements may be as much as 1 week smaller than expected based on late ovulation (Fig. 9–3).

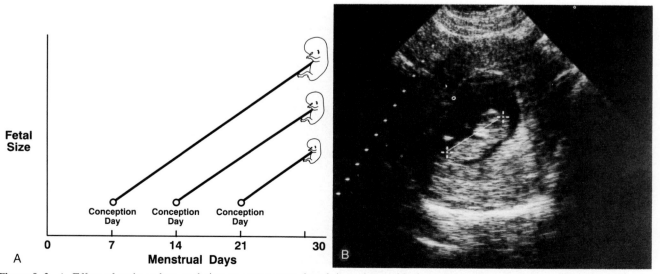

Figure 9–3. *A.* Effect of early or late ovulation on crown-rump length in patients with the same date for the last normal menstrual period. Fetuses that are conceived late in the menstrual cycle (day 21) are smaller than fetuses conceived in midcycle because they are 1 week younger, not because they are growing abnormally. *B.* Thus, measurements of crown-rump length growth in the first trimester should not be considered abnormal until size is more than 1 week less than expected for good dates, and follow-up evaluation is always necessary to confirm abnormal growth.

Beyond the first trimester of pregnancy, the choice of parameters for detection of IUGR is a problematic one. In severe IUGR at term, almost any sonographic parameter could prove useful as a diagnostic tool if the dates are known unequivocally; as Dicke and colleagues have demonstrated, this is especially true in chromosomal abnormalities such as trisomy 13 and trisomy 18 (Fig. 9–4).[26, 27] However, because the goal is to detect IUGR early enough for proper clinical management, my colleagues and I have developed a comprehensive fetal growth profile to optimize our chances for detecting this entity early in pregnancy. This profile, designed to provide the same type of information gained from neonatal evaluation at delivery, evaluates head size, trunk size, soft tissue mass, weight, length, and body proportionality.[36] This wealth of information can be gained from evaluation of three high-quality images of the fetal head, abdomen, and femur (Fig. 9–5).

HEAD SIZE

As outlined in Chapter 7 on fetal dating, the head is imaged in a transverse axial plane using the cavum septi pellucidi, thalamic nuclei, falx cerebri, and choroid plexus as landmarks.[37] Because the biparietal diameter of the head can be misleading in cases associated with head shape changes (e.g., dolichocephaly),[49] the head circumference is the measurement of choice for evaluation of head growth in utero.[46] Once a satisfactory image has been obtained (Fig. 9–6), the perimeter can be traced along the outer margin of the calvarium using a map measurer or electronic digitizer, or it can be calculated from the two outer-to-outer diameters using the formula for the perimeter of an ellipse. Our experience has indicated that these measurement techniques give equivalent results. In examining the fetal head for this measurement, it is very important to rule out anomalies, since these may be seen in association with some forms of growth retardation. The normalcy of fetal head growth can then be judged against population standards such as those in Table 9–2.

In symmetric IUGR, fetal head size will frequently be compromised early in pregnancy, and when dates are known unequivocally, a head circumference below the third percentile for age is cause for concern. This finding could be the result of a focal process such as

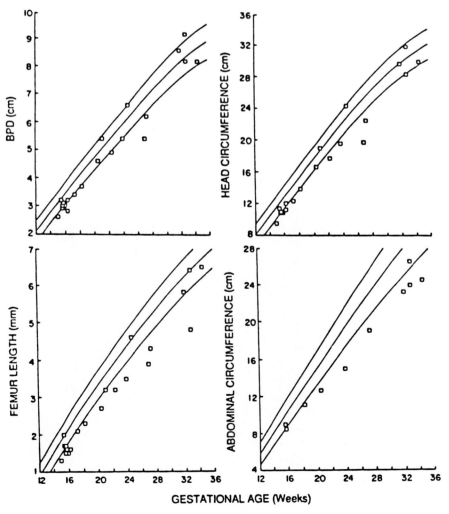

Figure 9–4. Biparietal diameter (BPD), head circumference, abdominal circumference, and femur length in a group of fetuses with trisomy 18 seen at varying stages in pregnancy. Note that in these chromosomally abnormal fetuses growth disturbances are evident in the early second trimester of pregnancy, particularly for the abdominal circumference. (From Dicke J, Crane JP: Sonographic recognition of major malformations and aberrant fetal growth in trisomic fetuses. J Ultrasound Med 10:433, 1991, with permission of the American Institute of Ultrasound in Medicine.)

GESTATIONAL AGE (Weeks)

TRISOMY 18

FETAL HEAD MEASUREMENTS (BPD, HC)

FETAL ABDOMINAL CIRCUMFERENCE

FETAL FEMUR LENGTH

Figure 9–5. Appropriate planes of section for measurement of the fetal head (biparietal diameter [BPD], head circumference [HC]), fetal abdomen, and fetal femur. The landmarks in the fetal head are the falx (F) anteriorly and posteriorly, the cavum septi pellucidi (CSP) anteriorly, the thalamic nuclei (T) in the midline, and the choroid plexus (CP) in the atria of the lateral ventricles. The landmarks in the abdomen are the portal vein (PV), the stomach (S), and the spine (SP). The femur is measured along the diaphyseal shaft, excluding the distal femoral epiphysis (DFE).

Table 9–2. PERCENTILE VALUES FOR FETAL HEAD CIRCUMFERENCE

Menstrual Week	Head Circumference (cm)				
	3rd	**10th**	**50th**	**90th**	**97th**
14	8.8	9.1	9.7	10.3	10.6
15	10.0	10.4	11.0	11.6	12.0
16	11.3	11.7	12.4	13.1	13.5
17	12.6	13.0	13.8	14.6	15.0
18	13.7	14.2	15.1	16.0	16.5
19	14.9	15.5	16.4	17.4	17.9
20	16.1	16.7	17.7	18.7	19.3
21	17.2	17.8	18.9	20.0	20.6
22	18.3	18.9	20.1	21.3	21.9
23	19.4	20.1	21.3	22.5	23.2
24	20.4	21.1	22.4	23.7	24.3
25	21.4	22.2	23.5	24.9	25.6
26	22.4	23.2	24.6	26.0	26.8
27	23.3	24.1	25.6	27.1	27.9
28	24.2	25.1	26.6	28.1	29.0
29	25.0	25.9	27.5	29.1	30.0
30	25.8	26.8	28.4	30.0	31.0
31	26.7	27.6	29.3	31.0	31.9
32	27.4	28.4	30.1	31.8	32.8
33	28.0	29.0	30.8	32.6	33.6
34	28.7	29.7	31.5	33.3	34.3
35	29.3	30.4	32.2	34.1	35.1
36	29.9	30.9	32.8	34.7	35.8
37	30.3	31.4	33.3	35.2	36.3
38	30.8	31.9	33.8	35.8	36.8
39	31.1	32.2	34.2	36.2	37.3
40	31.5	32.6	34.6	36.6	37.7

Adapted from Hadlock FP, Deter RL, Harrist RB, Park SK: Estimating fetal age: Computer-assisted analysis of multiple fetal growth parameters. Radiology 152:497–501, 1984.

microcephaly, or it may be seen in association with more generalized growth retardation, in which case other fetal parameters will also be small for age. When this finding is observed in early pregnancy, we prefer to proceed with genetic amniocentesis and amniotic fluid cultures to rule out the possibility of a chromosomal abnormality or intrauterine infection accounting for poor head growth. In asymmetric IUGR, the growth of the fetal head is typically normal until very late in pregnancy because of preferential blood flow to the brain at the expense of other organ systems such

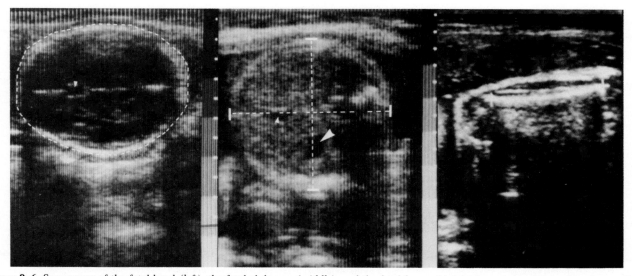

Figure 9–6. Sonograms of the fetal head *(left)*, the fetal abdomen *(middle)*, and the fetal femur *(right)* taken at the planes of section outlined in Figure 9–5. The head circumference and abdominal circumference can be measured directly along the outer perimeter with a digitizer (see fetal head), or they can be calculated from two diameters, as indicated for the fetal abdomen. The femur length is measured along the diaphyseal shaft (caliper markers) exclusive of the distal femoral epiphysis seen to the left of the femur shaft.

as the liver. For this reason, measurement of the fetal head in such cases will typically fail to diagnose IUGR early enough to impact clinical management.

TRUNK SIZE

Fetal trunk size and soft tissue mass are best analyzed by measurement of the fetal abdominal circumference. This measurement, first proposed by Campbell and Thoms[67] as a means of estimating fetal weight and ruling out growth retardation, is measured from a transverse axial section of the fetal abdomen at the level of the portal-umbilical venous complex (see Fig. 9–6). This measurement can be traced along the outer perimeter using a map measurer or electronic digitizer, or it can be calculated from two outer diameters, using the formula for the circumference of a circle (D1 + D2 × 1.57). In our laboratory, measurements using these two techniques have given equivalent results and our normal data for abdominal circumference have been very reproducible (Table 9–3).

One point to remember, however, is that the abdominal circumference measurement has the greatest inter-observer and intraobserver variability of all fetal measurements reported in the literature (Table 9–4). In addition to differences in imaging and measurement techniques, population differences and differences in mathematic modeling techniques may play a role in the significant differences reported in the literature for 10th percentile cutoff boundaries for abdominal circumference. For example, the data from Jeanty and coworkers are based on a longitudinal study of 46 white fetuses examined by one physician, and the perimeter measurements were calculated from mean abdominal diameters.[52] The data from Tamura and Sabbagha, on the other hand, are from a cross-sectional analysis of 197 women of different racial origins in whom the abdominal circumference was traced directly using an electronic digitizer.[53] The differences are dramatic, particular late in pregnancy (beyond 30 weeks)

Table 9–3. PERCENTILE VALUES FOR FETAL ABDOMINAL CIRCUMFERENCE

Menstrual Week	Abdominal Circumference (cm)				
	3rd	10th	50th	90th	97th
14	6.4	6.7	7.3	7.9	8.3
15	7.5	7.9	8.6	9.3	9.7
16	8.6	9.1	9.9	10.7	11.2
17	9.7	10.3	11.2	12.1	12.7
18	10.9	11.5	12.5	13.5	14.1
19	11.9	12.6	13.7	14.8	15.5
20	13.1	13.8	15.0	16.3	17.0
21	14.1	14.9	16.2	17.6	18.3
22	15.1	16.0	17.4	18.8	19.7
23	16.1	17.0	18.5	20.0	20.9
24	17.1	18.1	19.7	21.3	22.3
25	18.1	19.1	20.8	22.5	23.5
26	19.1	20.1	21.9	23.7	24.8
27	20.0	21.1	23.0	24.9	26.0
28	20.9	22.0	24.0	26.0	27.1
29	21.8	23.0	25.1	27.2	28.4
30	22.7	23.9	26.1	28.3	29.5
31	23.6	24.9	27.1	29.4	30.6
32	24.5	25.8	28.1	30.4	31.8
33	25.3	26.7	29.1	31.5	32.9
34	26.1	27.5	30.0	32.5	33.9
35	26.9	28.3	30.9	33.5	34.9
36	27.7	29.2	31.8	34.4	35.9
37	28.5	30.0	32.7	35.4	37.0
38	29.2	30.8	33.6	36.4	38.0
39	29.9	31.6	34.4	37.3	38.9
40	30.7	32.4	35.3	38.2	39.9

Adapted from Hadlock FP, Deter RL, Harrist RB, Park SK: Estimating fetal age: Computer-assisted analysis of multiple fetal growth parameters. Radiology 152:497–501, 1984.

when the 50th percentiles reported by Jeanty and coworkers are less than the 10th percentile values reported by Tamura and Sabbagha (see Table 9–4). It is critically important, therefore, when using data from another source, to duplicate the techniques of the original authors. Although one should theoretically choose tables from centers with similar population characteristics, our data have not shown significant

Table 9–4. A COMPARISON OF ABDOMINAL CIRCUMFERENCE PERCENTILES USING SONOGRAPHY

Menstrual Week	Abdominal Circumference (cm)					
	10th Percentile			90th Percentile		
	Jeanty et al*	Hadlock et al†	Tamura and Sabbagha‡	Jeanty et al*	Hadlock et al†	Tamura and Sabbagha‡
18	10.2	11.5	11.7	13.6	13.5	12.0
20	12.4	13.7	14.2	15.8	16.3	16.7
22	14.6	16.0	14.7	18.0	18.8	19.7
24	16.7	18.1	18.9	20.1	21.3	22.8
26	18.8	20.1	19.8	22.2	23.7	26.7
28	20.8	22.0	23.1	24.2	26.0	27.2
30	22.7	23.9	24.4	26.1	28.3	30.1
32	24.5	25.8	26.7	27.9	30.4	32.4
34	26.2	27.5	28.6	29.6	32.5	33.6
36	27.6	29.2	31.0	31.0	34.4	37.8
38	28.9	30.8	32.8	32.3	36.4	38.5
40	29.9	32.4	33.3	33.3	38.2	41.2

*Data from Jeanty P, Cousaert E, Cantraine F: Normal growth of the abdominal perimeter. Am J Perinatol 1:129, 1984.
†Data from Hadlock FP, Deter RL, Harrist RB, Park SK: Estimating fetal age: Computer-assisted analysis of multiple fetal growth parameters. Radiology 152:497, 1984.
‡Data from Tamura RK, Sabbagha RE: Percentile ranks of sonar fetal abdominal circumference measurements. Am J Obstet Gynecol 138:475, 1980.

Table 9–5. THE SENSITIVITY OF INDIVIDUAL SONOGRAPHIC PARAMETERS FOR DETECTING INTRAUTERINE GROWTH RETARDATION

Parameter	Sensitivity	
	Hadlock et al* (37.5 ± 2.1 wk)	Brown et al† (37.9 ± 1.9 wk)
Abdomen	100%	96%
Femur length	20%	45%
Head/abdomen	70%	No data
Femur/abdomen	63%	57%
Estimated weight percentile	87%	63%
Ponderal index	47%	54%

*Data from Hadlock FP, Deter RL, Harrist RB, et al: A date-independent predictor of intrauterine growth retardation: Femur length/abdominal circumference ratio. AJR 141:979, 1983.

†Data from Brown HL, Miller JM, Gabert HA, Kissling G: Ultrasonic recognition of the small-for-gestational-age fetus. Obstet Gynecol 69:693, 1987.

differences in patients of different race and socioeconomic origins.[43]

When fetal growth is compromised, the abdominal circumference is dramatically affected because of the reduction in adipose tissue and the depletion of glycogen stores in the liver. It is not surprising, then, that virtually all studies that have included this measurement have demonstrated it to be the most sensitive single indicator of growth retardation in both symmetric and asymmetric IUGR (Table 9–5). In our experience, measurements below the 10th percentile for known age are highly suspicious for growth abnormality, and measurements below the third percentile for age are considered unequivocal evidence of IUGR until proven otherwise. The limiting factor in the use of the abdominal circumference to predict IUGR is that dates must be known unequivocally for proper use of this measurement. If dates are not known, serial evaluation at 2-week intervals can be done to evaluate interval growth. For example, Divon and coworkers have demonstrated that abdominal circumference growth of less than 1 cm in 14 days is indicative of IUGR.[72]

FETAL LENGTH

Neonatal crown-heel length is an important measure of growth because of its role in the ponderal index, which describes the weight-for-length relationship of the neonate at delivery. Although we can measure fetal crown-rump length using ultrasound scanning in early pregnancy, it is virtually impossible to obtain a realistic measure of crown-heel length, particularly beyond 18 menstrual weeks. However, several authors have evaluated the fetal femur length using sonography and have demonstrated a consistent relationship between fetal femur length and neonatal crown-heel length.[69] Thus, sonographic measurement of femur length can be used as a substitute variable for crown-heel length in the sonographic growth profile (see Fig. 9–6).

There has been extensive sonographic evaluation of

the fetal femur length in utero, and the data across centers have been very reproducible (Table 9–6). Moreover, most authors have demonstrated no significant differences in femur lengths among patients of different racial and socioeconomic origins.[60] However, the degree to which the fetal femur is compromised in IUGR is less well established. Fetal femur length can be affected in early pregnancy in cases of early symmetric growth retardation related to chromosomal abnormalities or infection, but in general the fetal femur length is not affected until very late in pregnancy in asymmetric IUGR. For example, my colleagues and I reported the femur length to be below the 3rd percentile in 20% of third-trimester fetuses with IUGR,[70] and Brown and coworkers reported the femur length to be less than the 10th percentile in 45% of growth-retarded fetuses in the third trimester.[71] Perhaps the major role of the femur length in the growth profile is in the evaluation of fetal weight and body proportionality.

FETAL WEIGHT

Early efforts to evaluate fetal weight in utero demonstrated that the abdominal circumference could be used for predicting weight in normally growing fetuses at term. In preterm fetuses, however, and in fetuses with abnormalities of fetal growth, the variability associated with predicting fetal weight from abdominal circumference alone (2 SD = 24%) was too great for

Table 9–6. PERCENTILE VALUES FOR FETAL FEMUR LENGTH

Menstrual Week	Femur Length (cm)				
	3rd	10th	50th	90th	97th
14	1.2	1.3	1.4	1.5	1.6
15	1.5	1.6	1.7	1.9	1.9
16	1.7	1.8	2.0	2.2	2.3
17	2.1	2.2	2.4	2.6	2.7
18	2.3	2.5	2.7	2.9	3.1
19	2.6	2.7	3.0	3.3	3.4
20	2.8	3.0	3.3	3.6	3.8
21	3.0	3.2	3.5	3.8	4.0
22	3.3	3.5	3.8	4.1	4.3
23	3.5	3.7	4.1	4.5	4.7
24	3.8	4.0	4.4	4.8	5.0
25	4.0	4.2	4.6	5.0	5.2
26	4.2	4.5	4.9	5.3	5.6
27	4.4	4.6	5.1	5.6	5.8
28	4.6	4.9	5.4	5.9	6.2
29	4.8	5.1	5.6	6.1	6.4
30	5.0	5.3	5.8	6.3	6.6
31	5.2	5.5	6.0	6.5	6.8
32	5.3	5.6	6.2	6.8	7.1
33	5.5	5.8	6.4	7.0	7.3
34	5.7	6.0	6.6	7.2	7.5
35	5.9	6.2	6.8	7.4	7.8
36	6.0	6.4	7.0	7.6	8.0
37	6.2	6.6	7.2	7.9	8.2
38	6.4	6.7	7.4	8.1	8.4
39	6.5	6.8	7.5	8.2	8.6
40	6.6	7.0	7.7	8.4	8.8

Adapted from Hadlock FP, Deter RL, Harrist RB, Park SK: Estimating fetal age: Computer-assisted analysis of multiple fetal growth parameters. Radiology 152:497–501, 1984.

general clinical use.[41] For this reason, many authors have attempted to incorporate additional parameters into models for estimating fetal weight, and some have suggested that separate fetal weight models must be used for fetuses that are small or large for dates. In our own experience, the use of a model that incorporates head size, abdominal size, and femur length has proven remarkably accurate over the entire range of weights and ages (1 SD = ± 7.5%).[59] With the use of this technique, estimated fetal weights below the 10th percentile in our laboratory have successfully identified 87% of fetuses with IUGR scanned in the late third trimester of pregnancy (see Table 9–5).[70] Vintzileos and associates have reported similar results using this multiparameter approach to fetal weight estimates.[61]

A major problem in the evaluation of normal growth has been the application in utero of fetal weight charts developed postnatally.[56] In a comprehensive review of this problem, we demonstrated that postnatal weight charts are appropriate for use in the term fetus (38 to 42 weeks), since over 90% of the infants used for these large studies were born at term, but that the range of preterm weights is too broad to be clinically useful.[57] This is because the sample population below 38 weeks in postnatal studies is based on premature deliveries, and these fetuses may not have been growing normally before term. To resolve this issue, we have established normal weights and weight ranges in utero from 10 to 40 weeks and have demonstrated that the variability is constant when expressed as a percentage of the predicted value (Table 9–7). Because our preterm boundaries for normal and abnormal are so narrow compared with the postnatal studies, we recommend that in utero weight evaluations using our tables be applied only to fetuses that have had verification of fetal age using crown-rump length in the first trimester of pregnancy.[57]

BODY PROPORTIONALITY

The earliest application of sonography to the recognition of abnormal body proportionality was reported by Campbell and Thoms using the head circumference/abdominal circumference ratio to evaluate fetuses with asymmetric IUGR.[67] In our experience, this ratio is abnormal in approximately two thirds of all growth-retarded fetuses, generally failing to diagnose the one third of fetuses with symmetric IUGR (see Table 9–5).[70] A major limitation of this ratio is the fact that the normal values change with time, so that strict knowledge of menstrual age is required in the use of this ratio. The second reported problem has been a high number of false-positive results that could result, for example, from a fetus with a 75th percentile head size and a 50th percentile abdominal size (whose weight actually might be above the 50th percentile for age). In view of these findings, most authors believe that the use of abdominal circumference alone in patients with known menstrual age can be used effectively in place of this ratio.[70]

In an attempt to develop an in utero ponderal index for evaluating the weight-length relationship of the fetus, my colleagues and I[70] and Jeanty and coworkers[64]

Table 9–7. IN UTERO FETAL SONOGRAPHIC WEIGHT STANDARDS

Menstrual Week	Estimated Fetal Weight (g)				
	3rd	10th	50th	90th	97th
10	26	29	35	41	44
11	34	37	45	53	56
12	43	48	58	68	73
13	55	61	73	85	91
14	70	77	93	109	116
15	88	97	117	137	146
16	110	121	146	171	183
17	136	150	181	212	226
18	167	185	223	261	279
19	205	227	273	319	341
20	248	275	331	387	414
21	299	331	399	467	499
22	359	398	478	559	598
23	426	471	568	665	710
24	503	556	670	784	838
25	589	652	785	918	981
26	685	758	913	1068	1141
27	791	876	1055	1234	1319
28	908	1004	1210	1416	1513
29	1034	1145	1379	1613	1724
30	1169	1294	1559	1824	1949
31	1313	1453	1751	2049	2189
32	1465	1621	1953	2285	2441
33	1622	1794	2162	2530	2703
34	1783	1973	2377	2781	2971
35	1946	2154	2595	3036	3244
36	2110	2335	2813	3291	3516
37	2271	2513	3028	3543	3785
38	2427	2686	3236	3786	4045
39	2576	2851	3435	4019	4294
40	2714	3004	3619	4234	4524

From Hadlock FP, Harrist RB, Martinez-Poyer J: In utero analysis of fetal growth: A sonographic weight standard. Radiology 181:129–133, 1991.

independently proposed an evaluation of the relationship between abdominal circumference (as an indicator of fetal weight) and femur length (as an indicator of the fetal length). Subsequently, several authors have found this relationship to be relatively constant beyond 20 weeks, indicating that it could be used as an age-independent indicator of IUGR. We have found this ratio to be elevated in approximately two thirds of growth-retarded fetuses, generally failing to detect the one third of fetuses that are symmetrically growth retarded (see Table 9–5).[70] Given the low incidence of IUGR in the general population, we postulated that the positive predictive value of this ratio in screening the general population would be only approximately 25%, and this has been confirmed in subsequent studies.[71, 74] Because it is age independent, we believe this tool is especially useful in evaluating fetuses that present in the third trimester with no dates.

Vintzileos and coworkers have reported other age-independent indices of fetal growth (tibia/abdominal circumference ratio, femur/thigh circumference ratio, and tibia/calf circumference ratio) and have suggested their use in high-risk patients who present late in pregnancy with no dates.[76, 77] Unfortunately, there have been no follow-up data to demonstrate the usefulness of these ratios. Yagel and coworkers[80] evaluated an in utero ponderal index (IUPI) calculated using the estimated fetal weight (EFW) and the femur length (IUPI = EFW/FL^3). Interestingly, these authors found fetal and neonatal well-being were clearly compromised when IUGR was associated with a low in utero ponderal index. It is my bias that these more complicated approaches are less reproducible and offer no additional advantage to the femur length/abdominal circumference ratio.

INTRAUTERINE ENVIRONMENT

It is now well known that clues to the diagnosis of abnormal fetal growth reside in simple observations of the fetus and the intrauterine environment. For example, a reduction in amniotic fluid volume (oligohydramnios) is a common finding in pregnancies affected by IUGR,[94] and Manning and associates initially advocated using an estimate of amniotic fluid volume as a screening tool for IUGR. They had observed that when the largest pocket of amniotic fluid is less than 1 cm in its greatest dimension, there is a high probability that the fetus is growth retarded. However, this degree of oligohydramnios is unusual until very late in pregnancy. For example, Hill and coworkers[83] demonstrated oligohydramnios using this definition in only 3 of 66 growth-retarded fetuses in the third trimester of pregnancy. Moreover, Hill and coworkers demonstrated that even a subjective decrease in amniotic fluid volume was present in only 20 of 66 growth-retarded fetuses.[83] Because it is also common in post-dates pregnancies, oligohydramnios obviously cannot be specific for the detection of IUGR. Nevertheless, when one suspects oligohydramnios in patients with intact membranes and no fetal renal abnormalities, the possibility of IUGR is increased, and close monitoring of fetal growth and well-being is indicated.[97-99] Because the subjective identification of oligohydramnios requires a great deal of experience, I recommend use of the four-quadrant technique using the normal values reported by Moore and Cayle (Table 9–8).[96]

A second clue to the possible presence of IUGR is the finding of advanced placental senescence (grade 3 placenta).[100] Platt and Petrucha[101] have demonstrated that while 20% of normal patients will have a grade 3 placenta at term, it is rare to have a grade 3 placenta before 36 weeks; so it is possible that a grade 3 placenta at this stage of pregnancy could be a marker of early placental insufficiency. Subsequently, Kazzi and associates[102] demonstrated that when a grade 3 placenta is identified in the presence of a sonographic fetal weight estimate below 2700 g, there is a fourfold increase in the incidence of IUGR in comparison with fetuses of the same size with placental grades less than grade 3. Thus, the presence of oligohydramnios and a grade 3 placenta in fetuses weighing less than 2700 g should be considered evidence of IUGR until proven otherwise. In such cases, aggressive monitoring of the pregnancy to ensure fetal growth and well-being is indicated.[94, 95]

A third observation recommended as a potential tool in the diagnosis of IUGR is a delayed appearance of the distal femoral epiphyseal ossification center.[92, 93] It

Table 9–8. AMNIOTIC FLUID INDEX VALUES IN NORMAL PREGNANCY

Menstrual Week	Amniotic Fluid Index Percentile Values (mm)				
	3rd	5th	50th	95th	97th
16	73	79	121	185	201
17	77	83	127	194	211
18	80	87	133	202	220
19	83	90	137	207	225
20	86	93	141	212	230
21	88	95	143	214	233
22	89	97	145	216	235
23	90	98	146	218	237
24	90	98	147	219	238
25	89	97	147	221	240
26	89	97	147	223	242
27	85	95	146	226	245
28	86	94	146	228	249
29	84	92	145	231	254
30	82	90	145	234	258
31	79	88	144	238	263
32	77	86	144	242	269
33	74	83	143	245	274
34	72	81	142	248	278
35	70	79	140	249	279
36	68	77	138	249	279
37	66	75	135	244	275
38	65	73	132	239	269
39	64	72	127	226	255
40	63	71	123	214	240
41	63	70	116	194	216
42	63	69	110	175	192

Adapted from Moore TR, Cayle JE: The amniotic fluid index in normal human pregnancy. Am J Obstet Gynecol 162:1168, 1990.

is well established that this ossification center appears in normally growing fetuses at approximately 32 to 33 menstrual weeks (see Figs. 9–5 and 9–6). In 1984, Gentili and associates[93] found the appearance of this ossification center to be delayed in 36 pregnancies with IUGR, being most pronounced in cases of symmetric IUGR. In a subsequent study by Zilianti and coworkers in 1987,[92] the appearance of the distal femoral epiphyseal ossification center was delayed in 15 of 18 infants judged to be small for gestational age. Thus, in fetuses with well-established dates, this finding may serve as an additional clue to altered fetal growth.

New Developments

The latest developments in the sonographic identification of IUGR have focused on using a combination of factors to detect IUGR. Hill and colleagues[83] and Benson and coworkers,[81, 82] in independent studies, have suggested the use of models that incorporate clues from the maternal history with fetal measurements and/or amniotic fluid volume scores (Table 9–9). Hill and coworkers[83] combined the maternal history score with fetal measurements to produce a logistic IUGR score, which could define the probability of IUGR in a given case. Interestingly, these researchers found the probability of IUGR was directly related to the estimated weight percentile and inversely related to femur length. Unfortunately, they did not evaluate

Table 9–9. A COMPARISON OF MULTIPARAMETER MODELS FOR DETECTION OF INTRAUTERINE GROWTH RETARDATION (IUGR)

Benson Method*	Hill Method†
IUGR score = 39.2 (constant) + Maternal blood pressure score (normal = 0, high = 6.8) + Amniotic fluid score (normal = 0, mild = 9.1, moderate or severe = 14.8) − 13.1 × age standardized estimated weight (SD) *Example:* (High blood pressure, fluid mildly decreased, weight estimate 2 SD below mean for age) *Score* = 39.2 + 6.8 + 9.1 − (13.1 × −2 SD) = 81.3 (probable IUGR)	IUGR score = 15.24 (constant) + 1.2 Antenatal IUGR score (previous small for gestational age = 1, blood pressure >140/90 after 34 weeks = 1, history of renal disease = 1, smoking = 2, bleeding or preterm labor = 1, poor weight gain = 1, no fundal growth or decrease in fundal height = 3) − 2.0 (femur length in cm) − 0.35 (estimated weight percentile) *Example:* (Antenatal score 1, femur = 6.5 cm, 5th weight percentile) *Score:* 15.24 + 1.2 − 13.0 − 1.75 = 169 Probability of IUGR = $e^{1.69}/(1 + e^{1.69})$ = 84%

*Data from Benson CB, Boswell SB, Brown DL, et al: Improved prediction of intrauterine growth retardation with use of multiple parameters. Radiology 168:7, 1988.

†Data from Hill LM, Guzick D, Belfar HL, et al: A combined historic and sonographic score for the detection of intrauterine growth retardation. Obstet Gynecol 73:291, 1989.

abdominal circumference percentile as a potential variable in their model.

Benson and coworkers[81–83] designed an IUGR score (see Table 9–9) so that the combination of elevated maternal blood pressure, severe oligohydramnios, and an estimated fetal weight 3 SD below the mean for age yields a score of 100, whereas the combination of normal blood pressure, normal fluid volume, and an estimated weight 3 SD above the mean for age yields a score of 0. In their initial report, an IUGR score below 50 virtually excluded the diagnosis of IUGR with a negative predictive value of 99.1%. A score above 75 allowed confident prediction of IUGR, with a positive predictive value of 82%. A score of 50 to 75 was equivocal, in that it could be associated within a 24% likelihood of IUGR. In a subsequent follow-up study, the authors found that a score below 50 virtually excludes IUGR (3% probability), a score above 60

allows confident diagnosis (75% probability), and a score of 50 to 60 is intermediate (13% probability). It is possible that the use of an in utero–generated weight curve such as the one reported from our institution will further enhance the ability of these complex models to detect IUGR. It is unfortunate that neither Hill nor Benson evaluated abdominal circumference percentiles as a predictor of IUGR, since the sensitivity based on this measurement alone as reported in the literature appears to be equivalent to the sensitivity of these complex methods (Fig. 9–7).[81–83]

Other authors have compared the use of real-time ultrasound measurements with Doppler studies of the fetus or umbilical cord in detection of IUGR.[84–91] Some authors believe that Doppler studies become abnormal long before the measurements in the fetal growth profile become abnormal, but this has not been our experience using Doppler evaluation of the umbilical

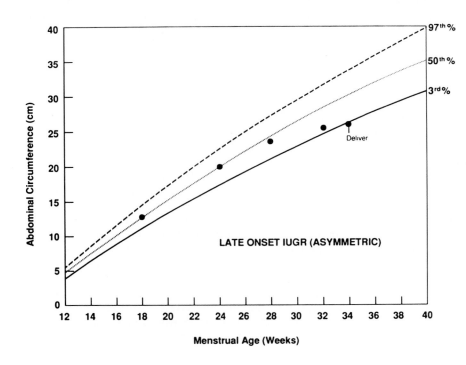

Figure 9–7. Abdominal circumference (AC) growth plotted against known menstrual age (MA) in a case of late-onset asymmetric intrauterine growth retardation (IUGR). Note that the abdomen growth began to decline at approximately 28 menstrual weeks, and that there was virtually no growth between 32 and 34 weeks. In such cases, intensive antenatal surveillance is mandatory and early delivery is often indicated.

artery systolic/diastolic ratio. Other authors have suggested that Doppler studies of the fetal cerebral circulation,[89–91] especially when used in comparison with the Doppler evaluation of the umbilical cord, provide strong evidence of intrauterine growth retardation. Data suggest that biometry is the best indicator of fetal size, while abnormal Doppler studies, particularly absent or reversed end-diastolic flow, are more predictive of poor outcome. Most authors, therefore, have concluded that the combination of fetal biometry and fetal Doppler studies is more useful than either tool used alone.[84–87]

It is clear that the diagnosis of IUGR requires attention to a number of details and that the diagnosis will be enhanced if one combines maternal history, fetal biometry, intrauterine observations, and fetal Doppler studies. Although such an approach would appear on the surface to be exceedingly time consuming and expensive, we routinely incorporate maternal history, fetal biometry (fetal growth profile), and intrauterine observations in every complete obstetrical ultrasound evaluation, and we find the studies can be done in most cases in 15 to 20 minutes. At the present time, we reserve the use of Doppler sonography for patients in whom an abnormality is suspected on the basis of a complete sonogram as described (low weight percentile, low amniotic fluid volume, placental or uterine abnormality) or an abnormal biophysical profile score. It is likely, however, that a Doppler sample of the umbilical cord will eventually become a routine part of a complete obstetrical ultrasound examination.

MACROSOMIA

Macrosomia refers to a condition in which accelerated fetal growth in utero results in an infant who at birth is large for gestational age. Macrosomia has generally been defined in the literature as a birthweight of 4000 g or more, and it occurs in approximately 10% of all infants weighing over 2500 g at birth.[114] Given this relationship, my colleagues and I consider macrosomia in utero to be any fetus whose estimated weight is greater than the 90th percentile for age at any point in pregnancy (Fig. 9–8).[36, 41] Perhaps the most common clinical association with macrosomia is that of maternal diabetes. However, although it is true that diabetics have a higher incidence of macrosomia than the nondiabetic population, only approximately 2% of macrosomic fetuses will be born to mothers with diabetes mellitus.[114] Probably the most significant risk factors for delivery of a macrosomic fetus are multiparity, age older than 35 years, maternal height exceeding 169 cm, prepregnant weight exceeding 70 kg, and delivery 7 days or more past term.[119]

Historically, macrosomic fetuses have generally been classified on their morphologic characteristics at birth.[114, 118] However, I believe that macrosomic fetuses can be loosely classified as symmetric or asymmetric based on their in utero and birth characteristics.[124] For example, fetuses that are macrosomic because of prolonged pregnancy or genetic factors tend to be more symmetric in their body proportions, while macrosomic fetuses born to diabetic patients tend to be more asymmetric, with the abdominal girth being disproportionately large in comparison with head size and overall length. Validation of this system of classification will require additional study.

Finally, and most importantly, we must consider the clinical significance of intrauterine growth acceleration. In these large fetuses, perinatal mortality is increased approximately one and one-half times the normal-weight peer population, but the major significance of macrosomia appears to be the morbidity related to birth trauma, birth asphyxia, and prolonged pregnancy.[114, 118] Moreover, the incidence of these compli-

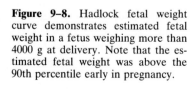

Figure 9–8. Hadlock fetal weight curve demonstrates estimated fetal weight in a fetus weighing more than 4000 g at delivery. Note that the estimated fetal weight was above the 90th percentile early in pregnancy.

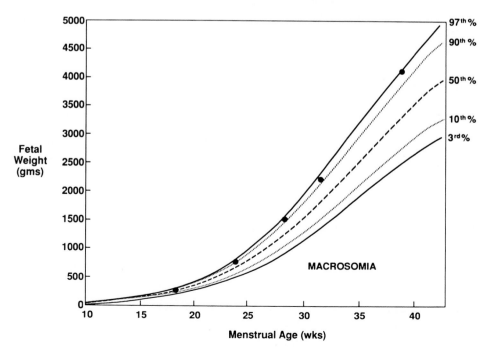

cations appears to be directly related to birthweight, being more common in the severely macrosomic fetus (birthweight greater than 4500 g). Thus, it is imperative that we recognize macrosomia in utero, with the hope that these fetuses can be delivered before the extremes of fetal weight develop (at approximately 38 weeks).

Sonographic Detection of Macrosomia

The sonographic growth profile used for identification of growth-retarded fetuses is equally useful in the recognition of the growth-accelerated fetus.[36] As indicated, although all individual growth parameters are usually increased in the macrosomic fetus, the abdominal circumference is definitely the most sensitive single indicator of macrosomia (Table 9–10).[120, 124, 127] The detection rate for macrosomia should approach that for IUGR for examinations done at 38 weeks, using the 90th percentile for age as a borderline between normal and abnormal (see Table 9–3). Head size and femur length will generally be less useful as individual predictors, although the femur length/abdominal circumference and head circumference/abdominal circumference ratios will frequently demonstrate early evidence of macrosomia.[124]

Sonographic estimates of fetal weight would appear to be a natural tool for the detection of macrosomia, and the development of an in utero fetal weight curve should allow diagnosis early in pregnancy (see Fig. 9–8 and Table 9–7). However, the experience in the literature has been less than successful, and most authors have questioned the validity of this technique.[130–134] One of the limitations of fetal weight estimates in macrosomic fetuses consists of the technical factors associated with obtaining the image, particularly in fetuses whose abdominal girth exceeds the field of the transducer. A second and perhaps more important factor is that most fetal weight models have been based on fetuses with normal body composition, whereas macrosomic fetuses typically have an increase

in adipose tissue.[135, 136] Because fat is less dense than muscle mass, one would postulate that estimates of weight based on models developed from normal weight populations would overestimate weight systematically in macrosomic fetuses. This has been a consistent finding in our laboratory, and in that of others, with a systematic overestimation of 3% to 4%. When this systematic bias is removed by developing models based on macrosomic fetuses, the variability in weight estimations in this group generally is comparable to those in normally grown and undergrown fetuses (1 SD = approximately 7.5% of the predicted weight).[133, 134] It remains to be seen whether use of such models will eliminate the high false-positive and false-negative diagnoses reported in the literature. This is particularly true in light of the report by Farmer and coworkers,[134] who found that the use of a neural network for the sonographic estimation of fetal weight in the macrosomic fetus resulted in an average error of 4.7% of actual birthweight.

THE FUTURE

We have made great strides in the identification of abnormal fetal growth in the past decade. This has been due primarily to the development of normal range data for a number of individual fetal growth parameters and can only be enhanced by the development of a normal in utero fetal weight curve standard.[57] Nonetheless, an inherent problem in the diagnosis of growth disturbances is not knowing the genetic growth potential of a given fetus, so the normalcy of the growth of any fetus has been judged to this point against population standards. Fortunately, great strides have been made in this area using sophisticated mathematic modeling of growth in longitudinal studies of normally growing fetuses. Deter and Rossavik[115] have demonstrated that a specific growth curve for any fetal growth parameter can be developed on an individualized basis from two ultrasound examinations obtained before the third trimester of pregnancy (preferably at 16 weeks and 26 weeks). Using these techniques, the authors have been able to predict birth characteristics with a high degree of accuracy 14 weeks before delivery in normally growing fetuses.[116] Based on these fetal measurements and actual birth measurements at delivery, a growth potential realization index can be calculated for fetal weight, head circumference, abdominal circumference, and thigh circumference. Deter and colleagues combined these growth potential realization index values to form a neonatal growth assessment score, which appears to be a sensitive indicator of third-trimester growth abnormalities.[117] Further validation of these exciting techniques will undoubtedly enhance our ability to recognize abnormalities of fetal growth both prenatally and postnatally.

References

1. Battaglia FC, Lubcheno LO: A practical classification of newborn infants by weight and gestational age. J Pediatr 71:159, 1967.

Table 9–10. COMPARISON OF FETAL PARAMETERS IN AGA AND LGA FETUSES

Parameter	Appropriate for Gestational Age Group (mean ± SD)	Large for Gestational Age Group (mean + SD)	P Value
Biparietal diameter (cm)	9.2 ± 0.4	9.6 ± 0.4	<.0001
Head circumference (HC) (cm)	33.7 ± 1.1	35.2 ± 1.3	<.0001
Abdominal circumference (AC) (cm)	33.6 ± 1.6	37.4 ± 1.3	<.0001
Femur length (FL) (cm)	7.4 ± 0.4	7.6 ± 0.3	<.0001
HC/AC	1.0 ± 0.05	0.94 ± 0.04	<.0001
FL/AC*	22.0 ± 1.0	20.5 ± 1.0	<.0001

*Expressed as femur length ÷ abdominal circumference × 100.
From Hadlock FP, Harrist RB, Fearneyhough TC, et al: Use of femur length/abdominal circumference ratio in detecting the macrosomic fetus. Radiology 154:503–505, 1985.

2. Gruenwald P: Growth of the human fetus. Am J Obstet Gynecol 94:1112, 1966.
3. Vorherr H: Factors influencing fetal growth. Am J Obstet Gynecol 142:577, 1982.
4. Lubchenco LO, Hansman C, Dressler M, Boyd E: Intrauterine growth as estimated from liveborn birth-weight data at 24 to 42 weeks of gestation. Pediatrics 32:793, 1963.
5. Brenner WE, Edelman DA, Hendricks CH: A standard of fetal growth for the United States of America. Am J Obstet Gynecol 126:555, 1976.
6. Williams RL, Creasy RK, Cunningham GC: Fetal growth and perinatal viability in California. Obstet Gynecol 59:624, 1982.
7. Ulrich M: Fetal growth patterns in normal newborn infants in relation to gestational age, birth order, and sex. Acta Paediatr Scand Suppl 292:5, 1982.
8. Robertson PA, Sniderman SH, Laros RK, et al: Neonatal morbidity according to gestational age and birth weight from five tertiary care centers in the United States, 1983 through 1986. Am J Obstet Gynecol 166:1629, 1992.
9. Altman DG, Coles EC: Nomograms for precise determination of birth weight for dates. Br J Obstet Gynaecol 87:81, 1980.
10. Forbes JF, Smalls MJ: A comparative analysis of birthweight for gestational age standards. Br J Obstet Gynaecol 99:297, 1983.
11. Kloosterman GJ: On intrauterine growth. Int J Gynaecol Obstet 8:895, 1970.
12. Galbraith RS, Karchmar EJ, Piercy WN, Low JA: The clinical prediction of intrauterine growth retardation. Am J Obstet Gynecol 133:281, 1979.
13. Hill RM, Verinaud WM, Deter RL, et al: The effect of intrauterine malnutrition on the human infant. Acta Paediatr Scand 73:482, 1984.
14. Patterson RM, Prihoda TJ, Gibbs CE, et al: Analysis of birth weight percentile as a predictor of perinatal outcome. Obstet Gynecol 68:459, 1986.
15. Patterson RM, Poudiot MR: Neonatal morphometrics and perinatal outcome: Who is growth retarded? Am J Obstet Gynecol 157:691, 1987.
16. Fitzhardinge PM, Steven EM: The small-for-date infant: II. Neurological and intellectual sequelae. Pediatrics 49:50, 1972.
17. Vohr BR, Oh W, Rosenfield AG, Cowett RM: The preterm small-for-gestational age infant: A two-year follow-up study. Am J Obstet Gynecol 133:425, 1979.
18. Soothill PW, Ajayi RA, Campbell S, et al: Relationship between fetal acidemia at cordocentesis and subsequent neurodevelopment. Ultrasound Obstet Gynecol 2:80, 1992.
19. Low JA, Galbraith RS, Muir DW, et al: Mortality and morbidity after intrapartum asphyxia in the preterm fetus. Obstet Gynecol 80:57, 1992.
20. Lin CC, Su SJ, River LP: Comparison of associated high-risk factors and perinatal outcome between symmetric and asymmetric fetal intrauterine growth retardation. Am J Obstet Gynecol 164:1535, 1991.
21. Low JA, Galbraith RS, Muir D, et al: Intrauterine growth retardation: A study of long-term morbidity. Am J Obstet Gynecol 142:670, 1982.
22. Sibai BM, Anderson GD, Abdella TN, et al: Eclampsia: III. Neonatal outcome, growth and development. Am J Obstet Gynecol 146:307, 1983.
23. Visser GHA, Huisman A, Saathof PWF, Sinnige HAM: Early fetal growth retardation: Obstetric background and recurrence rate. Obstet Gynecol 67:40, 1986.
24. Lang JM, Cohen A, Lieberman E: Risk factors for small-for-gestational-age birth in a preterm population. Am J Obstet Gynecol 166:1374, 1992.
25. Benacerraf BR: Intrauterine growth retardation in the first trimester associated with triploidy. J Ultrasound Med 7:153, 1988.
26. Dicke J, Crane JP: Sonographic recognition of major malformations and aberrant fetal growth in trisomic fetuses. J Ultrasound Med 10:433, 1991.
27. Dicke JM, Gray DL, Songster GS, et al: Fetal biometry as a screening tool for the detection of chromosomally abnormal pregnancies. Obstet Gynecol 74:724, 1989.
28. Thomas D, Makhoul J, Muller C: Fetal growth retardation due to massive subchorionic thrombohematoma: Report of two cases. J Ultrasound Med 11:245, 1992.
29. Daikoku NH, Johnson JWC, Graf C, et al: Patterns of intrauterine growth retardation. Obstet Gynecol 54:211, 1979.
30. Saintonge J, Cote R: Intrauterine growth retardation and diabetic pregnancy: Two types of fetal malnutrition. Am J Obstet Gynecol 146:194, 1983.
31. Villar J, Belizan JM: The timing factor in the pathophysiology of the intrauterine growth retardation syndrome. Obstet Gynecol Survey 37:499, 1982.
32. Miller HC, Hassanein K: Diagnosis of impaired fetal growth in newborn infants. Pediatrics 48:511, 1971.
33. Woods DL, Malan AF, de v Heese H: Patterns of retarded fetal growth. Early Hum Dev 3:257, 1979.
34. Keirse MJNC: Epidemiology and aetiology of the growth retarded baby. Clin Obstet Gynaecol 11:415, 1984.
35. Ott WJ: The diagnosis of altered fetal growth. Obstet Gynecol Clin North Am 15:237, 1988.
36. Hadlock FP, Deter RL, Harrist RB: Sonographic detection of abnormal fetal growth patterns. Clin Obstet Gynecol 27:342, 1984.
37. Hadlock FP, Deter RL, Harrist RB, Park SK: The use of ultrasound to determine fetal age—a review. Med Ultrasound 7:95, 1983.
38. Matsumoto S, Nogami Y, Ohkuri S: Statistical studies on menstruation: A criticism on the definition of normal menstruation. Gumma J Med Sci 11:294, 1962.
39. Waldenstrom U, Axelsson O, Nilsson S: A comparison of the ability of a sonographically measured biparietal diameter and the last menstrual period to predict the spontaneous onset of labor. Obstet Gynecol 76:336, 1990.
40. Hadlock FP, Shah YP, Kanon DJ, Lindsey JV: Fetal crown-rump length: Reevaluation of relation to menstrual age (5–18 weeks) with high-resolution real-time us. Radiology 182:501, 1992.
41. Hadlock FP: Sonographic estimation of fetal age and weight. Radiol Clin North Am 28:39, 1990.
42. Hadlock FP, Harrist RB, Martinez-Poyer J: How accurate is second trimester fetal dating? J Ultrasound Med 10:557, 1991.
43. Hadlock FP, Harrist RB, Shah YP, et al: Estimating fetal age using multiple parameters: A prospective evaluation in a racially mixed population. Am J Obstet Gynecol 156:955, 1987.
44. Hadlock FP, Harrist RB, Martinez-Poyer J: Fetal body ratios in second trimester: A useful tool for identifying chromosomal abnormalities? J Ultrasound Med 11:81, 1992.
45. Hadlock FP, Deter RL, Harrist RB, Park SK: Fetal biparietal diameter: A critical re-evaluation of the relation to menstrual age by means of real-time ultrasound. J Ultrasound Med 1:97, 1982.
46. Hadlock FP, Deter RL, Harrist RB, Park SK: Fetal head circumference: Relation to menstrual age. AJR 138:649, 1982.
47. Hadlock FP, Deter RL, Harrist RB, Park SK: Fetal abdominal circumference as a predictor of menstrual age. AJR 139:367, 1982.
48. Hadlock FP, Harrist RB, Deter RL, Park SK: Fetal femur length as a predictor of menstrual age: Sonographically measured. AJR 138:875, 1982.
49. Hadlock FP, Deter RL, Carpenter RJ, Park SK: Estimating fetal age: Effect of head shape on BPD. AJR 137:83, 1981.
50. Hadlock FP, Deter RL, Harrist RB, Park SK: Estimating fetal age: Computer-assisted analysis of multiple fetal growth parameters. Radiology 152:497, 1984.
51. Jeanty P, Cousaert E, Hobbins JC, et al: A longitudinal study of fetal head biometry. Am J Perinatol 1:118, 1984.
52. Jeanty P, Cousaert E, Cantraine F: Normal growth of the abdominal perimeter. Am J Perinatol 1:129, 1984.
53. Tamura RK, Sabbagha RE: Percentile ranks of sonar fetal abdominal circumference measurements. Am J Obstet Gynecol 138:475, 1980.
54. Tamura RK, Sabbagha RE, Pan WH, Vaisrub N: Ultrasonic fetal abdominal circumference: Comparison of direct versus calculated measurement. Obstet Gynecol 67:833, 1986.
55. Jeanty P, Cousaert E, Cantraine F, et al: A longitudinal study of fetal limb growth. Am J Perinatol 1:136, 1984.
56. Goldenberg RL, Cutter GR, Hoffman JH, et al: Intrauterine growth retardation: Standards for diagnosis. Am J Obstet Gynecol 161:271, 1989.
57. Hadlock FP, Harrist RB, Martinez-Poyer J: In utero analysis

of fetal growth: A sonographic weight standard. Radiology 181:129, 1991.

58. Deter RL, Harrist RB, Hadlock FP, et al: Longitudinal studies of fetal growth with the use of dynamic image ultrasonography. Am J Obstet Gynecol 143:545, 1982.

59. Hadlock FP, Harrist RB, Sharman RS, et al: Estimating fetal weight with the use of head, body and femur measurements: A prospective study. Am J Obstet Gynecol 151:333, 1985.

60. Ruvulo KA, Filly RA, Callen PW: Evaluation of fetal femur length for prediction of gestational age in a racially mixed population. J Ultrasound Med 6:417, 1987.

61. Vintzileos AM, Campbell WA, Rodis JF, et al: Fetal weight estimation formulas with head, abdominal, femur, and thigh circumference measurements. Am J Obstet Gynecol 157:410, 1987.

62. McLean FH, Boyd ME, Usher RH, Kramer MS: Post-term infants: Too big or too small? Am J Obstet Gynecol 164:619, 1991.

63. Secher NJ, Hansen PK, Lenstrup C, et al: Birthweight-for-gestational age charts based on early ultrasound estimation of gestational age. Br J Obstet Gynaecol 93:128, 1986.

64. Jeanty P, Cantraine F, Romero R, et al: A longitudinal study of fetal weight growth. J Ultrasound Med 3:321, 1984.

65. Ott WJ: Defining altered fetal growth by second-trimester sonography. Obstet Gynecol 75:1053, 1990.

66. Deter RL, Harrist RB, Hadlock FP, Carpenter RJ: The use of ultrasound in the detection of intrauterine growth retardation: A review. J Clin Ultrasound 10:9, 1982.

67. Campbell S, Thoms A: Ultrasound measurement of the fetal head to abdomen circumference ratio in the assessment of growth retardation. Br J Obstet Gynaecol 84:165, 1977.

68. Crane JP, Kopta MM: Prediction of intrauterine growth retardation via ultrasonically measured head/abdominal circumference ratios. Obstet Gynaecol 54:597, 1979.

69. Hadlock FP, Deter RL, Roecker E, et al: Relation of fetal femur length to neonatal crown-heel length. J Ultrasound Med 3:1, 1984.

70. Hadlock FP, Deter RL, Harrist RB, et al: A date-independent predictor of intrauterine growth retardation: Femur length/abdominal circumference ratio. AJR 141:979, 1983.

71. Brown HL, Miller JM, Gabert HA, Kissling G: Ultrasonic recognition of the small-for-gestational-age fetus. Obstet Gynecol 69:631, 1987.

72. Divon MY, Chamberlain PF, Sipos L, et al: Identification of the small for gestational age fetus with the use of gestational age-independent indices of fetal growth. Am J Obstet Gynecol 155:1197, 1986.

73. Ott WJ: Fetal femur length, neonatal crown-hell length, and screening for intrauterine growth retardation. Obstet Gynecol 65:460, 1984.

74. Benson CB, Doubilet PM, Saltzman DH, Jones TB: FL/AC ratio: Poor predictor of intrauterine growth retardation. Invest Radiol 20:727, 1985.

75. Benson CB, Doubilet PM, Saltzman DH: Intrauterine growth retardation: Predictive value of US criteria for antenatal diagnosis. Radiology 160:415, 1986.

76. Vintzileos AM, Neckles S, Campbell WA, et al: Three fetal ponderal indexes in normal pregnancy. Obstet Gynecol 65:807, 1985.

77. Vintzileos AM, Neckles S, Campbell WA, et al: Ultrasound fetal thigh-calf circumferences and gestational age-independent fetal ratios in normal pregnancy. J Ultrasound Med 4:287, 1985.

78. Hays D, Patterson RM: A comparison of fetal biometric ratios to neonatal morphometrics. J Ultrasound Med 6:71, 1987.

79. Eden RD, Seifert LS, Kodack LD, et al: A modified biophysical profile for antenatal fetal surveillance. Obstet Gynecol 71:365, 1988.

80. Yagel S, Zacut D, Igelstein S, et al: In utero ponderal index as a prognostic factor in the evaluation of intrauterine growth retardation. Am J Obstet Gynecol 157:415, 1987.

81. Benson CB, Boswell SB, Brown DL, et al: Improved prediction of intrauterine growth retardation with use of multiple parameters. Radiology 168:7, 1988.

82. Benson CB, Belville JS, Lentini JF, et al: Intrauterine growth retardation: Diagnosis based on multiple parameters—a prospective study. Radiology 177:499, 1990.

83. Hill LM, Guzick D, Belfar HL, et al: A combined historic and sonographic score for the detection of intrauterine growth retardation. Obstet Gynecol 73:291, 1989.

84. Gaziano E, Knox GE, Wager GP, et al: The predictability of the small-for-gestational-age infant by real-time ultrasound-derived measurements combined with pulsed Doppler umbilical artery velocimetry. Am J Obstet Gynecol 158:1431, 1988.

85. Miller JM, Gabert HA: Comparison of dynamic image and pulsed Doppler ultrasonography for the diagnosis of the small-for-gestational-age fetus. Am J Obstet Gynecol 166:1820, 1992.

86. Divon MY, Guidetti DA, Braverman JJ, et al: Intrauterine growth retardation—a prospective study of the diagnostic value of real-time sonography combined with umbilical artery flow velocimetry. Obstet Gynecol 72:611, 1988.

87. Berkowitz GS, Mehalek KE, Chitkara U, et al: Doppler umbilical velocimetry in the prediction of adverse outcome in pregnancies at risk for intrauterine growth retardation. Obstet Gynecol 71:742, 1988.

88. Ott WJ: Comparison of dynamic image and pulsed Doppler ultrasonography for the diagnosis of intrauterine growth retardation. J Clin Ultrasound 18:3, 1990.

89. Wladimiroff JW, Tonge HM, Stewart PA: Doppler ultrasound assessment of cerebral blood flow in the human fetus. Br J Obstet Gynaecol 93:471, 1986.

90. Cohn HE, Sacks EJ, Heymann MA, Rudolph AM: Cardiovascular response to hypoxemia and acidemia in fetal lambs. Am J Obstet Gynecol 120:817, 1974.

91. Mari G, Moise KJ, Deter RL, et al: Doppler assessment of the pulsatility index in the cerebral circulation of the human fetus. Am J Obstet Gynecol 160:698, 1989.

92. Zilianti M, Fernandez S, Azuaga A, et al: Ultrasound evaluation of the distal femoral epiphyseal ossification center as a screening test for intrauterine growth retardation. Obstet Gynecol 70:361, 1987.

93. Gentili P, Trasimeni A, Giorlandino C: Fetal ossification centers as predictors of gestational age in normal and abnormal pregnancies. J Ultrasound Med 3:193, 1984.

94. Manning FA, Hill LM, Platt LD: Qualitative amniotic fluid volume determination by ultrasound: Antepartum detection of intrauterine growth retardation. Am J Obstet Gynecol 139:254, 1981.

95. Vintzileos AM, Tsapanos V: Biophysical assessment of the fetus. Ultrasound Obstet Gynecol 2:133, 1992.

96. Moore TR, Cayle JE: The amniotic fluid index in normal human pregnancy. Am J Obstet Gynecol 162:1168, 1990.

97. Philipson EH, Sokol RJ, Williams T: Oligohydramnios: Clinical associations and predictive value for intrauterine growth retardation. Am J Obstet Gynecol 146:271, 1983.

98. Hoddick WK, Callen PW, Filly RA, et al: Ultrasonographic determination of qualitative amniotic fluid volume in intrauterine growth retardation. Am J Obstet Gynecol 149:758, 1984.

99. Rutherford SE, Phelan JP, Smith CV, Jacobs N: The four-quadrant assessment of amniotic fluid volume: An adjunct to antepartum fetal heart rate testing. Obstet Gynecol 70:353, 1987.

100. Grannum PA, Berkowitz RL, Hobbins JC: The ultrasonic changes in the maturing placenta and their relation to fetal pulmonic maturity. Am J Obstet Gynecol 133:915, 1979.

101. Petrucha RA, Platt LV: Relationship of placental grade to gestational age. Am J Obstet Gynecol 144:733, 1982.

102. Kazzi GM, Gross TL, Sokol RJ, Kazzi NJ: Detection of intrauterine growth retardation: A new use for sonographic placental grading. J Obstet Gynecol 145:733, 1983.

103. Wittmann BK, Robinson HP, Aitchison T, Fleming JEE: The value of diagnostic ultrasound as a screening test for intrauterine growth retardation: Comparison of nine parameters. Am J Obstet Gynecol 134:30, 1979.

104. Hughey MJ: Routine ultrasound for detection and management of the small-for-gestational-age fetus. Obstet Gynecol 64:101, 1984.

105. Ferrazzi E, Nicolini U, Kustermann A, Pardi G: Routine obstetric ultrasound: Effectiveness of cross-sectional screening for fetal growth retardation. J Clin Ultrasound 14:17, 1986.

106. Warsof SL, Cooper DJ, Little D, Campbell S: Routine ultrasound screening for antenatal detection of intrauterine growth retardation. Obstet Gynecol 67:33, 1986.

107. Waldenstrom U, Nilsson S, Fall O, et al: Effects of routine

one-stage ultrasound screening in pregnancy: A randomised controlled trial. Lancet 2:585, 1988.

108. Rosendahl H, Kivinen S: Routine ultrasound screening for early detection of small for gestational age fetuses. Obstet Gynecol 71:518, 1988.

109. Skovron ML, Berkowitz GS, Lapinski RH, et al: Evaluation of early third-trimester ultrasound screening for intrauterine growth retardation. J Ultrasound Med 10:153, 1991.

110. De Vore GR, Hebertson RM: The temporal association of the implementation of a fetal diagnostic and surveillance program and decreased fetal mortality in a private hospital. Obstet Gynecol 75:210, 1990.

111. Ferrazzi E, Nicolini U, Kustermann A, Pardi G: Routine obstetric ultrasound: Effectiveness of cross-sectional screening for fetal growth retardation. J Clin Ultrasound 14:17, 1986.

112. Grumbach K, Coleman BG, Arger PH, et al: Twin and singleton growth patterns compared using US. Radiology 158:237, 1986.

113. Parker AJ, Davies P, Mayho AM, Newton JR: The ultrasound estimation of sex-related variations of intrauterine growth. Am J Obstet Gynecol 149:655, 1984.

114. Boyd ME, Usher RH, McLean FH: Fetal macrosomia: Prediction, risks, proposed management. Obstet Gynecol 61:715, 1983.

115. Deter RL, Rossavik IK: A simplified method for determining individual growth curve standards. Obstet Gynecol 70:801, 1987.

116. Deter RL, Hill RM, Tennyson LM: Predicting the birth characteristics of normal fetuses 14 weeks before delivery. J Clin Ultrasound 17:89, 1989.

117. Deter RL, Harrist RB, Hill RM: Neonatal growth assessment score: A new approach to the detection of intrauterine growth retardation in the newborn. Am J Obstet Gynecol 162:1030, 1990.

118. Gordon HH: The infants of diabetic mothers. Am J Med Sci 244:129, 1962.

119. Spellacy WN, Miller S, Winegar A, Peterson PQ: Macrosomia: Maternal characteristics and infant complications. Obstet Gynecol 66:158, 1985.

120. Ogata ES, Sabbagha R, Metzger BE, et al: Serial ultrasonography to assess evolving fetal macrosomia. JAMA 243:2405, 1980.

121. Wladimiroff JW, Bloemsma CA, Wallenburg HCS: Ultrasonic diagnosis of the large-for-dates infant. Obstet Gynecol 52:285, 1978.

122. Elliott JP, Garite TJ, Freeman RK, et al: Ultrasonic prediction of fetal macrosomia in diabetic patients. Obstet Gynecol 60:159, 1982.

123. Deter RL, Hadlock FP: Use of ultrasound in the detection of macrosomia: A review. J Clin Ultrasound 13:519, 1985.

124. Hadlock FP, Harrist RB, Fearneyhough TC, et al: Use of femur length/abdominal circumference ratio in detecting the macrosomic fetus. Radiology 154:503, 1985.

125. Benson CB, Coughlin BF, Doubilet PM: Amniotic fluid volume in large-for-gestational-age fetuses of nondiabetic mothers. J Ultrasound Med 10:149, 1991.

126. Hill LM, Guzick D, Fries J, et al: The transverse cerebellar diameter in estimating gestational age in the large for gestational age fetus. Obstet Gynecol 75:981, 1990.

127. Tamura RK, Sabbagha RE, Depp R, et al: Diabetic macrosomia: Accuracy of third trimester ultrasound. Obstet Gynecol 67:826, 1986.

128. Miller JM, Korndorffer FA, Kissling GE, et al: Recognition of the overgrown fetus: In utero ponderal indices. Am J Perinatol 4:86, 1987.

129. Benson CB, Doubilet PM, Saltzman DH, et al: Femur length/abdominal circumference ratio: Poor predictor of macrosomic fetuses in diabetic mothers. J Ultrasound Med 5:141, 1986.

130. Miller JM, Korndorffer FA, Gabert HA: Fetal weight estimates in late pregnancy with emphasis on macrosomia. J Clin Ultrasound 14:437, 1986.

131. Benson CB, Doubilet PM, Saltzman DH: Sonographic determination of fetal weights in diabetic pregnancies. Am J Obstet Gynecol 156:441, 1987.

132. Sabbagha RE, Minogue J, Tamura RK, Hungerford SA: Estimation of birth weight by use of ultrasonographic formulas targeted to large-, appropriate-, and small-for-gestational-age fetuses. Am J Obstet Gynecol 160:854, 1989.

133. Hirata GI, Medearis AL, Horenstein J, et al: Ultrasonographic estimation of fetal weight in the clinically macrosomic fetus. Am J Obstet Gynecol 162:238, 1990.

134. Farmer RM, Medearis AL, Hirata GI, Platt LD: The use of a neural network for the ultrasonographic estimation of fetal weight in the macrosomic fetus. Am J Obstet Gynecol 166:1467, 1992.

135. Bernstein IM, Catalano PM: Influence of fetal fat on the ultrasound estimation of fetal weight in diabetic mothers. Obstet Gynecol 79:561, 1992.

136. Catalano PM, Tyzbir ED, Allen SR, et al: Evaluation of fetal growth by estimation of neonatal body composition. Obstet Gynecol 79:46, 1992.

137. Levine AB, Lockwood CJ, Brown B, et al: Sonographic diagnosis of the large for gestational age fetus at term: Does it make a difference? Obstet Gynecol 79:55, 1992.

138. Delpapa EH, Mueller-Heubach E: Pregnancy outcome following ultrasound diagnosis of macrosomia. Obstet Gynecol 78:340, 1991.

139. Pollack RN, Hauer-Pollack G, Divon MY: Macrosomia in post-dates pregnancies: The accuracy of routine ultrasonographic screening. Am J Obstet Gynecol 167:7, 1992.

CHAPTER 10

■ ■ ■ ■ ■ ■ # Ultrasound Evaluation of Normal Fetal Anatomy*

ROY A. FILLY, M.D.

Our understanding of normal fetal anatomy as seen on sonograms continues to be an area of considerable growth. Instrumentation has improved steadily, yielding both improved and more consistent image quality. Among the most significant advancements for fetal imaging has been the ability to choose the depth of the zone of best focus of the ultrasonic beam. With this capability, the area of anatomy being observed can be consistently inspected with the focused portion of the beam, a highly significant advantage.

Furthermore, sonologists have gradually improved their understanding of the anatomy portrayed on in utero sonograms. Unquestionably, clearer images have led the way to our improved understanding, but other factors have been involved. Not the least of these has been the surge in ultrasonic imaging of premature neonates.[1, 2] These tiny neonates are the equivalent of second-trimester fetuses as early, at times, as 24 weeks. Visualization of their head[1, 2] (Fig. 10–1) and body (Fig. 10–2) anatomy in the more ideal ex utero environment, which permits the use of higher-frequency transducers, a greater selection of planes of section, and comparison with other imaging modalities, has done much to improve our understanding of fetal anatomy. This newly won information can be, to a large extent, extrapolated to younger fetuses.

The ability of sonography to detect intrafetal structures depends on a balance between spatial resolution and contrast.[3] This balance, however, strongly favors contrast as the more important aspect of perception.

*This chapter is adapted from Filly RA: Sonographic anatomy of the normal fetus. *In* Harrison MA, Golbus MS, Filly RA (eds): The Unborn Patient: Prenatal Diagnosis and Treatment. Philadelphia, WB Saunders, 1991, pp 92–130.

For example, a large white dot on a white wall is difficult or impossible to see because no contrast differential exists even though the eye can spatially resolve easily a tiny black dot (high contrast) on the same wall. Structures possessing high levels of subject contrast can be consistently detected at a smaller size (often equating to an earlier age) than those displaying poor contrast. Sonologists, unfortunately, possess no agents to alter contrast of fetal organs and thus are totally dependent on subject contrast (inherent contrast) for visualization of internal fetal morphologic details. Clearly, spatial resolution is also a critical feature in defining morphology but has not been the limiting factor in demonstrating fetal anatomy.

Other parameters, important in fetal imaging, also cannot be controlled. Sonography is a tomographic technique. Appropriate positioning for obtaining the best tomographic plane is always desirable. However, we are unable to control fetal position to attain this end. We also cannot control maternal body habitus or the amount of amniotic fluid, both of which may dramatically alter our ability to discern fetal anatomy. Despite these problems, a large number of fetal structures are consistently visible sonographically.

High-resolution, real-time scanners with their flexible approach to imaging are mandatory for modern fetal sonography.[4–6] In the following sections, various aspects of fetal anatomy will be detailed as seen on such instrumentation. An estimate will be made of the ability of ultrasound instrumentation to consistently demonstrate the anatomic part under consideration as well as an attempt to estimate when the fetus has attained sufficient size such that the anatomic structure is large enough to be detected. It is important to recall that size and visualization may be relative at any given

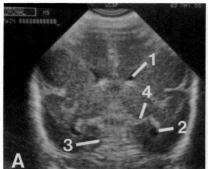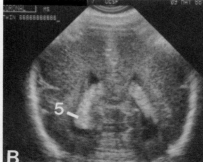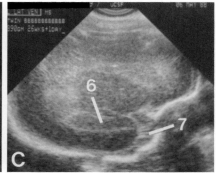

Figure 10–1. Neonatal head sonogram. Coronal *(A)*, axial *(B)*, and parasagittal *(C)* images enable correlation with fetal examinations. 1, lateral ventricular body; 2, temporal horn; 3, ambient cistern; 4, choroidal fissure; 5, glomus of choroid plexus; 6, temporal lobe; 7, cistern with linear bridging veins.

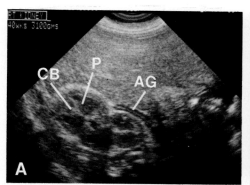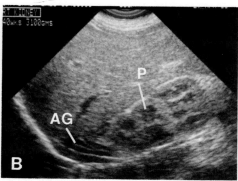

Figure 10–2. Neonatal abdominal sonogram. *A.* Transverse image. *B.* Parasagittal image. AG, adrenal gland, both cortex (thicker) and medulla (thinner); P, medullary pyramid of the kidney; CB, Bertin column.

stage of development. For example, in a small fetus whose urinary bladder is well distended, identification of the bladder is relatively easy. Alternatively, identification of the bladder will be difficult or impossible in a term fetus that has recently voided. The urine, in this instance, provides the "contrast" that ordinarily makes the urinary bladder an easy structure to perceive. If this "contrast agent" drains away, the size of the fetus (and thus its bladder) will not rescue one from the loss of contrast. Important, also, is the concept that the human eye sees best in the "relative" rather than the "absolute" sense of size. Thus, in a young fetus the cerebral ventricle is much more readily seen than in an older fetus because the relative size of the ventricle compared with overall brain size is larger early (even though the absolute size is larger later).

If the sonographer begins with a specific intent to image a particular fetal part, it is frequently possible to succeed.[3, 7] To accomplish this end, the sonographer must (1) assess the precise fetal position; (2) consider whether the anatomic part of interest is best visualized in planes perpendicular to the fetal long axis or parallel to the fetal long axis; and (3) adjust time gain compensation and transducer angulation to visualize the area to best advantage. Obviously, such rules are the same throughout all of sonography. The challenge of imaging intrafetal structures is to apply the above rules when fetal position is changing such that the current scanning plane is no longer applicable for the part one wishes to visualize.

The flexibility offered by real-time sonographic systems enables one to quickly survey the fetus to determine precise position. Second, the sonographic tomograms, which are rapidly generated (virtually "real-time" imaging), enable one to view a large volume of the fetus with closely spaced sections. Such a rapid look at many contiguous tomograms eliminates one of the basic flaws of tomographic imaging of a moving target. Finally, fetal movements are viewed directly, which enables one to quickly reorient the transducer to the optimal plane of section to image the structure of interest.

Fetal parts of interest to the sonologist fall into three major categories of subject contrast that subsequently, then, determine the relative ease with which the structure is sonographically visible. These categories are (1) structures that generate high-amplitude reflections (e.g., ossified bones); (2) structures that generate no

internal echoes (e.g., fluid-containing viscera); and (3) those that generate mid-range gray echoes (e.g., the parenchymal organs—lungs, brain, spleen, liver, kidneys, and muscles). The categories are listed from most visible to least visible. Within the last category one may anticipate seeing a spectrum of gray shades that will enable distinction between several parenchymal organs and intraorgan components. For example, the medullary portions of the fetal renal parenchyma generate lower-amplitude internal echoes than do the surrounding cortical tissues and septa of Bertin, thus enabling recognition of this separate component of renal tissue (Fig. 10–3).[8]

A feature of critical importance for organ imaging is the fetal position. Clearly, a prone fetus is in an optimal position for imaging the kidneys, ordinarily difficult to

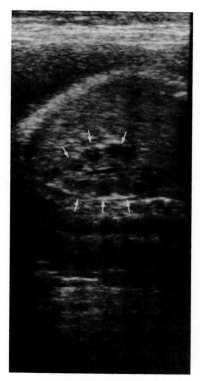

Figure 10–3. Sonogram of a fetal kidney *(arrows)*. The medullary pyramids are distinguished from surrounding cortical tissues and septa of Bertin. Bright echos surrounding the kidney represent perirenal fat.

A. Longitudinal Lie Cephalic Presentation

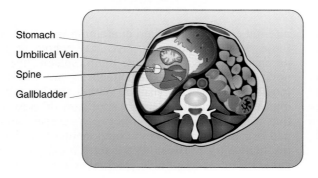

Stomach
Umbilical Vein
Spine
Gallbladder

B. Longitudinal Lie Breech Position

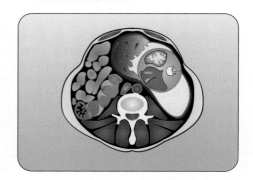

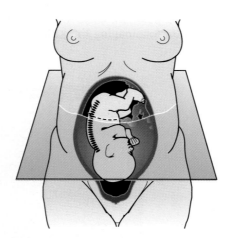

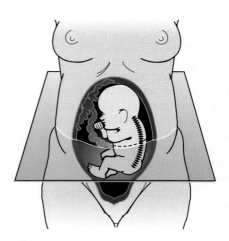

Figure 10–4. Knowledge of the plane of section across the maternal abdomen (longitudinal or transverse) as well as the position of the fetal spine and left-sided (stomach) and right-sided (gallbladder) structures can be used to determine fetal lie and presenting part. *A.* This transverse scan of the gravid uterus demonstrates the fetal spine on the maternal right with the fetus lying with its right side down (stomach anterior, gallbladder posterior). Since these images are viewed looking up from the patient's feet, the fetus must be in a longitudinal lie and in cephalic presentation. *B.* When the gravid uterus is scanned transversely and the fetal spine is on the maternal left, with the right side down, the fetus is in a longitudinal lie and in breech presentation.

C. Transverse Lie
Head, Maternal Left

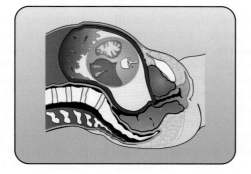

D. Transverse Lie
Head, Maternal Right

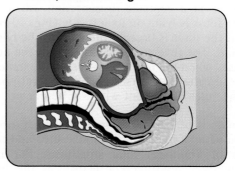

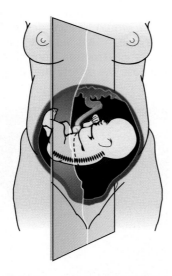

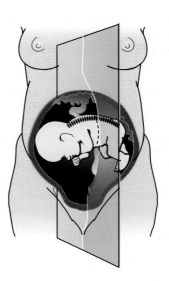

Figure 10–4 *Continued C.* When a longitudinal plane of section demonstrates the fetal body to be transected transversely and the fetal spine is nearest the lower uterine segment, with the fetal right side down, the fetus is in a transverse lie with the fetal head on the maternal left. *D.* When a longitudinal plane of section demonstrates the fetal body to be transected transversely and the fetal spine is nearest the uterine fundus with the fetal right side down, the fetus is in a transverse lie with the fetal head on the maternal right. Although real-time scanning of the gravid uterus quickly allows the observer to determine fetal lie and presentation, this maneuver of identifying specific right- and left-sided structures within the fetal body forces one to determine fetal position accurately and identify normal and pathologic fetal anatomy.

perceive, but in a poor position to demonstrate the urinary bladder, which is usually easy to image. Determination of fetal position should be accomplished in all obstetric sonographic examinations from the second trimester onward. The fetal position should be determined as precisely as possible before an interpretation of fetal anatomy is begun, because the position of a structure will often influence our interpretation. The general fetal orientation is first assessed, that is, cephalic, breech, oblique, or transverse. Once this is determined, the location of the fetal spine is noted. If, for example, the fetal spine is on the maternal left side and the fetus is in a cephalic presentation, one can judge that the fetus is lying on its left side (Fig. 10–4). Conversely, if the fetus is breech, then it must be lying on its right side. The reverse is the case for breech and cephalic fetuses when the fetal spine lies on the maternal right side. In the transverse or oblique fetal positions the same rules apply, but with a different orientation.

Such an analysis of fetal position is vital for proper interpretation of abdominal and thoracic situs and for identification of abnormal fetal structures. For instance, a rounded, fluid-filled structure in the left posterior portion of the upper fetal abdomen may be assumed to represent the fundus of the fetal stomach. However, a structure of identical appearance, but located on the right side of the upper fetal abdomen, must be interpreted as a pathologic lesion.

It is important to recall that pathologic structures are frequently more visible than their normal counterparts (i.e., dilated small bowel loops are easier to detect than normal small bowel loops). However, it is even more important to keep in mind that the most difficult pathologic observation is to recognize the "absence" of a structure that ordinarily could be visualized (i.e., a missing portion of an extremity, the inability to see the "stomach" when esophageal atresia without tracheoesophageal fistula is present).

SUPERFICIAL ANATOMY OF THE FETUS

Routine sonography for obstetric indications rarely requires a survey of superficial fetal structure. However, when an anomaly is suspected, a careful look at superficial features of the fetus becomes important or even mandatory. Superficial anatomy that will be considered in this section includes the face, ears, hair, and external genitalia.

The fetal face can be viewed with considerable clarity. Expectant mothers are often surprised to "see" their fetus so clearly (Figs. 10–5 and 10–6). The brow, cheeks, eyelids (and occasionally even eyelashes), nose, lips, and chin can be seen with consistency. The nose and lips are the more important to image in detail (to exclude clefting). The alae, column, and nares can be clearly depicted (Figs. 10–7 and 10–8). The upper lip is more important diagnostically than the lower lip and fortunately easier to see. Visualization is usually good enough to identify the philtrum. The cheeks are prominent, as expected, and the subcutaneous tissues

of the cheek, because of the presence of a large fat pad, are brightly echogenic.

The ears can be visualized quite well and their progressive maturation noted.[9] The external auditory canal, helix (and antihelix in older fetuses), lobule, and tragus can be depicted (Fig. 10–9), but the relative position of the ear (i.e., as in "low set" ears) is difficult to judge. The ear may be protuberant and can be mistaken for an abnormality, especially an encephalocele.[10]

Scalp hair is readily perceived in late fetuses (that have some). The bright linear echoes protruding from or paralleling the scalp and neck are quite conspicuous. Indeed, the only benefit of recognizing hair is not to be misled into mistaking long hair for a pathologic process, namely, an encephalocele or cystic hygroma, because longer hair, wet and matted by the amniotic fluid, may "trap" some of the fluid between it and the skin of the occiput or neck, creating the false impression of a cystic mass in this location (Fig. 10–10).

The external genitalia can be appreciated from early second trimester onward. Gender can be quite accurately assigned.[11–13] Ordinarily, this is not of clinical consequence. However, in certain circumstances gender should always be determined. These include all living twins where a single placental site is seen or when monozygotic twinning, other than for reasons of placentation, would be considered detrimental to pregnancy outcome.[14] All fetuses with suspected lower urinary tract obstruction should have gender determined, because the differential diagnosis is different in

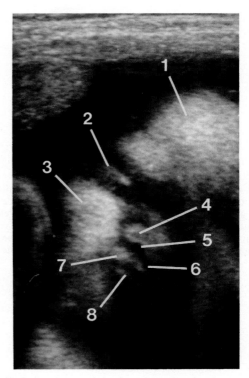

Figure 10–5. Sonogram of the fetal face. Despite the fact that this image is a tomogram with relatively little depth, facial features are seen well. Amniotic fluid surrounding the face provides the "contrast" for visualization. 1, brow; 2, eyelid; 3, cheek; 4, ala of nose; 5, nostril; 6, philtrum; 7, upper lip; 8, lower lip.

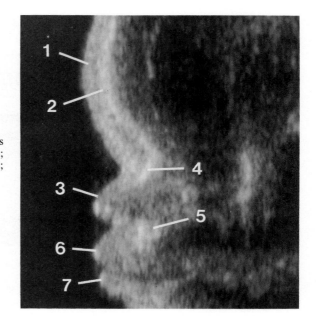

Figure 10–6. "Profile" view of the fetal face. Diagnostically this view offers substantially less information than that in Figure 10–5. 1, soft tissues of brow; 2, frontal bone; 3, soft tissues of nose; 4, nasal bone; 5, portion of hard palate; 6, upper lip; 7, lower lip.

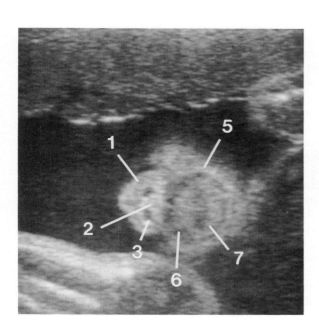

Figure 10–7. "Coronal" sonogram of the nose and mouth. Nasal structure is particularly well seen (1, ala; 2, nostril; 3, column). The mouth displays less detail, although consistent and characteristic layering of echoes is seen. These layers are (presumably) the subcutaneous (5) and muscular tissue (6), the orbicularis oris muscle, and (7) the mucosal tissue.

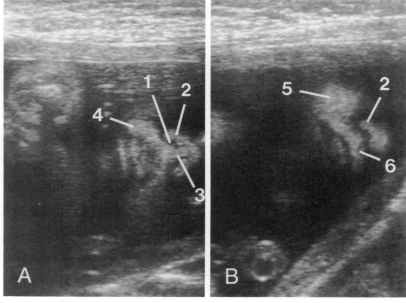

Figure 10–8. *A.* True coronal image of the nose and upper lip. 1, nostril; 2, column; 3, ala; 4, upper lip. *B.* Inclined coronal image demonstrates a slightly different perspective. 5, cheek; 6, philtrum.

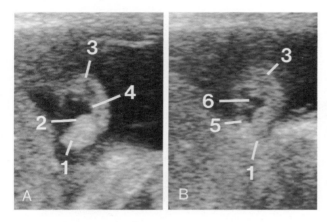

Figure 10–9. *A* and *B*. Fetal ear. 1, lobule; 2, antitragus; 3, helix; 4, antihelix; 5, tragus; 6, fossa triangularis.

males and females. Certain other circumstances would require gender determination if karyotyping were refused or impractical to perform. These would include, but are not limited to, risk for X-linked disorders or when the Turner syndrome is suspected due to a dysmorphic feature (e.g., cystic hygroma).

Female gender should be assigned only by identification of the major and minor labia (Fig. 10–11). Assigning female gender because of an inability to "see" a penis will result in many diagnostic errors. Male genitalia are readily seen (Fig. 10–12). The penis and scrotum are most obvious. Testes may be seen in the scrotal sac, sometimes as early as the beginning of the third trimester. Details of the penis, including the glans, urethra, and corpora cavernosa may be appreciated (Fig. 10–13). Even the foreskin is visible in some cases.

MUSCULOSKELETAL SYSTEM

Real-time ultrasonography provides the most appropriate format for imaging fetal bones. The resolution and flexibility offered by such systems enables one to rapidly survey the fetal skeleton. Of all structures within the fetus, the ossified portions of the skeleton possess the highest level of subject contrast and thus are seen earlier and more consistently than any other organ system.[4, 15–18] Indeed, sonography surpasses all other imaging modalities in fetal skeletal imaging. Although radiographs of abortuses demonstrate bony morphology more advantageously than would a sonogram,[19, 20] the reverse is true of fetuses in the womb where overlying maternal soft tissues and bones, fetal movement, and inappropriate fetal position defeat radiographic techniques in visualization of the early fetal skeleton.

Fetal position is extremely important. The posterior elements of the fetal spine may be clearly imaged with the fetus in a prone or decubitus position but are difficult to image when the fetus is supine.[21] Similarly, the extremities are imaged to excellent advantage when floating freely in the amniotic fluid. The same extremity tucked under the fetus will be quite difficult to image.

Despite these potential problems, fetal skeletal structures remain the earliest and most readily recog-

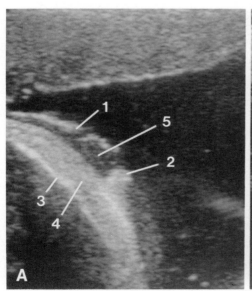
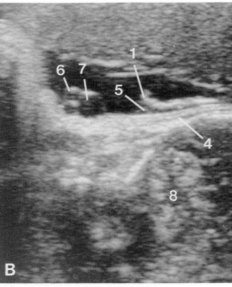

Figure 10–10. *A*. Hair (1) may be mistaken for the outer membrane of a cystic mass in an older fetus. 2, portion of ear; 3, occipital bone; 4, subcutaneous tissues and muscles in the occipital region; 5, "trapped" amniotic fluid. *B*. Scan at 90° to *A*. This image clarifies that the fetus is normal. 6, umbilical artery; 7, umbilical vein; 8, cerebellum.

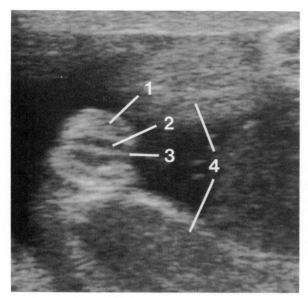

Figure 10–11. External female genitalia. 1, major labium; 2, minor labium; 3, vaginal cleft; 4, thighs.

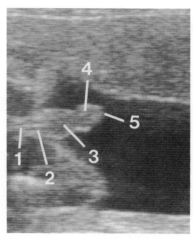

Figure 10–13. Details in an erect fetal penis. 1, urethra; 2, corpus cavernosum; 3, shaft; 4, glans; 5, foreskin.

nized. Indeed, the earliest structures seen with consistency are the ossification centers of the maxilla, mandible, and clavicle; the first bones of the human body to ossify.[4] The calvarium can be imaged from the late first trimester onward. The same is true of the long bones of the upper and lower extremity (Fig. 10–14). Visibility of bony detail rapidly increases and by 17 to 18 menstrual weeks (sometimes earlier) even phalanges can be visualized. Bones of only 2 to 3 mm in size can be consistently imaged by sonography provided that no unusual impediments to the scanning procedure exist (Fig. 10–15). Many specific bony structures can be depicted. Bones in both the appendicular and axial skeleton are well imaged.

It is important to clarify that sonography has the capacity to visualize not only the ossified portions of the fetal skeleton but also the cartilaginous portions.[4] Cartilaginous ends of the long bones may be seen by the early second trimester. Indeed, bones entirely in cartilage can be seen sonographically (Fig. 10–16). It is equally important to recognize that the full thickness of the ossified diaphysis of long bones is not seen sonographically.[22] This is due to acoustic shadowing. The cartilaginous ends of long bones help us to recognize this aberration. By matching up the width of the epiphysis, the full thickness of which can be seen, with the apparent "width" of the bony diaphysis, it is clear that these are unequal (Figs. 10–17 and 10–18). This observation helps to correct some perceptual errors that can lead to erroneous diagnoses. For example, the inability to see the full thickness of the

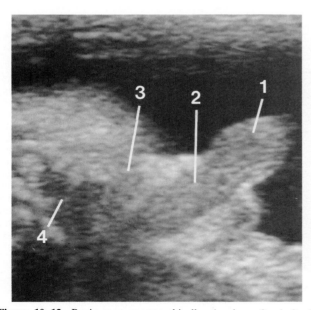

Figure 10–12. Penis seen sonographically. 1, glans; 2, shaft; 3, subcutaneous tissues of the groin; 4, pubic ramus.

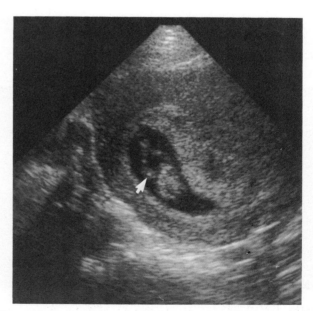

Figure 10–14. Sonogram of a 10.5-week embryo demonstrates the tiny (approximately 1 mm) primary ossification center of the femur *(arrow)*. (From Mahony BS, Filly RA: High-resolution sonographic assessment of the fetal extremities. J Ultrasound Med 3:489, 1984.)

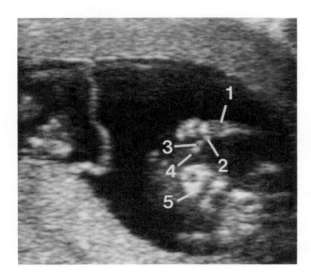

Figure 10–15. Sonogram of a 15-week fetal hand. 1, cartilaginous carpal bones seen as a conglomerate; 2, first metacarpal; 3, proximal phalanx of thumb; 4, distal phalanx of thumb; 5, maxilla.

Figure 10–16. Midsagittal sonogram through the leg of a fetus with a bone dysplasia. Note the bowed tibial diaphysis (1). The patella (2), an entirely cartilaginous bone, is clearly depicted. 3, proximal tibial epiphysis; 4, distal femoral epiphysis; 5, femoral diaphysis.

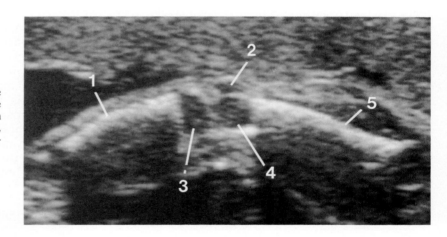

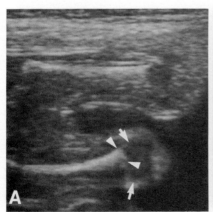
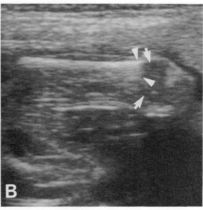

Figure 10–17. *A.* Sonogram best demonstrating the femur farther from the transducer. Arrows mark the edges of the distal epiphysis. Arrowheads mark the apparent "edges" of the distal femoral diaphysis. The more medial edge of the diaphysis matches the edge of the medial condyle, but the lateral edges of "diaphysis" and lateral condyle are widely disparate. *B.* The same exercise can be performed on the nearer femur. Again, arrows mark the edges of the distal epiphysis and arrowheads mark the "edges" of the femoral diaphysis. Shadowing, caused by the bone but not the cartilage, causes this deceptive appearance.

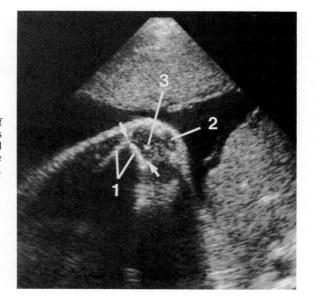

Figure 10–18. Sector sonogram of the distal femur taken such that the lines of sight from the transducer intersect the inferior end of the femoral metaphysis at the epiphyseal plate (1). By this maneuver, the full thickness of the distal ossified femur is seen sonographically (compare with Fig. 10–17). Now, the thickness of the epiphysis *(arrows)* and ossified femoral shaft match perfectly. 2, patella; 3, secondary ossification center of the distal femoral epiphysis.

femoral diaphysis creates the impression that the fetal femur farther from the transducer is bowed (Fig. 10–19).[22] This error is caused by visualization of only the medial cortex of the femoral diaphysis (which is normally curved) (Fig. 10–20). However, the inability to "visually correct" this normal curvature by simultaneous observation of the "straight" lateral cortex causes the perceptual error.

The majority of the bones of the appendicular skeleton can be seen in early to mid second trimester, although phalanges may be difficult to perceive in some instances. It is a general rule of appendicular skeletal imaging that the more proximal a bone, the more readily it is identified. This rule in one sense is untrue of the hands and feet, where the metacarpals and metatarsals are seen more readily and earlier than either the carpal or tarsal bones (see Figs. 10–15 and 10–21). This is because the metacarpals and metatarsals are well ossified at 4 months, while the carpals and tarsals (except for the tarsal calcaneus and talus) remain cartilaginous throughout pregnancy. The tarsal

calcaneus and talus ossify between the fifth and sixth months, while the remaining tarsals and carpals do not ossify until after birth (Figs. 10–22 and 10–23).

The scapula (Figs. 10–24 and 10–25), clavicle, humerus (see Figs. 10–24 and 10–26), radius (Figs. 10–26 and 10–27), ulna (see Figs. 10–26 and 10–27), metacarpals (see Figs. 10–15 and 10–27), and phalanges (see Fig. 10–15) can be imaged in most cases. Interestingly, the clavicle may be difficult to see, presumably because of the flexed position of the fetal neck, which draws the calvarium into a position that obscures the clavicle. Nonetheless, if one desires to see the clavicle, this can nearly always be accomplished. Indeed, measurements exist for normal clavicular length at various gestational ages.[23] Similarly, the femur (Figs. 10–28 through 10–31), tibia (Fig. 10–32), fibula (see Fig. 10–32), metatarsals (see Figs. 10–21 through 10–23), and phalanges (see Figs. 10–21 through 10–23) of the lower extremity can be appreciated well sonographically. The figures demonstrating the hip joint, femur, and knee (see Figs. 10–28 through

Text continued on page 158

Figure 10–19. *A.* The diaphysis of the femur nearer to the transducer appears straight *(arrows).* The full thickness of the diaphysis is not seen. (Match the edges of the epiphysis *[arrowheads]* as in Figures 10–17 and 10–18 and to the radiograph in Figure 10–20.) *B.* The diaphysis of the femur farther from the transducer appears curved *(arrows).* Compare with Figure 10–20. This is a normal shape of this aspect of the bone. However, the curvature is visually compensated by the straight lateral cortex in the radiograph but not the sonogram because the full thickness of bone is not perceived (compare again the diaphyseal "thickness" to the epiphyseal thickness *[arrowheads]*).

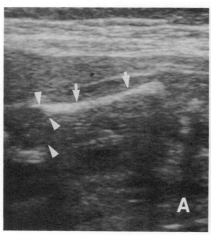
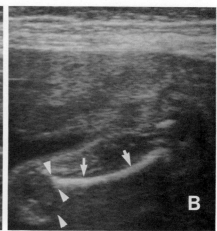

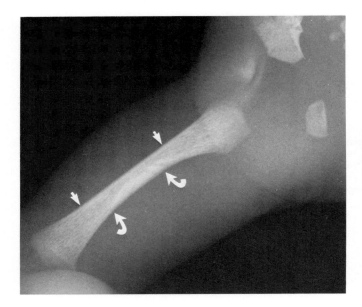

Figure 10–20. Radiograph of a mid-trimester fetal femur. Note that our eye compensates for the curvature of the medial diaphyseal cortex *(curved arrows)* by noting the straight lateral diaphyseal cortex *(straight arrows)*. Compare with Figure 10–19.

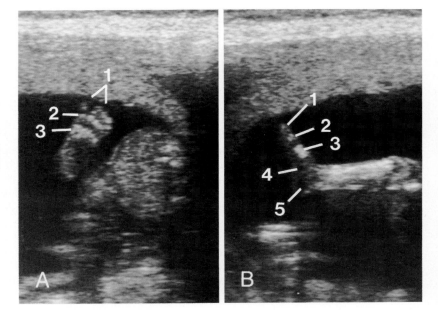

Figure 10–21. Fetal foot at 16 weeks' gestation in transverse axial *(A)* and parasagittal *(B)* planes. 1, toes; 2, proximal phalangeal ossification centers; 3, metatarsal ossification centers; 4, tarsal cuboid in cartilage; 5, tarsal calcaneus in cartilage.

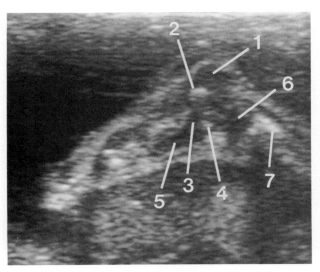

Figure 10–22. Midsagittal sonogram of the fetal foot in late mid trimester. 1, cartilagineous calcaneus; 2, primary ossification center of calcaneus; 3, cartilagineous talus; 4, primary ossification center of talus; 5, tarsal navicular in cartilage; 6, distal tibial epiphysis; 7, distal tibial diaphysis.

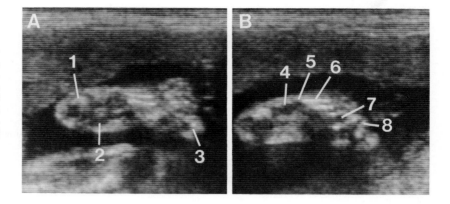

Figure 10–23. *A* and *B*. Transverse axial sonograms of the fetal foot, late second trimester. 1, calcaneus both ossified and nonossified; 2, talus, both ossified and nonossified; 3, great toe; 4, tarsal cuboid in cartilage; 5, proximal epiphysis of fifth metatarsal; 6, ossified diaphysis of fifth metatarsal; 7, distal epiphysis of second metatarsal; 8, ossification center of distal phalanx of second toe.

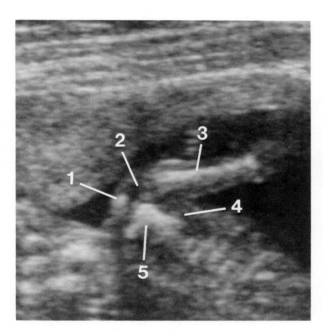

Figure 10–24. Coronal sonogram of the shoulder and upper arm. 1, distal clavicle; 2, cartilaginous humeral head; 3, ossified humeral diaphysis; 4, latissimus dorsi muscle; 5, scapula.

Figure 10–25. *A* and *B*. Parasagittal sonograms of the scapula. 1, infraspinous fossa; 2, infraspinatus muscle; 3, scapular spine; 4, supraspinatus muscle; 5, supraspinous fossa; 6, subscapularis muscle; 7, ribs in short axis.

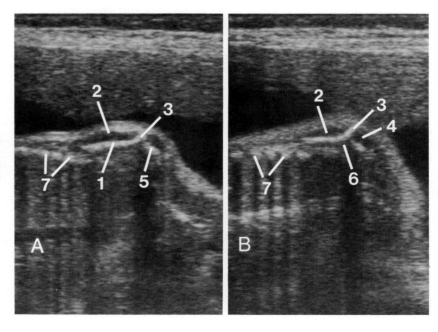

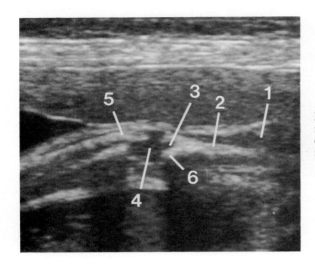

Figure 10–26. Fetal elbow, hand pronated, coronal sonogram. 1, triceps muscle; 2, ossified humeral diaphysis; 3, cartilaginous olecranon fossa; 4, conglomerate cartilages about the elbow joint; 5, proximal ulnar diaphysis; 6, medial humeral epicondyle.

Figure 10–27. *A* and *B*. Coronal sonograms of the forearm and wrist. 1, ulnar diaphysis; 2, olecranon in cartilage; 3, radial diaphysis; 4, distal ulnar epiphysis; 5, fifth metacarpal diaphysis; 6, distal third metacarpal epiphysis; 7, phalangeal ossification centers; 8, carpal arch seen as a conglomerate cartilage.

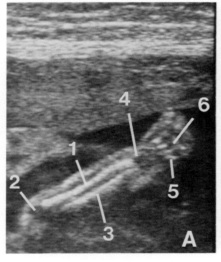
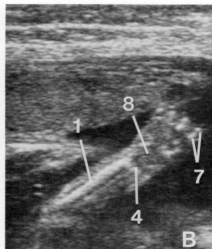

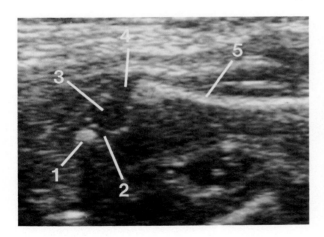

Figure 10–28. Coronal image of the fetal hip. 1, ischial ossification center; 2, cartilaginous acetabulum; 3, femoral head in cartilage; 4, greater trochanter in cartilage; 5, femoral diaphysis.

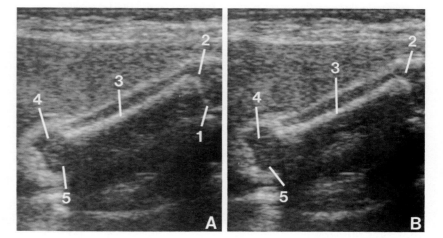

Figure 10–29. *A* and *B.* Longitudinal coronal sonograms of thigh. 1, posterior hip joint capsule; 2, greater trochanter; 3, femoral diaphysis; 4, lateral condyle; 5, medial condyle.

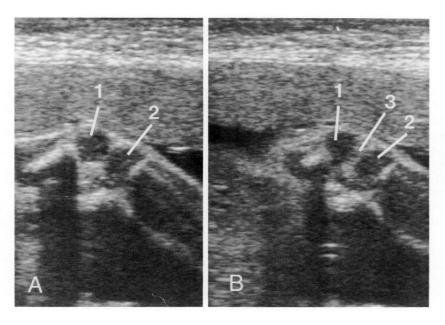

Figure 10–30. *A.* Parasagittal sonogram of the fetal knee. The femoral condyle (1) articulates with the tibial plateau (proximal tibial epiphysis [2]). *B.* Midsagittal sonogram of the fetal knee. Note the gap (3) between the distal femoral epiphysis (1) and the proximal tibial epiphysis (2). This is due to the intercondylar notch (see Fig. 10–31).

Figure 10–31. Transverse axial sonogram through the distal epiphysis of the femur (cartilaginous). 1, lateral condyle; 2, patellar groove; 3, medial condyle; 4, intercondylar notch.

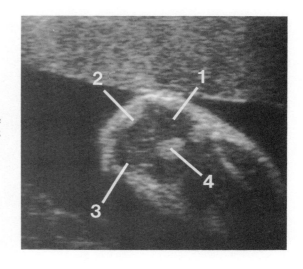

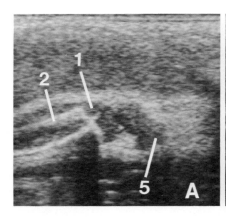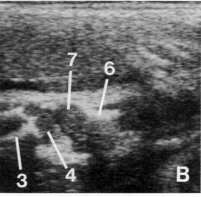

Figure 10–32. *A* and *B*. Coronal sonograms of the knee (off axis). 1, proximal fibular epiphysis; 2, fibular diaphysis; 3, tibial diaphysis; 4, proximal tibial epiphysis; 5, patella; 6, femoral metaphysis; 7, lateral femoral condyle.

10–30) may be reviewed to appreciate the remarkably detailed anatomy that can be achieved with high-resolution sonography.

The simplest way to identify the types of long bones of the extremity viewed on the sonogram is to obtain planes of section that traverse the short axis of the limb. Sonograms obtained in such a plane through the forearm and calf will demonstrate two bones. In the lower leg, the more lateral bone is the fibula, and the medial bone is the tibia (see Fig. 10–32). This method works as well in the forearm but is less precise because pronation may cause the radius and ulna to "cross." In the normal fetus, the tibia and fibula and radius and ulna end at the same level distally (see Fig. 10–27). Proximally, of course, the ulna is longer than the radius (see Fig. 10–26). This allows both ready differentiation of these two bony sets and of the radius from the ulna in the upper extremity set. That both paired long bones of the upper and lower extremity end at the same level distally is important in assessing possible limb reduction abnormalities.

The hand can be assessed more critically than the foot.[24–26] With patience one can usually discern all four fingers and the thumb. The hand is frequently clenched in a fistlike fashion, which can complicate the counting of fingers. However, even under this circumstance one

can frequently make the necessary observations. The toes, although smaller than the fingers, can be seen relatively well with modern equipment (see Fig. 10–21). If difficulty arises, it is usually the functionally less important fourth and fifth toes that are not seen.

It is possible in the late third-trimester fetus to identify the distal femoral (see Figs. 10–18 and 10–33) and proximal tibial (Fig. 10–33) epiphyseal ossification centers.[27, 28] Ossification of these epiphyses, as seen on radiographs, is known to be an indicator of fetal maturity. Identification of the epiphyseal ossification centers about the knee provides a different type of parameter that sonologists can use in the assessment of gestational age in the third trimester of pregnancy. One can obtain a high sensitivity, specificity, and accuracy of a positive prediction if one employs a 33-week cutoff point for the appearance of the distal femoral epiphysis (Figs. 10–34 through 10–36). Similarly, the same data suggest a threshold for the appearance of the proximal tibial epiphysis at 35 weeks. Statistical analysis of this threshold demonstrates that only a positive identification of the proximal tibial epiphysis appears to be clinically useful. A relatively large number of fetuses of greater than 35 menstrual weeks do not possess an identifiable proximal tibial epiphysis. These ossification centers appear earlier, on

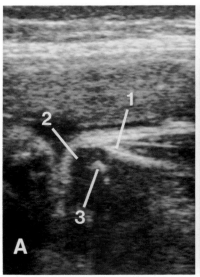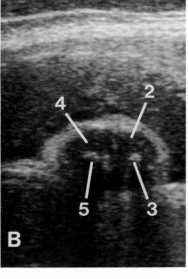

Figure 10–33. *A*. Coronal sonogram of the distal thigh in a term fetus. 1, femoral metaphysis; 2, lateral condyle; 3, ossification center of distal femoral epiphysis. *B*. Axial sonogram through the knee. Note the large and similar sizes of the ossification centers, a virtually certain sign of a near-term fetus. 4, proximal tibial epiphysis; 5, ossification center of the proximal tibial epiphysis.

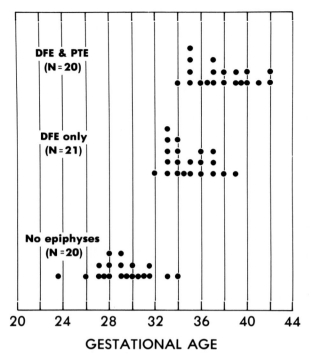

Figure 10–34. Appearance time of the distal femoral epiphysis (DFE) and proximal tibial epiphysis (PTE) in a mixed group of 61 fetuses when two of the following three dating parameters agreed: last menstrual period, early sonogram, Dubowitz scores. (From Chinn DH, Bolding DB, Callen PW, et al: Ultrasonographic identification of fetal lower extremity epiphyseal ossification centers. Radiology 147:815–818, 1983.)

ing length, this shortcoming is often compensated for by assuming the "longest" measurement obtained in several attempts to be the most accurate, an assumption that can lead to serious overestimates, as will shortly be discussed. However, if both cartilaginous ends of the desired bone to be measured are seen, this guarantees that the plane of section has passed through the longest axis of the bone (Fig. 10–37). The only remaining task to minimize error is to accurately position measurement cursors at the ends of the bone.

Another common misconception in measurement of the femur is that no other tissue in proximity to the bony termination will yield an echo of equal brightness to the bone. Thus, one "should always place measurement cursors" from the edge of the distal brightest reflection to the edge of the proximal brightest reflection. This long-standing belief is unfortunately erroneous especially in older fetuses, although younger fetuses are not exempt from this potentially significant error in femur length estimation.[29] Figure 10–38 demonstrates that a nonosseous, but nonetheless equally bright, reflection is returned from tissues distal to the epiphyseal plate but in immediate contiguity with the distal femoral metaphysis. This is called the "distal

average, in female fetuses (see Fig. 10–35).[28] The size of the distal femoral ossification center correlates with late gestational age (see Fig. 10–36).[28]

As stated earlier, many "bones" of the fetal appendicular skeleton are entirely cartilaginous. Some of these still can be imaged sonographically. Indeed, the patella can be seen rather commonly (see Figs. 10–16 and 10–18). This bone does not begin to ossify until after birth. All of the carpal and most of the tarsal bones are entirely cartilaginous (see Figs. 10–15, 10–21 through 10–23, and 10–27). The carpals cannot be seen discretely. Rather they are perceived as a conglomerate hypoechoic band spanning the gap from the distal radius and ulna to the proximal metacarpal ossification centers (see Fig. 10–27). Of course, this "gap" also includes the cartilaginous epiphyses of the long bones, as well. Conversely, some of the tarsal bones can be discretely identified from time to time (see Figs. 10–21 through 10–23). These include, most notably, the early tarsal calcaneus and talus (before 24 weeks) and the tarsal navicular and cuboid throughout gestation.

Visualization of the cartilaginous ends of the long bones assists in their measurement in two ways. The measurement of fetal long bones is confined to the ossified portion. A potential error is to foreshorten the bone by failing to obtain the plane of section through the true long axis of the bone. To avoid underestimat-

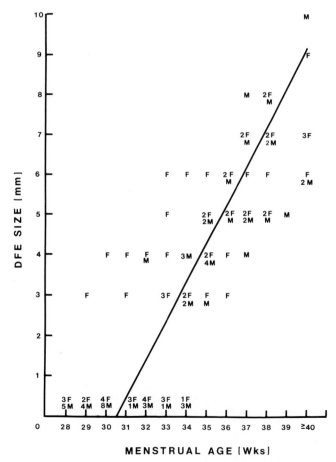

Figure 10–35. Variation in the distal femoral epiphysis (DFE) appearance time and size in male and female fetuses. (From Mahony SB, Callen PW, Filly RA: The distal femoral epiphyseal ossification center in the assessment of third trimester menstrual age: Sonographic identification and measurement. Radiology 155:201–204, 1985.)

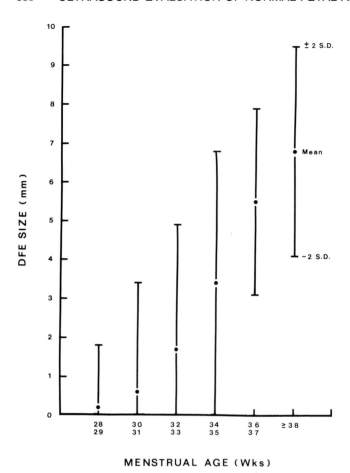

Figure 10–36. Mean diameter of the distal femoral epiphysis (DFE) with increasing age. (From Mahony SB, Callen PW, Filly RA: The distal femoral epiphyseal ossification center in the assessment of third trimester menstrual age: Sonographic identification and measurement. Radiology 155:201–204, 1985.)

femoral point" for lack of a more precise anatomic term.[29] That this "point" is not part of the ossified femur can be determined by noting its relationship to the cartilaginous lateral condyle. The femoral metaphysis ends at the beginning of the distal femoral epiphysis and does not overlap the edge of the epiphysis. Compare the radiograph of the fetal femur in Figure

10–20 with the sonogram of the fetal femur in Figure 10–38. No such *ossified* femoral point exists.

Sonography, from time to time, demonstrates rather extraordinary features of the musculoskeletal system of the extremities. At present, no known diagnostic usefulness for this information has been established nor is it possible to demonstrate such structures with the consistency necessary to employ their visualization in diagnostic pursuits. However, several of these remarkable features are demonstrated in Figures 10–39 through 10–41.

Many bones or components of bones of the axial skeleton are also routinely visualized. In the skull region one can perceive a number of bones individually or as a conglomerate. The greater wing of the sphenoid and petrous ridge are easily identified and define the anterior, middle, and posterior cranial fossae (Fig. 10–42). The orbits can be visualized without difficulty unless the more anteriorly positioned orbit severely shadows the more posteriorly positioned orbit (Fig. 10–43). Standards have been established for fetal interorbital distances to evaluate hypotelorism and hypertelorism.[30] In older fetuses, surprising detail of the intraorbital contents can be appreciated including the wall of the globe, lens, retrobulbar fat, optic nerve, and rectus muscles (Fig. 10–44). Portions of the maxilla and nearly all of the mandible can be identified, as well as the bony nasal ridge (see Fig. 10–43). Similarly, the frontal, parietal, and squama of the temporal and occipital bones, the bones making up the calvarium, can be seen clearly. The cartilaginous zones of articulation of these bones, the coronal, sagittal, and lambdoid sutures, are commonly visible (Fig. 10–45). The fontanelles may be seen as well (Fig. 10–46) and occasionally used as windows for brain imaging (Fig. 10–47).

The ribs, spine, and pelvis are easily imaged and serve as excellent anatomic landmarks. In the pelvis, the iliac ossification centers are easily observed from early second trimester onward (ossified at 2.5 to 3 fetal months). Ischial ossification (see Fig. 10–28) is present at 4 months, but pubic ossification is not present until 6 months.

The spine is an extremely important structure in

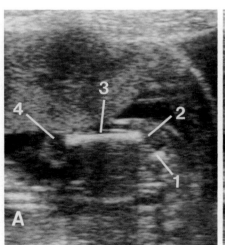
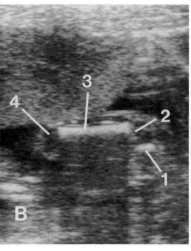

Figure 10–37. *A* and *B*. Two views of the femur for measurement. Visualization of the proximal (2) and distal (4) cartilaginous bone ensures that the plane of section is through the long axis of the diaphysis (3). Only proper positioning of the cursors remains to ensure an accurate measurement. 1, ischial ossification center.

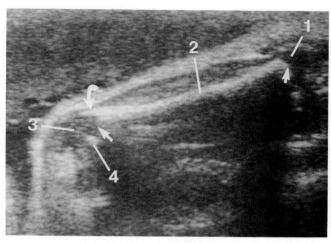

Figure 10–38. View of the fetal femur, third trimester. A bright reflector *(curved arrow)* is seen in continuity with the lateral femoral metaphysis. This structure is not part of the ossified femur. Endpoints of femur measurement are marked by straight arrows. 1, greater trochanter; 2, femoral diaphysis; 3, lateral condyle; 4, ossification center of the distal epiphysis.

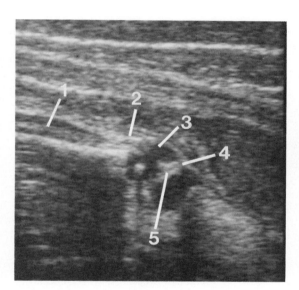

Figure 10–39. Midsagittal sonogram of the extended knee. In addition to structures pointed out in earlier figures, note the quadriceps muscle (1), the quadriceps tendon (2), the patella (3), the patella ligament (4), and synovium (5) contained by the knee joint.

Figure 10–40. Midsagittal sonogram of the fetal knee in flexion. The distal femoral epiphysis (1), patella, patella ligament (2), and proximal tibial epiphysis (3) define the knee joint boundaries. Within the knee joint is a large quantity of highly echogenic tissue, presumably synovium. Clearly outlined by the bright "synovium" is the cruciate ligament (4).

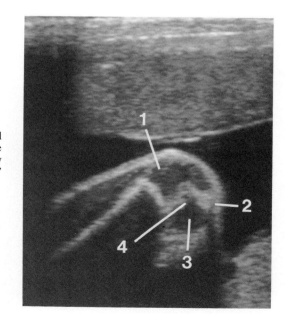

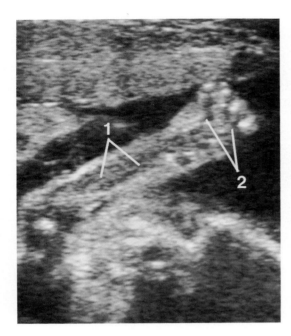

Figure 10–41. Coronal sonogram through the dorsal soft tissues of the forearm and hand. 1, extensor muscle group; 2, extensor tendons.

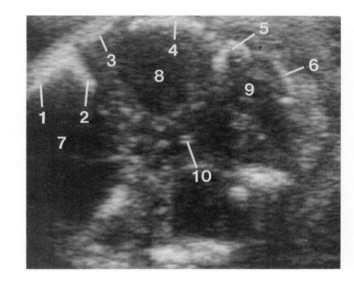

Figure 10–42. Transverse axial sonogram near the skull base. 1, frontal bone; 2, greater wing of sphenoid bone; 3, parietal bone; 4, temporal bone; 5, petrous ridge; 6, occipital bone; 7, anterior cranial fossa; 8, middle cranial fossa; 9, posterior cranial fossa; 10, basilar artery.

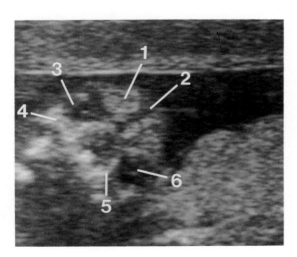

Figure 10–43. Fetal orbits, early second trimester. 1, frontal bone; 2, metopic suture; 3, orbit; 4, maxilla; 5, nasal bone; 6, lens.

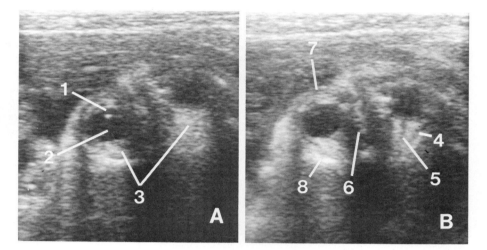

Figure 10–44. *A* and *B*. Orbits and contents. 1, lens; 2, globe; 3, retrobulbar fat; 5, optic nerve; 6, lateral rectus muscle; 7, eyelid; 8, lateral orbit wall.

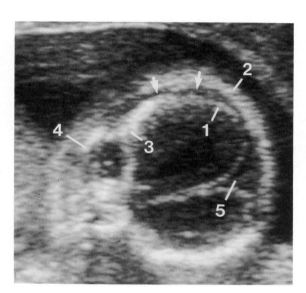

Figure 10–45. Oblique view demonstrating the coronal suture *(arrows)*. 1, frontal bone; 2, parietal bone; 3, greater wing of sphenoid bone; 4, maxilla; 5, interhemispheric fissure with brain edges showing brightly reflective covering of pia-arachnoid.

Figure 10–46. Transverse axial sonogram of the posterior fontanelle (1). 2, lambdoid suture; 3, sagittal suture; 4, parietal bone; 5, occipital bone.

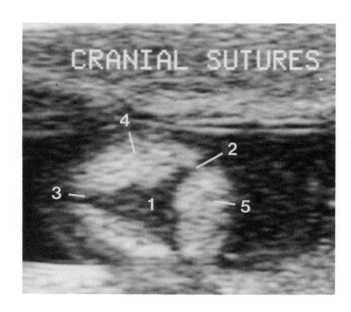

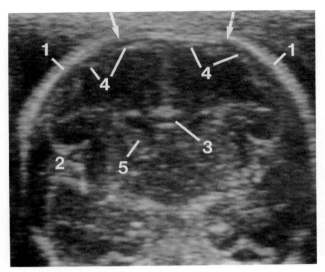

Figure 10–47. The sonographic beam was directed through the anterior fontanelle *(arrows)* in a mid-trimester fetus enabling recognition of striking detail in the fetal brain due to the "bone free window" 1, parietal bone; 2, lateral fissure; 3, corpus callosum; 4, brain edges over the most cephalic portions of the parietal lobes; 5, head of caudate nucleus.

fetal diagnosis.[21, 31–33] With the advent of maternal serum α-fetoprotein screening, as well as the concurrent development of sophisticated high-resolution ultrasound imaging technology, the potential exists to diagnose nearly all lesions of spina bifida before the 20th week of pregnancy.[34] These changes in obstetric care mandate that the morphology of the fetal spine be well understood by sonologists. The sequence of development of ossification centers in the fetal vertebral column has been extensively studied in the past with radiologic and histologic methods.[19, 20] Each vertebra usually has three primary ossification centers, one for the body (centrum) and one on each side of the posterior neural arch. The centra are ossified first in the lower thoracic and upper lumbar regions followed by progressive ossification in both the cephalic and caudal directions. By contrast and in general, the ossification centers for the posterior neural arch appear in a more standard cephalocaudal direction. The posterior neural arch first begins to ossify (sonographically recognizable high amplitude reflections) at the base of the transverse process (Fig. 10–48). Ossification proceeds from this center to progressively include the laminae and pedicles. The progression of ossification of the laminae is the more important for the diagnosis of neural tube defects, because spina bifida is the most consistently demonstrable dysmorphic lesion in open spinal defects. This abnormality is recognized sonographically by an abnormal outward flaring of the posterior neural arch ossification centers.

Varying degrees of maturation of spinal ossification are present at differing levels of the spine when we are most frequently called on to assess normalcy of the fetal spine.[21] Although there are some exceptions as noted previously, ossification in the neural arch first appears at the base of the transverse process. Early posterior neural arch ossification then progresses anteriorly into the pedicles, also contributing a portion of the vertebral body, and posteriorly into the laminae. Additionally, craniocaudal extension into the articular processes and lateral extension into the transverse process occurs. Because the critical observation in the diagnosis of open spinal neural tube defects is the demonstration of spina bifida (seen as an outward flaring of the posterior arch ossification centers), the ideal situation to confirm normalcy would be to observe the antithesis of this pathologic state (i.e., inward angulation of the laminae). This indeed is the case when visible ossification is present in the normal laminae (Fig. 10–49). Unfortunately, there is insufficient ossification of the laminae to perceive inward angulation of the posterior neural arch ossification centers in the lower spine to confirm normalcy of the fetal spine during the crucial stage of gestation when this sonographic diagnosis must be made (18 to 22 menstrual weeks) (see Fig. 10–48).[31, 34] This is particularly impor-

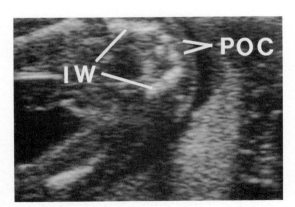

Figure 10–48. Early ossification centers in the sacral spine. Anteriorly is the centrum, and posteriorly (POC) the ossifications of the posterior arch appear near the base of the transverse processes. IW, iliac wings. (From Filly RA, Simpson GF, Linkowski G: Fetal spine morphology and maturation during the second trimester: Sonographic evaluation. J Ultrasound Med 6:631, 1987.)

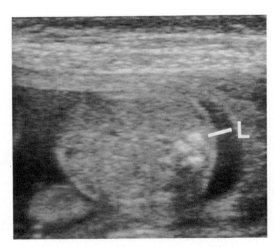

Figure 10–49. Lumbar vertebra, transverse axial sonogram. The laminae (L) demonstrate early ossification causing the appearance of "inward angulation" of the posterior arch. (From Filly RA, Simpson GF, Linkowski G: Fetal spine morphology and maturation during the second trimester: Sonographic evaluation. J Ultrasound Med 6:631, 1987.)

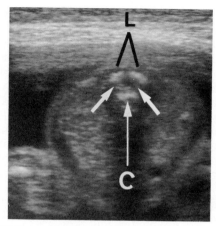

Figure 10–50. Lumbar spine, transverse axial sonogram, 23 weeks. Well-defined ossification of the laminae (L). C, centrum; arrows, neurocentral synchondroses. (From Filly RA, Simpson GF, Linkowski G: Fetal spine morphology and maturation during the second trimester: Sonographic evaluation. J Ultrasound Med 6:631, 1987.)

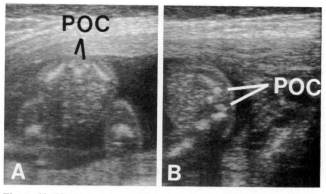

Figure 10–52. Transverse axial sonograms, sacral spine, same fetus in prone (A) and decubitus (B) positions. The posterior arch (POC) anatomy is seen well in either position. (From Filly RA, Simpson GF, Linkowski G: Fetal spine morphology and maturation during the second trimester: Sonographic evaluation. J Ultrasound Med 6:631, 1987.)

tant when considering the most common location of such lesions (i.e., lumbar and sacral regions).[31] Easily identifiable ossification of the laminae is visible in the cervical region in all fetuses by 18 to 19 menstrual weeks, while thoracic ossification of the laminae is only partially visible during the 18- to 19-menstrual week period.[21] There is no ossification of the laminae in the lumbar or sacral regions of fetuses examined before 19 menstrual weeks (see Fig. 10–48). The thoracic vertebrae consistently demonstrate partial ossification of the laminae in the range of 20 to 22 weeks, while the lumbar region does not demonstrate a similar degree of ossification until 22 to 24 weeks (Fig. 10–50). The sacral spine reveals no evidence of ossification in the laminae before 22 weeks. Only after 25 weeks is there consistently recognizable ossification of the arch in the sacral region (Fig. 10–51). Fetal position (either prone or decubitus) does not appear to affect appreciably the ability to discern the degree of neural arch ossification, although the prone position usually results in the clearest images (Fig. 10–52). If the fetus is supine, a

critical examination of the posterior neural arch cannot be carried out (Fig. 10–53).[21]

The spine may be seen in both longitudinal and transverse axial planes. Although both planes are important, the transverse axial plane demonstrates the anatomy to best advantage. On longitudinal planes of section the posterior elements are seen as "parallel" bands of echoes. In fact, they are not precisely parallel because they flair in the upper cervical region and converge in the sacrum and, in addition, careful scanning usually discloses a slight widening of the lumbar area. It is important not to mistake this slight lumbar widening as a pathologic event. Because the fetal spine is normally kyphotic, usually one cannot visualize the entire spine in a single longitudinal coronal plane. It is for this reason that transverse axial planes of section are necessary to be certain that the entire spine has been imaged on a segment-by-segment basis. Caution

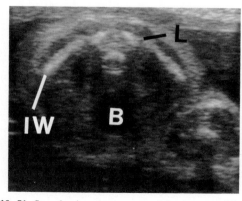

Figure 10–51. Sacral spine, transverse axial sonogram, 26 weeks. L, laminae; IW, iliac wing; B, bladder. (From Filly RA, Simpson GF, Linkowski G: Fetal spine morphology and maturation during the second trimester: Sonographic evaluation. J Ultrasound Med 6:631, 1987.)

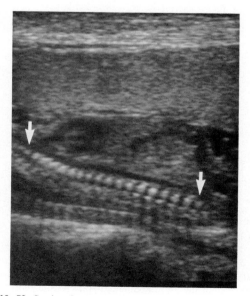

Figure 10–53. Supine fetus, second trimester. The vertebral bodies, lying between the arrows, are clearly seen but the posterior arch cannot be well appreciated.

must be exercised as well to ensure that the spine has been examined in its entirety on transverse planes. At the cephalic end, no problem arises because one encounters the calvarium. However, the caudal end is more difficult. One can successfully employ the ischial ossification centers as landmarks to ensure that the caudal end of the spine has been reached. In older fetuses, both spinal and spinal canal anatomy can often be quite dramatically depicted (Fig. 10–54).

Cartilaginous structure in the axial skeleton is less conspicuous than in the appendicular skeleton but nonetheless is visible in virtually all fetuses. The sutures of the calvarial vault already have been noted. The cartilaginous neurocentral synchondrosis of the spine (the junction of the centrum and the posterior ossification centers) is visible in all fetuses from the end of the first trimester onward (Figs. 10–48 through 10–52).[21] Similarly, the gaps between the vertebral body ossification centers are a composite of the unossified margin of the adjoining vertebral bodies plus the intervertebral disk (Fig. 10–53). The margin of cartilage in the vertebral body is best appreciated posteriorly, lying between the ossification center and the dura of the spinal canal (see the section on the central nervous system) (see Fig. 10–54C and D). As well, the spinous processes of the posterior neural arch are

occasionally seen, these structures again being entirely composed of cartilage in fetal life (see Fig. 10–54C).

One feature that cannot be well judged on sonograms is the degree of ossification of the bones. Thus, increased ossification, as in osteopetrosis, goes completely unrecognized on sonograms. Similarly, diminished ossification is poorly judged. Only in the most extremely osteopenic bone can one appreciate diminished ossification on sonograms. Examples would be the nearly nonossified calvarium in fetuses with recessive osteogenesis imperfecta or recessive hypophosphatasia[35–37] or the spine in fetuses with achondrogenesis.[38]

Little space will be devoted to the fetal muscular system even though many muscles and muscle groups may be seen quite well (see Figs. 10–24 and 10–25). In general, normal muscles are quite hypoechoic, at times so much so that they simulate fluid collections. This is most notable of the abdominal wall musculature, which may simulate ascites (pseudoascites) (Fig. 10–55).[39] Currently, high-resolution sonographic equipment decreases the propensity to "overcall" ascites caused by this artifactual situation because the layers of the abdominal wall can be seen quite clearly.[40]

The abdominal wall muscles, the internal and external oblique and the transversus abdominis, are, at

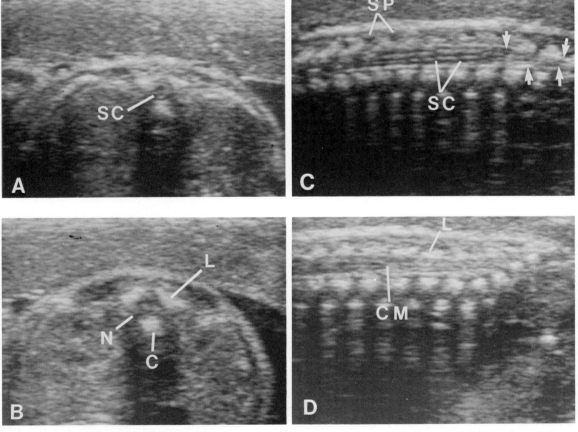

Figure 10–54. *A* and *B.* Lumbar spine of 27-week fetus, axial sections. L, 0 + 2 laminae; SC, spinal cord; C, centrum; N, neurocentral synchondrosis. *C* and *D.* Longitudinal scans of the thoracolumbar *(C)* and lumbosacral *(D)* spine. SP, spinous process (in cartilage); L, laminae; SC, spinal cord—note bright linear echo from central canal; CM, conus medullaris; arrows, dura. (From Filly RA, Simpson GF, Linkowski G: Fetal spine morphology and maturation during the second trimester: Sonographic evaluation. J Ultrasound Med 6:631, 1987.)

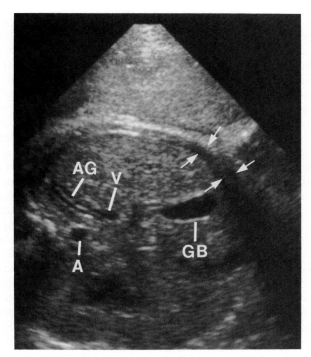

Figure 10–55. Transverse axial sonogram, fetal abdomen. Lucent abdominal wall musculature *(arrows)* may erroneously give the impression that ascites is present. A, aorta; AG, adrenal gland; V, vena cava; GB, gallbladder.

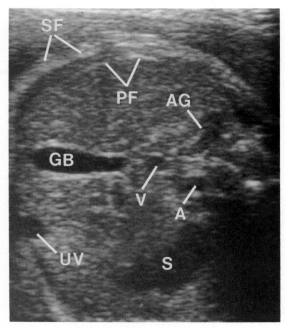

Figure 10–56. Abdominal wall musculature lies between the subcutaneous fat (SF) and the properitoneal fat (PF). Individual layers can be appreciated. AG, adrenal gland; GB, gallbladder; V, vena cava; A, aorta; S, stomach; UV, umbilical vein.

times, so clearly visible that the individual layers can be detected (Fig. 10–56). More commonly seen as a "single" layer of muscles, this tissue is easily recognized as lying within the abdominal wall by noting its position between the subcutaneous fat and the properitoneal fat. The latter is traced from the paranephric fat as it curves onto the flank. Furthermore, the abdominal wall muscles "meet" the ends of the lower thoracic ribs, while ascites would pass "between" the ribs and the abdominal viscera.[40]

CARDIOVASCULAR SYSTEM

The anatomy of the heart and great vessels will be discussed in detail in Chapter 14. In this section the focus is on those fetal vessels visible within the uterus and fetal corpus that are not covered elsewhere. Indeed, a surprisingly large number of individual fetal blood vessels can be seen. The list could be expanded substantially if one were to include arteries that are recognized only by the location of their pulsation, although the wall and lumen of the vessel remain undetected.

The fetal circulation begins in the placenta. In virtually all second- and third-trimester fetuses one can detect the surface (fetal) vessels of the placenta, and occasionally one can even appreciate that these vessels penetrate the placental substance. The surface vessels coalesce at the cord "insertion." The identification of the cord insertion has become important since the advent of percutaneous fetal blood sampling for diagnosis and management (see Chapter 2).[41] The cord

"insertion" is often easily seen, but if not, it is worthwhile to search for large placental surface vessels and trace these to the cord.

The normal umbilical cord is composed of two arteries and a vein (Fig. 10–57). The cord is virtually always coiled and sometimes extremely so. This leads to a variety of appearances of the cord when viewed with tomographic sections as generated by sonography.

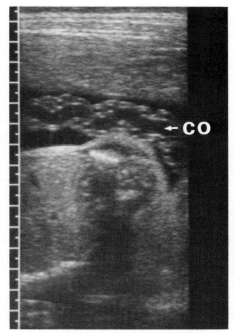

Figure 10–57. Longitudinal sonogram of a three-vessel umbilical cord (CO).

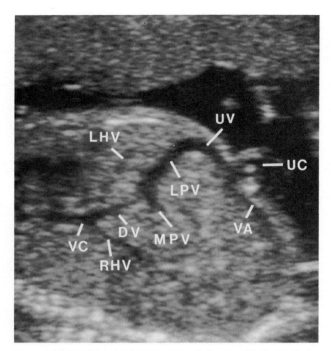

Figure 10–58. Midsagittal sonogram of the umbilical circulation. UC, umbilical cord; LPV, umbilical segment of left portal vein; DV, ductus venosus; VC, inferior vena cava; LHV, left hepatic vein; RHV, right hepatic vein; MPV, main portal vein; UA, umbilical artery.

Indeed, the "simple" task of counting cord vessels can be made quite frustrating by the coils. To consistently obtain the correct count of cord vessels, one must rely on a true transverse axial section of the cord vessels. Longitudinal or oblique views can be misleading.

These vessels enter the fetus, by definition, at the umbilicus and there immediately diverge.[42] The umbilical vein proceeds cephalically (Fig. 10–58); the umbilical arteries egress from a caudal direction. The umbilical arteries proceed along the margin of the urinary bladder from their origin at the iliac arteries in their course toward the umbilicus (Fig. 10–59). As they course along the bladder margin, they should not be mistaken for dilated ureters, a distinction easily made by taking a moment to notice their pulsation.

The umbilical vein joins the fetal portal circulation. The fetal portal circulation is seen with a high degree of consistency on sonograms. Obviously, the larger the fetus, the more readily one will see the smaller elements of this system. Importantly, many of the illustrations seen in the literature incorrectly interpret the fetal umbilical and portal venous anatomy. Confusion has led not only to improper nomenclature but also to use of inappropriate landmarks for obtaining important fetal measurements. With a clear understanding of fetal portal vein anatomy, one can avoid these pitfalls and better appreciate fetal and adult segmental hepatic anatomy.

The dynamics of maternal-fetal circulation determine the details of fetal hepatic portal venous and segmental anatomy.[43] Because there are no blood-diverting branches of the umbilical vein, the volume of placental blood entering the left portal venous system equals

that in the umbilical vein. Thus, the umbilical vein and the initial portion (umbilical segment) of the left portal vein have the same diameter (see Fig. 10–58). Thereby, the left portal vein of the fetus is larger than the right, the reverse of the situation seen in the child and adult. From this point there are several avenues through which blood may reach the right atrium. A common misconception of the maternal-fetal circulation is that the bulk of umbilical venous blood bypasses the liver capillary bed through a large patent ductus venosus. However, in utero, the ductus venous averages only one seventh the diameter of the umbilical vein[44] and even may be closed (see Fig. 10–58).[45] It should be remembered, however, that the peripheral resistance of the hepatic vascular bed is not present in the ductus venosus, enabling this smaller caliber vessel to carry a larger quantity of blood than might be expected. Nonetheless, a significant portion of umbilical venous blood, which carries the highest concentration of nutrients and oxygen in the fetus, actually circulates through the left lobe of the fetal liver through branches supplying the medial and lateral segments before entering the systemic venous system through the left and middle hepatic veins (Fig. 10–60). Although the right lobe of the liver receives a small amount of umbilical venous blood from the left portal vein, the bulk of blood entering the right portal vein is derived from the main portal vein, which, in the fetus, contains low concentrations of both nutrients and oxygen.[45] The unequal distribution of nutrients to the fetal liver partially accounts for the relatively large size of the left lobe of the fetal liver. Following closure of the umbilical vein at birth, the nutrient supply to the entire liver equalizes and the relative size of the left lobe decreases.

In the fetus, the umbilical vein courses cephalically in the free margin of the falciform ligament (see Fig. 10–58). As noted earlier, it joins the umbilical portion

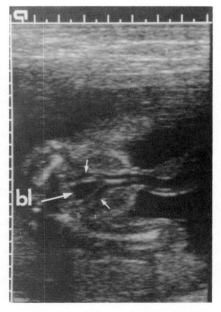

Figure 10–59. Umbilical cord insertion into the fetus. The umbilical arteries *(arrows)* egress from a caudal direction, coursing along the margin of the urinary bladder (bl).

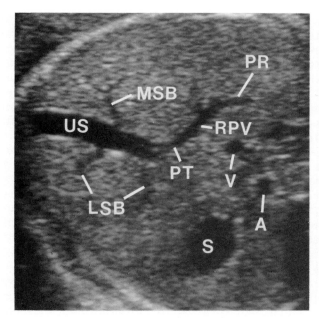

Figure 10–60. Fetal left portal circulation. US, umbilical segment of left portal vein; PT, pars transversa of left portal vein; MSB, medial segmental branch; LSB, lateral segmental branches; RPV, right portal vein; PR, posterior division of right portal vein; V, vena cava; A, aorta; S, stomach.

of the left portal vein at the caudal margin of the left intersegmental fissure of the liver.[46] After birth, the umbilical vein collapses and ultimately becomes the ligamentum teres hepatis.

The umbilical portion of the left portal vein has a predominantly posterior course but also courses superiorly in the left intersegmental fissure (see Fig. 10–58). Its branches supply the medial and lateral segments of the left lobe of the liver.[47] The left portal vein then courses abruptly to the right, exits the left intersegmental fissure, and forms the transverse por-

tion (pars transversa) of the left portal vein (see Figs. 10–60 and 10–61). The pars transversa joins imperceptibly with the right portal vein at the main lobar fissure. The ductus venosus originates from the pars transversa (but occasionally more rightward).[48] The ductus continues posteriorly but assumes a more cephalad course than the umbilical portion of the left portal vein (see Fig. 10–61). It continues as an unbranched structure to join the left or, less commonly, the middle hepatic vein. In this position it lies in the superior extension of the gastrohepatic ligament, which separates the developing caudate lobe posteriorly from the medial and lateral segments of the left hepatic lobe anteriorly. Following birth, the ductus venosus closes and becomes the fibrous ligamentum venosum.[46]

Sonograms of the upper portion of the fetal abdomen clearly demonstrate the anatomy described previously (Figs. 10–58 through 10–61). Because the umbilical vein courses cephalically, transversely oriented planes of section intersect this vessel's short axis (see Fig. 10–56). Slight cephalad movement of the transducer demonstrates a position at which this venous structure abruptly courses posteriorly (see Figs. 10–60 and 10–61). This posteriorly coursing vein represents the umbilical portion of the left portal vein rather than the cephalic portion of the umbilical vein as it is commonly mislabeled in the literature. That this vessel is indeed the left portal vein is easily observed in that branches to the medial and lateral segments of the left lobe arise from this vein (see Figs. 10–60 and 10–61). Recall that the umbilical vein has no branches. When the umbilical portion of the left portal vein is seen throughout its entire course, one can be certain that some angulation has been introduced into the scan plane because this venous structure courses not only posterior but slightly cephalad (see Fig. 10–58). A variety of branches of the umbilical segment of the left portal vein are occasionally imaged; these include the medial, superolateral, and inferolateral branches (see Fig. 10–60).

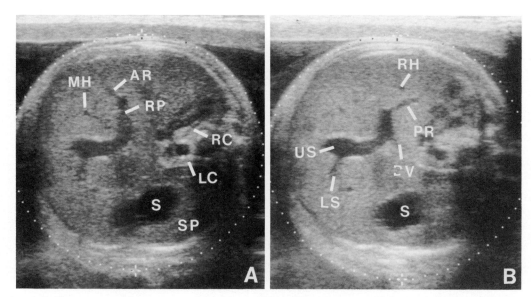

Figure 10–61. A and B. Transverse axial sonograms of fetal liver. US, umbilical segment of left portal vein; LS, lateral segmental branch; DV, ductus venosus; RP, right portal vein; AR, anterior division of right portal vein; PR, posterior division of right portal vein; MH, middle hepatic vein; RH, right hepatic vein; SP, spleen; S, stomach; RC and LC, right and left diaphragmatic crura.

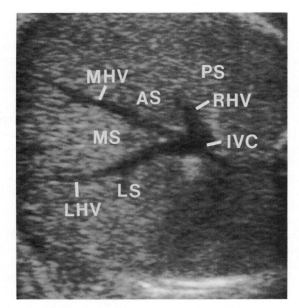

Figure 10–62. Sonogram through the long axis of the proximal fetal hepatic veins. MHV, middle hepatic vein; LHV, left hepatic vein; RHV, right hepatic vein; IVC, inferior vena cava. These veins divide the liver into lobes and segments. AS and PS, anterior and posterior segments of the right hepatic lobe; MS and LS, medial and lateral segments of the left hepatic lobe.

The right portal vein divides into anterior and posterior segmental branches, as in the adult (see Fig. 10–61). Each supplies a respective segment of the right hepatic lobe. The hepatic veins can be recognized by their relationship to portal veins[46] and can be seen to radiate toward the inferior vena cava, coalescing with this venous channel immediately before it enters the right atrium (Fig. 10–62). These veins divide the liver into lobes and segments. The hepatic veins are most easily sought near the level of the diaphragm where their caliber is the largest.[49] Nonetheless, the middle and right hepatic vein are commonly seen in more inferior planes of section by noting their relative position compared with the right portal vein divisions (see Fig. 10–61). The right hepatic vein (anterior branch)

passes between the anterior and posterior divisions of the right portal vein, while the middle hepatic vein always crosses anterior to the right portal vein (in the main lobar fissure). The aorta and inferior vena cava have a similar course in the lower abdomen but diverge in the upper abdomen where the aorta penetrates the diaphragm posteriorly (in contact with the spine), while the inferior vena cava turns anteriorly to join the right atrium (Fig. 10–63).

The great vessels near and around the heart are described in Chapter 14. The vessels arising from the transverse aorta are frequently visible and include the brachiocephalic, left common carotid, and left subclavian arteries. The common carotid arteries and jugular veins are also commonly seen in the neck of older fetuses. The brachial artery and vein are less frequently seen adjacent to the humerus when the arterial pulsation is sought.

Certain intracranial arterial structures are occasionally perceived as tubular vessels (Fig. 10–64). More commonly they are recognized by virtue of the location of their pulsation. These include the middle cerebral artery in the sylvian cistern, the posterior cerebral artery in the ambient cistern, the anterior cerebral arteries in the interhemispheric cistern (near the genu of the corpus callosum), and the basilar artery in the interpeduncular cistern. Pulsations from the circle of Willis are seen in the basilar cisterns caudal to the third ventricle.

The abdominal aorta and inferior vena cava are easily identified, as are the common iliac arteries and veins. Other branches of the abdominal aorta can be visualized, although inconsistently, and include the celiac axis, the superior mesenteric artery, and the renal arteries. Similarly, the renal veins are seen from time to time.

In the leg, the superficial femoral artery and vein (Fig. 10–65) may be visualized in older fetuses. When the knee is extended, it is not difficult to trace these vessels to the level of the popliteal artery and vein (Fig. 10–66), a virtually impossible task when the knee is flexed.

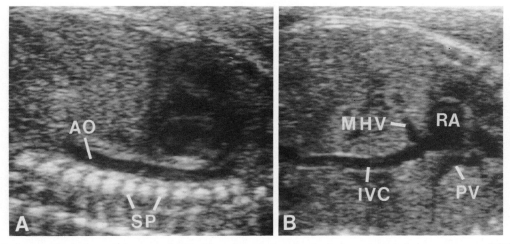

Figure 10–63. *A.* Longitudinal view of the aorta (AO). SP, spine. *B.* Longitudinal view of the inferior vena cava (IVC). MHV, middle hepatic vein; RA, right atrium; PV, pulmonic vein.

Figure 10–64. Transverse axial sonogram through the basal cisterns demonstrates the internal carotid arteries (CA) and the basilar artery (BA).

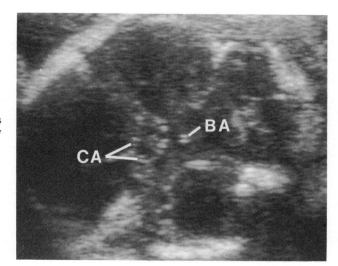

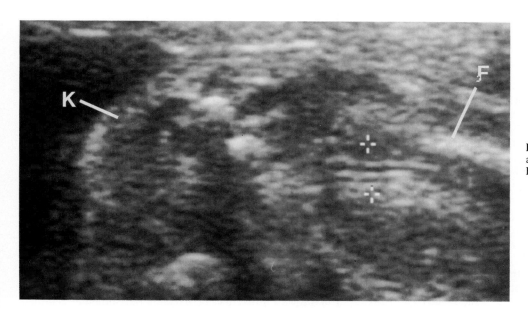

Figure 10–65. Superficial femoral artery and vein marked by cursors. F, femur; K, knee.

Figure 10–66. *A.* Posterior aspect of knee in extension. Popliteal artery and vein are visible. *B.* More anterior plane for reference. T, tibia; F, femur.

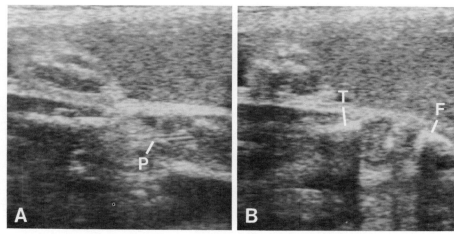

GASTROINTESTINAL SYSTEM

Many components of the gastrointestinal system can be seen sonographically, some as early as the end of the first trimester.[50] The largest parenchymal organ of the system and of the torso, the liver, is seen consistently from the second trimester onward, although its margins are often indistinct in the earlier phases of pregnancy. Conversely, the other major parenchymal organ of the gastrointestinal system, the pancreas, is only uncommonly seen even in third-trimester fetuses. For lack of a better section in which to include it, the spleen will be considered with the gastrointestinal tract. This organ is also visible consistently in the second trimester, but, like the liver, each of its margins is rarely distinct. Conversely, those portions of the fetal gastrointestinal system that consistently contain fluid, the stomach (see Figs. 10–56, 10–60, and 10–61) and gallbladder (see Figs. 10–55 and 10–56), are among the earliest and most consistently seen of fetal structures.

The components within and about the oral cavity are seen relatively well on sonography.[51] The lips and cheeks have been described in the section on superficial anatomy (see Figs. 10–7 and 10–8). Also consistently seen is the tongue (Fig. 10–67). The tongue is seen to best advantage during the swallowing movements. The gingival ridge with tooth buds is seen not uncommonly in older fetuses (see Fig. 10–67A). The hard palate is difficult to define consistently, but with practice can be detected (see Fig. 10–6). For this reason cleft palate (independent of cleft lip) is a difficult diagnosis to establish sonographically. The soft palate cannot be recognized discretely. The oropharynx and laryngeal pharynx frequently contain fluid and thus are seen relatively often when sought (Figs. 10–67 and 10–68). Transverse axial scans through the upper neck are quite successful for visualization of the pharynx, but longitudinal coronal images, more difficult to obtain, display the anatomy to greater advantage. In longitudinal coronal planes, the continuity of the pharyngeal zones can be appreciated as well as the larynx protruding into the pharynx (see Fig. 10–68). The pyriform sinuses, valleculae, and glottis may be appreciated.

The mid and distal esophagus may be seen surprisingly often when sought (Fig. 10–69).[51] The proximal esophagus is extraordinarily difficult, if not impossible, to visualize in the normal fetus. The mid and distal esophagus may be seen, although inconsistently, in both longitudinal coronal and transverse axial images. The key to identification of this structure is the descending thoracic aorta, a structure easily seen. The mid and distal esophagus lie immediately anterior to the descending thoracic aorta. The aorta is first visualized in a longitudinal coronal plane. The transducer is then slowly moved anteriorly. As the aorta disappears from view the esophagus comes into "view" but is much more difficult to recognize. It is seen as five parallel linear echoes. These are created by the hyperechoic serosa and lumen and the hypoechoic muscular wall (see Fig. 10–69). Conceptually, one could apply a similar strategy to visualization of the upper third of the esophagus. In this instance, one would image the trachea (see subsequent section) in a longitudinal coronal plane, then slowly move the transducer posteriorly. As the trachea disappears the esophagus should again come into "view." Unfortunately, this concept, while anatomically correct, is practically unsuccessful.

The stomach and gallbladder are the only portions of the subdiaphragmatic fetal gastrointestinal system that normally contain fluid (see Figs. 10–55, 10–56, 10–60, and 10–61).[50, 52, 53] Thus, any fluid-containing small bowel should be viewed with suspicion, although in late fetuses one may occasionally see very small amounts of normal succus entericus in the small bowel lumen, usually made more obvious by accompanying peristalsis.

Fluid contained within the normal fetal stomach is almost entirely imbibed. The fetus begins to swallow amniotic fluid at approximately 16 weeks.[52, 53] The volume that the fetus swallows increases dramatically throughout pregnancy and reaches 400 to 500 mL by term. There is a relative proportionality between the volume of urine produced and the amount of amniotic fluid imbibed by the fetus. In the absence of a patent esophagus the stomach will be empty (invisible) except in two circumstances. First, and most common, is the concomitant presence of a tracheoesophageal fistula, enabling the fetus to "breath" amniotic fluid into the esophagus and thence to the stomach.[54] This inefficient method is almost universally associated with polyhydramnios in late pregnancy but not always before 24

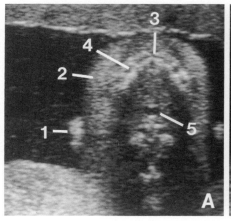
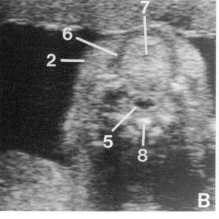

Figure 10–67. *A* and *B*. Transverse axial sonograms of the oral cavity. 1, ear; 2, cheek fat pads (Bichat's); 3, mandible; 4, tooth buds; 5, oropharynx; 6, buccal musculature; 7, tongue; 8, cervical vertebral centrum.

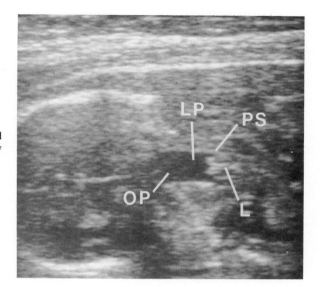

Figure 10–68. Coronal sonogram of the fetal hypopharynx. The fluid-filled oropharynx (OP) and laryngopharynx (LP) are well seen. Fluid slightly distends the pyriform sinuses (PS). L, larynx.

weeks. Second, the association of esophageal atresia without tracheoesophageal fistula but with a second proximal gastrointestinal tract atresia or obstruction will allow secretions from the stomach to accumulate within the gastric lumen.

The stomach varies considerably in size depending, presumably, on how much amniotic fluid has been recently imbibed by the fetus.[52, 53] A prominent stomach never should be taken as sole evidence of obstruction. When the stomach is well distended, its various parts (i.e., the fundus, body, and antrum) can be identified. The fundus is most posterior while the antrum is most anterior. The incisura angularis can be noted when the stomach is well distended. The incisura angularis is a notch of variable depth that is usually found along the lesser curvature between the body and antrum of the stomach.[55]

Small bowel becomes progressively more visible through the second and third trimesters. Meconium accumulating in the small bowel during early and mid second trimester begins to impart an appearance of a "conglomerate" zone of increased echogenicity in the mid and lower abdomen of the fetus. This should not be mistaken either for an abnormal mass (pseudomass of bowel)[56–58] or of a bowel abnormality. With passage of time, and somewhat dependent on ease of imaging,

discrete small bowel loops become visible (Fig. 10–70). As with the esophagus, the lumen tends to be brighter relative to the hypoechoic muscular wall. The serosa is again greater in echogenicity than the muscular layer. Late in pregnancy, the deposition of small amounts of fat in the mesentery probably accentuates this feature. Ultimately, in late pregnancy, discrete small bowel containing small amounts of fluid (succus entericus) can be visualized in nearly all fetuses.[59]

The colon tends to become visible near the beginning of the third trimester and, again, is seen progressively better with increasing gestational age.[59, 60] The colon tends to be relatively hypoechoic (Figs. 10–71 and 10–72). As such, colon should not be mistaken for dilated small bowel. It is the characteristic course of the colon that most readily permits distinction from pathologically dilated small bowel. The ascending colon courses along the right flank (see Fig. 10–71A) in relation to the right kidney. As it approaches the liver it bends leftward, the hepatic flexure (see Fig. 10–71A). The transverse colon courses along the free edge of the liver (see Figs. 10–71A and 10–72A) and passes inferior to the stomach. At the splenic flexure the colon turns posteriorly and again comes into intimate relationship with the kidney; of course in this instance it is the left kidney. Frequently, when imaging the kidneys, the

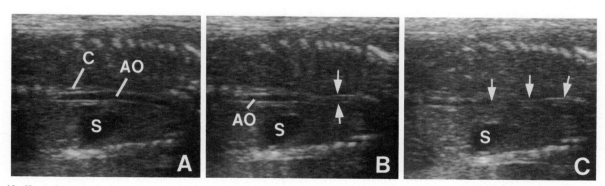

Figure 10–69. A through C. Coronal sonograms depicting demonstration of the esophagus. First (A), the descending aorta (AO) is localized. C, diaphragmatic crura; S, stomach. As the transducer is moved anteriorly (B and C) the esophagus (arrows) comes into view.

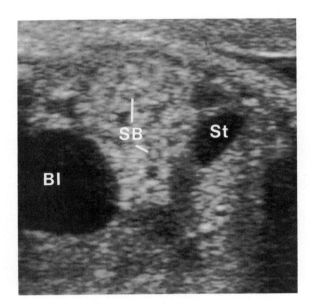

Figure 10–70. Small bowel (SB) in a late third-trimester fetus. St, stomach; Bl, bladder.

colon is detected. Indeed, when a kidney is absent, the colon occupies the renal fossa and should not be misinterpreted as a normal or abnormal kidney. Finally, the sigmoid colon arcs over the urinary bladder to join the rectum (see Figs. 10–71B and 10–72B). Occasionally, haustral markings can be noted in the colon wall. A redundant sigmoid colon (see Fig. 10–72B) should not be mistaken for dilated small bowel.

The liver, as noted earlier, is proportionately larger in the fetus than in the child or adult.[61] Similarly, in the early second trimester, the liver constitutes 10% of the total fetal weight, but only 5% of the total weight at term. The fetal liver, in addition, has a substantially larger left lobe. Indeed, the fetal liver spans the entire width of the abdomen throughout pregnancy, the left lobe always contacting the left

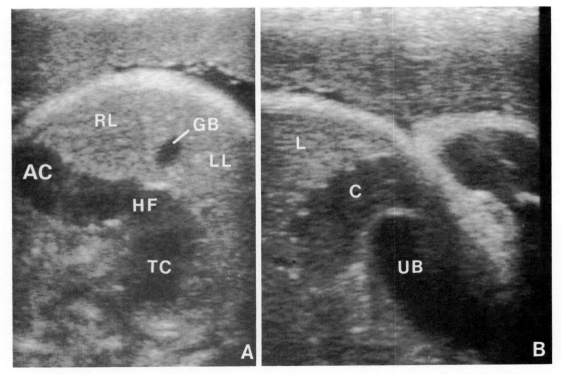

Figure 10–71. A. Transverse axial sonogram of the fetal abdomen demonstrates, by position, the ascending (AC) and transverse (TC) colon with the hepatic flexure (HF) between. RL, right hepatic lobe; GB, gallbladder; LL, left hepatic lobe. B. Off-axis coronal sonogram of the lower abdomen. The sigmoid colon (C) arches over the urinary bladder (UB). Note the haustral markings at the edge of the bowel loop. L, liver.

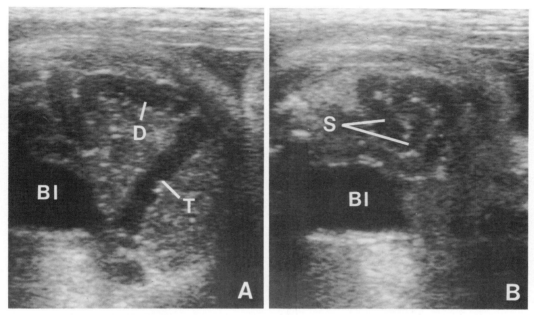

Figure 10–72. *A.* Coronal sonogram demonstrates the transverse colon (T) and descending colon (D). Unlabeled is the splenic flexure. *B.* A markedly looped sigmoid colon (S) is noted. Bl, bladder.

abdominal wall. This would be unusual in an adult, although this relationship can be seen in adults, as well.

The two major segments of each hepatic lobe can be seen in older fetuses (see Fig. 10–62) and to some extent even in early second-trimester fetuses.[43, 46] The lateral segment of the left lobe extends to the left of the umbilical segment of the left portal vein (see Figs. 10–60 and 10–61). The medial segment of the left lobe is the tissue lying between the gallbladder (or middle hepatic vein more superiorly) and the umbilical segment of the left portal vein or the intersegmental fissure more caudally (Fig. 10–73). The right lobe is all of the

hepatic tissue lying to the right of the gallbladder, middle hepatic vein, and the inferior vena cava (see Figs. 10–56 and 10–61). These latter three structures all reside in the main lobar fissure. The left portal vein and left hepatic vein mark the left intersegmental fissure. Finally, the right intersegmental fissure is marked by the right hepatic vein cephalically and its anterior branch inferiorly.

The pancreas, as noted, is difficult to perceive at any gestational age. The pancreatic tissue lies posterior to the stomach, an area that can be visualized consistently in the fetus. However, discrete perception of the pancreas requires demonstration of the splenic vein

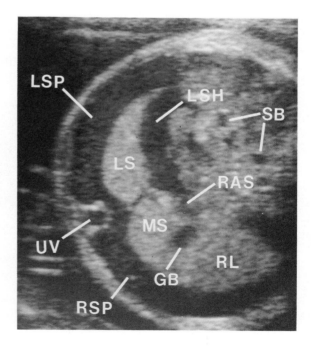

Figure 10–73. Transverse axial sonogram of the fetal abdomen following an intraperitoneal transfusion for Rh isoimmunization enables recognition of many peritoneal spaces, including the right (RSP) and left (LSP) subphrenic spaces and the right anterior (RAS) and left subhepatic spaces. Segmental anatomy of the fetal liver is also well seen, including the medial (MS) and lateral (LS) segments of the left hepatic lobe. GB, gallbladder; RL, right hepatic lobe; SB, small bowel; UV, umbilical vein.

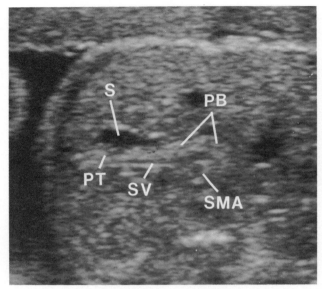

Figure 10–74. Fetal pancreas is not commonly seen discretely but, as depicted in this unusual example, lies between the splenic vein (SV) and the posterior stomach wall (S). PB, pancreatic body; PT, pancreatic tail; SMA, superior mesenteric artery.

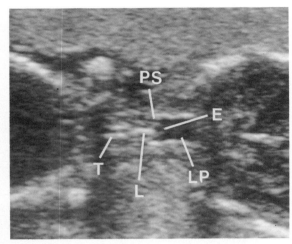

Figure 10–75. Fetal larynx (L) and epiglottis (E). LP, laryngopharynx; PS, pyriform sinus; T, trachea.

and origin of the superior mesenteric artery in a transverse axial plane of section (Fig. 10–74). The pancreas then is the band of tissue between these vessels and the posterior gastric wall.

The spleen is not truly a gastrointestinal organ (see Fig. 10–61). The spleen is bounded superiorly by the diaphragm, laterally by the lower ribs, medially by the stomach, and posteriorly by both the diaphragm and kidney. It is only the inferior margin that is difficult to delimit. In the fetus the spleen echogenicity is similar to the liver. In the adult the liver is slightly less echogenic than the spleen.[62–65] The spleen grows progressively through fetal life, and nomograms of splenic size are available in the literature.[62]

RESPIRATORY SYSTEM

The upper respiratory tract system is seen partially. The nose has been previously illustrated (see Figs. 10–

7 and 10–8). The nasal cavity, septum, and palate can be detected with practice. As noted earlier, portions of the pharynx and hypopharynx are commonly visible because of the presence of fluid.[51] The pyriform sinuses are seen when fluid filled (see Fig. 10–68). When relatively large amounts of fluid are present in the pharynx of an older fetus, the epiglottis may be seen protruding into the fluid (Fig. 10–75). The epiglottis is particularly visible during swallowing.

The larynx is virtually always visible when the hypopharynx is fluid filled (see Figs. 10–68 and 10–75). Details of laryngeal anatomy are not particularly evident, but the larynx itself is easily recognized as a superior constriction of the tracheal fluid column protruding into the hypopharynx and flanked by the pyriform sinuses. If the head is markedly flexed, the overlying mandible frequently defeats efforts to visualize the larynx and hypopharynx.

The trachea is a relatively easy structure to visualize (see Figs. 10–75 through 10–77).[51] Again, this is predominantly because it is consistently fluid filled. Not only do the lungs produce fluid that is expelled into the amniotic sac through the trachea, but the fetus intermittently and frequently "breathes" amniotic fluid

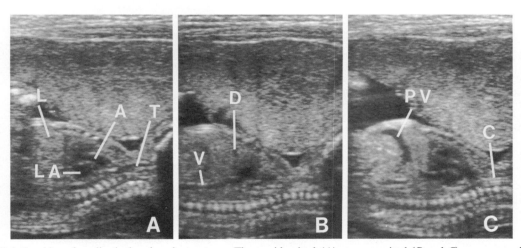

Figure 10–76. Relationships of mediastinal and neck structures. Three midsagittal *(A)* or parasagittal *(B* and *C)* sonograms demonstrate the trachea (T) down to the level of the aortic arch (A). The carotid (C) arteries lie adjacent to the trachea in the neck. L, liver; LA, left atrium; V, inferior vena cava; D, diaphragm; PV, left portal vein.

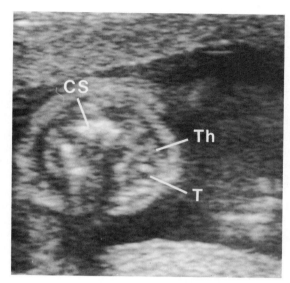

Figure 10–77. Transverse axial sonogram of the fetal neck. T, trachea; Th, thyroid lobe; CS, cervical spine.

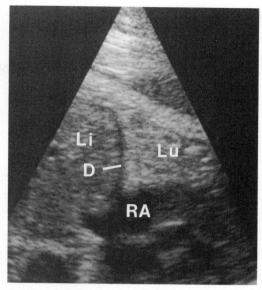

Figure 10–79. Echogenicity difference between lung (Lu) and liver (Li) in an older fetus. D, diaphragm; RA, right atrium.

into the trachea. Additionally, the trachea, along much of its length, is flanked by the conspicuous pulsations of the common carotid arteries. The trachea usually can be traced to its distal end, passing posterior to the aortic arch (see Fig. 10–76A), but the carina and bronchi are quite difficult to perceive. Because mainstem bronchi are usually invisible, smaller ramifications of the bronchi are, for all intents and purposes, universally invisible at this time in the development of fetal sonography.

The right and left pulmonary arteries and several pulmonary veins (see Figs. 10–63 and 10–78) are visible in a large percentage of older fetuses. However, one generally pursues visualization of these major vessels during examination of the heart rather than the lungs. Details of the pulmonary arterial and venous anatomy will be found in Chapter 14.

The lung (at least lung tissue) can be seen from late first trimester onward. Early in pregnancy, definition of the lung is drawn more from the structures that surround it. These include, predominantly, the ribs superolaterally and the heart (and to a lesser extent other mediastinal structures) medially. Inferiorly, the early lung blends imperceptibly with the liver. These two organs are equal in echogenicity throughout the second trimester and the early third trimester.

As pregnancy progresses, the lung becomes more echogenic than the liver (Fig. 10–79). The reason for this is unknown. It was speculated that this difference may signal pulmonary maturity, a notion that never has been proven and that is likely erroneous.[66, 67] Furthermore, the muscular portion of the diaphragm becomes progressively more visible with fetal growth (Fig. 10–80).

These markers of the inferior extent of the lung improve pulmonary tissue visibility with advancing gestational age. Discrete pulmonary lobes are not visible in the normal fetus, but when a pleural effusion is present, insinuation of fluid into the major fissures (and the minor fissure on the right) marks lobar boundaries.

GENITOURINARY SYSTEM

Although the extreme variability of fetal positioning and the lack of subject contrast between kidney and the surrounding tissues do not permit consistent identification of both fetal kidneys, normal fetal kidneys may be identified in their paraspinous location as early as at 15 to 16 menstrual weeks. Visualization does not become consistent until the 20th week.[68] In longitudinal section, fetal kidneys appear as bilateral elliptical structures, and in transverse section they have a circular appearance adjacent to the lumbar spinal ossification centers bilaterally. Later in pregnancy, echogenic ret-

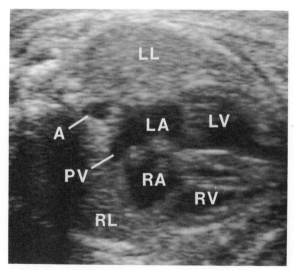

Figure 10–78. Transverse axial sonogram of the fetal thorax. A, descending aorta; LA, left atrium; LV, left ventricle; RA, right atrium; RV, right ventricle; PV, pulmonary vein; LL, left lung; RL, right lung.

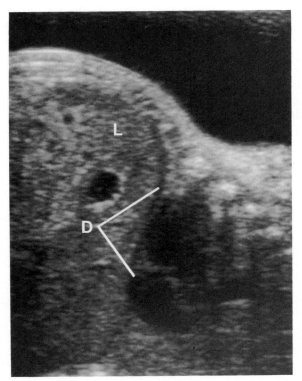

Figure 10–80. The muscular diaphragm (D) is relatively hypoechoic. L, liver.

roperitoneal fat, which surrounds the kidneys, assists in their sonographic visualization (see Figs. 10–3 and 10–81). The echopenic fetal renal pyramids can frequently be discriminated from the surrounding cortex and columns of Bertin in older fetuses and are arranged in an anterior and posterior row (see Fig. 10–3) in a configuration corresponding to the calyces that contact the apices of the pyramids (the papillae).[69] The echotexture of the normal fetal renal cortex, which usually approximates or may even be slightly greater than that of the surrounding tissues, highlights the relatively echopenic pyramids. The characteristic position of the pyramids avoids any potential confusion with renal parenchymal cysts. Confusion with dilated calyces is avoided by noting the interspaced columns of Bertin and the lack of communication with dilated infundibula and pelvis. Within the renal sinus of fetuses there is generally a paucity of fat. Intrarenal collecting structures, the pelvis and infundibula, are commonly seen in fetuses because they frequently contain fluid,[70, 71] a topic that will be addressed in Chapter 18.

The fetal kidneys grow throughout gestation. Standards for renal length width, thickness, volume, and circumference have been established as a function of menstrual age and correspond with measurements of renal size obtained on stillborn fetuses postnatally.[72–74] Throughout pregnancy the ratio of kidney circumference to abdominal circumference remains relatively constant at 0.27 to 0.30. Such measurements are more efficient for detecting enlarged kidneys than small ones. Diminution in renal size is more difficult to detect because the exact renal border, especially of small kidneys, may be partially obscured, because the plane

of section may not be through the longest renal axis, and because of the wide standard deviation in renal size.[72–74]

The normal fetal ureter cannot be identified. Rarely one may see a normal ureter, but visualization of a fetal ureter should always suggest pathologic dilatation. However, as early as 15 menstrual weeks the normal fetal urinary bladder can be identified (see Fig. 10–59). Only a few cubic centimeters of bladder urine would be needed to allow ready visualization in such a young fetus. Because the fetus normally fills and empties the urinary bladder every 30 to 45 minutes, the bladder will frequently be seen to increase in size and to empty during the course of a sonographic examination.[75–77] Similarly, fetuses in whom the urinary bladder is not visualized can be examined at intervals for bladder filling. If the bladder cannot be seen in the presence of oligohydramnios, sequential imaging to test for bladder filling is mandatory.

At 32 weeks of gestation the maximum fetal bladder volume measures 10 mL. By term the normal fetal bladder volume quadruples (see Fig. 10–70). Similarly, fetal urine production, as calculated by determination of change in bladder volume with time, increases from 9.6 mL/h at 30 weeks to 27.3 mL/h at 40 weeks menstrual age.[75, 76] Of course, term fetuses void, thus the bladder may be empty.[77] Filling and emptying of the fetal urinary bladder confirms that the fetus produces urine but does not indicate the "quality" of urine produced. The normal fetal urinary bladder, the wall of which is very thin and virtually invisible when the bladder is well distended (see Fig. 10–70), occupies a midline position within the fetal pelvis. Changes in volume of the urinary bladder with time differentiate it from cystic pathologic pelvic structures.

The normal fetal urethra may be identified, from

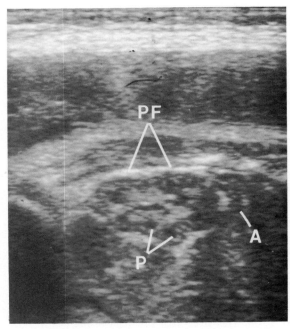

Figure 10–81. Sagittal sonogram of the fetal kidney marginated by perirenal fat (PF). Pyramids (P) can be discretely seen. The adrenal gland (A) caps the upper pole.

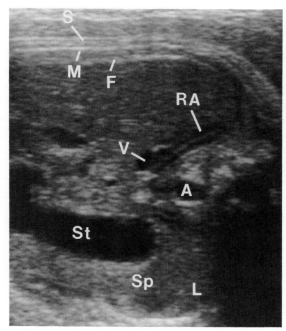

Figure 10–82. Sonogram of the right adrenal gland (RA), although much anatomy can be seen on this image of the upper fetal abdomen. Note both limbs of the right adrenal gland immediately posterior to the inferior vena cava (V) and a portion of the left adrenal gland (unlabeled) to the left of the aorta (A). Posterior and lateral to the stomach (St) the spleen (Sp) is well seen. A slight echogenicity change discriminates the lung (L) lying above the diaphragm in the posterior costophrenic sulcus from the spleen below the diaphragm. The abdominal wall, including the subcutaneous fat (S), muscle layers (M), and properitoneal fat (F), is well seen.

genitourinary system, is seen quite routinely when searching for the kidneys (Figs. 10–81 and 10–82).[78, 79] Indeed, even in the presence of agenesis of one or both kidneys, the adrenal glands can be appreciated in their expected paraspinous locations. Lewis and co-workers believe that the fetal adrenal glands can be consistently imaged after 30 menstrual weeks. The adrenal glands have a specific size, shape, and echogenicity. The echo pattern is so characteristic that the cortex and medulla can be appreciated separately (see Figs. 10–55, 10–56, 10–61A, and 10–82). In the fetus, both adrenal glands cap the upper renal poles (in the adult the left adrenal gland most often lies anterior to the upper pole).[79] The right adrenal is seen more consistently. Its upper portion lies immediately posterior to the proximal inferior vena cava (see Fig. 10–82).

CENTRAL NERVOUS SYSTEM

The fetal brain was one of the first areas of investigational interest in the diagnosis of fetal anomalies.[80] This was a result of two factors: (1) the fetal head was imaged routinely to obtain a biparietal diameter for the determination of gestational age; and (2) central nervous system anomalies are among the most common birth defects. At first, only gross morphologic aberrations such as anencephaly or advanced hydrocephalus were discovered prenatally. As instrumentation has improved to the present day, many malformations of the brain can be diagnosed with accuracy even before 20 weeks of development.[81–86]

The path to the diagnosis of anomalous development, as always, begins with a firm grasp of normal developmental anatomy. Initially, many errors were made when interpreting normal fetal intracranial anatomy as seen by sonography.[87–89] This was due to the unusual circumstance that "fluid" and "solid" areas of the brain did not behave in an anticipated fashion. It was initially expected that the sonographic appearance of the lateral ventricles would be dominated by cerebrospinal fluid, which would render them echolucent.

time to time, as an echogenic line extending the length of an erect penis (see Fig. 10–13). In females and males examined at a time when the penis is flaccid, the normal urethra is difficult or impossible to identify. The uterus and ovaries cannot be visualized in normal female fetuses. The testes can be visualized in male fetuses only after they have descended into the scrotum. The prostate cannot be visualized. The external genitalia were discussed previously in the section on superficial anatomy.

The fetal adrenal gland, although not part of the

Figure 10–83. *A.* Transverse axial scan at the level of the lateral ventricular atria. The brain parenchyma (P) is very lucent. C, choroid plexus; IF, interhemispheric fissure. *B.* Slightly lower scan demonstrates well-developed thalami (T) and midbrain (M) (biparietal diameter of 27 mm at 14 weeks). The frontal horns (F) are large and filled with cerebrospinal fluid.

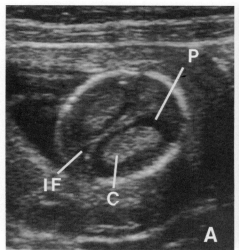
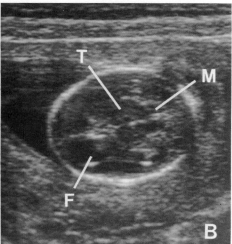

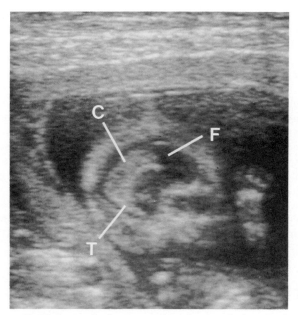

Figure 10–84. Parasagittal sonogram in early second trimester shows choroid filling the early ventricle. The frontal horn (F) is demarcated by specular reflectors. The early temporal horn is seen (T). Note absence of an occipital horn. Choroid (C) fills the body, atrium, and early temporal horn.

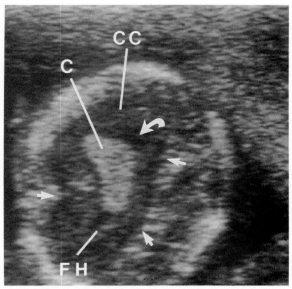

Figure 10–85. Parasagittal sonogram through the ventricle of an 18-week fetus. The choroid (C) defines the ventricular size. Note the substantial increase in cortical brain (CC) thickness compared with fetuses only a few weeks younger (see Fig. 10–84). Bright echoes marginate the edge of the telencephalon *(straight arrows)*. Note the beginnings of an occipital horn *(curved arrow)*. FH, frontal horn.

Instead, their appearance was dominated by highly echogenic choroid plexus (Figs. 10–83 through 10–85).[90, 91] Conversely, the bulk of neural tissue, the telencephalon, diencephalon, and mesencephalon, is quite echopenic compared with other solid tissues in the human body (see Fig. 10–83).[90, 92] The more recent entrant into the area of diagnostic sonography can well imagine the potential for misinterpretation among early researchers when the largest fluid-containing areas of the brain yielded the greatest amplitude echoes while the solid tissue yielded the lowest. To further complicate matters, dramatic changes occur as brain development progresses, resulting in ever-changing positions of certain "landmarks." These changes had never been observed in vivo, and postmortem examination of the brain can be at variance with its appearance during life.

A series of key observations led to the clear delineation of normal developmental neuroanatomy as viewed sonographically. These observations included recognition of the fetal third ventricle, the brightly echogenic choroid plexus,[90] and pulsating vasculature in several cisterns.[92] The first two identified the supratentorial ventricular system. The last enabled identification of the sylvian cistern (middle cerebral artery pulsation), interpeduncular cistern (basilar artery pulsation), and ambient cisterns (posterior cerebral artery pulsations). The landmarks established by these observations provided a framework for subsequent identification of other specific neural structures.

Later in the course of the development of sonography, the neonatal brain came under study (see Figs. 10–1 and 10–86).[1, 2, 91] Interestingly, this resulted in much greater understanding of the appearance of the

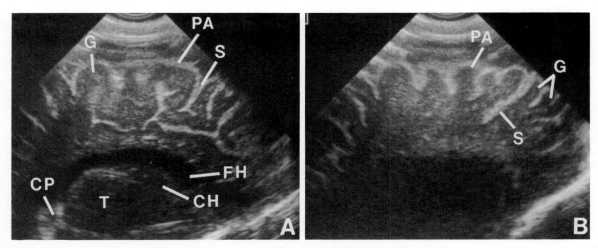

Figure 10–86. *A* and *B.* Parasagittal sonograms of the brain of a 6-month-old child. Gyri (G) are well developed. Pia-arachnoid (PA) tissues cover the surface of the brain and make the sulci (S) highly conspicuous. Careful inspection of gyri shows that cortical gray matter is less echogenic than the white matter. T, thalamus; CH, caudate head; FH, frontal horn; CP, choroid plexus.

fetal brain because examination of "newborn children" now begins commonly at 25 to 26 weeks of development (essentially a second-trimester fetus). Investigators then began to apply neuroanatomy as learned from the neonatal brain, which was imaged with great clarity through the anterior fontanelle, to the developing fetal brain. The following analysis of fetal intracranial anatomy is presented on the basis of these observations.

The fetal head can be clearly discriminated from the fetal torso when an embryo reaches a crown-rump length of 10 to 15 mm. By the 10th to 11th weeks following the last normal menstrual period, one can already begin to appreciate symmetric anatomy inside the developing fetal calvarium. At this point, the intracranial tissue components consist almost entirely of the thalamus and corpus striatum which yield the symmetric appearance of the brain as these structures narrow the developing third ventricle into a midline specular reflector.

By the end of the first trimester, the thalamus, third ventricle, midbrain, brain stem, and cerebellar hemispheres have achieved an appearance that will remain largely unchanged, other than progressive enlargement, throughout the remaining period of sonographic observation of the fetus (see Fig. 10–83). Therefore, the vast majority of the changes that are observed (and they are substantial) relate to the growth and development of the telencephalon. As mentioned, by the end of the first and beginning of the second trimesters, the sonographic appearance of the telencephalon is dominated by the lateral ventricles (see Figs. 10–83*A*, 10–84, and 10–85). These, in turn, are dominated by the brightly echogenic choroid plexus. By 12 to 13 weeks, the lateral ventricles can be clearly seen, appear ovoid, and are largely filled with choroid plexus. Only the frontal horns are devoid of choroid plexus as they are throughout life (see Figs. 10–83*B*, 10–84, and 10–86). At this stage of development, only the rudiments of a temporal horn (see Fig. 10–84) and an occipital horn (see Fig. 10–85) are present. The frontal horn, body of the ventricle, and atrium of the ventricle are large and easily detected. The choroid is the easiest structure to recognize because of its size and high-amplitude echogenicity. Conversely, the mantle of developing cerebral cortex surrounding the lateral ventricle is more difficult to delineate because of its low-amplitude echogenicity, but a demarcation between the lateral ventricle and the cerebral mantle can be appreciated from specular reflections arising from the walls of the lateral ventricle (see Fig. 10–84). These, of course, are seen where the acoustic beam intersects the ventricular wall perpendicularly. By 18 weeks the mantle of developing cortical tissue has thickened appreciably (compare Figures 10–84 and 10–85).

The relative echogenicity of structures, which will be viewed throughout the remainder of gestation, is largely established at this time. Two types of tissue are brightly echogenic and therefore most easily seen during the examination of the fetal brain. These tissues are the choroid plexus, as noted earlier, and the brain coverings: the dura (pachymeninx) and pia-arachnoid

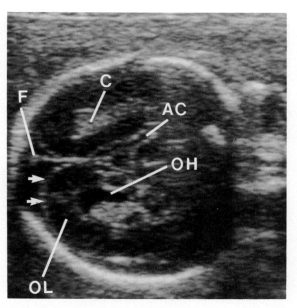

Figure 10–87. Transverse axial sonogram of the occipital lobes (OL) and occipital horn (OH). The brain edge is marginated by bright echoes (pia-arachnoid) *(arrows)*. The cisterns over the brain surface have visible cerebrospinal fluid. F, falx; AC, ambient cistern; C, choroid plexus.

(leptomeninx). Interestingly, the choroid develops from the vascular pia. The leptomeninges demarcate the edges of the brain with a brightly reflective margin of echoes (see Figs. 10–86 and 10–87). Peripheral to this echogenic margin are the subarachnoid spaces that contain cerebrospinal fluid (Figs. 10–87 and 10–88). A feature that confounds the inexperienced sonologist is the relative lack of change in echogenicity between the peripheral (i.e., cortical brain) tissue and the cerebrospinal fluid space as seen across the brightly reflecting marginal echo from the pia-arachnoid (indeed, the cerebrospinal fluid–containing space may be more echogenic) (see Figs. 10–88 and 10–89). This perceptual problem originates from the anticipation that the subarachnoid spaces should be anechoic while the brain parenchyma should be echogenic. This reasonable assumption is untrue in many instances. Recall that these spaces have both cerebrospinal fluid and pia-arachnoid tissue within them. *It is the relative amount of these two components that determines the sonographic appearance of the subarachnoid spaces.* Small subarachnoid cisterns (such as the basal and perimesencephalic cisterns) have an appearance dominated by pia-arachnoid and thus are seen as brightly echogenic spaces (see Fig. 10–89). This is not to say that these cisterns are devoid of cerebrospinal fluid, but the fluid does not significantly influence their sonographic appearance. Conversely, larger subarachnoid spaces, such as those over the convexities of the hemispheres (see Fig. 10–87) and the cisterna magna (see Fig. 10–89), have an appearance dominated by cerebrospinal fluid. Thus, they behave, in the sonographic sense, as one would anticipate for a fluid-containing cavity. Intermediate-sized subarachnoid spaces will have both anechoic zones from visible cerebrospinal fluid and brightly

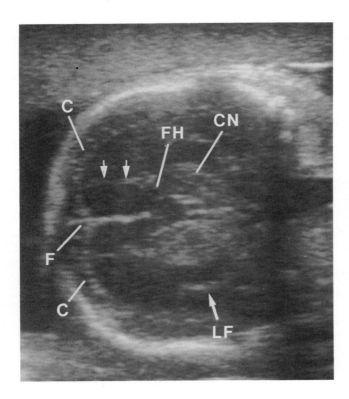

Figure 10–88. Coronal section through the heads of the caudate nuclei (CN). The frontal horn (FH), which is not well seen, drapes over the caudate. Extending between the ventricular margin and the edge of the brain are linear echoing structures previously mistaken for ventricles *(arrows)*. Also seen are bridging strands of pia-arachnoid through the cistern (C) over the convexities (probably bridging veins covered with pia-arachnoid). F, falx; LF, lateral fissure.

echogenic zones from visible pia-arachnoid tissues (Fig. 10–90*A*).

As noted earlier, brightly reflecting structures dominate the appearance of the fetal brain as seen by the sonologist. The choroid plexus and brain coverings (pia-arachnoid and dura) are the two major compo-

nents within the developing calvarium that produce bright reflections. The important dural structures from the perspective of sonographic fetal brain anatomy are the falx and tentorium (see Figs. 10–88 through 10–90). However, the choroid and meninges are not exclusively the bright reflectors. An occasional neural

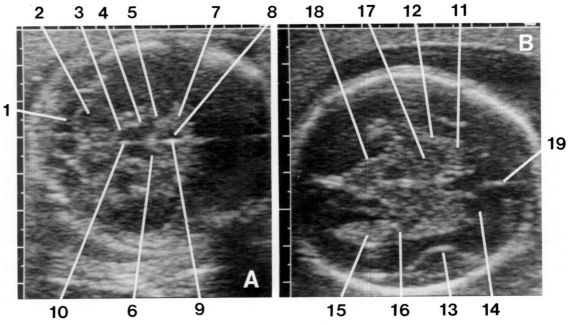

Figure 10–89. *A* and *B*. Transverse axial sonograms demonstrating many discrete neural structures. Note the varying echogenicities of the cisterns. Large cisterns (1, cistern magna) have an appearance dominated by cerebrospinal fluid. Small cisterns (7, basal cisterns) are dominated by pia-arachnoid. 2, cerebellar hemisphere; 3, quadrigeminal cistern; 4, ambient cistern; 5, crural cistern; 6, interpeduncular cistern (note walls of basilar artery centrally in this cistern); 8, hypothalamus; 9, inferior recess of third ventricle; 10, sylvian aqueduct; 11, head of caudate; 12, lentiform nuclei, 13, lateral fissure; 14, frontal horn; 15, atrial choroid; 16, posterior limb of internal capsule; 17, thalamus; 18, tentorial hiatus; 19, falx.

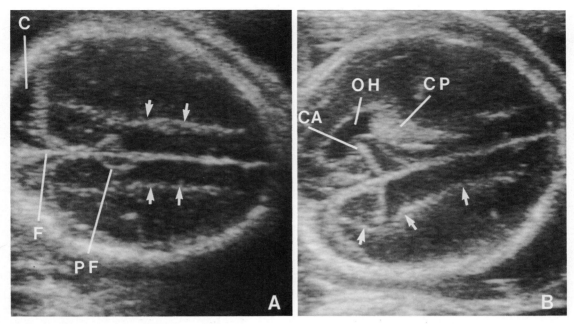

Figure 10–90. *A.* Transverse axial sonogram near the vertex. Bright linear echoes *(arrows)* often mistaken for lateral ventricles are clearly seen. Note that these echoes extend to the brain edge. PF, parieto-occipital fissure; F, falx; C, convexity cistern with cerebrospinal and hair like bridging veins covered by brightly echogenic pia-arachnoid. *B.* Off-axis scan through both the lateral ventricle and the linear echo *(arrow)* seen in *A.* The occipital horn (OH) is now well seen. Note again that the linear echo extends to the brain edge while the occipital horn is entirely marginated by brain tissue. CP, choroid; CA, calcar avis.

structure generates high-amplitude reflections. Most common in this regard is the cerebellar vermis.

Also important as high-amplitude echoing structures are specular reflections from the walls of the ventricular systems (see Figs. 10–84 and 10–87). Such reflections occur when the ultrasonic beam strikes the smooth ventricular wall perpendicularly or nearly so. Thus, one would assume that points and lines of brightness so produced might vary from moment to moment depending on the direction the transducer was pointed. This, however, is not the case for two reasons. First, fetal brain images are predominantly produced in transverse axial planes (appropriate for both biparietal diameter and head circumference measurements) and less commonly coronal planes. In both of these planes, the beam tends to intersect the ventricular system perpendicularly at the same interfaces. Second, the curvature of the bony calvarium limits the number of axial and coronal planes that can be achieved due to significant beam divergence when curved portions of calvarium are intersected by the beam. Thus, the specular reflections from the ventricular walls tend to be seen in stable locations and can be employed as important and reproducible anatomic landmarks.

Additionally, within the substance of the brain, most notably in the region of the cerebral white matter tracks, other bright reflections are noted (see Figs. 10–88 through 10–90). Earlier, these reflectors were mistaken for the lateral ventricular walls, with which they are contiguous.[89, 92, 93] The exact origin of these reflections remains undecided, but the most likely candidates are blood vessels supplying the deeper white matter regions, particularly venous structures.

The sonographic ''skeleton'' of the developing fetal brain originates from the brightly reflective structures just considered. Employing these structures as the framework, numerous discrete neural tissue areas are discernible sonographically (see Figs. 10–89 and 10–91 through 10–95).[1, 2] As the brain develops, multiple areas of the telencephalon, diencephalon, midbrain, pons, and cerebellum become anatomically identifiable. These are recognized by variations in the echogenicity of specific nuclei and tracts that pass through

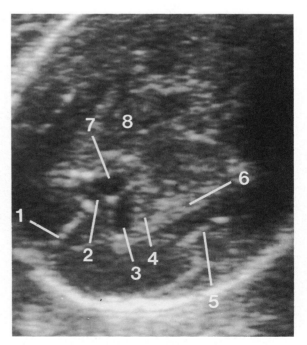

Figure 10–91. Transverse axial sonogram. 1, falx; 2, corpus callosum; 3, frontal horn; 4, caudate nucleus; 5, lateral fissure; 6, lentiform nuclei; 7, cavum septi pellucidi; 8, thalamus.

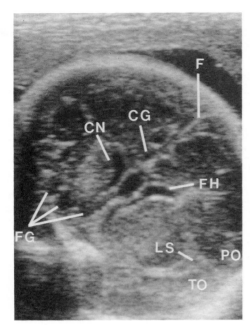

Figure 10–92. Coronal sonogram, anteriorly. F, falx; CG, cingulate gyrus; FH, frontal horn; CN, caudate nucleus; FG, frontal gyri; LS, lateral sulcus; PO, parietal operculum; TO, temporal operculum.

these zones. Several brain nuclei, as well as some other areas of neural tissue, demonstrate a moderate increase in echo amplitude compared with surrounding brain elements. These nuclei demonstrate lower-amplitude signals than choroid or leptomeninges. Among these structures are the caudate and lenticular nuclei, separated by the internal capsule. Less commonly, the claustrum, marginated by the extreme and external capsules, is visible. Similarly, the substantia nigra in the midbrain and dentate nuclei of the cerebellum are discernible. Also, the pars ventralis (belly) of the pons is seen as a zone of moderate echogenicity, as opposed

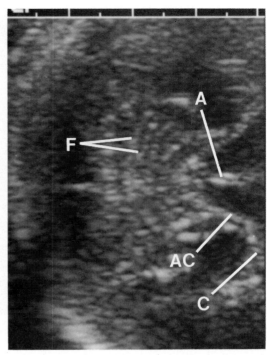

Figure 10–94. Posterior fossa view (axial) demonstrating folia (F) of the cerebellum. AC, ambient cistern; A, sylvian aqueduct; C, choroidal fissure.

to the pars dorsalis (tegmentum), which returns low-amplitude echoes.[1]

It is important for sonologists to be familiar with the appearance of the lateral ventricles as they change throughout growth and development of the fetal brain. By 18 to 20 weeks, easily recognizable occipital horns and temporal horns are visible. The lateral ventricles

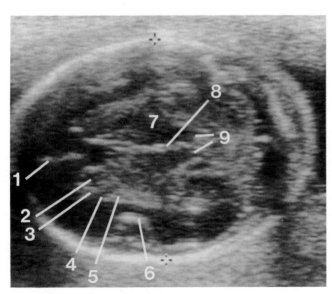

Figure 10–93. Transverse axial sonogram. 1, falx; 2, frontal horn; 3, caudate head; 4, anterior limb of internal capsule; 5, lentiform nuclei; 6, lateral sulcus; 7, thalamus; 8, third ventricle; 9, quadrigeminal bodies.

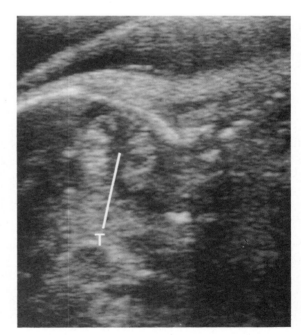

Figure 10–95. Parasagittal sonogram of the posterior fossa. Cerebellar white matter tracts (T) are well seen. Bright margin is most likely due to reflections from pia-arachnoid drawn into the cerebellum by folia formation. (Gray matter is hypoechoic.)

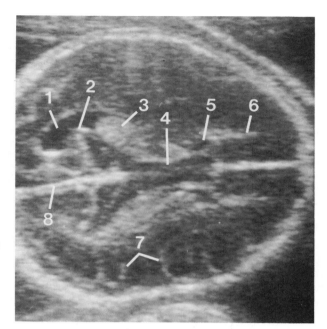

Figure 10–96. Transverse axial sonogram. 1, occipital horn; 2, calcar avis; 3, atrial choroid; 4, corpus callosum; 5, frontal horn; 6, linear echo in white matter (see Figs. 10–88 and 10–90A); 7, sulci; 8, falx.

have achieved their adult components. From this point onward, the lateral ventricles change in shape and proportion as influenced by neural tissues growing adjacent to their walls. For example, the growth of the caudate nucleus markedly reshapes the lateral ventricles.[94] However, throughout the period of observation of fetal lateral ventricles (from 13 to 40 weeks) the size of the atria remains largely unchanged. The transverse diameter of the ventricular atrium at the level of the glomus of the choroid plexus shows an average dimension of 8 mm and a range of 6 to 10 mm throughout the second and third trimesters.[95] This is the most convenient area to recognize fetal ventricular enlargement, as is discussed in detail in the section on ventriculomegaly in Chapter 11.[90, 91, 95] It is important to note that the anterior and occipital horns of the lateral ventricles do not possess choroid plexus. Between 24 weeks and term, the telencephalon undergoes little structural change other than increased cortical growth and the consequent increase in convolutions (and thus sulcal markings), which can be recognized adjacent to the convexities (Fig. 10–96).[96] The increase in brain volume causes the lateral ventricles, which are more stable in volume, to become progressively less conspicuous.

As opposed to sulci, which are narrow and develop later as gyri form, fissures are present earlier in development and can be seen before 20 weeks. Of the two that are commonly seen, the parieto-occipital fissure is smaller and less important (see Fig. 10–90). The lateral fissure is a deep groove in the margin of the developing telencephalon.[95, 97, 98] This important fissure results in frequent confusion because it causes a portion of the brain surface to be invaginated deeply into the hemisphere (see Figs. 10–88, 10–89, and 10–93). The pia-arachnoid on the surface of the insula, the tissue at the base of the lateral fissure, generates a curvilinear

reflection that appears to lie within the brain substance rather than at its "edge." This echo is often mistaken for a specular reflection from the lateral wall of the lateral ventricle, an error leading to misdiagnoses of hydrocephalus. With progressive growth of the temporal and parietal lobes this fissure progressively closes, burying the previously exposed insular cortex behind the developing temporal and parietal opercula (see Fig. 10–92). By term (38 to 42 weeks) the lateral fissure closes and ultimately becomes the sylvian cistern complex.

One of the difficulties in mastering the sonographic anatomy of intracranial structures is the usual inability to see both hemispheres of the brain symmetrically.[99] The hemisphere nearest to the transducer is virtually always "clouded" over by reverberation artifacts generated as the acoustic beam passes through the near calvarial wall. Calvarial ossification appears to be at the root of this artifact since the artifact is markedly reduced in fetuses with recessive osteogenesis imperfecta or other bone dysplasias wherein calvarial ossification is nearly absent (Fig. 10–97). Unfortunately, essentially all other fetuses possess calvarial ossification. The following rule should always be applied: *the sonologist must assume that the intracranial anatomy of the fetus is symmetric, whether normal or abnormal, unless images document an asymmetry.*

As noted earlier, the fetal spine is seen well from 15 to 16 weeks onward. However, evaluation for suspected myelomeningocele is often delayed until 18 to 22 weeks of gestation. This is due to significant and favorable maturational changes in the spine that occur during this period. The posterior ossification centers begin at the base of the transverse processes (see Figs. 10–48 through 10–54). As ossification progresses, the laminae become visible (see Figs. 10–49 through 10–

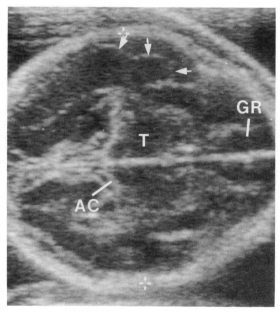

Figure 10–97. Transverse axial sonogram of a fetus with little calcification of the calvarium (recessive osteogenesis imperfecta). Note the lack of near calvarial reverberation artifact. T, thalamus; GR, gyrus rectus; AC, ambient cistern; arrows, near edge of temporal lobe.

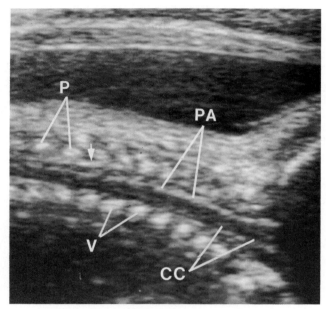

Figure 10–98. Longitudinal sonogram at the craniocervical junction demonstrating the cervical cord (CC). PA, pia-arachnoid; V, vertebral body ossification centers; arrow, dura; P, posterior arch ossification centers.

51 and 10–54). The inward angulation of the normal laminae is the opposite of the outward splaying of the laminae seen in spina bifida, an optimal situation for detecting this anomaly. Spina bifida, of course, is the bony anomaly seen in all myelomeningoceles. The spinal cord neural tissue, like that of most brain tissue, is echopenic (see Fig. 10–54). The conus medularis (see Fig. 10–54D) and the craniocervical junction (Fig. 10–98) can be seen, albeit inconsistently, in older fetuses. The tissues surrounding the cord (leptomeninges) are brightly echogenic, as are those that surround the brain, and the dura is usually also seen discretely as a linear bright reflector (see Fig. 10–54C and D).

References

1. Yousefzadeh DK, Naidich TP: US anatomy of the posterior fossa in children: Correlation with brain sections. Radiology 156:353, 1985.
2. Naidich TP, Gusnard DA, Yousefzadeh DK: Sonography of the internal capsule and basal ganglia in infants: I. Coronal sections. AJNR 6:909, 1985.
3. Filly RA, Callen PW: Ultrasonographic evaluation of normal fetal anatomy. In Sanders R, James E (eds): Ultrasonography in Obstetrics and Gynecology, 2nd ed. New York, Appleton-Century-Crofts, 1980.
4. Mahony BS, Filly RA: High-resolution sonographic assessment of the fetal extremities. J Ultrasound Med 3:489, 1984.
5. Cooperberg PL, Chow T, Kite V, et al: Biparietal diameter: A comparison of real-time and conventional B-scan techniques. J Clin Ultrasound 4:421, 1976.
6. Docher MF, Sellatree RS: Comparison between linear array, real-time ultrasonic scanning and conventional compound scanning in the measurement of the fetal biparietal diameter. Br J Obstet Gynecol 84:924, 1977.
7. Filly RA: Sonographic anatomy of the normal fetus. In Harrison MR, Golbus MS, Filly RA (eds): The Unborn Patient: Prenatal Diagnosis and Treatment. Philadelphia, WB Saunders, 1991.
8. Bowie JD, Rosenberg ER, Andreotti MD, et al: The changing sonographic appearance of the fetal kidneys during pregnancy. J Ultrasound Med 2:505, 1983.
9. Birnholz JC: The fetal external ear. Radiology 147:819, 1983.
10. Fink IJ, Chinn DH, Callen PW: A potential pitfall in the ultrasonographic diagnosis of fetal encephalocele. J Ultrasound Med 2:313, 1983.
11. Elejalde BR, de Elejalde MM, Heitman T: Visualization of the fetal genitalia by ultrasonography: A review of the literature and analysis of its accuracy and ethical implications. J Ultrasound Med 4:633, 1985.
12. Birnholz JC: Determination of fetal sex. N Engl J Med 309:942, 1983.
13. Natsuyama E: Sonographic determination of fetal sex from 12 weeks of gestation. Am J Obstet Gynecol 149:748, 1984.
14. Mahony BS, Filly RA, Callen PW: Amnionicity and chorionicity in twin pregnancies: Prediction using ultrasound. Radiology 155:205, 1985.
15. Filly RA, Golbus MS: Ultrasonography of the normal and pathologic fetal skeleton. Radiol Clin North Am 20:311, 1982.
16. Filly RA, Golbus MS, Carey JC, et al: Short-limbed dwarfism: Ultrasonic diagnosis by mensuration of fetal femoral length. Radiology 138:653, 1981.
17. O'Brien GB, Queenan JT, Campbell S: Assessment of gestation age in the second trimester by real-time ultrasound measurement of the femur length. Am J Obstet Gynecol 139:540, 1981.
18. Jeanty P, Kirkpatrick C, Dramaix-Wilmet M, et al: Ultrasonic evaluation of fetal limb growth. Radiology 140:165, 1981.
19. O'Rahilly R, Meyer DB: Roentgenographic investigation of the human skeleton during early fetal life. AJR 76:455, 1956.
20. Bagnall KM, Harris PF, James RM: A radiographic study of the human fetal spine: II. The sequence of development of ossification centers in the vertebral column. J Anat 124:791, 1977.
21. Filly RA, Simpson GF, Linkowski G: Fetal spine morphology and maturation during the second trimester: Sonographic evaluation. J Ultrasound Med 6:631, 1987.
22. Abrams SL, Filly RA: Curvature of the fetal femur: A normal sonographic finding. Radiology 156:490, 1985.
23. Yarkoni S, Schmidt W, Jeanty P, et al: Clavicular measurement: A new biometric parameter for fetal evaluation. J Ultrasound Med 4:467, 1985.
24. Jeanty P, Romero R, d'Alton M, et al: In utero sonographic detection of hand and foot deformities. J Ultrasound Med 4:595, 1985.
25. Bernacerraf BR, Frigoletto FD: Prenatal ultrasound diagnosis of clubfoot. Radiology 155:211, 1985.
26. Hashimoto BE, Filly RA, Callen PW: Sonographic diagnosis of clubfoot in utero. J Ultrasound Med 5:81, 1986.
27. Chinn DH, Bolding DB, Callen PW, et al: Ultrasonographic identification of fetal lower extremity epiphyseal ossification centers. Radiology 147:815, 1983.
28. Mahony SB, Callen PW, Filly RA: The distal femoral epiphyseal ossification center in the assessment of third trimester menstrual age: Sonographic identification and measurement. Radiology 155:201, 1985.
29. Goldstein RB, Filly RA, Simpson G: Pitfalls in femur length measurement. J Ultrasound Med 6:203, 1987.
30. Jeanty P, Cantraine F, Cousaert E, et al: The binocular distance: A new way to estimate fetal age. J Ultrasound Med 3:241, 1984.
31. Dennis MA, Drose JA, Pretorius DH, Manco-Johnson ML: Normal fetal sacrum simulating spina bifida: Pseudodysraphism. Radiology 155:751, 1985.
32. Abrams SL, Filly RA: Congenital vertebral malformations: Prenatal diagnosis using ultrasonography. Radiology 155:762, 1985.
33. Birnholz JC: Fetal lumbar spine: Measuring axial growth with ultrasound. Radiology 158:805, 1986.
34. Hashimoto BE, Mahony BS, Filly RA, et al: Sonography, a complementary examination to alpha-fetoprotein testing for neural tube defects. J Ultrasound Med 4:307, 1985.
35. Brown BS: The prenatal diagnosis of osteogenesis imperfecta lethalis. J Can Assoc Radiol 35:63, 1984.

36. Kousseff BG, Mulivor RA: Prenatal diagnosis of hypophosphatasia. Obstet Gynecol 57:9, 1981.
37. Merz E, Goldhofer W: Sonographic diagnosis of lethal osteogenesis imperfecta in the second trimester: Case report and review. J Clin Ultrasound 14:380, 1986.
38. Mahony BS, Filly RA, Cooperberg PL: Antenatal sonographic diagnosis of achondrogenesis. J Ultrasound Med 3:333, 1984.
39. Rosenthal SJ, Filly RA, Callen PW, et al: Fetal pseudoascites. Radiology 131:195, 1979.
40. Hashimoto BE, Filly RA, Callen PW: Fetal pseudoascites: Further observations. J Ultrasound Med 5:151, 1986.
41. Daffos F: Fetal blood sampling under ultrasound guidance. In Harrison MR, Golbus MS, Filly RA (eds): The Unborn Patient: Prenatal Diagnosis and Treatment, 2nd ed. Philadelphia, WB Saunders, 1991.
42. Moore KL: The placenta and fetal membranes. In The Developing Human: Clinically Oriented Embryology, 4th ed. Philadelphia, WB Saunders, 1988.
43. Chinn DH, Filly RA, Callen PW: Ultrasonic evaluation of fetal umbilical and hepatic vascular anatomy. Radiology 144:153, 1982.
44. Barron DH: The changes in the fetal circulation at birth. Physiol Rev 24:277, 1944.
45. Emery JL: Functional asymmetry of the liver. Ann NY Acad Sci 111:37, 1963.
46. Marks WM, Filly RA, Callen PW: Ultrasonic anatomy of the liver: A review with new applications. J Clin Ultrasound 7:137, 1979.
47. Gupta SC, Gupta CD, Arora AK: Intrahepatic branching patterns of portal veins: A study by corrosion cast. Gastroenterology 72:621, 1977.
48. Rosen MS, Reich SB: Umbilical venous catheterization in the newborn: Identification of correct positioning. Radiology 95:335, 1970.
49. Hattan RA, Rees GK, Johnson ML: Normal fetal anatomy. Radiol Clin North Am 20:271, 1982.
50. Goldstein RB, Callen PW: Ultrasound evaluation of the fetal thorax and abdomen. In Callen PW (ed): Ultrasonography in Obstetrics and Gynecology, 2nd ed. Philadelphia, WB Saunders, 1988.
51. Cooper C, Mahony BS, Bowie JD, et al: Ultrasound evaluation of the normal fetal upper airway and esophagus. J Ultrasound Med 4:343, 1985.
52. Pritchard JA: Fetal swallowing and amniotic fluid volume. Obstet Gynecol 28:606, 1966.
53. Abramovich DR: Fetal factors influencing the volume and composition of liquor amnii. J Obstet Gynecol Br Commonw 77:865, 1970.
54. Pretorius DH, Meier PR, Johnson ML: Diagnosis of esophageal atresia in utero. J Ultrasound Med 2:475, 1983.
55. Gross BH, Filly RA: Potential for a normal fetal stomach to simulate the sonographic "double bubble" sign. J Can Assoc Radiol 33:39, 1982.
56. Grand RJ, Watkins JB, Torti FM: Development of the human gastrointestinal tract. Gastroenterology 70:790, 1976.
57. Manco LG, Nunan FA, Sohnen H, et al: Fetal small bowel simulating abdominal mass at sonography. J Clin Ultrasound 14:404, 1986.
58. Fakhry J, Reiser M, Shapiro LR, et al: Increased echogenicity in the lower fetal abdomen: A common normal variant in the second trimester. J Ultrasound Med 5:489, 1986.
59. Zilianti M, Fernandez A: Correlation of ultrasonic images of fetal intestine with gestational age and fetal maturity. Obstet Gynecol 62:569, 1983.
60. Nygerg DA, Mack LA, Patten RM, et al: Fetal bowel, normal sonographic findings. J Ultrasound Med 6:3, 1987.
61. Crelin ES: Functional Anatomy of the Newborn, pp 47–69. New Haven, CT, Yale University Press, 1973.
62. Schmidt W, Yarkoni S, Jeanty P, et al: Sonographic measurements of the fetal spleen: Clinical implications. J Ultrasound Med 4:667, 1985.
63. Potter EL: Pathology of the Fetus and Infant. Chicago, Year Book Medical Publishers, 1961.
64. Gruenwald P, Minh HN: Evaluation of body and organ weights in perinatal pathology. Am J Clin Pathol 34:247, 1960.
65. Mittlestaedt CA: Ultrasound of the spleen. Semin Ultrasound 2:233, 1981.
66. Fried AM, Loh FK, Umer MA, et al: Echogenicity of fetal lung: Relation to fetal age and maturity. AJR 145:591, 1985.
67. Cayea PD, Grant DC, Doubilet PM, et al: Prediction of fetal lung maturity: Inaccuracy of study using conventional ultrasound instruments. Radiology 155:473, 1985.
68. Lawson TL, Foley WD, Berland LL, et al: Ultrasonic evaluation of fetal kidneys: Analysis of normal size and frequency of visualization as related to stage of pregnancy. Radiology 138:153, 1981.
69. Bowie JD, Rosenberg ER, Andreotti MD, et al: The changing sonographic appearance of fetal kidneys during pregnancy. J Ultrasound Med 2:505, 1983.
70. Hoddick WK, Filly RA, Mahony BS, Callen PW: Minimal fetal renal pyelectasis. J Ultrasound Med 4:85, 1985.
71. Arger PH, Coleman BG, Mintz MD, et al: Routine fetal genitourinary tract screening. Radiology 156:485, 1985.
72. Grannum P, Bracken M, Silverman R, et al: Assessment of fetal kidney size in normal gestation by comparison of ratio of kidney circumference to abdominal circumference. Am J Obstet Gynecol 136:249, 1980.
73. Jeanty P, Dramaix-Wilmet M, Elkhazen N: Measurement of fetal kidney growth on ultrasound. Radiology 144:159, 1982.
74. Bertagnoli L, Lalatta F, Gallicchio MD, et al: Quantitative characterization of the growth of the fetal kidney. J Clin Ultrasound 11:349, 1983.
75. Wladimiroff JW, Campbell S: Fetal urine-production rates in normal and complicated pregnancy. Lancet 1:151, 1974.
76. Campbell S, Wladimiroff JW, Dewhurst CJ: The antenatal measurement of fetal urine production. J Obstet Gynecol Br Commonw 80:680, 1973.
77. Chamberlain P, Manning FA, Morrison I, et al: Circadian rhythm in bladder volumes in the term human fetus. Obstet Gynecol 64:657, 1984.
78. Rosenberg ER, Bowie JD, Andreotti RF, et al: Sonographic evaluation of fetal adrenal glands. AJR 139:1145, 1982.
79. Co S, Filly RA: Normal fetal adrenal gland location. J Ultrasound Med 5:117, 1986.
80. Goldberg BB, Isard HJ, Gershon-Cohen J, et al: Ultrasonic fetal cephalometry. Radiology 87:328, 1966.
81. Hidalgo H, Bowie J, Rosenberg ER, et al: In utero sonographic diagnosis of fetal cerebral anomalies. AJR 139:143, 1982.
82. Fiske CE, Filly RA: Ultrasound evaluation of the normal and abnormal fetal neural axis. Radiol Clin North Am 20:285, 1982.
83. Pasto ME, Kurtz AB: The prenatal examination of the fetal cranium, spine, and central nervous system. Semin Ultrasound CT MR 5:170, 1984.
84. Filly RA: Ultrasonography. In Harrison MR, Golbus MS, Filly RA (eds): The Unborn Patient: Prenatal Diagnosis and Treatment, pp 33–123. Orlando, FL, Grune & Stratton, 1984.
85. Carrasco CR, Stierman ED, Harnsberger HR, Lee TG: An algorithm for prenatal ultrasound diagnosis of congenital CNS abnormalities. J Ultrasound Med 4:163, 1985.
86. Edwards MSD, Filly RA: Diagnosis and management of fetal disorders of the central nervous system. In Hoffman HJ, Epstein F (eds): Disorders of the Developing Nervous System: Diagnosis and Treatment, pp 55–73. Boston, Blackwell Scientific Publications, 1986.
87. Young GB: The arrow pattern: A new anatomical fetal biparietal diameter. Radiology 137:445, 1980.
88. Jeanty P, Chervenak FA, Romero R, et al: The Sylvian fissure: A commonly mislabeled cranial landmark. J Ultrasound Med 3:15, 1984.
89. Denkhaus H, Winseberg F: Ultrasonic measurement of the fetal ventricular system. Radiology 131:781, 1979.
90. Chinn DH, Callen PW, Filly RA: The lateral cerebral ventricle in early second trimester. Radiology 148:529, 1983.
91. Fiske CE, Filly RA, Callen PW: The normal choroid plexus: Ultrasonographic appearance of the neonatal head. Radiology 141:467, 1981.
92. Johnson ML, Dunne MG, Mack LA, Rashbaum CL: Evaluation of fetal intracranial anatomy by static and real-time ultrasound. J Clin Ultrasound 8:311, 1980.
93. Jeanty P, Dramaix-Wilmet M, Delbeke D, et al: Ultrasonic

evaluation of fetal ventricular growth. Neuroradiology 21:127, 1981.

94. Day WR: Casts of the foetal lateral ventricles. Brain 82:109, 1959.

95. Seidler DE, Filly RA: Relative growth of the higher fetal brain structures. J Ultrasound Med 6:573–576, 1987.

96. Worthen NJ, Gilbertson V, Lau C: Cortical sulcal development seen on sonography: Relationship to gestational parameters. J Ultrasound Med 5:153, 1986.

97. Pilu G, DePalma L, Romero R, et al: The fetal subarachnoid cisterns: An ultrasound study with report of a case of congenital communicating hydrocephalus. J Ultrasound Med 5:365, 1986.

98. Laing FC, Stamler CE, Jeffrey RB: Ultrasonography of the fetal subarachnoid space. J Ultrasound Med 2:29, 1983.

99. Reuter KG, D'Orsi CJ, Ratopoulos VD, et al: Sonographic pseudoasymmetry of the prenatal cerebral hemispheres. J Ultrasound Med 1:91; 1982.

CHAPTER 11

Ultrasound Evaluation of the Fetal Neural Axis

ROY A. FILLY, M.D.

Among the various fetal anomalies that can be diagnosed by sonography, central nervous system (CNS) abnormalities are probably the most devastating in their clinical consequences and, therefore, it is important that these abnormalities be recognized at an early stage. Each year in the United States, approximately 6000 neonates are afflicted with one of these congenital anomalies.[1] Early in the use of prenatal sonography, only defects producing gross anatomic distortions were detected.[2] Recent rapid technologic advances now allow early and accurate diagnosis of numerous CNS malformations.[3–7] As a result, the sonologist, by observation and diagnosis, frequently initiates a decision-making process that involves the obstetrician and the prospective parents with regard to making difficult choices. Consequently, the sonologist must provide accurate and reliable information on which these decisions can be based. Knowledge of normal and abnormal developmental neuroanatomy is essential to identify specific malformations.

With widespread use of prenatal sonography, increasing numbers of fetal CNS anomalies are being detected.[3–6] In certain circumstances, a patient may be referred so that a search can be made for a specific anatomic malformation. An example of such a case would be a pregnant woman who had previously been delivered of a child with an open neural tube defect. Her present fetus has an increased risk of having the same or a similar anomaly. However, in most cases, fetal neural defects are identified serendipitously during examinations performed for obstetric indications. Although it is uncertain whether the diagnosis of a CNS defect in utero can influence the eventual outcome for the fetus, recognition of structural abnormalities before birth helps to provide time to counsel the family and may significantly affect obstetric management.[7]

When severe anomalies, which are incompatible with postnatal survival, are diagnosed in utero (e.g., anencephaly), the parents may choose to terminate the pregnancy. When lesions that require surgical correction at, or soon after, birth are diagnosed (e.g., myelomeningocele), arrangements can be made for delivery at a hospital where immediate repair is possible. Hydrocephalus and certain other CNS anomalies frequently cause dystocia and therefore require either a planned cesarean section or cephalocentesis to allow a vaginal delivery. Increasing hydrocephalus may cause progressive neurologic damage that may necessitate early delivery to hasten treatment in an ex utero environment. Finally, some abnormalities may cause progressive harm or may interfere with normal development before fetal viability (e.g., potentially some cases of progressive hydrocephalus). In this latter case, sonographically guided techniques are available for intervention before birth.[8]

A great deal can be learned with regard to the natural history of certain CNS anomalies that have been diagnosed prenatally. Furthermore, the area of sonographic CNS diagnosis is still in its early stages, and even the most experienced sonologists realize that, despite the sophisticated techniques available, it is still quite possible to miss subtle but life-threatening anomalies that could alter the expected outcome and make certain choices of treatment inappropriate. Therefore, as our knowledge of these disorders increases and as our techniques for their diagnosis and management become more reliable, the decision-making process preceding and after diagnosis will undoubtedly change. In this chapter, the development of the fetal brain and spinal cord, as well as the diagnosis of CNS anomalies, is discussed in detail.

EMBRYOLOGIC DEVELOPMENT OF THE BRAIN*

Sonologists have an opportunity to visualize the developing brain with some degree of clarity from the latter portion of the first trimester onward. Despite this long period of observation and an ability to examine the human brain earlier than with any other available modality, it is important to recall that most specific brain structures have already developed before sonologists have an opportunity to begin observations.

The CNS develops from a thickened area of embryonic ectoderm called the neural plate.[9] The neural plate develops at 18 to 20 days after conception or 4.5 weeks after the beginning of the last normal menstrual period (LNMP). Promptly thereafter, the neural plate begins to alter and forms both the neural tube and the neural crest (Fig. 11–1). The neural tube differentiates into the CNS, consisting of both the brain and the spinal cord. The neural crest gives rise to most of the structures in the peripheral nervous system.

The neural tube is open temporarily at both the cranial and the caudal ends (see Fig. 11–1). The cranial opening or the rostral neuropore closes about 24 days after conception (38 days after the LNMP). The caudal

---

*This section has been excerpted mainly from Moore KL: The nervous system. In The Developing Human, 4th ed, pp 364–401. Philadelphia, WB Saunders, 1988.

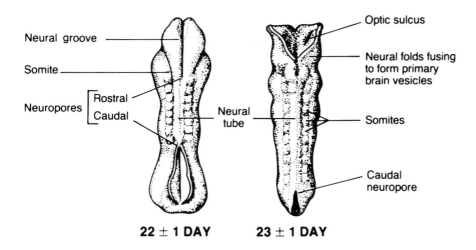

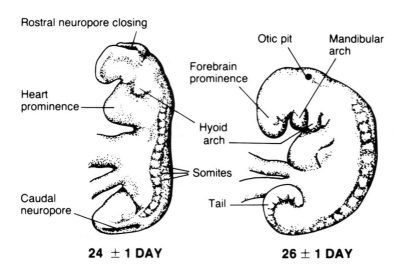

Figure 11–1. Development of the neural tube (22 to 26 days). (From Moore KL, Persaud TVN: The Developing Human: Clinically Oriented Embryology, 5th ed. Philadelphia, WB Saunders, 1993.)

neuropore closes slightly later (26 days after conception, 40 days after the LNMP). The walls of the tube thicken to form various portions of the brain and the spinal cord. The lumen of the neural tube becomes the ventricular system of the brain cranially and the central canal of the spinal cord caudally.

Growth and differentiation of the neural tube are greatest at the cranial end. Toward the end of the fourth week after conception (6 menstrual weeks), the cranial end of the neural tube differentiates into three primary brain vesicles (Fig. 11–2). These vesicles consist of the prosencephalon (forebrain), the mesencephalon (midbrain), and the rhombencephalon (hindbrain). During the ensuing week the forebrain further differentiates into the telencephalon (end brain), which is the most rostral portion of the embryonic brain, and the diencephalon (intermediate brain). Similarly, the hindbrain divides into the metencephalon and myelencephalon. As a result of these partial divisions, five secondary brain vesicles now exist. In addition to the aforementioned process of diverticulation, flexion of the developing brain further discriminates among these discrete areas of early brain morphology.

The diencephalon is positioned centrally, whereas the telencephalon consists of lateral expansions (i.e.,

the right and left cerebral vesicles) (see Fig. 11–2). The diencephalon develops from the tissues of the walls of the third ventricle that form three discrete swellings; the epithalamus, the thalamus, and the hypothalamus. The thalamus is the dominant portion of the diencephalon and enlarges rapidly. While this enlargement occurs, the thalami bulge into the cavity of the third ventricle and reduce the ventricular lumen to a narrow cleft, an event that has occurred by the time the developing brain can be visualized sonographically with any degree of clarity. The thalami usually meet and fuse in the midline. The bridge formed by this fusion is called the massa intermedia. The hypothalamus gives rise to the adult structure of the same name, whereas the epithalamus gives rise predominantly to the pineal gland.

The telencephalic or cerebral vesicles, when these first arise, communicate widely with the cavity of the third ventricle (see Fig. 11–2). Along the choroidal fissure, the medial wall of the developing cerebral hemisphere becomes thin. Invaginations of vascular pia form the choroid plexus of the lateral ventricles at this site. The expanding hemispheres progressively cover the surfaces of the diencephalon, the midbrain, and, ultimately, the hindbrain (Fig. 11–3). As the

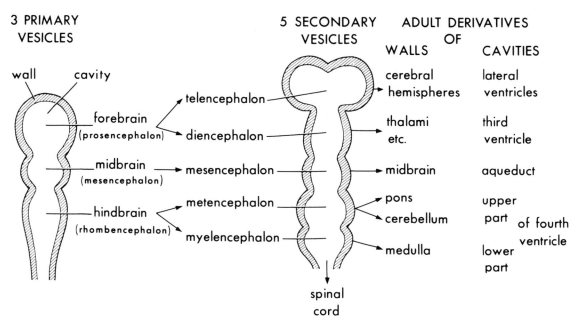

Figure 11–2. Early development of the human fetal brain, with the adult derivatives of the fetal precursors. (From Moore KL, Persaud TVM: The Developing Human: Clinically Oriented Embryology, 5th ed. Philadelphia, WB Saunders, 1993.)

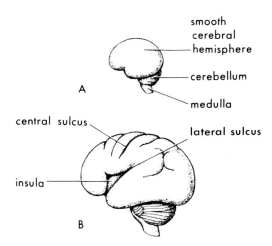

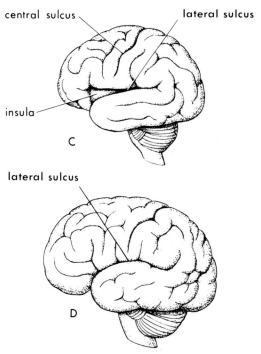

Figure 11–3. *A* through *D.* Development of the telencephalon, demonstrating dramatic growth with progressive development of the fissures and sulci. The open lateral sulcus matures into the sylvian cistern. The exposed insula "disappears" behind the temporal and parietal opercula. (From Moore KL, Persaud TVM: The Developing Human: Clinically Oriented Embryology, 5th ed. Philadelphia, WB Saunders, 1993.)

hemispheres grow and meet in the midline, mesenchyme is trapped and gives rise to the falx cerebri. This sequence discretely separates the lateral ventricles from the third ventricle. At this early stage only the frontal horns, bodies, and atria of the lateral ventricles exist (Fig. 11–4). Growth of the temporal and occipital lobes eventuates in the formation of discrete occipital and temporal horns.[10] These horns are not clearly demarcated until between 16 and 18 weeks of development.

Returning to the sixth week of development (8 menstrual weeks), a swelling appears in the floor of each cerebral vesicle. This structure is known as the corpus striatum. As the cerebral cortex develops further, fibers pass to and from the developing hemispheres through the corpus striatum and divide it into

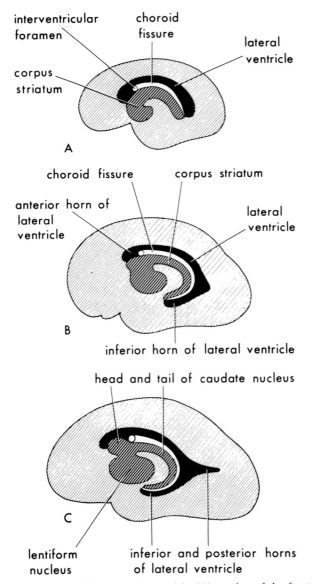

interventricular foramen
choroid fissure
lateral ventricle
corpus striatum

A

choroid fissure
corpus striatum
anterior horn of lateral ventricle
lateral ventricle

B

inferior horn of lateral ventricle

head and tail of caudate nucleus

C

lentiform nucleus
inferior and posterior horns of lateral ventricle

Figure 11–4. The early lateral ventricle *(A)* consists of the frontal horn, body, and atrium. Later, temporal *(B)* and occipital *(C)* horns develop; sonography can visualize the fetal ventricular system before these structures develop. (From Moore KL, Persaud TVM: The Developing Human: Clinically Oriented Embryology, 5th ed. Philadelphia, WB Saunders, 1993.)

the caudate and lentiform nuclei. This fiber path is the internal capsule.

The mesencephalon undergoes less change than do other parts of the developing brain. The lumen of this vesicle narrows to form the sylvian aqueduct. Four large groups of neurons form in the roof of the midbrain, which are known as the superior and inferior colliculi (quadrigeminal body). In the basal portion of the midbrain, fibers passing from the growing cerebrum form the cerebral peduncles. A broad layer of gray matter adjacent to these large fiber tracts is known as the substantia nigra.

The rhombencephalon undergoes flexion (pontine flexure), which divides the hindbrain into the metencephalon and myelencephalon. The myelencephalon changes little and becomes the medulla, whereas the metencephalon changes dramatically and gives rise to the pons and the cerebellum. The cerebellum originates from paired, symmetric swellings positioned dorsally. The fourth ventricle forms from the cavity of the hindbrain and, like the lateral and third ventricles, contains choroid plexus derived from an invagination of vascular pia into the ependyma-lined cavity of the hindbrain.

A substantial number of brain anomalies are already present when the early process of brain development is complete (e.g., anencephaly, holoprosencephaly, Dandy-Walker malformation, encephalocele) but are usually not recognizable on sonograms until later in gestation. Further growth of the calvaria and progressive aberration of brain development do, however, enable sonologists to recognize some of these abnormalities near the end of the first trimester and at the beginning of the second trimester.

INFRATENTORIAL ANOMALIES

Dandy-Walker Syndrome

The Dandy-Walker syndrome is a spectrum of disorders resulting from abnormal development of the cerebellum with associated maldevelopment of the fourth ventricle.[11–20] The fundamental features include enlargement of the fourth ventricle, atresia of the Luschka and Magendie foramina (although these may be patent), agenesis or hypoplasia of the cerebellar vermis, and a variable degree of hydrocephalus.

The enlargement of the fourth ventricle is often so dramatic that a large cyst occupies and expands the posterior fossa (the Dandy-Walker cyst) (Fig. 11–5). The expansion elevates the tentorium and the torcula.[11, 12] The former can be easily seen sonographically, but the latter cannot. The cyst covering is the posterior medullary velum that bulges upward in the presence of the vermal defect. Thus, the inner cellular layer of the cyst is ependyma, and the outer layer is pia-arachnoid.[12] There is a potential for great variation in both the size of the fourth ventricle and in the degree of dysgenesis of the vermis. These features affect the ease of detection of this anomaly in utero. This anomaly is established early in the development

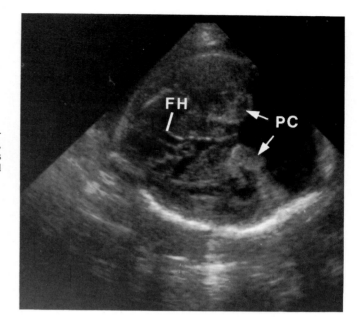

Figure 11–5. Transverse axial sonogram of a fetus with Dandy-Walker syndrome. Arrows indicate cerebellar hemispheres. FH, frontal horn; PC, posterior fossa cyst. (From Harrison MR, Golbus MS, Filly RA [eds]: The Unborn Patient: Prenatal Diagnosis and Treatment, 2nd ed. Philadelphia, WB Saunders, 1990.)

of the fetus and can often be detected before 20 menstrual weeks (Fig. 11–6).

Dandy-Walker syndrome is commonly associated with hydrocephalus (Fig. 11–7) and agenesis of the corpus callosum (Fig. 11–8).[11, 12] Hydrocephalus may dominate the dysmorphic appearance. Importantly, colpocephaly, associated with callosal agenesis, may yield the mistaken impression that hydrocephalus complicates a Dandy-Walker malformation (see Fig. 11–8 and the section on agenesis of the corpus callosum). The degree of supratentorial ventricular enlargement does not correlate with the patency of the foramina, the vermal hypoplasia, or the size of the fourth ventricular cyst (see Fig. 11–7). When the defect in the vermis is small (usually inferior), the fourth ventricle bulges into the void provided by the cisterna magna. This space may only appear slightly larger than average under these circumstances. The enlarged fourth ventricle generates no mass effect. An evaluation of the "large" cisterna magna is discussed in detail subsequently.

The structures involved in this complex malformation include the vermis, posterior medullary velum, fourth ventricle, and corpus callosum, which are all midline structures. This anomaly appears most appropriately to be categorized with other midline anomalies. However, because the major dysmorphic features reside in the posterior fossa, it tends to be treated independently in differential diagnostic considerations.

Although the features of this malformation are often "classic" and easily recognized,[14, 15] its differential diagnosis from other posterior fossa aberrations is important because the prognosis varies from normal to marked disability depending on the severity of the brain malformation and on the association of anomalies outside the CNS.[11, 12] The sine qua non for the firm diagnosis of Dandy-Walker syndrome is the separation of the cerebellar hemispheres by the enlarged fourth ventricle (see Figs. 11–5 through 11–8). Thus, it is not the presence of the large posterior fossa fluid collection that enables the diagnosis to be made but the effect of the fluid collection on the cerebellum. When the Dandy-Walker cyst is large, the cerebellar hemispheres are widely displaced and compressed against the tentorium (see Figs. 11–5 and 11–6). Additionally, the hemispheres are small both from compression by the cyst and in absolute mass. Thus, they must be sought carefully.

The major competing diagnosis when a large posterior fossa cyst is seen is an arachnoid cyst (Fig. 11–9).[14] A retrocerebellar arachnoid cyst is a less common and more benign abnormality than Dandy-Walker syndrome, because the underlying brain is normally formed. This lesion always generates a mass effect, but

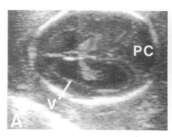
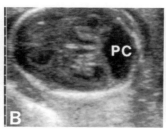
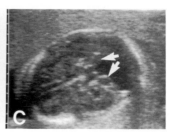

Figure 11–6. *A.* Transverse axial sonogram demonstrating a posterior fossa cyst (PC) and ventricular enlargement (V). *B.* Large posterior fossa cyst (PC). *C.* Small and separated cerebellar hemispheres *(arrows).*

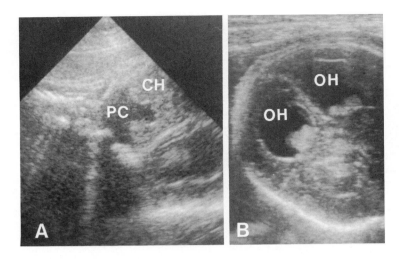

Figure 11–7. *A.* Sonogram of the posterior fossa. A relatively small posterior fossa cyst (PC) is shown. CH, cerebellar hemisphere. *B.* Note the marked dilatation of the occipital horns (OH).

instead of the cystic mass separating the cerebellar hemispheres it displaces these hemispheres en bloc (see Fig. 11–9). Such a mass may well elevate the tentorium. Thus, this feature is not differentially diagnostic.

It is important in the evaluation of a fetus with a posterior fossa cyst to carefully examine the supertentorial compartment. As noted earlier, ventriculomegaly may be present and may represent true hydrocephalus or colpocephaly associated with agenesis of the corpus callosum. Features of agenesis of the corpus callosum should be sought. Large retrocerebellar arachnoid cysts may also produce ventricular enlargement by compression, but these cysts are not associated with agenesis of the corpus callosum or colpocephaly.

Other Infratentorial Abnormalities

In the preceding section, the diagnosis of Dandy-Walker syndrome and its distinction from a retrocere-bellar arachnoid cyst was considered. These entities appear to be similar when a large cyst is generated by the underlying abnormality. However, the most difficult situation arises when the cisterna magna appears to be large.[21–23] Because several congenital posterior fossa lesions alter the size of the cisterna magna, an evaluation of the fetal cisterna magna is important in assessing infratentorial anatomy and pathology.[21] The cisterna magna consists of a portion of the subarachnoid space that bathes the posterior fossa with cerebrospinal fluid (CSF). It arches around the cerebellum posteriorly and is normally deepest in the midline, where invagination of the space occurs between the two cerebellar hemispheres. Antenatal sonography readily demonstrates the normal cisterna magna, especially between 16 and 28 menstrual weeks (Fig. 11–10). An evaluation of the cisterna magna in utero has documented that its depth measures 5 ± 3 mm; the largest cisterna magna measured was 10 mm in depth.[21] However, overzealous inclination of the plane of sec-

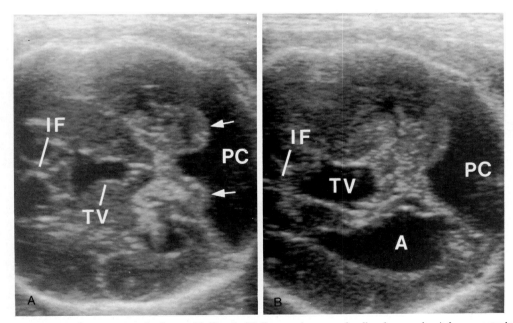

Figure 11–8. *A.* Transverse axial sonogram of a fetus with Dandy-Walker syndrome and callosal agenesis. A large posterior fossa cyst (PC) insinuates between the cerebellar hemispheres *(arrows).* TV, enlarged and abnormally shaped third ventricle. *B.* Transverse axial sonogram showing colpocephaly (enlarged atrium [A]). The third ventricle (TV) lies in a high position and insinuates into the interhemispheric fissure (IF).

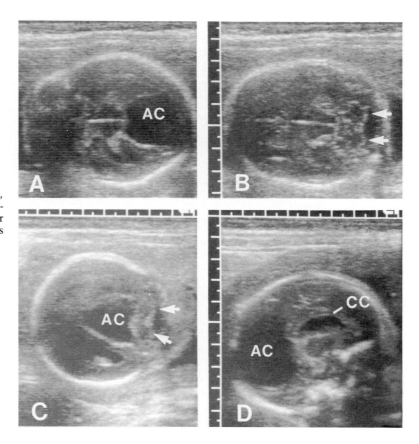

Figure 11–9. Transverse axial *(A and B)*, coronal *(C)*, and midsagittal *(D)* sonograms of a fetus with a retrocerebellar arachnoid cyst (AC). Note that the cerebellar hemispheres *(arrows)* are not separated. CC, corpus callosum.

tion through the posterior fossa can increase this measurement (Fig. 11–11), sometimes to a dimension as great as 13 or 14 mm in normal subjects. As expected, this does not differ significantly in preterm neonates.[13]

When the cisterna magna is enlarged, the examiner must distinguish among competing diagnoses of normal variant (Fig. 11–12), communicating hydrocephalus, cerebellar hypoplasia (Fig. 11–13), and Dandy-Walker or retrocerebellar arachnoid cyst (see Fig. 11–9). Cerebellar hypoplasia can be excluded by measuring the

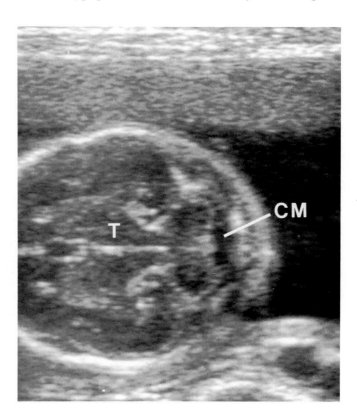

Figure 11–10. Transverse axial sonogram demonstrates a normal fetal cisterna magna (CM) dimension. T, thalamus.

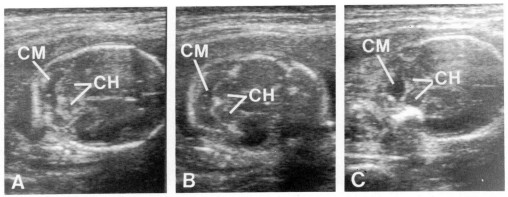

Figure 11–11. Normal cisterna magna (CM). Note that the inclination of the planes of the section (*A, B,* and *C*) alters the apparent depth of the cistern. CH, cerebellar hemispheres. (From Harrison MR, Golbus MS, Filly RA [eds]: The Unborn Patient: Prenatal Diagnosis and Treatment, 2nd ed. Philadelphia, WB Saunders, 1990.)

diameter of the cerebellar hemispheres and by comparing this measurement with published standards of size versus menstrual age.[22] Exclusion of cerebellar hypoplasia is important because chromosomal anomalies are associated with this entity, and a fetal karyotype is therefore required.

Communicating hydrocephalus is rare in fetuses and is excluded when an absence of ventricular dilatation is noted. Usually, in the case under consideration, only the enlarged cisterna magna is evident. Finally, a close examination of the junction of the cerebellar hemi-

spheres is indicated to look for clefting, which may be seen with small Dandy-Walker malformations. An enlarged cisterna magna (see Fig. 11–12), as a normal variant, or a small retrocerebellar arachnoid cyst constitutes a diagnosis of exclusion. Because it is essentially impossible to exclude subtle vermian dysgenesis with in utero sonography alone, these benign presumptive diagnoses are unsettling. Some consolation may be taken from the relatively benign course of mild cases of Dandy-Walker syndrome; patients affected by this syndrome may develop normally. Indeed, inferior

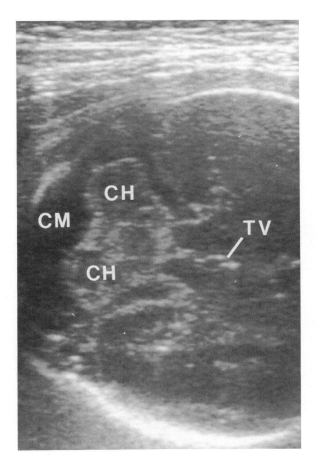

Figure 11–12. Transverse axial sonogram of a large, but normal, cisterna magna (CM). Note that the fluid collection does not affect the junction of the cerebellar hemispheres (CH). TV, third ventricle.

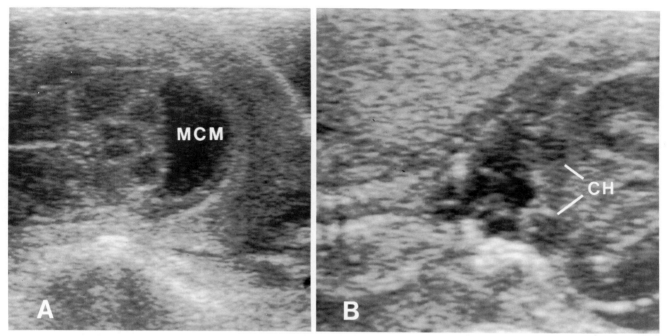

Figure 11–13. *A* and *B.* Two views of the posterior fossa. A chromosomally anomalous fetus in a severely oligohydramniotic sac has a large cisterna magna (MCM). Normally joined but small cerebellar hemispheres (CH) indicate the presence of cerebellar hypoplasia.

vermian agenesis may differ entirely from Dandy-Walker syndrome.

SUPRATENTORIAL ANOMALIES

Agenesis of the Corpus Callosum

The corpus callosum is the largest fiber tract within the CNS.[24–26] The fetal corpus callosum is much smaller than that found in the adult. However, sonographic resolution is sufficiently good that this structure can be detected occasionally in fetuses less than 20 weeks' gestational age (see Fig. 11–9D). This fiber tract consists of commissural fibers that radiate among symmetric regions of the cerebral cortex and serves a function both in learning and memory that is shared between cerebral hemispheres.[24]

Development of the corpus callosum does not begin until the 12th week and is incomplete until the 17th week.[27] Therefore, by comparison with most CNS structures, its development is late. Development begins anteriorly (rostrum and genu) and proceeds posteriorly (splenium). Partial interruption of callosal development, therefore, tends to affect the posterior aspect of this large fiber tract. The septum pellucidum is formed concomitantly with the corpus callosum, stretching between the corpus callosum and the fornices, which is an important feature in the exclusion of anomalous development of this structure on sonographic images.

Dysgenesis of the corpus callosum ranges from complete to partial absence. When partially absent, the abnormality usually lies in the region of the splenium (the most dorsal portion).[24–27] Up to the present time, only complete agenesis of the corpus callosum has been diagnosed in utero by sonography.[28] The appearance of complete agenesis of the corpus callosum is typical on sectional imaging studies of the neonate, such as computed tomography, transfontanelle sonography, and magnetic resonance imaging.[29–33] The characteristic features seen at birth extrapolate appropriately to the fetus.

The striking dysmorphic features relate to the changed appearance of the supratentorial ventricular system when the corpus callosum fails to develop. The presence of the corpus callosum does a great deal to shape the ventricles, such as they are seen in normal fetuses. When the corpus callosum is absent, the fibers that were destined to cross in this tract have still developed, although these fibers now run in thick longitudinal (Probst) bundles along the medial walls of the lateral ventricles (Figs. 11–14B and 11–15B).[25] The effects of these bundles on the appearance of the lateral

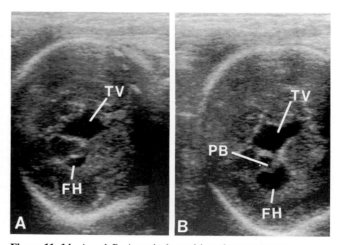

Figure 11–14. *A* and *B.* Anteriorly positioned coronal sonograms of a fetus with agenesis of the corpus callosum. Enlarged and high-riding third ventricle (TV). The frontal horns (FH) are indented medially by the Probst bundles (PB).

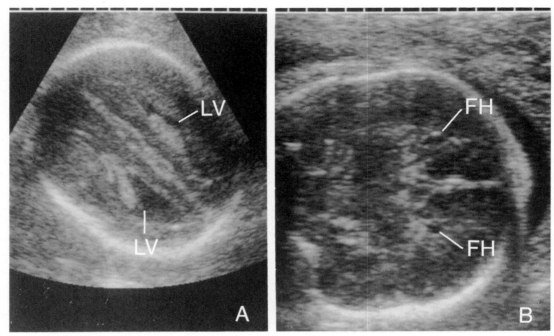

Figure 11–15. Transverse axial *(A)* and coronal *(B)* sonogram of a fetus with agenesis of the corpus callosum. The lateral ventricles (LV) are more laterally and superiorly positioned and the frontal horn (FH) is indented.

ventricles are (1) the ventricles are "displaced" more laterally (Fig. 11–15*A*); and (2) the medial walls are "indented," resulting in the characteristic shape seen on coronal sections when this anomaly is present (see Fig. 11–14). This latter appearance causes the ventricles to have a crescentic shape, and this appearance has been compared with the horns of a steer, especially when seen on coronal planes in the frontal regions.

The absence of the large callosal tract over the roof of the ventricles allows the latter to extend more cranially. This is most evident when viewing the third ventricle but is also true of the lateral ventricles (Fig. 11–16). The third ventricle may, in some cases, expand dramatically, herniating upward between the hemispheres. This produces the "interhemispheric cyst," which is not infrequently seen in this anomaly (Fig. 11–17).

Deep white matter of the cerebrum is poorly developed in this condition and results in the feature that first draws attention to possible maldevelopment of the brain. The poorly developed white matter surrounding the atria and occipital horns of the lateral ventricles results in a measurable enlargement of these portions of the lateral ventricles (called colpocephaly) (see Figs. 11–8 and 11–17). This type of ventriculomegaly is important because it initiates a critical evaluation of the CNS anatomy that one hopes ends in the correct diagnosis of callosal agenesis and also because it is an excellent example that ventricular enlargement does not always result from ventricular obstruction. Although fetuses with agenesis of the corpus callosum may develop true hydrocephalus, colpocephaly is not aided by shunting procedures.[26] When ventriculomegaly is noted in the atrial and occipital regions (i.e., possible colpocephaly), the association of midline developmental anomalies should be excluded. Ordinarily,

if one suspects callosal agenesis, an attempt would be made to demonstrate the corpus callosum. Unfortunately, this is a difficult structure to document consistently. However, the development of the corpus cal-

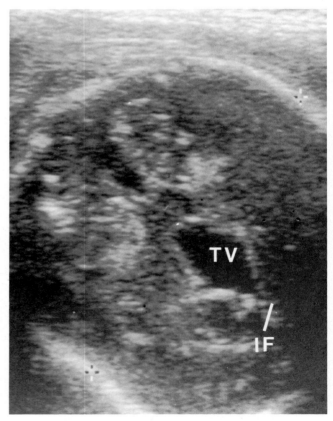

Figure 11–16. Transverse axial sonogram of the high-riding third ventricle (TV) insinuating into the interhemispheric fissure (IF).

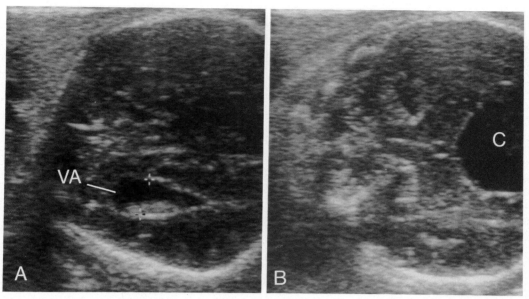

Figure 11–17. Transverse axial *(A)* and coronal *(B)* sonograms of a fetus with agenesis of the corpus callosum. The ventricular atrium (VA) has a "teardrop" configuration. A large interhemispheric cyst (C) is seen.

losum is related integrally to the development of the septum pellucidum and to the cavum septi pellucidi.[24, 27] The cavum septi pellucidi is readily demonstrated in all fetuses with normal development of midline structures. Thus, documentation of the cavum septi pellucidi excludes complete agenesis of the corpus callosum.

The elevation of the third ventricle described earlier, the medial indentation of the frontal horns, and the abnormal axis of the lateral ventricles should be sought sonographically to confirm the diagnosis of callosal agenesis. Finally, the missing corpus callosum results in an abnormal pattern of gyral development along the interhemispheric fissure that can be seen sonographically.[24] The sulci radiate toward the third ventricle and create a wavy appearance of the midline in transverse axial planes of section. Unfortunately, because gyri do not develop until late in pregnancy, this feature is not useful in the early diagnosis of callosal agenesis.

Although agenesis of the corpus callosum may be seen as an isolated lesion, it is also associated with various other CNS malformations and syndromes.[24] Associated CNS malformations include the holoprosencephalies. In alobar holoprosencephaly, callosal agenesis does not dominate the appearance of the CNS malformation, although it is always present. Conversely, in the lesser (lobar) form of holoprosencephaly, this feature may dominate the sonographic picture. Interestingly, fetuses with isolated agenesis of the corpus callosum may have the same type of central clefting of the lip that is commonly associated with lesser forms of holoprosencephaly. Callosal agenesis also often accompanies the Dandy-Walker malformation (see Fig. 11–8). Other CNS malformations that may be present include dysgenesis or hypoplasia of the falx, cranial lipoma, and heterotopic gray matter. Trisomy 13 may be present, and fetal karyotyping is indicated. Trisomy 8 and trisomy 18 have also been reported with callosal agenesis. Female fetuses with callosal agenesis are at risk for Aicardi syndrome,

which includes mental retardation and chorioretinopathy.

The prognosis in agenesis of the corpus callosum may depend more on the associated abnormalities than on the callosal agenesis itself. Importantly, some of these important associated malformations may not be indicated by sonography. Although it is true that isolated agenesis may be asymptomatic, low intelligence occurs in 70% and seizures occur in 60% of these patients.[24] Hydrocephalus, distinct from colpocephaly, may require ventricular shunting. There may also be disturbances of hypothalamic function.

Isolated complete agenesis of the corpus callosum and minor forms of holoprosencephaly have some obvious similarities. Although they can be distinguished pathologically, one must assume, at present, that they cannot be accurately discriminated in utero. Thus, features suggesting one should result in a differential diagnosis that includes both. Pathologically, agenesis of the corpus callosum has an absence of the lamina terminalis, but fornices are usually present, whereas in lobar holoprosencephaly the lamina terminalis is thickened and fornices are never present. In agenesis of the corpus callosum, the thalami are separated and usually more so than normal (i.e., enlarged third ventricle), whereas in lobar holoprosencephaly they may be fused. Furthermore, the frontal lobes may be fused in lobar holoprosencephaly, a feature not present in callosal agenesis. Most of these discriminatory features cannot be seen on in utero sonograms. However, fusion of the thalami may be discernible and, in some cases, differentiates these anomalies.

Holoprosencephaly

The term *holoprosencephaly* refers to a group of disorders arising from a failure of normal forebrain development during early embryonic life.[34–44] The reported incidence of holoprosencephaly is approximately 0.6/1000 live births. The term *holoprosencephaly* includes a series of complex disorders that range broadly in severity. In these disorders, a single embryologic defect affects the development of both the brain and the face.[34] Normally, the processes of cleavage and diverticulation divide the prosencephalon into the diencephalon and telencephalon (cerebral vesicles). The latter eventually grows to meet in the midline and forms the falx and interhemispheric fissure. The optic vesicles and olfactory bulbs that evaginate from the prosencephalon early in development are frequently abnormal in holoprosencephaly. In the most severe form of this disease (alobar holoprosencephaly), none of these developmental processes has taken place.

The degree of disordered prosencephalic development determines the classification and clinical severity of holoprosencephaly.[34–37] In alobar holoprosencephaly, the brain is small. Instead of a ventricular system with distinct lateral and third ventricles, a monoventricular cavity communicating with a dorsal sac is present. The thalamus and corpus striatum are fused. The corpus callosum, fornix, falx cerebri, optic tracts, and olfactory bulbs are absent. The midbrain, brain stem, and cerebellum are structurally normal. However, if hydrocephalus ensues, the significant mass effect of the large monoventricular cavity and dorsal sac may cause the contents of the posterior fossa to be hypoplastic.

With less severe developmental abnormalities of the prosencephalon, an intermediate form, semilobar holoprosencephaly, results.[34–37, 43] A monoventricular cavity with rudimentary occipital horns is present. A rudimentary falx and interhemispheric fissure form caudally, resulting in partial formation and separation of discrete occipital lobes. The olfactory bulbs and corpus callosum are usually absent. Again, the thalami and basal ganglia tend to be fused.

At the milder end of the spectrum is lobar holoprosencephaly, in which the appearance of the brain is more normal.[35, 44] Two hemispheres are usually well separated in this form of the disease, except in the rostral portion where fusion occurs. The lateral ventricles are enlarged, although not necessarily obstructed, and frequently communicate broadly owing to the absence of the septum pellucidum. However, the atria, occipital horns, and temporal horns are separate and individualized. The corpus callosum may be present, hypoplastic, or absent. The septum pellucidum does not form in any type of holoprosencephaly, even the most mild lobar variety. Therefore, identification of a septum pellucidum or cavum septi pellucidi excludes all forms of holoprosencephaly. However, when ventricular dilatation occurs in obstructive hydrocephalus, it is not always possible to demonstrate a septum pellucidum with confidence. The septum pellucidum is also absent in cases of complete agenesis of the corpus callosum. Therefore, the inability to demonstrate a septum pellucidum does not confirm a diagnosis of lobar holoprosencephaly.

Holoprosencephaly frequently involves the face, and the facial deformations are commonly severe.[34, 36] Facial anomalies include cyclopia, ethmocephaly, cebocephaly, and median cleft lip. Cyclopia is a facial deformity characterized by median monophthalmia, synophthalmia, or anophthalmia. There is no nose or median facial bones. A proboscis is usually present and may be double (Figs. 11–18 and 11–19). Hypognathia is seen in some cases. Ethmocephaly is the combination of ocular hypotelorism, usually severe, often associated with a proboscis. Cebocephaly consists of ocular hypotelorism with the nose present. However, the nose has a single nostril. Less severe forms of facial dysmorphia include hypotelorism with a flat nose and median cleft lip. The more severe forms of facial dysmorphology are usually associated with alobar

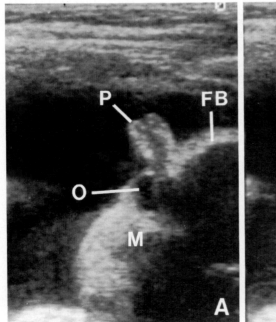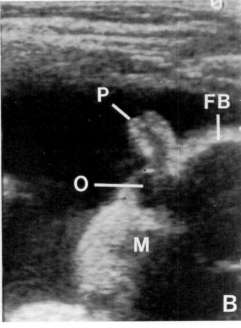

Figure 11–18. *A* and *B*. Midsagittal sonograms of a fetus with cyclopia. FB, frontal bone; M, absent maxillary bones; O, orbit; P, proboscis.

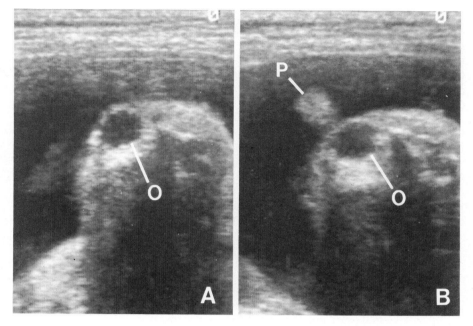

Figure 11–19. *A* and *B*. Transverse axial sonograms of the same fetus that is shown in Figure 11–18. The single orbit (O) and the proboscis (P) are seen in the midline.

holoprosencephaly. Cyclopia and ethmocephaly are almost always seen with the alobar variety.[34] Ceboce-phaly and the other less severe forms of facial dysmor-phology are also seen in alobar holoprosencephaly and in the milder varieties. Facial anomalies, however, are not universally present even in the severe alobar form of the disease. This finding has led to the dictum that "the face predicts the brain but the brain does not always predict the face."

The reader is referred to the excellent review of holoprosencephaly by Manelfe and Sevely on which the following description of imaging dysmorphology in this anomaly is based.[35] The sonologist is immediately impressed by gross malformation of the brain, even after a cursory examination of a fetus with alobar holoprosencephaly. The calvaria appears to be filled mainly with fluid (Figs. 11–20 through 11–22). This collection of fluid represents the large monoventricular cavity in the cerebral midline that communicates pos-teriorly with a "dorsal" sac (see Figs. 11–20 and 11–21). It is prognostically not important to draw an accurate line of distinction between the monoventri-cular cavity and the dorsal sac that communicate very broadly in the alobar form of this disease process. In fact, the two structures appear to be a single structure in most cases. The importance of visualizing the line of junction between these entities, the hippocampal ridge, is that this ridge of tissue generates one of the most characteristic and differentially diagnostic fea-tures of this process (see Fig. 11–22), a differential diagnosis that includes severe hydrocephalus and hy-dranencephaly in addition to the lesser forms of holo-prosencephaly.

The remaining cerebral tissue that surrounds the large monoventricular cavity is reduced in quantity and cephalically displaced and commonly forms a wedge of tissue anteriorly. The cephalically displaced tissue re-sembles a "boomerang" (see Figs. 11–20 and 11–22)

or "horseshoe" (see Fig. 11–21). No cortical mantle is seen about the dorsal cyst (see Figs. 11–20 through 11–22). The basal ganglia and thalami are fused in the midline (Figs. 11–23 and 11–24). This important fea-ture immediately excludes hydrocephalus from the differential diagnosis. In hydrocephalus the thalami should be widely separated due to the enlarged third ventricle, which leaves hydranencephaly as being the most important differential diagnostic possibility. How-ever, from a practical perspective, both hydranenceph-

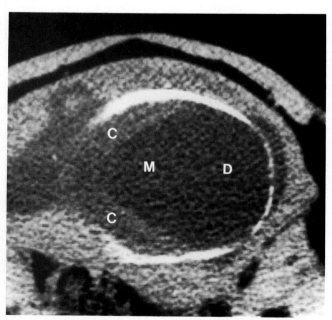

Figure 11–20. Transverse axial in utero computed tomographic scan of a fetus with alobar holoprosencephaly, demonstrating the classic features of this anomaly. The monoventricle (M) communicates with the dorsal sac (D). The line of demarcation *(arrows)* is the hippo-campal ridge. The cerebral cortex (C) is displaced anteriorly.

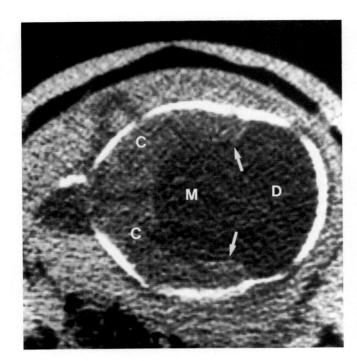

Figure 11–21. A more cephalic section of the same fetus that is seen in Figure 11–20. The boomerang-shaped anteriorly displaced cerebral cortex (C) is shown. D, dorsal sac; M, monoventricular cavity.

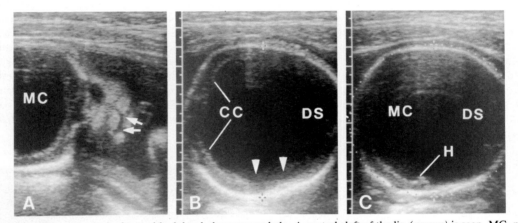

Figure 11–22. *A.* Coronal sonogram of a fetus with alobar holoprosencephaly. A central cleft of the lip *(arrows)* is seen. MC, monoventricular cavity. *B.* The hippocampal ridge is obscured by a side lobe artifact *(arrowheads),* but the symmetric, anteriorly displaced cerebral cortex (CC) is revealed and is unobscured by near-calvarial reverberation. *C.* Reorientation of the transducer discloses the hippocampal ridge (H), but the near-calvarial reverberation artifact now obscures the symmetry of the cerebral cortex. Varying transducer angulations are important to "bring out" specific differentially diagnostic features. The features shown are now *specific* for alobar holoprosencephaly. DS, dorsal sac.

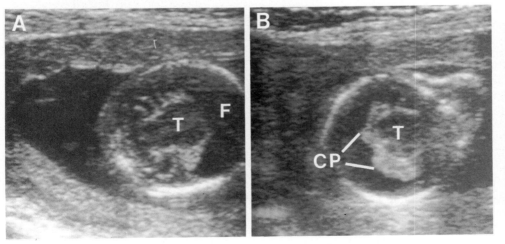

Figure 11–23. *A* and *B.* Early fetus with a presumptive diagnosis of a severe form of holoprosencephaly (semilobar). Note the fluid-filled supratentorial compartment (F) and the fused thalami (T). The absence of a dilated third ventricle excludes hydrocephalus. Hydranencephaly is still a differential diagnostic possibility. However, both have an extremely dismal prognosis. The parents chose to terminate the pregnancy by dilatation and extraction. No postmortem examination of the brain was possible. CP, choroid plexus.

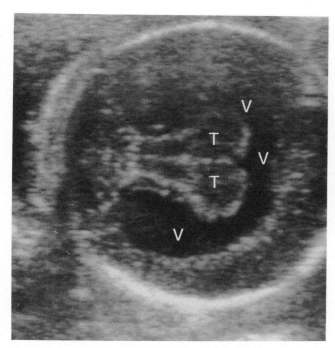

Figure 11–24. Transverse axial sonogram of a fetus with semilobar holoprosencephaly demonstrating a monoventricle (V) and fused thalami (T). (Courtesy of Beth Kleiner, M.D., San Mateo, CA.)

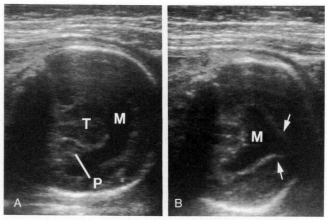

Figure 11–25. *A.* Fetus with semilobar holoprosencephaly. Symmetry is obscured by near-calvarial reverberation but can be assumed to be present. Note the fused thalami (T). The monoventricle (M) arches over the thalami. The parahippocampal gyrus (P) is in its normal position and excludes alobar holoprosencephaly. *B.* The monoventricle extends between the hemispheres as an interhemispheric or dorsal cyst *(arrows).* Agenesis of corpus callosum with an interhemispheric cyst can be excluded by the fused thalami (no third ventricular enlargement).

aly and alobar holoprosencephaly have profound consequences for future mental development, and stillbirth or short survival is the rule. Other than pragmatic considerations, hydranencephaly is excluded by demonstration of either the symmetric and rostrally displaced cerebral mantle or the hippocampal ridge.

The posterior fossa is usually small, which causes difficulty in sonographic imaging of this space. However, if visible, the posterior fossa structures are normal or only mildly hypoplastic. No falx cerebri is present. A great deal has been made of this feature in the diagnosis of alobar holoprosencephaly. However, various artifacts may simulate the appearance of a falx when the cranium is expanded with fluid. Furthermore, the major competing differential diagnostic possibility, hydranencephaly, frequently also lacks a visible falx.

In semilobar holoprosencephaly the occipital lobes tend to be formed, thus a falx and separated ventricles are seen dorsally. Fused thalami exclude hydrocephalus, and the visible occipital brain mantle or frontal brain mantle surrounding the unseparated central ventricular cavity excludes hydranencephaly (Fig. 11–25). Fetuses with complete agenesis of the corpus callosum associated with a large interhemispheric cyst may closely simulate the appearance of semilobar holoprosencephaly. Segregation of these entities may be difficult. Differential diagnostic features include the ability to see frontal horns and a large fluid-filled third ventricle between the thalami in callosal agenesis (see Fig. 11–14); these features are almost never seen in semilobar holoprosencephaly (see Fig. 11–25).*

Lobar holoprosencephaly may be mimicked by callosal agenesis and hydrocephalus with a fenestrated septum (Figs. 11–26 and 11–27). Demonstration of any convincing portion of the septum pellucidum excludes lobar holoprosencephaly and complete agenesis of the corpus callosum. The latter two entities should always be considered simultaneously when examining fetuses with dilated atria and occipital horns of the lateral ventricles and an inability to demonstrate a septum pellucidum or cavum septi pellucidi.

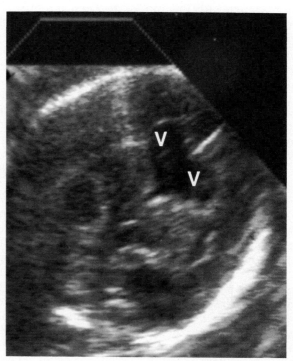

Figure 11–26. Sonogram of a fetus with ventriculomegaly (V). Note the inability to show a septum pellucidum. No definitive diagnosis was possible.

---

*Some cases of semilobar holoprosencephaly demonstrate a small third ventricle.

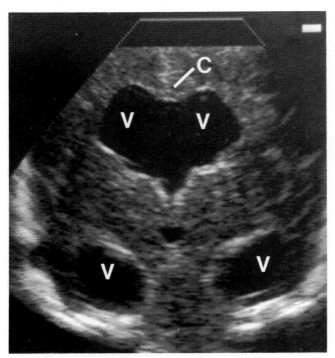

Figure 11–27. Neonatal sonogram of the fetus shown in Figure 11–26. Ventriculomegaly (V), absence of septum pellucidum, and small corpus callosum (C) are shown. A neurologic evaluation and follow-up confirmed lobar holoprosencephaly.

Fetuses with holoprosencephaly may have a head size that is normal, smaller than normal, or enlarged. The enlargement results from hydrocephalus. In addition to the ventricular malformation, severe ventricular dilatation may also occur. Because cases diagnosed during routine obstetric scanning tend to be the more severe varieties of this disease process, the prognosis is uniformly poor and most fetuses discovered with this anomaly die in utero before or not long after birth. Survivors usually have severe mental retardation. The poor prognosis is reflected in the experience of most authors.[38, 44] Nonetheless, prognosis for lobar holoprosencephaly is less severe. A normal life span has been reported for some patients, but many are severely retarded. It is presumed that the rare persons who have normal mentation and a form of holoprosencephaly likely demonstrate the least structural brain disorganization and therefore have the most subtle dysmorphic features. Thus, these fetuses are least likely to be detected.

All varieties of holoprosencephaly have been diagnosed in utero by sonography.[38–44] The more severe forms have predominated,[38, 43] but lobar holoprosencephaly has also been recognized.[44] Obstetric management in cases of holoprosencephaly depends on the gestational age at the time of diagnosis and on the severity of the abnormality.[42] If this condition is detected before 24 weeks' gestation, the parents may choose to terminate the pregnancy. In the third trimester, macrocephaly due to ventricular enlargement may well prevent vaginal delivery. Thus, to avoid cesarean section in hopeless cases, cephalocentesis is usually recommended. An effective cephalocentesis should

significantly reduce the size of the cranium. An analysis of the fetal karyotype should be considered in almost any CNS anomaly. Karyotyping is clearly indicated in cases of holoprosencephalies in which a high incidence of chromosomal abnormalities has been discovered.[34, 36] Trisomy 13 is particularly common; however, other chromosomal anomalies may be detected.

Hydranencephaly, Porencephaly, and Schizencephaly

Purists would argue that grouping these three entities together has no basis in fact. Conversely, pragmatists would see no reason to overly debate the incorporation of these entities into a single section of such a chapter. Hydranencephaly and porencephaly are unambiguously destructive lesions of the fetal brain.[45–52] Schizencephaly is not as unambiguously a destructive process, and many researchers consider that this entity is developmental.[53–56] Sonographic evidence supports the hypothesis that schizencephaly, like hydranencephaly and porencephaly, is the result of a destructive process.[49, 56] Probably all three entities represent the sequelae of in utero vascular accidents that differ only in timing and in degree.[48] The timing element probably accounts for the variations in development of other CNS structures that confuse the etiologic categorization of these entities.

Hydranencephaly is complete or almost complete destruction of the cerebral cortex and basal ganglia (Figs. 11–28 and 11–29).[45, 46] The thalami and lower brain centers are usually preserved, although the thalami may be involved in the destructive process.[47] The head size is often small. However, the choroid plexus may be preserved and functional; hydrocephalus may ensue. That normally developed brain tissue was present and was then destroyed has been sonographically documented in utero.[49] Bilateral internal carotid artery occlusion may result in this abnormality, but this hypothesis is difficult to prove because these vessels are usually patent when an autopsy is done.[45–47] Nonetheless, if one works from the premise that massive brain infarction, which may occur from occlusion of the internal carotid arteries, results in hydranencephaly, all the morphologic features seen sonographically in utero can be anticipated.

Severe increases in ventricular size and pressure over prolonged periods also destroy the cortical mantle. However, hydranencephaly is clearly distinct from this process, and the two can be easily separated pathologically, if not clinically, in all cases.[57] In hydranencephaly the telencephalon is replaced by fluid-filled cavities covered only by leptomeninges. In prolonged massive hydrocephalus, a thin rim of abnormal, but identifiable, cortical brain tissue persists.

The abnormalities seen sonographically in hydranencephaly are so striking that detection is not a problem (see Figs. 11–28 and 11–29); unfortunately, differential diagnoses are. Alternative diagnostic possibilities include massive hydrocephalus, alobar holoprosencephaly, and brain atrophy that result in thinned, but

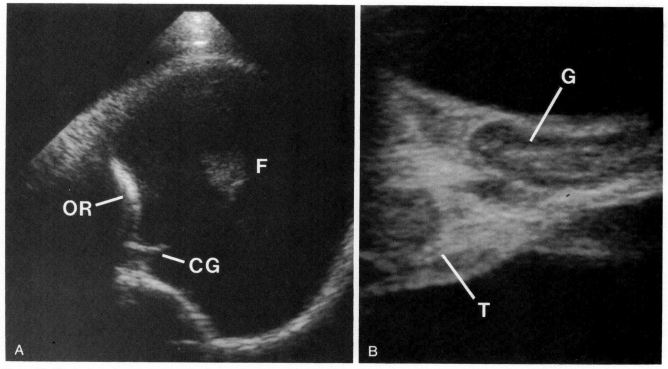

Figure 11–28. *A.* Anterior coronal scan is shown of a fetus with hydranencephaly. No brain tissue or dural structure (falx) is seen. Only fluid (F) is present. However, the crista galli (CG) is apparent. OR, orbital roof. *B.* A posterior scan identifies a "preserved" gyrus (G) of the occipital lobe. T, tentorium.

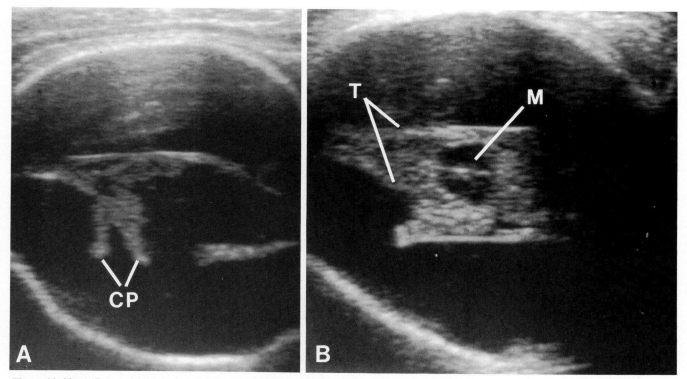

Figure 11–29. *A.* Fetus with hydranencephaly. The calvarial contents are almost totally fluid. Little structure is visible, but a dangling choroid plexus (CP) is seen. *B.* Note that infratentorially (T) the midbrain–pons (M) junction appears to be entirely normal.

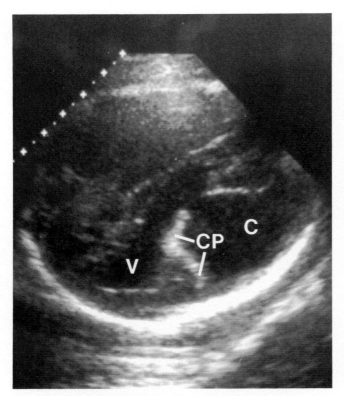

Figure 11–30. A porencephalic cyst in a fetus is shown in a transverse axial sonogram. The large cyst (C) is located in the supply distribution of the middle cerebral artery. Despite its large size, the cyst has no mass effect. The ipsilateral ventricle (V) is enlarged. The cyst communicates with the ventricle; note that the choroid plexus (CP) hangs from the ventricle into the cyst.

usually into the adjacent ventricular lumen or the subarachnoid space (Fig. 11–30). The residuum, then, is a cystic lesion that is in free communication with the ventricle, or less commonly, the subarachnoid cisterns at the external brain surface.* Because the ischemic event is often more widespread than the focal infarction that eventuates in the porencephaly, the hemisphere tends to be small and is manifested by enlargement of the ipsilateral ventricle. The porencephalic cyst is an ex vacuo event; thus, it never produces a mass effect. This is an important differential diagnostic point between arachnoid cysts and interhemispheric cysts (Fig. 11–31), such as that seen in agenesis of the corpus callosum. Furthermore, ischemic injury may cause degenerative cysts that do not communicate with the ventricles (periventricular leukomalacia, cystic encephalomalacia) (Fig. 11–32).

Schizencephaly, or bilateral clefts in the cerebral cortex, has been considered to be the result of bilateral middle cerebral artery infarction with subsequent development of symmetric porencephalic cysts or clefts (Fig. 11–33).† Depending on the timing of this event (early versus late), the interruption of blood supply may also result in abnormal brain growth and development. These cysts are always lined by gray matter, a feature that contradicts the inclusion of this entity with hydranencephaly and porencephaly. However, the dysmorphic features in "classic" cases strongly simulate the expected location of bilateral middle cerebral artery distribution of porencephalic cysts.[53-56] The fluid collections communicate with the ventricular lumen bilat-

---

*Areas of cystic necrosis within the brain substance that do not communicate with the subarachnoid space or the ventricular lumen are called "false porencephalies" or cystic leukomalacia.

†More strictly, the cyst (or cleft) must extend from the ependyma of the ventricle to the brain surface (leptomeninges) and must be lined by gray matter. The clefts are not necessarily bilateral and may be so narrow that they do not contain any CSF.

not absent, cerebral hemispheres. Features that distinguish these entities have been considered in other sections. However, a few additional and important features are appropriately discussed here. First, there may be scattered, preserved zones of cerebral cortical tissue in cases of hydranencephaly, although histologically the tissue is usually gliotic (see Fig. 11–28B). These zones occur where tissue might be preserved by collateral arterial flow. Preserved brain tissue includes medial occipital lobe tissue, presumably preserved through the posterior communicating arteries, and, occasionally, areas of frontal lobe tissue, presumably preserved through ophthalmic artery collaterals. The hippocampus and parahippocampal gyrus may be preserved; and when this occurs, they lie in immediate contiguity with the ambient cistern, which is their normal location. This position of the hippocampal tissues is distinct from alobar holoprosencephaly, wherein the hippocampal ridge is located peripherally. The third ventricle is present and visible but is not enlarged in hydranencephaly compared with severe hydrocephalus that enlarges the third ventricle. Fusion of the thalami, which is seen invariably in alobar holoprosencephaly, is never present in hydranencephaly.

Porencephaly is at the milder end of a continuum from hydranencephaly and develops when infarction of or hemorrhage into brain parenchyma occurs. The destroyed area necroses and is gradually evacuated,

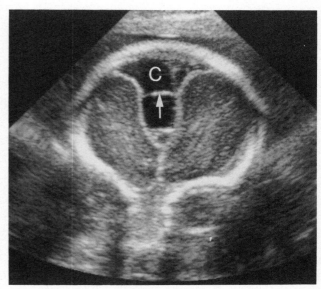

Figure 11–31. Coronal sonogram of an interhemispheric cyst (C) in a fetus with agenesis of the corpus callosum. Note the septation *(arrow)* within the cyst, which is not an uncommon feature.

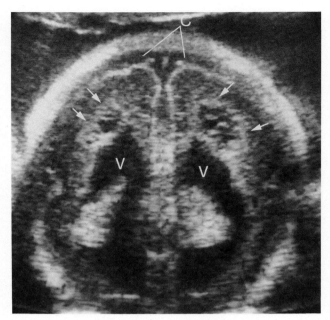

Figure 11–32. Transverse axial sonogram of a fetus with brain atrophy and periventricular leukomalacia *(arrows)*. C, subarachnoid cisterns; V, ventricle. (Courtesy of Harris Finberg, M.D., Phoenix, AZ.)

Hydrocephalus Versus Nonobstructive Ventriculomegaly

The preceding sections have documented that multiple anomalies of brain development result in ventricular enlargement. The term *hydrocephalus* should be reserved for that dynamic process resulting in a progressive increase in ventricular volume due to either a relative or a complete obstruction between sites of production and absorption of CSF or, much less commonly, overproduction.[58, 59] Therefore, in hydrocephalus there is an increase in relative pressure between the CSF and the intracranial venous system.

Obstructive hydrocephalus is the more common form. This type may be further subdivided into communicating versus noncommunicating hydrocephalus.[59] In the former, the site of obstruction is extraventricular, most often at the arachnoid granulations, whereas in the latter, the obstruction is within the ventricular system itself. Among fetuses, communicating hydrocephalus is distinctly uncommon. Neonates and young children have a higher incidence of communicating hydrocephalus that is seen most commonly after intraventricular hemorrhage in premature children or as a result of meningitis in older children; both conditions are rare in fetuses.

By the aforementioned definition, the term *hydrocephalus ex vacuo* should be avoided, because in this entity the enlarged ventricles originate from a loss of surrounding brain parenchyma. Awareness of the subtleties of these definitions is, unfortunately, important. For example, in hydranencephaly there is a profound loss of brain tissue surrounding the ventricles (hydrocephalus ex vacuo). The ventricular edge extends to the calvarial wall with no intervening brain tissue.

erally and extend to the calvaria. A major problem sonographically is that symmetry is difficult to demonstrate due to the near-calvarial reverberation artifact (see Fig. 11–33). The unwary examiner may be content to have observed and characterized the "down side" lesion as an isolated, unilateral porencephaly.

As would be expected, the prognosis with the disorders under consideration depends on which portion of the brain has been destroyed and to what extent other areas of the brain can compensate for the lost tissue. Hydranencephaly, of course, has a grim prognosis because almost all of the higher brain centers have been destroyed. Interestingly, hydranencephalic neonates may appear to be quite normal and escape early clinical detection only to be discovered a few months later.[46, 49] Early clinical detection appears to depend more on the absence of hypothalamic function than on the cortical brain function. If the hypothalamus is intact, the newborn appears to be relatively normal. However, electroencephalography shows no cortical activity, and hyperreflexia and clonus are generally present.

In porencephaly and schizencephaly, the disability is likely to be more severe than expected based on the observed abnormalities. More brain tissue may have been involved in the hypoxic event than can be documented sonographically. Experience with the later entities is small. However, extrapolation from more common CNS anomalies suggests that the more severe cases, with correspondingly poorer prognoses, tend to be detected in utero. A poor prognosis cannot be accurately predicted in fetuses with a porencephalic cyst.

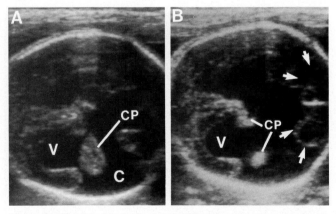

Figure 11–33. *A* and *B*. Schizencephaly is shown in paired transverse axial sonograms. A large cleft (or cyst) (C) is seen in the hemisphere farther from the transducer. Choroid plexus (CP) dangles into the cyst. The ipsilateral ventricle (V) is enlarged and has an abnormal shape. The lateral ventricles communicate broadly. No septum is seen (the near-ventricular choroid plexus hangs down into the opposite ventricle). A near-calvarial reverberation artifact obscures the symmetry of this anomaly, but careful inspection of *B (arrows)* shows the bilaterality of the anomaly. (Courtesy of L. Mack, M.D., University of Washington.)

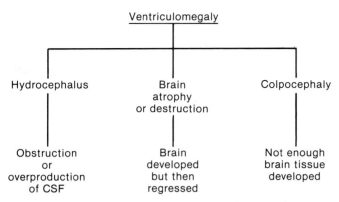

Figure 11–34. Pathologic causes of ventriculomegaly.

These enlarged "ventricles" should not be classified as hydrocephalus. However, in a hydranencephalic fetus the normal- to small-sized head may begin to expand owing to an obstruction of CSF flow (true hydrocephalus). Furthermore, the true hydrocephalus may be either communicating or noncommunicating.

Once enlarged ventricles are noted, the sonologist must make all efforts to determine whether the ventricular enlargement represents true hydrocephalus or ventriculomegaly from another cause (i.e., colpocephaly or brain atrophy) (Fig. 11–34). If one suspects hydrocephalus, further efforts should be made to determine whether it is isolated or associated with other anomalies of CNS or extra-CNS development, a chal-

lenge that, in some cases, may be beyond our current capabilities (Fig. 11–35). Among these anomalies, the most important are neural tube defects.[60–75] One third of all cases of hydrocephalus will be associated with myelomeningocele or encephalocele (the former being the more common). The hydrocephalus in these cases is due to the Chiari malformation. A careful search of the spine by an experienced sonologist is necessary in all cases of ventricular enlargement.

Other etiologies include aqueductal stenosis (Figs. 11–36 and 11–37), either X-linked or idiopathic, holoprosencephaly (see Fig. 11–22), hydranencephaly (see Fig. 11–28), Dandy-Walker malformation (see Fig. 11–6), and cloverleaf skull deformity (Fig. 11–38).[60–75] The posterior fossa must be examined carefully for evidence of the Dandy-Walker syndrome because the supratentorial ventricular enlargement does not depend on the size of the fourth ventricular cyst (see Fig. 11–7).

There is a great temptation for the inexperienced examiner to blame aqueductal stenosis as being the cause of ventricular enlargement for several reasons. First, enlargement of the lateral and third ventricles is

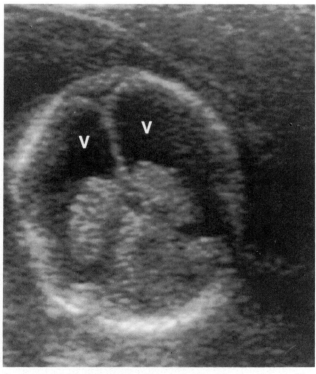

Figure 11–35. Ventriculomegaly associated with a syndrome. Ventriculomegaly (V) was noted at 16 weeks in a fetus with a genetic risk of Walker-Warburg syndrome. Ventriculomegaly is only one manifestation of this severe syndrome but was the only feature that could be documented. A ventricular shunt, either before or after birth, would not provide a cure for this fetus.

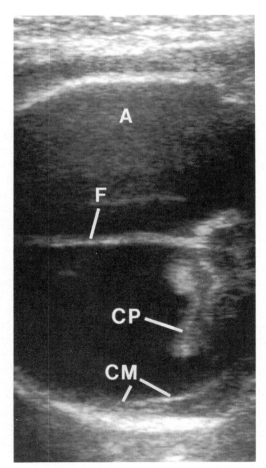

Figure 11–36. Transverse axial sonogram of a fetus that was difficult to examine. Severe ventriculomegaly from aqueductal stenosis is noted. A near-calvarial reverberation artifact (A) obscures most of the anatomy of the hemisphere closer to the transducer. The thinned contralateral cortical mantle (CM) can be seen. Symmetry can be assumed. Note that the choroid plexus (CP) dangles at a 90° angle. F, falx.

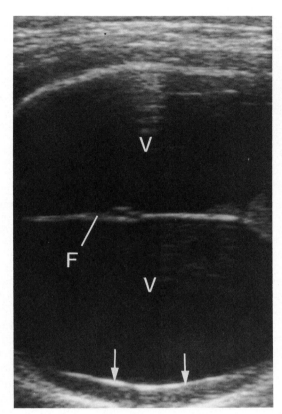

Figure 11–37. Transverse axial sonogram of a fetus with aqueductal stenosis and massive hydrocephalus. V, ventricles; F, falx; arrows, parenchyma.

easier to perceive than enlargement of the subarachnoid spaces (Fig. 11–39) (brain atrophy with large ventricles), enlargement of the fourth ventricle (communicating hydrocephalus or Dandy-Walker syndrome), and spinal dysraphism (Chiari II malformation associated with myelomeningocele). Second, ventricular enlargement (with or without hydrocephalus) caused by anomalies, such as agenesis of the corpus callosum or lobar holoprosencephaly, may require sub-

tle observations of brain maldevelopment. Third, aqueductal stenosis is a diagnosis of exclusion, even when made by the most sophisticated examiner. The inexperienced examiner who fails to meticulously search out these manifold possibilities often presumes their absence and may thus erroneously conclude that aqueductal stenosis (isolated) is the correct etiology of the observed ventricular enlargement.

There are significant unsolved problems in managing a fetus with ventriculomegaly. We are only now beginning to understand the natural history of such cases.[76] The relationship between hydrocephalus detected in utero and that seen in neonates is only speculative. Current evidence demonstrates that the accuracy of prenatal ultrasound evaluation in discriminating true hydrocephalus from nonobstructive ventriculomegaly is less than perfect even when determined by an expert.[76–82] Furthermore, there is a clear potential to fail to diagnose associated CNS and life-threatening extra-CNS anomalies.

Pragmatically, prenatal ultrasound evaluation recognizes three patterns of ventriculomegaly,[76] including fetuses who have ventriculomegaly associated with severe abnormalities that would be fatal (e.g., Meckel syndrome). In such cases, the parents may be counseled and the pregnancy may be terminated (depending on their decision). The second group includes fetuses with marked ventriculomegaly detected serendipitously late in gestation, which is associated with abnormalities that are severe but not invariably fatal. In this case, parents commonly choose vaginal delivery following cephalocentesis. Because the latter is usually a destructive procedure and the vaginal delivery is a further trauma to the fetus, neonatal death is almost always the outcome. Finally, there is the most difficult group. This group consists of fetuses with isolated ventriculomegaly in whom there is no sonographically evident associated anomaly or an anomaly that is not particularly severe (e.g., unilateral hydronephrosis). One could include in this group of fetuses those with an anomaly such as myelomeningocele, which is not usu-

Figure 11–38. *A.* Fetus with a cloverleaf skull deformity (transverse axial sonogram taken only of the frontal region). The dilated frontal horns (F) are devoid of choroid plexus. Note the compressed cavum septi pellucidi (C). This observation excludes midline anomalies. *B.* This parasagittal sonogram shows the frontal bossing and flattened nose found in such fetuses. F, dilated frontal horn; FC, frontal cortex. (*B* from Harrison MR, Golbus MS, Filly RA [eds]: The Unborn Patient: Prenatal Diagnosis and Treatment, 2nd ed. Philadelphia, WB Saunders, 1990.)

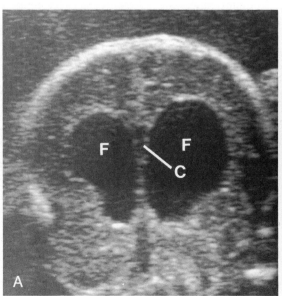

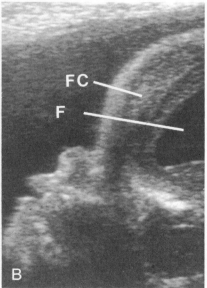

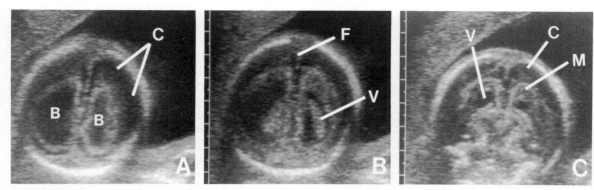

Figure 11–39. Transverse axial (*A* and *B*) and coronal *(C)* sonograms of a twin who had a brain infarction after the death in utero of its sibling (from twin transfusion syndrome). Brain tissue (B) is shrinking and is causing abnormally large cisterns (C). The edge of the brain is well marked by the brightly echogenic pia-arachnoid. F, falx; M, mantle of brain; V, ventricle. (From Harrison MR, Golbus MS, Filly RA [eds]: The Unborn Patient: Prenatal Diagnosis and Treatment, 2nd ed. Philadelphia, WB Saunders, 1990.)

ally associated with subsequent mental retardation although it is associated with disability.

In the first two groups a poor outcome is easily predicted. In the last group it is not easily predicted. Furthermore, in this group it is most difficult to segregate true hydrocephalus from nonobstructive ventriculomegaly, and there is invariably a suspicion that subtle, but significant, CNS or extra-CNS anomalies may have been missed. This group of fetuses requires an aggressive investigation that includes serial sonograms, determination of karyotype, α-fetoprotein (AFP) analysis, and viral cultures and titers. Because it is impossible to determine intraventricular pressure safely in utero, hydrocephalus should not be diagnosed in this group unless the head is enlarged or serial sonograms document increasing ventricular and head size. Importantly, the lack of the aforementioned two features does not, however, exclude true hydrocephalus with high pressure.

Independent of the ability of sonography to discriminate nonobstructive ventricular enlargement from true hydrocephalus, the prognosis for fetal ventriculomegaly is clearly poor.[65–69] Only about one case in four of fetuses with enlarged ventricles survive, as presently reported in the literature. The most frequent cause of death is iatrogenic (pregnancy termination, cephalocentesis). The mortality rate is high even if these interventions are not used. Moreover, only half of the survivors are intellectually normal. The high mortality rate is likely due to the frequent association of CNS abnormalities with anomalous development of other important organs.[63, 69] There is an 80% incidence of associated abnormalities. The anomalies are often severe and can affect many organ systems, including the cardiovascular, gastrointestinal, and renal system. Other CNS aberrations are also common.

As stated earlier, the prognosis for normal intellectual outcome is poor.[63–69] Survivors tend to represent a select group that generally has less severe associated anomalies. Included in this group is a subset of persons who have mild ventriculomegaly.[70, 71] Mild ventriculomegaly, just like fetal ventriculomegaly in general, is often associated with a wide range of serious concomitant abnormalities.[70] Mortality, as well, remains high.

However, fetuses with isolated mild ventriculomegaly appear to have a much better prognosis. Mortality is less than half that of the group with other anomalies, and chances for normal mental development are also improved.[70] Unfortunately, the degree of ventriculomegaly is not uniformly predictive of outcome.[63] Infants may have moderate-to-severe ventricular enlargement and demonstrate normal intellectual development after postnatal shunting. Conversely, fetuses with mild-to-moderate ventriculomegaly may show significantly delayed development. Rather than the degree of ventricular enlargement, it is most often the presence of other abnormalities that worsens the prognosis for the fetus.[69] It is therefore important that these anomalies be identified. Unfortunately, even in the hands of highly experienced sonologists, all abnormalities may not be identified. Almost all major series dealing with the evaluation of fetal ventricular enlargement have shown false-negative rates in the range of 20% to 39%.[63–69] However, among fetuses with mild ventriculomegaly, 98% have been correctly categorized as isolated versus associated with other anomalies.[70] Once another anomaly was detected, there remained a high likelihood that a third or fourth anomaly may go undetected. In fetuses with abnormal ventricles, it is more likely that experienced sonologists will miss anomalies outside the CNS than associated anomalies within the CNS.

SONOGRAPHIC DIAGNOSIS OF VENTRICULAR ENLARGEMENT

The sonographic diagnosis of ventricular enlargement has been well described in the literature.[72, 73] Considerable work has been done by using measurements of frontal horns and lateral ventricular "widths" to define the normal limits for ventricular size at different stages of development. A set of ratio measurements comparing the distance of the lateral wall of the lateral ventricle from the midline to the hemispheric width (LVW/HW ratio) has been proposed as a method for diagnosing hydrocephalus.[72] However, the accuracy of the ratio measurement suffers not only

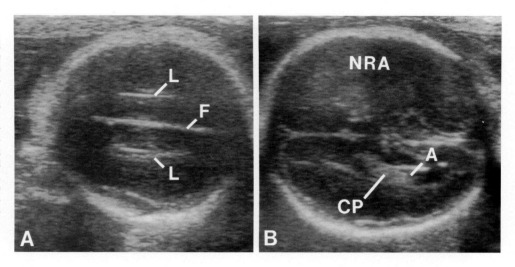

Figure 11–40. *A.* Transverse axial sonogram taken relatively near the vertex. Linear echoes (L) were previously thought to be reflections from the ventricular wall. F, falx. *B.* Transverse axial sonogram through the ventricular atria (A). The near atrium is totally obscured by near-calvarial reverberation artifact (NRA). The atrium is well marked by the choroid plexus (CP). (From Harrison MR, Golbus MS, Filly RA [eds]: The Unborn Patient: Prenatal Diagnosis and Treatment, 2nd ed. Philadelphia, WB Saunders, 1990.)

from technical difficulties that considerably alter the ratio value (depending on the plane of section in which the scan is performed) but also from a wide standard deviation that renders it insensitive to identification of early dilatation.[74] Not the least problem with this approach is the fact that the normal data are based on measurements from a linear echoing structure that does not actually represent the lateral ventricular wall (see Chapter 10).

It is preferable to determine ventricular enlargement by direct observations of the ventricle. These observations are best carried out in the region of the ventricular atrium where, in the normal fetus, the choroid plexus fills (or almost fills) the transverse dimension of this component of the ventricular system (Figs. 11–40 and 11–41). This relationship is important because in early hydrocephalus the first recognizable aberration is a relative shrinkage of the normally prominent choroid plexus within the body of the lateral ventricle. The apparent frontal horn size may seem to be prominent in the early second trimester, but as long as the choroid plexus can be seen filling the lateral ventricular body in its transverse dimension, hydrocephalus is not present. One should never assume that a normal head size (biparietal diameter or head circumference) excludes either ventriculomegaly or true hydrocephalus.[75, 76]

The atrial diameter is a particularly important measurement to determine normalcy of ventricular size.[73] Evidence has shown that there is little, if any, change in the diameter of the lateral ventricular atrium from 15 to 35 weeks. The transverse diameter of the ventricular atrium measures approximately 7 mm, and 10 mm is the upper limit of normal (see Fig. 11–41). No measurement is necessary if the choroid fills the atrial lumen. If a modest amount of fluid lies between the choroid and the ventricular wall, a measurement is advisable (Fig. 11–42).

The lack of apparent growth in the diameter of the atrium is particularly useful to sonologists. The volume of the ventricle increases throughout the second and third trimesters and is dramatically reshaped by the marked growth of the adjacent brain. The adjacent brain does not markedly reshape the atrium, which

accounts for the relative stability of both the atrial diameter and the ratio of choroidal width to atrial width.[73]

The reverberation from the near-calvarial wall often obscures the lateral ventricle that lies closer to the transducer (see Fig. 11–41). Thus, in most cases, the ventricles appear to be asymmetric when enlarged. The temptation to diagnose ventricular asymmetry should be avoided (see Figs. 11–36 and 11–41). Although unilateral ventricular enlargement and unilateral ventricular hydrocephalus are possibilities, they are distinctly uncommon (see Fig. 11–42).[77]

Recognition of ventricular enlargement is relatively

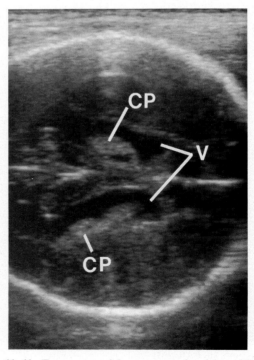

Figure 11–41. Transverse axial sonogram of a fetus with mildly dilated ventricles (V). The atrial diameter exceeds 10 mm. The choroid plexus (CP) fails to fill the atrium and is a visual clue to ventricular enlargement. (From Harrison MR, Golbus MS, Filly RA [eds]: The Unborn Patient: Prenatal Diagnosis and Treatment, 2nd ed. Philadelphia, WB Saunders, 1990.)

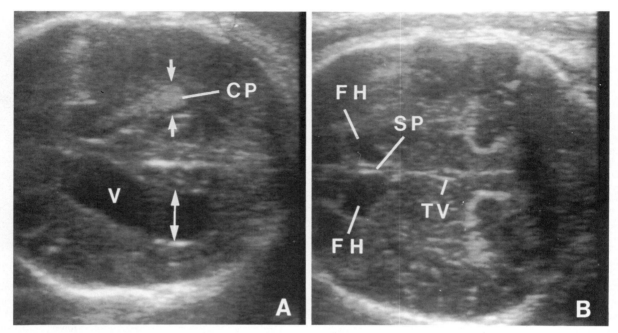

Figure 11–42. Unilateral ventriculomegaly in a fetus is seen in a transverse axial sonogram. *A.* The near-ventricular atrium has a normal diameter *(inward-pointing arrows)* and is "filled" by choroid plexus (CP). The more distant ventricle (V) is enlarged. The atrial diameter exceeds 10 mm. The ventricle is enlarged sufficiently that this plane of section clearly cuts through the atrium without simultaneously visualizing the choroid plexus, which is almost an impossible task in a normal ventricle. *B.* The frontal horns (FH) are also asymmetric. Note the preserved septum pellucidum (SP). TV, normal third ventricle. (From Harrison MR, Golbus MS, Filly RA [eds]: The Unborn Patient: Prenatal Diagnosis and Treatment, 2nd ed. Philadelphia, WB Saunders, 1990.)

straightforward by observing the appearance of the ventricular atrium. Conversely, there is a true potential to frequently overstate the presence of hydrocephalus because of the poorly echogenic adjacent brain parenchyma that may be mistakenly interpreted as CSF surrounding the atrial choroid (pseudohydrocephalus) (Fig. 11–43).[78] This appearance is augmented by the technical error of applying insufficient gain when ex-

amining the brain.* Pseudohydrocephalus is recognized easily by remembering that the choroid plexus always rests in a gravitationally dependent position (Fig. 11–

---

*When examining the head of the fetus, the ultrasonic beam passes through the attenuating calvaria. Therefore, overall gain and time-gain compensation must be increased compared with the examination of the torso.

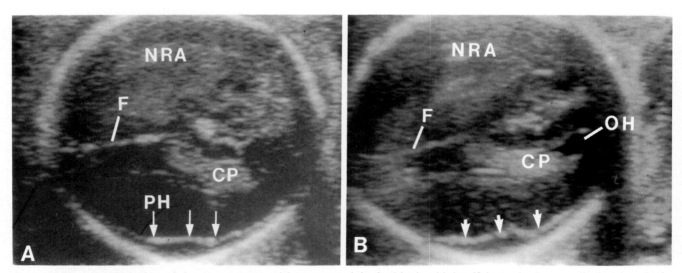

Figure 11–43. *A.* Pseudohydrocephalus. A transverse axial sonogram of the fetal brain with insufficient gain. Low-amplitude echoes in the far parenchyma of the hemisphere (PH) drop out and create an echolucency that simulated an enlarged, fluid-filled ventricle. Additionally, the bright echoes from pia-arachnoid *(arrows)* that are found at the edge of the brain enhance the erroneous interpretation, because they simulate the ventricular wall echo. Note, however, that the choroid plexus (CP) appears to be "suspended" in the "ventricle"—a physical impossibility confirming this technical error. NRA, near-reverberation artifact. *B.* Readjustment of the time-gain compensation documents normalcy. F, falx; OH, occipital horn. (From Harrison MR, Golbus MS, Filly RA [eds]: The Unborn Patient: Prenatal Diagnosis and Treatment, 2nd ed. Philadelphia, WB Saunders, 1990.)

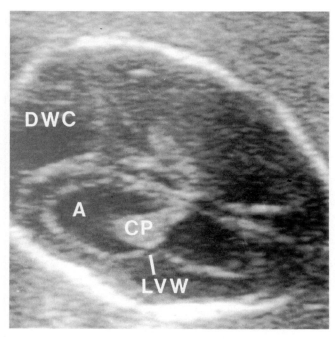

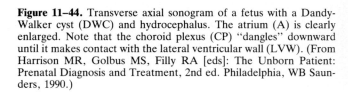

Figure 11-44. Transverse axial sonogram of a fetus with a Dandy-Walker cyst (DWC) and hydrocephalus. The atrium (A) is clearly enlarged. Note that the choroid plexus (CP) "dangles" downward until it makes contact with the lateral ventricular wall (LVW). (From Harrison MR, Golbus MS, Filly RA [eds]: The Unborn Patient: Prenatal Diagnosis and Treatment, 2nd ed. Philadelphia, WB Saunders, 1990.)

44). Therefore, the choroid plexus always rests against the lateral ventricular wall unless the lateral ventricle is so large that the choroid plexus, tethered at the Monro foramen, is simply not long enough to reach the lateral wall. The choroid, a highly echogenic structure, may help to obscure the lateral ventricular wall where it lies in contact with this structure (Fig. 11-45). Therefore, if the choroid plexus appears to be "suspended" in an "enlarged ventricle," one can predict that it is a case of pseudohydrocephalus and one can increase the gain and produce the appropriate images that document the error. Using the knowledge that the choroid plexus always assumes a gravitationally dependent position also helps to recognize true ventricular enlargement, "the dangling choroid sign" (Figs. 11-46 and 11-47).[79] The greater the degree of angulation of the choroid from the midline, the larger is the ventricle.

Space-Occupying Lesions (Neoplasm, Arteriovenous Malformation, Arachnoid Cyst, and Choroid Plexus Cyst)

Fortunately, congenital brain tumors are rare abnormalities.[80-104] They account for approximately 0.3% of neonatal deaths at younger than 28 days of age.[80]

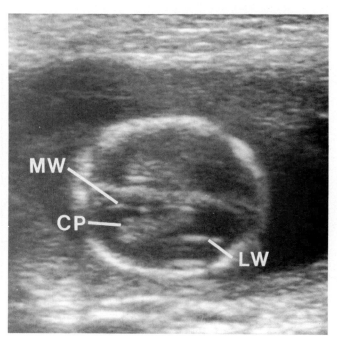

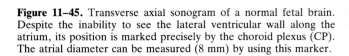

Figure 11-45. Transverse axial sonogram of a normal fetal brain. Despite the inability to see the lateral ventricular wall along the atrium, its position is marked precisely by the choroid plexus (CP). The atrial diameter can be measured (8 mm) by using this marker.

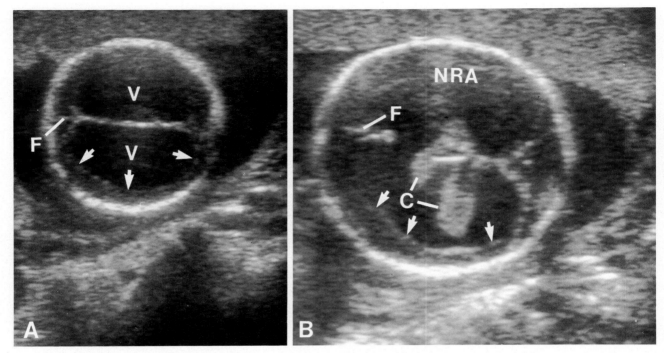

Figure 11–46. *A.* Transverse axial sonogram of a fetus with severe ventricular enlargement (V) and marked thinning of cortex, especially medially. The etiology was a large myelomeningocele. F, falx. *B.* Transverse axial sonogram that is more inferior than in *A.* The "dangling choroid" (C) sign is shown. Note that the choroid of the ventricle nearer to the transducer "dangles" through the open septum into the ventricle farther from the transducer (whose choroid dangles to the limit of its length but cannot reach the lateral ventricular wall, which is marked by arrows).

Various lesions may be found, but the most common is the teratoma, which accounts for approximately 50% of all congenital intracranial neoplasms.[81] This lesion may be seen at any time during life, but it is often present in the neonate and rapidly decreases in incidence with increasing age.[82] Teratomas may be either benign or malignant, although even the benign lesions tend to have devastating consequences. Glial tumors are second in frequency and include glioblastomas, astroblastomas, and spongioblastomas. Glioblastomas

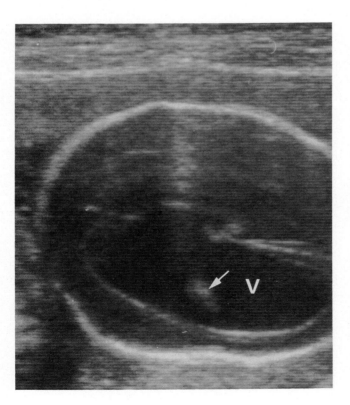

Figure 11–47. Transverse axial sonogram of a fetus with hydrocephalus. The ventricle (V) is enlarged. Choroid plexus is seen "dangling" within the labeled ventricle *(arrow).*

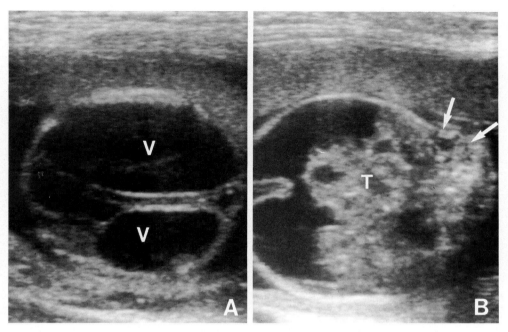

Figure 11–48. *A.* Transverse axial sonogram showing asymmetric hydrocephalus. V, ventricle. *B.* Coronal sonogram showing a heterogeneous tumor mass (T) that extensively involves the base of the entire supratentorial compartment and extends out of the orbit *(arrows)*. The mass was a teratoma.

predominate. Any of these lesions can produce hydrocephalus by ventricular obstruction, which is a common event.[82] Teratomatous lesions tend to be mixed, solid, and cystic lesions, and they usually have a great degree of disorganization (Fig. 11–48). However, the cystic component may occasionally predominate, and there is some potential to misdiagnose this neoplastic lesion as being an arachnoid cyst. The only reported sonographic case of glioblastoma diagnosed prenatally presented as diffusely increased echoes throughout the tumor mass.[83] The appearance was similar to that seen in a large hemorrhage or hemorrhagic infarct.

Dystocia may occur during vaginal delivery and may be due both to the size of the tumor mass that can greatly expand the cranium and to the secondary hydrocephalus (see Fig. 11–48). Lesions are more commonly supratentorial than infratentorial, although distortion may be too great to make this distinction. Cephalocentesis may be worthwhile if severe hydrocephalus or a large cystic component is dominant.[82] Unfortunately, in many cases delivery must be by cesarean section because vaginal delivery is often impossible even after cephalocentesis. Although such lesions may be small and potentially resectable,[86] until now only large lesions have been detected prenatally.[82–85, 87–89] In each case the fetus has been stillborn or has died in the neonatal period. Thus, it may be prudent to assume a fatal prognosis and manage cases with this outcome in mind. Necrotic brain tissue in developing hydranencephaly may simulate the appearance of an intracranial teratoma.[90] Of course, the prognosis in this situation is equally if not more dismal.

At the opposite end of the spectrum is a mass lesion that is both common and essentially benign.[84–86, 94–97] This lesion is the choroid plexus cyst (Fig. 11–49). It is common to identify choroid plexus cysts if this lesion is actively sought in all fetuses of the correct gestational age.[97] These lesions are seen almost exclusively in fetuses between 16 and 21 weeks of gestational age

and are always located in the lateral ventricle near the glomus of the choroid plexus. By the 23rd week they are clearly regressing, and it would be unusual to see such a lesion after 25 to 26 weeks.

Because of the ability of ultrasonography to scan large numbers of fetuses at the appropriate age range and to resolve even tiny cysts in the choroid plexus, these lesions, which were previously thought to be rare, are now known to be common.[97] Choroid plexus cysts are probably the most common aberration of fetal development observed sonographically in utero. These cysts may be unilateral or bilateral. However, bilateral recognition is difficult owing to near-side reverberation caused by the calvaria.

Choroid plexus cysts typically range from 0.5 to 2 cm. Commonly, they are multilocular (see Fig. 11–49). Only the larger lesions expand the walls of the lateral ventricle (Fig. 11–50). The lesions appear to be

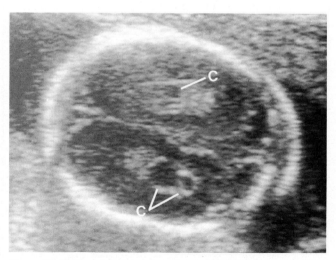

Figure 11–49. Transverse axial sonogram of bilateral choroid plexus cysts (C). The larger cyst is bilocular.

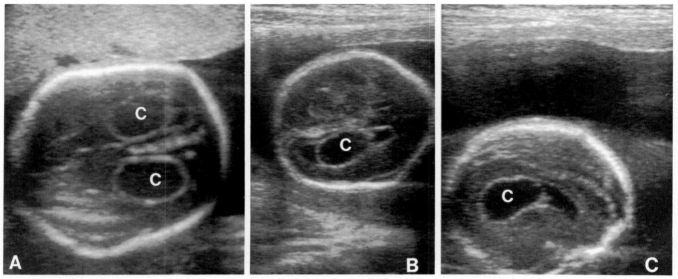

Figure 11–50. *A.* Very large choroid plexus cysts (C) seen in a transverse axial sonogram. *B.* A somewhat off-axis axial sonogram. *C.* Parasagittal planes. These cysts are so large that they expand the ventricles *(A).* Polyhydramnios and other anomalies were present. Trisomy 18 was found on karyotype. (*A* from Harrison MR, Golbus MS, Filly RA [eds]: The Unborn Patient: Prenatal Diagnosis and Treatment, 2nd ed. Philadelphia, WB Saunders, 1990.)

benign and transient. There have been several reports of an association of these cysts with chromosomal abnormalities.[94–97] There is considerable dispute regarding the practicality of recommending second-trimester amniocentesis when a choroid plexus cyst is seen. On one side of the argument is the observation that fetuses who demonstrate no other anomalies still carry a risk of karyotype anomaly greater than the risk of amniocentesis.[94, 96] Others dispute this observation.[95, 97] Previously it was thought that large size (> 1 cm) or bilaterality favored an abnormal karyotype. It is now clear that small, unilateral lesions may be seen in chromosomally anomalous fetuses.[94] At the present time, all fetuses with choroid plexus cysts should undergo detailed sonographic examination by a person skilled in prenatal diagnosis. This should be followed by unbiased counseling. Again, the expectation is that almost all cysts will regress.

A more important, although less common, supratentorial cyst is the arachnoid cyst.[98, 99] This lesion is the supratentorial analogue of the retrocerebellar arachnoid cyst described earlier (see Fig. 11–9). However, in the larger supratentorial compartment, more variety in appearance may be anticipated. Arachnoid cysts may be either congenital or acquired.[100, 101] The acquired cysts are more common. As a group of lesions seen at any time during life these cysts constitute only 1% of all intracranial masses. Thus, the congenital variety is indeed rare. Congenital arachnoid cysts are likely to be formed by maldevelopment of the leptomeninges and are located between the pia-arachnoid layers. The lesion originally communicates with the subarachnoid space. Acquired arachnoid cysts may follow hemorrhage or infection. Because these pathologic processes occur in utero, as well as after birth, some "congenital" arachnoid cysts are likely to be "acquired."

Arachnoid cysts probably grow in a partially walled off zone between the pia-arachnoid, which has a ball-valve communication with the subarachnoid space.[102] Thus, a fluid-filled mass is formed that may grow progressively. Alternatively, there may be heterotopic choroid plexus–like tissue within the cyst.[103] This tissue presumably secretes CSF into a closed space and results in cyst formation. These lesions produce their ill effects by pressure and mass effect that may result in hydrocephalus. However, they do not cause brain maldevelopment, and, if treated before irreversible brain damage occurs, a good outcome may be anticipated.

Arachnoid cysts must be distinguished from other supratentorial cysts that include choroid plexus cysts, porencephalic (schizencephalic) cysts, cystic tumors, midline cysts associated with agenesis of the corpus callosum, dorsal cysts of holoprosencephaly, and arteriovenous malformations (vein of Galen aneurysms). Arachnoid cysts create a mass effect and never communicate with the lateral ventricle, whereas porencephalic cysts create no mass effect and usually communicate with the lateral ventricle. A cyst in the quadrigeminal plate cistern may simulate the appearance of a vein of Galen aneurysm.[99] However, no Doppler flow is seen in arachnoid cysts while high-velocity signals return from a dilated Galen vein. Choroid plexus cysts are easily discriminated by location. Cystic tumors (teratomas) usually have relatively large amounts of disorganized solid tissue associated with the cystic component, which is a feature that is not shared with arachnoid cysts. Distinction of arachnoid cysts from cysts seen in callosal agenesis and holoprosencephaly is based on the lack of associated brain maldevelopment seen invariably in these other disorders.

The supratentorial arteriovenous malformation or vein of Galen aneurysm is another rare "cystic" space-occupying supratentorial mass (Fig. 11–51).[104] This "cystic" lesion, unlike choroid plexus cysts or arachnoid cysts, is associated with severe cardiovascular hemodynamic abnormalities. Associated CNS disturbances are the rule. Cardiac failure manifested in utero by hydrops fetalis (nonimmune) may be evident. The basic lesion is the arteriovenous communication that results in marked dilatation of the venous component (vein of Galen). The "cyst" is the enlarged vein. In addition to the stress placed on the heart by the arteriovenous malformation, cerebral perfusion is compromised by diversion of blood from brain tissue directly to the venous limb ("steal" phenomenon). This results in brain infarction and in the development of leukomalacia.

The features of this lesion are characteristic and are easily diagnosed by prenatal sonography. The supratentorial cyst is located in or near the tentorial hiatus (the quadrigeminal plate cistern, cistern of the velum interpositum). A high-frequency, turbulent Doppler signal is readily obtained from the lesion (see Fig. 11–51). The carotid arteries and jugular veins are enlarged and similarly show high flow signals. The heart is enlarged, and hydrops fetalis may be seen. Thus, this constellation of findings enables a specific prenatal diagnosis. Unfortunately, little can be done postnatally to prevent death and morbidity. Both are the rule rather than the exception.

Intracranial Hemorrhage

Intracranial hemorrhage is a common event in preterm neonates, especially in those who weigh less than 1500 g and who are born earlier than 32 weeks.[105, 106] The incidence of such hemorrhage is 40% to 50%. The hemorrhages tend to originate in the germinal matrix, which is a highly vascular tissue located in the subependymal region of the lateral ventricles. The germinal matrix is the source of neurons migrating to the cerebral cortex.

Studies in premature infants using computed tomography and real-time sonography show that most hemorrhages occur 1 to 7 days after birth.[106] Although the pathophysiology of neonatal intracranial hemorrhage is unknown, the consensus is that sudden changes in blood pressure of the premature neonate may cause subependymal hemorrhages that may subsequently rupture into the ventricular lumen (intraventricular hemorrhage).

Hypoxic events tend to trigger such fluctuations in blood pressure, resulting in subependymal (germinal matrix) hemorrhage in preterm neonates.[105] Because fetuses have copious germinal matrix and are also susceptible to hypoxemia, one would hypothesize that such hemorrhages could also be common in utero. In fact, intracranial hemorrhage in utero appears to be a peculiarly uncommon event. No series has been reported; only isolated cases appear in the literature.

Intracranial hemorrhages are most commonly categorized by the classification of Papile[106]:

- Type I: Confined to the germinal matrix (i.e., subependymal hemorrhage)
- Type II: Subependymal hemorrhage with rupture into the ventricle, but no dilatation of the ventricle
- Type III: Same as type II, but now the ventricle is dilated with blood
- Type IV: Extension of the hemorrhage into the brain parenchyma

Because hypoxia is a common preceding event in the development of hemorrhages, it is important to remember that infarction and other anoxic brain injuries may be present but may be detected less readily by sonography.

All cases discovered in utero have been types III or IV (Fig. 11–52).[107, 108] These types have the worst prognosis. In preterm neonates types I and II are the more common varieties. On the one hand, this suggests that minor grades of in utero hemorrhage are undetected on prenatal sonograms and are more common

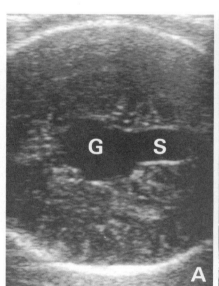

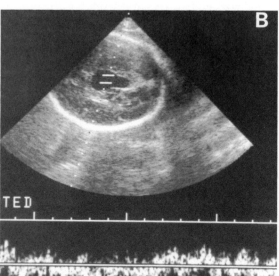

Figure 11–51. *A.* Transverse axial sonogram of the fetal brain showing a central and posterior midline fluid collection. The larger, central component is the dilated Galen vein (G) (the so-called aneurysm). The smaller, posterior component is the dilated straight sinus (S). *B.* That the pathologic structure is a dilated vein is easily shown with pulse-gated Doppler sonography that demonstrates the turbulent flow in the venous side of the arteriovenous malformation. (From Harrison MR, Golbus MS, Filly RA [eds]: The Unborn Patient: Prenatal Diagnosis and Treatment, 2nd ed. Philadelphia, WB Saunders, 1990.)

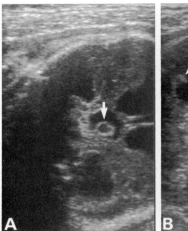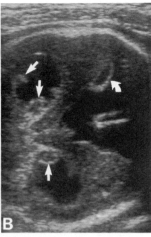

Figure 11–52. *A* and *B*. Transverse axial sonograms showing numerous, maturing blood clots *(arrows)* in the dilated ventricles of a fetus whose mother had severe preeclampsia. The "clot" at the frontal horn margin abutting the caudate head is likely to be a subependymal hematoma *(curved arrow)*. This is a grade III intracranial hemorrhage by Papile's classification. (From Harrison MR, Golbus MS, Filly RA [eds]: The Unborn Patient: Prenatal Diagnosis and Treatment, 2nd ed. Philadelphia, WB Saunders, 1990.)

than the literature documents.* It is well known that even small hemorrhages detected sonographically remain visible for weeks after the inciting event. Thus, if intracranial hemorrhages were very common in the 3 to 4 weeks preceding birth, one would expect to find residual evidence frequently by sonography in the neonate. This is not the case.

A feature that is commonly seen in case reports of fetal intracranial hemorrhage is severe illness in the mother; case reports have included evidence of severe hepatitis,[109] severe hypertension,[110] eclampsia,[108] and acute pancreatitis.[111] However, several cases lacked significant maternal disease. In one of these cases, the fetus was anomalous.[112] In a second case, there was a previous history of two stillbirths of male fetuses.[107] The fetus with intracranial hemorrhage was also male. Nonetheless, in a few cases, the pregnancy appeared to be uncomplicated except for the hemorrhage.[113–115] Especially in cases in which there is no apparent predisposing factor, a diagnosis of alloimmune thrombocytopenia should be considered.[116] In this disorder the mother is sensitized to the fetal platelets, and her antibodies attack and destroy the fetal platelets similar to Rh isoimmunization and the destruction of fetal red blood cells. Other potential causes of fetal thrombocytopenia are infection, thrombocytopenia–absent radius (TAR) syndrome, and maternal idiopathic thrombocytopenic purpura, among others.[116] Even among cases in which illness in the mother is suspected as the etiology of intracranial hemorrhage, some consideration should be given to disorders that can recur in subsequent pregnancies (i.e., alloimmune thrombocytopenia, TAR syndrome).

---

*Postnatal sonograms, obtained through the anterior fontanelle, enable resolution of much greater detail more consistently than in utero sonograms that generally require the beam to pass through the calvaria.

As in the neonate, intracranial hemorrhage, when recent, appears as a brightly echogenic focus, either within the parenchyma of the brain or within the ventricular system. Blood in the ventricular system may show a fluid-fluid level. Intraparenchymal hemorrhage may show progressive liquefaction and excavation that result in a typical porencephalic cyst.

OPEN NEURAL TUBE DEFECTS

General Principles

Neural tube defects are among the most common congenital anomalies in the United States.[116–120] The prevalence of these malformations has been estimated to be as high as 16 per 10,000 births in the eastern United States.[116] The recurrence risk is much higher for a woman who has previously given birth to a child with a neural tube defect. In the United States, the risk of recurrence after one child with a neural tube anomaly is 2% to 3%, and after a second abnormal child the risk is approximately 6%.[118] Women who have previously given birth to a child with a neural tube defect have usually had emotional as well as financial hardship. These women, who have increased risk of having another child with a neural tube defect, frequently seek prenatal testing at an early stage in pregnancy to detect a recurrence of this defect. This has been accomplished generally with measurement of amniotic fluid levels of AFP (see Chapter 3).

α-Fetoprotein is a glycoprotein that is synthesized by the normal fetal liver but is not normally produced by adult hepatocytes.[117–120] AFP is not an abnormal "marker" protein generated by exposed neural tissues. It is a normal protein found in high concentrations in fetal serum. Serum levels are measured in milligrams per milliliter. Under normal circumstances, some of the AFP finds its way into the amniotic fluid. The normal quantity of AFP in amniotic fluid has a much lower level of concentration (measured in micrograms per milliliter) than fetal serum. The mechanism by which AFP normally passes from the fetal circulation into the amniotic fluid is not fully understood, although two likely pathways are through fetal proteinuria (probably a normal event in very early pregnancy) and transudation of plasma proteins across immature fetal epithelium. The AFP found in amniotic fluid normally demonstrates a unimodal concentration curve that peaks early in the second trimester and then declines to very low levels by the end of the pregnancy. Very small but measurable quantities (nanograms per milliliter) of this protein enter the maternal circulation from the amniotic fluid compartment.

If all women who had previously been delivered of a child with an open neural tube defect were screened by measuring amniotic fluid AFP, only 10% of all fetuses with a neural tube defect would be detected.[118] Ninety percent of such anomalies occur as first-time events to women who have not previously been delivered of a child with a neural tube defect. The only practical and safe method for large-scale screening of all pregnant women requires the measurement of maternal serum AFP levels. Measurement of AFP in amniotic fluid has been used successfully for more than two decades to detect open neural tube defects in fetuses. Serum AFP testing is a more recent technique.

When an open neural tube defect is present, a portion of the fetus lacks its normal integumentary covering. For example, in anencephaly there is no skin covering the abnormality. The cranial surface is covered instead by a thick angiomatous stroma. In meningocele, encephalocele, or myelomeningocele, only a membranous covering (or no covering at all) is present. This allows abnormally large quantities of AFP to "leak" into the amniotic fluid and thus, from the amniotic fluid compartment, into the maternal serum.

The results of maternal serum AFP testing have been very encouraging. Almost all pregnant women in the United States are offered AFP screening. When large numbers of women are screened, almost all sonologists doing obstetric scanning will encounter cases referred specifically for "elevation of maternal serum AFP." One must be aware of the problems encountered in such testing.[120–122] First, the maternal serum AFP level may be spuriously elevated. An erroneous LNMP, a common problem, causes the measured AFP to be compared for normalcy with standards for the wrong gestational age. Twins and fetal death also cause elevations of maternal serum AFP without a specific anomaly being present.

Second, such tests detect abnormalities other than open neural tube defects. For example, omphalocele and particularly gastroschisis are also anomalies associated with integumentary defects and leak AFP into the amniotic fluid.[123, 124] Although these fetuses are abnormal, a fetus with gastroschisis has a better prognosis than does a fetus with an encephalocele. Knowledge that a fetus has one defect rather than another (found by sonographic discrimination) could clearly affect a parental decision regarding subsequent management of the pregnancy (i.e., termination versus continued gestation with surgical repair of the anomaly after birth).

Third, and most important, normal, living, singleton fetuses may be incorrectly judged to be abnormal by either maternal serum or amniotic fluid AFP testing.[118–123] For example, fetal serum contains many times more AFP than does amniotic fluid. Thus, slight contamination of the amniotic fluid with fetal blood spuriously elevates amniotic fluid AFP levels into the abnormal zone. Additionally, a problem that one often neglects to consider in a diagnostic setting must be strongly considered in a screening study. Statistically, a small percentage of normal fetuses have amniotic fluid or maternal serum AFP levels greater than 2 or even 3 standard deviations (SD) above the mean.[122] For example, 2 SD above the mean implies that, in a gaussian distribution, approximately 2.5% of normal persons will fall above this cutoff. Even if we assume that every abnormal fetus will fall above 2 SD, the following situation occurs in 10,000 samples tested:

2.5% of normals > 2 SD = 250 normals
100% of abnormals > 2 SD = 16 abnormals

In this example, there would be 266 tests with an abnormal result, but only 16 of the fetuses would have a neural tube defect. A partial solution is to raise the "normal" cutoff to 3, 4, or even 5 SD above the mean. However, each time that one does this, the risk of "missing" an abnormal fetus increases. Unfortunately, even if one were to go as high as 5 SD above the mean and test many thousands of women, there would still be a small but significant number of false-positive diagnoses.

What is clearly needed in such a situation is a second level of testing that discriminates the normal from the abnormal case. Sonography adequately serves as the second level of testing.[123–126] The first level of testing (AFP analysis) works with a very large group of fetuses that has a very low prevalence of disease. The second level of testing (sonography) works with a small group of fetuses with a high prevalence of disease. This statistical situation can greatly improve diagnostic accuracy with the second testing system. Additionally, the sonologist is provided with a "list" of potential abnormalities that could be identified. Using this "road map," specific areas of the fetus may be preferentially examined for the presence of anomalies, providing a set of circumstances that can lead to extremely accurate sonographic results.[124]

Anencephaly

This severe defect is the most common of the open neural tube defects and is also the most common anomaly affecting the CNS.[117–119] It shows a clear female predominance with a female-to-male ratio of 4:1. An increased familial incidence has been established, such as with all other neural tube defects.

Even though anencephaly means absence of the brain, functioning neural tissue is always present.[127] The telencephalon is usually absent, whereas the brain stem and portions of the mesencephalon are usually present. Absence of the cranial vault (the bones formed in membrane) is a constant finding (acrania). However, bones formed in cartilage at the base of the skull, including the orbits, are usually present.

Anencephaly results from a failure of the neural tube to completely close at its cephalic end.[9] This occurs between the second and third week of development when the neural folds at the cranial end of the neural plate normally fuse to form the forebrain. The defect is covered by a thick membrane of angiomatous stroma but never by bone or normal skin.

Anencephaly was the earliest fetal malformation to be recognized by sonography[128] and can be consistently detected.[123–126, 129, 130] Most often, anencephaly is discovered sonographically at the time of attempted biparietal diameter determination for fetal age. However, more recently, it is being discovered with increasing frequency in patients referred for elevated AFP levels. Almost all cases of this universally fatal anomaly can be discovered at an early stage in pregnancy with widespread AFP testing programs.

The finding that draws the attention of the observer to the presence of a severe abnormality is the absence

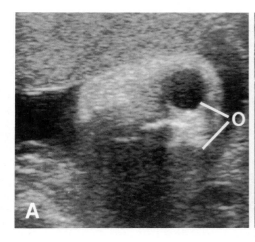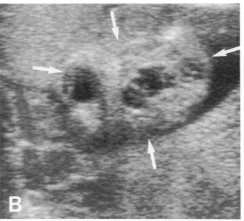

Figure 11–53. Anencephaly in the mid-second trimester. *A.* Coronal sonogram through the face shows the "classic" appearance of anencephaly (symmetric absence of calvaria above the orbits [O]). *B.* Oblique section through the angiomatous stroma *(arrows)* overlying the base of the skull. The tissue is partially solid and partially cystic.

of the normal cephalic outline (acrania). Although this may be recognizable toward the end of the first trimester, the calvarial bones are so small before the 13th week that they may be unnoticed during a routine examination. The symmetric absence of the calvarial bone enables a specific diagnosis of anencephaly to be made by sonography—a feature that is best demonstrated on a coronal image of the fetal face (Fig. 11–53), although sagittal images are dramatic as well (Fig. 11–54). Relatively copious amounts of tissue may be present above the orbits when this anomaly is seen at an early stage (Fig. 11–55). This tissue may represent either abnormally exposed brain tissue (exencephaly)[131] or buoyant angiomatous stroma. Many cases of anencephaly have been recognized as showing a typical configuration by the 16th week, whereas a fetus examined during the 12th week with this anomaly failed to show classic features.[132] Identification of the "head" is not sufficient to exclude anencephaly. The bony skull base and orbits are generally present and may give the impression of a cranial structure if they are viewed hurriedly. Failure to identify normal bony structure

and brain tissue cephalad to the bony orbits is the most reliable feature of this anomaly. Equally important, the absence of the bony calvaria should be symmetric (see Fig. 11–55).

Common associated anomalies include spinal defects that occur in 50% of anencephalic fetuses. Severe rachischisis (spina bifida), with or without myelomeningocele, can often be demonstrated by sonography. Other associated anomalies may also be seen. However, because anencephaly is a uniformly fatal abnormality, effort should be concentrated on confirming its presence. Once a fetus has a confirmed fatal abnormality, the identification of additional anomalies is superfluous. Polyhydramnios is present in 40% to 50% of cases but does not occur usually until after 26 weeks of gestation. Oligohydramnios is encountered occasionally.

A distinction should be made between anencephaly and other conditions that may be confused with it. Any similar-appearing anomaly that has caused the cranium and brain to be sufficiently small, by either abnormal growth or destruction, should be judged to carry the same fatal prognosis. However, the risk of recurrence for the mother may vary considerably (ranging from no risk of recurrence up to a 25% risk of recurrence). The precise nature of the abnormality may not be detectable by ex utero examination of an abortus if dilatation and extraction were the methods used to evacuate the uterus. Thus, the in utero sonographic examination may be the only opportunity to establish the true nature, and thus the potential recurrence risk, of the anomaly.

When severe, microcephaly may mimic the appearance of anencephaly. However, one can always identify a cranial vault when microcephaly is present. Frequently, cortical brain tissue is identified in microcephaly, although it may be very small in quantity. If microcephaly is extremely severe, one must rely solely on identification of the cranial vault to distinguish this entity from anencephaly. In anencephaly, of course, both the cranial vault and cortical brain tissue are absent. Depending on the etiology, microcephalic disorders may have a 25% risk of recurrence. Amniotic band syndrome involving the head may present a confusing picture, because this entity may destroy most

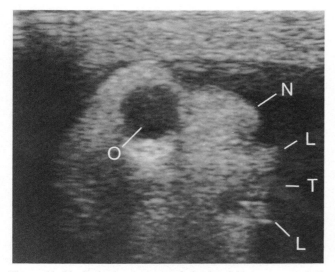

Figure 11–54. Sagittal sonogram of the head in an anencephalic fetus. Note the absence of calvarial structure above the orbit (O). N, nose; L, lip; T, tongue.

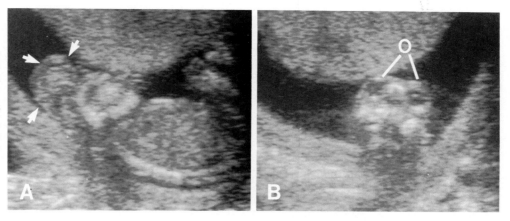

Figure 11–55. Anencephaly in the early second trimester. *A.* Sagittal sonogram shows a large amount of angiomatous stroma *(arrows)* cephalad to the base of the skull. *B.* However, the coronal image of the face demonstrates the symmetric absence of calvaria above the orbits (O), thus confirming the diagnosis of anencephaly.

of the cranial vault and the brain.[133] However, amniotic band syndrome tends to destroy the cranium asymmetrically. In anencephaly, the absence of the cranial vault is symmetric. There is no known risk of recurrence for amniotic band syndrome. The rare occurrence of the holoacardious "acephalic" twin can be a true anencephalic aberration. In this case, the entire cranial structure may be lacking, or severe microcephaly may be present. This condition occurs only in identical twins.[134] The acephalic acardiac twin is a parasite on the sibling. However, true anencephaly can occur asynchronously in twins without association of parabiotic vascular communications in the placenta. Presumably this later situation, unlike the holoacardious identical twin, has a risk of recurrence in subsequent singleton pregnancies.

Encephalocele

This condition is the least common open neural tube defect.[123–125, 135–138] Encephalocele results from failure of the surface ectoderm to separate from the neuroectoderm.[9] This results in a mesodermal (bony calvarial) defect that allows herniation of the meninges alone (cranial meningocele) or the brain and the meninges (true encephalocele) through the bony defect. The most common site of occurrence is the occipital midline (75%) (Figs. 11–56 and 11–57) followed by the frontal midline (13%). Parietal lesions are noted in approximately 12% of cases.[139, 140] However, lesions located off of the midline are almost always the result of the amniotic band syndrome (Fig. 11–58). Although AFP screening programs have further improved the prenatal detection of fetal cephaloceles, most cephaloceles are skin covered and therefore not associated with AFP elevation.

Encephaloceles are recognized as being spherical, fluid-filled, or brain-filled sacs (Fig. 11–59) that extend from the bony calvaria in the occipital or frontal region.[5, 6, 135–137] Identification of the encephalocele sac is usually not difficult. Identification of the associated bony defect is more difficult (see Fig. 11–56). Importantly, acoustic shadowing may produce a spurious "defect" in the calvaria. In the suspect gestation with elevated AFP levels, a systematic and detailed approach should be used to evaluate the calvaria for these defects in the typical locations described earlier.

Absence of brain tissue within the cranial meningocele sac is the single most favorable prognostic feature for survival.[141] Visualization of solid brain elements within the sac is usually straightforward. However, it is difficult to exclude incorporated brain tissue in sacs that appear completely filled with fluid. Small amounts

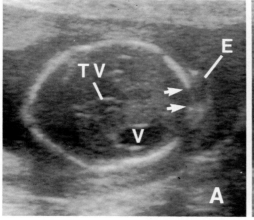
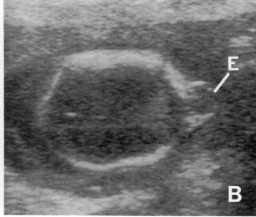

Figure 11–56. Small occipital encephalocele. *A* and *B.* Paired transverse axial sonograms. Arrows indicate bony defect. E, encephalocele sac; TV, enlarged third ventricle; V, prominent ventricle.

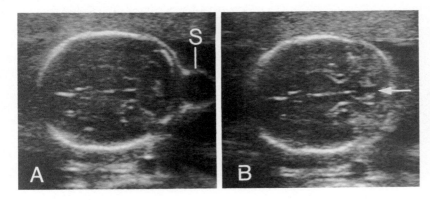

Figure 11–57. *A.* Transverse axial sonogram demonstrating a small encephalocele sac (S). *B.* Additionally there is partial agenesis of the vermis *(arrow)* (a Dandy-Walker syndrome variant).

Figure 11–58. *A.* Transverse axial sonogram through the calvaria of a fetus with an encephalocele (E) that does not lie in the midline *(arrow)*. This feature should suggest the amniotic band syndrome. *B.* A further search discloses numerous bands *(arrowheads)* attached to the extremities of the fetus.

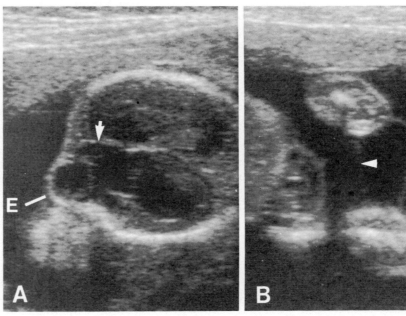

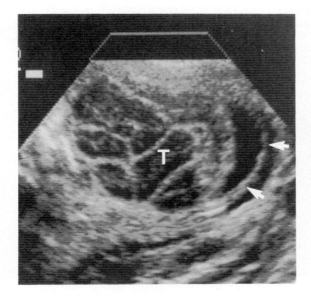

Figure 11–59. Sector real-time sonogram of a large, fetal encephalocele. Arrow indicates sac margin. T, disorganized brain tissue. Avoid the temptation to call the swirled tissue in the sac "gyri and sulci." This type of structure is poorly developed in young *normal fetuses*. It is unlikely that this process is more advanced in fetuses with maldeveloped brain tissue.

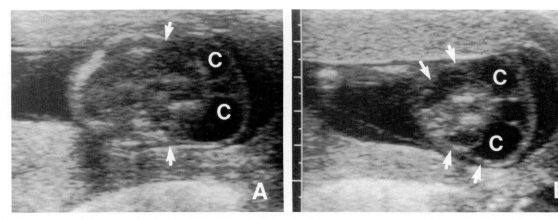

Figure 11–60. Transverse axial sonograms through the basiocciput *(A)* and neck *(B)* in a fetus with a large nuchal cystic hygroma (C). Margins of these lesions "line up" with the adjacent cutaneous tissues *(arrows)*. Adjacent subcutaneous tissues are almost always abnormal and can be recognized as such.

of incorporated brain tissue may be present toward the periphery of the sac. Associated anomalies include hydrocephalus (from the concomitant Chiari malformation), agenesis of the corpus callosum, Dandy-Walker syndrome, and the Meckel syndrome (encephalocele, microcephaly, polydactyly, cystic kidneys).

Some lesions may be mistaken for encephaloceles. The most common of these lesions is the cystic hygroma (Fig. 11–60). Cystic hygromas have no cranial defect, and careful scanning confirms that the lesion is continuous with abnormal skin and subcutaneous tissues adjacent to the cystic cavity (Fig. 11–61). Care is required because a spurious calvarial defect may be caused by reflective shadowing, resulting in an erroneous diagnosis of encephalocele. Nasal teratomas must be distinguished from frontal encephaloceles. The

teratoma is usually more irregularly shaped and heterogeneous in its architecture. A cloverleaf skull deformity also simulates the appearance of an encephalocele. A distinction can be made in this case by observing the presence of calvaria surrounding the three cephalic protrusions of fetuses that have the clover-leaf skull deformity.

Finally, dacryocystoceles, cysts of the tear duct, could potentially be confused with frontal encephaloceles. However, their typical location medial to the globe and simple cystic appearance help to distinguish this benign entity (Fig. 11–62).

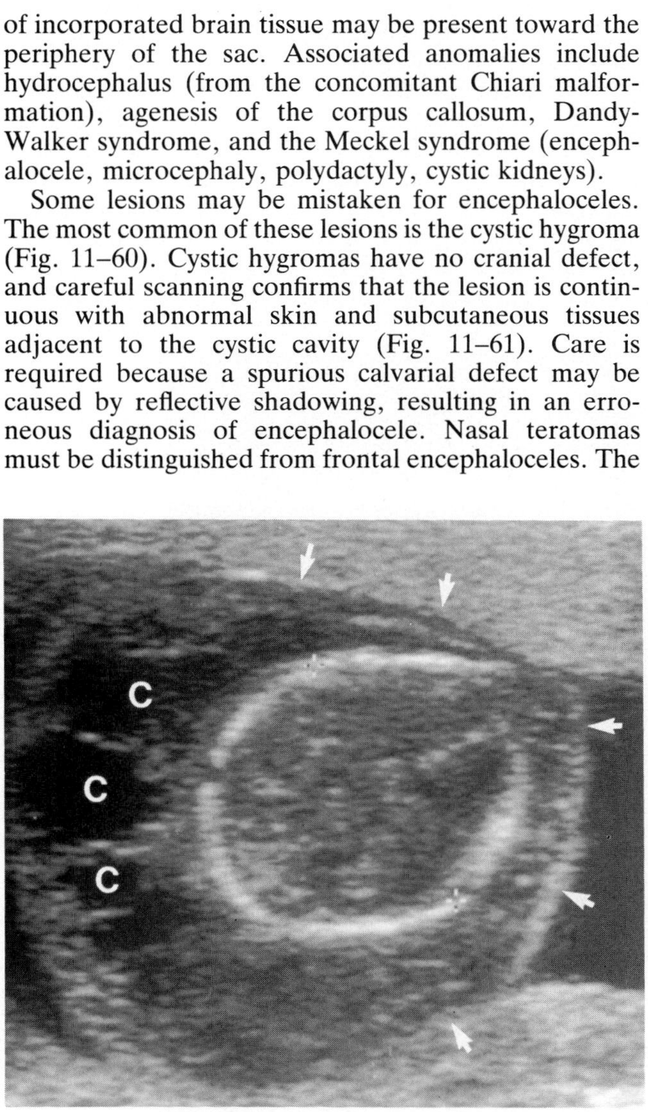

Myelomeningocele—Spina Bifida

Myelomeningocele is the second most common open neural tube defect.[118] As with the calvaria, it is possible to have a spinal meningocele without incorporated nerve roots or cord within it. However, isolated me-

Figure 11–61. Transverse axial sonogram showing diffuse lymphangiectasia with cystic hygroma formation. The cystic spaces (C) shown posteriorly should not be misinterpreted as being encephaloceles. Note that all the subcutaneous tissues *(arrows)* are abnormal. (From Harrison MR, Golbus MS, Filly RA [eds]: The Unborn Patient: Prenatal Diagnosis and Treatment, 2nd ed. Philadelphia, WB Saunders, 1990.)

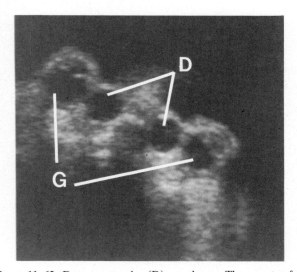

Figure 11–62. Dacryocystoceles (D) are shown. These cysts of the tear duct apparatus sit medial to the globes (G) of the eyes. They are generally benign and should not be confused with frontal encephaloceles. (From Harrison MR, Golbus MS, Filly RA [eds]: The Unborn Patient: Prenatal Diagnosis and Treatment, 2nd ed. Philadelphia, WB Saunders, 1990.)

ningoceles are rare by comparison with myelomeningoceles. These lesions may occur anywhere along the spine but are most common in the lumbar and sacral regions. The malformation results from failure of closure of the neural tube (caudal neuropore) at 3 to 4 weeks, resulting in an exposed neural plate.[9] The defect varies in size and content. Neurologic defects range from minor anesthesia to complete paraparesis and death. Prognosis is worse the higher the lesion or the larger the lesion and if the lesion is associated with other anomalies.[142]

The fetal spine is easily and clearly evaluated by 16 to 17 weeks of development.[143] The normal posterior ossification centers are seen as two closely spaced parallel lines of echoes that widen normally in the cervical region. The distance between the posterior ossification centers is tantamount to the interpediculate distance.[5, 6, 143] In the transverse plane of section three ossification centers are identified, all within close proximity surrounding the spinal cord. In spina bifida (Fig. 11–63), which is the bony accompaniment to myelomeningocele, there is separation on the transverse and longitudinal scans of the posterior ossification centers (Figs. 11–64 through 11–68). Normally in transverse planes the posterior ossification centers are parallel to each other or angle toward one another. Spina bifida can be diagnosed when the posterior ossification centers splay outward and are further apart than the ossification centers above or below the defect (see Figs. 11–65 and 11–66). The latter is noted on longitudinal images (Fig. 11–67). The cleft in the soft tissues can almost always be seen with modern high-resolution equipment. Indeed, the cleft is recognized more easily in some cases than the bony defect itself (see Fig. 11–64). Spinal defects are easily diagnosed if three or more vertebral segments are involved.[123, 124] If two or fewer spinal segments are involved, the diagnosis becomes more difficult. Abnormal morphology of the posterior ossification centers of the spine must be used to make the diagnosis if the myelomeningocele sac is not intact or if it is flattened (see Figs. 11–66 and 11–69). When the sac is intact and bulges into the amniotic cavity, the anomaly is recognized more easily as being a cystic extension off of the posterior aspect of the spine, which in real time may have a shimmering quality with fetal movement. Fetal movement may be quite active, even in the lower extremities of fetuses with myelomeningoceles, although a neurologic effect on the lower extremity can be seen not uncommonly (clubfoot deformity) (Fig. 11–70).

When a specific search is made for a myelomeningocele (i.e., elevated AFP level), very small lesions can be detected (Fig. 11–71A). This is especially true when a sac is present and is in contact with amniotic fluid (see Fig. 11–71B). When the fetal spine abuts the myometrium or placenta, the sac, even when present, may be obscured (see Figs. 11–65 and 11–66). When the skin is intact over a myelomeningocele, no AFP

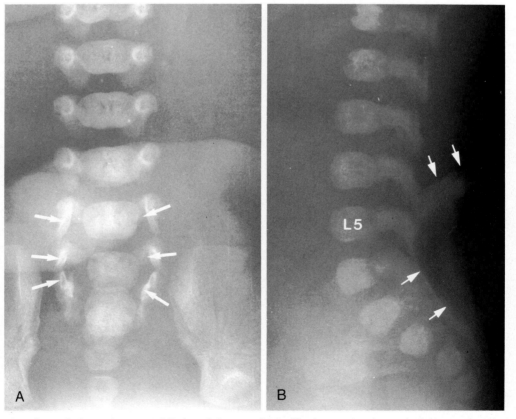

Figure 11–63. *A.* A radiograph shows the outward flaring of the posterior ossification centers *(arrows)* of the vertebrae in spina bifida. This increases the interpediculate distance. *B.* A lateral radiograph demonstrates the sac margins *(arrows)*. (From Harrison MR, Golbus MS, Filly RA [eds]: The Unborn Patient: Prenatal Diagnosis and Treatment, 2nd ed. Philadelphia, WB Saunders, 1990.)

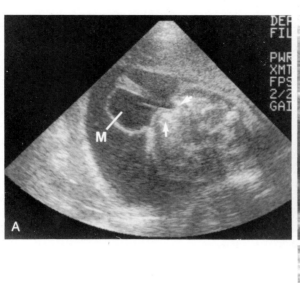

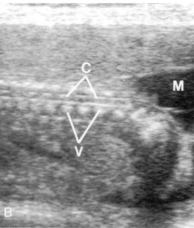

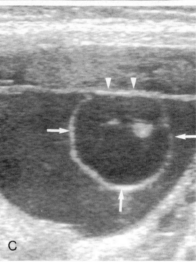

Figure 11–64. *A.* Transverse axial sonogram of the sacrum in a fetus with a myelomeningocele (M). Abnormal posterior ossification centers are seen *(arrows)*. *B.* Longitudinal sonogram demonstrating the myelomeningocele (M) extending from the spine. The spinal cord (C) ends at an abnormally low level (tethered cord). V, vertebral bodies. *C.* Scan oriented through the sac of the myelomeningocele. The sac margin is easily seen where it makes contact with the amniotic fluid *(arrows)* but almost disappears *(arrowheads)* where the sac makes contact with the placental surface.

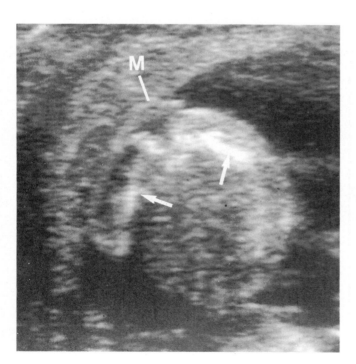

Figure 11–65. Transverse axial scan through the iliac wings *(arrows)* showing a small myelomeningocele (M). Note that the sac is obscured mainly by contact with the myometrium.

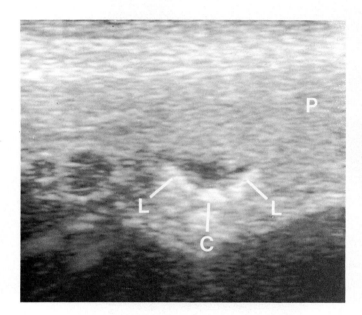

Figure 11–66. Transverse axial sonogram of the lumbar spine showing a spina bifida lesion. This fetus with an open spinal lesion had no sac. Additionally, profound oligohydramnios was present. Thus, the only opportunity to detect this lesion is by demonstration of the flared laminae (L), which are characteristic of spina bifida. C, centrum; P, placenta.

Figure 11–67. Coronal sonogram through the posterior ossification centers (POC) of the lumbosacral spine showing a small myelomeningocele. Abnormal spacing *(arrows)* of the POC is seen; this is the spina bifida lesion.

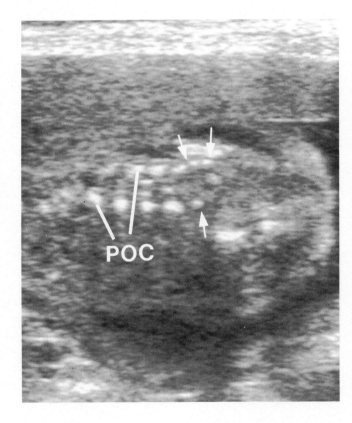

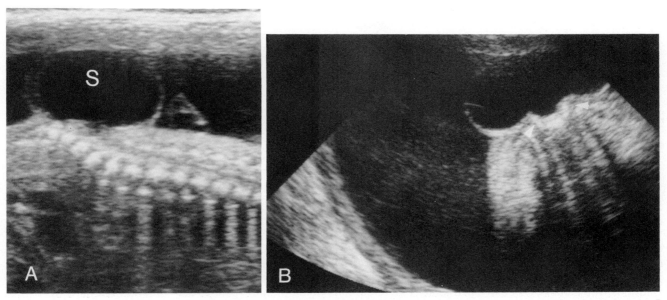

Figure 11–68. *A.* Parasagittal sonogram of the spine demonstrates a myelomeningocele sac (S) beginning at L5 and extending inferiorly. *B.* Transverse axial sonogram demonstrates the splayed posterior elements *(arrowheads).*

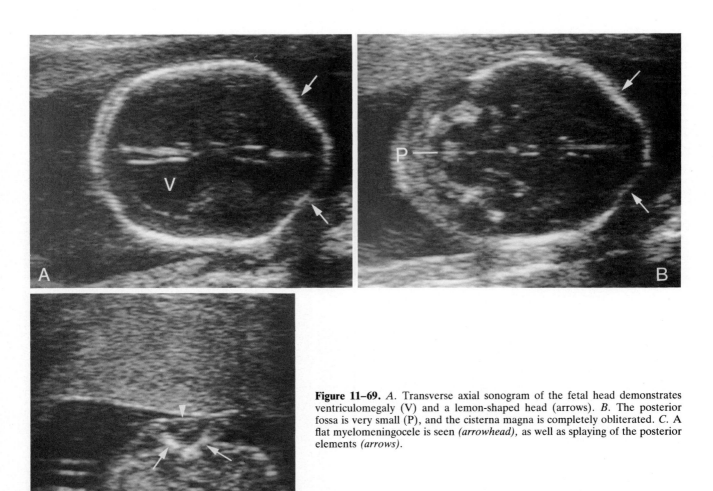

Figure 11–69. *A.* Transverse axial sonogram of the fetal head demonstrates ventriculomegaly (V) and a lemon-shaped head (arrows). *B.* The posterior fossa is very small (P), and the cisterna magna is completely obliterated. *C.* A flat myelomeningocele is seen *(arrowhead),* as well as splaying of the posterior elements *(arrows).*

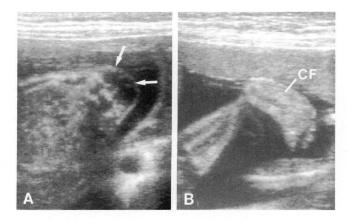

Figure 11–70. *A.* Fetus with a lumbar myelomeningocele *(arrows)*. *B.* Clubfoot deformity (CF) secondary to the myelomeningocele.

elevation will occur. In this situation, only sonography has an opportunity to detect the anomaly (Fig. 11–72).

As with encephaloceles, associated abnormalities are commonly present. Ventricular enlargement secondary to the Arnold-Chiari (type II) malformation is very common (see Fig. 11–69A).[142] Although not all fetuses with myelomeningocele display the Chiari (type II) malformation, the percentage of fetuses afflicted with this malformation at the craniocervical junction is very high. Furthermore, almost every fetus with a myelomeningocele has an abnormal posterior fossa, although the abnormality may not fulfil the morphologic requirements to diagnose the Chiari (type II) malformation (Figs. 11–73 and 11–74B).[144] Myelomeningocele is the most common single etiology of hydrocephalus in a fetus; the hydrocephalus develops secondary to the Chiari malformation. Thus, the presence of ventricular enlargement and an abnormally small or absent cisterna magna is an observation that should always

engender an extremely careful search of the spine for the presence of an open neural tube defect. An additional feature that is a signal for the presence of a myelomeningocele is the so-called lemon sign.[145] This is a scalloping of the frontal bones (see Figs. 11–69A and 11–74A). The lemon sign, however, is also seen in normal fetuses and in cephaloceles.[138] However, the diagnosis of myelomeningocele should always be based on direct observation of the spinal anomaly and not on secondary signs.

Detection of CNS Anomalies: A Practical Level of Effort for a "Routine" Sonogram

Sonography is an extraordinarily powerful technology that enables detection and characterization of numerous CNS malformations, some of which cause

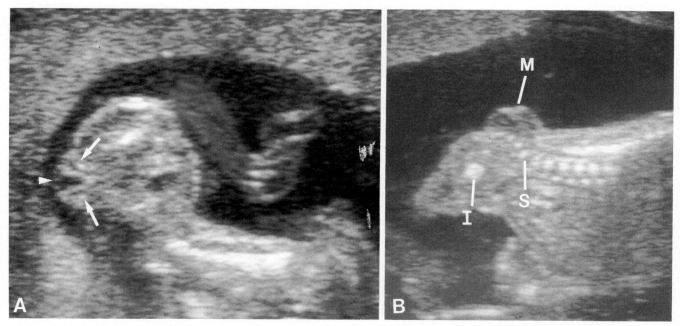

Figure 11–71. *A.* Transverse axial sonogram of the sacrum showing a very small myelomeningocele. A characteristic sac *(arrowhead)* and "splaying" of posterior ossification centers *(arrows)* are shown. *B.* Longitudinal sonogram of the same fetus. The myelomeningocele sac (M) is slightly greater than 1 cm but is seen very easily. Although smaller lesions are more difficult to detect, visualization does not depend strictly on size. I, ischial ossification center; S, sacral promontory.

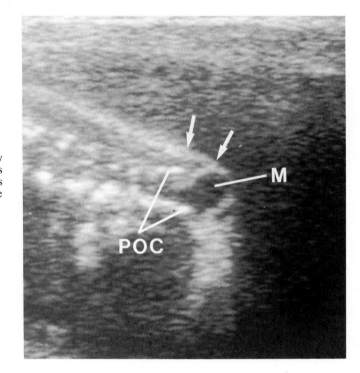

Figure 11–72. Longitudinal sonogram of sacrum showing a very small myelomeningocele (M). This unusual myelomeningocele is covered with skin *(arrows)* (compare with Fig. 11–71). Despite its small size (< 1 cm), it is easily seen. Note the splaying of the posterior ossification centers (POC).

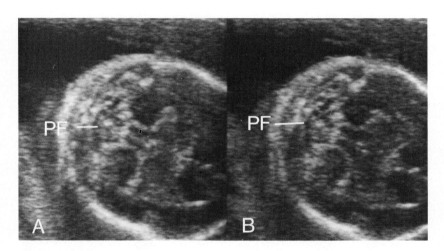

Figure 11–73. *A* and *B*. Transverse axial sonograms demonstrating an extremely small posterior fossa (PF) in a fetus with a myelomeningocele. The cisterna magna is completely obliterated.

Figure 11–74. *A* and *B*. Transverse axial sonogram of the fetal brain demonstrating a "lemon" sign *(arrows)*, enlargement of the ventricular atrium *(cursors)*, and effacement of the cisterna magna *(curved arrow)* in a fetus with a myelomeningocele.

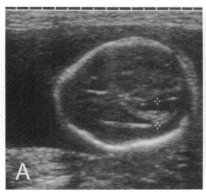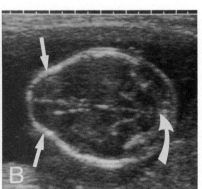

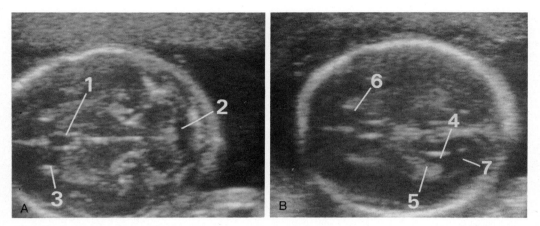

Figure 11–75. *A* and *B*. Transverse axial sonograms of the fetal brain demonstrating the cavum septi pellucidi (1), the cisterna magna (2), and the ventricular atrium (4). Also demonstrated are the frontal horn (3 and 6), the glomus of the choroid plexus (5), and the occipital horn (7).

only subtle aberrations in morphology. As physicians, we must balance our desire to do the utmost for each of our patients with the practicality that performing detailed evaluations of the brain and spinal cord in every case is simply impossible.

Fortunately, there are a few simple observations that can be made while measuring a biparietal diameter or head circumference that will exclude most anomalies of both the brain and the spine. Three structures, namely, the cavum septi pellucidi, the ventricular atrium, and the cisterna magna, are easily demonstrated even by inexperienced examiners (Fig. 11–75).[146] What is substantially more difficult is understanding how demonstration of these normal structures is so effective at excluding many CNS malformations, especially those of the spinal cord. Importantly, this

scheme helps one to recognize that an abnormality may be present but does not help to make specific diagnoses. If these three structures appear well within normal limits, the chances that the fetus has a neural axis anomaly of any type (including myelomeningocele) are very small.

Open neural tube defects are the most common CNS malformations. Anencephaly, which is the single most common open neural tube defect, is so severe that it is immediately detected when attempting to perform biometry of the fetal head. Not even one of the three recommended observations could possibly be made, even mistakenly, in an anencephalic fetus. Unfortunately, the second most common type is myelomeningocele, the opening of which can be so subtle and difficult to detect that even the most skilled examiners

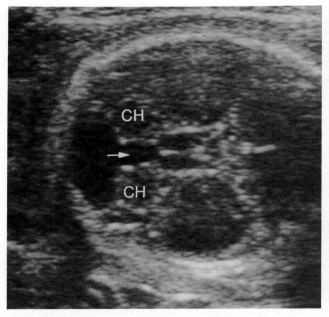

Figure 11–76. Transverse axial sonogram demonstrating an "enlarged cisterna magna" (actually an enlarged fourth ventricle) in a fetus with inferior vermian agenesis *(arrow)*. Ch, cerebellar hemispheres.

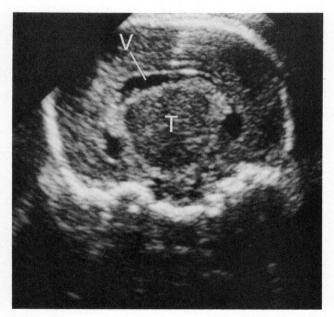

Figure 11–77. Coronal sonogram of a fetus with lobar holoprosencephaly. There is a single ventricle (V), but it is not enlarged. The thalami are fused (T). No cavum septi pellucidi would be demonstrable in such a case.

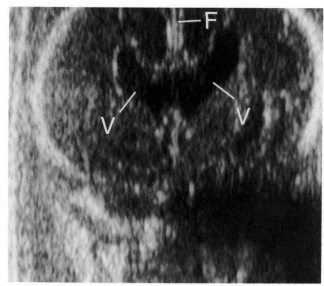

Figure 11–78. Coronal sonogram demonstrating absence of the cavum septi pellucidi in a fetus with agenesis of the corpus callosum. F, falx; V, frontal horn of the ventricle.

are afraid of false-negative results. However, this entity is almost always associated with the Chiari malformation. The Chiari malformation invariably effaces and most often obliterates the cisterna magna (see Fig. 11–73). An easily demonstrated cisterna magna with a clearly normal depth (4 to 10 mm) will be present rarely, if ever, in a fetus with a myelomeningocele. The alternative method to diagnose myelomeningoceles requires a careful evaluation of every vertebral segment. Almost 100% of myelomeningoceles can be detected with this approach. However, it is an approach that is entirely impractical for daily use. Furthermore, a normal cisterna magna excludes all but the mildest forms of Dandy-Walker syndrome (Fig. 11–76), cerebellar hypoplasia, and retrocerebellar arachnoid cyst.

Gross abnormalities of the supratentorial CNS (hydranencephaly, alobar holoprosencephaly, and massive hydrocephalus) are easily detected when attempting head measurements, although a differential diagnosis is substantially more difficult to make. However, less morphologically severe anomalies such as agenesis of the corpus callosum and lobar holoprosencephaly or brain atrophy can easily escape detection (Fig. 11–77). Complete agenesis of the corpus callosum and lobar holoprosencephaly are always associated with absence of the septum pellucidum and, thus, the cavum septi pellucidi (Fig. 11–78). Therefore, demonstration of the cavum septi pellucidi excludes almost every subtle malformation of midline development of the brain.

Similarly, visualization of the ventricular atrium enables detection of very early ventricular enlargement. Importantly, enlargement of the atrium detects both obstructive hydrocephalus from any cause (communicating [rare] or noncommunicating) and nonobstructive ventricular enlargement, including developmental (colpocephaly) and destructive (brain atrophy) etiologies.

The cavum septi pellucidi should be visible in the plane in which the biparietal diameter is measured. Only minor alterations in angulation of the transducer relative to the base of the skull are required to visualize the ventricular atrium and the cisterna magna. Once practiced, this procedure takes only seconds to accomplish. This brief effort to demonstrate these three structures leaves the examiner with a high level of confidence that most lesions in the development of the CNS, even some of the most difficult lesions to detect, are not present.

References

1. Carrasco CR, Stierman ED, Harnsberger HR, Lee TG: An algorithm for prenatal ultrasound diagnosis of congenital CNS abnormalities. J Ultrasound Med 4:163, 1985.
2. Goldberg BB, Isard JH, Gershon-Cohen J, et al: Ultrasonic fetal cephalometry. Radiology 87:328, 1966.
3. Hidalgo H, Bowie J, Rosenberg ER, et al: In utero sonographic diagnosis of fetal cerebral anomalies. AJR 139:143, 1982.
4. Pasto ME, Kurtz AB: The prenatal examination of the fetal cranium, spine, and central nervous system. Semin Ultrasound CT MR 5:170, 1984.
5. Fiske CE, Filly RA: Ultrasound evaluation of the normal and abnormal fetal neural axis. Radiol Clin North Am 20:285, 1982.
6. Filly RA: Ultrasonography. In Harrison MR, Golbus MS, Filly RA (eds): The Unborn Patient: Prenatal Diagnosis and Treatment, pp 33–123. Orlando, FL, Grune & Stratton, 1984.
7. Edwards MSD, Filly RA: Diagnosis and management of fetal disorders of the central nervous system. In Hoffman HJ, Epstein F (eds): Disorders of the Developing Nervous System: Diagnosis and Treatment, pp 55–73. Boston, Blackwell Scientific Publications, 1986.
8. Clewell WH, Johnson ML, Meier PR, et al: A surgical approach to the treatment of fetal hydrocephalus. N Engl J Med 306:1320, 1982.
9. Moore KL: The nervous system. In The Developing Human, 3rd ed, pp 375–412. Philadelphia, WB Saunders, 1982.
10. Day WR: Casts of the foetal lateral ventricles. Brain, 82:109, 1959.
11. Masdeu JC, Dobben GD, Azar-Kia B: Dandy-Walker syndrome studies by computed tomography and pneumoencephalography. Radiology 147:109, 1983.
12. Gardner E, O'Rahilly R, Prolo D: The Dandy-Walker and Arnold-Chiari malformations. Arch Neurol 23:393, 1974.
13. Goodwin L, Quisling RG: The neonatal cisterna magna: Ultrasonic evaluation. Radiology 149:691, 1974.
14. Dempsey PJ, Koch HJ: In utero diagnosis of the Dandy-Walker syndrome: Differentiation from extra-axial posterior fossa cyst. J Clin Ultrasound 9:403, 1981.
15. Lipton HL, Preiosi TJ, Moses H: Adult onset of the Dandy-Walker syndrome. Arch Neurol 35:672, 1978.
16. Lee TG, Newton BW: Posterior fossa cyst: Prenatal diagnosis by ultrasound. J Clin Ultrasound 4:29, 1976.
17. Hatjis CG, Horbar JD, Anderson GG: The in utero diagnosis of a posterior fossa intracranial cyst (Dandy-Walker cyst). Am J Obstet Gynecol 140:473, 1981.
18. Kirkinen P, Jouppila P, Valkeakari T, Saukkonen AL: Ultrasonic evaluation of the Dandy-Walker syndrome. Obstet Gynecol 59:18S, 1982.
19. Newman GC, Buschi AI, Sugg NK, et al: Dandy-Walker syndrome diagnosed in utero by ultrasonography. Neurology 32:180, 1982.
20. Depp R, Sabbagha RE, Brown T, et al: Fetal surgery for hydrocephalus: Successful in utero ventriculoamniotic shunt for Dandy-Walker syndrome. Obstet Gynecol 61:710, 1983.
21. Comstock H, Boal DB: Enlarged fetal cisterna magna: Appearance and significance. Obstet Gynecol 66:25S, 1985.
22. McCleary R, Kuhns L, Barr M: Ultrasonography of the fetal cerebellum. Radiology 151:439, 1984.

23. Archer C, Darwish H, Smith K: Enlarged cisternae magnae and posterior fossa cysts simulating Dandy-Walker syndrome on computed tomography. Radiology 127:681, 1978.
24. Kendall E: Dysgenesis of the corpus callosum. Neuroradiology 25:239, 1983.
25. Probst FP: Congenital defects of the corpus callosum: Morphology and encephalographic appearances. Acta Radiol (Diag) 331:1S, 1973.
26. Harwood-Nash DC: Absence of the corpus callosum. In Harwood-Nash DC (ed): Neuroradiology in Infants and Children, vol 3, p 1019. St. Louis, CV Mosby, 1976.
27. Rakic P, Yakovlev PI: Development of the corpus callosum and cavum septi in man. J Comp Neurol 132:45, 1968.
28. Comstock CH, Culp D, Gonzalez J, Boal DB: Agenesis of the corpus callosum in the fetus: Its evolution and significance. J Ultrasound Med 4:613, 1985.
29. Gebarski SS, Gebraski KS, Bowerman RA, Silver TM: Agenesis of the corpus callosum: Sonographic features. Radiology 151:443, 1984.
30. Mok PM, Gunn TR: The diagnosis of absence of the corpus callosum by ultrasound. Australas Radiol 26:121, 1982.
31. Skeffington F: Agenesis of the corpus callosum: Neonatal ultrasound appearance. Arch Dis Child 57:713, 1982.
32. Skidmore MB, Dolfin T, Becker LE, et al: The sonographic diagnosis of agenesis of the corpus callosum. J Ultrasound Med 2:55, 1983.
33. Babcock DS: The normal, absent and abnormal corpus callosum: Sonographic findings. Radiology 151:449, 1984.
34. Cohen MM, Jirasek JE, Guzman RT, et al: Holoprosencephaly and facial dysmorphia: Nosology, etiology and pathogenesis. Birth Defects 7:125, 1971.
35. Manelfe C, Sevely A: Neuroradiologic study of holoprosencephalies. J. Neuroradiol 9:15, 1982.
36. Warkany J, Lemire R, Cohen M: Holoprosencephaly: Cyclopia series. In Warkany J: Mental Retardation and Congenital Malformations of the Central Nervous System, pp 176–190. Chicago, Year Book Medical Publishers, 1981.
37. Cohen MM: An update on the holoprosencephalic disorders. J Pediatr 101:865, 1982.
38. Filly RA, Chinn DH, Callen PW: Alobar holoprosencephaly: Ultrasonographic prenatal diagnosis. Radiology 151:455, 1984.
39. Chervenak FA, Isaacson G, Hobbins JC, et al: Diagnosis and management of fetal holoprosencephaly. Obstet Gynecol 66:322, 1985.
40. Greene MF, Benacerraf BR, Frigoletto FD: Reliable criteria for the prenatal sonographic diagnosis of alobar holoprosencephaly. Am J Obstet Gynecol 156:687, 1987.
41. Toth Z, Csecsei K, Szeifert G, et al: Early prenatal diagnosis of cyclopia associated with holoprosencephaly. J Clin Ultrasound 14:550, 1986.
42. Chervenak FA, Isaacson G, Mahoney MJ, et al: The obstetric significance of holoprosencephaly. Obstet Gynecol 63:115, 1984.
43. Cayea PD, Balcar I, Alberti O, Jones TB: Prenatal diagnosis of semilobar holoprosencephaly. Am J Radiol 142:401, 1984.
44. Hoffman-Tretin JC, Horoupian DS, Koenigsberg M, et al: Lobar holoprosencephaly with hydrocephalus: Antenatal demonstration and differential diagnosis. J Ultrasound Med 5:691, 1986.
45. Muir CS: Hydranencephaly and allied disorders. Am J Dis Child 34:231, 1959.
46. Lemire RJ, Loeser JD, Leech RW, Alvord EC: Normal and Abnormal Development of the Human Nervous System, p 251. Hagerstown, MD, Harper & Row, 1975.
47. Friede RL: Developmental Neuropathology, p 109. New York, Springer-Verlag, 1975.
48. Jung JH, Graham JM, Schultz N, Smith DW: Congenital hydranencephaly/porencephaly due to vascular disruption in monozygotic twins. Pediatrics 73:467, 1984.
49. Green MF, Benacerraf B, Crawford J: Hydranencephaly: US appearance during in utero evolution. Radiology 156:779, 1985.
50. Straus S, Bouzouki M, Goldfarb A, et al: Antenatal ultrasound diagnosis of an unusual case of hydranencephaly. J Clin Ultrasound 12:420, 1984.
51. Fleischer A, Brown M: Hydramnios associated with fetal hydranencephaly. J Clin Ultrasound 5:41, 1977.
52. Lee TG, Warren BH: Antenatal diagnosis of hydranencephaly by ultrasound: Correlation with ventriculography and computed tomography. J Clin Ultrasound 5:271, 1977.
53. Page LK, Brown SB, Gargano FP, Shortz RW: Schizencephaly: A clinical study and review. Childs Brain 1:348, 1975.
54. Miller GM, Stears JC, Guggenheim MA, Wilkening GR: Schizencephaly: A clinical and CT study. Neurology 34:997, 1984.
55. Williams JP, Blalock CP, Dunaway CL, Chalhub EG: Schizencephaly. J Comput Assist Tomogr 7:135, 1983.
56. Klingensmith WC, Cioffi-Ragan DT: Schizencephaly: Diagnosis and progression in utero. Radiology 159:617, 1986.
57. Sutton LN, Bruce DA, Schut L: Hydranencephaly versus maximal hydrocephalus: An important clinical distinction. Neurosurgery 6:35, 1980.
58. Chuang S: Perinatal and neonatal hydrocephalus. Perinatology 9:8, 1986.
59. Harwood-Nash DC, Fitz CR: Neuroradiology in Infants and Children, pp 609–677. St. Louis, CV Mosby, 1976.
60. McElroy DB: Hydrocephalus in children. Nurs Clin North Am 15:23, 1980.
61. Shannon MW, Nadler HL: X-linked hydrocephalus. J Med Genet 5:326, 1968.
62. Carter LO: Clues to the etiology of neural tube malformations. Dev Med Child Neurol 16:3, 1976.
63. Hudgins RJ, Edwards MJB, Goldstein R, et al: Natural history of fetal ventriculomegaly. Pediatrics 82:692, 1988.
64. Glick PL, Harrison MR, Nakayama DK, et al: Management of ventriculomegaly in the fetus. J Pediatr 105:97, 1984.
65. Chervenak FA, Berkowitz RL, Tortura M, Hobbins JL: The management of fetal hydrocephalus. Am J Obstet Gynecol 151:933, 1985.
66. Serlo W, Kirkinen P, Jouppila P, Herva R: Prognostic signs in fetal hydrocephalus. Childs Nerv Syst 2:93, 1986.
67. Cochrane DD, Miles ST, Nimrod C, et al: Intrauterine hydrocephalus and ventriculomegaly: Associated anomalies and fetal outcome. Can J Neurol Sci 12:51, 1984.
68. Pretorious DW, Davis K, Manco-Johnson ML, et al: Clinical course of fetal hydrocephalus: 40 cases. Am J Radiol 144:827, 1985.
69. Nyberg DA, Mack LA, Hirsch J, et al: Fetal hydrocephalus: Sonographic detection and clinical significance of associated anomalies. Radiology 163:187, 1987.
70. Goldstein RB, Lapidus AS, Filly RA, Cardoza J: Mild lateral cerebral ventricular dilatation in utero: Clinical significance and prognosis. Radiology 176:237, 1990.
71. Mahony BS, Nyberg DA, Hirsch JH, et al: Mild idiopathic lateral cerebral ventricular dilatation in utero: Sonographic evaluation. Radiology 169:715, 1988.
72. Pretorius DH, Drose JA, Manco-Johnson ML: Fetal lateral ventricular ratio determination during the second trimester. J Ultrasound Med 5:121, 1986.
73. Cardoza JD, Goldstein RB, Filly RA: Exclusion of fetal ventriculomegaly with a single measurement: The width of the lateral ventricular atrium. Radiology 169:711, 1988.
74. Fiske CE, Filly RA, Callen PW: Sonographic measurement of lateral ventricular width in early ventricular dilatation. J Clin Ultrasound 9:303, 1981.
75. Gillieson MS, Hickey NM: Prenatal diagnosis of fetal hydrocephalus with a normal biparietal diameter. J Ultrasound Med 3:227, 1984.
76. Callen PW, Chooljian D: The effect of ventricular dilatation upon biometry of the fetal head. J Ultrasound Med 5:17, 1986.
77. Hartung RW, Yiu-Chiu V: Demonstration of unilateral hydrocephalus in utero. J Ultrasound Med 2:369, 1983.
78. Case KJ, Hirsch J, Case MJ: Simulation of significant pathology by normal hypoechoic white matter in cranial ultrasound. J Clin Ultrasound 11:281, 1983.
79. Cardoza J, Filly RA, Podrasky AE: The dangling choroid plexus: A sonographic observation of value in excluding ventriculomegaly. AJR 15:167, 1988.
80. Fraumeni JR, Miller RW: Cancer deaths in the newborn. Am J Dis Child 117:186, 1969.
81. Koos WT, Miller MH: Intracranial Tumors of Infants and Children, pp 12–14. St. Louis, CV Mosby, 1971.
82. Lipman SP, Pretorius DH, Rumack CM, Manco-Johnson ML:

Fetal intracranial teratoma: US diagnosis of three cases and a review of the literature. Radiology 157:491, 1985.

83. Riboni G, DeSimoni M, Leopardi O, Molla R: Ultrasound appearance of a glioblastoma in a 33 week fetus in utero. J Clin Ultrasound 13:345, 1985.

84. Hoff NR, Mackay IM: Prenatal ultrasound diagnosis of intracranial teratoma. J Clin Ultrasound 8:247, 1980.

85. Shawker TH, Schwartz RM: Ultrasound appearance of a malignant fetal brain tumor. J Clin Ultrasound 11:35, 1983.

86. Whittle IR, Simpson DA: Surgical treatment of neonatal intracranial teratoma. Surg Neurol 15:268, 1981.

87. Crade M: Ultrasonic demonstration in utero of an intracranial teratoma. JAMA 247:1173, 1982.

88. Jon RS, Ilana L, Lorraine M, et al: Antenatal ultrasound diagnosis of an intracranial neoplasm (craniopharyngioma). J Clin Ultrasound 14:304, 1986.

89. Ross AC, Lee EP, Sue H, et al: Sonographic diagnosis of lipoma of the corpus callosum. J Ultrasound Med 6:449, 1987.

90. Hanae LB, Jeffrey AK, Lyndon MH, et al: Evolving fetal hydranencephaly mimicking intracranial neoplasm. J Ultrasound Med 10:237, 1991.

91. Chudleigh P, Pearce JM, Campbell S: The prenatal diagnosis of transient cysts of the fetal choroid plexus. Prenat Diagn 4:135, 1984.

92. Ostlere SJ, Irving HC, Lilford RJ: Choroid plexus cysts in the fetus. Lancet 1:1491, 1987.

93. Ricketts NEM, Lowe EM, Patel NB: Prenatal diagnosis of choroid plexus cysts. Lancet 1:213, 1987.

94. Perpignano MC, Cohen HL, Klein VR, et al: Fetal choroid plexus cysts: Beware the smaller cyst. Radiology 182:715, 1992.

95. Benacerraf BR, Harlow B, Frigoletto FO: Are choroid plexus cysts an indication for second-trimester amniocentesis? Am J Obstet Gynecol 162:1001, 1990.

96. Platt LD, Carlson DE, Medearis AL, et al: Fetal choroid plexus cysts in the second trimester: A cause for concern. Am J Obstet Gynecol 164:1652, 1991.

97. Chinn DH, Miller EI, Worthy LM, Towers CV: Sonographically detected fetal choroid plexus cysts: Frequency and association with aneuploidy. J Ultrasound Med 10:255, 1991.

98. Diakoumakis EE, Weinberg B, Mollin J: Prenatal sonographic diagnosis of a suprasellar arachnoid cyst. J Ultrasound Med 5:529, 1986.

99. Mack LA, Rumack CM, Johnson ML: Ultrasound evaluation of cystic intracranial lesions in the neonate. Radiology 137:451, 1980.

100. Oliver LC: Primary arachnoid cysts. Br Med J 1:1147, 1958.

101. Starkman SP, Brown TC, Linell EA: Cerebral arachnoid cysts. J Neuropathol Exp Neurol 17:484, 1958.

102. Williams B, Guthkelch DL: Why do central arachnoid pouches expand? J Neurol Neurosurg Psychol 37:1085, 1974.

103. Koto A, Horoupians DS, Shulman K: Choroidal epithelial cyst. J Neurosurg 47:955, 1977.

104. Reiter AA, Huhta JC, Carpenter JR, et al: Prenatal diagnosis of arteriovenous malformation of the vein of Galen. J Clin Ultrasound 14:623, 1986.

105. Morales WJ: Effect of intraventricular hemorrhage on the one-year mental and neurologic handicaps of the very low birth-weight infant. Obstet Gynecol 70:11, 1987.

106. Papile T, Burstein J, Burstein R, et al: Incidence and evolution of subependymal and intraventricular hemorrhage: A study of infants with birth weights less than 1,500 grams. J Pediatr 92:529, 1978.

107. Lustig-Gillman I, Young BK, Silverman F, et al: Fetal intraventricular hemorrhage: Sonographic diagnosis in clinical implications. J Clin Ultrasound 11:277, 1983.

108. Minkoff H, Schaffer RM, Delke I, Grunebaum AN: Diagnosis of intracranial hemorrhage in utero after a maternal seizure. Obstet Gynecol 65:22, 1985.

109. Chinn DH, Filly RA: Extensive intracranial hemorrhage in utero. J Ultrasound Med 2:285, 1983.

110. Bondurant S, Boehm FH, Fleischer AC, Machin JE: Antepartum diagnosis of fetal intracranial hemorrhage by ultrasound. Obstet Gynecol 63:255, 1984.

111. Kim MS, Elyaderani MK: Sonographic diagnosis of cerebral ventricular hemorrhage in utero. Radiology 142:479, 1982.

112. Mintz MC, Arger P, Coleman BG: In utero sonographic diagnosis of intracerebral hemorrhage. J Ultrasound Med 4:375, 1985.

113. Donn SM, DiPietro MA, Faix RG, Bowerman RA: The sonographic appearance of old intraventricular hemorrhage present at birth. J Ultrasound Med 2:283, 1983.

114. Donn SM, Barr M, McLeary RD: Massive intracerebral hemorrhage in utero: Sonographic appearance and pathologic correlation. Obstet Gynecol 63:28, 1984.

115. McGahan JP, Haesslein HC, Meyers M, Ford KB: Sonographic recognition of in utero intraventricular hemorrhage. Am J Radiol 142:171, 1984.

116. Greenberg F, James LM, Oakley GP: Estimates of birth prevalence rates of spina bifida in the United States from computer-generated maps. Am J Obstet Gynecol 145:570, 1983.

116. Levine AB, Berkowitz RL: Neonatal alloimmune thrombocytopenia. Semin Perinatol 15:35, 1991.

117. Kimball ME, Milunsky A, Alpert E: Prenatal diagnosis of neural tube defects: III: A reevaluation of alphafetoprotein assay. Obstet Gynecol 49:532, 1977.

118. Main DM, Mennuti MT: Neural tube defects: Issues in prenatal diagnosis and counseling. Obstet Gynecol 67:1, 1986.

119. U.K. collaborative study on alpha-fetoprotein in relation to neural tube defects: Maternal serum alpha-fetoprotein measurement in antenatal screening for anencephaly and spina bifida in early pregnancy. Lancet 1:1323, 1977.

120. Milunsky A, Alpert E: Prenatal diagnosis of neural tube defects: I. Problems and pitfalls: Analysis of 2495 cases using the alpha-fetoprotein assay. Obstet Gynecol 48:1, 1976.

121. Milunsky A, Alpert E: Prenatal diagnosis of neural tube defects: II. Analysis of false positive and false negative alpha-fetoprotein results. Obstet Gynecol 48:6, 1976.

122. Goldberg MF, Oakley GP: Interpreting elevated amniotic fluid alpha-fetoprotein levels in clinical practice: Use of the predictive value positive concept. Am J Obstet Gynecol 133:126, 1979.

123. Slotnick N, Filly RA, Callen PW, et al: Sonography as a procedure complementary to alphafetoprotein testing for neural tube defects. J Ultrasound Med 1:319, 1982.

124. Hashimoto BE, Mahony BS, Filly RA, et al: Sonography: A complementary examination to alphafetoprotein testing for neural tube defects. J Ultrasound Med 4:307, 1985.

125. Linkfors KK, McGahan JP, Tennant FP, et al: Midtrimester screening for open neural tube defects: Correlation of sonography with amniocentesis results. Am J Radiol 149:141, 1987.

126. Roberts CJ, Evans KT, Hibbard BM, et al: Diagnostic effectiveness of ultrasound in detection of neural tube defect. Lancet 2:1068, 1983.

127. Warkany J: Anencephaly. In Warkany J: Congenital Malformations: Notes and Comments, pp 189–200. Chicago, Year Book Medical Publishers, 1971.

128. Sunden B: On the diagnostic value of ultrasound in obstetrics and gynecology. Acta Obstet Gynecol Scand 43:1, 1964.

129. Campbell S, Johnstone FD: Anencephaly: Early ultrasonographic diagnosis and active management. Lancet 2:1226, 1972.

130. Johnson A, Losure TA, Weiner S: Early diagnosis of fetal anencephaly. J Clin Ultrasound 13:503, 1985.

131. Cox GG, Rosenthal SJ, Holsapple JW: Exencephaly: Sonographic findings and radiologic-pathologic correlation. Radiology 155:755, 1985.

132. Goldstein RB, Filly RA, Callen PW: Sonography of anencephaly: Pitfalls in early diagnosis. J Clin Ultrasound 17:397, 1989.

133. Mahony BS, Filly RA, Callen PW, Golbus MS: The amniotic band syndrome: Antenatal sonographic diagnosis and potential pitfalls. Am J Obstet Gynecol 152:63, 1985.

134. Mahony BS, Filly RA, Callen PW: Amnionicity and chorionicity in twin pregnancy: Prediction using ultrasound. Radiology 155:205, 1985.

135. Graham D, Johnson TRB, Winn K, Sanders RC: The role of sonography in the prenatal diagnosis and management of encephalocele. J Ultrasound Med 1:111, 1982.

136. Chervenak FA, Isaacson G, Mahoney MJ, et al: Diagnosis and management of fetal cephalocele. Obstet Gynecol 64:86, 1984.

137. Chatterjee MJ, Bondoc B, Adhate A: Prenatal diagnosis of occipital encephalocele. Obstet Gynecol 153:646, 1985.
138. Goldstein RB, Lapidus AS, Filly RA: Fetal cephaloceles: Diagnosis with us. Radiology 180:803, 1991.
139. Ingraham FD, Swah H: Spina bifida and cranium bifidum: A survey of 546 cases. N Engl J Med 228:559, 1943.
140. Suwanwela C, Suwanwela N: A morphological classification of sincipital encephalomeningoceles. J Neurosurg 36:201, 1972.
141. Mealey J, Ozenitis AJ, Hockley AA: The prognosis of encephaloceles. J Neurosurg 32:209, 1970.
142. Lorber J: Results of treatment of myelomeningocele: An analysis of 524 unselected cases, with special reference to possible selection for treatment. Dev Med Child Neurol 13:279, 1971.
143. Filly RA, Simpson GF, Linkowski GD: Fetal spine morphology and maturation during the second trimester. J Ultrasound Med 6:631, 1987.
144. Naidich TP: Personal communication, 1989.
145. Campbell J, Gilbert WM, Nicolaides KH, Campbell S: Ultrasound screening for spina bifida: Cranial and cerebellar signs in a high risk population. Obstet Gynecol 70:247, 1987.
146. Filly RA, Cardoza JD, Goldstein RB, Barkovich AJ: Detection of fetal central nervous system anomalies: A practical level of effort for a routine sonogram. Radiology 172:403, 1989.

CHAPTER 12

Ultrasound Evaluation of the Fetal Face

BERYL R. BENACERRAF, M.D.

Modern sonographic technology and user experience have made it possible to identify an increasingly large number of fetal malformations. Imaging of the fetal face is not routinely included in second- and third-trimester obstetric ultrasound evaluations in all ultrasound laboratories; however, anomalies of the fetal face are readily recognizable and may have a significant impact on obstetric management and outcome. Although facial defects such as cleft lip and palate can be an isolated occurrence, most facial abnormalities seen sonographically are associated with abnormal karyotypes and/or multiple congenital abnormalities.[1–4] Facial anomalies may, at times, be more readily recognizable sonographically than other defects and may be a clue to the presence of an associated syndrome. It is therefore crucial that the face be imaged in several planes to search for dysmorphology, which may possibly lead to the discovery of chromosomal anomalies and other fundamental fetal malformations. The sonographic identification of isolated fetal facial clefts, even in the absence of other fetal abnormalities, can be enormously helpful to reduce parental distress at birth.

EMBRYOLOGY

To understand the mechanism of facial malformations requires familiarity with the embryology of facial development. The fetal face forms between the fourth to eighth gestational weeks and arises from the first branchial arch.[5] The branchial arches appear in the fourth to fifth weeks of development and consist of a core of mesenchymal tissue derived from intraembryonic mesoderm covered by ectoderm and containing endoderm. Neural crest cells migrate into the branchial arches and proliferate, resulting in swellings that demarcate each arch. The neural crest cells will contribute to the skeletal components of the face while the mesoderm of each arch gives rise to the musculature of the face and neck.[5, 6]

The first branchial arch gives rise to the maxillary prominences, which grow cranially just under the eyes, and the mandibular prominence which grows inferiorly. The primitive mouth is a slight depression on the surface of the ectoderm called stomodeum. By the fifth week of gestation, five prominences are identified: the frontal nasal prominence, forming the upper boundary of the stomodeum; the paired maxillary prominences of the first branchial arch, forming the lateral boundaries of the stomodeum; and the paired mandibular prominences forming the caudal boundary. The surface ectoderm then thickens into the nasal placodes on each side of the frontal nasal prominence, and these placodes invaginate to form the nasal pits. The edges around the nasal pits are called the nasal prominences (medial and lateral). Until 24 to 26 days of gestation, the stomodeum is separated from the pharynx by a membrane that ruptures by about 26 days, putting the primitive gut in communication with the amniotic cavity.[5–7]

Between 5 and 8 gestational weeks, the maxillary prominences grow medially, compressing the medial nasal prominences together toward the midline. The two medial nasal prominences and the two maxillary prominences lateral to them fuse together, forming the upper lip (Fig. 12–1). The medial nasal prominences form the intermaxillary segment of the upper lip (the medial aspect of the lip), which is the origin of the labial component (philtrum) of the lip, the upper incisor teeth, and the anterior aspect of the primary palate. The lateral nasal prominences form the alae of the nose. The maxillary prominences and lateral nasal prominences are separated by the nasolacrimal groove. The ectoderm in the floor of this groove forms the nasolacrimal duct and lacrimal sac.[5–7]

The nose is formed in three parts. The bridge of the nose originates from the frontal prominence, the two medial nasal prominences form the crest and tip of the nose, and the lateral nasal prominences form the sides or alae.[5] The mandibular prominences merge at the end of the fourth to fifth week and form the lower lip, chin, and mandible.[5]

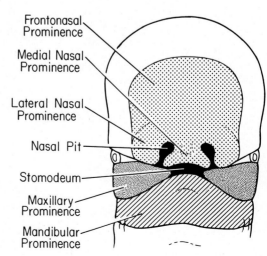

Figure 12–1. Diagram showing the embryology of the fetal face.

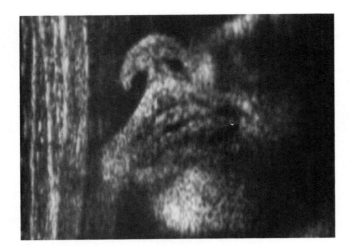

Figure 12–2. Modified coronal view of the lower face in a third-trimester fetus, showing the normal appearance of the upper lip and nose.

Abnormalities of the first branchial arch are caused by insufficient migration of the neural crest cells into the first branchial arch during the fourth gestational week, resulting in abnormalities of the lower face and mandible, such as Treacher Collins (mandibulofacial dysostosis) and Pierre Robin syndromes.[5, 6]

THE NORMAL FACE AND EXAMINATION TECHNIQUES

By 10 to 11 menstrual weeks, features of the fetal face can be identified sonographically. In particular, the orbits are visualized along with the midline structures in the developing brain. By 13 to 14 menstrual weeks, the fetal profile can be seen in a sagittal view, showing development of the nose, mandible, maxilla, as well as the orbits. One can image the face throughout the second and third trimesters of pregnancy using several planes. The modified coronal view is the most useful view to visualize cleft lip and palate. This view includes the soft tissues of the upper lip and fulcrum of the nose (Figs. 12–2 and 12–3). Moving posteriorly into a true coronal orientation, one can examine the integrity of the maxilla and the formation of the orbits. The lens of the eye is identifiable as a small echogenic circle within the bony orbit (Fig. 12–4). The longitudinal view demonstrates the nasal bones and soft tissues as well as the mandible and is most useful to rule out micrognathia, anterior encephalocele, or nasal bridge defects (Fig. 12–5). The upper lip should also be examined in profile for the presence of clefts. Lastly, the transverse view through the face can reveal orbital abnormalities and examines the intraorbital distances. Various transverse planes through the face evaluate the maxilla, the mandible, and the region of the tongue. Behind the tongue, one can identify the oropharynx and its connection to the larynx.

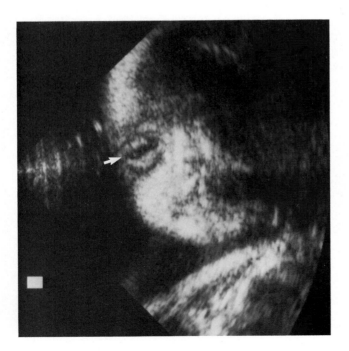

Figure 12–3. Coronal view through the soft tissues of the fetal face in the third trimester, showing normal appearance of the partly open eye *(arrow)*. Shadows obscure the appearance of the half of the face distal to the transducer.

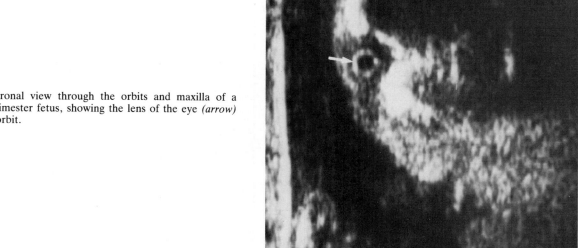

Figure 12–4. Coronal view through the orbits and maxilla of a normal second-trimester fetus, showing the lens of the eye *(arrow)* within the bony orbit.

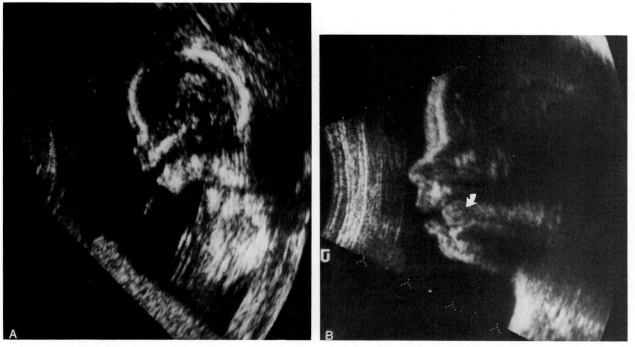

Figure 12–5. *A.* Sagittal view of a normal fetal face in the second trimester, showing the normal relationship between the maxilla, mandible, and forehead. *B.* Sagittal view of a normal fetal profile in the third trimester, showing the normal relationship between the frontal bone, maxilla, and mandible, as well as soft tissues. Note the normal position of the fetal tongue when in the mouth *(arrow)*.

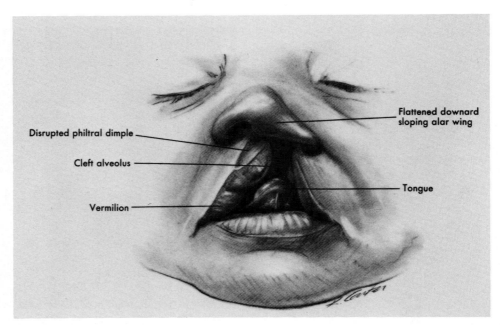

Figure 12–6. Unilateral cleft lip. (From Jurkiewicz MJ, Krizek TJ, Mathes SJ, Ariyan S [eds]: Plastic Surgery: Principles and Practice. St. Louis, CV Mosby, 1990.)

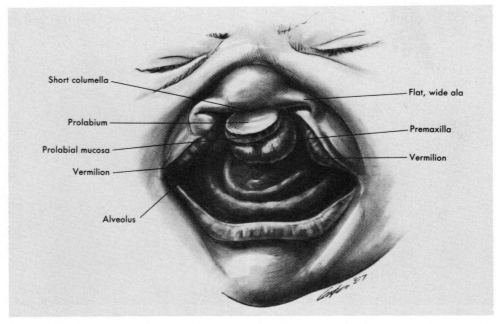

Figure 12–7. Bilateral cleft lip. (From Jurkiewicz MJ, Krizek TJ, Mathes SJ, Ariyan S [eds]: Plastic Surgery: Principles and Practice. St. Louis, CV Mosby, 1990.)

FACIAL CLEFTS

Cleft lip and palate constitutes the most common congenital facial malformation and is usually paramedian, extending between the lateral incisors and canine teeth (Figs. 12–6 through 12–8).[5] The cleft probably results from the arrest of mesenchymal proliferation, leading to failure of the maxillary prominence to merge with the intermaxillary segment (formed by the medial nasal prominences). The medial cleft lip (central) is caused by incomplete merging of the two medial nasal prominences in the midline and is a much rarer abnormality. Oblique facial clefts occur uncommonly and result from failure of the maxillary prominence to merge with the lateral nasal swelling, with exposure of the nasolacrimal duct.[5]

A complete bilateral cleft lip and palate was one of the earliest fetal facial defects to be identified sonographically.[2–4, 8–12] This defect is easily recognized owing to the large gap in the upper lip seen on modified coronal view of the lip and nose as well as the mass effect formed by the free intermaxillary portion of the upper lip bulging forward (Figs. 12–9 through 12–11).[3, 9] In addition, the nose is usually flattened and widened.

The incidence of cleft lip and palate is approximately 1 in 1000 births, although it rises to 4% for a sibling of a previously affected fetus and to 9% to 10% for a sibling of two previously affected infants (Table 12–1). In families in which one parent and a child have cleft lip, subsequent children have up to a 17% risk of being affected.[6] Associated congenital abnormalities occur in more than 50% of fetuses with facial clefts, depending on the type of cleft.[1] In addition, there is a high incidence of chromosomal abnormalities among fetuses with facial clefts, in particular trisomies 13 and 18.[12, 13]

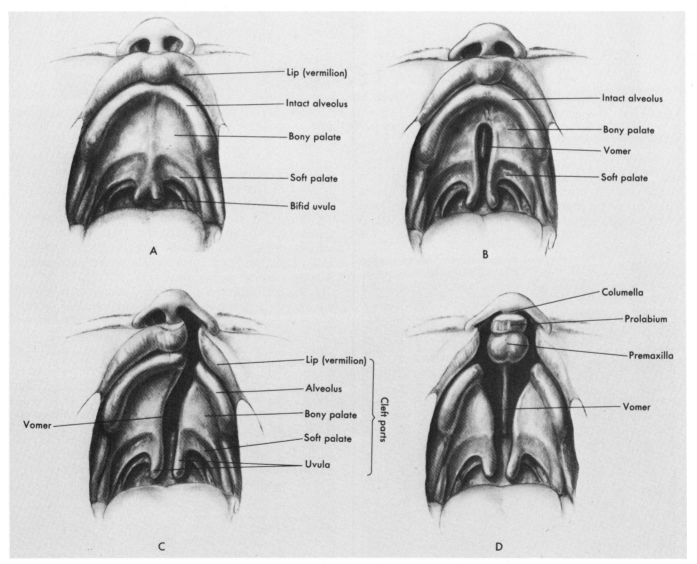

Figure 12–8. Variations in cleft palate anatomy. *A.* Bifid uvula, the most common cleft palate presentation. *B.* Incomplete cleft of secondary palate with intact premaxillary structures. *C.* Unilateral complete cleft lip and palate. *D.* Bilateral complete cleft lip and palate. (From Jurkiewicz MJ, Krizek TJ, Mathes SJ, Ariyan S [eds]: Plastic Surgery: Principles and Practice. St. Louis, CV Mosby, 1990.)

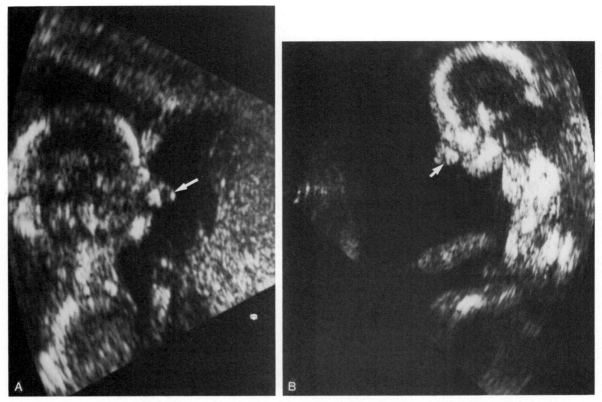

Figure 12–9. *A.* Sagittal view of a second-trimester fetal profile showing a major midface cleft in a fetus with trisomy 13. Note the protrusion in the nasal area *(arrow).* *B.* Sagittal view of an early second-trimester fetus with complete bilateral cleft lip and palate showing anterior displacement of the intermaxillary portion of the upper lip bulging forward *(arrow).*

The incidence of associated defects in children with facial clefts is much lower (<25%) than in fetuses, since many pregnancies with fetuses who have facial clefts end in spontaneous abortion.[1] Cleft lip and palate are associated with many hereditary syndromes, and patients at risk for these defects often seek prenatal diagnosis (Table 12–2).[14–16]

Complete bilateral cleft lip and palate disrupts the appearance of the face sufficiently, even in the early second trimester, to be easily recognizable sonographically. Unilateral cleft lip and palate or even incomplete cleft lip may be more subtle (Fig. 12–12). Unilateral cleft lip and palate results from incomplete fusion of the maxillary prominence to the medial nasal prominence on one side, with the other side being intact.[5]

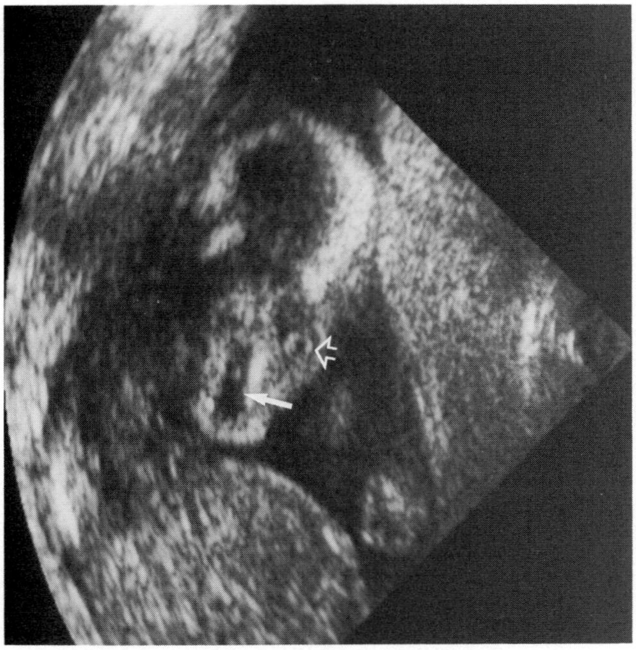

Figure 12–10. Coronal view through the fetal maxilla of a second-trimester fetus with a midface cleft showing disruption of the maxilla *(arrow).* The lens of the eye is shown by the open arrow.

Table 12–1. INCIDENCE OF DEFORMITY IN SUBSEQUENT OFFSPRING

	Cleft Lip ± Palate (%)	Cleft Palate Alone (%)
Unaffected Parents		
No affected offspring	0.1	0.04
No affected offspring + one affected first cousin	0.4	0.09
One affected offspring	4	2
Two affected offspring	9	1
One affected offspring + one affected relative	4	7
Affected Parents		
One parent + no affected offspring	4	6
One parent + one affected offspring	10–17	15
Two parents + one affected offspring	60	60

From Jurkiewicz MJ, Krizek TJ, Mathes SJ, Ariyan S (eds): Plastic Surgery: Principles and Practice. St. Louis, CV Mosby, 1990.

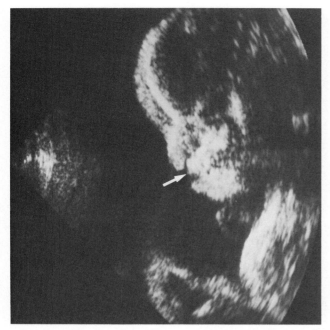

Figure 12–11. Sagittal view of a fetus with trisomy 18 who has a major midface cleft. Note the flattened nose and distorted upper lip *(arrow)*.

The unilateral complete cleft lip and palate may not be as obvious in the parasagittal plane of the fetal profile unless the plane is moved to the side of the cleft, because the intermaxillary portion of the upper lip does not form a mass as it does when the cleft is bilateral. The modified coronal view of the lip is the best orientation to demonstrate unilateral cleft lip and palate, owing to the flattened appearance of one side

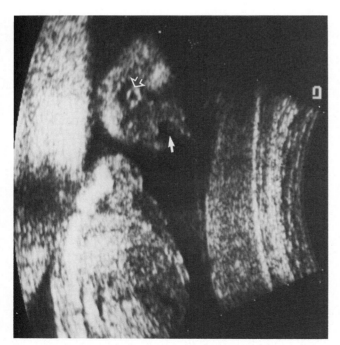

Figure 12–12. Modified coronal view of the lateral aspect of the fetal face in the second trimester, showing a complete cleft lip and palate *(solid arrow)*. The orbit is indicated by the open arrow.

Table 12–2. FETAL-NEONATAL CLEFT LIP AND PALATE

Entity	Genetics
Chromosomal Errors	
Trisomy 13	
Trisomy 18	
Triploidy	Sproadic (unless parental translocation)
Trisomy 4p	
4p deletion	
Trisomy 9	
5p deletion	
Early amnion rupture sequence	Sporadic
Teratogenic Effects	
Fetal hydantoin effect	
Fetal trimethadione effect	
Fetal valproate effect	Sproadic
Fetal alcohol effect	
Maternal phenylketonuria fetal effect	
Hyperthermia-induced defects	
Syndromes, Sequences, and Associations	
Holoprosencephaly sequence	Sporadic/AD
Caudal dysplasia sequence	Sporadic
CHARGE association	?
MURCS association	Sporadic
Short-rib polydactyly syndrome	AR
Kniest dysplasia	Sporadic/AD
Meckel-Gruber syndrome	AR
Larsen syndrome	? AR, ? AD
Neu-Laxova syndrome	AR
Child syndrome	X-linked D
Roberts SC phocomelia syndrome	AR
Cleft lip sequence	?
Oral-facial-digital syndrome	X-linked D or AD
Miller syndrome	AR
Mohr syndrome	? AR
Facial-auriculovertebral spectrum	Sporadic
Frontonasal dysplasia sequence	? Sporadic
Robinow syndrome	?
Pallister-Hall syndrome	? Sporadic
Oculodentodigital syndrome	AD
Adams-Oliver syndrome	AD
Aase syndrome	? AR
Van de Woude syndrome	AD
Rapp-Hodgkin ectodermal dysplasia	AD
Ectodactyly-ectodermal dysplasia-clefting syndrome	? AD
Hay-Wells syndrome	AD
Popliteal pterygium syndrome	AD

AD, autosomal dominant; AR, autosomal recessive; X-linked D, X-linked dominant.

From Dimmick JE, Kalousek DK (ed): Developmental Pathology of the Embryo and Fetus. Philadelphia, JB Lippincott, 1992.

with widening of the nostril and communication between the nostril and the mouth (Fig. 12–13). Incomplete cleft lip is considerably more subtle and may not be detectable until late in the second or third trimester of pregnancy. The incomplete cleft is visualized only in the modified coronal view of the lip since, in many cases, it does not disturb the integrity of the nose sufficiently to be recognized in other orientations (Fig. 12–14). Incomplete cleft lip is less likely to be associated with chromosomal defects and is readily surgically correctable, yielding excellent results.

The median cleft lip is a rare form of clefting that occurs when there is incomplete merging of the two medial nasal prominences in the midline. This type of

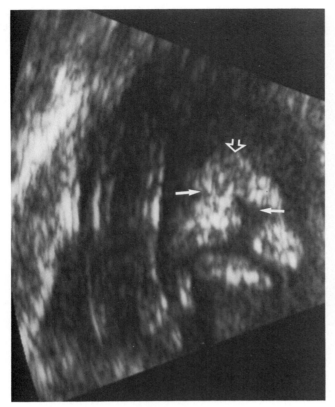

Figure 12–13. View of the soft tissues of a third-trimester fetus with complete unilateral cleft lip and palate. The tip of the nose (midline) is shown by the open arrow. The solid arrows indicate the nostrils. Note that the cleft involves only one nostril, which is splayed laterally.

clefting can be associated with forms of holoprosencephaly and is often accompanied by intracranial anomalies (Figs. 12–15 and 12–16).[5, 17, 18]

Isolated cleft palate may be exceedingly difficult to identify since the lip is intact. In many cases, only the soft palate is affected and the cleft cannot be recog-

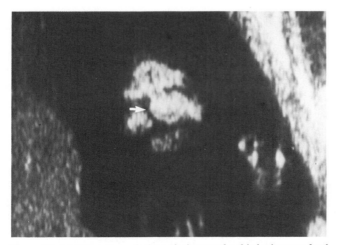

Figure 12–14. View through the soft tissues of a third-trimester fetal face, showing a unilateral incomplete cleft lip. The arrow indicates the discontinuity of the upper lip on one side, although the fetal nose does not appear distorted.

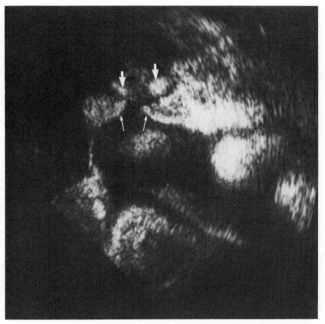

Figure 12–15. Third-trimester fetus with trisomy 13 and a median cleft lip and palate. The nose *(solid arrows)* is deformed and widened. The upper lip *(thin arrows)* is disrupted in the midline.

nized prenatally. Only hard palate clefting is detectable prenatally (see Fig. 12–10).[19]

Cleft lip and palate can be repaired postnatally with a good prognosis unless accompanied by associated defects. When a fetal facial cleft is identified sonographically, karyotyping, as well as a thorough search for other structural defects (such as clubfoot, hand abnormalities, and congenital heart disease), should be undertaken.[1–4]

Abnormalities of the mouth also include masses protruding from the mouth, such as alveolar ridge tumors, hemangiomas, and teratomas (Fig. 12–17).[20]

FETAL MANDIBLE

Major mandibular malformations result from abnormalities of the first branchial arch and are caused by deficiency or insufficient migration of the neural crest cells in the fourth week of fetal development.[5–7] Because neural crest cells also contribute to the aortic and pulmonary artery formation, first arch syndromes are often accompanied by congenital heart defects.[6] Treacher Collins syndrome (mandibulofacial dysostosis) is an autosomal dominant disorder that affects the ears and mandible as well as the palate. The eyes are often slanted downward, the mandible is small, and the chin recedes (micrognathia), resulting in a considerable overbite.[21–24] The ears may be low lying and the auricles malformed and either large or small. Other abnormalities resulting in abnormal mandibular development include Goldenhar syndrome (hemifacial microsomia), Pierre Robin syndrome, Seckel syndrome, lethal multiple pterygium syndrome, as well as several of the autosomal trisomies (Figs. 12–18 through 12–

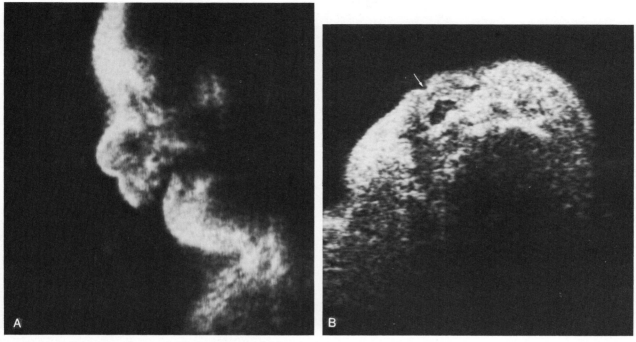

Figure 12–16. Sagittal *(A)* and coronal *(B)* views of the fetal face in the second trimester, showing a median cleft lip. The fetus had multiple congenital abnormalities, including major intracranial anomalies. Note the indentation of the upper lip in the midline *(arrow)*.

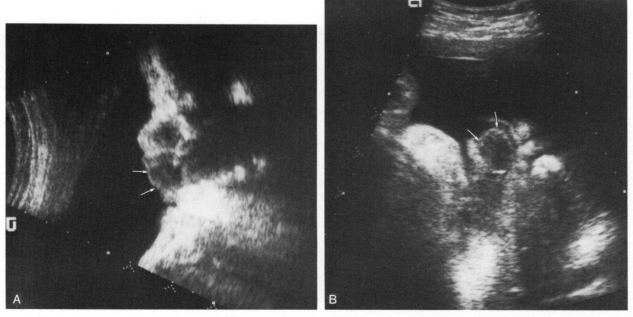

Figure 12–17. Sagittal *(A)* and modified coronal *(B)* views of the lower face of a third-trimester fetus, with a mass protruding from the oropharynx *(arrows)*. The fetus is unable to close the mouth around this solid mass, which, at birth, was a gingival tumor.

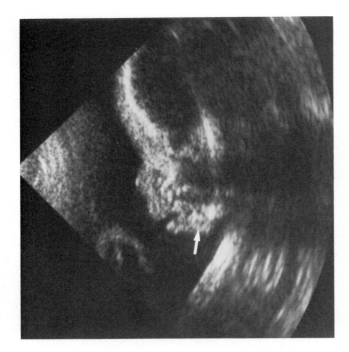

Figure 12–18. Sagittal view of a third-trimester fetus with trisomy 18, showing micrognathia. The small chin is indicated by the arrow.

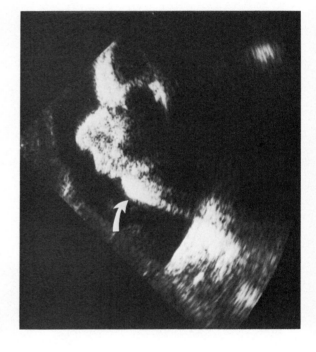

Figure 12–19. Sagittal view of the profile of a third-trimester fetus with trisomy 13, showing severe micrognathia *(arrow).* (From Benacerraf B, Miller W, Frigoletto F: Sonographic detection of fetuses with trisomy 13 and 18: Accuracy and limitations. Am J Obstet Gynecol 158:404, 1988.)

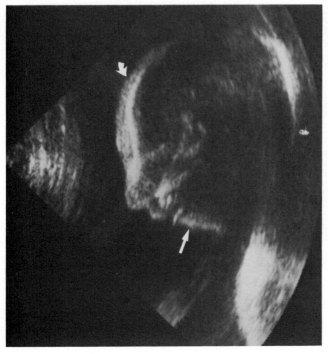

Figure 12–20. Sagittal view of a fetus with multiple congenital abnormalities. Note the severe micrognathia *(arrow)* as well as the sloping forehead *(curved arrow),* indicating microcephaly.

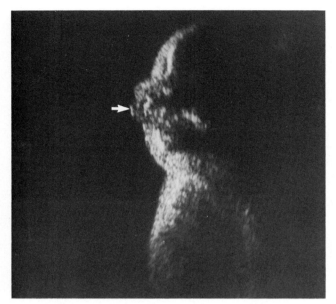

Figure 12–21. Sagittal view of the profile of a third-trimester fetus with lethal multiple pterygium syndrome. The fetus had multiple contractures of the extremities and severe polyhydramnios. Note the protruding upper lip *(arrow)*, as well as the micrognathia.

21).[25–28] Some of the osteochondrodysplasias, such as camptomelic dysplasia or achondrogenesis, and limb reduction syndromes such as Nager acrofacial dysostosis or oromandibular limb hypogenesis syndromes have associated micrognathia.[26, 29, 30] Harlequin syndrome, a lethal familial defect of the skin and soft tissues (congenital ichthyosis), is another cause of micrognathia (Fig. 12–22).[31, 32]

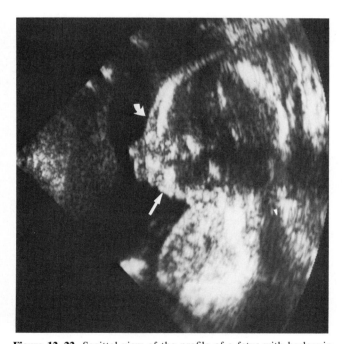

Figure 12–22. Sagittal view of the profile of a fetus with harlequin syndrome. Note the edema of the soft tissues of the nose and maxillary region *(curved arrow)*, as well as the small mandible *(arrow)*. The patient had a fetus previously with harlequin syndrome.

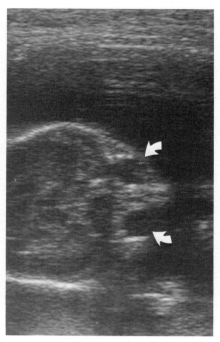

Figure 12–23. Oblique coronal view through the fetal orbits *(arrows)* of a second-trimester fetus with hypotelorism and other morphologic abnormalities.

The midline sagittal or profile view of the fetal face is the most helpful to evaluate the size of the mandible versus the rest of the face.[21–25] One can also image the mandible in a transverse view of the lower face, although this orientation is not as helpful for comparing the mandible with the rest of the face. The presence of micrognathia is often a clue that the fetus has multiple congenital abnormalities and/or a chromosomal defect and should prompt a careful structural survey of the fetus as well as karyotyping.

FETAL ORBITS

Charts for normal intraorbital and interorbital diameters exist to help differentiate between normal size, hypertelorism, and hypotelorism (Table 12–3).[33, 34] The evaluation of the size and location of orbits is usually done subjectively during real-time ultrasonography, although quantitative measurements can be helpful when a fetus is at particular risk for a genetic abnormality. Causes of hypertelorism include the craniosynostoses syndromes, such as Apert and Crouzon syndromes, Pena-Shokeir syndrome, cleft lip and palate, frontal encephaloceles, and teratogens such as phenytoin.[26]

Hypotelorism is usually a manifestation of a severe brain malformation (Figs. 12–23 and 12–24). Holoprosencephaly is the most commonly associated brain anomaly and can result in a continuum of orbital defects ranging from mild hypotelorism to cyclopia. Anophthalmia and cryptophthalmos have been described sonographically in the fetus and result in absence of the eyes.[35–37] Varying degrees of ocular de-

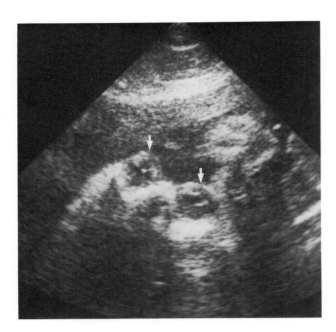

Figure 12–24. Transverse view through the fetal orbits *(arrows)* in the third trimester, showing hypotelorism. The intraorbital distance was reduced.

Table 12–3. PREDICTED BIPARIETAL DIAMETER AND WEEKS' GESTATION FROM THE INNER AND OUTER ORBITAL DISTANCES

BPD (cm)	Gestation (wk)	IOD (cm)	OOD (cm)	BPD (cm)	Gestation (wk)	IOD (cm)	OOD (cm)
1.9	11.6	0.5	1.3	5.8	24.3	1.6	4.1
2.0	11.6	0.5	1.4	5.9	24.3	1.6	4.2
2.1	12.1	0.6	1.5	6.0	24.7	1.6	4.3
2.2	12.6	0.6	1.6	6.1	25.2	1.6	4.3
2.3	12.6	0.6	1.7	6.2	25.2	1.6	4.4
2.4	13.1	0.7	1.7	6.3	25.7	1.7	4.4
2.5	13.6	0.7	1.8	6.4	26.2	1.7	4.5
2.6	13.6	0.7	1.9	6.5	26.2	1.7	4.5
2.7	14.1	0.8	2.0	6.6	26.7	1.7	4.6
2.8	14.6	0.8	2.1	6.7	27.2	1.7	4.6
2.9	14.6	0.8	2.1	6.8	27.6	1.7	4.7
3.0	15.0	0.9	2.2	6.9	28.1	1.7	4.7
3.1	15.5	0.9	2.3	7.0	28.6	1.8	4.8
3.2	15.5	0.9	2.4	7.1	29.1	1.8	4.8
3.3	16.0	1.0	2.5	7.3	29.6	1.8	4.9
3.4	16.5	1.0	2.5	7.4	30.0	1.8	5.0
3.0	16.5	1.0	2.6	7.5	30.6	1.8	5.0
3.6	17.0	1.0	2.7	7.6	31.0	1.8	5.1
3.7	17.5	1.1	2.7	7.7	31.5	1.8	5.1
3.8	17.9	1.1	2.8	7.8	32.0	1.8	5.2
4.0	18.4	1.2	3.0	7.9	32.5	1.9	5.2
4.2	18.9	1.2	3.1	8.0	33.0	1.9	5.3
4.3	19.4	1.2	3.2	8.2	33.5	1.9	5.4
4.4	19.4	1.3	3.2	8.3	34.0	1.9	5.4
4.5	19.9	1.3	3.3	8.4	34.4	1.9	5.4
4.6	20.4	1.3	3.4	8.5	35.0	1.9	5.5
4.7	20.4	1.3	3.4	8.6	35.4	1.9	5.5
4.8	20.9	1.4	3.5	8.8	35.9	1.9	5.6
4.9	21.3	1.4	3.6	8.9	36.4	1.9	5.6
5.0	21.3	1.4	3.6	9.0	36.9	1.9	5.7
5.1	21.8	1.4	3.7	9.1	37.3	1.9	5.7
5.2	22.3	1.4	3.8	9.2	37.8	1.9	5.8
5.3	22.3	1.5	3.8	9.3	38.3	1.9	5.8
5.4	22.8	1.5	3.9	9.4	38.8	1.9	5.8
5.5	23.3	1.5	4.0	9.6	39.3	1.9	5.9
5.6	23.3	1.5	4.0	9.7	39.8	1.9	5.9
5.7	23.8	1.5	4.1				

From Mayden KL, Tortora M, Berkowitz RL, et al: Orbital diameters: A new parameter for prenatal diagnosis and dating. Am J Obstet Gynecol 144:289, 1982.

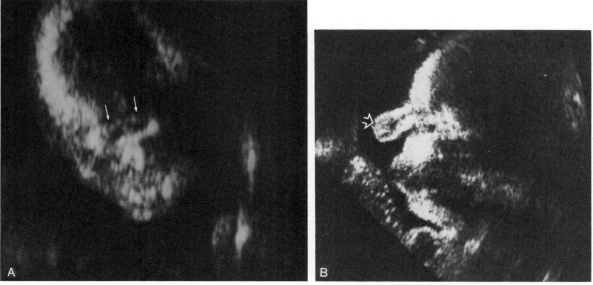

Figure 12–25. Coronal *(A)* and sagittal *(B)* views of the fetal face of a fetus with cyclopia. The two orbits *(thin arrows)* are side by side. The proboscis *(open arrow)* is shown directly above the level of the orbit. *(A,* from Benacerraf BR, Frigoletto FD, Greene MF: Abnormal facial features and extremities in human trisomy syndromes: Prenatal ultrasound appearance. Radiology 159:243–246, 1986; *B,* from Benacerraf B: Use of sonography for antenatal detection of aneuploidy. Clin Diagn Ultrasound 25:21, 1989. New York, Churchill Livingstone, 1989.)

fects, including cataracts, have been described prenatally by astute observers, although routine identification of orbital, globe, or lens defects is difficult.[35] Fetal cyclopia is usually associated with holoprosencephaly and occurs when the orbits are side by side, with a single midline orbital fossa containing either a single optical vesicle or two vesicles side by side. The nose is almost always abnormal and is a tubular appendage attached to the upper aspect of the face, above the orbit (proboscis) (Fig. 12–25).[10, 13, 17, 18, 38, 39] In less severe forms of hypotelorism, the nose may attach in normal position and may have only one nostril (cebocephaly) (Fig. 12–26).

Lacrimal duct cysts appear sonographically as small

Figure 12–26. Modified coronal views of the face of a fetus with trisomy 13 and holoprosencephaly. *A.* Note the hypotelorism with the orbits *(closed arrows)* close together. *B.* The nose has only one nostril *(arrow)*. *C.* Monoventricular cavity *(asterisk)* typical of holoprosencephaly.

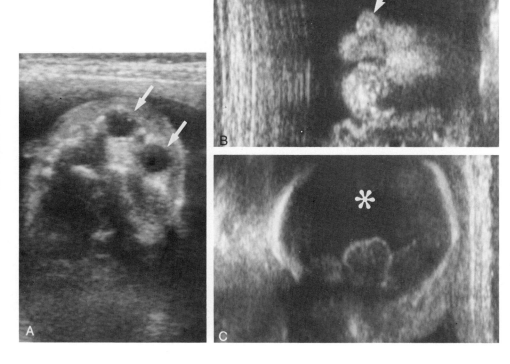

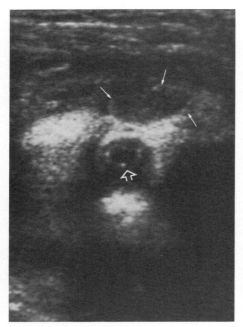

Figure 12–27. Magnified view of the region of the fetal orbit near term, showing a soft tissue mass *(thin arrows)* in the region of the corner of the eye *(open arrow)*, just between the orbit and the nose. This mass was shown at birth to be a glioma.

fluid collections adjacent to the orbits, medially. Masses in and around the orbits may be related to the lacrimal duct or can represent encephaloceles, gliomas, or hemangiomas (Fig. 12–27).[40]

OTHER FACIAL DEFECTS

Current ultrasound equipment enables us to identify dysmorphic features of the face, such as a low nasal bridge. Down syndrome, bone dysplasias such as thanatophoric dysplasia or achondroplasia, as well as effects of drugs such as phenytoin may result in maxillary hypoplasia (Figs. 12–28 and 12–29).[26] Frontal bossing and/or hypertelorism can also be seen in fetuses affected with achondroplasia or craniosynostoses, such as Cruzon or Apert syndrome (Fig. 12–30).[25, 41] The extremities should be examined carefully in cases in which frontal bossing is present sonographically. Protrusion of the tongue can be a sign of congenital malformations (i.e., Beckwith-Wiedemann syndrome, Down syndrome, or other chromosomal defects) (Fig. 12–31). Osteogenesis imperfecta results in diminished ossification of the skull and may affect the appearance of the face as well (Fig. 12–32). The skull may lose its shape, giving the face and eyes a more prominent appearance (Fig. 12–33). Microcephaly may produce a slanted forehead and bulging eyes, which is characteristic of diminished skull growth. Acrania or anencephaly result from a lack of formation of the cranium, with prominence of the orbits as being the highest bony structure of the head (Fig. 12–34). Hydrops with edema of the fetal facial soft tissues can result in an abnormal facial profile (Fig. 12–35).

Malformations of the face, such as face duplication, can occur secondary to abnormal twinning. In this rare form of conjoined twins, a central orbit is identified,

Text continued on page 253

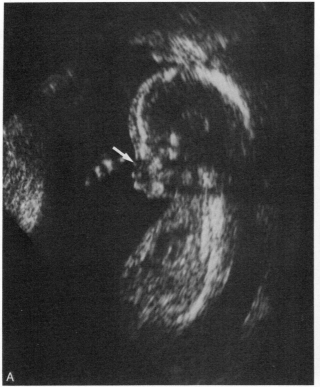

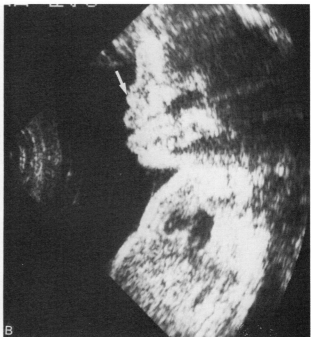

Figure 12–28. Sagittal views of two fetuses. *A.* Second-trimester fetus. *B.* Third-trimester fetus with Down syndrome. Note the small nose and hypoplasia of the maxillary region *(arrow)*, as well as prominent lips.

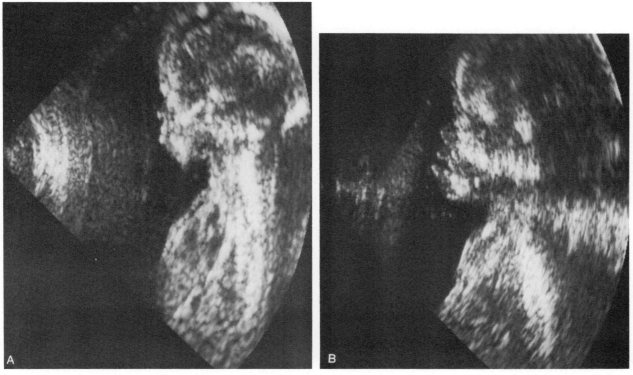

Figure 12–29. Facial profile in two fetuses with maxillary hypoplasia. *A.* Patient had a seizure disorder and was taking antiseizure medication. *B.* Fetus had an osteochondrodysplasia, with abnormalities of the tubular long bones, as well as midface hypoplasia and multiple intracranial abnormalities.

Figure 12–30. Sagittal view of a third-trimester fetus with heterozygous achondroplasia. Note the frontal bossing and the depression of the nasal bridge *(arrow).*

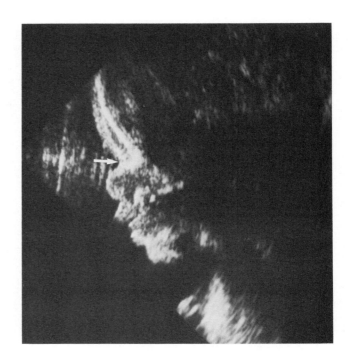

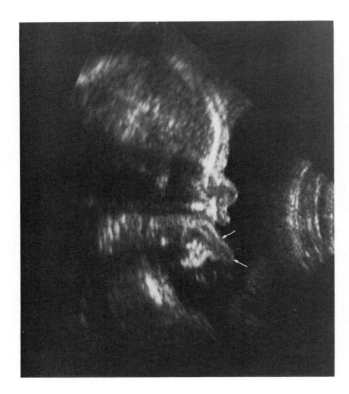

Figure 12–31. Fetal profile in the third trimester, showing protrusion of the fetal tongue *(arrows)*. This fetus had multiple congenital abnormalities and was chromosomally abnormal. The fetus spent much of its time with its tongue protruding in this fashion.

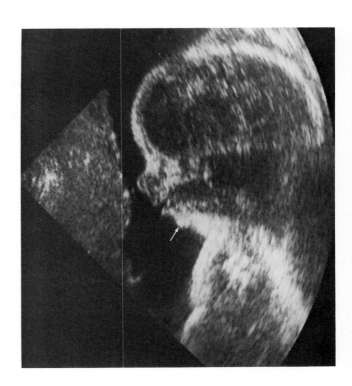

Figure 12–32. Sagittal view of the face of a fetus with osteogenesis imperfecta. Note the small mandible *(arrow)*.

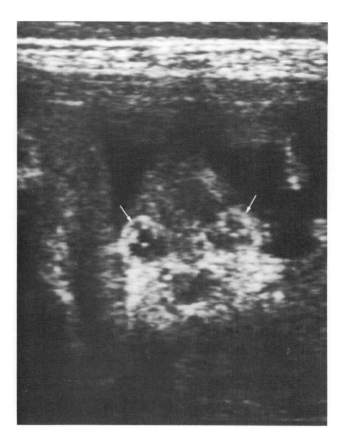

Figure 12–33. Modified coronal view of the fetal orbits in a case of osteogenesis imperfecta. The orbits *(arrows)* are prominent because of the lack of ossification of the cranium.

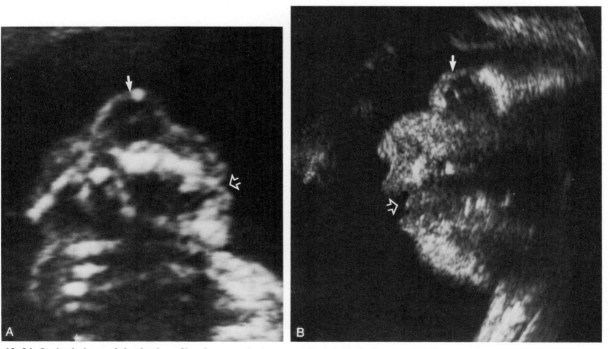

Figure 12–34. Sagittal views of the fetal profile of a second-trimester *(A)* and third-trimester *(B)* fetus with anencephaly. Note that the fetal orbits *(solid arrows)* are the highest structures of the fetal head. The open arrow indicates the mouth.

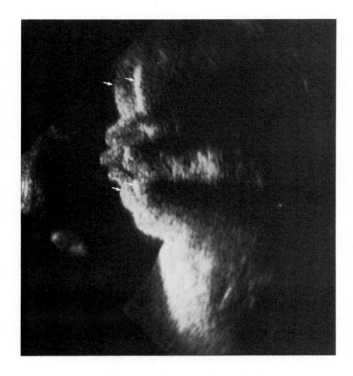

Figure 12–35. Sagittal view of a third-trimester fetus with nonimmune hydrops. Note the swelling of the soft tissues of the entire face, with increased space between the bony structures and the outer aspect of the fetal face *(arrows)*.

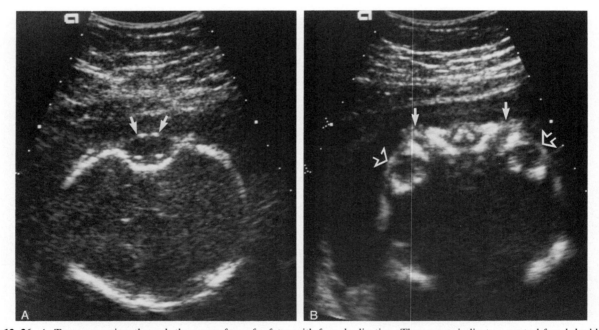

Figure 12–36. *A.* Transverse view through the upper face of a fetus with face duplication. The arrows indicate a central fused double orbit. *B.* In a slightly different plane, one can observe the two noses extending laterally *(solid arrows)* and two additional orbits lateral to the fetal noses *(open arrows)*. This fetus had craniofacial duplication, or diprosopus, at 22 weeks' gestation.

with a nose on either side of it, and an additional orbit lateral to each nose (Fig. 12–36).[42–44] The intracranial anatomy is usually severely distorted, with two falces and four lateral ventricles.

Although examination of the face is not yet part of the American Institute of Ultrasound in Medicine endorsed guidelines for second- and third-trimester fetal sonography, the appearance of the face is intimately related to intracranial anatomy and the features of the face can be evaluated as part of the examination of the head in most second- and third-trimester fetuses.

References

1. Kraus BS, Kitamura H, Ooe T: Malformations associated with cleft lip and palate in human embryos and fetuses. Am J Obstet Gynecol 86:321, 1963.
2. Saltzman DH, Benacerraf BR, Frigoletto FD: Diagnosis and management of fetal facial clefts. Am J Obstet Gynecol 155:377, 1986.
3. Seeds JW, Cefalo RC: Technique of early sonographic diagnosis of bilateral cleft lip and palate. Obstet Gynecol 62:2S, 1983.
4. Pilu G, Reece EA, Romero R, et al: Prenatal diagnosis of craniofacial malformations with ultrasonography. Am J Obstet Gynecol 155:45, 1986.
5. Moore KL: The Developing Fetus, 4th ed, pp 189–206. Philadelphia, WB Saunders, 1988.
6. Sadler TW: Langman's Medical Embryology, 6th ed, pp 297–305. Baltimore, Williams & Wilkins, 1990.
7. Moore KL: Essentials of Human Embryology, pp 75–85. Philadelphia, BC Decker, 1988.
8. Hegge FN, Prescott GH, Watson PT: Fetal facial abnormalities identified during obstetric sonography. J Ultrasound Med 5:679, 1986.
9. Chevenak FA, Tortora M, Mayden K, et al: Antenatal diagnosis of median cleft face syndrome: Sonographic demonstration of cleft lip and hypertelorism. Am J Obstet Gynecol 149:94, 1984.
10. Benacerraf BR, Frigoletto FD, Bieber FR: The fetal face: Ultrasound examination. Radiology 153:495, 1984.
11. Christ JE, Meininger MG: Ultrasound diagnosis of cleft lip and palate before birth. Plast Reconstruct Surg 68:854, 1981.
12. Savoldelli G, Schmid W, Schinzel A: Prenatal diagnosis of cleft lip and palate by ultrasound. Prenat Diagn 2:313, 1982.
13. Benacerraf BR, Frigoletto FD, Greene MF: Abnormal facial features and extremities in human trisomy syndromes: Prenatal ultrasound appearance. Radiology 159:243, 1986.
14. Stioui S, Privitera O, Brambati B, et al: First-trimester prenatal diagnosis of Roberts syndrome. Prenat Diagn 12:145, 1992.
15. Kohler R, Sousa P, Jorge CS: Prenatal diagnosis of the ectrodactyly, ectodermal dysplasia, cleft palate syndrome. J Ultrasound Med 8:337, 1989.
16. Robinow M, Johnson GF: The Gordon syndrome: Autosomal dominant cleft palate, camptodactyly and clubfeet. Am J Med Genet 9:139, 1981.
17. Martin AO, Perrin JCS, Muir WA, et al: An autosomal dominant midline cleft syndrome resembling familial holoprosencephaly. Clin Genet 12:65, 1977.
18. Greene MF, Benacerraf BR, Frigoletto FD: Reliable criteria for the prenatal sonographic diagnosis of alobar holoprosencephaly. Am J Obstet Gynecol 156:687, 1987.
19. Bundy AL, Saltzman DH, Emerson D, et al: Sonographic features associated with cleft palate. J Clin Ultrasound 14:486, 1986.
20. Chervenak FA, Tortora M, Moya FR, et al: Antenatal sonographic diagnosis of epignathus. J Ultrasound Med 3:235, 1984.
21. Meizner I, Carmi R, Katz M: Prenatal ultrasonic diagnosis of mandibulofacial dysostosis (Treacher Collins syndrome). J Clin Ultrasound 19:124, 1991.
22. Crane JP, Beaver HA: Midtrimester sonographic diagnosis of mandibulofacial dysostosis. Am J Med Genet 25:251, 1986.
23. Nicolaides KH, Johansson D, Donnai D, et al: Prenatal diagnosis of mandibulofacial dysostosis. Prenat Diagn 4:201, 1984.
24. Behrents RG, McNamara JA, Avery JK: Prenatal mandibulofacial dysostosis (Treacher Collins syndrome). Cleft Palate J 14:13, 1977.
25. Tamas DE, Mahony BS, Bowie JD, et al: Prenatal sonographic diagnosis of hemifacial microsomia (Goldenhar-Gorlin syndrome). J Ultrasound Med 5:461, 1986.
26. Jones KL: Smith's Recognizable Patterns of Human Malformations, 4th ed, pp 725–728. Philadelphia, WB Saunders, 1988.
27. Pilu G, Romero R, Reece EA, et al: The prenatal diagnosis of Robin anomalad. Am J Obstet Gynecol 154:630, 1986.
28. Cayea PD, Bieber FR, Ross MJ, et al: Sonographic findings in otocephaly (synotia). J Ultrasound Med 4:377, 1985.
29. Benson CB, Pober BR, Hirsh MP, et al: Sonography of Nager acrofacial dysostosis syndrome in utero. J Ultrasound Med 7:163, 1988.
30. Shechter SA, Sherer DM, Geilfuss CJ, et al: Prenatal sonographic appearance and subsequent management of a fetus with oromandibular limb hypogenesis syndrome associated with pulmonary hypoplasia. J Clin Ultrasound 18:661, 1990.
31. Mihalko M, Lindfors KK, Grix AW, et al: Prenatal sonographic diagnosis of harlequin ichthyosis. AJR 153:827, 1989.
32. Meizner I: Prenatal ultrasonic features in a rare case of congenital ichthyosis (harlequin fetus). J Clin Ultrasound 20:132, 1992.
33. Jeanty P, Dramaix-Wilmet M, VanGansbeke D, et al: Fetal ocular biometry by ultrasound. Radiology 143:513, 1982.
34. Mayden KL, Tortora M, Berkowitz RL, et al: Orbital diameters: A new parameter for prenatal diagnosis and dating. Am J Obstet Gynecol 144:289, 1982.
35. Bronshtein M, Zimmer E, Gershoni-Baruch R, et al: First and second trimester diagnosis of fetal ocular defects and associated anomalies: Report of eight cases. Obstet Gynecol 77:443, 1991.
36. Levine RS, Powers T, Rosenberg HK, et al: The cryptophthalmos syndrome. AJR 143:375, 1984.
37. Feldman E, Shalev E, Weiner E, et al: Microphthalmia—prenatal ultrasonic diagnosis: A case report. Prenat Diagn 5:205, 1985.
38. Lev-Gur M, Maklad NF, Patel S: Ultrasonic findings in fetal cyclopia: A case report. J Reprod Med 28:554, 1983.
39. Persutte WH, Lenke RR, DeRosa RT: Prenatal ultrasonographic appearance of agnathia malformation complex. J Ultrasound Med 9:725, 1990.
40. Davis WK, Mahony BS, Carroll BA, et al: Antenatal sonographic detection of benign dacrocystoceles (lacrimal duct cysts). J Ultrasound Med 6:461, 1987.
41. Leo MV, Suslak L, Ganesh VL, et al: Crouzon syndrome: Prenatal ultrasound diagnosis by binocular diameters. Obstet Gynecol 78:906, 1991.
42. Chervenak FA, Pinto MM, Heller CI, et al: Obstetric significance of fetal craniofacial duplication: A case report. J Reprod Med 30:74, 1985.
43. Strauss S, Tamarkin M, Engelberg S, et al: Prenatal sonographic appearance of diprosopus. J Ultrasound Med 6:93, 1987.
44. Okazaki JR, Wilson JL, Holmes SM, et al: Diprosopus: Diagnosis in utero. AJR 149:147, 1987.

CHAPTER 13

Ultrasound Evaluation of the Fetal Musculoskeletal System

BARRY S. MAHONY, M.D.

In recent years, high-resolution real-time ultrasonography has become the primary, most sensitive, and most accurate prenatal method for detecting fetal musculoskeletal abnormalities. These abnormalities are neither rare nor esoteric and, as a group, are among the most amenable to sonographic diagnosis during the second trimester of pregnancy.[1-8] Ultrasonography permits the sonologist to play a central role in the antenatal diagnosis and subsequent management of affected pregnancies. Other methods for prenatally confirming or elucidating abnormalities of the extremities (e.g., fetoscopy, amniography, radiography, amniocentesis, umbilical blood sampling) may provide adjunctive information in some cases but usually yield less information than the sonogram.

Documentation of each fetal bone is neither necessary nor practical in the vast majority of obstetric sonograms. Nevertheless, the relatively simple maneuver of measuring the fetal femur will lead to the accurate identification of many fetal skeletal abnormalities, especially the lethal syndromes.[6] Measurement of the femur length, therefore, must be a routinely documented part of the obstetric examination.[9]

The amount of amniotic fluid and fetal positioning may occasionally limit the portions of the extremities that can be well imaged. Restriction of fetal motion by oligohydramnios, for example, may limit the evaluation of one or more extremities. Conversely, extreme polyhydramnios may make a detailed survey of the extremities difficult and time consuming because of increased distance from the transducer surface and frequent fetal movements. With practice, however, adequate visualization can be obtained in most cases to predict the presence or absence of many extremity abnormalities.

A formidable number of abnormalities may affect the fetal musculoskeletal system.[1-4, 10-13] However, the list of abnormalities usually recognized prenatally is much more manageable. For example, despite the vast number of potential skeletal dysplasias and published case reports documenting their sonographic features, the cases presented in published series are most commonly thanatophoric dysplasia, osteogenesis imperfecta, achondrogenesis, or achondroplasia.

This chapter provides an approach to categorize and minimize the number of diagnostic possibilities when confronted by one of the numerous and varied fetal musculoskeletal abnormalities. Although prenatal ultrasound evaluation may not always permit an exact diagnosis, thorough evaluation usually limits the diagnostic possibilities to one of several entities and pro-

vides useful prognostic information for management of the pregnancy.

NORMAL PRENATAL DEVELOPMENT

By the end of the embryonic period (10 menstrual weeks) the extremities have differentiated into structures with relative position and form identical to those of an adult (Fig. 13–1).[14] The remainder of gestation and postnatal development involves increasing size and complexity of structures already present by the end of the first trimester of pregnancy.

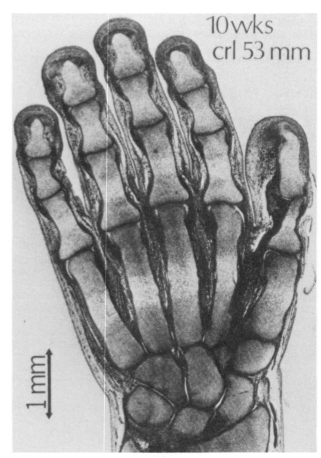

Figure 13–1. Histologic section of the fetal hand at approximately 12 menstrual weeks (10 weeks after conception) shows adult proportions. By 10 menstrual weeks the musculoskeletal system has differentiated into structures with adult form and proportions. (From Garn SM: Contribution of the radiographic image to our knowledge of human growth. AJR 137:231, 1981. Copyright 1981, American Roentgen Ray Society.)

Endochondral ossification of the midshaft of the long bones begins toward the end of the embryonic period.[15] These primary ossification centers can be imaged sonographically simultaneously with or shortly after their inception, especially with endovaginal probes in close proximity to the imaged structures. Limb joint structures and musculature also develop during embryogenesis. By the middle to end of the embryonic period muscular activity has begun and all large joints have complete joint cavities.[1, 16] Ultimate joint structure and function depend on extremity movement in utero, and failure of extremity motion during development may result in a variety of malformations and postural deformities. Attention to extremity motion, therefore, may prove useful in predicting eventual limb function.

The first bones to ossify are the clavicle and mandible, which begin to ossify at 8 menstrual weeks. All of the appendicular long bones, phalanges, ilium, and scapula have begun to ossify by the end of the first trimester. The metacarpals and metatarsals ossify at between 12 and 16 weeks' gestation, and the pubis, talus, and calcaneus ossify during the fifth and sixth months. Ossification of all of the carpal bones and the remaining tarsals does not occur until after birth. The secondary ossification centers within the epiphyseal cartilages of the distal femur, proximal tibia, and occasionally the proximal humerus appear prenatally.[17–21] The remaining secondary epiphyseal ossification centers do not ossify until after birth.

NORMAL APPENDICULAR SKELETON

The ossification centers of the shoulder and pelvis provide excellent landmarks to orient imaging of the

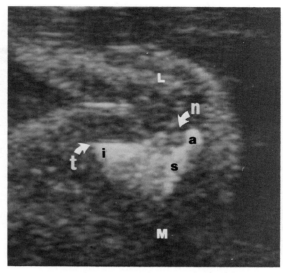

Figure 13–3. Posterior view of the scapula at 19 menstrual weeks demonstrates the scapular tip (t), inferior angle (i), spine (s), notch (n), and acromion (a). M, medial; L, lateral.

appendicular skeleton.[22] The clavicle and scapula define the shoulder girdle (Fig. 13–2). The scapula has a triangular shape when imaged posteriorly, and when imaged coronally it has a characteristic shape resembling a "Y" with the supraspinatus, subscapularis, and infraspinatus muscles in their respective fossae. (Fig. 13–3). If not obscured by flexion of the fetal head, the clavicles can be seen and measured. They grow at a linear rate of approximately 1 mm/wk, reaching a length of 20 mm at 20 weeks and 40 mm at 40 weeks.[23]

The echopenic humeral head epiphyseal cartilage localizes between the ossified scapula, distal clavicle, and proximal humeral diaphysis. The nonossified coronoid fossa of the distal humerus delineates the medial and lateral humeral epicondyles (Fig. 13–4). The more

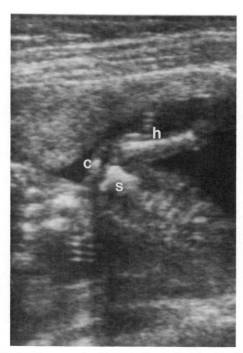

Figure 13–2. The scapula (s) and distal clavicle (c) define the shoulder girdle and are separated from the ossified humeral diaphysis (h) by the echopenic proximal humeral epiphyseal cartilage.

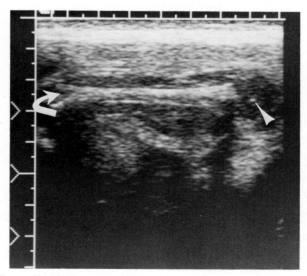

Figure 13–4. The coronoid fossa of the distal humerus (curved arrow) delineates the medial and lateral epicondyles. Note the small secondary epiphyseal ossification center centrally positioned within the echopenic cartilage of the humeral head (arrowhead) in this fetus near term.

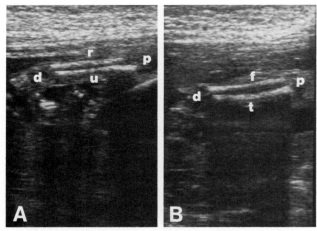

Figure 13–5. Longitudinal scans of the forearm *(A)* and lower leg *(B)* show that the radius and ulna end distally at the same level, as do the tibia and fibula. At the elbow, however, the ulna extends more proximally, whereas the tibia and fibula begin at the same level at the knee. r, radius; u, ulna; f, fibula; t, tibia; p, proximal; d, distal.

proximal extent of the ulna at the elbow distinguishes the ulna from the radius, but at the wrist the ulna and radius end at the same level. Demonstration of this relationship effectively excludes many radial ray defects that characteristically foreshorten the distal radius (Fig. 13–5). The carpals produce a conglomerate zone of gray echoes because they do not ossify prenatally, but the ossified metacarpal and phalanges are readily visualized if the fetus extends the hand.

In the lower extremities, the echopenic femoral head epiphyseal cartilage localizes between the ossified ischium and femoral diaphysis (Fig. 13–6). The proximal

and distal ends of the ossified femoral diaphysis flare slightly to join the larger echopenic epiphyseal cartilages and may give the femur a slightly bowed appearance especially evident medially.[24] Acoustic shadowing caused by the diaphyseal ossification produces a false impression that the femoral diaphysis is too thin for the width of the epiphyseal cartilages, but the width of the epiphyseal cartilage enables extrapolation of the true diaphyseal width.[22]

The echogenic material in and about the knee clearly defines the echopenic cartilages of the patella, distal femur, and proximal tibia and fibula (Figs. 13–7 and 13–8).[22] The secondary epiphyseal ossification centers of the distal femur and then of the proximal tibia become visible centrally positioned within their respective cartilages during the third trimester of pregnancy.[17–21, 25] These secondary epiphyseal ossification centers enlarge centrifugally as term approaches. Since the proximal tibial epiphyseal ossification center grows more rapidly than the distal femoral epiphyseal ossification center grows, their sizes are approximately equal near term.[19]

Unlike the radius and ulna, the tibia and fibula end at approximately the same level proximally as well as distally. The cartilaginous tips of the bones create echopenic gaps between the ossified diaphyses of these bones as well as of the ossified metatarsals and phalanges (see Fig. 13–5).

The epiphyseal ossification centers of the knee and shoulder appear and enlarge at variable rates but in a predictable sequence. The epiphyseal ossification center of the distal femur appears at 28 to 35 weeks, followed 2 to 3 weeks later by the proximal tibial center, then the proximal humeral epiphyseal ossification center at greater than 38 weeks (see Figs. 13–7 and 13–9). Intrauterine growth retardation may delay

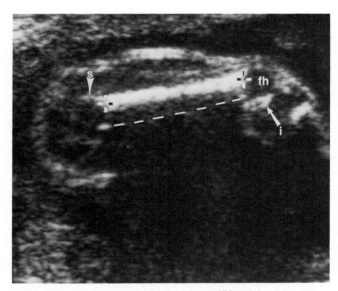

Figure 13–6. The echopenic femoral head (fh) epiphyseal cartilage separates the ossified femoral diaphysis from the ischium (i). Note that the sonographic femur length *(cursors)* measures only the ossified femoral diaphysis and does not include the proximal and distal nonossified cartilages. In addition, the measurements do not include the specular reflection (s) arising from the surface of the distal epiphyseal cartilage. The shadowing from the ossified diaphysis makes the femur look narrower than it is; the dashed line indicates the approximate location of the medial margin of this femur.

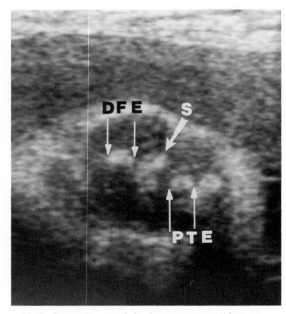

Figure 13–7. Coronal scan of the knee near term demonstrates the echogenic distal femoral (DFE) and proximal tibial (PTE) epiphyseal ossification centers within their respective hypoechoic epiphyseal cartilages. The echogenic synovium (S) within the intercondylar notch should not be confused with an epiphyseal center.

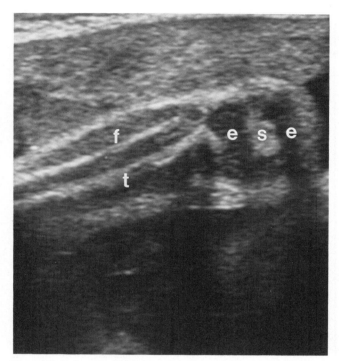

Figure 13–8. Longitudinal view of the knee and lower leg shows the echogenic synovium (s) within the knee joint outlined by the echopenic cartilages of the distal femur and proximal tibia (e). The synovium should not be confused with an epiphyseal ossification center because it is not centrally positioned within the epiphyseal cartilage of either the distal femur or the proximal tibia. f, fibula; t, tibia.

this sequence.[25] Since effectively all fetuses born after 38 weeks have mature lungs, identification of the proximal humeral epiphyseal ossification center provides useful information regarding lung maturity, although not all fetuses with mature lungs have a visible proximal humeral epiphyseal ossification center.[20]

EXTREMITY MEASUREMENTS

Numerous studies correlate the length of the ossified femoral diaphysis with menstrual age and yield consistent and well-defined results (Table 13–1).[26-35] The sonologist should use only charts that relate extremity length to menstrual age when predicting menstrual age based on extremity length. Estimation of menstrual age based on extremity lengths should use menstrual age as the independent variable[26, 27]; that is, charts that relate extremity length to menstrual age may be used to predict menstrual age. Conversely, one should employ charts that correlate extremity length with other parameters of gestational age assessment (biparietal diameter, head circumference, and similar measurements) in detecting whether a fetus suffers from a short-limb dysplasia. In other words, for prediction of a short-limbed bone dysplasia extremity measurements should be compared with other growth parameters.

Attention to technical detail in fetal bone measurement maximizes reproducibility and minimizes meas-

urement error.[36-38] Published measurements of fetal bone lengths correspond to measurement of the ossified diaphyses and exclude the epiphyseal cartilages (see Fig. 13–6).[22] Since the ossified diaphysis may be artifactually foreshortened by scanning obliquely through the shaft, the longest measurement showing both proximal and distal epiphyseal cartilages simultaneously is usually most accurate. Conversely, one may overestimate the diaphyseal length by including in the measurement a portion of the bone width at the end of the diaphysis if the bone orients obliquely through the scan plane.[22] The specular echo arising from the edge of the epiphyseal cartilage should not be included in diaphyseal measurement.[37]

Measurements of the femur length and humeral length during the second trimester of pregnancy have been suggested as screening methods in the detection of Down syndrome.[39-42] The positive predictive value of a short femur (< 90% of predicted value) is reported to be approximately 1% for a high-risk population (prevalence of Down syndrome, 1 in 250) and 0.3% for a low-risk population (prevalence of Down syndrome, 1 in 700).[41] Humeral shortening may be more predictive of trisomy 21 than is femur length. The positive predictive value of a short humerus (< 90% of predicted value) is reported to be approximately 3% for a high-risk population and 1% to 2% for a low-risk population.[42]

The foot length can be accurately measured during the second and third trimesters. Measurements can be made either on the plantar or on the sagittal image of the foot and extend from the heel to the tip of the longest toe (Fig. 13–10). The foot length remains nearly equal to the femur length throughout gestation, such that the normal femur length/foot length ratio remains near unity.[43-45] The femur length/foot length ratio for fetuses with skeletal dysplasia tends to be less

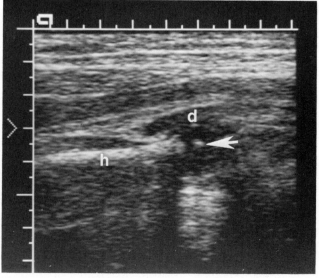

Figure 13–9. The proximal humeral epiphyseal ossification center *(arrow)* appears near term centrally positioned within the humeral head epiphyseal cartilage. h, ossified humeral diaphysis; d, deltoid muscle.

Table 13–1. NORMAL EXTREMITY LONG BONE LENGTHS AND BIPARIETAL DIAMETER AT DIFFERENT MENSTRUAL AGES*

Menstrual Age (wk)	Biparietal Diameter	Bone					
		Femur	Tibia	Fibula	Humerus	Radius	Ulna
13	2.3 (0.3)	1.1 (0.2)	0.9 (0.2)	0.8 (0.2)	1.0 (0.2)	0.6 (0.2)	0.8 (0.3)
14	2.7 (0.3)	1.3 (0.2)	1.0 (0.2)	0.9 (0.3)	1.2 (0.2)	0.8 (0.2)	1.0 (0.2)
15	3.0 (0.1)	1.5 (0.2)	1.3 (0.2)	1.2 (0.2)	1.4 (0.2)	1.1 (0.1)	1.2 (0.1)
16	3.3 (0.2)	1.9 (0.3)	1.6 (0.3)	1.5 (0.3)	1.7 (0.2)	1.4 (0.3)	1.6 (0.3)
17	3.7 (0.3)	2.2 (0.3)	1.8 (0.3)	1.7 (0.2)	2.0 (0.4)	1.5 (0.3)	1.7 (0.3)
18	4.2 (0.5)	2.5 (0.3)	2.2 (0.3)	2.1 (0.3)	2.3 (0.3)	1.9 (0.2)	2.2 (0.3)
19	4.4 (0.4)	2.8 (0.3)	2.5 (0.3)	2.3 (0.3)	2.6 (0.3)	2.1 (0.3)	2.4 (0.3)
20	4.7 (0.4)	3.1 (0.3)	2.7 (0.2)	2.6 (0.2)	2.9 (0.3)	2.4 (0.2)	2.7 (0.3)
21	5.0 (0.5)	3.5 (0.4)	3.0 (0.4)	2.9 (0.4)	3.2 (0.4)	2.7 (0.4)	3.0 (0.4)
22	5.5 (0.5)	3.6 (0.3)	3.2 (0.3)	3.1 (0.3)	3.3 (0.3)	2.8 (0.5)	3.1 (0.4)
23	5.8 (0.5)	4.0 (0.4)	3.6 (0.2)	3.4 (0.2)	3.7 (0.3)	3.1 (0.4)	3.5 (0.2)
24	6.1 (0.5)	4.2 (0.3)	3.7 (0.3)	3.6 (0.3)	3.8 (0.4)	3.3 (0.4)	3.6 (0.4)
25	6.4 (0.5)	4.6 (0.3)	4.0 (0.3)	3.9 (0.4)	4.2 (0.4)	3.5 (0.3)	3.9 (0.4)
26	6.8 (0.5)	4.8 (0.4)	4.2 (0.3)	4.0 (0.3)	4.3 (0.3)	3.6 (0.4)	4.0 (0.3)
27	7.0 (0.3)	4.9 (0.3)	4.4 (0.3)	4.2 (0.3)	4.5 (0.2)	3.7 (0.3)	4.1 (0.2)
28	7.3 (0.5)	5.3 (0.5)	4.5 (0.4)	4.4 (0.3)	4.7 (0.4)	3.9 (0.4)	4.4 (0.5)
29	7.6 (0.5)	5.3 (0.5)	4.6 (0.3)	4.5 (0.3)	4.8 (0.4)	4.0 (0.5)	4.5 (0.4)
30	7.7 (0.6)	5.6 (0.3)	4.8 (0.5)	4.7 (0.3)	5.0 (0.5)	4.1 (0.6)	4.7 (0.3)
31	8.2 (0.7)	6.0 (0.6)	5.1 (0.3)	4.9 (0.5)	5.3 (0.4)	4.2 (0.3)	4.9 (0.4)
32	8.5 (0.6)	6.1 (0.6)	5.2 (0.4)	5.1 (0.4)	5.4 (0.4)	4.4 (0.6)	5.0 (0.6)
33	8.6 (0.4)	6.4 (0.5)	5.4 (0.5)	5.3 (0.3)	5.6 (0.5)	4.5 (0.5)	5.2 (0.3)
34	8.9 (0.5)	6.6 (0.6)	5.7 (0.5)	5.5 (0.4)	5.8 (0.5)	4.7 (0.5)	5.4 (0.5)
35	8.9 (0.7)	6.7 (0.6)	5.8 (0.4)	5.6 (0.4)	5.9 (0.6)	4.8 (0.6)	5.4 (0.4)
36	9.1 (0.7)	7.0 (0.7)	6.0 (0.6)	5.6 (0.5)	6.0 (0.6)	4.9 (0.5)	5.5 (0.3)
37	9.3 (0.9)	7.2 (0.4)	6.1 (0.4)	6.0 (0.4)	6.1 (0.4)	5.1 (0.5)	5.6 (0.4)
38	9.5 (0.6)	7.4 (0.6)	6.2 (0.3)	6.0 (0.4)	6.4 (0.3)	5.1 (0.5)	5.8 (0.6)
39	9.5 (0.6)	7.6 (0.8)	6.4 (0.7)	6.1 (0.6)	6.5 (0.6)	5.3 (0.5)	6.0 (0.6)
40	9.9 (0.8)	7.7 (0.4)	6.5 (0.3)	6.2 (0.1)	6.6 (0.4)	5.3 (0.3)	6.0 (0.5)
41	9.7 (0.6)	7.7 (0.4)	6.6 (0.4)	6.3 (0.5)	6.6 (0.4)	5.6 (0.4)	6.3 (0.5)
42	10.0 (0.5)	7.8 (0.7)	6.8 (0.5)	6.7 (0.7)	6.8 (0.7)	5.7 (0.5)	6.5 (0.5)

*Mean values (cm); value of 2 SD in parentheses.

From Merz E, Mi-Sook KK, Pehl S: Ultrasonic mensuration of fetal limb bones in the second and third trimesters. J Clin Ultrasound 15:175, 1987. Copyright © 1987. Reprinted by permission of John Wiley & Sons, Inc.

than 0.9, whereas the ratio tends to be greater than 0.9 for fetuses that are constitutionally small or symmetrically growth retarded but without skeletal dysplasia. These observations may prove useful in distinguishing fetuses with dwarfism from those that are constitutionally small or symmetrically growth retarded.[43]

SONOGRAPHIC APPROACH TO MUSCULOSKELETAL ABNORMALITIES

Many fetal musculoskeletal abnormalities occur in a sporadic or autosomal recessive pattern. Therefore, the sonologist is usually the first to detect an unexpected problem. However, in the vast majority of reported cases, musculoskeletal abnormalities have occurred in the setting of polyhydramnios, concomitant fetal structural anomalies, or a positive family history for a recurrent syndrome. The presence of any of these risk factors should signal the sonologist to examine the extremities.[6] Pedigree analysis, assessment of amniotic fluid volume, and fetal survey are essential for prenatal detection of, and distinction among, the various abnormalities involving the musculoskeletal system.

Many fetuses with lethal musculoskeletal abnormalities present with severe manifestations readily apparent on the prenatal ultrasound evaluation (Fig. 13–11). Because the nonlethal syndromes typically manifest as milder manifestations, the sensitivity and specificity of ultrasound detection of these syndromes would be expected to be lower than for the lethal syndromes, especially in the absence of genetic risk.

Assessment of the following questions assists in prenatal diagnosis of many abnormalities of the fetal musculoskeletal system (Table 13–2):

- *Are the extremity bones abnormally short or are portions of the bones absent?* Shortening of the extremity bones indicates the presence of skeletal dysplasia. Focal absence of extremity bones usually indicates amputation, radial ray defect, or sirenomelia.
- *Are the extremities immobile or anomalously postured?* Anomalous posturing or immobility suggests the presence of contractures and potential neuromuscular defects.
- *Are subtle hand and foot deformities present?* Polydactyly and syndactyly in the setting of other severe and more obvious abnormalities may indicate the presence of a syndrome or chromosome abnormality.

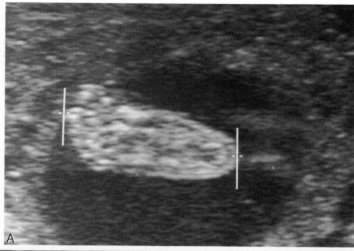

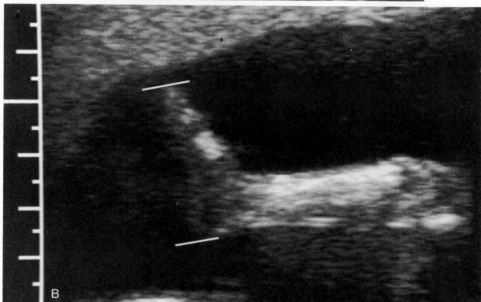

Figure 13–10. The foot length may be measured either on the plantar *(A)* or on the sagittal *(B)* view. The foot is measured *(between lines)* from the heel to the tip of the longest toe.

Table 13–2. NOMENCLATURE REGARDING MORE COMMON FETAL LIMB ABNORMALITIES

Disorder	Description
Bone Shortening (Micromelia)	
Acromelia	Shortening of distal segments
Mesomelia	Shortening of middle segments
Rhizomelia	Shortening of proximal segments
Focal Absence	
Ectrodactyly	Absence of fingers or toes
Hemimelia	Absence of extremity below the knee or elbow
Phocomelia	Absent or deficient development of middle segment of an extremity with preservation of proximal and distal segments
Sirenomelia	Fusion of the legs
Contractures and Postural Deformities	
Arthrogryposis	Extremity contractures
Clinodactyly	Overlapping digits
Equinus	Extension of the foot
Pterygium	Web of skin across a joint
Talipes	Clubfoot
Valgus	Bent outward
Varus	Bent inward

Skeletal Dysplasia

An abnormally shortened bone length signifies the presence of skeletal dysplasia. Although some bone dysplasias (especially heterozygous achondroplasia) do not produce shortened bone lengths early in gestation, a fetus whose bones measure shorter than 2 standard deviations (SD) below the mean for a known menstrual age should be considered at risk for dwarfism.[46–48] Many dwarf syndromes cause the extremity bones to measure significantly shorter than 2 SD below the mean by 22 weeks (see Fig. 13–11), and, occasionally, limb shortening can be recognized as early as 12 to 13 weeks' gestation when sonography can first measure the femur length reliably. However, normal limb lengths early in the second trimester do not exclude the presence of a dwarf syndrome.[49]

If the femur length measures 2 to 4 SD below the mean for a known menstrual age and no other abnormalities are evident on the prenatal sonogram, a follow-up ultrasound examination in 3 to 4 weeks is

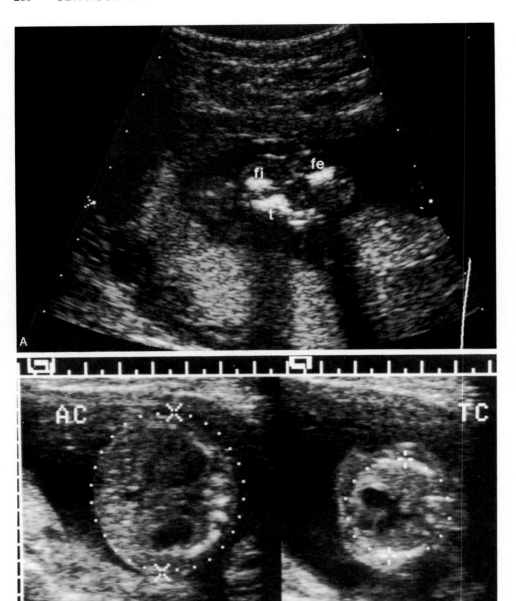

Figure 13–11. Severe micromelia and small thorax indicate a high probability for a lethal skeletal dysplasia in this 20-week fetus. *A.* The femur (fe), tibia (t), and fibula (fi) are all markedly shortened with lengths mean for 12 to 13 weeks. *B.* The thoracic circumference (TC) is unmistakably small relative to the normal abdominal circumference (AC). This fetus had thanatophoric dysplasia.

recommended to evaluate interval growth.[46] Normal interval growth indicates a high likelihood that the fetus does not have a skeletal dysplasia. Deviation further from the mean by at least 1 SD suggests the presence of skeletal dysplasia but can also be seen with growth retardation in the absence of skeletal dysplasia. If the femur length is markedly short (shorter than 4 SD below the mean for a known menstrual age), skeletal dysplasia is likely, especially in the presence of other abnormalities, including polyhydramnios.[46]

Severe intrauterine growth retardation predominantly affecting extremity length can occur and may be difficult to distinguish from skeletal dysplasia.[50] However, this is an unusual and atypical form of intrauterine growth retardation. Assessment of amniotic fluid volume (polyhydramnios versus oligohydramnios) and umbilical arterial Doppler velocimetry may assist in distinction between skeletal dysplasia and atypical intrauterine growth retardation.

Sonographic screening for extremity abnormalities has detected skeletal dysplasia in 0.075% to 0.1% of pregnancies, and fetuses with skeletal dysplasia represent 1% to 3.5% of fetuses with sonographically detectable abnormalities.[6, 8] The prenatal prevalence of skeletal dysplasias probably exceeds the prevalence at birth because many fetuses with skeletal dysplasia do not survive (Table 13–3).[5, 7]

Following the detection of shortened extremity bones, evaluation of the following sonographic parameters and questions permits accurate prenatal diagnosis of many skeletal dysplasias:

- *How severely shortened are the bones?* The severity of bone shortening varies from mild to moderate

Table 13–3. APPROXIMATE BIRTH PREVALENCE OF SHORT-LIMBED SKELETAL DYSPLASIAS

Dysplasia	Approximate Birth Prevalence
Lethal (Severe Micromelia)	
Thanatophoric dysplasia	1/10,000
Achondrogenesis	1/40,000
Osteogenesis imperfecta type II	1/60,000
Others	<1/100,000
Variable Prognosis (Mild-to-Moderate Rhizomelic Bone Shortening)	
Heterozygous achondroplasia	1/30,000
Asphyxiating thoracic dysplasia	1/70,000
Others	<1/200,000
Total	1/4,000

Table 13–4. COMMON CAUSES FOR EXTREMITY FRACTURES OR BOWING OF FETAL EXTREMITY BONES

Osteogenesis imperfecta type II
Achondrogenesis
Campomelic dysplasia
Hypophosphatasia
Thanatophoric dysplasia

(with a relatively normal orientation of the limbs to the fetal trunk) to extreme (bone length many standard deviations below the mean with the limbs oriented at approximately right angles to the fetal trunk).

- *Are bones fractured or bowed* (Table 13–4)? Fractures usually indicate osteogenesis imperfecta, especially when involving the ribs. Extremity bowing may indicate the presence of fracture, campomelic dysplasia, or a rare dysplasia. Thanatophoric dysplasia may produce a "telephone receiver" appearance of the extremity bones.
- *Is the thorax abnormally small* (Table 13–5)?[51] A small thorax indicates a high probability of pulmonary hypoplasia and a lethal prognosis. Rib fractures with concavity of the thoracic cage characterize os-

teogenesis imperfecta type IIA. Otherwise, the thoracic shape usually does not assist in defining a specific diagnosis.

- *Does the degree of ossification appear normal* (Table 13–6)? Hypomineralization usually indicates osteogenesis imperfecta, hypophosphatasia, or achondrogenesis.
- *What is the calvarial shape?* Cloverleaf skull deformity with severe micromelia and a small thorax typically indicates thanatophoric dysplasia.

Additional parameters that, in my experience, have not proven to be as useful in the prenatal ultrasound evaluation as they are on the postnatal evaluation include the following:

- *Distribution of bone shortening* (Table 13–7). Rhizomelic, mesomelic, or acromelic bone shortening occurs with different dysplasias.
- *Appearance of the spine.* Severe platyspondyly is characteristic of thanatophoric dysplasia, and lack of normal increase in the interpedicular distance of the lumbar spine with thoracolumbar kyphosis typifies achondroplasia.

Table 13–5. NORMAL THORACIC CIRCUMFERENCE (CM) CORRELATED WITH MENSTRUAL AGE

Gestational Age (wk)	No.	Predictive Percentiles								
		2.5	5	10	25	50	75	90	95	97.5
16	6	5.9	6.4	7.0	8.0	9.1	10.3	11.3	11.9	12.4
17	22	6.8	7.3	7.9	8.9	10.0	11.2	12.2	12.8	13.3
18	31	7.7	8.2	8.8	9.8	11.0	12.1	13.1	13.7	14.2
19	21	8.6	9.1	9.7	10.7	11.9	13.0	14.0	14.6	15.1
20	20	9.5	10.0	10.6	11.7	12.9	13.9	15.0	15.5	16.0
21	30	10.4	11.0	11.6	12.6	13.7	14.8	15.8	16.4	16.9
22	18	11.3	11.9	12.5	13.5	14.6	15.7	16.7	17.3	17.8
23	21	12.2	12.8	13.4	14.4	15.5	16.6	17.6	18.2	18.8
24	27	13.2	13.7	14.3	15.3	16.4	17.5	18.5	19.1	19.7
25	20	14.1	14.6	15.2	16.2	17.3	18.4	19.4	20.0	20.6
26	25	15.0	15.5	16.1	17.1	18.2	19.3	20.3	21.0	21.5
27	24	15.9	16.4	17.0	18.0	19.1	20.2	21.3	21.9	22.4
28	24	16.8	17.3	17.9	18.9	20.0	21.2	22.2	22.8	23.3
29	24	17.7	18.2	18.8	19.8	21.0	22.1	23.1	23.7	24.2
30	27	18.6	19.1	19.7	20.7	21.9	23.0	24.0	24.6	25.1
31	24	19.5	20.0	20.6	21.6	22.8	23.9	24.9	25.5	26.0
32	28	20.4	20.9	21.5	22.6	23.7	24.8	25.8	26.4	26.9
33	27	21.3	21.8	22.5	23.5	24.6	25.7	26.7	27.3	27.8
34	25	22.2	22.8	23.4	24.4	25.5	26.6	27.6	28.2	28.7
35	20	23.1	23.7	24.3	25.3	26.4	27.5	28.5	29.1	29.6
36	23	24.0	24.6	25.2	26.2	27.3	28.4	29.4	30.0	30.6
37	22	24.9	25.5	26.1	27.1	28.2	29.3	30.3	30.9	31.5
38	21	25.9	26.4	27.0	28.0	29.1	30.2	31.2	31.9	32.4
39	7	26.8	27.3	27.9	28.9	30.0	31.1	32.2	32.8	33.3
40	6	27.7	28.2	28.8	29.8	30.9	32.1	33.1	33.7	34.2

From Chitgara U, Rosenberg J, Chevenak FA, et al: Prenatal sonographic assessment of the fetal thorax: Normal values. Am J Obstet Gynecol 156:1069, 1987.

Table 13–6. COMMON CAUSES OF HYPOMINERALIZATION OF FETAL BONE

Osteogenesis imperfecta
Hypophosphatasia
Achondrogenesis

- *Polydactyly.* Polydactyly with skeletal dysplasia usually indicates short-rib polydactyly syndrome, chondrodysplasia punctata, or asphyxiating thoracic dysplasia. However, polydactyly with severe growth retardation may also occur with chromosome abnormalities, such as trisomy 13.

Even in the absence of a family history for a recurrent skeletal dysplasia, careful assessment of these criteria may permit accurate diagnosis of a specific skeletal dysplasia in over 50% of cases on the basis of sonography alone and enables accurate assessment of prognosis in approximately 85% of lethal dwarfism.[52]

Focal Absence of Extremity Bone

Focal absence of an extremity bone ranges in severity from loss of a single bone or segment of bone to loss of an entire extremity. The focal absence of bone contrasts to the skeletal dysplasias in which the bones may be extremely foreshortened but remain present. The following questions may be helpful in the evaluation of a fetus with focal limb loss:

- *What portions of the limbs are absent?* Asymmetric amputations in nonembryologic distributions indicate the amniotic band sequence or limb–body wall complex. Symmetric absence of a segment of a limb (phocomelia) with preservation of distal components often suggests the Roberts syndrome. Fusion of the entire lower extremity indicates sirenomelia.
- *Is the hand oriented at an acute angle with the wrist?* Sharp radial angulation of the hand at the wrist with absence of the distal radius indicates a radial ray deformity.

Anomalous Posture and Hand and Foot Deformities

Extremity contractures often occur in conjunction with musculoskeletal or neurologic disorders that limit fetal mobility. In some affected cases fetal contractures and persistent lack of mobility are so striking that they are unmistakable during ultrasound evaluation. In other cases, however, the contractures may be quite subtle and require meticulous attention to fetal positioning and limb motion to be detected.

Clinodactyly, polydactyly, syndactyly, and other subtle hand and foot deformities also often occur as a manifestation of a syndrome. Their detection requires meticulous attention to detail. Prenatal detection of these deformities may facilitate diagnosis of a lethal syndrome or chromosome abnormality and permit proper parental counseling and early neonatal treatment.

Prediction of Outcome

The prognosis varies widely among the vast range of musculoskeletal abnormalities amenable to prenatal sonographic diagnosis. Some entities have an invariably fatal prognosis, while others have a variable or good prognosis but one that is certainly not uniformly fatal in early infancy. Especially during the third trimester of pregnancy, the most crucial dwarf syndromes for the sonologist to identify include those for which the fetus has little or no chance for survival; accurate assessment of prognosis in these cases will obviate heroic procedures to save the fetus.

If examined with prenatal sonography even before 24 menstrual weeks, fetuses with a lethal short-limbed dysplasia typically exhibit striking micromelia or other severe manifestations or characteristic features that permit accurate distinction from nonlethal syndromes (Table 13–8; see Fig. 13–11). The combination of severe micromelia and an unmistakably small thorax correlates with a high probability for a lethal skeletal dysplasia.

Some of the dysplasias that are not invariably fatal have variable expressivity of phenotype. As a general rule (and with inevitable exceptions), however, those dysplasias that manifest later and with less severe features have a better prognosis than do the lethal syndromes (Tables 13–9 and 13–10).

In general, the prognosis for a fetus with focal absence of an extremity bone or extremity contractures also tends to obey this rule. For example, the Roberts syndrome and the pseudothalidomide syndrome may represent variations in phenotypic expression of the same entity. Severely affected fetuses have a high perinatal mortality rate, unlike those with mild manifestations of the syndrome. On the other hand, the degree of subtlety created by hand and foot deformities often associated with chromosome abnormalities does not correlate with the prognosis in many cases.

Table 13–7. MORE COMMON SHORT-LIMBED DWARFISMS IDENTIFIABLE AT BIRTH, CATEGORIZED BY DISTRIBUTION OF SHORTENING

Diffuse Shortening
Achondrogenesis
Thanatophoric dysplasia
Osteogenesis imperfecta types II and III
Rhizomelia
Asphyxiating thoracic dysplasia
Heterozygous achondroplasia
Mesomelia
Acromesomelic dysplasias
Mesomelic dysplasias

Table 13–8. HELPFUL SONOGRAPHIC FEATURES IN THE DIFFERENTIAL DIAGNOSIS OF THE MORE COMMON LETHAL SKELETAL DYSPLASIAS THAT MAY PRESENT PRENATALLY, LISTED IN APPROXIMATE ORDER OF PREVALENCE

Dysplasia	Inheritance Pattern	Helpful Sonographic Features	Comments
Common			
Thanatophoric dysplasia	Sporadic, ? AR if cloverleaf skull	Cloverleaf skull (14% cases); narrow spine; platyspondyly	
Achondrogenesis	AR	± Absent vertebral body and sacral ossification	Ossified calvarium distinguishes from hypophosphatasia
Osteogenesis imperfecta type II	AR	Multiple fractures; rib fractures; hypomineralized calvarium; "thick" bones	
Rare			
Congenital hypophosphatasia	AR	Thin, delicate or absent bones; ± fractures; ± decreased bone echogenicity	Decreased alkaline phosphatase in amniocytes
Campomelic dysplasia	?AR	Anterior bowing of femur, tibia, and fibula but of overall normal length	
Chondrodysplasia punctata, rhizomelic type	AR	Stippled epiphyses; rhizomelic shortening; contractures; dorsal and ventral ossification of vertebral bodies	
Homozygous dominant achondroplasia	AD	Resembles thanatophoric dysplasia	Both parents achondroplastic dwarfs
Short-rib polydactyly syndrome	?AR	Polydactyly; ± cleft lip, renal cysts	Micromelia, more severe than chondroectodermal dysplasia or asphyxiating thoracic dysplasia

AR, autosomal recessive; AD, autosomal dominant.

Table 13–9. NONLETHAL SHORT-LIMBED OSTEOCHONDRODYSPLASIAS

Dysplasia	Inheritance Pattern	Characteristic or Distinctive Sonographic Features	Comments
Variable Prognosis			
Chondroectodermal dysplasia (Ellis-van Creveld)	AR variable expressivity	Postaxial hexadactyly, 50% have large atrial septal defect	Very frequent in one Amish group
Asphyxiating thoracic dystrophy	AR	Narrow thorax; ± rhizomelic shortening; ± polydactyly, renal cysts	Almost always in whites, may be very similar to chondroectodermal dysplasia
Metatrophic dysplasia	Heterogeneous	Narrow thorax, kyphoscoliosis, relatively long trunk	± Characteristic taillike appendage over sacrum
Roberts syndrome, pseudothalidomide syndrome	AR, variable expressivity	Tetraphocomelia, midline facial clefts	Pseudothalidomide syndrome, much less severe manifestations
Diastrophic dysplasia	AR	Multiple contractures, "hitchhiker" thumb	More muscle mass than arthrogryposis
Good Prognosis			
Heterozygous achondroplasia	AD, over 80% spontaneous mutation	Rhizomelic micromelia	Characteristic fetal growth curve, narrow interpedicular distance of lumbar spine (subtle)
Spondyloepiphyseal dysplasia congenita	AD, variable expressivity	Short, bowed femora; short spine and trunk	Delayed ossification of epiphyseal centers, calcaneus, and talus
Kniest dysplasia	Probably AD	Kyphoscoliosis, short trunk, broad thorax	
Mesomelic and acromesomelic dysplasia	AR or AD (depends on type)	Micromelia of middle or distal segments	Distribution of shortening distinguishes from lethal syndromes

AR, autosomal recessive; AD, autosomal dominant.

Table 13–10. OSTEOCHONDRODYSPLASIAS WITH NORMAL BODY PROPORTIONS

Dysplasia	Inheritance Pattern	Prognosis	Characteristic or Distinctive Sonographic Features	Comments
Osteogenesis imperfecta (types I, III, IV)	AD or sporadic	Variable	± Several fractures with normal or near-normal bone lengths	
Cleidocranial dysplasia	AD; wide expressivity, high penetrance	Good	Clavicular hypoplasia/aplasia, brachycephaly	One third occur by spontaneous mutation
Otopalatodigital syndrome	AD in males	Mild mental retardation	Hypoplasia of proximal radius, short thumbs	Not manifest at birth in females
Larsen syndrome	Sporadic	Good	Talipes, hypertelorism, multiple dislocations, ± kyphoscoliosis	
Osteopetrosis congenita	AR	Variable	Hepatosplenomegaly	Probably requires radiography for diagnosis

AD, autosomal dominant; AR, autosomal recessive.

LETHAL DYSPLASIAS

In the past 25 years a large number of lethal skeletal dysplasias have been recognized and categorized and many more remain unclassified. Nevertheless, thanatophoric dysplasia, osteogenesis imperfecta, and achondrogenesis account for the vast majority of cases associated with lethal short-limbed dysplasia seen prenatally. The remaining lethal cases occur only rarely, and new syndromes are frequently being described. Because almost all lethal skeletal dysplasias (except homozygous achondroplasia) occur in a sporadic or autosomal recessive inheritance pattern, the sonologist most often serendipitously discovers these lethal syndromes.

Thanatophoric Dysplasia

Probably the most common lethal skeletal dysplasia, thanatophoric dysplasia, occurs in approximately 1 in 4,000 to 15,000 births.[5, 7, 8] The term derives from the Greek *thanatos*, meaning "death bearing."

Approximately 50% of cases with thanatophoric dysplasia present as large for dates measurements secondary to polyhydramnios. The extremities are markedly foreshortened such that the fetus holds its extremities at approximately right angles with its trunk. Other features associated with this lethal dysplasia include the cloverleaf skull deformity, bowed limbs, soft tissue redundancy, narrow thorax, and flattened vertebral bodies (platyspondyly) with a narrow spinal canal.[13, 52–54] Although the platyspondyly is a characteristic feature of thanatophoric dysplasia, it often requires radiography for confirmation.[52, 54]

Because of the absence of familial risk in most cases with thanatophoric dysplasia, the majority of reported cases with thanatophoric dysplasia were scanned for obstetric reasons, usually large for dates measurements during the third trimester of pregnancy. Numerous cases have been detected during the second trimester, however, implying that screening ultrasonography can detect this abnormality at or before 24 weeks' gestation, but one report documents a normal sonogram at 13 weeks of a fetus subsequently shown to have thanatophoric dysplasia.[49]

Identification of the cloverleaf skull deformity provides a useful finding that enables accurate prenatal diagnosis of thanatophoric dysplasia in the setting of severe micromelia and polyhydramnios (Fig. 13–12). Although this deformity only occurs in approximately 14% of cases with thanatophoric dysplasia and may occur with a variety of other nondwarf syndromes, it typically occurs in short-limbed dwarfs who have either thanatophoric dysplasia or homozygous achondroplasia.[55] Since the parents of a fetus with homozygous achondroplasia are readily recognizable as achondroplasts and homozygous achondroplasia is exceedingly rare, no confusion should exist between these two lethal syndromes.

The cloverleaf skull (Kleeblattschadel) deformity, often associated with hydrocephaly and cranial enlargement, results from premature craniosynostosis and creates a distinctive trilobed appearance of the skull. The absence of calvarial defect distinguishes the cloverleaf skull deformity from encephalocele.[56] Some authors suggest that thanatophoric dwarfism with the cloverleaf skull deformity may be transmitted in an autosomal recessive pattern, unlike the sporadic transmission of the dysplasia without the skull deformity.[57, 58] Furthermore, cases with the cloverleaf skull deformity and thanatophoric dysplasia may also have agenesis of the corpus callosum (Fig. 13–13).[52, 59]

In the absence of these characteristic features, other very rare lethal short-limbed dysplasias (e.g., atelosteogenesis, fibrochondrogenesis, San Diego dysplasia, Schneckenbecken dysplasia, Torrance dysplasia) may mimic thanatophoric dysplasia and require postnatal radiographic and histologic evaluation for diagnosis. Nevertheless, the general rule holds true that severe manifestations of skeletal dysplasia signify a poor prognosis.

Achondrogenesis

Probably the second most common lethal short-limbed dwarfism, achondrogenesis occurs in approximately 1 in 40,000 births.[5, 7] Achondrogenesis is inherited as an autosomal recessive trait. Although parents with an affected child have a 25% chance of recurrence, the rarity of the syndrome dictates that most cases

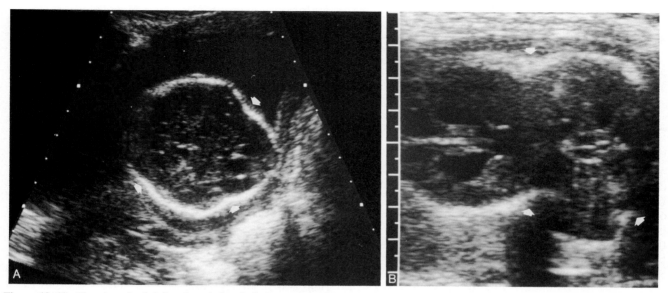

Figure 13–12. The cloverleaf deformity of the skull *(arrows)* exhibits a trilobed appearance. The combination of severe dwarfism and cloverleaf skull deformity provides convincing prenatal evidence for thanatophoric dysplasia. The degree of calvarial distortion may vary at different stages of gestation. For example, the calvarial distortion (arrows) in one affected fetus at 20 menstrual weeks *(A)* is much less apparent than for another affected fetus near term *(B).*

detected by the sonographer will probably not include a positive family history.

The hallmarks of achondrogenesis include severely retarded or absent skeletal ossification with profound limb length reduction of all extremity tubular bones caused by disorganization of cartilage and absence of normal bony architecture.[60] The affected fetus also has a short trunk and thorax because of the absent or severely delayed vertebral body and sacral ossification. The absence of vertebral body ossification permits unusually clear sonographic visualization of the relatively lucent spinal column on longitudinal sonograms, even as early as the middle of the second trimester (Fig. 13–14). Only two vertebral ossification centers per spinal segment are visible on cross-sectional sonograms of the spine.[52, 61]

Two types of achondrogenesis occur: type I (Parenti-Fraccaro) and type II (Langer-Saldino).[12] Three distinct prototypes of type II achondrogenesis also exist (Table 13–11).[62] Approximately 80% of achondrogenesis is type II, and half of these are of one of the three prototypes. Degrees of ossification vary among the different types and prototypes of achondrogenesis.[62, 63] For example, all prototypes of type II achon-

Figure 13–13. Approximately 25% of thanatophoric dwarfs with cloverleaf skull deformity also have agenesis of the corpus callosum, as this coronal scan of the head shows (same fetus as in Fig. 13–12B). lv, lateral cerebral ventricle; 3, third cerebral ventricle.

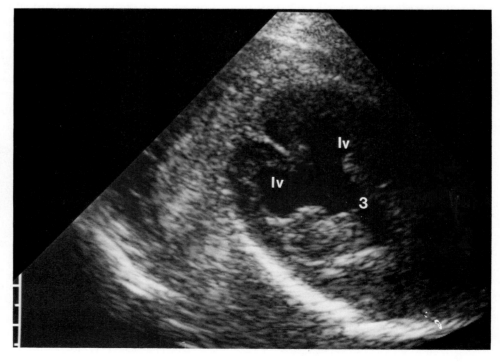

Table 13–11. CLASSIFICATION AND SONOGRAPHIC FEATURES OF ACHONDROGENESIS

Type	Prototype	% of Cases	Degree of Extremity Shortening	Rib Fractures	Calvarial Ossification	Vertebral Body Ossification
I		20	Severe	Yes	Poor	Poor
II	II	20	Severe	No	Good	Poor
	III	40	Moderate to severe	No	Good	Poor
	IV	20	Moderate	No	Good	Good

From Mahony BS: The extremities. In Nyberg DA, Mahony BS, Pretorius DH (eds): Diagnostic Ultrasound of Fetal Anomalies: Text and Atlas. Chicago, Mosby-Year Book, 1990.

drogenesis have normal calvarial ossification but type I may have diminished calvarial mineralization. On the other hand, virtual absence of vertebral body ossification occurs in all types except prototype IV, in which the vertebral bodies may only be underdeveloped. In other words, all cases of achondrogenesis have diminished or absent vertebral body ossification except prototype IV (approximately 20% of cases); all cases of type II achondrogenesis (approximately 80% of cases) have normal calvarial ossification; and prototypes II and III (approximately 60% of achondrogenesis cases) have normal calvarial ossification but severely diminished or absent vertebral body ossification. Only prototype IV may have both normal calvarial and vertebral body ossification.

Although other lethal dysplasias (thanatophoric dysplasia, homozygous achondroplasia, short-rib polydactyly) may have variable underdevelopment of the vertebral bodies, none of these dysplasias also have concomitant calvarial underossification.[12, 63] In addition, severe hypophosphatasia may also result in severe delay in calvarial and spinal ossification (similar to type I achondrogenesis) but severe hypophosphatasia tends to have diffuse underossification, rather than the more focal lack of ossification in achondrogenesis.[12, 63] Therefore, the combination of absent vertebral body ossification and normal calvarial ossification differentiates achondrogenesis from other lethal short-limbed dwarf syndromes even though not all fetuses with achondrogenesis have both of these features.[61]

Osteogenesis Imperfecta

Characterized by repeated fractures of brittle bones, osteogenesis imperfecta encompasses a group of clini-cally and genetically heterogeneous disorders having defective collagen.[64–67] Although the classification of osteogenesis imperfecta has changed several times in the past, the Sillence classification first proposed in 1979 with subsequent modifications is probably the most widely accepted (Table 13–12).[65] This classification recognizes two severe or lethal types (II and III) and two relatively mild forms (I and IV). Types I and IV are subdivided into A and B subtypes based on the presence or absence of dentinogenesis imperfecta, and type II is also divided into subtypes A, B, and C. Type III may only represent a heterogeneous subtype of type IIB.[67, 68]

Type IIA osteogenesis imperfecta, the classic subtype with innumerable fractures, severe extremity shortening ("accordian" or "telescoped" bones), and decreased bone echogenicity, occurs with a frequency of approximately 1 in 60,000 births (Fig. 13–15). Most cases arise as a new mutation.[65] Type II osteogenesis imperfecta represents the large majority of cases of osteogenesis imperfecta detected with prenatal sonography, and the majority (approximately 80%) of these cases probably involved type IIA. The diagnosis of lethal osteogenesis imperfecta has been suggested as early as at 13.5 weeks and made definitively as early as at 15 weeks.[69, 70] Since many cases are scanned for obstetric reasons, however, the diagnosis is often not made until the third trimester.

The features of type IIB osteogenesis imperfecta include moderately shortened femurs with visible isolated fractures. This is a severe but not necessarily fatal syndrome. The sonographic distinction between type IIB and IIC osteogenesis imperfecta is quite subtle, but the lethal type IIC has shortening of all limbs, unlike the isolated femoral shortening of type

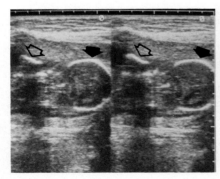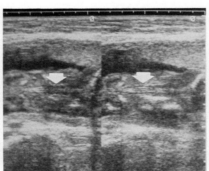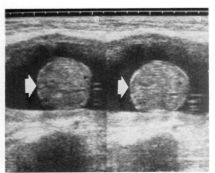

Figure 13–14. Documentation of severe limb shortening, absent vertebral ossification, and normal calvarial ossification permitted antenatal diagnosis of achondrogenesis in this case of approximately 19 menstrual weeks. Open arrows indicate shortened humerus, solid black arrows indicate normal calvarial ossification, and solid white arrows indicate absent vertebral ossification that permits visualization of the spinal cord. (Courtesy of Roy A. Filly, M.D., University of California, San Francisco, CA.)

Table 13–12. CLASSIFICATION AND SONOGRAPHIC FEATURES OF OSTEOGENESIS IMPERFECTA

| Type | Usual Inheritance Pattern | Typical Prenatal Sonographic Features | | | Usual Outcome |
		Bone Shortening	Fractures	Bone Echogenicity	
I	Autosomal dominant	No	Isolated in 5% of cases; otherwise none	Normal	Good; deafness in 35%
IIA	Autosomal dominant; many new mutations	Severe	Innumerable	± Decreased	Fatal
IIB	Autosomal recessive	Moderate of femur only	Numerous	Normal	Fatal
IIC	Autosomal recessive	Moderate of all extremity bones	Numerous	Normal	Fatal
III	Autosomal recessive	Moderate of femur only	Numerous	± Decreased	Severe handicaps
IV	Autosomal dominant	No	Occasional, isolated	Normal	Good

From Mahony BS: The extremities. In Nyberg DA, Mahony BS, Pretorius DH (eds): Diagnostic Ultrasound of Fetal Anomalies: Text and Atlas. Chicago, Mosby-Year Book, 1990.

IIB.[65] Furthermore, the distinction between type IIB and type III is also quite subtle.

The classic sonographic features of type IIA osteogenesis imperfecta include the following:

1. Severe micromelia with deformity secondary to fractures (discontinuity of the bone, sharp angulation or bowing) and apparent thickening of the limb bones, secondary to numerous fractures with the exuberant callus formation typical of this disorder (Figs. 13–16 and 13–17)

2. Hypomineralization of bone, especially of the calvarium, characterized by decreased echogenicity of the skeleton with abnormally increased through-transmission of the ultrasound beam through the skeleton. Skull hypomineralization permits abnormally clear visualization of the brain and ventricular system because of the absence of reverberation artifact and may lead to the impression of "pseudohydrocephalus." The calvarium may also be abnormally compressible (Fig. 13–18). Isolated bones may exhibit normal mineralization.

3. Multiple rib fractures with collapse of the thoracic cage (Fig. 13–19)

4. Platyspondyly may also be seen with osteogenesis

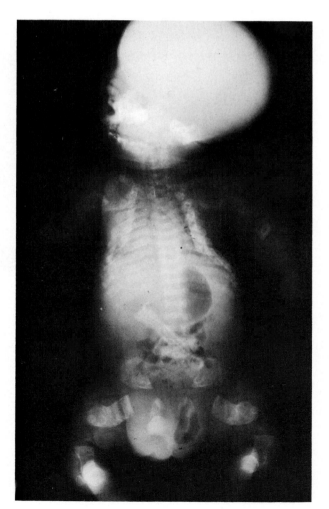

Figure 13–15. Postmortem radiograph of infant with osteogenesis imperfecta type IIA demonstrates the innumerable fractures with limb shortening ("accordian effect") and angulation. Also note the concavity of the thorax and irregular contour of the ribs secondary to the numerous fractures.

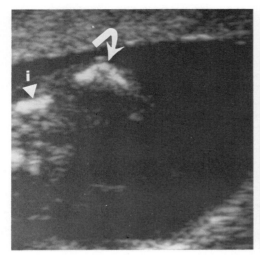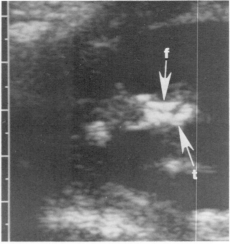

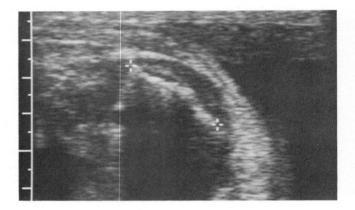

Figure 13–16. A and B. Even at approximately 14 menstrual weeks, acute angulation of the femur and tibia may indicate fractures of recurrent homozygous recessive osteogenesis imperfecta (type II). Curved arrow indicates femur. t, tibia; f, fibula; i, iliac wing.

Figure 13–17. The innumerable bone fractures with exuberant callus formation typical of osteogenesis imperfecta type IIA later in gestation tend to give the shortened femur (cursors) a thickened, irregular appearance.

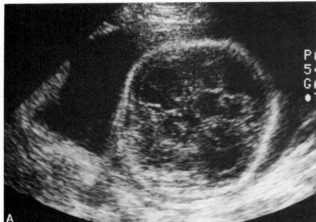

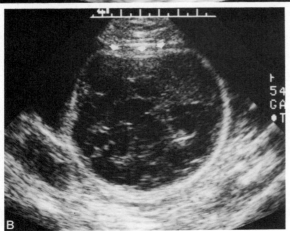

Figure 13–18. Poor calvarial mineralization in osteogenesis imperfecta type IIA can be documented with very gentle compression of the maternal abdomen by the transducer. Without gentle compression (A) the head configuration is slightly rounded but gentle compression of the head with the transducer (B) produces obvious distortion (arrows) of the head configuration.

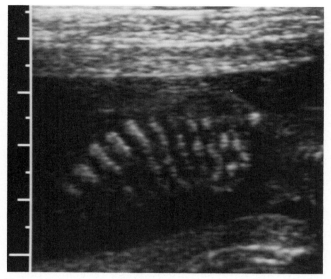

Figure 13–19. Sagittal scan of the thorax in a fetus with osteogenesis imperfecta type IIA shows multiple rib deformities with areas of decreased rib echogenicity indicating poorly ossified bones with multiple fractures.

imperfecta type IIA, but this is an inconsistent finding (Fig. 13–20). In a retrospective review, Munoz and associates distinguished osteogenesis imperfecta type II from other fetal skeletal abnormalities on the basis of micromelia, extremity fractures, and demineralization of the calvaria.[71] Among eight fetuses with osteogenesis imperfecta type II, all had micromelia, extremity fractures (one had isolated femoral fractures), and calvarial hypomineralization (detected in one only following postnatal radiograph). In this series, a normal sonogram after 17 menstrual weeks excluded osteogenesis imperfecta type II.

Other Lethal Short-Limbed Dwarf Syndromes

Prenatal ultrasonography can also detect a variety of other rare lethal short-limbed dwarf syndromes. In the absence of familial risk, sonographic features of these syndromes often would be expected to be detectable but probably not distinctive enough in most cases to permit a specific prenatal diagnosis.

CAMPOMELIC DYSPLASIA

Campomelic dysplasia occurs with a frequency of approximately 1 in 150,000 births. Like many other skeletal dysplasias, it probably includes a heterogeneous group of disorders, with some cases being more severely affected than others.[13, 72] Campomelic dysplasia has been considered to be uniformly fatal, but in a review of 97 reported cases Houston and coworkers described six patients who survived beyond 1 month of age and three who were documented to be alive beyond 1 year with one patient alive at 17 years.[72] The nonsurvivors tended to have more severe manifestations of the syndrome than the survivors.

The features of campomelic ("bent bone") dysplasia include ventral bowing of shortened tibia and femora with severe talipes equinovarus, absent or hypoplastic fibulae, extremely small scapulae, narrow thorax, and hypoplastic pedicles of the thoracic vertebrae.[3, 12, 13, 72, 73] The bowing of the tibiae and femora probably results from a primary shortness of the calf and hamstring musculature, which, in turn, leads to the talipes equinovarus deformity.[72, 74] Affected fetuses also frequently have cerebroventricular dilation, cleft palate, congenital heart disease, midthoracic scoliosis, and pelvocaliectasis but die of complications from laryngotracheomalacia.[72]

CHONDRODYSPLASIA PUNCTATA— RHIZOMELIC TYPE

The rhizomelic type of chondrodysplasia punctata is usually inherited in an autosomal recessive manner.[13, 75, 76] It occurs in approximately 1 in 110,000 births and results in neonatal death or severe mental retardation with death in early childhood.[5]

In a fetus at risk for recurrence of the rhizomelic form of chondrodysplasia punctata, certain features may manifest on the prenatal sonogram and permit confident antenatal diagnosis.[3, 12, 13] This dysplasia results in severe micromelia, especially of the humeri but also of the femora, with multiple joint contractures. In the absence of familial risk, the severity of the symmetric rhizomelic shortening may help to distinguish this entity from others with less severe rhizomelia and a variable prognosis (i.e., heterozygous achondroplasia and asphyxiating thoracic dystrophy). Late in the third trimester the characteristic stippling of the humeral and femoral cartilaginous epiphyses may be visible and

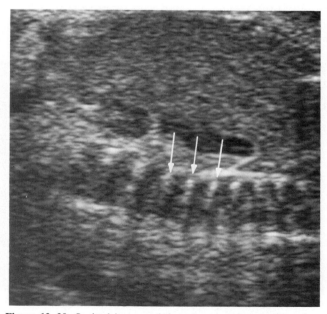

Figure 13–20. Sagittal images of the spine may demonstrate platyspondyly *(arrows)* in osteogenesis imperfecta type IIA. This is an inconsistent finding in osteogenesis imperfecta type II, more commonly seen with thanatophoric dysplasia. (Courtesy of Peter W. Callen, M.D., University of California, San Francisco, CA.)

enable confident prenatal diagnosis, although epiphyseal stippling is not present in all cases (Fig. 13–21).[76, 77] The vertebral bodies in chondrodysplasia punctata (rhizomelic type) are reported to have distinctive ventral and dorsal ossification centers separated by a bar of cartilage.[12]

CONGENITAL HYPOPHOSPHATASIA

Congenital (lethal) hypophosphatasia occurs with an incidence of approximately 1 in 100,000 births and recurs in an autosomal recessive manner probably with more than one allele.[78, 79] It is characterized by abnormal bone mineralization with a deficiency of alkaline phosphatase.[78, 80, 81]

The sonographic features of congenital hypophosphatasia include moderate to severe micromelia and diffuse hypomineralization, the degree of which may resemble that in osteogenesis imperfecta IIA. However, in contrast to the thickened bones of osteogenesis imperfecta IIA, the extremity bones in congenital hypophosphatasia tend to be delicate or may even be absent.[82] De Lange and Rouse reported a case of congenital hypophosphatasia without a family history of the condition diagnosed based on the prenatal sonographic findings of micromelia, generalized underossification, and absent ossification of the hands, spinal neural arches, and groups of vertebral bodies (Fig. 13–22).[83]

HOMOZYGOUS DOMINANT ACHONDROPLASIA

This rare lethal dysplasia may manifest many of the same features as thanatophoric dysplasia, including severe micromelia and cloverleaf skull.[84] Since it occurs only in the setting of at least one parent (and usually both parents) being affected with heterozygous achondroplasia, homozygous achondroplasia is rare and should be readily distinguishable from thanatophoric dysplasia.[84, 85] The micromelia of homozygous achondroplasia may occur earlier in gestation and to a more severe degree than with heterozygous achondroplasia, although the prenatal features of this dysplasia are not known with certainty because of the paucity of reported cases. One case seen at approximately 18 weeks already had micromelia,[85] but I followed an affected fetus who had normal femur length until 21 menstrual weeks followed by virtual absence of subsequent femoral growth (Fig. 13–23).

SHORT-RIB POLYDACTYLY SYNDROME

This rare and lethal skeletal dysplasia with several different types is probably inherited in an autosomal recessive manner. Characteristic features include micromelia, short ribs with a narrow thorax, and polydactyly with frequent cardiovascular or genitourinary anomalies, especially cystic renal dysplasia. Three different types have been recognized with additional variants.[86] The distinguishing features among the three types are as follows: the Saldino-Noonan type has narrow metaphyses; the Majewski type has cleft lip/cleft palate and disproportionately shortened tibiae; and the Naumoff type has wide metaphyses with spurs.

These distinctions, although real, are of little clinical utility to the sonographer since in most cases a positive family history will signal a careful search for recurrence. In the absence of familial risk, the features may not be sufficiently distinctive to permit distinction among the types of the syndrome. Nevertheless, the severity and distribution of abnormalities help to distinguish the short-rib polydactyly syndrome from other entities. For example, the micromelia and narrow chest resemble thanatophoric dysplasia but polydactyly is not a feature of thanatophoric dwarfism. On the other hand, chondroectodermal dysplasia exhibits limb shortening, a small thorax, and polydactyly, but the degree

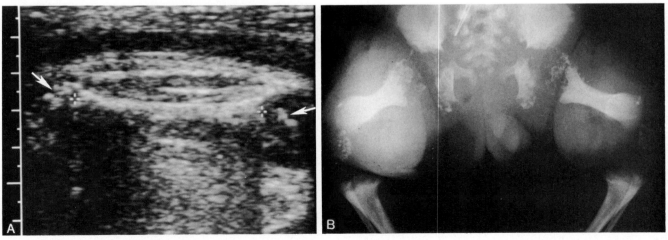

Figure 13–21. *A.* Longitudinal scan of the femur in a fetus with the rhizomelic form of chondrodysplasia punctata at 37 menstrual weeks shows stippled calcification within the epiphyseal cartilages *(arrows)*. The femoral length *(cursors)* was mean for 27 weeks. The humeral length was mean for 20 weeks, and the humeri also showed similar epiphyseal findings. Other extremity bone lengths were normal. *B.* The postnatal radiograph confirms the prenatal findings. (From Mahony BS: The extremities. In Nyberg DA, Mahony BS, Pretorius DH [eds]: Diagnostic Ultrasound of Fetal Anomalies: Text and Atlas. Chicago, Mosby-Year Book, 1990.)

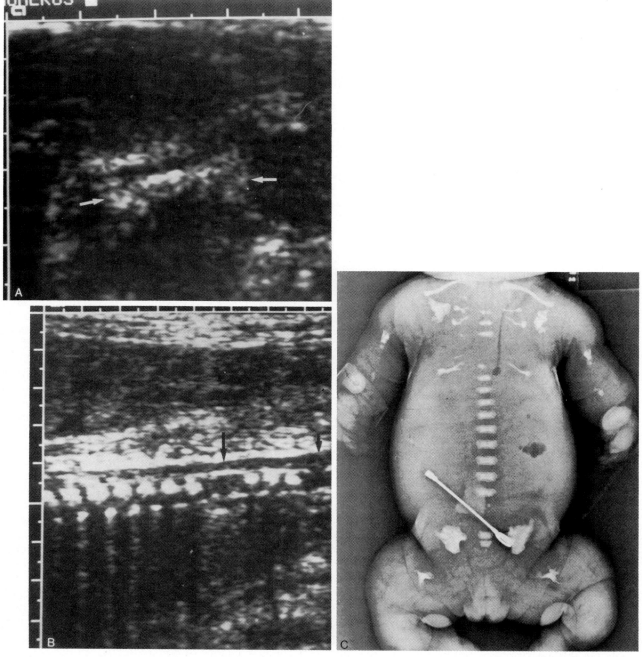

Figure 13–22. *A* through *C.* This fetus with congenital hypophosphatasia at 27 weeks' gestation shows poor ossification of shortened extremity bones and unossified thoracic vertebral bodies *(black arrows)* confirmed with postnatal radiograph. White arrows indicate humerus. (From DeLange M, Rouse GA: Prenatal diagnosis of hypophosphatasia. J Ultrasound Med 9:115, 1990.)

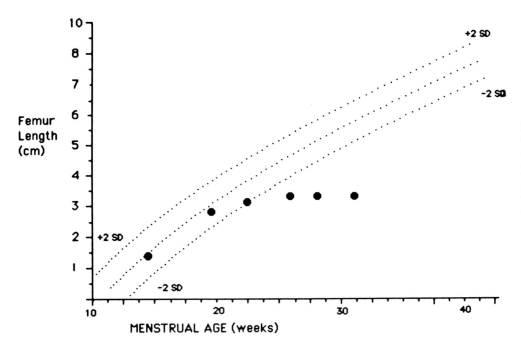

Figure 13–23. Graph correlating the femur length with menstrual age in a fetus with homozygous achondroplasia. The femur length was normal until approximately 21 menstrual weeks, after which time the femur length remained unchanged.

of involvement is much less severe than in short-rib polydactyly syndrome. Similarly, asphyxiating thoracic dysplasia may resemble chondroectodermal dysplasia but the limb shortening is only mild to moderate and occurs in only 60% of cases and polydactyly occurs in only 14% of cases.

DYSPLASIAS WITH A VARIABLE OR GOOD PROGNOSIS

The dysplasias with a variable or good prognosis (or at least one that is not almost uniformly fatal in early infancy) tend to present later in gestation and with milder features than the uniformly fatal syndromes. The sensitivity and specificity of sonography for detection of many of the nonlethal dysplasias would be expected to be less than for the lethal dysplasias, especially in the absence of familial risk and before 24 weeks when many parents request accurate diagnosis. Far fewer reports of sonographic detection of nonlethal dysplasias exist than of lethal dysplasias.

Heterozygous Achondroplasia

Heterozygous achondroplasia, which occurs in approximately 1 in 30,000 births, results in retardation of endochondral bone formation but normal life span and mentation.[5, 8, 12, 48] Approximately 80% of cases result from a spontaneous mutation, with the remainder being inherited in an autosomal dominant mode.[13] The cardinal signs of heterozygous achondroplasia postnatally include moderate rhizomelic shortening, a large calvarium but small skull base and saddle-nose deformity, thoracolumbar kyphosis with lack of normal increase in interpedicular distance caudally, squared-off iliac wings, and relatively short proximal and middle phalanges (trident hands).[3, 12, 13]

Reports of prenatal detection of heterozygous achondroplasia concentrate on the discrepancy between head size and femur length.[47, 48] This discrepancy becomes progressively more apparent during the third trimester (Fig. 13–24). Among affected fetuses scanned because one parent is affected by heterozygous achondroplasia, the fetal femur lengths become progressively more disproportionately shortened relative to the biparietal diameter during the third trimester. Affected fetuses have a normal femur length relative to biparietal diameter during the second trimester, but the femur length falls below the 99% confidence limit for a biparietal diameter corresponding to approximately 27 weeks. This progressive discrepancy during the third trimester presumably results from a combination of less than anticipated femoral growth and relative head enlargement. The absence of this discrepant growth pattern helps to exclude recurrence, but one cannot exclude heterozygous achondroplasia on the basis of a normal femur length before approximately 27 weeks.[47, 48]

In the absence of an affected parent with heterozygous achondroplasia, on the other hand, fetuses without heterozygous achondroplasia may show this same growth pattern. Therefore, although the correlation between biparietal diameter and femur length provides reliable evidence for the presence or absence of recurrent heterozygous achondroplasia when the fetus carries a 50% chance of being affected, in the absence of this recurrence risk I caution against the relative lack of specificity of the biparietal diameter/femur length graph.

Asphyxiating Thoracic Dysplasia

Asphyxiating thoracic dysplasia occurs with a prevalence of approximately 1 in 70,000 births and recurs by autosomal recessive transmission, but the phenotype manifests with variable expressivity.[5, 12, 13] Consequently, the clinical manifestations vary widely from perinatal death from respiratory failure to latent phenotypes without respiratory symptoms and a good prognosis.[13] The characteristic features include mild-to-moderate rhizomelic limb shortening, small thorax, and renal dysplasia.[12, 13] Approximately 14% of patients also have polydactyly. In cases with a positive family history, the 25% recurrence risk alerts the sonologist to search for these features. The growth pattern may mimic that of heterozygous achondroplasia.

Although the key factor leading to the diagnosis of asphyxiating thoracic dysplasia may be an abnormally small thorax, this feature often does not help distinguish asphyxiating thoracic dysplasia from other entities since many of the patients with osteochondrodysplasia (and all those reported in one series) had a small thorax.[52, 87] Nevertheless, it may be a helpful sign to search for and, when unmistakably severe, helps to predict a poor prognosis secondary to pulmonary hypoplasia.

Chondroectodermal Dysplasia

Chondroectodermal dysplasia (Ellis-van Creveld syndrome) occurs in approximately 1 in 200,000 births with a high prevalence among an Amish community. It recurs as an autosomal recessive trait.[5, 11] It closely resembles asphyxiating thoracic dysplasia except that almost all patients with chondroectodermal dysplasia have polydactyly.[88, 89] The manifestations of chondroectodermal dysplasia are much less severe than in the short-rib polydactyly syndrome and correspond with its better prognosis.[86] The predominant features of chondroectodermal dysplasia include mild-to-moderate limb shortening and postaxial polydactyly. Approximately 50% of patients also have congenital heart disease, mainly atrial septal defect.[13]

Diastrophic Dysplasia

Diastrophic ("distorted") dysplasia is a rare autosomal recessive disorder with variable expression of phenotype, ranging from mild to severe.[90–92] Severely affected patients typically have micromelia, talipes, cleft palate, extension limitation of the elbows and hips, flexion limitations of finger joints (resulting in the characteristic fixed lateral positioning of the thumb, termed the *hitchhiker thumb*), progressive scoliosis, and micrognathia.[11, 13, 92] Diastrophic dysplasia causes increased infant mortality, but affected cases who survive infancy have normal intellectual development and a normal expected life span if the progressive kyphoscoliosis does not compromise cardiac and pulmonary function.[12, 92] For this reason, diastrophic dysplasia is included here among dysplasias with a variable prognosis, recognizing that the general rule holds that severe manifestations of dysplasia signify a poor prognosis, even in syndromes with variable phenotypes.

Osteogenesis Imperfecta, Types I and IV

Type I osteogenesis imperfecta, which occurs in approximately 1 in 28,500 births, is probably the most

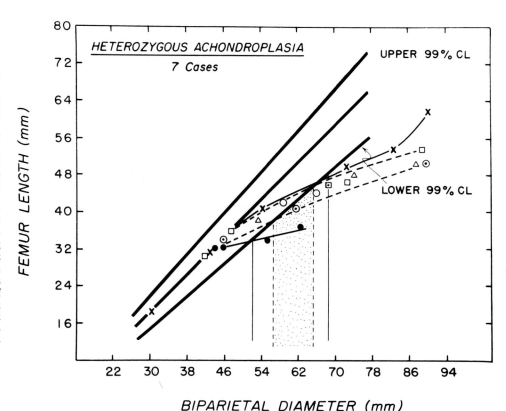

Figure 13–24. This graph compares the femur length and biparietal diameter in seven cases of recurrent heterozygous achondroplasia and demonstrates the characteristic progressive shortening of the femur length relative to the biparietal diameter during the second and third trimesters. The femur length falls below the 99% confidence limit (CL) by the time the biparietal diameter corresponds with approximately 27 menstrual weeks. The symbols on the graph indicate individual cases seen at advancing stages of gestation. (From Kurtz AB, Filly RA, Wapner RJ, et al: In utero analysis of heterozygous achondroplasia: Variable time of onset as detected by femur length measurements. J Ultrasound Med 5:137, 1986. Copyright 1986, American Institute of Ultrasound in Medicine.)

common type of osteogenesis imperfecta, although affected fetuses have overall normal limb lengths and only approximately 5% of neonates have a bone fracture at birth.[65] Therefore, it is only rarely detected prenatally (Fig. 13–25). Since it recurs by autosomal dominant transmission and only rarely by spontaneous mutation, most affected cases of this type will have an affected parent. Extremity bone bowing with fracture and diminished echogenicity may occur late in gestation.[93, 94] Type IV osteogenesis imperfecta resembles type I except it does not produce deafness or blue sclerae. Vaginal delivery of a fetus with nonlethal osteogenesis imperfecta has been reported with only minimal fetal morbidity attributable to the mode of delivery.[94]

Other Rare Dysplasias

The Second International Nomenclature of Constitutional Diseases of Bone also lists numerous other rare defects of growth of tubular bones and/or spine identifiable at birth and, therefore, potentially detectable at least in the latter stages of gestation (Fig. 13–26).[10] Prenatal ultrasound evaluation rarely detects any of these, and the sonographic features may be very subtle.[95–97]

FOCAL LIMB LOSS OR ABNORMALITY

Entities that manifest on the prenatal sonogram as focal absence of an extremity bone, segment, or entire limb or as fusion of the limbs include radial ray defects, the amniotic band sequence, the limb–body wall complex, Roberts syndrome, proximal focal femoral deficiency, and sirenomelia. These disorders do not represent bone dysplasias.

Radial Ray Defects

A wide variety of disorders may result in aplasia or hypoplasia of the radius and thumb, including (but not limited to) the VACTERL association (*v*ertebral defects, *a*nal atresia, *c*ardiac defects, *t*racheo*e*sophageal atresia, and *r*enal and *l*imb anomalies), trisomy 18 and trisomy 13, the Holt-Oram syndrome, thrombocytopenia–absent radius syndrome, Fanconi syndrome, and de Lange syndrome.[3, 11, 13] The characteristic sonographic features of a radial ray defect are sharp radial deviation of the hand and absence of visualization of the distal radius at the same level as the ulna. In contrast to other conditions characterized by radial absence, in thrombocytopenia–absent radius syndrome the thumb is always present (Fig. 13–27).[98] The ulna

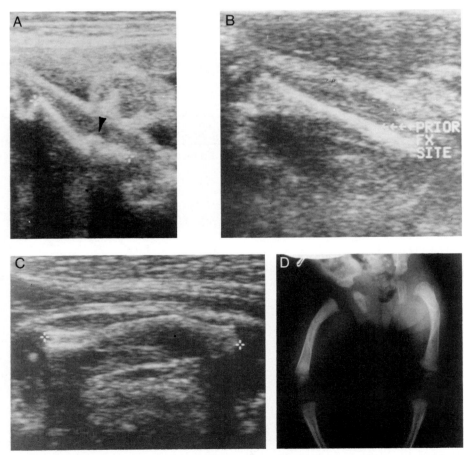

Figure 13–25. This fetus with osteogenesis imperfecta, type I (the autosomal dominant form with blue sclerae) has normal extremity bone lengths. At 29 menstrual weeks, however, a left tibial fracture *(A)* with some callus formation is evident *(arrowhead)*. Nineteen days later, the left tibial fracture has healed *(B)*, but the femur angulates *(C)* at the junction of its proximal and middle thirds, indicative of fracture deformity. A postnatal radiograph *(D)* confirms the antenatal findings.

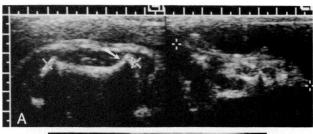

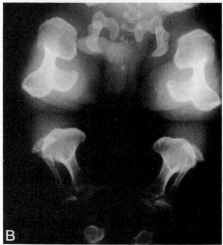

Figure 13–26. *A.* Dual-image scan of a fetus with metatropic dwarfism at term shows a short femur (left portion of scan) measuring only 45 mm in length (mean for 24.5 weeks). Other extremity long bones were also proportionately short. However, the foot length of 75 mm (right portion of scan) was near mean for term. Therefore, the femur length–foot length ratio was abnormally decreased at 60%. The femoral metaphyses flare markedly *(arrow). B.* Postnatal radiograph confirms the lower-extremity findings. (From Mahony BS: The extremities. In Nyberg DA, Mahony BS, Pretorius DH [eds]: Diagnostic Ultrasound of Fetal Anomalies: Text and Atlas. Chicago, Mosby-Year Book, 1990.)

and humerus may also be shortened or absent, in which case the five-fingered hand attaches at the shoulder.

In the absence of familial risk for a radial ray defect, most cases detected prenatally will probably have concomitant and more obvious anomalies that signal a careful search for an extremity abnormality.[99–101] However, serendipitous detection of a radial ray defect probably warrants search for other manifestations of the VACTERL association and chromosomal analysis. Detection during the third trimester probably justifies fetal umbilical blood sampling to assess platelet count.

Amniotic Band Sequence and Limb–Body Wall Complex

The amniotic band sequence and the limb–body wall complex often produce variable but frequently striking abnormalities of the fetal musculoskeletal system. The amniotic band sequence occurs sporadically with an incidence of as high as 1 in 1200 births and 1 in 56 spontaneous abortions.[102–104] Most authors ascribe to the hypothesis elucidated by Torpin, who asserted that rupture of the amnion leads to transient oligohydramnios and subsequent entanglement of embryonic or fetal tissue by fibrous bands emanating from the chorionic side of the amnion (Fig. 13–28).[105] Depending on the time of rupture and the distribution and the orientation of the bands slashing across the developing fetus, deformities occur ranging from subtle amputation or lymphedema to amputation of large portions of the fetus. Following disruption of the amnion, the

fetus may adhere to and fuse with the chorion, producing maldevelopment of the subjacent fetal tissue.

The amniotic band sequence causes variable patterns of fetal deformity but a propensity for certain anomalies, including extremity amputation, lymphedema or constriction rings, facial clefts in bizarre and nonembryologic distributions, large abdominal wall or chest wall defects, and encephaloceles occurring in locations other than the midline.[105, 106]

Extremity amputations may result from teratogenic or genetic causes, but several distinguishing features help identify amputations related to the amniotic band sequence from those related to teratogenic or genetic causes (Fig. 13–29).[105, 106] Constriction ring defects occur in most, if not all, unequivocal examples of the amniotic band sequence (Fig. 13–30).[104, 107] Identification of a band of tissue within a constriction ring with distal lymphedema or protrusion of uncovered bone distal to the soft tissue at the site of an amputation constitutes convincing evidence for the amniotic band sequence. In addition, amputations resulting from this sequence typically occur asymmetrically, unlike the characteristic bilaterally symmetric genetic or teratogenic amputations (Fig. 13–31).

Among reported cases of the amniotic band sequence detected sonographically between 16 and 31 weeks, commonly detected abnormalities included extremity anomalies (50% to 60%), asymmetric encephalocele or discordant anencephaly (45%), large body wall defects, (40%), amniotic bands (40%), and facial cleft (22%).

The limb–body wall complex occurs sporadically, with an incidence of approximately 1 in 4000 births.[108]

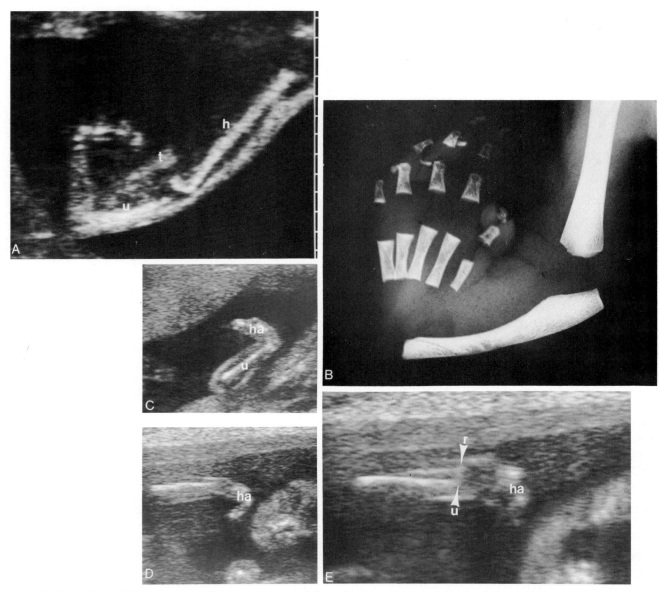

Figure 13–27. *A.* Scan of the upper extremity shows absence of the radius but presence of the thumb in this fetus with thrombocytopenia and absent radius syndrome. *B.* The postnatal radiograph confirms the prenatal findings. *C* through *E.* Another fetus held its hand flexed at the wrist throughout the examination. Although the positioning suggested radial ray anomaly, identification of the distal radius and ulna extending to the same level at the wrist excluded a radial ray anomaly. u, ulna; r, radius; h, humerus; t, thumb; ha, hand. (*A* and *B* from Mahony BS: The extremities. In Nyberg DA, Mahony BS, Pretorius DH [eds]: Diagnostic Ultrasound of Fetal Anomalies: Text and Atlas. Chicago, Mosby-Year Book, 1990.)

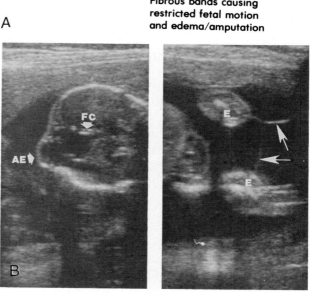

Figure 13–28. *A*. In the amniotic band syndrome, rupture of the amnion causes variable malformations ranging from subtle to severe. The bands may create bizarre slash defects across the face, cause gastropleural schisis, or entangle the extremities, resulting in edema or amputation. *B* and *C*. Adherence of the fetus to the chorion may cause asymmetric encephalocele (AE) and numerous bands *(arrows)* attached to the extremities (E). FC, falx cerebri. (From Mahony BS, Filly RA, Callen PW, Golbus MS: The amniotic band syndrome: Antenatal sonographic diagnosis and potential pitfalls. Am J Obstet Gynecol 152:63, 1985.)

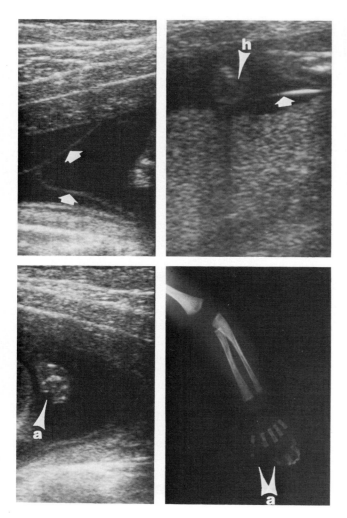

Figure 13–29. In this pregnancy numerous bands *(arrows)* were attached to the fetal extremities and there were subtle amputations (a), indicative of the amniotic band sequence. h, hand.

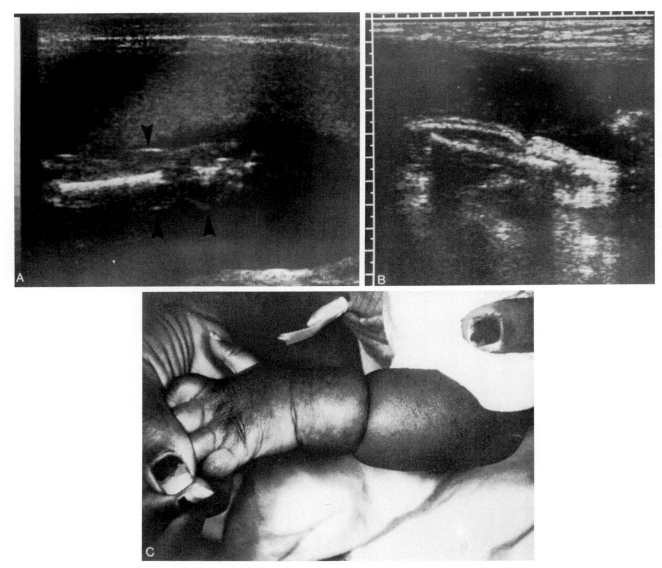

Figure 13–30. Amniotic band causes subcutaneous edema of the hand *(arrowheads)* at 18 menstrual weeks *(A)* and constriction of the forearm at 38 menstrual weeks *(B)* as well as at 6 weeks after birth *(C)*. (From Hill LM, Kislak S, Jones N: Prenatal ultrasound diagnosis of a forearm constriction band. J Ultrasound Med 7:293, 1988.)

This entity produces a similar but invariably severe and lethal set of fetal malformations as the amniotic band sequence and is also characterized by a high incidence of marked scoliosis and defects involving the internal organs (see Fig. 13–31).[109, 110] Van Allen and associates reviewed 25 cases of the limb–body wall complex and found limb abnormalities in 95%, internal organ defects in 95%, marked scoliosis in 77%, thoracoabdominal schisis in 64%, neural tube defects in 60%, and facial clefts in 40%.[108, 109] Only 40% had amniotic bands. The limb deformities detected prenatally have included absent extremities, bilateral clubfeet or positional abnormalities, discrepant femur lengths, and syndactyly.

The etiology of this complex remains uncertain. Some authors assert that it results from rupture of the amnion between the third and fifth weeks of embryogenesis, while others argue that it results from systemic alteration of embryonic blood supply or short umbilical cord.[108–110] The marked scoliosis probably results from decreased or absent paraspinous or thoracolumbar musculature on the same side as the body wall defect.[109]

Roberts Syndrome

The Roberts syndrome and the pseudothalidomide syndrome may represent separate conditions or variations in phenotypic expression of one rare autosomal recessive disorder.[3, 111, 112] Severely affected patients with severe manifestations have the Roberts syndrome with high perinatal mortality, whereas those with significantly less severe phenotype have the pseudothalidomide syndrome and a better prognosis. The characteristic features of the Roberts syndrome include tetraphocomelia, bilateral cleft lip and palate, hypertelorism, microcephaly, and growth retardation. The phocomelia typically involves the upper extremities more severely than the lower limbs and occurs symmetrically (Fig. 13–32). In severe cases, a three-digit hand attaches to the shoulder. Bowing of the legs, flexion contractures, clubfoot, and syndactyly also occur. Cytogenetic findings of amniocytes from affected pregnancies often show characteristic centromeric separation and puffing.[111] The extremity malformations of the Roberts syndrome resemble those of the thalidomide syndrome and the femur-fibula-ulna syndrome.

Proximal Focal Femoral Deficiency

The proximal focal femoral deficiency occurs in approximately 1 in 50,000 births, usually sporadically but with an increased incidence in infants of diabetic mothers. It produces shortening or absence of the femur and has been documented on the basis of an isolated unilateral finding of an abnormally short femur at 32 to 33 weeks.[113, 114]

Sirenomelia

The "mermaid syndrome" of lower extremity fusion, which occurs in approximately 1 in 60,000 births, is a severe manifestation of the caudal regression syndrome.[115] It frequently occurs in the setting of severe oligohydramnios, usually from fatal bilateral renal agenesis or multicystic dysplasia. The lower extremity fusion ranges from a membrane fusing the thighs but separate lower legs to total fusion of the lower legs with one midline femur and fibula (Fig. 13–33).[116] Intermediate between these two extremes is soft tissue fusion with two femora but one midline fibula.

The extreme oligohydramnios with resultant limitation of fetal motion and of extremity visualization limit the sensitivity of sonography in the prenatal detection of sirenomelia.[117–119] However, in the setting of bilateral renal agenesis or multicystic dysplastic kidneys with severe oligohydramnios, demonstration of a single lower extremity or femora consistently held in a side-by-side relationship enables prenatal diagnosis of sirenomelia.

CONTRACTURES AND POSTURAL DEFORMITIES

Normal development of the embryonic and fetal musculoskeletal system requires extremity movement as early as at 7 to 8 menstrual weeks. Absence of normal prenatal joint movement results in extremity contractures or deformity (Fig. 13–34).[120, 121] The four major causes of decreased fetal movement include (1) structural limitation of fetal movement (e.g., oligohydramnios, multiple gestation, extrauterine pregnancy, bicornuate uterus), (2) abnormalities of fetal nerve function or innervation, (3) intrinsic abnormalities of fetal musculature, and (4) defective fetal connective tissue. Terms referring to fetuses with a wide spectrum of heterogeneous disorders characterized by decreased fetal movement include arthrogryposis multiplex congenita, fetal akinesia deformation sequence, pterygium syndromes, and Pena-Shokeir phenotype.

Arthrogryposis multiplex congenita describes a fetus with multiple extremity contractures.[122] The outcome and recurrence risks for arthrogryposis multiplex congenita vary widely dependent on the underlying etiology of the movement disorder as well as on the concomitant anomalies.

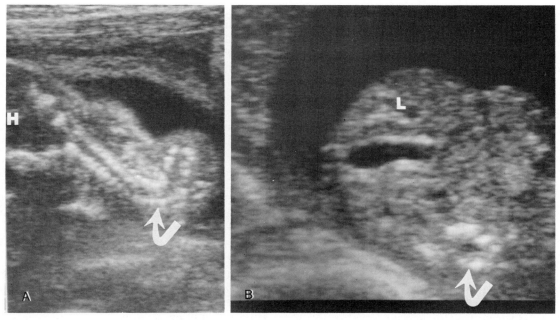

Figure 13–31. Limb–body wall complex probably results from early amnion rupture and produces very severe and lethal malformations, including severe scoliosis *(A)* and gastropleural schisis *(B)*. H, head; arrows, spine; L, liver exteriorized through gastropleural schisis. (Courtesy of Jack H. Hirsch, M.D., Swedish Hospital Medical Center, Seattle, WA.)

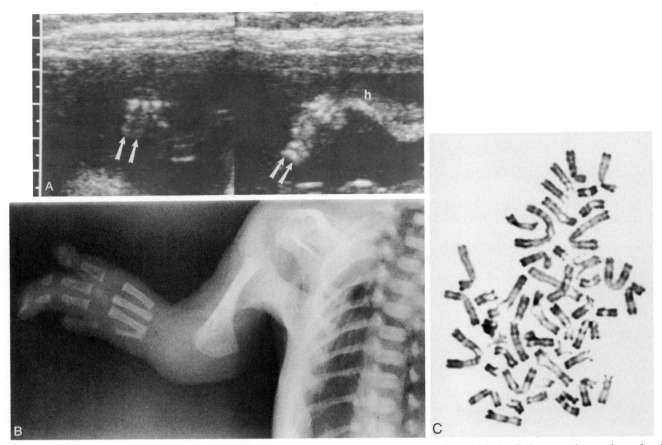

Figure 13–32. *A.* This dual-image scan of the upper extremity at 20 menstrual weeks in a fetus with the Roberts syndrome shows fused fingers *(right portion of the scan)* and absence of the radius and ulna with the hand attached at a right angle to the upper arm *(left portion of the scan)*. Throughout the entire course of the examination two of the fingers *(arrows)* remained fused bilaterally, indicative of syndactyly. Other scans showed shortened tibiae but absent fibulae, mild polyhydramnios, and mild dilatation of the lateral cerebral ventricles. *B.* Postmortem radiograph confirms the prenatal findings. *C.* C-banded chromosomes from cultured fibroblasts postnatally exhibit the extreme centromere separation indicative of the Roberts syndrome. h, humerus. (From Mahony BS: The extremities. In Nyberg DA, Mahony BS, Pretorius DH [eds]: Diagnostic Ultrasound of Fetal Anomalies: Text and Atlas. Chicago, Mosby-Year Book, 1990; chromosomal analysis performed by Children's Hospital Cytogenetics Laboratory, Seattle, WA.)

Abnormalities of any system leading to decreased fetal movement may result in the *fetal akinesia deformation sequence*, characterized by intrauterine growth retardation, micrognathia, depressed nasal tip, limb anomalies, pulmonary hypoplasia, short umbilical cord, and polyhydramnios.[120, 121, 123] Limb anomalies include limitation of joint movement, abnormal shape and position, and deficient bone growth and calcification. Oligohydramnios need not exist to produce the fetal akinesia deformation sequence. For example, paralysis with curare during the latter half of fetal development in an animal model produces this phenotype.[120, 121] These anomalies imply that normal fetal bone growth, ossification, and position require normal extremity function.[123]

Pterygium is a term referring to webbing of the skin across a joint.[124] Limb pterygia at birth signify reduced intrauterine mobility of the webbed joints, probably occurring in the first trimester as a sequela of the fetal akinesia deformation sequence.[120, 124] Numerous limb pterygium syndromes exist of varying severity, prognosis, and inheritance pattern.[124] The popliteal pterygium syndrome is the most common dominantly inher-

ited limb pterygium syndrome, although most cases occur sporadically.[124] Predominant manifestations include cleft lip and palate, popliteal pterygium, syndactyly, and equinovarus foot deformity.

The *Pena-Shokeir phenotype* includes a set of malformations produced by the fetal akinesia deformation sequence and characterized by arthrogryposis multiplex congenita.[123] Approximately 20% of cases also have limb pterygia. Its severe and lethal manifestations include polyhydramnios, intrauterine growth retardation, pulmonary hypoplasia, short umbilical cord, and facial deformities correlating with the phenotype produced by the fetal akinesia deformation sequence.[123] Many patients with the Pena-Shokeir phenotype also have thin, underossified bones that fracture easily.[123] This underscores the important role that normal limb motion plays in development of extremities.

In the absence of familial risk for a specific syndrome that may result in fetal contractures, the sonographic features are not sufficiently distinctive to permit differentiation among a wide variety of syndromes with similar phenotypes. For example, recurrent autosomal dominant distal arthrogryposis produces overriding,

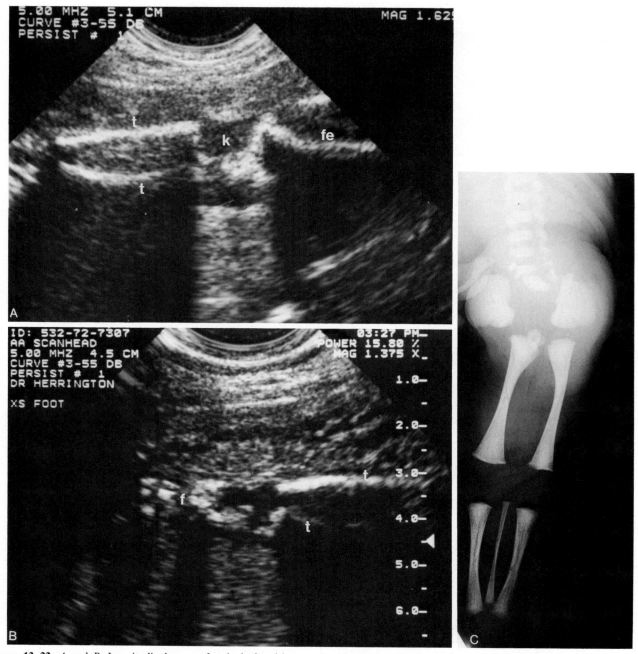

Figure 13–33. *A* and *B*. Longitudinal scans of a single fused lower extremity in sirenomelia shows the single femur (fe) and knee (k) with separate tibiae (t) leading to a single foot (f). *C*. Postmortem radiograph of a different fetus with sirenomelia shows a dysplastic sacrum, two femora and tibiae but a single midline fibula and soft tissue fusion. This breech fetus had anhydramnios and bilateral multicystic dysplastic kidneys at 27 weeks. These limitations precluded prenatal visualization of sirenomelia. (From Mahony BS: The extremities. In Nyberg DA, Mahony BS, Pretorius DH [eds]: Diagnostic Ultrasound of Fetal Anomalies: Text and Atlas. Chicago, Mosby-Year Book, 1990.)

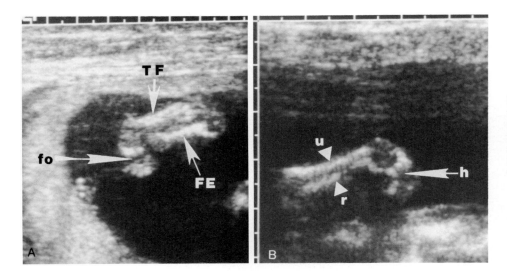

Figure 13–34. *A* and *B*. This fetus with arthrogryposis multiplex had multiple joint contractures. It remained motionless and contorted during the examination. FE, femur; TF, tibia and fibula; fo, foot; r, radius; u, ulna; h, hand.

clenched fingers, but overriding fingers may also occur in a variety of other entities, including trisomy 13 or trisomy 18.[11, 13, 125–130] Nevertheless, prenatal sonography can detect fetuses with extremity contractures, especially in the setting of familial risk. In the absence of familial risk, the accuracy of prenatal sonography in detection of these fetuses may be much lower, especially if the manifestations are subtle.

HAND AND FOOT DEFORMITIES

Prenatal sonography can detect numerous deformities of the hands and feet, especially during a targeted examination of these structures because of familial risk for deformity or based on identification of concomitant anomalies.[6] In the absence of these predisposing factors, the yield for screening ultrasound evaluation of the hands and feet would be expected to be low.

Clubfoot (Talipes)

Talipes occurs in approximately 1 in 250 to 1000 births, often as a component of a syndrome characterized by multiple other congenital anomalies, especially those resulting from the fetal akinesia deformation sequence. It may occasionally occur as an isolated entity.[131–133] In most cases of talipes the foot is plantarflexed and inverted (talipes equinovarus), but a variety of other talipes deformities may occur (Fig. 13–35).[134]

The sonographic features of talipes depend on the type of deformity, but the diagnosis can be made as early as 13 menstrual weeks.[135] In talipes equinovarus the foot deviates medially at the ankle and remains fixed at a right angle to the distal tibia and fibula. This causes the long axis of the foot to reside in the same longitudinal plane of section as the tibia and fibula. Normally in this plane of section the ankle and foot are seen in short axis (Figs. 13–36 and 13–37).[133, 136] The sonologist should exercise caution in making the

diagnosis of isolated clubfoot since the fetus may hold the foot in a position suggesting talipes in the absence of structural deformity at birth.[133]

Clinodactyly and Overlapping Digits

A variety of syndromes may result in contractures of the hands and feet and produce abnormally fisted or overlapping digits (clinodactyly). Although detection of overlapping digits or clinodactyly may suggest the presence of trisomy 13, 18, or 21, it is not pathognomonic for a chromosomal aberration, and other more obvious anomalies typically dominate the sonographic picture in these syndromes (Fig. 13–38).[137–139] Subtle phalangeal hypoplasias have been detected when specifically sought based on a known genetic risk, but routine search for these deformities would be exceedingly time consuming and nonproductive (Figs. 13–39 through 13–41).[139]

Polydactyly and Syndactyly

Diligent search for polydactyly or syndactyly may assist in narrowing the differential diagnosis in a variety of syndromes. For example, detection of polydactyly in a fetus with micromelia and a small thorax implies the short-rib polydactyly syndrome rather than thanatophoric dysplasia. In a fetus with moderate limb shortening and a small thorax, the polydactyly suggests chondroectodermal dysplasia instead of asphyxiating thoracic dysplasia. Detection of polydactyly alerts the sonologist to search for other findings and may assist in suggesting chromosome abnormality (see Fig. 13–38).

Syndactyly may be suspected when the digits remain persistently together, but syndactyly occurring as an isolated anomaly would be expected to be very difficult to confirm (see Fig. 13–32). One can exclude the presence of syndactyly only if the fetus splays open the digits or interdigitates the fingers.

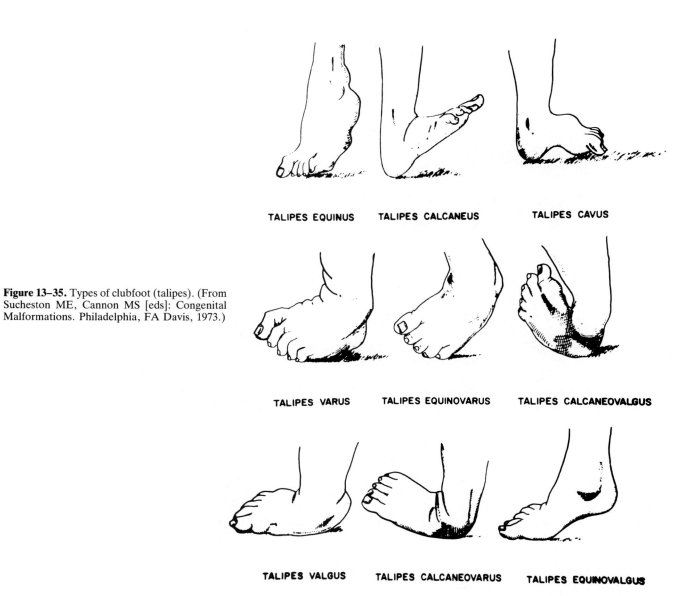

Figure 13–35. Types of clubfoot (talipes). (From Sucheston ME, Cannon MS [eds]: Congenital Malformations. Philadelphia, FA Davis, 1973.)

TALIPES EQUINUS   TALIPES CALCANEUS   TALIPES CAVUS

TALIPES VARUS   TALIPES EQUINOVARUS   TALIPES CALCANEOVALGUS

TALIPES VALGUS   TALIPES CALCANEOVARUS   TALIPES EQUINOVALGUS

A   B

Figure 13–36. *A.* Sagittal drawing of the lower leg and foot shows the normal relationships. *B.* Coronal drawing of the lower leg shows the abnormal relationships of talipes in which the metatarsals are visible in the same plane of section as the tibia and fibula but orient roughly perpendicularly to these two long bones. (From Jeanty P, Romero R, D'Alton M, et al: In utero sonographic detection of hand and foot deformities. J Ultrasound Med 4:595, 1985.)

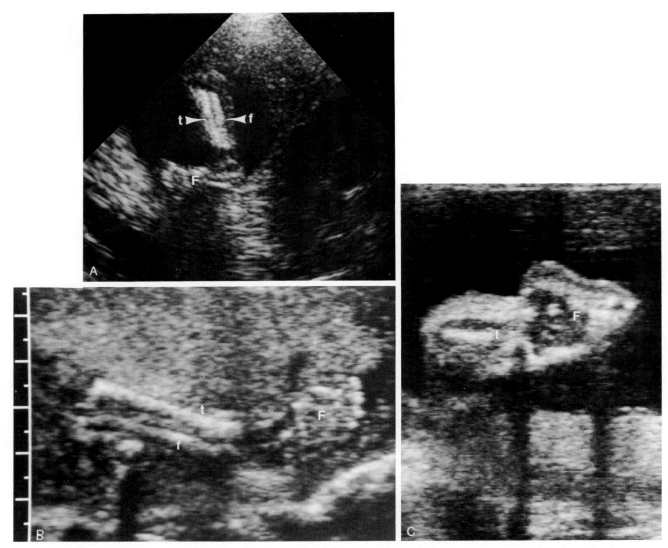

Figure 13–37. *A* and *B.* In talipes equinovarus the foot deviates medially at the ankle such that the frontal image of the lower leg demonstrates the tibia and fibula simultaneously with the long axis of the foot. *C.* In talipes equinus, however, the foot remains pointed but not medially deviated throughout the examination. Note that the amniotic fluid volume in *A* and *C* is not decreased. F, foot; t, tibia; f, fibula.

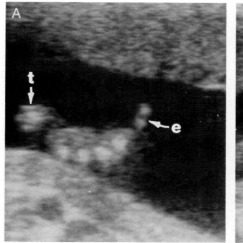

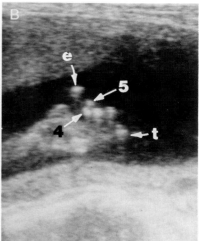

Figure 13–38. Transverse scan *(A)* through the hand, at the level of the metacarpals, demonstrates a supernumerary digit. This antenatal sonogram *(B)* and corresponding postnatal radiograph *(C)* show polydactyly and overlapping of the fifth (5) over the fourth (4) digit. On this basis, given the presence of holoprosencephaly, the correct antenatal sonographic diagnosis of trisomy 13 was made. t, thumb; e, supernumerary digit.

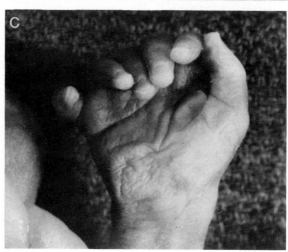

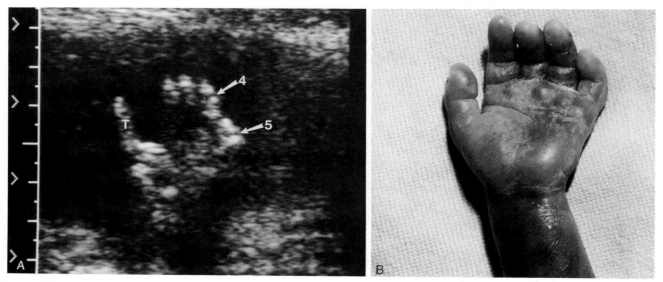

Figure 13–39. *A* and *B*. The fifth finger abnormally curves toward the fourth finger and is relatively short. This fetus also had abnormal nuchal thickening and echogenic bowel, and the karyotype confirmed the presence of trisomy 21. 5, fifth finger; 4, fourth finger; T, thumb.

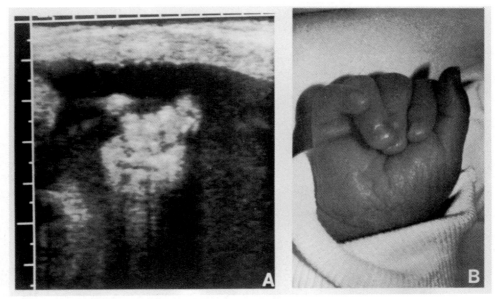

Figure 13–40. *A.* Sonogram of the right hand at 29 weeks shows persistent fisting of the hand with overriding fingers in this fetus with distal arthrogryposis type I. The overlapping fingers closely resemble the hand positioning frequently seen in trisomy 13. *B.* Postnatal photograph at 37 weeks confirms the prenatal findings. (From Baty BJ, Cubberley D, Morris C, et al: Prenatal diagnosis of distal arthrogryposis. Am J Med Genet 29:501–510, 1988. Copyright © 1988. Reprinted by permission of Wiley-Liss, a division of John Wiley & Sons, Inc.)

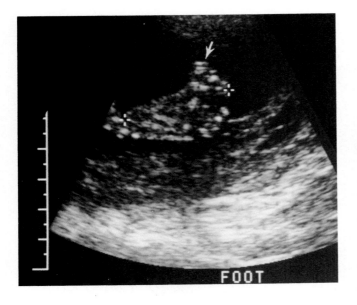

Figure 13–41. Fetal survey at 22 weeks detected polydactyly *(arrow)* of the foot as an isolated and unexpected finding. Cursors show foot length.

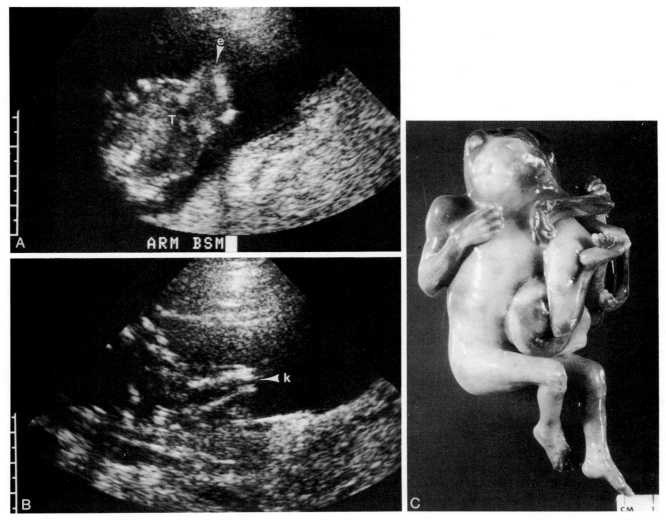

Figure 13–42. *A* and *B*. Sonograms of a fetus with anencephaly revealed an omphalocele and additional flexed arms and legs extending from the left thorax (T) indicative of a bizarre form of conjoined twins. *C.* Postnatal photograph confirms the prenatal findings. e, elbow of extra arm; k, knee of extra leg.

EXTREMITY ENLARGEMENT

Enlargement of an extremity usually represents a manifestation of readily apparent concomitant deformities, such as edema from hydrops fetalis or constriction bands with distal lymphedema from the amniotic band syndrome.[107] Prenatal detection of other causes for extremity enlargement are uncommon and include cutaneous hemangioma, asymmetric limb hypertrophy with the Klippel-Trenaunay-Weber syndrome, and unmistakably long extremity bones in a fetus with 50% risk for having Marfan syndrome, an autosomal dominant disorder.[140–142] Detection of unilateral limb enlargement may imply the presence of the Beckwith-Wiedemann syndrome, especially if a familial risk for the disorder exists and there is concomitant polyhydramnios, visceromegaly, macroglossia, and large for dates measurements. Detection of an accessory extremity is also unusual but indicates strong evidence for conjoined twinning (Fig. 13–42).

References

1. Mahony BS: The extremities. In Nyberg DA, Mahony BS, Pretorius DH (eds): Diagnostic Ultrasound of Fetal Anomalies: Text and Atlas, pp 492–562. Chicago, Year Book Medical Publishers, 1990.
2. Buyse ML (ed): Birth Defects Encyclopedia. Dover, MA, Blackwell Scientific, 1990.
3. Bergsma D (ed): Birth Defects Compendium, 2nd ed. New York, Alan R. Liss, 1979.
4. Poznanski AK: Bone dysplasias: Not so rare, definitely important. AJR 142:427, 1984.
5. Camera G, Mastroiacovo P: Birth prevalence of skeletal dysplasias in the Italian multicentric monitoring system for birth defects. In Papadatos CJ, Bartsocas CS (eds): Skeletal Dysplasias, pp 441–449. New York, Alan R. Liss, 1982.
6. Hegge FN, Prescott GH, Watson PT: Utility of a screening examination of the fetal extremities during obstetrical sonography. J Ultrasound Med 5:639, 1986.
7. Oriole IM, Castilla EE, Barbosa JG: Birth prevalence rates of skeletal dysplasias. J Med Genet 23:328, 1986.
8. Weldner B-M, Persson P-H, Ivarsson SA: Prenatal diagnosis of dwarfism by ultrasound screening. Arch Dis Child 60:1070, 1985.

9. American Institute of Ultrasound in Medicine: Guidelines for the Performance of the Antepartum Obstetrical Ultrasound Examination. J Ultrasound Med 10:577, 1991.
10. International nomenclature of constitutional diseases of bone. Am J Radiol 131:352, 1978.
11. Smith DW: Recognizable Patterns of Human Malformation, 3rd ed. Philadelphia, WB Saunders, 1982.
12. Spranger JW, Langer LO, Weidemann HR: Bone Dysplasias: An Atlas of Constitutional Disorders of Skeletal Development. Philadelphia, WB Saunders, 1974.
13. Taybi H: Radiology of Syndromes and Metabolic Disorders, 2nd ed. Chicago, Year Book Medical Publishers, 1983.
14. Garn SM, Burdi AR, Babler WJ, et al: Early prenatal attainment of adult metacarpal-phalangeal rankings and proportions. Am J Phys Anthrop 43:327, 1975.
15. O'Rahilly R, Gardner E: The initial appearance of ossification in staged human embryos. Am J Anat 134:291, 1972.
16. Sledge CB: Developmental anatomy of joints. In Resnick D, Niwayama G (eds): Diagnosis of Bone and Joint Disorders, vol 1, pp 2–20. Philadelphia, WB Saunders, 1981.
17. Chinn DH, Bolding DB, Callen PW, et al: Ultrasonographic identification of fetal lower extremity epiphyseal ossification centers. Radiology 147:815, 1983.
18. Mahony BS, Callen PW, Filly RA: The distal femoral epiphyseal ossification center in the assessment of third trimester age: Sonographic identification and measurement. Radiology 155:201, 1985.
19. Pyle SI, Hoerr NL: A Radiographic Standard of Reference for the Growing Knee. Springfield, IL, Charles C Thomas, 1969.
20. Mahony BS, Bowie JD, Killam AP, et al: Epiphyseal ossification centers in the assessment of fetal maturity: Sonographic correlation with the amniocentesis lung profile. Radiology 159:521, 1986.
21. Goldstein I, Lockwood CJ, Reece EA, Hobbins JC: Sonographic assessment of the distal femoral and proximal tibial ossification centers in the prediction of pulmonic maturity in normal women and women with diabetes. Am J Obstet Gynecol 159:72, 1988.
22. Mahony BS, Filly RA: High-resolution sonographic assessment of the fetal extremities. J Ultrasound Med 3:489, 1984.
23. Yarkoni S, Schmidt W, Jeanty P, et al: Clavicular measurement: A new biometric parameter for fetal evaluation. J Ultrasound Med 4:467, 1985.
24. Abrams SL, Filly RA: Curvature of the fetal femur: A normal sonographic finding. Radiology 156:490, 1985.
25. Zilianti M, Fernandez S, Azuaga A, et al: Ultrasound evaluation of the distal femoral epiphyseal ossification center as a screening test for intrauterine growth retardation. Obstet Gynecol 70:361, 1987.
26. Deter RL: Evaluation of studies of normal growth. In Deter RL, Harrist RB, Birnholz JC, Hadlock FP (eds): Quantitative Obstetrical Ultrasonography. New York, John Wiley & Sons, 1986.
27. Deter RL, Rossavik IK, Hill RM, et al: Longitudinal studies of femur growth in normal fetuses. J Clin Ultrasound 15:299, 1987.
28. Hill LM, Breckle R, Gehrking WC, et al: Use of femur length in estimation of fetal weight. Am J Obstet Gynecol 152:847, 1985.
29. Jeanty P, Rodesch F, Delbeke D, et al: Estimation of gestational age from measurements of fetal long bones. J Ultrasound Med 3:75, 1984.
30. Merz E, Kim-Kern M-S, Pehl S: Ultrasonic mensuration of fetal limb bones in the second and third trimester. J Clin Ultrasound 15:175, 1987.
31. Merz E, Grubner A, Kern F: Mathematical modeling of fetal limb growth. J Clin Ultrasound 17:179, 1989.
32. Ruvolo KA, Filly RA, Callen PW: Evaluation of fetal femur length for prediction of gestational age in a racially mixed obstetric population. J Ultrasound Med 6:417, 1987.
33. Shalev E, Feldman E, Weiner E, et al: Assessment of gestational age by ultrasonic measurement of the femur length. Acta Obstet Gynecol Scand 64:71, 1985.
34. Warda AH, Deter RL, Rossavik IK, et al: Fetal femur length: A critical reevaluation of the relationship to menstrual age. Obstet Gynecol 66:69, 1985.
35. Exacoustos C, Rosati P, Rizzo G, Arduini D: Ultrasound measurements of fetal limb bones. Ultrasound Obstet Gynecol 1:325, 1991.
36. Abramowicz J, Jaffe R: Comparison between lateral and axial ultrasonic measurements of the fetal femur. Obstet Gynecol 159:921, 1988.
37. Goldstein RB, Filly RA, Simpson G: Pitfalls in femur length measurements. J Ultrasound Med 6:203, 1987.
38. Krook PM, Wawrukiewicz AS, Hackethorn JC: Caveats in the sonographic determination of fetal femur length for estimation of gestational age. Radiology 154:823, 1985.
39. Benacerraf BR, Gelman R, Frigoletto FD: Sonographic identification of second-trimester fetuses with Down's syndrome. N Engl J Med 317:1371, 1987.
40. Perella R, Duerinckx AJ, Grant EG, et al: Second trimester sonographic diagnosis of Down syndrome: Role of femur-length shortening and nuchal-fold thickening. AJR 151:981, 1988.
41. Nyberg DA, Resta RG, Hickok DE, et al: Femur length shortening in the detection of Down syndrome: Is prenatal screening feasible? Am J Obstet Gynecol 162:1247, 1990.
42. Benacerraf BR, Nenberg D, Frigoletto FD: Humeral shortening in second trimester fetuses with Down syndrome. Obstet Gynecol 77:223, 1991.
43. Campbell J, Henderson A, Campbell S: The fetal femur/foot length ratio: A new parameter to assess dysplastic limb reduction. Obstet Gynecol 72:181, 1988.
44. Mercer BM, Sklar S, Shariatmadar A: Fetal foot length as a predictor of gestational age. Am J Obstet Gynecol 156:350, 1987.
45. Platt LD, Medearis AL, DeVore GR, et al: Fetal foot length: Relationship to menstrual age and fetal measurements in the second trimester. Obstet Gynecol 71:526, 1988.
46. Kurtz AB, Needleman L, Wapner RJ, et al: Usefulness of a short femur in the in utero detection of skeletal dysplasias. Radiology 177:197, 1990.
47. Filly RA, Golbus MS, Carey JC, et al: Short-limbed dwarfism: Ultrasonographic diagnosis by mensuration of fetal femoral length. Radiology 138:653, 1981.
48. Kurtz AB, Filly RA, Wapner RJ, et al: In utero analysis of heterozygous achondroplasia: Variable time of onset as detected by femur length measurements. J Ultrasound Med 5:137, 1986.
49. Macken MB, Grantmyre EB, Rimoin DL, Lachman RS: Normal sonographic appearance of a thanatophoric dwarf variant fetus at 13 weeks' gestation. AJR 156:149, 1991.
50. Pastarelli P, Pretorius DH, Edwards DK: Intrauterine growth retardation mimicking skeletal dysplasia on antenatal sonography. J Ultrasound Med 9:737, 1990.
51. Chitkara U, Rosenberg J, Chervenak FA, et al: Prenatal sonographic assessment of the fetal thorax: Normal values. Am J Obstet Gynecol 156:1069, 1987.
52. Pretorius DH, Rumack CM, Manco-Johnson ML, et al: Specific skeletal dysplasias in utero: Sonographic diagnosis. Radiology 159:237, 1986.
53. Maroteaux P, Lamy M, Robert JM: Le nasisme thanatophore. Presse Med 75:2519, 1967.
54. Rouse GA, Filly RA, Toomey F, Grube GL: Short-limb skeletal dysplasias: Evaluation of the fetal spine with sonography and radiography. Radiology 174:177, 1990.
55. Mahony BS, Filly RA, Callen PW, et al: Thanatophoric dwarfism with the cloverleaf skull: A specific antenatal sonographic diagnosis. J Ultrasound Med 4:151, 1985.
56. Fink IJ, Filly RA, Callen PW, et al: Sonographic diagnosis of thanatophoric dwarfism in utero. J Ultrasound Med 1:337, 1982.
57. Elejalde BR, de Elejalde MM: Thanatophoric dysplasia: Fetal manifestations and prenatal diagnosis. Am J Med Genet 22:669, 1985.
58. Partington MW, Gonzales-Crussi F, Khakee SG, et al: Cloverleaf skull and thanatophoric dwarfism. Arch Dis Child 46:656, 1971.
59. Stamm ER, Pretorius DH, Rumack CM, et al: Kleeblattschadel anomaly: In utero sonographic appearance. J Ultrasound Med 6:319, 1987.
60. Saldino RM: Lethal short-limbed dwarfism: Achondrogenesis and thanatophoric dwarfism. AJR 112:185, 1971.

61. Mahony BS, Filly RA, Cooperberg PL: Antenatal sonographic diagnosis of achondrogenesis. J Ultrasound Med 3:333, 1984.

62. Whitley CB, Gorlin RJ: Achondrogenesis: New nosology with evidence of genetic heterogeneity. Radiology 148:693, 1983.

63. Sillence DO, Rimoin DL, Lachman R: Neonatal dwarfism. Pediatr Clin North Am 25:453, 1978.

64. Byers PH, Tsipouras P, Bonadio JF, et al: Perinatal lethal osteogenesis imperfecta (OI type II): A biochemically heterogeneous disorder usually due to new mutations in the genes for type I collagen. Am J Hum Genet 42:237, 1988.

65. Sillence DO, Senn A, Danks DM: Genetic heterogeneity in osteogenesis imperfecta. J Med Genet 16:101, 1979.

66. Spranger J, Cremin B, Beighton P: Osteogenesis imperfecta congenita. Pediatr Radiol 12:21, 1982.

67. Spranger J: Osteogenesis imperfecta: A pasture for splitters and lumpers. Am J Med Genet 17:425, 1984.

68. Sillence DO, Barlow KK, Garber AP, et al: Osteogenesis imperfecta type II: Delineation of the phenotype with reference to genetic heterogeneity. Am J Med Genet 17:407, 1984.

69. Brons JTJ, Van der Harten HJ, Wladimiroff JW, et al: Prenatal ultrasonographic diagnosis of osteogenesis imperfecta. Am J Obstet Gynecol 159:176, 1988.

70. Stephens JD, Filly RA, Callen PW, et al: Prenatal diagnosis of osteogenesis imperfecta type II by real-time ultrasound. Hum Genet 64:191, 1983.

71. Munoz C, Filly RA, Golbus MS: Osteogenesis imperfecta type II: Prenatal sonographic diagnosis. Radiology 174:181, 1990.

72. Houston CS, Opitz JM, Spranger JW, et al: The campomelic syndrome: Review, report of 17 cases, and follow-up on the currently 17 year old boy first reported by Maroteaux et al in 1971. Am J Med Genet 15:3, 1983.

73. Hall BD, Spranger JW: Campomelia dysplasia: Further elucidation of a distinct entity. Am J Dis Child 134:285, 1980.

74. Lazjuk GI, Shved IA, Cherstvoy ED, et al: Campomelic syndrome: Concepts of the bowing and shortening in the lower limbs. Teratology 35:1, 1987.

75. Gilbert EF, Opitz JM, Spranger JW, et al: Chondrodysplasia punctata—rhizomelic form: Pathologic and radiologic studies of three infants. Eur J Pediatr 123:89, 1976.

76. Duff P, Harlass FE, Milligan DA: Prenatal diagnosis of chondrodysplasia punctata by sonography. Obstet Gynecol 76:497, 1990.

77. Curry CJR, Magenis RE, Brown M, et al: Inherited chondrodysplasia punctata due to a deletion of the terminal short arm of an X chromosome. N Engl J Med 311:1010, 1984.

78. Mulivor RA, Mennuti M, Zackai EH, et al: Prenatal diagnosis of hypophosphatasia: Genetic, biochemical, and clinical studies. Am J Hum Genet 30:271, 1978.

79. Rattenbury JM, Blau K, Sandler M, et al: Prenatal diagnosis of hypophosphatasia. Lancet 1:306, 1976.

80. Benzie R, Doran TA, Escoffery W, et al: Prenatal diagnosis of hypophosphatasia. Birth Defects 12(6):271, 1976.

81. Rudd NL, Miskin M, Hoar DI, et al: Prenatal diagnosis of hypophosphatasia. N Engl J Med 295:146, 1976.

82. Wladimiroff JW, Niermeijer MF, Van der Harten JJ, et al: Early prenatal diagnosis of congenital hypophosphatasia: Case report. Prenat Diagn 5:47, 1985.

83. DeLange M, Rouse GA: Prenatal diagnosis of hypophosphatasia. J Ultrasound Med 9:115, 1990.

84. Langer LO, Spranger JW, Greinacher I, et al: Thanatophoric dwarfism: A condition confused with achondroplasia in the neonate, with brief comments on achondrogenesis and homozygous achondroplasia. Radiology 92:285, 1969.

85. Filly RA, Golbus MS: Ultrasonography of the normal and pathologic fetal spine. Radiol Clin North Am 20:311, 1982.

86. Meizner I, Bar-Ziv J: Prenatal ultrasonic diagnosis of short-rib polydactyly syndrome (SRPS) type III: A case report and a proposed approach to the diagnosis of SRPS and related conditions. J Clin Ultrasound 13:284, 1985.

87. Skiptunas SM, Weiner S: Early prenatal diagnosis of asphyxiating thoracic dysplasia (Jeune's syndrome): Value of fetal thoracic measurement. J Ultrasound Med 6:41, 1987.

88. Bui T-H, Marsk L, Eklof O: Prenatal diagnosis of chondroectodermal dysplasia with fetoscopy. Prenat Diagn 4:155, 1984.

89. Mahoney MJ, Hobbins JC: Prenatal diagnosis of chondroec-todermal dysplasia (Ellis-van Creveld syndrome) with fetoscopy and ultrasound. N Engl J Med 297:258, 1977.

90. Gollop RR, Eigier A: Prenatal ultrasound diagnosis of diastrophic dysplasia at 16 weeks. Am J Med Genet 27:321, 1987.

91. Horton WA, Rimoin DL, Lachman RS, et al: The phenotypic variability of diastrophic dysplasia. J Pediatr 93:609, 1978.

92. Kaitila I, Ammala P, Karjalainen D, et al: Early prenatal detection of diastrophic dysplasia. Prenat Diagn 3:237, 1983.

93. Chervenak FA, Romero R, Berkowitz RL, et al: Antenatal sonographic findings of osteogenesis imperfecta. Am J Obstet Gynecol 143:228, 1982.

94. Kuller J, Bellantoni J, Dorst J, et al: Obstetric management of a fetus with nonlethal osteogenesis imperfecta. Obstet Gynecol 74:477, 1988.

95. Kirk JS, Comstock CH: Antenatal sonographic appearance of spondyloepiphyseal dysplasia congenita. J Ultrasound Med 9:173, 1990.

96. Bromley B, Miller W, Foster SC, Benacerraf BR: The prenatal sonographic features of Kneist syndrome. J Ultrasound Med 10:705, 1991.

97. Romero R, Ghidini A, Eswara MS, et al: Prenatal findings in a case of spondylocostal dysplasia type I (Jarcho-Levin syndrome). Obstet Gynecol 71:988, 1988.

98. Hall JG: Thrombocytopenia and absent radius (TAR) syndrome. J Med Genet 24:79, 1987.

99. Benson CB, Pober BR, Hirsch MP, et al: Sonography of Nager acrofacial dysostosis syndrome in utero. J Ultrasound Med 7:163, 1988.

100. Brons JTJ, Van Geijn HP, Wladimiroff JW, et al: Prenatal ultrasound diagnosis of the Holt-Oram syndrome. Prenat Diagn 8:175, 1988.

101. Meizner I, Bar-Ziv J, Barki Y, et al: Prenatal ultrasonic diagnosis of radial-ray aplasia and renal anomalies (acro-renal syndrome). Prenat Diagn 6:223, 1986.

102. Kalousek DK, Bamforth S: Amnion rupture sequence in previable fetuses. Am J Med Genet 31:63, 1988.

103. Rushton DI: Amniotic band syndrome. Br Med J 286:919, 1983.

104. Seeds JW, Cefalo RC, Herbert WNP: Amniotic band syndrome. Am J Obstet Gynecol 144:243, 1982.

105. Torpin R: Fetal malformations caused by amnion rupture during gestation. Springfield, IL, Charles C Thomas, 1968.

106. Mahony BS, Filly RA, Callen PW, et al: The amniotic band syndrome: Antenatal sonographic diagnosis and potential pitfalls. Am J Obstet Gynecol 152:63, 1985.

107. Hill LM, Kislak S, Jones N: Prenatal ultrasound diagnosis of a forearm constriction band. J Ultrasound Med 7:293, 1988.

108. Van Allen MI, Curry C, Gallagher L: Limb body wall complex: I. Pathogenesis. Am J Med Genet 28:529, 1987.

109. Van Allen MI, Walden CE, Gallagher L, et al: Limb–body wall complex: II. Limb and spine defects. Am J Med Genet 28:549, 1987.

110. Patten RM, Allen MV, Mack LA, et al: Limb–body wall complex: In utero sonographic diagnosis of a complicated fetal malformation. AJR 146:1019, 1986.

111. Tomkins D, Hunter A, Roberts M: Cystogenetic findings in Roberts-SC phocomelia syndrome(s). Am J Med Genet 4:17, 1979.

112. Grundy HO, Burlbaw J, Walton S, et al: Roberts syndrome: Antenatal ultrasound: A case report. J Perinat Med 16:71, 1988.

113. Graham M: Congenital short femur: Prenatal sonographic diagnosis. J Ultrasound Med 4:361, 1985.

114. Jeanty P, Kleinman G: Proximal femoral focal deficiency. J Ultrasound Med 8:639, 1989.

115. Duhamel B: From the mermaid to anal imperfection: The syndrome of caudal regression. Arch Dis Child 36:152, 1961.

116. Sonek JD, Gabbe SG, Landon MB, et al: Antenatal diagnosis of sacral agenesis syndrome in a pregnancy complicated by diabetes mellitus. Am J Obstet Gynecol 162:806, 1990.

117. Sirtori M, Ghidini A, Romero R, et al: Prenatal diagnosis of sirenomelia. J Ultrasound Med 8:83, 1989.

118. Honda N, Shimokawa H, Yamaguchi Y, et al: Antenatal diagnosis of sirenomelia (sympus apus). JCU 16:675, 1988.

119. Chenoweth CK, Kellogg SJ, Abu-Yousef MM: Antenatal so-

nographic diagnosis of sirenomelia. J Clin Ultrasound 19:167, 1991.

120. Davis JE, Kalousek DK: Fetal akinesia deformation sequence in previable fetuses. Am J Med Genet 29:77, 1988.

121. Moessinger AC: Fetal akinesia deformation sequence: An animal model. Pediatrics 72:857, 1983.

122. Goldberg JD, Chervenak FA, Lipman RA, et al: Antenatal sonographic diagnosis of arthrogryposis multiplex congenita. Prenat Diagn 6:45, 1986.

123. Hall JG: Invited editorial comment: Analysis of Pena-Shokeir phenotype. Am J Med Genet 25:99, 1986.

124. Hall JG, Reed SD, Rosenbaum KN, et al: Limb pterygium syndromes: A review and report of eleven patients. Am J Med Genet 12:377, 1982.

125. Baty BJ, Cubberley D, Morris C, et al: Prenatal diagnosis of distal arthrogryposis. Am J Med Genet 29:501, 1988.

126. Lockwood C, Irons M, Troiani J, et al: The prenatal sonographic diagnosis of lethal multiple pterygium syndrome: A heritable cause of recurrent abortion. Am J Obstet Gynecol 159:474, 1988.

127. Gorzyca DP, McGahan JP, Lindfors KK, et al: Arthrogryposis multiplex congenita: Prenatal ultrasonographic diagnosis. J Clin Ultrasound 17:40, 1989.

128. Genkins SM, Hertzberg BS, Bowie JD, Blow O: Pena-Shokeir type I syndrome: In utero sonographic appearance. J Clin Ultrasound 17:56, 1988.

129. Ohlsson A, Fong KW, Rose TH, et al: Prenatal sonographic diagnosis of Pena-Shokeir syndrome type I, or fetal akinesia deformation sequence. Am J Med Genet 29:59, 1988.

130. Pursutte WH, Lenke RR, Kurezynski TW, et al: Antenatal diagnosis of Pena-Shokeir syndrome (type I) with ultrasonography and magnetic resonance imaging. Obstet Gynecol 72:472, 1988.

131. Chervenak FA, Tortora M, Hobbins JC: Antenatal sonographic diagnosis of clubfoot. J Ultrasound Med 4:49, 1985.

132. Cowell HR, Wein BK: Genetic aspects of clubfoot. J Bone Joint Surg 62:1381, 1980.

133. Hashimoto BE, Filly RA, Callen PW: Sonographic diagnosis of clubfoot in utero. J Ultrasound Med 5:81, 1986.

134. Sucheston ME, Cannon MS (eds): Congenital Malformations. Philadelphia, FA Davis, 1973.

135. Bronshtein M, Zimmer EZ: Transvaginal ultrasound diagnosis of fetal clubfeet at 13 weeks menstrual age. J Clin Ultrasound 17:518, 1989.

136. Jeanty P, Romero R, d'Alton M, et al: In utero sonographic detection of hand and foot deformities. J Ultrasound Med 4:595, 1985.

137. Benacerraf BR, Frigoletto FD, Greene MF: Abnormal facial features and extremities in human trisomy syndromes: Prenatal ultrasonographic appearance. Radiology 159:243, 1986.

138. Bundy AL, Saltzman DH, Pober B, et al: Antenatal sonographic findings in trisomy 18. J Ultrasound Med 5:361, 1986.

139. Benacerraf BR, Osathanondh R, Frigoletto FD: Sonographic demonstration of hypoplasia of the middle phalanx of the fifth digit: A finding associated with Down syndrome. Am J Obstet Gynecol 159:181, 1988.

140. Shalev E, Romero S, Nseir T, et al: Klippel-Trenaunay syndrome: Ultrasonic prenatal diagnosis. J Clin Ultrasound 16:268, 1988.

141. Suma V, Marini A, Gamba PG, Luzzatto C: Giant hemangioma of the thigh: Prenatal sonographic diagnosis. J Clin Ultrasound 18:421, 1990.

142. Koenigsberg M, Factor S, Cho S, et al: Fetal Marfan syndrome: Prenatal ultrasound diagnosis with pathological confirmation of skeletal and aortic lesions. Prenat Diagn 1:241, 1981.

CHAPTER 14

Ultrasound Evaluation of the Fetal Heart

NORMAN H. SILVERMAN, M.D.
KLAUS G. SCHMIDT, M.D.

Because of the technologic advances complemented by the increasing ability of sonographers to recognize normal and abnormal fetal anatomy, the use of ultrasonography as a diagnostic obstetric tool continues to expand. Although structural abnormalities of the heart and great vessels are fairly common congenital abnormalities, occurring in approximately 8 in 1000 live neonates,[1, 2] fetal cardiac ultrasonography, or fetal echocardiography, has only recently attracted more attention. Because the fetal heart is small and beats rapidly, it could be imaged reliably only after high-resolution real-time ultrasound scanners became available. Since the advent of cross-sectional scanners, which provide real-time directed M-mode and pulsed Doppler echocardiography and color-coded Doppler flow mapping, the sonographer is able to recognize congenital heart defects,[3–11] arrhythmias,[12–17] or disturbed cardiac function in utero.[18–20] The information from fetal echocardiography has augmented genetic counseling, has permitted sophisticated monitoring of cardiac arrhythmias during transplacental treatment, and may help determine a site and route of delivery when a serious cardiac abnormality has been recognized. In the future, acquisition of such information may allow decisions about cardiac surgery in utero.[21, 22]

CLINICAL INDICATIONS

Indications for fetal echocardiography include the previous occurrence of congenital heart disease in siblings or parents; a maternal disease known to affect the fetus, such as diabetes mellitus or connective tissue disease; and the maternal use of drugs that might cause cardiac abnormalities in the fetus, such as lithium or alcohol.[23] Obstetric examinations indicating abnormal cardiac findings due to chromosomal abnormalities, diaphragmatic hernia, omphalocele, hydrops, excessive or very little amniotic fluid volume, or a very fast or slow fetal heart rate are other reasons for referral. The most common indication is a family history of congenital heart disease (Table 14–1). Although in our experience, and in that of others,[24] the rate of recurrence is low when there is one previously affected child, this rate might be considerably higher when there is more than one previously affected child or when a parent has congenital heart disease.[24–26] We have found several examples in which the mother, father, or siblings have had congenital heart disease. Most repetitions have

been of the same type, but with some variation. Most of the women who are referred because their disease puts them at risk for cardiac abnormalities have insulin-dependent diabetes mellitus. Euglycemic control in diabetics at the time of conception and in early pregnancy may diminish the risk, and we have not found cardiac abnormalities in the offspring of such diabetic women. Structural cardiac defects are encountered more frequently when other fetal abnormalities have been detected previously on obstetric ultrasound examination, especially when there is nonimmune hydrops, omphalocele, or diaphragmatic hernia.

In the presence of a very slow fetal heart rate (< 80 beats per minute), the fetus is at high risk of associated heart disease; fetal echocardiography should be performed not only to evaluate the arrhythmia but also to rule out the presence of a structural cardiac defect. The association of complete heart block with structural cardiac defects appears to have an extremely poor prognosis, presumably because of their adverse interaction and the atrioventricular valve regurgitation that frequently complicates the condition. In fetuses with complete heart block but without structural cardiac defect, the mother frequently suffers from a connective tissue disorder.[27, 28] Other arrhythmias have, in our experience, no association with any structural abnormality of the heart. All incidences found reflect a trend, but the individual numbers are too small to extrapolate a true incidence of fetal cardiac disease. Although these clues have been useful, continuously expanding experience makes hard and fast indications difficult to articulate.

We prefer to perform the initial study between 18 and 22 weeks of gestation because the valves are well developed, the size of the heart is adequate for study, and the fetal size and position usually allow best access

Table 14–1. INDICATIONS FOR ECHOCARDIOGRAPHY AND INCIDENCE OF STRUCTURAL CARDIAC ABNORMALITIES IN 1650 FETUSES

Indication	%
Family history of congenital heart disease	44.3
Maternal disease affecting the fetus	7.0
Maternal ingestion of drugs or teratogens	4.5
Fetal abnormalties and dysmaturity	11.7
Nonimmune fetal hydrops	7.5
Abnormal amniotic fluid volume	1.5
Fetal arrhythmias	23.6

to the heart. If necessary, however, it is possible to display the fetal cardiac anatomy and to analyze cardiac rhythm and function from 16 weeks to term.

EQUIPMENT

The cornerstone of fetal echocardiography is high-resolution imaging with cross-sectional (two-dimensional) echocardiography. When studying the fetal heart, it is also desirable to use ultrasound systems equipped with M-mode, pulsed Doppler, and continuous wave Doppler ultrasonography. We have gained additional information using color Doppler flow mapping. The ability to recognize valvular regurgitation and flow direction has led us to incorporate this modality as a standard routine. The technique allows rapid identification of flow disturbance and is even helpful for recognizing morphologic abnormalities. The transducer frequency for cardiac imaging should be as high as possible; we prefer 7.5- or 5-MHz transducers but have also used transducers with a 3-MHz frequency. Both linear array and sector scanners may be used to image the fetal heart. We prefer the sector scanner because it provides easier access to the fetal heart. Since this format is commonly used in pediatric or adult cardiology, the additional modalities of ultrasonography, such as M-mode, conventional Doppler, or color Doppler flow mapping, are usually available. Image magnification and cineloop facilities that allow one to image the beating heart in real time or in slow motion have augmented our diagnostic ability. Recording the studies on videotape for later playback and analysis is, we believe, essential. The video recorder used for replay of the study should have slow motion, forward and reverse playing, and single frame advance capabilities. This facilitates analysis, especially when studies are recorded and interpreted subsequently by different people. We have also used an off-line computer-assisted analysis system with cineloop and full measurement facilities.

M-mode echocardiography can be most easily understood as a true display of information under the single cursor or scan line. This provides an "ice pick" view of the heart, but because the sample rate runs at between 1000 and 2000 Hz (cycles per second), accurate measurements of the dimensions of walls, cavities, and vessels can easily be made. It also provides exquisite detail of structural motion that is too fast to be perceived by sector scanning, which has a frame rate of 20 to 60 Hz. For example, the rapid motion of valve opening and closure, the fine flutter of valve leaflets, the small motion of atrial contraction, and the rates of change in muscle thickening or cavity size diminution are clearly displayed.

Pulsed Doppler ultrasonography demonstrates the direction and characteristics of the blood flow within the fetal heart and the great vessels and allows the qualitative and quantitative definition of flow disturbances such as those that occur with valvular stenotic or regurgitant lesions. As is our practice after birth, pulsed Doppler ultrasonography can also be used as a form of flow mapping or "intracardiac stethoscope."

Doppler scanning uses the change in frequency (the so-called Doppler shift) of sound waves reflected from the red blood cells within the cardiovascular system. If the red blood cells are traveling toward the transducer, the pitch increases; and if the cells are traveling away from the transducer, the pitch is lowered. These Doppler signals are displayed above or below the baseline, respectively. By timing the receiving period, it is possible to "listen" at a specific distance from the transducer (range gating). This is displayed by a small line or box (the so-called sample volume) on the cursor, which can be steered through any sector line or depth of the image. The size of the sample volume may vary from 1.5 to 9 mm in axial depth. Lateral resolution varies depending on the focal length of the transducer. The angle between the blood flow and the path of the Doppler sound is called the angle of insonance (angle θ). The more perpendicular the sound wave is to the blood flow, the less is the frequency (or velocity) change. The ideal approach for sampling, then, is axial to the blood flow. For practical purposes of measurement, it is desirable to keep the angle θ to less than 25°. The Doppler carrier frequency used is 3 or 5 MHz, preferably the higher frequency to ensure lower ultrasound exposure of the fetus. Current state of the art pulsed Doppler studies employing fast Fourier analysis have become accepted as standard. Most ultrasound systems convert the frequency shift into a velocity display automatically through the formula:

$$v = (f_d \times c)/(2f_o \times \cos \theta)$$

where v is the velocity (m/s), f_d is the frequency shift (Hz), c is the conducting velocity of sound in water (1560 m/s), f_o is the carrier frequency of the transducer (e.g., 3 or 5 MHz), and θ is the angle of insonance. One problem with pulsed Doppler ultrasonography is that high-velocity flow cannot be determined accurately because of the finite sampling rate. The frequency shift from range gating techniques can only be sampled at a rate that depends on the number of pulses of sound emitted by the transducer. If the frequency shift of the red blood cell targets exceeds the sampling frequency, aliasing of the signal occurs. This is analogous to observing a wagon wheel apparently spinning backward as it is moving forward, which relates to the optic sampling frequency (27 cycles/s for the human eye) being exceeded. To measure high velocities of flow, two alternatives are available: high pulse repetition frequency or continuous wave Doppler ultrasonography. High pulse repetition frequency Doppler imaging has an advantage in the fetus because the beam and the sample volume can be guided through the sector image to define the origin of the flow disturbance. With the systems we have used, continuous wave Doppler ultrasonography cannot be directed through the image and therefore is of limited value in the fetus. In other systems, the problem is eliminated with continuous wave Doppler imaging that is steerable through the sector image. Nevertheless, with high-velocity signals, a blind aligning of the transducer at the site of the flow disturbance may be an efficacious way of determining the peak velocity.

Doppler ultrasonography exposes the fetus to higher

levels of ultrasonic energy than M-mode or cross-sectional imaging. Although echocardiography has not been reported to have harmful effects on the developing fetus, Doppler ultrasonic energy should be kept at or below a 100 mW/cm^2 spatial peak-temporal average, and Doppler interrogation should be limited to as short a time as possible.* On the other hand, Doppler ultrasonography provides information unavailable with other techniques in the fetus and, despite the concern as to its bioeffects, remains a most valuable technique.

Color-coded Doppler flow mapping may aid in detecting flow disturbance and flow direction (see Figs. 14–26 and 14–54) and should be used when appropriate. This technique has become an essential part of the fetal cardiac examination. The color Doppler map, besides indicating flow disturbances and direction of blood flow, permits demonstration of cardiac and vascular morphology. Color Doppler flow mapping is a multigate Doppler technique in which sampling along all the scan lines and depths in the field occurs simultaneously. No hard and fast standard of color Doppler display is in use; however, flow toward the transducer is commonly depicted as warm colors (orange and red), and flow away from the transducer is depicted as cold colors (blue). Disturbed flow signals are depicted by adding the color green. As these colors are displayed across the cross-sectional image in real time, not only can the direction of blood flow be mapped in time but the direction and magnitude of flow disturbances resulting from leaks and stenoses can also be assessed. This technique has been valuable for the assessment of congenital heart disease in utero. Unfortunately, the energy levels of this ultrasound method are higher than those of older established methods and have led to certain manufacturers recommending that this technique should not be used in the fetus.

We limit color Doppler examination to brief periods of time and consider the information it provides an important addition to ultrasound evaluation in general. Some investigators have suggested that the use of this Doppler technique may allow more rapid identification of a pathologic condition, thereby limiting the time of examination and the exposure of the fetus to further ultrasound examination.

TECHNIQUE

Cross-Sectional Imaging

To define the cardiac position and situs, it is necessary to orient the cross-sectional image to the fetal body by noting the position of the head, body, and limbs. It is also important to estimate fetal age using head or femoral length measurements, because cardiac dimensions relate to gestational age and fetal weight.[5, 29–31] The best access to the heart is through

---

*For more details on the bioeffects of ultrasonography, see NIH Publication 84-667: Diagnostic Ultrasound Imaging In Pregnancy. US Department of Health and Human Services, 1984.

the fetal abdomen, but imaging is also possible through the rib cage and from the back, because the fetal lungs are filled with fluid and are not a barrier to the passage of the ultrasound beam, as they are postnatally. In later gestation, however, when the fetal back may be very close to the maternal abdominal wall, much of the ultrasonic energy is absorbed by the vertebral bodies, scapulae, and ribs, which have become ossified, resulting in poorer imaging potential from this direction. To improve imaging, it may be necessary to turn the mother onto one or another side or to elevate her chest or pelvis. We have often found it helpful to have the mother walk around or empty her bladder, or to delay the examination for hours or even days. In the presence of polyhydramnios, the fetus may lie at some distance from the transducer when the mother is recumbent. The fetus can be brought closer to the transducer by having the mother rest on her knees and elbows.

Once the fetal heart is located, only slight movements of the transducer are needed to display the cardiac structures because, with the fetal heart being at some distance from the transducer, small movements subtend great angle changes. We consider a complete cardiac examination to encompass scanning of the fetal heart from side to side and from top to bottom. Reference planes similar to those obtained postnatally are gathered, namely, four-chamber, long- and short-axis views (Fig. 14–1). These terms are derived from traditional cardiac reference planes established postnatally.

Although the four-chamber view (see Fig. 14–1A) is very valuable for defining the comparative sizes of the chambers, it allows the display of only the atrioventricular connections. It does not pass through a plane that allows recognition of the aorta and pulmonary arteries and therefore will not define the complexes of transposition of the great arteries, tetralogy of Fallot, truncus arteriosus, or a double-outlet right ventricle. It also does not pass through the outlet part of the ventricular septum and will not define outlet ventricular septal defects and aortic override as found in tetralogy of Fallot, truncus arteriosus, or a double-outlet right ventricle. It may not pass through a plane where most ventricular septal defects lie. The arterial valve anatomy is not defined in the four-chamber view, so aortic and pulmonic stenosis cannot be detected from this plane. Abnormalities of the aortic arch, such as interruption and coarctation, will not be identified either. We therefore recommend that the mere display of a four-chamber view is not adequate for a fetal cardiac examination. It should be appreciated that when the four-chamber view is obtained from a subcostal equivalent view, simply rotating the transducer along its axis by approximately 90° brings the great veins and great arteries into view, allowing one to establish the venoatrial, atrioventricular, and ventriculoarterial connections.

The cardiac segments should be assessed sequentially in a manner similar to that performed postnatally.[32] In utero, the left and right sides of the body must be established to define the cardiac position within the

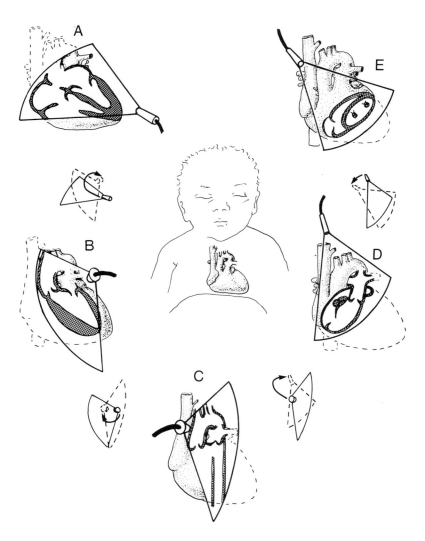

Figure 14–1. Schematic representation of the different views and approaches used to image the fetal heart and great vessels. The fetal heart has a more horizontal axis compared with its postnatal lie in the chest *(center)*. Note that all the views are shown as being obtained from the chest or the abdominal wall; however, it is also possible to achieve all these imaging planes from the back. *A.* Four-chamber view showing both atria and the foramen ovale within the atrial septum, both ventricles, and the atrioventricular valves. *B.* After slight clockwise rotation and tilt of the transducer toward the fetal left shoulder, the long axis comes into view. *C.* Further clockwise rotation and tilt of the transducer results in sagittally oriented planes, which are valuable for depicting the aortic arch and the "ductus arch." *D.* Perpendicular to the long axis, the short axis views are obtained. At the base of the heart, the aorta lies centrally and is surrounded by the structures of the right ventricle and the pulmonary artery, as postnatally. *E.* Further toward the apex, the left ventricular structure with two papillary muscles can be seen.

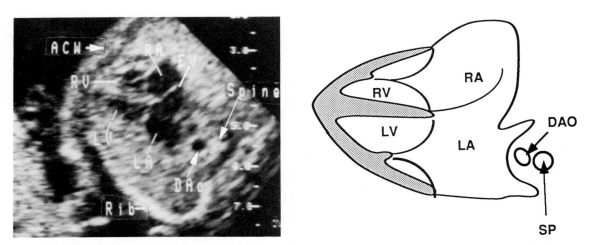

Figure 14–2. Magnified horizontal section through the fetal heart (four-chamber view) and thorax. The right ventricle (RV) is seen close to the anterior chest wall (ACW), whereas the left atrium (LA) lies more posteriorly in front of the descending aorta (DAo) and the spine. The eustachian valve (EV) is noted within the right atrium (RA). LV, left ventricle. In this and most subsequent echocardiographic images, a centimeter-scale marker is included on the right of the figure. The diagram on the right represents the important anatomic features of the echocardiogram.

chest. Inappropriate identification or the assumption of levocardia and situs solitus can lead to basic errors. Although the echocardiographic views might be obtained from unusual transducer planes, the reference to cardiac position and situs (atrial arrangement) is facilitated by noting that the left atrium lies closer to the vertebral column and the right ventricle lies closer to the anterior chest wall (Fig. 14–2). Furthermore, in situs solitus, the fluid-filled stomach is left-sided, whereas the hepatic veins and the inferior vena cava, as well as the superior vena cava, drain into the right-sided atrium (Fig. 14–3). Magnifying the image considerably aids the recognition of anatomic details (Fig. 14–4B).

The definition of the atrial situs requires the identification of the venous connections and atrial structures. Usually the venous connections can be distinguished in utero (see Fig. 14–3). Sometimes even the specific structures of the atrial appendages may be visible, thus substantiating the atrial situs (see Fig. 14–3). More often, however, the atrial structures are identified indirectly by the presence of the valve of the inferior

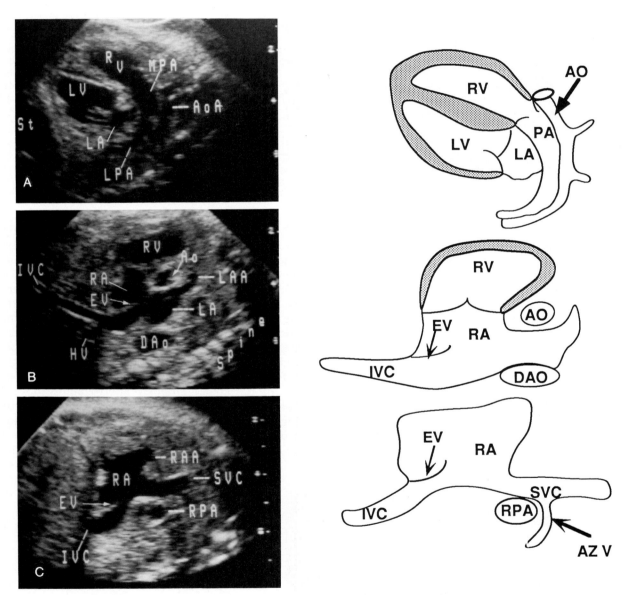

Figure 14–3. Series of magnified parasagittal views in the fetus, representing a sweep from the left to the right side. *A.* The fluid-filled stomach (St) is seen inferior to the left ventricle (LV). The right ventricle (RV) lies anteriorly and is in continuation with the main pulmonary artery (MPA), which gives rise to the left pulmonary artery (LPA). A part of the aortic arch (AoA) can be seen above the pulmonary "arch." The left atrium (LA) lies between the left pulmonary artery and the left ventricle. *B.* In a sagittal view obtained to the right of the previous section, the inferior vena cava (IVC) and a hepatic vein (HV) draining into the right atrium (RA) are demonstrated. The eustachian valve (EV) separates the inferior vena cava from the rest of the right atrium and is pointing toward the atrial septum. Note the narrow-based, fingerlike left atrial appendage (LAA) lying behind the aortic root (Ao). The descending aorta (DAo) is seen lying between the left atrium (LA) and the spine. *C.* This section was obtained by directing the transducer farther to the fetal right side in a sagittal orientation demonstrating the entry of the inferior (IVC) and superior (SVC) vena cava into the right atrium (RA). The right atrium is characterized by the presence of the eustachian valve (EV) and of a broad-based right atrial appendage (RAA). The right pulmonary artery (RPA) is visible in cross section, posterior to the superior vena cava. The diagrams on the right represent the important anatomic features of the echocardiogram. AZ V, azygos vein.

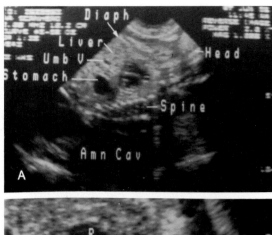

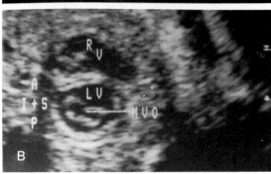

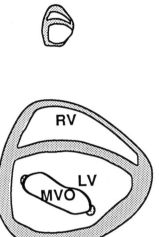

Figure 14–4. Short-axis view of a fetal heart at 22 weeks' gestation. *A.* This frame shows the position of the head, spine, and abdominal organs (stomach, liver), indicating the superior, inferior, anterior, and posterior directions. Amn Cav, amniotic cavity; Diaph, diaphragm; Umb V, umbilical vein. The depth in the panel is up to 11 cm. *B.* After magnification (3×), this frame shows the heart, which lies between 2.5 and 4.5 cm away from the transducer. The cardiac structures are better demonstrated than in *A;* the left ventricle (LV), the mitral valve orifice (MVO), and the right ventricle (RV) can be identified. A, anterior; I, inferior; P, posterior; S, superior. The diagrams on the right represent the important anatomic features of the echocardiogram.

vena cava (eustachian valve) within the right atrium and by the demonstration of the flap valve of the foramen ovale, which is the septum primum, within the left atrium (Fig. 14–5). When the situs is ambiguous, these atrial structures may be absent or vestigial. In these situations, one has to rely on additional scanning of the abdomen for the relative positions of the aorta and the azygos, hemiazygos, or inferior caval veins to define the nature of any ambiguous situs, as has been reported after birth.[33, 34] In situs solitus (the usual atrial arrangement), the aorta is more posterior and leftward, whereas the inferior vena cava is more anterior and on the right of the spine (Fig. 14–6). The identification of these vessels can be complemented by interrogation with pulsed Doppler ultrasonography. In situs inversus there is a mirror image arrangement of

these vessels, with the aorta posterior and to the right, the inferior vena cava anterior and to the left, and the stomach on the right. When the situs is ambiguous, there is either left atrial isomerism (polysplenia syndrome or double left-sidedness) or right atrial isomerism (asplenia syndrome or double right-sidedness). In left atrial isomerism, the inferior vena cava is usually interrupted above the renal veins and lower body venous drainage is achieved by means of azygos or hemiazygos veins. These veins are identified posterior to the aorta, either on the same or on the opposite side of the spine. Doppler interrogation allows the rapid differentiation of arterial and venous structures (Fig. 14–7). In right atrial isomerism, there is almost invariably juxtaposition of the abdominal aorta and the inferior vena cava on the same side of the spine,

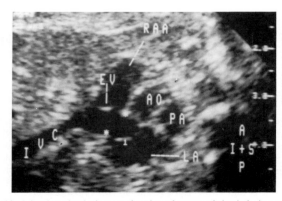

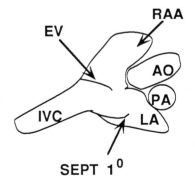

Figure 14–5. Magnified fetal sagittal view at the site of entry of the inferior vena cava (IVC) into the right atrium with its broad-based right atrial appendage (RAA). The eustachian valve (EV) is seen within the right atrium, and the flap valve of the foramen ovale or septum primum (1) is seen within the left atrium (LA). The asterisks indicate the boundaries of the foramen ovale. AO, aorta; PA, pulmonary artery; A, anterior; I, inferior; P, posterior; S, superior. The diagram on the right represents the important anatomic features of the echocardiogram. SEPT 1°, septum primum.

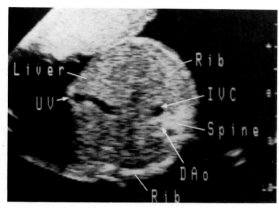

Figure 14–6. Horizontal section at the umbilical level in a fetus of 22 weeks' gestation demonstrating normal situs. The liver and umbilical vein (UV) lie anterior; the spine lies posterior. Note the inferior vena cava (IVC) more anterior and to the right of the spine, whereas the descending aorta (DAo) can be seen more posterior and to the left of the spine.

either side by side or in an anteroposterior relationship, the posterior vessel being the aorta. Again, in this situation it has been extremely valuable to confirm which vascular structure is which by pulsed Doppler interrogation of these vessels.

Having established the situs, the atrioventricular and ventriculoarterial connections are determined using a variety of examining planes. The four-chamber view (see Fig. 14–1A) is easily obtained by tracing the inferior vena cava to the right atrium and then angling the transducer slightly cranially until the four chambers are visualized (Fig. 14–8). The relatively large fetal liver and the noninflated lungs keep the diaphragm at a higher level within the chest, making the heart lie more horizontal than it does after birth. The four-chamber view usually allows identification of the prominent eustachian valve within the right atrium and the flap valve of the foramen ovale (septum primum) within the left atrium. In real time, the septum primum moves forward to the left atrial cavity and back toward the atrial septum twice during each cardiac cycle. The phasic movement of this interatrial valve appears to mirror the interatrial flow dynamics in the fetus. Both atrioventricular valves are seen in the normal heart,

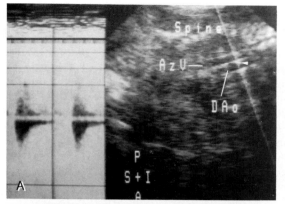

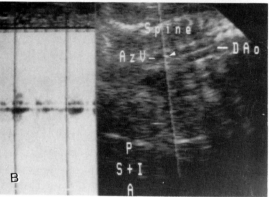

Figure 14–7. Abdominal sagittal view in a fetus of 23 weeks' gestation with left atrial isomerism (polysplenia syndrome) and complete heart block. *A.* In the right panel, two parallel vessels are recognized on the same side of the spine. The Doppler sample volume is placed in the anterior vessel *(arrowhead)*. The Doppler display *(left)* shows an arterial flow signal at a rate of 57 beats per minute, thus identifying the descending aorta (DAo). *B.* In the right panel, the Doppler sample volume is now seen in the posterior vessel *(arrowhead)*. The Doppler display *(left)* demonstrates a low-velocity venous flow signal, thus indicating an azygous vein (AzV). This finding strongly suggests the presence of an interrupted inferior vena cava with azygous continuation of the lower body veins. A, anterior; I, inferior; P, posterior; S, superior.

and the tricuspid valve lies closer to the cardiac apex than the mitral valve does. The right ventricle often shows the septal attachment of the tricuspid valve leaflets, the moderator band, or the associated large

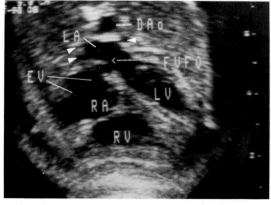

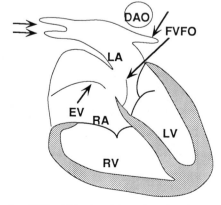

Figure 14–8. Magnified fetal four-chamber view demonstrating the eustachian valve (EV) within the right atrium (RA) and the flap valve of the foramen ovale (FVFO) (i.e., the septum primum) within the left atrium (LA). The arrowheads indicate pulmonary veins entering the left atrium. DAo, descending aorta; LV, left ventricle; RV, right ventricle. The diagram on the right represents the important anatomic features of the echocardiogram.

anterior papillary muscle. The right ventricle may also appear slightly larger than the left ventricle.[5]

The four-chamber view allows the definition of atrioventricular connections, the evaluation of atrioventricular valve malformations, the comparative assessment of chamber size, and the identification of some positions of ventricular septal defects. Scanning more cranially toward the outflow tracts in the four-chamber view may also display the ventriculoarterial connections (Fig. 14–9). This is not always possible, and other planes should also be used to define these connections. The definition of the fetal four-chamber view requires one to define the connection between the specific ventricle and its artery. The crossing of the outflow tracts and display of the vessels traveling at right angles to one another is important for the definition of normal connections. Furthermore, the identification of the coronary arteries and the arch vessels defines the aorta, whereas identifying the bifurcating vessels and arterial duct defines the pulmonary trunk (see Figs. 14–9 and 14–10).

By rotating the transducer clockwise from the four-chamber view and tilting it slightly toward the fetal left shoulder, the scan plane is oriented in the long axis of the heart, similar to that of long-axis views observed postnatally (see Fig. 14–1B). These views allow a better definition of venoatrial, atrioventricular, and ventriculoarterial connections. The crossing of the right

and the left ventricular outflow tracts, as well as the perpendicular relationship of the aorta (posterior) and the pulmonary artery (anterior), can be defined (see Fig. 14–10). This crossing of the great arteries will be absent when they are transposed. Furthermore, long-axis planes demonstrate the left-sided structures of the heart just as they would postnatally (see Fig. 14–10 A). With slight motion of the scan plane toward the fetal left side, the right ventricular outflow tract, pulmonary valve, main pulmonary artery, and descending aorta can also be demonstrated (see Fig. 14–10B). From the long axis, slight clockwise rotation allows one to display the aortic root and the entire aortic arch (see Fig. 14–1C), including the origin of the head and neck arteries, the aortic isthmus, the innominate vein, and the right pulmonary artery (Fig. 14–11). This plane is important because the origin of the head and neck vessels may help to identify the laterality of the aortic arch. Moving the plane slightly farther leftward shows the main pulmonary artery and its continuation into the descending aorta, where the ductus arteriosus is defined as that vessel connecting the pulmonary trunk, at the site of the origin of its branches, to the descending aorta (the ductus arch, Fig. 14–12). Aortic isthmus narrowing is a normal feature in utero (Fig. 14–13) but may be distinguished from coarctation.

From these classic long-axis planes, views in the short axis, similar to those obtained postnatally, can

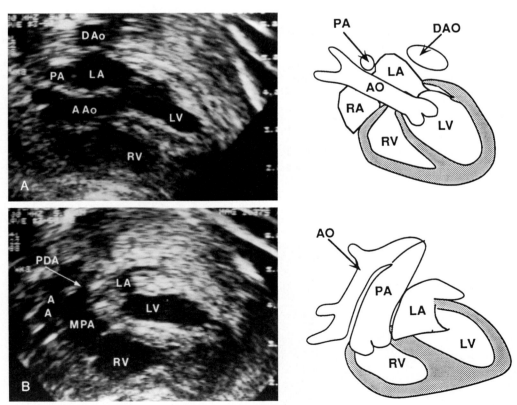

Figure 14–9. From the fetal four-chamber view, with anterior angulation of the transducer, the ventriculoarterial connections are imaged. *A.* The ascending aorta (AAo) is seen arising from the left ventricle (LV). The circular pulmonary artery (PA) lies above the left atrium (LA) and behind the ascending aorta. DAo, descending aorta; RV, right ventricle. *B.* With even further anterior angulation of the ultrasonic beam, the main pulmonary artery (MPA) is displayed arising from the right ventricle (RV), as it lies below the aortic arch (AA). The ductus arteriosus (PDA) is seen arising from the distal end of the main pulmonary artery. The diagrams on the right represent the important anatomic features of the echocardiogram.

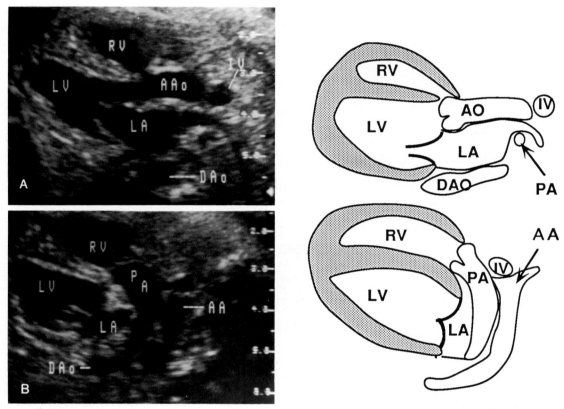

Figure 14–10. Magnified fetal long-axis view demonstrating the left atrioventricular and both ventriculoarterial connections. *A.* The left atrium (LA) drains into the left ventricle (LV) by way of the mitral valve. The ascending aorta (AAo) arises from the left ventricle. The innominate vein (IV) is seen coursing anterior to the aorta. The descending aorta (DAo), running posterior to the left atrium, is imaged in cross section. *B.* With slight angulation of the scan plane to the fetal left side, the pulmonary artery (PA) is seen arising from the right ventricle (RV) and running below the aortic arch (AA). The diagrams on the right represent the important anatomic features of the echocardiogram.

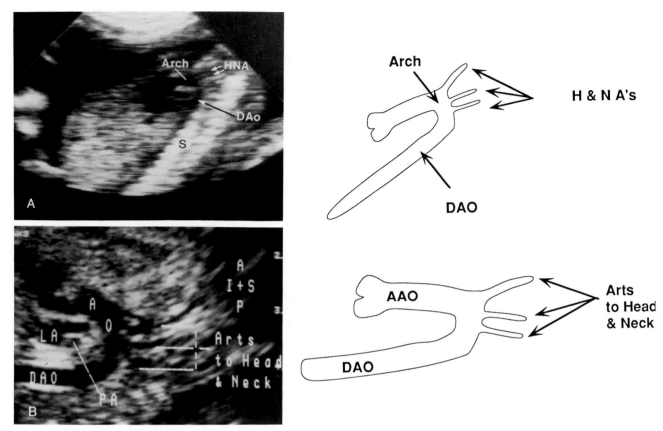

Figure 14–11. Fetal sagittal view of the entire aortic arch in an 18-week fetus. *A*. The arch, with the head and neck arteries (HNA), can be seen; the descending aorta (DAo) lies in front of the spine (S). *B*. This magnified view, obtained from a different fetus, shows three arteries (Arts) to the head and neck, arising from the aortic arch (AO). These arteries are the innominate, the left carotid, and the left subclavian. In the concavity of this arch, the left atrium (LA) and the right pulmonary artery (PA) are seen. Note that the "ductus arch" cannot be seen in this plane. A, anterior; I, inferior; P, posterior; S, superior. The diagrams on the right represent the important anatomic features of the echocardiogram.

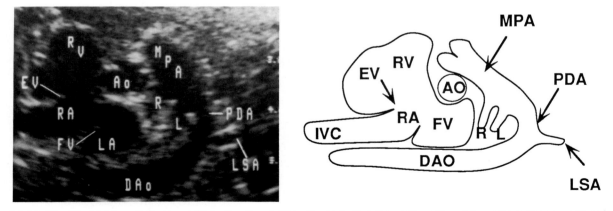

Figure 14–12. Magnified fetal sagittal view at 36 weeks of gestation, demonstrating the continuation of the main pulmonary artery (MPA), ductus arteriosus (PDA), and descending aorta (DAo), the so-called ductus arch. The ascending aorta (Ao) is seen in cross section; the main pulmonary artery gives rise to the right (R) and left (L) branch pulmonary arteries. The ductus begins after the branch pulmonary arteries are given off and ends where the left subclavian artery (LSA) arises from the descending aorta. Note that the ductus at this stage of gestation appears to be narrower than the pulmonary artery or the descending aorta. The other structures identified in this view are the eustachian valve (EV) within the right atrium (RA), the flap valve of the foramen ovale (FV) within the left atrium (LA), and the right ventricle (RV). The diagram on the right represents the important anatomic features of the echocardiogram.

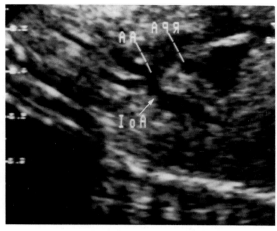

Figure 14–13. Magnified fetal sagittal view of the aortic arch (AA), demonstrating the normal aortic isthmus (AoI), which is relatively narrow. RPA, right pulmonary artery.

be acquired (see Fig. 14–1D and E). The short axis here refers to images obtained perpendicular to the long axis of the heart. Because of the horizontal lie of the fetal heart, the long- and short-axis views are often at right angles to or parallel to the fetal spine, respectively. The short-axis views allow the visualization of the fetal heart from the level of the cardiac apex through the level of the ventricles (where the papillary muscle architecture in the left ventricle is best displayed) and more cranially (where the mitral valve morphology is characteristic [see Fig. 14–4B]) up to the level of the great arteries (where the right ventricular outflow tract, the pulmonary trunk with its bifurcation into the branch pulmonary arteries [Fig. 14–14], and the ductus arteriosus can be seen). In this plane, obstructive lesions of the right ventricular outflow tract and of both semilunar valves can be displayed, and the size and position of the great arteries assessed. With high-resolution equipment, even the proximal coronary arteries may be displayed in this plane, thus helping to define the aortic vessel (Fig. 14–15).

M-Mode Echocardiography

Real-time directed M-mode echocardiography is a useful addition to cross-sectional imaging in the evaluation of fetal ventricular cavity dimension and wall thickness or valve and wall motion, as well as cardiac arrhythmias.[12, 15, 18, 29–31, 35, 36] Both long- and short-axis views at the level of the atrioventricular valves allow the assessment of ventricular size (Fig. 14–16). Previous studies have provided percentiles of ventricular sizes and arterial diameters from which comparisons can readily be made (Figs. 14–17 and 14–18). At the base of the heart, the movement of both semilunar valves can be seen, and the diameter of the great arteries measured (Fig. 14–19). Pericardial effusions, especially when small, are best substantiated by M-mode display, which demonstrates the separation of the parietal and visceral pericardium, better distinguishing a pericardial effusion from a pleural effusion in the hydropic fetus (Fig. 14–20). For the exploration of fetal arrhythmias, M-mode recordings can be obtained from any plane, which allows the simultaneous display of movements of an atrial and a ventricular wall or of a semilunar and an atrioventricular valve. The start of an atrial contraction is defined either by the onset of contraction of the atrial wall or by the F-point of an atrioventricular valve motion (Fig. 14–21). The start of a ventricular contraction is defined by the onset of ventricular wall motion, by the closure of an atrioventricular valve (C-point), or by the opening of a semilunar valve (see Fig. 14–21). Since the electromechanical delay differs between these points, one should consistently use the same markers in each study.

Imaging of the atrial wall motion may be difficult because of its small amplitude, but this technique is most valuable because the direct result of atrial contraction can be seen in most cases by careful examination (Fig. 14–22). If the M-mode recordings are obtained from the posterior fetal aspect, their display is inverted with respect to conventional M-mode display. The M-mode tracings can be read more easily by

Text continued on page 306

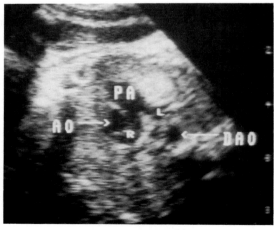

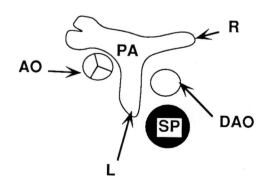

Figure 14–14. Fetal short-axis view at the level of the aortic root (AO), depicting the pulmonary artery (PA) and its bifurcation into the right (R) and left (L) pulmonary arteries. The descending aorta (DAO) is seen in cross section behind the bifurcating pulmonary branches. SP, spine. The diagram on the right represents the important anatomic features of the echocardiogram.

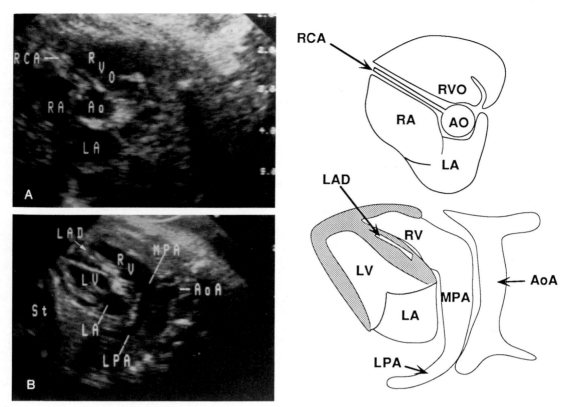

Figure 14–15. *A.* A magnified fetal short-axis view displays the right coronary artery (RCA), which arises from the aortic root (Ao). RVO, right ventricular outflow tract; LA, left atrium; RA, right atrium. *B.* A long-axis view of the right ventricular (RV) outflow tract shows the left anterior descending coronary artery (LAD) running on the ventricular septum. AoA, aortic arch; LA, left atrium; LPA, left pulmonary artery; LV, left ventricle; MPA, main pulmonary artery; St, stomach. The diagrams on the right represent the important anatomic features of the echocardiogram.

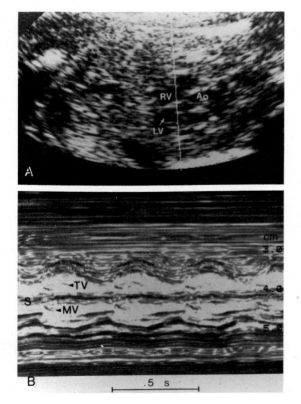

Figure 14–16. Real-time directed M-mode echocardiography at ventricular level in the fetus. *A.* In this cross-sectional image, the M-mode cursor line crosses the right (RV) and left (LV) ventricles, seen in long axis. Ao, aorta. *B.* The M-mode recording shows normal contractions and thickening of both ventricular walls in systole. The movement of the tips of the tricuspid (TV) and mitral (MV) valves is seen. The ventricular septum (S) and both ventricular free walls have about the same thickness.

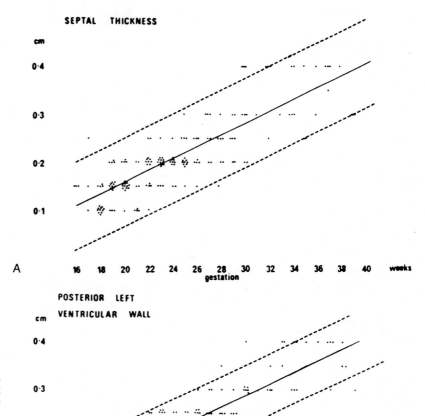

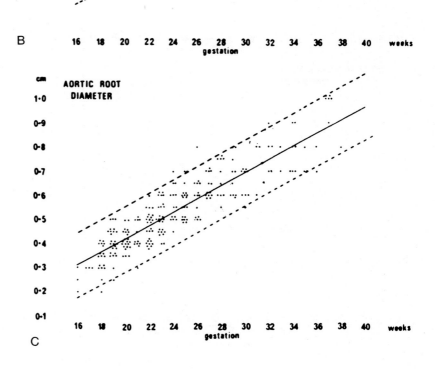

Figure 14–17. Graphic display of normal M-mode measurements of septal thickness *(A),* posterior left ventricular wall thickness *(B),* and aortic root diameters *(C)* in fetuses from 16 weeks' gestation to term. Values in centimeters (*y*-axis) are plotted against gestational age (*x*-axis); the dotted lines represent twice the standard error of the mean *(straight line).* (From Allan LD, Joseph MC, Boyd EGC, et al: M-mode echocardiography in the developing human fetus. Br Heart J 47:573, 1982.)

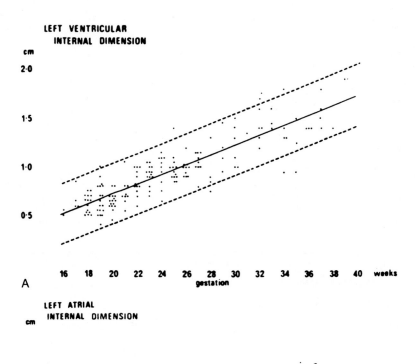

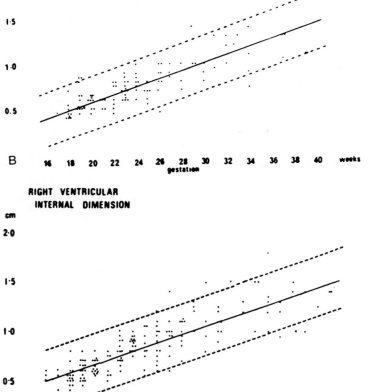

Figure 14–18. Graphic display of normal M-mode measurements of left ventricular *(A),* left atrial *(B),* and right ventricular *(C)* internal diameters in fetuses from 16 weeks' gestation to term. (From Allan LD, Joseph MC, Boyd EGC, et al: M-mode echocardiography in the developing human fetus. Br Heart J 47:573, 1982.)

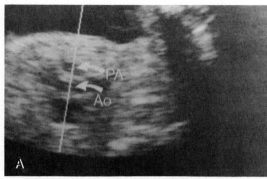

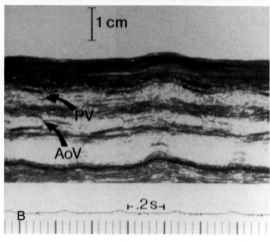

Figure 14–19. M-mode echocardiogram at the level of both great arteries. *A.* At the base of the heart, the M-mode reference line crosses the pulmonary artery (PA) and the aortic root (Ao). *B.* The typical systolic motion of both semilunar valves as open boxes is demonstrated. The black arrows indicate the closure of the pulmonary valve (PV) and of the aortic valve (AoV). The diameters of both great vessels can easily be measured from this M-mode recording.

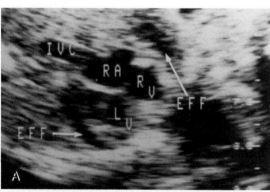

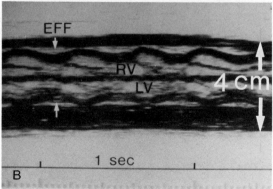

Figure 14–20. *A.* Magnified cross-sectional image of the heart at 22 weeks' gestation in a fetus with nonimmune hydrops. Although the pericardial effusion (EFF, *arrows*) may be seen, it can better be substantiated from the M-mode recording in the same fetus *(B).* The dense echoes of the pericardium and the rhythmically contracting ventricular myocardium are separated by the echo-free area of the effusion. IVC, inferior vena cava; LV, left ventricle; RA, right atrium; RV, right ventricle.

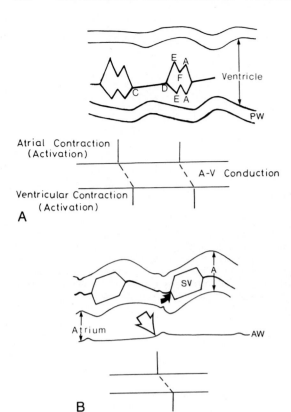

Figure 14–21. Schematic representation depicting the motion of cardiac structures as visualized by M-mode echocardiography, and ladder diagrams from these recordings. *A.* The ultrasound beam passes through a ventricle and an atrioventricular valve within it. The atrioventricular valve leaflets can be seen opening in early diastole (D-E portion), moving toward each other in mid diastole (E-F), and moving away from each other again in late diastole during atrial contraction (F-A). The beginning of this second opening (F-point) indicates the onset of atrial contraction. The closure of the valve leaflets (C-point) or the beginning of the forward motion of the posterior ventricular wall (PW) indicates the onset of the ventricular contraction. The ladder diagram *(below)* marks these events; the delay between atrial and ventricular activation is the atrioventricular (AV) conduction time. *B.* The ultrasound beam passes through the root of a great artery (A) and the semilunar valve within it, then through an atrium behind that vessel. The M-mode recording shows the onset of the forward motion of the atrial wall (AW, *open arrow*) that defines the beginning of atrial contraction. The opening of the semilunar valve (SV, *black arrow*) defines the beginning of the ventricular contraction. The ladder diagram *(below)* demonstrates these events as in the top panel.

inverting the recording and viewing it through a mirror (Fig. 14–23). These two maneuvers allow an orientation and pattern recognition similar to that achieved postnatally.

When structural abnormalities of the heart are coupled with an arrhythmia, such as with complete heart block[13, 15, 16] or, less frequently, with a tachyarrhythmia,[37] M-mode echocardiography is especially valuable. Even with direction of the cursor through the cardiac image, the variable fetal position may not allow a standardized beam orientation such as is possible postnatally, which makes the quantitative interpretation of M-mode echocardiography more difficult.

Doppler Echocardiography

Pulsed Doppler echocardiography is obtained by guiding the sample volume through the cross-sectional reference image. Doppler interrogation within vascular structures, either at the level of the umbilical cord or within the fetal body, identifies arterial or venous flow (see Figs. 14–8 and 14–24), assisting the sonographer to distinguish arteries and veins and to evaluate the direction of blood flow in complex cardiovascular malformations. Normal flow velocity profiles across both the atrioventricular and the semilunar valves have been defined in the fetus (Fig. 14–25)[38–41]; normal values for

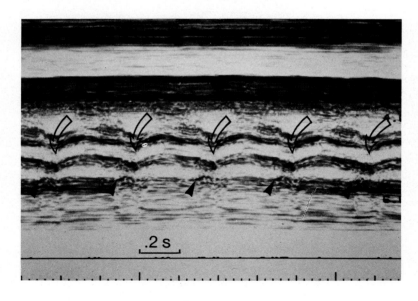

Figure 14–22. M-mode echocardiogram from a 24-week fetus with normal heart. The ultrasound beam passes through the right atrioventricular junction, the aortic root, and the left atrium. Atrial contraction *(arrowheads)* can be seen preceding ventricular contraction, which is indicated by aortic valve opening *(open arrows)* in this example.

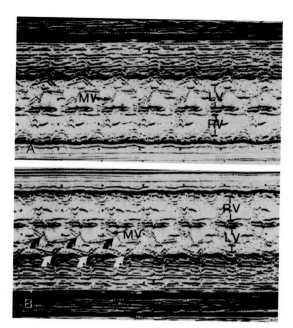

Figure 14–23. Fetal M-mode recording at ventricular level; the fetus is lying with its back toward the ultrasound transducer. *A.* The original display appears inverted compared with conventional M-mode display. Pattern recognition, therefore, becomes difficult. The M-mode recording shows the left ventricle (LV) on top and runs from right to left. *B.* Inverting the recording and viewing it in a mirror allows an orientation as seen postnatally. The same effect was achieved in this example by turning the negative of the original photograph backward, to display the appropriate lateral inversion, and printing it upside down. The onset of atrial contraction *(black arrows)* and of ventricular contraction *(white arrows)* can now easily be defined in the correct temporal sequence. MV, mitral valve; RV, right ventricle.

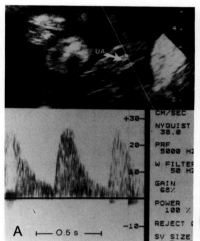

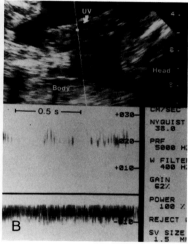

Figure 14–24. Pulsed Doppler interrogation at the site of the umbilical cord. *A.* The Doppler sample volume lies within the umbilical artery (UA, *arrow*). In the lower panel, a characteristic umbilical arterial signal is displayed above the baseline, demonstrating flow toward the transducer. *B.* The Doppler sample volume is now seen within the umbilical vein (UV, *arrow*); the fetal body and head are also shown. In the lower panel, a venous flow signal of fairly uniform low velocity throughout systole and diastole is demonstrated below the baseline; this flow is directed away from the transducer and toward the fetal body. Because the wall filter was set at 400 Hz, compared with 50 Hz in *A*, the origin of the spectral signals is blanked out.

Figure 14–25. Normal fetal Doppler flow profiles across an atrioventricular and a semilunar valve are shown. *A.* In a four-chamber view *(top)*, the left atrium (LA), the right atrium (RA), the left ventricle (LV), and the right ventricle (RV) are seen. The sample volume lies below the tricuspid valve. The Doppler display *(bottom)* shows the diastolic inflow into the right ventricle above the baseline, indicating its direction toward the transducer. A biphasic signal is seen with a smaller v-component resulting from rapid venous filling, followed by a larger a-component *(black arrowheads)* resulting from atrial contraction. This pattern with predominant a-waves is typical for the fetus. The mirrorlike display below the baseline is an artifact caused by too high a gain setting. *B.* In a fetal short-axis view *(top)*, the right atrium (RA), right ventricle (RV), pulmonary artery (PA), and aorta (Ao) are seen. The sample volume lies distal to the pulmonary valve within the pulmonary artery. The Doppler flow signal below the baseline is directed away from the transducer *(bottom)*.

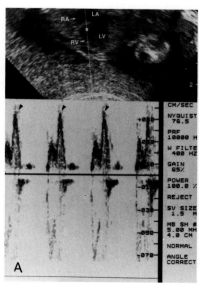

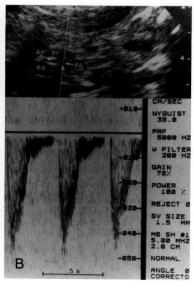

Table 14–2. FLOW MEASUREMENT IN THE NORMAL FETAL HEART

	Peak Velocity (cm/s)	Mean Temporal Velocity (cm/s)
Tricuspid valve*	51 ± 9.1	11.8 ± 3.1
Mitral valve*	47 ± 8.3	11.2 ± 2.3
Pulmonary valve*	60 ± 12.9	16 ± 4.1
Aortic valve*	70 ± 12.2	18 ± 3.3
Right ventricular output†	307 ± 127 mL/kg/min	
Left ventricular output†	232 ± 106 mL/kg/min	

*Angle-corrected maximal and mean temporal flow velocities across the cardiac valves are expressed as mean ± SD.

†Cardiac output derived from tricuspid and mitral valve area and mean velocities (mean ± SD).

Adapted from Reed KL, Meijboom EJ, Sahn DJ, et al: Cardiac Doppler flow velocities in human fetuses. Circulation 73:41, 1986.

peak and mean temporal flow velocities, as well as for volume flow across these valves, have been established (Table 14–2). The flow velocity curve across a fetal atrioventricular valve is normally characterized by a v-component (due to venous filling), which is followed by a higher a-component (due to atrial contraction) (see Fig. 14–25A). This pattern is different from that observed postnatally and in the adult when the v-component is higher than the a-component; this difference may relate to the fetal ventricular size or to diminished ventricular compliance. Because the flow through the atrioventricular orifice relates to filling in that portion of diastole, the high a-component in the fetus suggests that a substantial amount of filling occurs as a result of atrial contraction. This may explain why fetal tachycardia is so poorly tolerated in the fetus and may lead to the development of fetal hydrops.

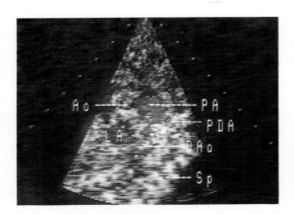

Figure 14–26. Doppler color-flow map taken in a short-axis view in a fetus of 34 weeks' gestation, with complete heart block and a structurally normal heart. The red and blue color bars indicate flow directed toward and away from the transducer, respectively. Normal flow directed away from the transducer is seen in the pulmonary artery (PA) indicated by blue color, but a change in color occurs in the ductus arteriosus (PDA) and in the descending aorta (DAo). This color change into yellow and turquoise represents a phenomenon called aliasing. Aliasing occurs when the velocity of the blood flow exceeds the equipment's ability to recognize the velocity accurately. In this case, the acceleration of the flow velocity is related to the narrowing of the ductus arteriosus that occurs as the fetus matures. Ao, aorta; LA, left atrium; Sp, spine.

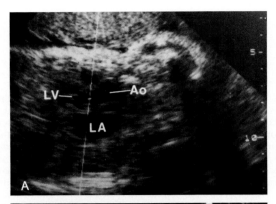

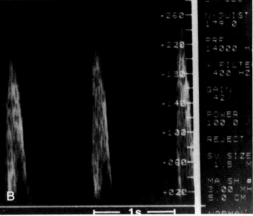

Figure 14–27. *A.* Long-axis view of a fetal heart at 32 weeks' gestation, with mild subaortic obstruction and complete heart block. The Doppler sample volume lies just above the aortic valve in the ascending aorta (Ao). The left atrium (LA) and left ventricle (LV) are also seen. *B.* Although the angle at the site of Doppler interrogation is more than 25 degrees, thus underestimating the flow velocity, high pulse repetition frequency Doppler demonstrates a jet velocity of 2.5 m/s. Some of this increase in velocity is related to the increased stroke volume associated with complete heart block.

The highest velocity in the fetal heart is recorded within the ductus arteriosus[42]; color-coded Doppler flow mapping demonstrates flow within the fetal ductus with the peak velocities exceeding the Nyquist limit. (Fig. 14–26). By using Doppler interrogation in a direction where the velocity of blood flow is axial to the sample volume, one may obtain high-velocity profiles across stenotic or regurgitant atrioventricular and semilunar valves, which permits estimation of the pressure difference across these valves (Fig. 14–27). For this purpose, the modified Bernoulli equation is used, which states that the pressure drop (measured in millimeters of mercury) across an orifice is proportional to four times the squared peak velocity (measured in meters per second) across that valve:

$$P = 4V_d^2$$

where V_d is the high velocity in the stenotic area or just distal to it.[43, 44]

Doppler ultrasonography also aids in the analysis of cardiac rhythm disturbances. Sampling in any arterial vessel provides a measurement of heart rate, and sampling within the region of an atrioventricular valve provides information about valve opening and closure. By increasing the size of the sample volume, it is possible to obtain signals from two chambers or vessels simultaneously, for example, from both the descending aorta and left atrial wall in complete heart block, demonstrating the asynchronous contraction of atria and ventricles (Fig. 14–28). The characteristics of the pulse in the umbilical artery have been used to demonstrate altered flow dynamics in growth-retarded fetuses. The ratio of the peak systolic velocity divided by the minimal diastolic velocity is called the S/D or A/B ratio; it changes normally during gestation.[45, 46] Higher ratios suggest a decreased flow to the placenta that may be due to a higher resistance of the placental vascular bed such as seems to occur in growth-retarded fetuses.[47] With ratios, the measurements may be less dependent on the angle of insonance. In our experience, Doppler ultrasonography is an essential technique that enables us to demonstrate stenotic and regurgitant lesions[48] and to diagnose arrthythmias in a fetus with congenital heart disease. The use of this modality allows the detection of cardiac lesions (e.g., mitral regurgitation in cardiomyopathy) not possible by other methods.

Doppler Color Flow Mapping

Doppler color flow mapping has provided a substantial addition to the diagnostic armamentarium. This procedure is essentially a pulsed Doppler technique, in which flow is represented as traveling toward or away from the baseline at a particular velocity at a particular point in time. The same is true with color flow, where the direction of flow is represented by colors; usually, hotter colors represent higher velocities

of flow toward the transducer and colder colors represent flow velocities away from the transducer, with higher velocities represented in increasing shades of lightness. We prefer to use velocity flow maps, as are generally used in pediatric or adult echocardiography, in which low velocities traveling toward the transducer are represented in red and increasing velocities toward the transducer are represented in shades of orange to yellow and the velocities traveling away from the transducer are represented in blue, with the higher velocities represented in lighter shades. The pulsed Doppler technique aliases when its Nyquist limit is exceeded (i.e., the signal wraps around the display). Similarly, color flow mapping exhibits the same response, but because of the lower sampling rates the Nyquist limit is substantially lower. High-velocity flow exceeding the Nyquist limits is thus represented by ambiguous or mixed color, another form of aliasing. This usually involves mixing of yellow and blue to form green or alternating shades of yellow and blue in the Doppler signal.

We have found the technique useful for defining normal flow events as well as abnormal flow events. Because of the speed with which these flow events can be determined and the opportunity for an accurate alignment based on the direction of blood flow, a much more rapid evaluation of the fetal cardiovascular system can be achieved using Doppler ultrasonography than with the pulsed or continuous wave modalities alone. In fact, after cross-sectional imaging, this modality is the next technique we now use, with pulsed and continuous wave Doppler imaging being reserved for more specific effects and for accurate measurement of velocity.

The Doppler signal can be used to identify usual flow in organs (Figs. 14–29 through 14–31). In addi-

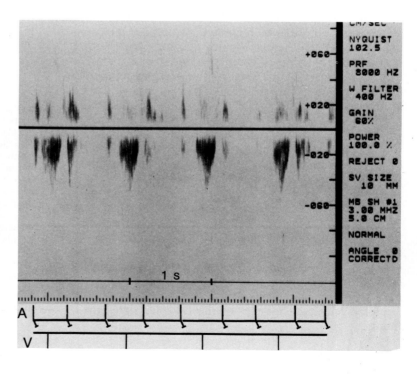

Figure 14–28. Pulsed Doppler recording from a fetus with complete heart block. Note in the right-hand side of the figure that the sample volume (SV) size has been increased to 10 mm. It has been placed astride the descending aorta and the left atrium in such a way as to allow simultaneous sampling of aortic flow and left atrial wall motion. The aortic flow is seen as the broader signal below the baseline. The smaller signals above and below the baseline indicate the wall "knock" of the left atrial contractions. The ladder diagram *(below)* demonstrates a ventricular rate of 65 beats per minute but an atrial rate of about 130 beats per minute; both chambers beat independently of each other.

tion, the flow signal is often very helpful for defining regular morphology when it is not easily visible using cross-sectional imaging alone (see Fig. 14–30). The technique is also helpful for defining defects or confirming their presence (Figs. 14–32 through 14–34). For example, the presence of a flow disturbance across an area of dropout, as identified in Figure 14–32, provides additional information as to the presence of a ventricular septal defect. In addition, the presence of shunting between the two ventricles provides additional physiologic information as to the timing of slight pressure differences between the ventricles (the pressures in both ventricles in the fetus are nearly identical). However, the presence of valvular stenosis permits observation of flow direction between the various chambers. Atrioventricular valve regurgitation or stenosis can be detected easily (see Fig. 14–33); in addition, color flow mapping allows one to determine whether a pulsed Doppler evaluation of velocity, in which axial alignment is necessary, can be achieved from a particular angle of interrogation (see Fig. 14–33). The presence of abnormal flow patterns also can be determined. Figure 14–34 shows a left-to-right shunt through the ductus arteriosus, the reverse of the expected direction in the fetus. Such a signal would need to be confirmed by means of pulsed Doppler or continuous wave Doppler imaging, but with reference to the real-time events in this instance, one could clearly see that the flow in the ductus arteriosus occurred after the aortic arch had been filled. This direction of flow indicates the presence of some obstruction to forward flow across the pulmonary valve. In this instance the fetus was confirmed to have an atretic pulmonary valve and the pulmonary arteries were filled exclusively through the ductus arteriosus.

The direction of flow can also be defined in structures the position of which is normal but in which flow was reversed. For example, in Figure 14–35, in a patient with total anomalous pulmonary venous return, flow in the vertical vein was identified as occurring in an abnormal direction for a venous channel. Placement of the pulsed Doppler sample within this structure (Fig. 14–35, *left panel*) showed the presence of flow toward the transducer, indicating that this venous structure carried abnormal flow, likely due to the presence of total anomalous pulmonary venous return with a vertical vein carrying blood toward the superior vena cava. In addition to this superimposition of color on cross-sectional imaging, color also can be superimposed on M-mode recordings (Fig. 14–36). This allows acute observation of timing, such as the temporal relationship of the regurgitant jet over the course of systole or the separation between the various parts of the circulation. Once a flow disturbance or flow event has been defined by color flow, appropriate selection of either continuous wave, pulsed wave, or M-mode superimposition can be used to define more specifically the questions one needs to answer with regard to Doppler velocity, character of the Doppler signal, or timing.

INTERPRETATION

Detection of Structural Defects

Of the 1650 fetuses we have now studied, a structural cardiac abnormality was found in 9.4% (Table 14–3). Normal cardiac anatomy with a cardiac rhythm disturbance was present in 18%. The remaining studies were within normal limits. The diagnosis of the structural cardiac defect was confirmed postnatally in all except two fetuses.

The most common structural abnormality in our experience was an atrioventricular septal defect, 1.5% of our total number of cases (see Table 14–3; Fig. 14–37). Often this defect was part of a complex cardiac lesion including left atrial isomerism, complete heart block, and nonimmune hydrops. Three of these pregnancies were terminated because of a fetal chromosomal defect. Seventy-five percent of the remaining fetuses with atrioventricular septal defect died either in utero or during the neonatal period. Although there were many referrals for examination because of trisomy 21 found at amniocentesis, one fetus was found to have duodenal atresia on ultrasound evaluation. The mother had refused amniocentesis. This fetus was also found to have an atrioventricular septal defect after birth.

Ventricular septal defects were also found frequently (Fig. 14–38), in 1.5% of our total number of cases. Occasionally the spontaneous closure of ventricular septal defects was observed on subsequent fetal ex-

Text continued on page 315

Table 14–3. STRUCTURAL ABNORMALITIES AND SURVIVORS

	n (% of Total)	Survivors (% of n)
Atrioventricular septal defect (including four with left atrial isomerism and complete heart block)	1.5	18.2
Ventricular septal defect (including one with left atrial isomerism and complete heart block)	1.5	45.5
Cardiomyopathy (including three with familial cardiomyopathy)	0.9	28.6*
Pulmonary atresia/stenosis without ventricular septal defect	0.8	33.3
Double-outlet right ventricle (including one with pulmonary stenosis)	0.7	0
Hypoplastic left heart syndrome	0.7	0
Univentricular atrioventricular connection (three left-sided, one right-sided)	0.5	0
Ebstein anomaly	0.4	0
Aortopulmonary transposition with ventricular septal defect	0.3	0
Truncus arteriosus/tetralogy of Fallot	0.3	0
Multiple rhabdomyoma	0.3	50.0
Thoracopagus	0.4	0
Others	1.1	37.5
Total	9.4	

*One after heart transplant at 6 months of age.

Figure 14–29. In the left-hand frame, the ductus venosus (DV), inferior vena cava (IVC), left atrium (LA), superior vena cava (SVC), and right ventricle (RV) are identified. The example on the right shows the superimposition of color flow, with red flow directed toward the transducer and blue flow directed away from the transducer. Flow from the inferior vena cava and ductus venosus is highlighted in blue, whereas atrial and right ventricular flow is seen as red in this diastolic frame. RA, right atrium.

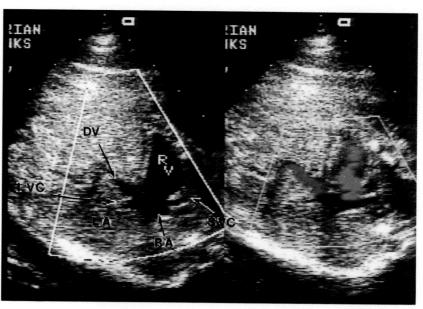

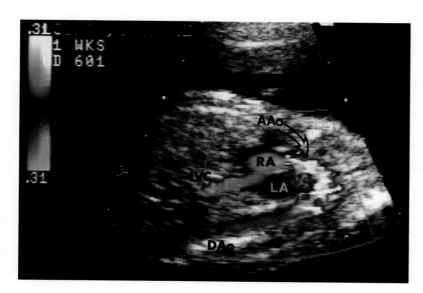

Figure 14–30. In this example, taken in a fetal sagittal body plane, the chest wall lies anteriorly and the spine posteriorly. The neck is on the viewer's right, and the abdomen is on the viewer's left. The scale bar on the left indicates the Nyquist limit range of flow velocity, which can be detected at 31 cm/s. Increasing velocities to 31 cm/s coming toward the transducer are in shades of red and yellow, and velocities away from the transducer to 31 cm/s (the Nyquist limits) are in increasingly light shades of blue and azure. In this frame, the red flow can be seen within the inferior vena cava (IVC) and right atrium (RA). In the sagittal plane, the entire aortic arch (AAo) is imaged with high velocities aliased above the 31-cm/s limit traveling away from the transducer in the proximal aorta, where the flow direction within the vessel is axial to ultrasound flow, ranging to darker blue, where the angle of insonification is almost parallel to the direction of flow. Nevertheless, this technique highlights the inferior vena cava, right atrium, aortic arch, and the origins of vessels to the head and neck, as well as flow in the descending aorta (DAo). LA, left atrium.

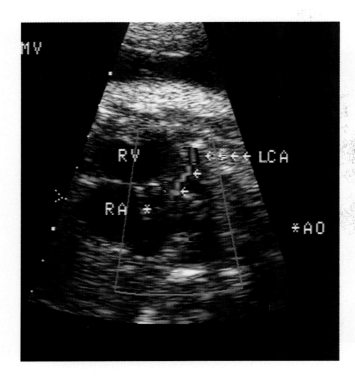

Figure 14–31. In this example, the aorta (∗) is identified in cross section, and flow in the left coronary artery (LCA), indicated by arrows, arising from the left sinus of Valsalva can be seen clearly directed toward the transducer. RA, right atrium; RV, right ventricle.

Figure 14–32. In this color-flow example of a midmuscular ventricular septal defect taken in a 25-week fetus, the defect (VSD) can be identified, with flow demonstrated between the two chambers (RV, LV).

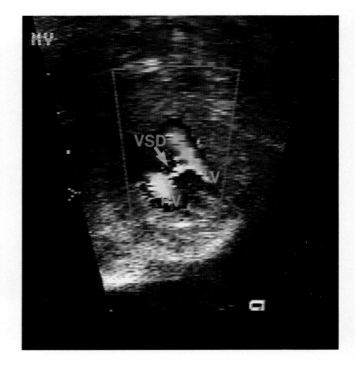

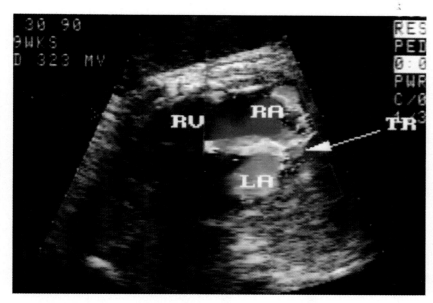

Figure 14–33. In this example of tricuspid regurgitation noted in a patient with pulmonary atresia during fetal life, a prominent stream of tricuspid regurgitation (TR) between the right ventricle (RV) and right atrium (RA) can be seen. The jet travels along the septum between the left atrium (LA) and right atrium, then fans along the posterior margin of the right atrium toward the transducer. Aliased flow at an almost horizontal angle of insonification suggests high-velocity tricuspid regurgitation consistent with the diagnosis of pulmonary atresia.

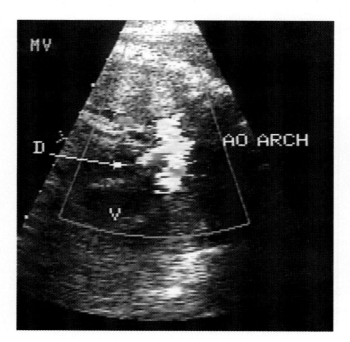

Figure 14–34. Color flow is identified within the aorta arising from the ventricle (V) and traveling toward the transducer. In addition, high-velocity flow into the ductus arteriosus (D, *arrow*) is identified, indicating the reverse direction of flow from that expected in the fetus, suggesting obstruction to right ventricular outflow.

Figure 14–35. In this patient, in whom findings strongly indicated the presence of abnormal situs and transposition of the great arteries, a Doppler color-flow map identified venous flow *(right panel)* in a vertical vein. The pulsed Doppler sample placed within this vessel indicated that the direction of the venous flow was toward the transducer, that is, away from the heart, indicating that this was a vertical vein (VV) associated with total anomalous pulmonary venous return. AO, aorta; DAO, descending aorta; RV, right ventricle.

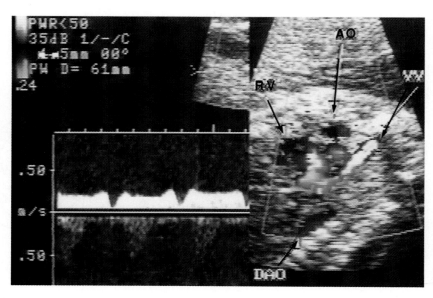

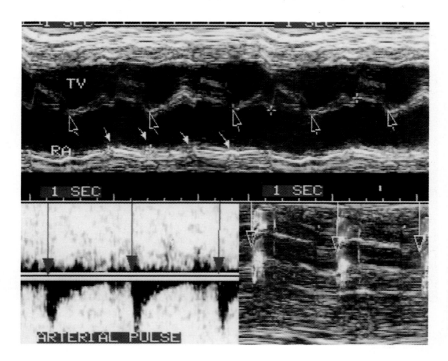

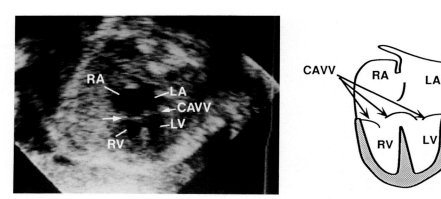

Figure 14–36. This example, from a fetus who had complete heart block, is a composite of M-mode echocardiography taken in a four-chamber view and passing through the right ventricular tricuspid valve (TV) and right atrium (RA) *(top)*, pulsed Doppler ultrasound from the umbilical artery *(bottom left),* and a Doppler color-flow map superimposed upon M-mode echocardiography through the pulmonary valve and identifying pulmonary ejection *(bottom right)*. The M-mode shows the right atrial contractions at approximately 150/min *(closed arrows),* whereas the ventricular rate *(open arrows),* judged from the tricuspid valve closure (TV) indicating the onset of ventricular systole, indicates one ventricular contraction per second. The time markers are identical, five markers being equivalent to 1-second intervals. In all these modalities, the ventricular rate is approximately 60 beats per minute, or 1-second intervals, whereas only the M-mode echocardiogram demonstrates the atrial rate, at approximately 150 beats per minute (400 ms). The Doppler color-flow map superimposed upon the M-mode echocardiogram allows easy recognition of the timing events.

Figure 14–37. Fetal four-chamber view at 32 weeks' gestation. An atrioventricular (canal) septal defect is demonstrated. The common atrioventricular valve (CAVV, *white arrows*) straddles a common atrioventricular orifice dividing the large defect seen in this view into an atrial and a ventricular component. LA, left atrium; LV, left ventricle; RA, right atrium; RV, right ventricle. DAO, descending aorta. The diagram on the right represents the important anatomic features of the echocardiogram.

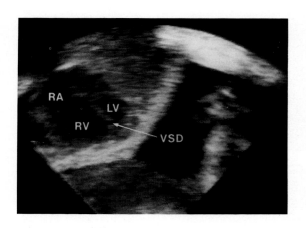

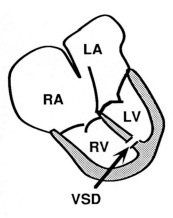

Figure 14–38. Fetal four-chamber view in a 32-week fetus. An isolated ventricular septal defect (VSD) is depicted in the apical muscular part of the ventricular septum. LV, left ventricle; RA, right atrium; RV, right ventricle. The diagram on the right represents the important anatomic features of the echocardiogram.

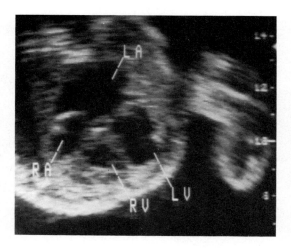
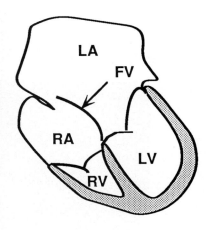

Figure 14–39. Magnified four-chamber view in a 31-week fetus with cardiomyopathy, severe mitral regurgitation, and hydrops. In this end-systolic frame, the left atrium (LA) and the left ventricle (LV) are considerably dilated, whereas the right atrium (RA) and the right ventricle (RV) appear to be of normal size. The diagram on the right represents the important anatomic features of the echocardiogram. FV, flap-valve of the foramen ovale.

aminations when there was no additional lesion. Nine cases of cardiomyopathy were encountered, more often the congestive form with a dilated, poorly contracting ventricle and atrioventricular valve regurgitation associated with fetal hydrops (Figs. 14–39 and 14–40). One fetus presented with a hypertrophic cardiomyopathy (Fig. 14–41) and was clinically identified to have Noonan syndrome at birth. Two fetuses appeared to have normal cardiac function at 20 weeks' gestational age but shortly after birth were recognized to have

congestive cardiomyopathy, suggesting that it may not always be possible to detect this abnormality prenatally and that myocardial dysfunction may occur either after examination in utero or after birth.

Complex forms of cardiac defects were diagnosed, such as univentricular atrioventricular connection in four fetuses, presenting in one as an absent right-sided atrioventricular connection with ventriculoarterial discordance (Figs. 14–42 and 14–43), and in three as an absent left-sided atrioventricular connection, a double-outlet right ventricle, and a hypoplastic or an interrupted aortic arch (Figs. 14–44 and 14–45). Ebstein anomaly was detected in five fetuses (Figs. 14–46 and 14–47); one of them died in utero with severe hydrops, and two others died during the first week of life. One of these fetuses was the product of a mother who had the same lesion; another one was born to a mother who had taken high doses of lithium, a known cardiac teratogen,[23, 49] during early pregnancy.

Five fetuses were found to have transposition of the great arteries with a ventricular septal defect; one also had pulmonary atresia (Fig. 14–48). In a thoracopagus twin detected as early as 16 weeks, we noted the hearts to be fused with shared atria and shared ventricles, one common atrioventricular valve, and only one dilated great artery in each body (pulmonary atresia in one, aortic hypoplasia with interrupted arch in the other) (Fig. 14–49). Several other lesions were encountered once, including absent pulmonary valve complex (Figs. 14–50 and 14–51), persistent truncus arteriosus (Fig. 14–52), and multiple intracardiac rhabdomyoma due to tuberous sclerosis (Fig. 14–53).

Using pulsed Doppler imaging, we detected severe atrioventricular valve regurgitation in 10 fetuses (Figs. 14–33, 14–40, and 14–54). All of these presented with fetal hydrops but with different cardiac defects, such as Ebstein anomaly, aortic or pulmonary atresia, atrioventricular septal defect, cardiomyopathy, or double-outlet right ventricle with atretic left-sided atrioventricular valve. Doppler echocardiography also aided the detection of pulmonary regurgitation (see Fig. 14–51) and disturbed flow in both left and right ventricular outflow tract obstructions (see Fig. 14–27). Display of an abnormal flow pattern indicating valvular stenosis and regurgitation was augmented using color-coded

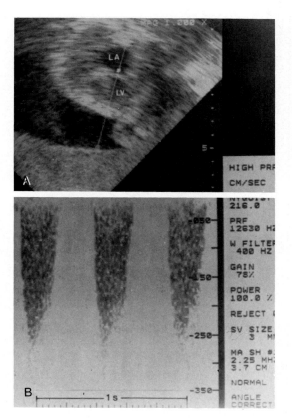

Figure 14–40. *A.* In a four-chamber view of a 28-week fetus with cardiomyopathy, the Doppler sample volume is above the mitral valve within the left atrium, which is considerably dilated. A turbulent jet of high velocity, directed away from the transducer, is displayed on high pulse repetition frequency Doppler in systole *(B),* indicating mitral insufficiency.

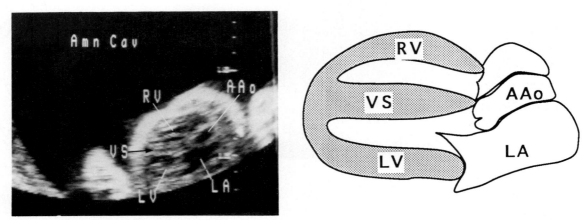

Figure 14–41. Long-axis view in a fetus with hypertrophic cardiomyopathy. This fetus was examined because of polyhydramnios. The ventricular septum (VS) and the right ventricular (RV) and the left ventricular (LV) free wall are thickened, and both ventricular cavities are diminutive. AAo, ascending aorta; Amn Cav, amniotic cavity; LA, left atrium. The diagram on the right represents the important anatomic features of the echocardiogram.

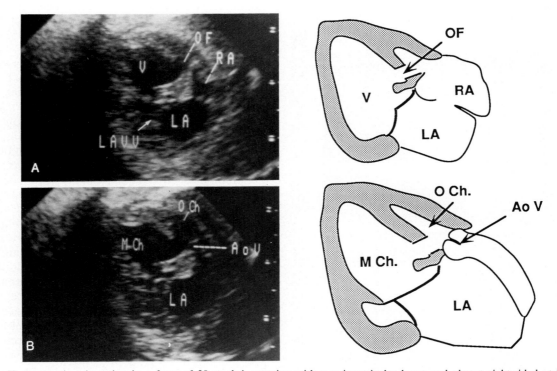

Figure 14–42. Long-axis orientation in a fetus of 38 weeks' gestation with a univentricular heart and absent right-sided atrioventricular connection ("tricuspid atresia"). *A.* Instead of a right atrioventricular valve, there is echodense tissue between the right atrium (RA) and the dilated ventricle (V). The left atrium (LA) is enlarged and drains through a left atrioventricular valve (LAVV) into the ventricle. An outlet foramen (OF) is displayed anteriorly, leading into an outlet chamber, which can better be appreciated in *B. B.* This frame demonstrates a semilunar valve connected to the outlet chamber (OCh). Since the aorta arises anteriorly from that outlet chamber (see Fig. 14–43), this is the aortic valve (AoV). The single atrioventricular valve is demonstrated lying between the left atrium (LA) and main chamber (MCh) or ventricle. The diagrams on the right represent the important anatomic features of the echocardiogram.

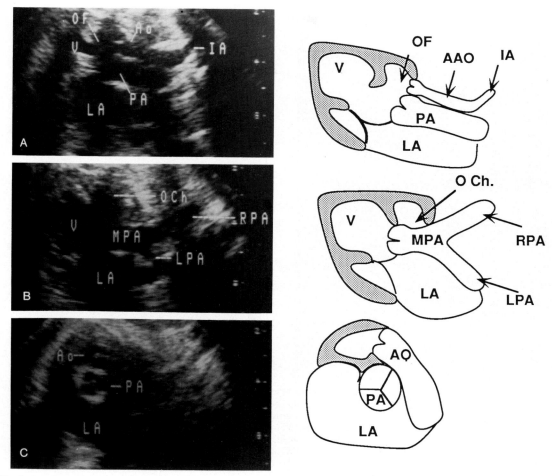

Figure 14–43. *A.* In a long-axis view of the same fetus as in Figure 14–42, the aorta (Ao) and the pulmonary artery (PA) are seen exiting the heart in parallel, indicating transposition. The aorta, which arises from the outlet chamber and runs anterior to the pulmonary artery, can easily be defined as such because it gives rise to an innominate artery (IA). The pulmonary artery can be seen to arise from the main ventricular chamber (V) posteriorly. *B.* In this view obtained by tilting the transducer slightly to the fetus' right side, the pulmonary artery (PA), which arises posteriorly from the ventricle (V) and branches into the right (RPA) and left (LPA) pulmonary arteries, is seen. *C.* In a short-axis view at the base of the heart, both tricuspid semilunar valves are seen. LA, left atrium; OF, outlet foramen; OCh, outlet chamber; AAo, ascending aorta; MPA, main pulmonary artery. The diagrams on the right represent the important anatomic features of the echocardiogram.

Doppler flow mapping (see Figs. 14–33, 14–40, and 14–54). Color Doppler flow imaging has been of immeasurable value in defining atrioventricular valve insufficiency, including that found in Ebstein anomaly.

Although Doppler imaging readily defines stenotic and regurgitant lesions, there are pitfalls of which one has to be aware. Because of beam divergence, ambiguity in the position of the sample volume may occur in closely situated structures; for example, sampling within the right atrium close to the aorta may lead to the misinterpretation of tricuspid regurgitation because, in fact, the signal of a normal flow in the ascending aorta was sampled. This becomes particularly important when short-focused high-frequency transducers are used. Unfavorable fetal position or great distance from the transducer, such as in cases of polyhydramnios, may limit the Doppler technique in certain cases. Attempts have been made to calculate the fetal cardiac output from blood flow velocity profiles,[38–41] but, unfortunately, this calculation requires accurate measurement of valve or vessel diameters;

inaccuracy of even 1 mm may yield an unacceptable high error in the calculation of fetal cardiac output, particularly when the flow vessel diameter is small. Color-coded flow mapping may facilitate the Doppler display, thereby shortening the study time, but in the fetus, color flow mapping also appears to have significant technical limitations due to aliasing and depth resolution. Off-axis signals may also not be well defined by color flow mapping.

Diagnostic Errors

In spite of the increased experience with fetal echocardiography, errors in interpretation are still possible. We have made a false-negative diagnosis of a structurally normal heart in four fetuses of our series. One had a ventricular septal defect, one had aortic coarctation coupled with double-orifice mitral valve, one had mild pulmonary stenosis, and one had situs inversus (mirror image dextrocardia). The last error should

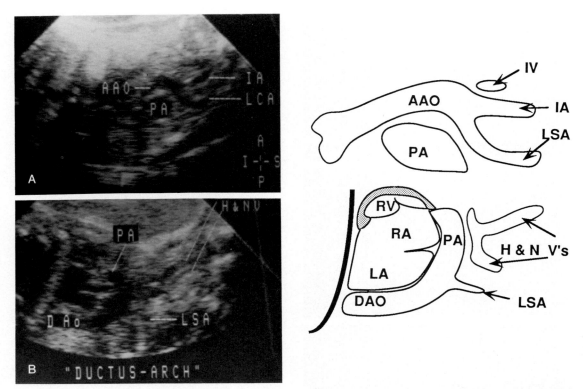

Figure 14–44. Sagittal view in a fetus of 34 weeks' gestation with absent left-sided atrioventricular connection, double-outlet right ventricle, and interrupted aortic arch. *A.* The ascending aorta (AAo) and the proximal arch, which runs on top of the right pulmonary artery (PA), are seen giving rise to the innominate artery (IA) and to the left carotid artery (LCA). A, anterior; I, inferior; P, posterior; S, superior. *B.* After slight angulation of the transducer to the fetus' left side, the dilated pulmonary artery (PA) and its continuation by way of the ductus arteriosus into the descending aorta (DAo) come into view (the so-called ductus arch). The left subclavian artery (LSA) can be seen arising from the descending aorta, which is separated from the arch and the head and neck vessels (H&NV). The diagrams on the right represent the important anatomic features of the echocardiogram.

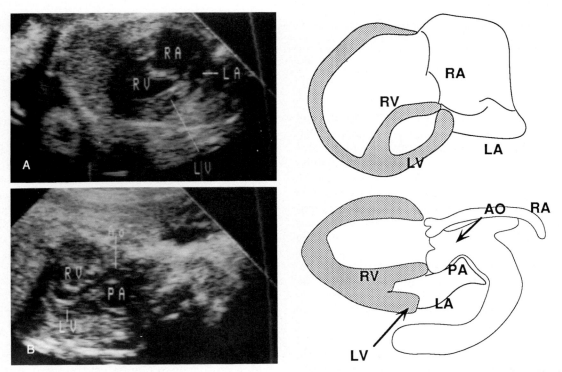

Figure 14–45. Four-chamber view in the same fetus as in Figure 14–44. *A.* The dilated right-sided structures and the hypoplastic left-sided structures of the heart are demonstrated: LA, left atrium; LV, left ventricle; RA, right atrium; RV, right ventricle. *B.* In a long-axis view, the aorta (Ao) and the pulmonary artery (PA) are seen to arise from the large right ventricle (RV); no vessel arises from the hypoplastic left ventricle (LV). The diagrams on the right represent the important anatomic features of the echocardiogram.

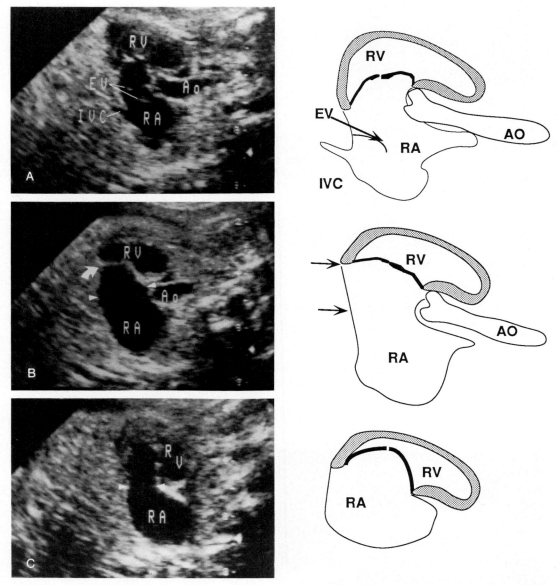

Figure 14–46. Magnified sagittal views in a fetus of 20 weeks' gestation with Ebstein's anomaly. *A.* The inferior vena cava (IVC) drains into the dilated right atrium (RA); the eustachian valve (EV) can be seen marking the approximate position of the atrioventricular groove. The right ventricle (RV) and aorta (Ao) are also seen. *B.* The displacement of the valve leaflets, especially of the posteroinferior leaflet *(curved arrow),* is demonstrated during systole when the leaflets are apposed. The tricuspid valve ring, which is part of the atrioventricular groove, is marked by small arrowheads. *C.* In a diastolic frame, the displaced posteroinferior leaflet is shown tethered to the diaphragmatic surface of the right ventricular wall. The diagrams on the right represent the important anatomic features of the echocardiogram.

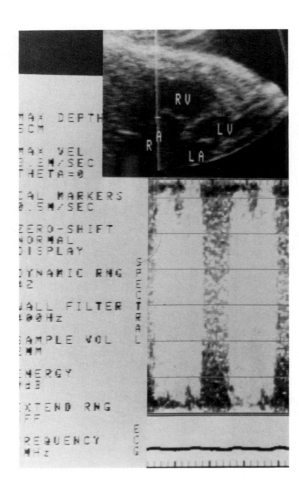

Figure 14–47. In this 26-week fetus with Ebstein's anomaly, a short-axis reference view *(top)* shows the Doppler sample volume within the right atrium (RA), proximal to the tricuspid valve. A turbulent regurgitant jet of high velocity, exceeding 3.2 ms, is demonstrated on Doppler display *(bottom)*. LA, left atrium; LV, left ventricle; RV, right ventricle.

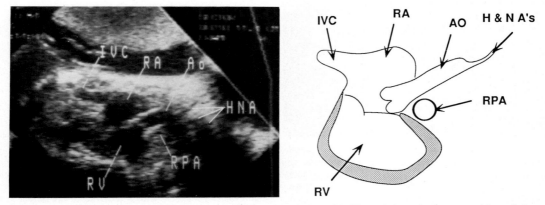

Figure 14–48. Sagittal view in a fetus presenting with the back lying anteriorly. This 32-week fetus had transposition of the great arteries, with ventricular septal defect and pulmonary atresia. The inferior vena cava (IVC) is seen draining into the right atrium (RA), which is connected to the right ventricle (RV). The aorta (Ao) arises anteriorly from the right ventricle and gives rise to the head and neck arteries (HNA). The right pulmonary artery (RPA) is diminutive, indicating severe obstruction of the pulmonary outflow tract. The diagram on the right represents the important anatomic features of the echocardiogram.

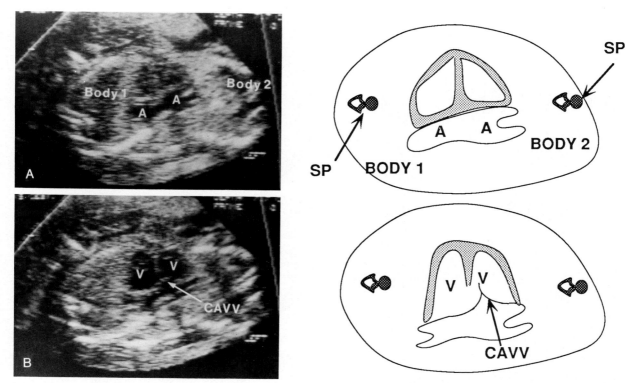

Figure 14–49. *A* and *B*. Thoracopagus twins at 24 weeks' gestation. Both bodies are visualized; the fused hearts share the atria (A) and the ventricles (V). Only one common atrioventricular valve (CAVV), shared between the two hearts, can be seen. SP, spine. The diagrams on the right represent the important anatomic features of the echocardiogram.

not be made if the correct position of the heart within the chest is determined first. In complex cardiac defects, the main lesion may be recognizable, but secondary lesions may be missed unless careful attention is paid to the entire examination. In general, experience suggests that prenatal findings in complex congenital defects tend to underestimate the severity of the spectrum of abnormalities.

Both false-negative and false-positive findings have been reported previously.[7, 8, 11, 50] When evaluating the cause of errors, we found that most of the serious ones had been made using older equipment that had poor resolution and no magnification or Doppler facilities. Other errors unrelated to equipment are beyond the sonographer's control, including technical factors such as suboptimal imaging, which may occur with maternal obesity, polyhydramnios, or fetal lie. Because the resolution of echocardiographic imaging is limited to distances of 1 to 1.5 mm, structural abnormalities such as relatively small ventricular septal defects may be technically impossible to image. Mild aortic or pulmonic stenosis may be difficult to detect because valve morphology may not be distorted, and blood flow velocity may be lower than after birth owing to low ventricular pressures present in fetal life. Other defects, such as mild aortic coarctation or a secundum atrial septal defect, may be indistinguishable from similar conditions in the normal fetus. Furthermore, cardiac lesions may develop or worsen later in pregnancy, as we have observed in cases of cardiomyopathy, and may require serial studies during the second and third trimesters. On the other hand, some lesions may disappear on subsequent studies, such as ventricular septal defects closing spontaneously.

Outcome of Fetuses with Structural Cardiac Defects

Reports that the overall outcome of a fetus with a structural cardiac abnormality is unfavorable[10, 48, 50, 51] were confirmed in our series (see Table 14–3). A report by Smythe and coworkers[52] showed the remarkably poor outcome for fetuses who have congenital heart disease detected in utero. Of 3016 fetuses, these authors identified 170 who had congenital cardiac abnormalities. Seventy-seven patients, or 45%, underwent termination of pregnancy. The remaining 93 (55%) continued the pregnancies, which resulted in 15 still births (9%) and 78 live births (46%). Of the 78 live births, 43 neonates died (25%), and only 35 neonates (21%) survived. The period of follow-up has been between 1 and 80 months. Of the 43 deaths, poor cardiac function was always associated, with nonimmune hydrops in 4 fetuses, severe chromosomal abnormalities in 5 fetuses, or extracardiac malformations in 13 fetuses. In descending order of frequency, the extracardiac malformations were intracranial ventricular abnormalities, neurologic abnormalities, duodenal atresia, cystic hygroma, renal disorders, conjoined twinning, esophageal atresia, biliary atresia, and multiple systemic abnormalities. The numbers in our series are really quite similar to those of Smythe and coworkers. The incidence of death in those fetuses pre-

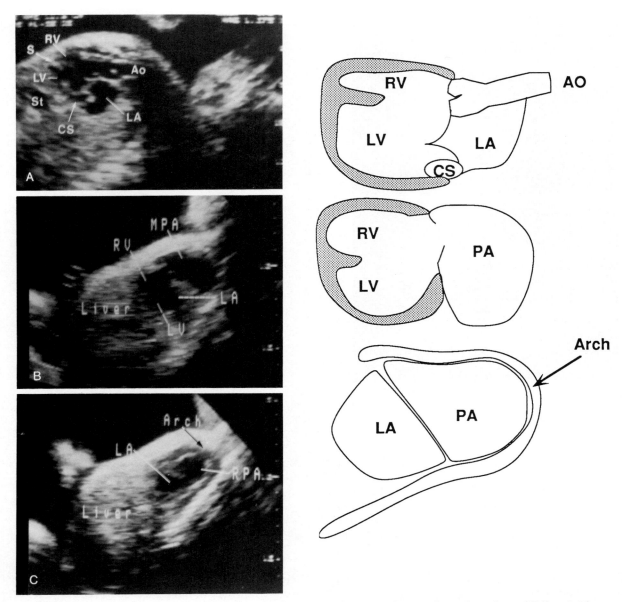

Figure 14–50. Sagittal views in a fetus of 31 weeks' gestation, with absent pulmonary valve complex and tetralogy of Fallot. *A.* The ascending aorta (Ao) is seen overriding a large ventricular septal defect. CS, coronary sinus; LA, left atrium; LV, left ventricle; RV, right ventricle; S, ventricular septum; St, stomach. *B.* With the scan plane directed more to the left, the dysplastic pulmonary valve and the markedly dilated main pulmonary artery (MPA) are demonstrated. *C.* More to the right, the aortic arch is shown. Note the discrepancy between the size of the aortic arch and the right pulmonary artery (RPA), which lies underneath it. The diagrams on the right represent the important anatomic features of the echocardiogram.

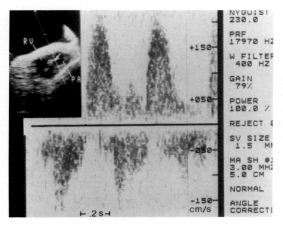

Figure 14–51. Pulsed Doppler ultrasound examination in the same fetus as in Figure 14–50. In the top left reference image, the Doppler sample volume lies in the pulmonary artery (PA), distal to the dysplastic pulmonary valve *(arrow);* the right ventricle (RV) is also seen. The spectral Doppler display is not corrected for angle. A diastolic signal of disturbed flow at a high velocity is demonstrated above the baseline (directed toward the transducer) and reflects pulmonary regurgitation, whereas the systolic signal below the baseline (directed away from the transducer) indicates pulmonary stenosis.

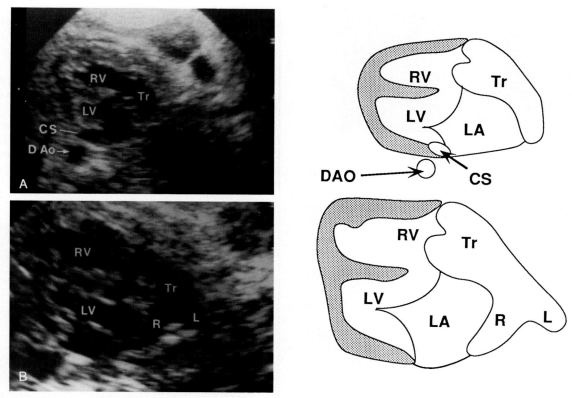

Figure 14–52. Long-axis orientation in a fetus of 32 weeks' gestation with truncus arteriosus. *A.* The single truncal vessel (Tr) is seen overriding a ventricular septal defect. The coronary sinus (CS) is dilated because of a left superior vena cava connection. DAo, descending aorta; LV, left ventricle; RV, right ventricle. *B.* After magnification and slight movement of the transducer to the fetal left side, the common origin of a pulmonary artery from the truncus and its division into right and left pulmonary branches (R, L) can be seen. The diagrams on the right represent the important anatomic features of the echocardiogram.

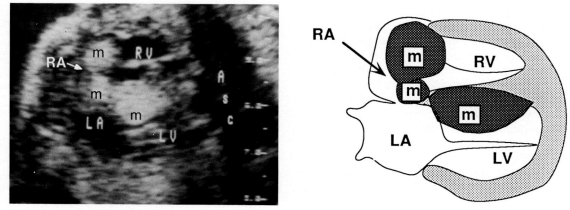

Figure 14–53. Magnified four-chamber view in a 29-week fetus presenting with nonimmune hydrops. A considerable amount of ascites (Asc) is demonstrated. Echo-dense masses (m) are depicted in the ventricular septum between the right ventricle (RV) and the left ventricle (LV), but they can also be seen at the right atrial (RA) level. These masses are multiple rhabdomyoma due to tuberous sclerosis. LA, left atrium. The diagram on the right represents the important anatomic features of the echocardiogram.

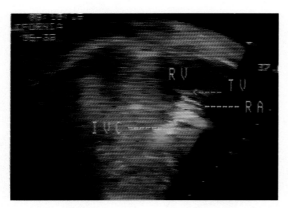

Figure 14–54. Doppler color-flow map taken in a short-axis view of a 29-week fetus with tricuspid regurgitation due to a structural cardiac defect (univentricular atrioventricular connection, aortic arch hypoplasia). In this systolic frame, the tricuspid valve (TV) can be seen between the right ventricle (RV) and the right atrium (RA). A regurgitant jet, refluxing all the way back into the inferior vena cava (IVC), is depicted in red and yellow colors, indicating its direction toward the transducer.

senting with nonimmune hydrops and cardiac defects was high (16 of 18 cases). In 10 of these, there was severe atrioventricular regurgitation, and all of them died either before birth or within the first week of life. Cardiac defects coupled with complete atrioventricular block were present in eight fetuses; in this group, there were seven prenatal or neonatal deaths.[53] The prognosis for fetal survival appears to be poor in the presence of structural abnormalities coupled with atrioventricular valve regurgitation, complete heart block, or fetal hydrops. Because the technique is in its early stages, those defects most likely to be symptomatic are more likely to be recognized.

Fetal Cardiac Arrhythmias

Analysis and comprehension of fetal cardiac arrhythmias using M-mode or Doppler ultrasonography is facilitated by the construction of ladder diagrams (see Fig. 14–21). Ladder diagrams allow the definition of the sequence of atrial and ventricular events and are used in electrophysiology for delineating arrhythmias. The horizontal lines indicate the division between the atria, the atrioventricular node, and the ventricles. With normal conduction, atrial (sinus) activity precedes atrioventricular nodal activity, which precedes ventricular activity (see Fig. 14–22). Echocardiography cannot identify the electrical events but only the mechanical events that succeed them. Mechanical events are less precise and less easy to define, underscoring the limitations of the technique. Despite these limitations, fetal echocardiography is the most practical method available for analyzing fetal arrhythmias and has proved to be remarkably valuable.

Most frequently, an irregular fetal heart rate results from isolated premature atrial contractions (Fig. 14–55 and Table 14–4). These are characterized by a compensatory pause that is almost invariably an incomplete one. Compensatory pauses are the same phenom-

enon seen in electrocardiography after birth; if they are complete, they account for two intervals of regular heartbeats. Isolated premature atrial contractions are fairly common, accounting for about two thirds of fetal arrhythmias noted in our series; they are benign and usually transient, and they do not require any treatment.[12–16] We do, however, recommend that mothers abstain from smoking and ingesting caffeine-containing products. This rhythm disturbance should be followed by the primary physician, because supraventricular tachycardia may develop on rare occasion; however, it does not require further routine echocardiographic examination, although frequent heart rate monitoring by the primary health care providers may be prudent if these atopic beats are frequent. Isolated premature ventricular contractions are characterized by a compensatory pause that is usually complete (Fig. 14–56);

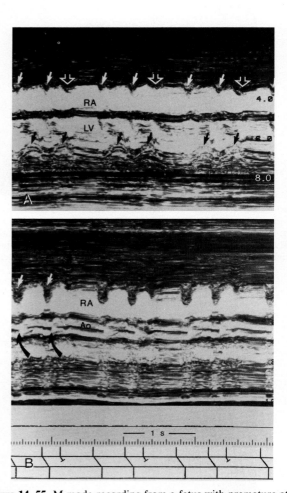

Figure 14–55. M-mode recording from a fetus with premature atrial contractions. *A.* The ultrasound beam passes through the right atrium (RA), the atrioventricular junction, and the left ventricle (LV). After two regular atrial beats *(white arrows)*, there is an ectopic beat *(open arrows)*. This premature atrial contraction is not conducted, since it is not followed by a ventricular contraction *(black arrows)*. The compensatory pause is 720 ms; it is an incomplete compensatory pause, because a complete one would last twice the atrial interval (900 ms). *B.* In the same patient, the ultrasound beam now passes through the right atrium (RA) and the aortic root (Ao). The white arrows indicate atrial contraction, and the black arrows mark the opening of the aortic valve, indicating the effect of ventricular contraction. Two ventricular beats are followed by an incomplete compensatory pause due to premature atrial beats.

Table 14–4. FETAL ARRHYTHMIAS DETECTED BY ULTRASOUND (n = 297)

	% of Total	Therapy	% of Neonatal Survivors
Premature atrial contractions	85.0		100
Premature ventricular contractions	1.0		100
Supraventricular tachycardia	6.0	All but 1*	94
Atrial flutter	1.7	†	100
Complete heart block	6.4‡	1§	58

Note: Two fetuses were noted to have premature atrial contractions, which degenerated into paroxysmal atrial tachycardia. One manifested after birth and has been successfully managed. One fetus developed paroxysmal junction reentrant tachycardia and was partially controlled on digoxin and flecainide.

*Effective treatment: digoxin alone in seven, digoxin and verapamil in one, digoxin and procainamide in one. In one fetus severe bradycardia occurred after administration of digoxin and verapamil leading to emergency cesarean section; this arrhythmia was controlled after birth. Three fetuses have been controlled on flecainide in addition to digoxin. In one fetus, digoxin, verapamil, propranolol, procainamide, and amiodarone failed to convert the cardiac rhythm; this fetus died. One fetus was not treated because of severe additional abnormalities and died subsequently.

†Effective treatment with digoxin alone in all except one fetus, in whom the arrhythmia was controlled with digoxin, quinidine, and verapamil.

‡Failed medical management; intrauterine placement of pacemaker was attempted but fetus died during attempt. Postmortem examination showed endocardial fibroelastosis.

§Pacemaker implanted in neonatal period.

they are, in our experience, much rarer than premature atrial contractions, but others have noted a higher incidence.[17] Premature ventricular beats are also benign and do not require treatment.

Tachyarrhythmias were present in 15% of our cases with a fetal cardiac rhythm disturbance. Most common is a supraventricular tachycardia (Fig. 14–57), which may lead to fetal cardiac failure, hydrops, and death. Doppler echocardiography demonstrates the reduction of stroke volume during runs of supraventricular tachycardia (Fig. 14–58). On rarer occasions, fetal tachyarrhythmia is caused by atrial flutter (Fig. 14–59), usually presenting with variable degrees of atrioventricular block. Atrial flutter may also lead to fetal cardiac failure and hydrops. When the survival of the fetus would be compromised by early delivery, intrauterine treatment by administering medications to the mother should be used, since it has been successful on numerous occasions.[12, 13, 19, 54, 55] It is now established practice to use the transplacental route for antiarrhythmic drug administration. Since supraventricular tachycardia is most likely the result of atrioventricular reentry (see Fig. 14–57), as experience with this arrhythmia in infancy suggests, digoxin is the drug of first choice.[12, 13, 19, 54–56] If digoxin fails to convert the fetal heart rate

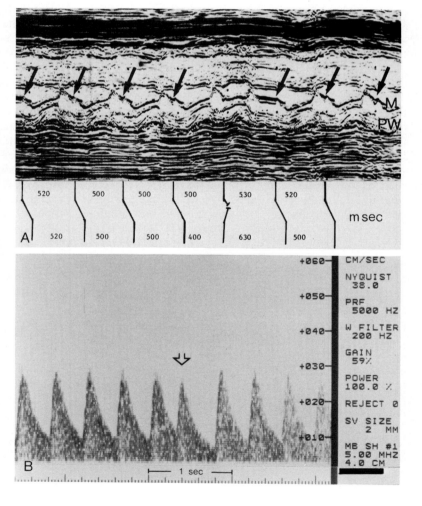

Figure 14–56. Fetal premature contractions that are more likely to be premature junctional or ventricular contractions. *A.* In this M-mode display, the movements of the mitral valve (M) and of the left ventricular posterior wall (PW) can be seen. The irregularity in the rhythm is caused by a premature fifth beat. Whereas all other beats are preceded by an atrial kick, seen on the mitral valve echo *(arrows),* the premature beat is not. Furthermore, the compensatory pause is complete, because two intervals of regular beats also last approximately 1020 ms, as seen in the ladder diagram below. This favors the diagnosis of a premature junctional or ventricular contraction. *B.* Pulsed Doppler sampling within the umbilical artery in a different fetus reveals a similar pattern of irregularity. The premature beat *(open arrow)* is followed by a complete compensatory pause and, therefore, is more likely to be of ventricular origin.

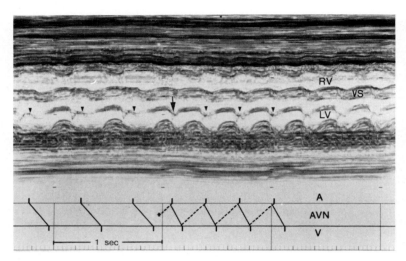

Figure 14–57. M-mode recording of a 30-week fetus with a supraventricular tachycardia. This example demonstrates the atrioventricular reentry mechanism at the onset of the tachycardia. To the left of the recording there is a normal sinus rhythm; note that the atrial click *(black arrowheads)* on the mitral valve echo, indicating atrial contraction, is fairly separated from the preceding valve movement during early diastolic filling. After three regular beats, a premature atrioventricular nodal depolarization causes retrograde atrial and antegrade ventricular activation, thus starting a reentry cycle. The first atrial click on the mitral valve echo appears at the same time as the early diastolic filling deflection *(black arrow);* during the tachycardia, it then can be seen in a different position, closer to the early filling wave than during the sinus rhythm. A, atrial contraction; AVN, atrioventricular node activation; LV, left ventricle; RV, right ventricle; V, ventricular contraction; VS, ventricular septum.

to sinus rhythm, we administer flecainide, verapamil, procainamide, quinidine, or propranolol, in that order (Table 14–5).

Our dosage schedule for these drugs is based on loading doses for the conversion of cardiac arrhythmias in adults (see Table 14–5). Except for digoxin, which may be given orally, other antiarrhythmic drugs carry some risk, and most are administered intravenously in a delivery set-up room. The mother remains in a position where rapid obstetric intervention is possible. Direct echocardiographic monitoring of the fetal heart should be performed during such cardioversion. Enteral absorption of digoxin may be limited during pregnancy, and additional administration of other drugs, such as verapamil, may decrease its clearance.[54] Therefore, the maintenance therapy should be monitored by maternal serum concentrations. Besides our own experience of antiarrhythmic medication administration, other drugs, such as amiodarone, have also been reported to be successful for converting supraventricular tachycardia.[56] Newer antiarrhythmic agents, such as mexiletine and tocainide have not yet been used in fetal tachyarrhythmias. We would like to stress that, except for digoxin, other agents are best admin-

istered in a tertiary care facility by a team consisting of pediatric cardiologists, electrophysiologists, obstetricians, anesthesiologists, and support personnel, since these antiarrhythmic drugs may have serious side effects to the mother and fetus.

Prolonged fetal bradyarrhythmia may result from several mechanisms, including the frequent occurrence of nonconducted premature atrial contractions, group beating, or complete heart block. Group beating may occur because of different electrophysiologic mechanisms, the most common of which is Wenckebach's phenomenon (usually second-degree atrioventricular block). We have also observed group beating with bradycardia and junctional or ventricular escape beats (Fig. 14–60). Doppler ultrasonography is valuable for distinguishing these different conditions (see Figs. 14–60 and 14–61).

Bradyarrhythmia due to complete heart block was present in 15% of our cases of fetal arrhythmia (Figs. 14–28 and 14–62). In our large, multicenter, collaborative study, we found 55 fetuses with complete atrioventricular block detected by prenatal ultrasound examination.[53] In 53% of these fetuses, the atrioventricular block was associated with structural heart de-

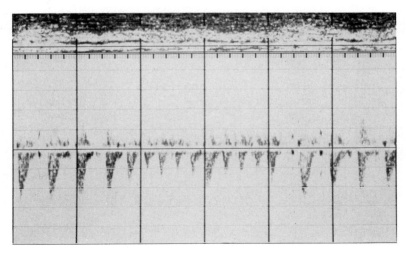

Figure 14–58. Pulsed Doppler interrogation within the pulmonary artery of a fetus with short runs of supraventricular tachycardia. Note the reduction in stroke volume at the onset of tachycardia, after the first four regular beats. Ten beats in tachycardia are followed by a pause and resumption of the normal sinus rhythm. Horizontal lines are markers of frequency shift (1 kHz or 0.25 m/s); vertical lines are time markers (1 second).

Table 14–5. DOSAGE SCHEDULE FOR ANTIARRHYTHMIC TRANSPLACENTAL TREATMENT

Drug	Loading		Maintenance			Plasma Level	
	Dose	Route	Dose	Route	Interval	Therapeutic	Toxic
Digoxin	0.5 mg (initial) + 0.25 mg q6h (total: 1.25–1.5 mg)	IV					
	or 1.5–2 mg (in 24–48 h)	PO	0.25–0.75 mg	PO	24 h	1–2 ng/mL	>2.5 ng/mL
Verapamil*†	0.1–0.2 mg/kg	IV (1–2 min)	80–120 mg	PO	6–8 h	80–300 ng/mL	>300 ng/mL
Propranolol*	0.1–0.2 mg/kg	IV	10–40 mg	PO	8–6 h	50–100 ng/mL	
Procainamide	15 mg/kg, max: 1 g	IV‡	0.5–1.0 g	PO	4 h	3–6 µg/mL	>8 µg/mL
Quinidine sulfate§			0.3–0.4 g	PO	6–8 h†	2–6 µg/mL	>8 µg/mL
Flecainide			100–150 mg	PO	bid		

*Do not use verapamil and propranolol at the same time!
†Atropine (0.5–1.0 mg) should be on hand for managing the side effect of maternal or fetal bradycardia due to atrioventricular block.
‡As infusion, about 50 mg/min.
§PO only.

fects (usually left atrial isomerism or, less frequently, discordant atrioventricular connection); 47% had normal cardiac anatomy, of whom 19 patients tested positive for connective tissue disease or antinuclear antibodies. Six fetuses showed progression from sinus rhythm to second-degree atrioventricular block. Of the 55 pegnancies, 5 underwent termination, and 24 fetuses or neonates died. At the end of the postnatal period, 26 neonates were still alive. Fetal and neonatal death correlated with the presence of structural heart disease. Of 29 fetuses with structural heart disease, only 4 survived. When hydrops was present in association, there were no survivors. An atrial rate of less than 120 beats per minute or a ventricular rate of less than 55 beats per minute appears to be a poor prognostic feature. The 4 fetuses treated with transplacental administration of sympathomimetic agents showed a variable response, with only a limited degree of success in increasing ventricular rate. Postnatally, permanent pacemakers were implanted in 13 neonates, of whom 9 survived the neonatal period. Complete heart block may occur coupled with structural cardiac defects—affected fetuses often present with nonimmune hydrops—but it may also be an isolated finding. In fetuses without structural defects, the mother often suffers from connective tissue disease. These women almost always have antibodies to soluble tissue ribonucleoprotein antigens (Ro[SS-A] and La[SS-B]) that may pass

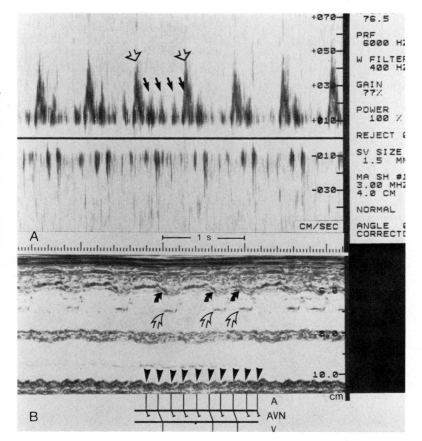

Figure 14–59. Atrial flutter with varying degrees of atrioventricular block in a 36-week fetus. *A*. The sample volume is placed across the descending aorta and the left atrial wall. Pulsed Doppler interrogation demonstrates atrial contractions (smaller flow signals, *black arrows*) and ventricular contractions (bigger flow signals, *open arrows*). In this recording, there is constantly a 4:1 atrioventricular block. This results in an apparently regular heart rate of about 100 beats per minute. *B*. M-mode recording from the same fetus. The ultrasound beam passes through the right ventricle anteriorly and the left atrium posteriorly. At the back of the heart, rapid atrial contractions at about 400 beats per minute can be seen *(black arrowheads)*. Ventricular activation is inferred from either the tricuspid valve closure *(open arrows)* or the onset of ventricular wall motion *(black arrows)*. The ladder diagram demonstrates the presence of a 4:1 atrioventricular block on the left side, with one following beat showing a 2:1 block. These varying degrees of atrioventricular block result in an irregular heart rate. A, atrium; AVN, atrioventricular node; V, ventricle.

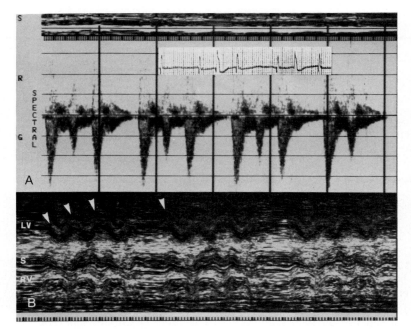

Figure 14–60. Group beating in a 38-week fetus with bradycardia and junctional or ventricular escape beats, demonstrated by pulsed Doppler study *(A)* and M-mode echocardiography *(B)*. *A.* The pulsed Doppler interrogation (paper speed: 50 mm/s) in the descending aorta demonstrates a less effective stroke volume from the second beat when compared with the first and the third beat of each group. Whereas group beating with three beats followed by a pause is usually noted with second-degree atrioventricular block (Wenckebach type), the less effective second beat strongly suggests that this is due to premature contractions rather than to atrioventricular block. The inset shows a scalp electrode electrocardiogram (paper speed: 25 mm/s) obtained after a rupture of the membranes had occurred. Premature junctional escape beats are seen, confirming the echocardiographic diagnosis. *B.* The M-mode tracing (paper speed: 75 mm/s), obtained from the same fetus, demonstrates the motion of the left ventricular (LV) wall, ventricular septum (S), and right ventricular (RV) wall. The same group-beating phenomenon is seen *(arrowheads)*, but the less effective nature of the premature beat cannot be noted.

the placental barrier and may be found in the affected neonate.[28, 57] No therapeutic approach is presently available for the sick fetus with heart block. Attempted direct fetal cardiac pacing has failed to prevent death.[58] We have attempted transabdominal stimulation with an extracardiac pacemaker applied to the maternal abdominal wall, with the same outcome. The prognosis of complete heart block in the fetus is especially poor when structural heart disease or hydrops is also present. However, most fetuses with complete heart block survive when this is an isolated phenomenon, regardless of any association with maternal connective tissue disease. In patients without structural heart disease and heart block, short-term success for pacing the heart block has been achieved by Carpenter and colleagues.[58] Following this experience, we attempted direct implantation of a pacemaker. This met with a similar, brief success at pacing, but the fetus died on the operating table.

It is a useful rule of thumb that in fetal arrhythmias, rapid (> 200 beats per minute) and slow (< 80 beats per minute) heart rates require further evaluation, whereas isolated irregular beats are of little concern. Should irregularities of fetal rhythm be associated with runs of tachycardia or bradycardia, they are of more concern. Isolated irregularities of fetal cardiac rhythm do not, in our experience, occur together with specific structural cardiac abnormalities; only complete heart block has this association.

COMMENTS

Incidence

The spectrum of abnormalities we found does not reflect the common incidence of the different types of congenital cardiac defects.[1, 2, 59, 60] On the contrary, rarer and more complex forms of congenital cardiac defects are detected, presumably because they are more likely to be symptomatic. Both the frequent diagnosis of complex lesions and the high incidence of structural cardiac defects may relate to the criteria we set for evaluating the population for the development of congenital heart defects. The risk of developing congenital heart disease has been thought to increase when there is a family history of either congenital heart defects or extracardiac malformations.[24–26, 61, 62] Maternal congenital heart disease appears to carry a risk factor as great as 10% to 15% for subsequent pregnancies, whereas the recurrence of congenital heart disease with one affected sibling is about 2%.

Impact of Fetal Echocardiography on Obstetric Management

Decisions on the further obstetric management of the pregnancy may be influenced by fetal echocardiography. Because of its potential for prenatal distinction of simple and complex structural abnormalities of the heart, this information is now made available for counseling, aiding the decision for elective termination of the pregnancy, or planning for treatment before or after birth. The detection of serious cardiac defects may become a much more frequent reason for terminating pregnancy as our experience and that of Smythe and coworkers are generally applied. The role of fetal echocardiography in detecting severe structural abnormalities is therefore comparable with that of amniocentesis or fetal blood sampling, which is used as a diagnostic tool for the assessment of severe chromosomal or inborn metabolic disorders. When terminating the pregnancy is not an alternative, fetal echocardiog-

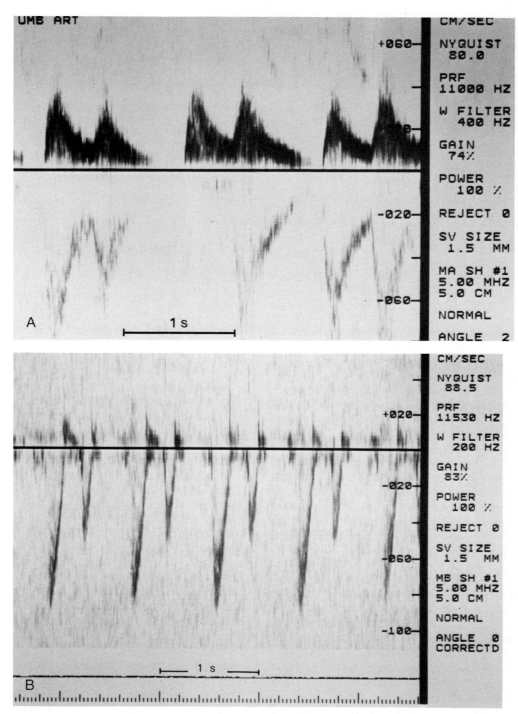

Figure 14–61. Doppler ultrasound recording showing group beating (bigeminal rhythm) in two fetuses with premature contractions. *A.* In this example taken from the umbilical artery (umb art), the mother had received digoxin because supraventricular tachycardia occurred in the fetus. Therefore, fetal group beating may well be related to fetal digitalis intoxication (either because of digoxin-induced atrioventricular block of the Wenckebach type or because of bigeminal premature ventricular contractions) but may result from nonconducted premature atrial contractions as well. Although the Doppler interrogation did not allow the distinction between these possible causes, the M-mode recording obtained from the same fetus (see Fig. 14–55) clearly showed nonconducted premature atrial contractions as being the cause of this bigeminal rhythm and indicated a satisfactory therapeutic response to the digoxin therapy. *B.* In this example taken from another fetus' pulmonary artery, the less effective ejection of every second beat is likely to result from premature contractions. Since this rhythm was so persistent that no sequence of regular beats could be recorded, it was not possible to distinguish between an atrial and a ventricular origin of the premature contractions. Postnatal follow-up demonstrated a normal sinus rhythm.

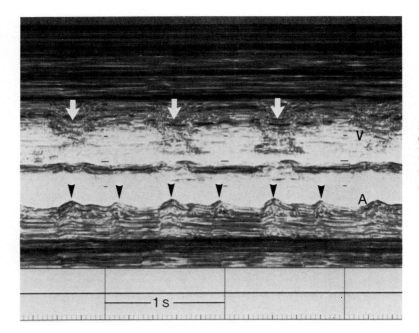

Figure 14–62. M-mode tracing of a 32-week fetus with complete atrioventricular block. The beam passes through the right ventricle (V) and the left atrium (A). Ventricular contractions *(white arrows)* at a rate of 68 beats per minute are seen occurring independently of atrial contractions *(black arrowheads);* the atrial rate is 142 beats per minute.

raphy plays an important role in determining the course of appropriate management.[63, 64] If immediate neonatal support is contemplated, the delivery can also be planned at a center with facilities for medical and surgical cardiac treatment of these neonates. The detection of cardiac defects may also influence the route of delivery; for example, when prolonged labor may cause myocardial ischemia, cesarean section might be contemplated.[64]

In our series, most fetuses with major cardiac defects had previously had an ultrasound examination by an obstetric sonographer who recognized some cardiac disturbance. The impact of fetal echocardiography will be greater when it becomes an accepted and familiar technique for primary care sonographers. Since it appears that fetal echocardiography is considerably more complex than obtaining a fairly "normal-looking" four-chamber view, obstetric sonographers will require further training in the recognition of structural abnormalities of the fetal heart. When cardiac examination of the fetus becomes a routine part of the primary ultrasound examination, it is conceivable that an entirely new perspective may emerge on congenital heart disease, including diagnosis and physiology, which may shift the emphasis for early treatment to the prenatal period. Cardiac examination is also important in making a decision about management of extracardiac abnormalities such as diaphragmatic hernia and omphalocele, in which the presence of a severe cardiac defect may change the overall outlook for the fetus.

Outlook

New therapeutic strategies may develop because of fetal echocardiography. Prenatal surgery, already an established treatment of hydronephrosis, may become an alternative approach to the treatment of congenital heart defects. Experimental data indicate the potential of performing certain forms of fetal cardiovascular surgery to palliate or remove severe right-sided cardiac obstructive lesions,[21, 22] which may allow better development of these malformed hearts. For the same reason, interventional catheterization in the fetus has been proposed as a possible therapeutic approach in the future.[51] Fetal echocardiography is the only technique currently available as a prenatal test for congenital heart defects. We have attempted placement of a pacemaker in a fetal heart. Although the initial result was unfavorable, we maintain that the technique may be useful in the future. Allan and colleagues[68] have reported balloon angioplasty of the aortic valve in critical aortic stenosis, although the results have not been satisfactory. In the fetus with such heart disease, surgical valvotomy may be an alternative. Although magnetic resonance imaging has been used to demonstrate fetal cardiac anatomy,[65] there are obviously limitations to its applicability.

Monitoring of the fetal cardiovascular function by echocardiography during treatment of arrhythmias or congestive heart failure with medication administered by both a maternal[12–15, 18–20, 54–56, 66, 69] and a direct fetal route[66, 67] may be expanded considerably in the future. Moreover, fetal echocardiography may allow the detection of undesired side effects of drugs taken for maternal indications, such as the constriction of the ductus arteriosus after indomethacin therapy in the mother.[42]

Ultrasonic monitoring of the fetus who has undergone surgery is vital. In all of our patients who have undergone fetal surgery for diaphragmatic hernia or sacrococcygeal teratoma, we have monitored fetal heart rate, umbilical flow, arterial pulsatility index in the cord and abdominal aorta, and the effects of indomethacin on the production of ductus constriction and tricuspid regurgitation.

Fetal echocardiography provides new information about the development of the heart in the presence of structural or functional disease[37, 48, 51, 68]; this knowledge will contribute to a better understanding of the natural history of congenital heart disease.

ACKNOWLEDGMENT

We are indebted to Dr. Melvin Scheinman (Division of Cardiology) for his advice concerning antiarrhythmic therapy and to many of our obstetric colleagues, especially Drs. Mitchell Golbus and James Goldberg (Division of Genetic Counseling and Prenatal Diagnosis) and Drs. Roy Filly and Peter Callen (Division of Radiology), for their help, advice, and support. We wish to thank Mrs. Heather Silverman for editorial assistance with this manuscript and Mrs. Mary Helen Briscoe for artwork.

References

1. Mitchell SC, Korones SB, Berendes HW: Congenital heart disease in 56,109 births: Incidence and natural history. Circulation 43:323, 1971.
2. Hoffman JIE, Christianson R: Congenital heart disease in a cohort of 19,502 births with long-term follow-up. Am J Cardiol 42:641, 1978.
3. Allan LD, Tynan MJ, Campbell S, et al: Echocardiographic and anatomical correlates in the fetus. Br Heart J 44:444, 1980.
4. Lange LW, Sahn DJ, Allen HD, et al: Qualitative real-time cross-sectional echocardiographic imaging of the human fetus during the second half of pregnancy. Circulation 62:799, 1980.
5. Sahn DJ, Lange LW, Allen HD, et al: Quantitative real-time cross-sectional echocardiography in the developing normal human fetus and newborn. Circulation 62:588, 1980.
6. Huhta JC, Hagler DJ, Hill LM: Two-dimensional echocardiographic assessment of normal fetal cardiac anatomy. J Reprod Med 29:162, 1984.
7. Allan LD, Crawford DC, Anderson RH, Tynan MJ: Echocardiographic and anatomical correlations in fetal congenital heart disease. Br Heart J 52:542, 1984.
8. Silverman NH, Golbus MS: Echocardiographic techniques for assessing normal and abnormal fetal cardiac anatomy. J Am Coll Cardiol 5(suppl):20S, 1985.
9. Fermont L, deGeeter B, Aubry MC, et al: A close collaboration between obstetricians and pediatric cardiologists allows antenatal detection of severe cardiac malformations by two-dimensional echocardiography. In Doyle EF, Engle MA, Gersony WM, et al (eds): Pediatric Cardiology, Proceedings of the Second World Congress, pp 34–37. New York, Springer, 1986.
10. Allan LD, Crawford DC, Anderson RH, Tynan M: Spectrum of congenital heart disease detected echocardiographically in prenatal life. Br Heart J 54:523, 1985.
11. Sandor GGS, Farquarson D, Wittmann B, et al: Fetal echocardiography: Results in high-risk patients. Obstet Gynecol 67:358, 1986.
12. Kleinman CS, Donnerstein RL, Jaffe CC, et al: Fetal echocardiography: A tool for evaluation of in utero cardiac arrhythmias and monitoring of in utero therapy: Analysis of 71 patients. Am J Cardiol 51:237, 1983.
13. Allan LD, Anderson RH, Sullivan ID, et al: Evaluation of fetal arrhythmias by echocardiography. Br Heart J 50:240, 1983.
14. DeVore GR, Siassi B, Platt LD: Fetal echocardiography: III. The diagnosis of cardiac arrhythmias using real-time-directed M-mode ultrasound. Am J Obstet Gynecol 146:792, 1983.
15. Silverman NH, Enderlein MA, Stanger P, et al: Recognition of fetal arrhythmias by echocardiography. J Clin Ultrasound 13:255, 1985.
16. Strasburger JF, Huhta JC, Carpenter RJ, et al: Doppler echocardiography in the diagnosis and management of persistent fetal arrhythmias. J Am Coll Cardiol 7:1386, 1986.
17. Steinfeld L, Rappaport HL, Rossbach HC, Martinez E: Diagnosis of fetal arrhythmias using echocardiographic and Doppler techniques. J Am Coll Cardiol 8:1425, 1986.
18. Kleinman CS, Donnerstein RL, DeVore GR, et al: Fetal echocardiography for evaluation of in utero congestive heart failure. N Engl J Med 306:568, 1982.
19. Wiggins JW, Bowes W, Clewell W, et al: Echocardiographic diagnosis and intravenous digoxin management of fetal tachyarrhythmias and congestive heart failure. Am J Dis Child 140:202, 1986.
20. Simpson PC, Trudinger BJ, Walker A, Baird PJ: The intrauterine treatment of fetal cardiac failure in a twin pregnancy with an acardiac, acephalic monster. Am J Obstet Gynecol 147:842, 1983.
21. Turley K, Vlahakes GJ, Harrison MR, et al: Intrauterine cardiothoracic surgery: The fetal lamb model. Ann Thorac Surg 34:422, 1982.
22. Slate RK, Stevens MB, Verrier ED, et al: Intrauterine repair of pulmonary stenosis in fetal sheep. Surg Forum 36:246, 1985.
23. Zierler S: Maternal drugs and congenital heart disease. Obstet Gynecol 65:155, 1985.
24. Allan LD, Crawford DC, Chita SK, et al: Familial recurrence of congenital heart disease in a prospective series of mothers referred for fetal echocardiography. Am J Cardiol 58:334, 1986.
25. Whittemore R, Hobbins JC, Engle MA: Pregnancy and its outcome in women with and without surgical treatment of congenital heart disease. Am J Cardiol 50:641, 1982.
26. Nora JJ, Nora AH: Maternal transmission of congenital heart diseases: New recurrence risk figures and the questions of cytoplasmic inheritance and vulnerability to teratogens. Am J Cardiol 59:459, 1987.
27. McCue CM, Mantakas ME, Tingelstad JB, Ruddy S: Congenital heart block in newborns of mothers with connective tissue disease. Circulation 56:82, 1977.
28. Scott JS, Maddison PJ, Taylor PV, et al: Connective tissue disease, antibodies to ribonucleoprotein, and congenital heart block. N Engl J Med 309:209, 1983.
29. Allan LD, Joseph MC, Boyd EGC, et al: M-Mode echocardiography in the developing human fetus. Br Heart J 47:573, 1982.
30. St John Sutton MG, Gewitz MH, Shah B, et al: Quantitative assessment of growth and function of the cardiac chambers in the normal human fetus: A prospective longitudinal echocardiographic study. Circulation 69:645, 1984.
31. DeVore GR, Siassi B, Platt LD: Fetal echocardiography: IV. M-mode assessment of ventricular size and contractility during the second and third trimesters of pregnancy in the normal fetus. Am J Obstet Gynecol 150:981, 1984.
32. Anderson RH, Becker AE, Freedom RM, et al: Sequential segmental analysis of congenital heart disease. Pediatr Cardiol 5:281, 1984.
33. Silverman NH, de Araujo LML: An echocardiographic method for the diagnosis of cardiac situs and malpositions. Echocardiography 4:35, 1987.
34. De Araujo LML, Silverman NH, Filly RA, et al: Prenatal detection of left atrial isomerism by ultrasound. J Ultrasound Med 6:667, 1987.
35. Stewart PA, Tonge HM, Wladimiroff JW: Arrhythmia and structural abnormalities of the fetal heart. Br Heart J 50:550, 1983.
36. Kleinman CS, Donnerstein RL: Ultrasonic assessment of cardiac function in the intact human fetus. J Am Coll Cardiol 5(suppl):84S, 1985.
37. Birnbaum SE, McGahan JP, Janos GG, Meyers M: Fetal tachycardia and intramyocardial tumors. J Am Coll Cardiol 6:1358, 1985.
38. Reed KL, Meijboom EJ, Sahn DJ, et al: Cardiac Doppler flow velocities in human fetuses. Circulation 73:41, 1986.
39. Huhta JC, Strasburger JF, Carpenter RJ, et al: Pulsed Doppler fetal echocardiography. J Clin Ultrasound 13:247, 1985.
40. Reed KL, Sahn DJ, Scagnelli S, et al: Doppler echocardiographic studies of diastolic function in the human fetal heart: Changes during gestation. J Am Coll Cardiol 8:391, 1986.
41. Maulik D, Nanda NC, Saini VD: Fetal Doppler echocardiography: Methods and characterization of normal and abnormal hemodynamics. Am J Cardiol 53:572, 1984.
42. Huhta JC, Moise KJ, Fisher DJ, et al: Detection and quantita-

tion of constriction of the fetal ductus arteriosus by Doppler echocardiography. Circulation 75:406, 1987.

43. Hatle L, Brubakk A, Tromsdal A, Angelsen B: Noninvasive assessment of pressure drop in mitral stenosis by Doppler ultrasound. Br Heart J 40:131, 1978.

44. Hatle L, Angelsen BA, Tromsdal A: Non-invasive assessment of aortic stenosis by Doppler ultrasound. Br Heart J 43:284, 1980.

45. Stuart B, Drumm J, FitzGerald DE, Duignan NM: Fetal blood velocity waveforms in normal pregnancy. Br J Obstet Gynaecol 87:780, 1980.

46. Schulman H, Fleischer A, Stern W, et al: Umbilical velocity wave ratios in human pregnancy. Am J Obstet Gynecol 148:985, 1984.

47. Trudinger BJ, Giles WB, Cook CM, et al: Fetal umbilical artery flow velocity waveforms and placental resistance: Clinical significance. Br J Obstet Gynaecol 92:23, 1985.

48. Silverman NH, Kleinman CS, Rudolph AM, et al: Fetal atrioventricular valve insufficiency associated with nonimmune hydrops: A two-dimensional echocardiographic and pulsed Doppler ultrasound study. Circulation 72:825, 1985.

49. Weinstein MR, Goldfield MD: Cardiovascular malformations with lithium use during pregnancy. Am J Psychiatry 132:529, 1975.

50. Huhta JC, Strasburger JF, Carpenter RJ, Reiter A: Fetal echocardiography: Accuracy and limitations in the diagnosis of cardiac disease. (Abstract) J Am Coll Cardiol 5:387, 1985.

51. Allan LD, Crawford DC, Tynan MJ: Pulmonary atresia in prenatal life. J Am Coll Cardiol 8:1131, 1986.

52. Smythe JF, Copel JA, Kleinman CS: Outcome of prenatally detected cardiac malformations. Am J Cardiol 69:1471, 1992.

53. Schmidt KG, Ulmer HE, Silverman NH, et al: Perinatal outcome of fetal complete atrioventricular block: A multicenter experience. J Am Coll Cardiol 17:1360, 1991.

54. Kleinman CS, Copel JA, Weinstein EM, et al: Treatment of fetal supraventricular tachyarrhythmias. J Clin Ultrasound 13:265, 1985.

55. Dumesic DA, Silverman NH, Tobias S, Golbus MS: Transplacental cardioversion of fetal supraventricular tachycardia with procainamide. N Engl J Med 307:1128, 1982.

56. Arnoux P, Seyral P, Llurens M, et al: Amiodarone and digoxin for refractory fetal tachycardia. Am J Cardiol 59:166, 1987.

57. Taylor PV, Scott JS, Gerlis LM, et al: Maternal antibodies against fetal cardiac antigens in congenital complete heart block. N Engl J Med 315:667, 1986.

58. Carpenter RJ, Strasburger JF, Garson A, et al: Fetal ventricular pacing for hydrops secondary to complete atrioventricular block. J Am Coll Cardiol 8:1434, 1986.

59. Scott DJ, Rigby ML, Miller GAH, Shinebourne EA: The presentation of symptomatic heart disease in infancy based on 10 years' experience (1973–82). Br Heart J 52:248, 1984.

60. Fyler DC, Buckley JP, Hellenbrand WE, et al: Report of the New England Regional Infant Cardiac Program. Pediatrics 65(suppl):375, 1980.

61. Copel JA, Pilu G, Kleinman CS: Congenital heart disease and extracardiac anomalies: Associations and indications for fetal echocardiography. Am J Obstet Gynecol 154:1121, 1986.

62. Nora JJ, Nora AH: The evolution of specific genetic and environmental counseling in congenital heart diseases. Circulation 57:205, 1978.

63. Sanders SP, Chin AJ, Parness IA, et al: Prenatal diagnosis of congenital heart defects in thoracoabdominally conjoined twins. N Engl J Med 313:370, 1985.

64. Huhta JC, Carpenter RJ, Moise KJ, et al: Prenatal diagnosis and postnatal management of critical aortic stenosis. Circulation 75:573, 1987.

65. Lowe TW, Weinreb J, Santos-Ramos R, Cunningham FG: Magnetic resonance imaging in human pregnancy. Obstet Gynecol 66:629, 1985.

66. Redel DA, Hansmann M: Prenatal diagnosis and treatment of heart disease. In Dellenbach P (ed): Symposium International d'Echocardiologie Foetale, pp 127–134. Strasbourg, Milupa Dietetique, 1982.

67. Hansmann M, Redel DA: Prenatal symptoms and clinical management of heart disease. In Dellenbach P (ed): Symposium International d'Echocardiologie Foetale, pp 137–149. Strasbourg, Milupa Dietetique, 1982.

68. Allan LD, Crawford DC, Tynan M: Evolution of coarctation of the aorta in intrauterine life. Br Heart J 52:471, 1984.

69. Spinnato JA, Shaver DC, Flinn GS, et al: Fetal supraventricular tachycardia: In utero therapy with digoxin and quinidine. Obstet Gynecol 64:730, 1984.

CHAPTER 15

Ultrasound Evaluation of the Fetal Thorax

RUTH B. GOLDSTEIN, M.D.

With the advent of high-resolution real-time ultrasonography, there has been a dramatic improvement in the ability to observe congenital anomalies prenatally. Along with anomalies of the central nervous and skeletal systems, anomalies of the thorax constitute a major group of fetal abnormalities currently detectable with prenatal ultrasound evaluation. Many of the fetal chest abnormalities that can now be observed are potentially life threatening, either at the time they are observed or by virtue of their potential to grow and produce fetal hydrops. Thus, the sonographer should be aware of these important observations since knowledge of the natural history of the malformation and of options for prenatal or perinatal therapy greatly influences parental counseling and obstetric management.

THE NORMAL FETAL CHEST

By the second and third trimesters of pregnancy, the pleural, pericardial, and peritoneal cavities are morphologically distinct,[1] and the contents of these spaces, as well as their relationships, can be studied during real-time ultrasonography. During routine survey of the fetal chest, coronal, transverse axial, and sagittal views may be useful in confirming the normal intrathoracic relationships. The position of the fetus is usually flexed, and transverse scanning through the fetal chest may require stepwise correction in the transducer's angulation relative to the skin surface. At the level of the pulmonary apices, the clavicles are a distinguishing landmark, just as the diaphragm is a caudal one (Fig. 15–1). The fetal diaphragm can be discretely observed as a smooth hypoechoic muscular margin between the fetal lungs and the liver or spleen (Fig. 15–2). By using routine transverse scanning of the chest in this way, much useful information can be quickly obtained regarding chest shape, size, and symmetry; cardiac size and morphology; and pulmonary echotexture (Figs. 15–3 and 15–4).

The mediastinum is centrally positioned in the chest, and the majority of the cardiac volume is positioned to the left of the midline. A simple four-chamber view of the heart, which can be visualized in all fetuses in the second and third trimesters, should be a part of routine obstetric scanning. This view is relatively easily obtained in a transverse imaging plane through the lower fetal thorax, at right angles to the spine. The ventricular chambers should be assessed for symmetry (Fig. 15–5). Nomograms for overall cardiac size and left/right ventricular ratios have been published. In most examinations, however, a subjective impression of ventricular symmetry and cardiac size is sufficient. This view of the heart will also encourage detection of chest masses or pleural effusions, which tend to cause mediastinal shift, as well as the rare occurrence of cardiac masses (e.g., a rhabdomyoma in tuberous sclerosis [Fig. 15–6] or a pericardial teratoma). Reported sensitivities for detection of significant cardiac malformations are variable, although hypoplastic left or right heart, large ventricular septal defects, and atrioventricular canals are often detected on the four-chamber view of the fetal heart. The right and left ventricles of the normal heart can be easily identified in the transverse axial plane/four-chamber view based on their position in the chest: the more anteriorly positioned chamber is the right ventricle, and the more posteriorly positioned chamber is the left atrium (see Fig. 15–5). The superior and inferior venae cavae are seen as anechoic tubular structures that may be followed to their confluence in the right atrium. Blood flow from the right to the left atrium results in regular opening and closing of the foramen ovale, which may occasionally be seen during real-time scanning but should not be confused with a pathologic septal defect. Several authors have reported that a small amount of pericardial fluid may be a normal finding.[2, 3] Mediastinal structures, such as the aortic arch, ductus arteriosus, and great vessels, can be visualized with regularity (Fig. 15–7).[4] With effort and color Doppler studies, even small structures such as the fetal pulmonary

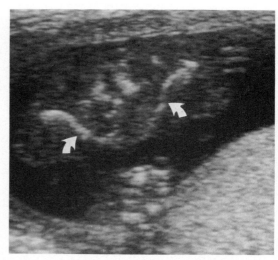

Figure 15–1. The clavicles (*arrows*) are sufficiently mineralized to provide a reliable anatomic marker in the fetus.

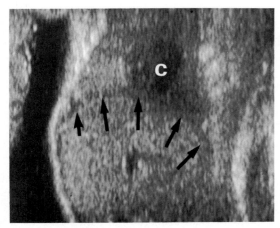

Figure 15–2. The fetal diaphragm (*arrows*) is a smooth hypoechoic band of tissue separating the thoracic and abdominal cavities. c, heart.

arteries and veins (see Fig. 15–5), fetal trachea, esophagus, and thyroid gland may be observed.[5]

Fetal Lung Development

One of the most important determinants of whether the fetus can survive as a neonate in the air-filled, ex utero environment is the adequate biochemical and structural development and maturity of the lungs. The adequacy of pulmonary development is probably the single most important determinant for fetal viability, and pulmonary immaturity is the major reason why fetuses younger than 24 weeks' gestation are generally considered nonviable. Buds from the early trachea form and penetrate the mesenchymal masses destined to become the lungs. Through a series of divisions and budding, bronchi give rise to bronchioles, and each terminal bronchiole gives rise to a number of alveolar ducts and alveoli; the latter are responsible for the bulk of gas exchange. By 16 to 20 weeks, the normal

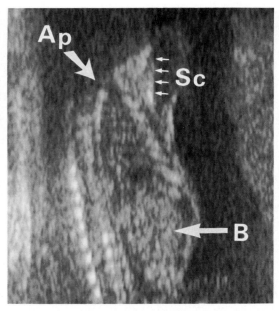

Figure 15–4. Parasagittal image. The polarity of the bell-shaped thorax is helpful in determining the fetal lie. Ap, thoracic apex; Sc, scapula; B, collapsed bowel.

number of bronchi have formed. However, for survival in postnatal life, the development and number of bronchi have less impact than the development of the parenchymal architecture (alveolar ducts and alveoli) destined for gas exchange. Between 16 and 24 weeks' gestation there is a dramatic increase in the number and complexity of air spaces, large blood vessels, and capillaries. After 24 weeks, another important developmental phenomenon occurs: progressive flattening of the epithelial cells lining the air spaces. This allows closer apposition of capillaries to the fluid-filled air-space lumen and results in further development of the air–blood barrier, necessary for efficient gas exchange after birth (Fig. 15–8). The number of alveoli continues to grow during childhood,

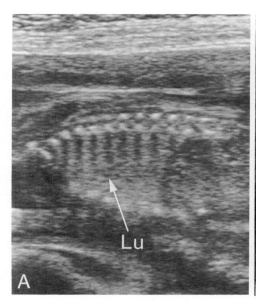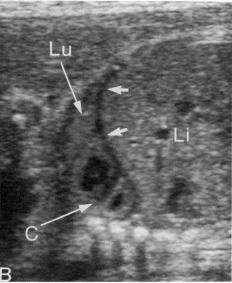

Figure 15–3. The normal echogenicity of the fetal lung may be similar to or even slightly greater than the echogenicity of the abdominal viscera. *A.* Sagittal scan demonstrates moderate amplitude echogenicity of the pulmonary parenchyma (Lu). *B.* Oblique coronal image in mid-gestation fetus demonstrates similar echogenicity of liver (Li) and lung (Lu). Arrows indicate diaphragm. C, heart.

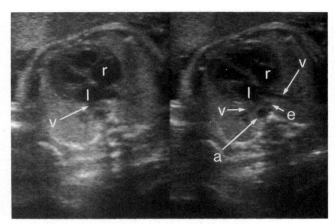

Figure 15–5. Four-chamber view of the heart. Pulmonary veins (v) are observed entering the left atrium (l). r, right atrium; a, aorta; e, esophagus.

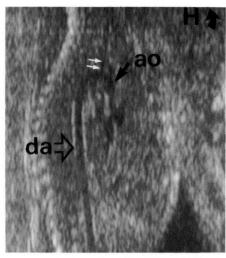

Figure 15–7. Aortic arch. The ascending aorta (ao) and descending aorta (da) are readily visualized. The origin of the great vessels is marked by small arrows. H, fetal head.

after which alveolar expansion becomes the major means of lung growth until adolescence.[6]

Three factors are most important for normal lung development during fetal life: (1) adequate thoracic space for growth, (2) fetal breathing movements, and (3) adequate amniotic fluid volume. Grossly hypoplastic lungs weigh less than expected for a given gestational age (low lung/body weight ratio). Histologically, hypoplastic lungs show reduced numbers of alveoli and often of bronchi as well. Pathologic conditions (both naturally occurring and experimentally produced in animals) that interfere with any of these three components have been associated with pulmonary hypoplasia. In fetal lambs, transection of the phrenic nerve (which inhibits breathing movements) or insertion of a large intrathoracic mass (which interferes with adequate thoracic volume for lung growth) results in pulmonary hypoplasia.[7, 8] In human fetuses, large space-occupying chest masses (i.e., congenital diaphragmatic hernia, large pleural effusion) with fixed volumes are routinely associated with ipsilateral and often contralateral pulmonary hypoplasia, likely due to the compression effect on the developing lung.

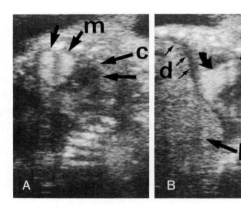

Figure 15–6. Fetus at risk for tuberous sclerosis. *A.* Oblique scan through the fetal chest and heart (c). An echogenic cardiac mass (m) is a rhabdomyoma. *B.* Oblique coronal image through the abdomen and chest of the same fetus. The echogenic cardiac rhabdomyoma (m) extends to the diaphragmatic surface of the heart. The hypoechoic diaphragm (d) and liver (L) are indicated by arrows.

Neuromuscular disorders such as the Pena-Shokeir syndrome, which interfere with the mechanism of fetal breathing, are also often associated with pulmonary hypoplasia despite normal overall chest circumference measurements.[9]

Fluid within the lung has an important influence on fetal lung development. Fluid is both secreted and absorbed within the primitive air spaces. It is generally thought that more fluid is secreted than absorbed, and in experiments with fetal lambs a net efflux of fluid from the trachea has been demonstrated.[10] Several animal experiments as well as "experiments in nature" confirm the importance of amniotic and lung fluid as an important stimulus for lung development.[10, 11] If lung fluid is drained through a tracheostomy in the fetal lamb, pulmonary hypoplasia results. Similarly, when oligohydramnios is chronic and severe, due to chronic amniotic fluid leakage or severe genitourinary abnormalities, lung development is retarded and severe (lethal) pulmonary hypoplasia results.[12]

It is postulated that lung fluid acts as an internal stent required for normal lung development. Although extrinsic compression of the chest may play a role in the occurrence of pulmonary hypoplasia in the setting of oligohydramnios, Nicolini and coworkers suggest that a net loss of lung fluid in association with the decreased amniotic pressure in this situation is the more likely explanation of oligohydramnios-related pulmonary hypoplasia.[13] For example, during fetal breathing periods there is an abnormally large efflux of lung fluid into the amniotic space in fetal lambs when oligohydramnios is present. These authors postulate that the loss of fluid from the lung, caused by the abnormal amniotic/alveolar pressure gradient in oligohydramnios, is probably responsible for the loss of this important fluid stent within the lungs and, therefore, that the loss of lung fluid is responsible for the pulmonary hypoplasia.

The opposite phenomenon has also been observed in animals and abnormal fetuses. Tracheal ligation or

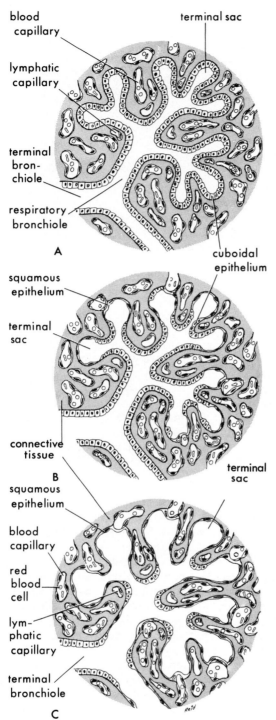

Figure 15–8. Progressive stages of lung development. *A.* Approximately 24 menstrual weeks. *B.* Early terminal sac period (approximately 26 menstrual weeks). Note the thinner squamous epithelium lining the air spaces and closer apposition of capillaries to the air sacs. *C.* Neonate. Note the thin alveolar-capillary membrane. Note also that some of the capillaries have begun to bulge into the terminal sacs (future alveoli). (From Moore KL: Development of body cavities, primitive mesenteries, and the diaphragm. In: The Developing Human: Clinically Oriented Embryology, 4th ed. Philadelphia, WB Saunders, 1988.)

balloon occlusion in fetal lambs prevents pulmonary hypoplasia, presumably at least in part by blocking the outflow of lung fluid.[10] Furthermore, fetuses with tracheal or laryngeal atresia develop lungs that are larger

and histologically hypertrophic, not hypoplastic.[14, 15] The pathophysiology of lung hypoplasia, as well as conditions that produce it and avert it, may be important for counseling patients, in addition to the future development of interventions to treat pulmonary hypoplasia in utero.

Sonography of the Normal Fetal Thorax

The fetal lungs appear homogeneous and of moderate echogenicity on the sonogram (see Fig. 15–3). Early in gestation, the pulmonary parenchyma appears similar to or slightly less echogenic than the liver, and as gestation progresses there is a trend toward increased pulmonary echogenicity relative to the liver. Although some investigators have attempted to correlate increasing pulmonary echogenicity, coarsening of the lung echotexture, and increasing through-sound transmission with pulmonary maturity, these attempts have largely been unsuccessful.[16, 17] Some have even suggested pulmonary maturity might be assessed through visual cues (i.e., pulmonary "squishiness"), suggesting developing lung compliance.[18] Of all the observations associated with pulmonary hypoplasia, however, among normal fetuses, *gestational age* most closely correlates with the degree of pulmonary development. In the presence of oligohydramnios, however, the degree to which the fetal lungs are underdeveloped or hypoplastic may be more severe than predicted by gestational age. Although sonographic features ("small" lungs, echogenic lungs, and similar findings) in the fetal chest alone cannot accurately predict pulmonary function, a correlation between pulmonary hypoplasia and a small chest circumference has been noted.[19, 20] Chest circumference measurements are obtained in the transverse plane at the level of the four-chamber view of the heart. Nomograms have been published for normal chest circumferences as a function of gestational age (Table 15–1) or compared with biometric parameters such as femur length, head, and abdominal circumference.[19–22] Although sensitivity, specificity, and normal and abnormal predictive values are fairly high (i.e., >80%, 80% to 90%, 85% to 90%, respectively), chest circumference measurements suffer from a number of potential pitfalls in predicting or excluding pulmonary hypoplasia:

1. Lungs may be hypoplastic despite a normal or larger than average thoracic cavity. This may occur in conditions that adversely influence lung growth but do not result in a smaller than expected chest circumference (i.e., pleural effusion,[22] congenital diaphragmatic hernia).

2. False-negative predictions can occur at the time of first presentation in the second trimester when the chest is not growing normally but the chest circumference has not yet fallen below the fifth percentile for a given gestational age. Alternatively, if the patient is examined soon after ruptured membranes have occurred in the second trimester, it is likely that the chest size will be normal.

3. The gestational age may not be known or femur length measurements may be unreliable.

Table 15–1. FETAL THORACIC CIRCUMFERENCE MEASUREMENTS*

Gestational Age (wk)	No.	Predictive Percentiles								
		2.5	5	10	25	50	75	90	95	97.5
16	6	5.9	6.4	7.0	8.0	9.1	10.3	11.3	11.9	12.4
17	22	6.8	7.3	7.9	8.9	10.0	11.2	12.2	12.8	13.3
18	31	7.7	8.2	8.8	9.8	11.0	12.1	13.1	13.7	14.2
19	21	8.6	9.1	9.7	10.7	11.9	13.0	14.0	14.6	15.1
20	20	9.5	10.0	10.6	11.7	12.8	13.9	15.0	15.5	16.0
21	30	10.4	11.0	11.6	12.6	13.7	14.8	15.8	16.4	16.9
22	18	11.3	11.9	12.5	13.5	14.6	15.7	16.7	17.3	17.8
23	21	12.2	12.8	13.4	14.4	15.5	16.6	17.6	18.2	18.8
24	27	13.2	13.7	14.3	15.3	16.4	17.5	18.5	19.1	19.7
25	20	14.1	14.6	15.2	16.2	17.3	18.4	19.4	20.0	20.6
26	25	15.0	15.5	16.1	17.1	18.2	19.3	20.3	21.0	21.5
27	24	15.9	16.4	17.0	18.0	19.1	20.2	21.3	21.9	22.4
28	24	16.8	17.3	17.9	18.9	20.0	21.2	22.2	22.8	23.3
29	24	17.7	18.2	18.8	19.8	21.0	22.1	23.1	23.7	24.2
30	27	18.6	19.1	19.7	20.7	21.9	23.0	24.0	24.6	25.1
31	24	19.5	20.0	20.6	21.6	22.8	23.9	24.9	25.5	26.0
32	28	20.4	20.9	21.5	22.6	23.7	24.8	25.8	26.4	26.9
33	27	21.3	21.8	22.5	23.5	24.6	25.7	26.7	27.3	27.8
34	25	22.2	22.8	23.4	24.4	25.5	26.6	27.6	28.2	28.7
35	20	23.1	23.7	24.3	25.3	26.4	27.5	28.5	29.1	29.6
36	23	24.0	24.6	25.2	26.2	27.3	28.4	29.4	30.0	30.6
37	22	24.9	25.5	26.1	27.1	28.2	29.3	30.3	30.9	31.5
38	21	25.9	26.4	27.0	28.0	29.1	30.2	31.2	31.9	32.4
39	7	26.8	27.3	27.9	28.9	30.0	31.1	32.2	32.8	33.3
40	6	27.7	28.2	28.8	29.8	30.9	32.1	33.1	33.7	34.2

*Measurements in centimeters.
From Chitkara U, Rosenberg J, Chervenak FA, et al: Prenatal sonographic assessment of the fetal thorax: Normal values. Am J Obstet Gynecol 156:1069, 1987.

4. Rarely, normal lung weights are associated with lethal pulmonary dysplasia.[23]

5. In a busy practice, using a series of published charts can be cumbersome, and these charts may not reflect the expected norms of the examiner's population.

For these reasons, and for the slightly better sensitivities reported when the thoracic/abdominal circumference (TC:AC) ratio is used, as well as its reliability and relative stability across gestational ages, a number of investigators have recommended use of the TC:AC ratio to sonographically assess adequacy of fetal thorax growth. The TC:AC ratio is greater than 0.80 (mean 0.89,[22] 0.85[24]) in nearly all normal pregnancies beyond 20 weeks.[23] In a study reported by D'Alton and colleagues,[23] the TC:AC ratio had a 75% sensitivity and a 100% specificity for the prediction of neonatal death from pulmonary disease following premature rupture of membranes in otherwise normal fetuses. It has been suggested that measurement of lung *lengths* may be similarly sensitive for the detection of pulmonary hypoplasia.[25] These measurements, however, may be less convenient than the TC:AC because the measurement of lung length may be technically more difficult than either thoracic or abdominal circumference. Finally, despite all of these theoretical and quantitative considerations, two points should be emphasized: (1) in most cases in clinical patients, measurements of any sort are only used to confirm the initial subjective impression of a small fetal chest; and (2) despite the work of many qualified investigators, at this time, amniocentesis accompanied by analysis of lecithin/sphingomyelin ratios

and phosphatidylglycerol remains the most reliable method for the important determination of fetal lung maturity (see Chapter 21).

INTRATHORACIC ABNORMALITIES

Chest masses in the fetus may appear echogenic and solid or cystic. In general, by the time they are large enough to be identified sonographically, they exert mass effect, with lung compression and deviation of the mediastinum and heart. The differential diagnosis of a fetal chest mass includes congenital diaphragmatic hernia (CDH), congenital cystic adenomatoid malformation (CCAM), pulmonary sequestration, bronchogenic or neurenteric cyst, congenital lobar emphysema, or bronchial atresia and, rarely, teratoma. If bilateral, consider laryngeal or tracheal atresia or *very* rarely, bilateral CCAM. The sonographic appearance of these entities may be very similar, and thus prenatal differentiation may be difficult. As a general rule, however, regardless of the precise identity of a fetal chest mass, poor fetal outcome is associated with fetal hydrops and maternal polyhydramnios. Nonimmune hydrops probably results from the mass effect of the mass (due to compression of heart and great vessels) with resultant elevation in fetal central venous pressure. Because each of these entities may be associated with concomitant malformations and chromosomal abnormalities, careful survey of the fetus for other anomalies, as well as chromosomal analysis of the fetus, is warranted when a lesion of this nature is suspected.

CONGENITAL DIAPHRAGMATIC HERNIA

The muscular diaphragm forms between the 6th and 14th menstrual weeks as a result of a complicated chain of events involving the fusion of four structures: (1) the septum transversum (future central tendon), (2) pleuroperitoneal membranes, (3) dorsal mesentery of the esophagus (future crura), and (4) body wall. The most posterior aspect of the diaphragm, derived from the body wall, forms last.[1] By the end of the 8th menstrual week, the primitive diaphragm is intact.

A failure of fusion of one of these processes results in a diaphragmatic defect that potentiates the herniation of abdominal viscera into the thorax. CDH is the most common developmental abnormality of the diaphragm and occurs in approximately 1 in 2000 to 5000 live births[1, 26]; 92% are posterolateral defects. These abnormalities are usually unilateral (97%) and on the left (75% to 90%).[26] In 3% to 4%, the posterolateral defects are bilateral, and in 1.5% the diaphragm is completely absent.[27] Much rarer diaphragmatic defects include eventrations (5%) and right-sided or retrosternal defects. Associated malformations occur in 20% to 53% of fetuses with CDH, most notably cardiac defects (9% to 23%),[28, 29] neural tube defects (28%), spinal defects, trisomies, and certain well-defined syndromes.[30–32] Trisomy 21 and trisomy 18 are found in 4%.

Congenital diaphragmatic hernia is virtually always associated with mass effect, which manifests in the fetus as mediastinal shift, lung compression, and near-universal reduction in functional lung tissue.[33] Compression of lung tissue before 16 weeks (at which time bronchial development is complete) results in reduction of the number of bronchi and alveoli in the developing lung. The latter is the cause of the pulmonary hypoplasia that is so commonly observed in neonates or abortuses with CDH. In addition to an increase in arterial medial wall thickness, muscular hypertrophy develops and extends along the small preacinar arteries, promoting pulmonary hypertension and persistent fetal circulation, the latter of which cannot be surgically corrected postnatally. These changes are most dramatic in the ipsilateral lung but also are observed in the contralateral lung presumed secondary to lung compression.

Patients carrying a fetus with a CDH are often first referred for sonography because of suspected polyhydramnios. The definitive sonographic diagnosis of fetal CDH relies on the visualization of abdominal organs in the chest, and the sonographic hallmark of a CDH is a fluid-filled mass just behind the left atrium and ventricle in the lower thorax as seen on a transverse view (Fig. 15–9). Even if a specific viscus is not identified, other sonographic features should raise strong suspicion of a CDH. These include absence of a stomach in the abdomen,[34] shift of the mediastinum, small fetal abdominal circumference, and polyhydramnios. In the more common left-sided lesion, the stomach, the small and large bowel, and the left lobe of liver may herniate into the chest (Fig. 15–10). With real-time ultrasonography, peristalsis of the bowel in

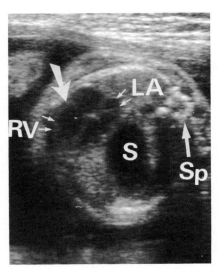

Figure 15–9. Congenital diaphragmatic hernia. Transverse view of the thorax. The stomach (S) has herniated into the chest, behind the four-chamber heart (*large arrow*). RV, right ventricle; LA, left atrium; Sp, spine.

the fetal chest may even be detected. The detection of the liver in the chest may be more difficult.

Occasionally an oblique section through a normal fetal chest results in an image that may be confused

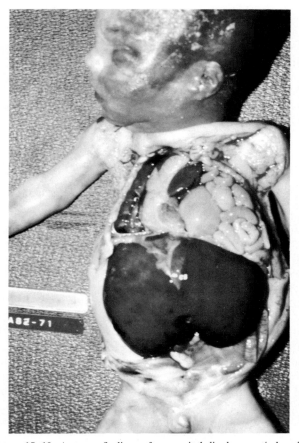

Figure 15–10. Autopsy findings of congenital diaphragmatic hernia. This neonate died of respiratory failure shortly after birth. The stomach, spleen, and intestines have herniated into the left chest and compressed the lungs. The mediastinum has shifted far to the right.

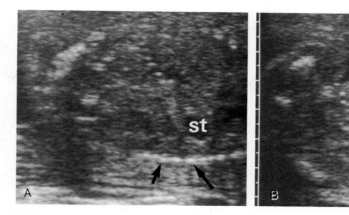

Figure 15–11. Oblique image simulates congenital diaphragmatic hernia (false positive). *A.* Fluid-filled stomach (st) is imaged in an area surrounded by ribs (*arrows*), simulating the location of the stomach in the fetal thorax. *B.* A more direct coronal image demonstrates normal relationships: intact hypoechoic diaphragm (*arrows*), stomach (st) below the diaphragm, and heart (c) in the fetal thorax.

with a CDH. This occurs because infradiaphragmatic structures such as bowel and liver are included in the same image as the lower thorax (Fig. 15–11). As a general rule, however, no bowel should be identified in the chest on the same image as the four-chamber view of the heart (see Fig. 15–5).[35] Thus, whenever this confusion arises, the four-chamber view of the heart, as well as the appropriate parasagittal or coronal views of the chest that include the fetal diaphragm and the infradiaphragmatic abdominal anatomy, should be sought to exclude or confirm the presence of a CDH. In most fetuses with large, clinically significant CDHs there is usually sufficient shift of the heart and mediastinum (and possibly a pleural effusion) to suggest the diagnosis.

The herniation of bowel through the defect may occur as an intermittent event, and thus the size and contents of the hernia may change from one examination to another. This phenomenon may explain why small hernias may not be diagnosed until late in gestation despite the fact that the diaphragmatic defect occurred much earlier.

In right-sided hernias, which occur less commonly but are associated with a worse prognosis, the right lobe of the liver alone may herniate. Although this type of hernia may be associated with other suggestive findings, such as hydrothorax and ascites,[36] right-sided lesions may be more difficult to identify, owing to the similar echotexture of the liver and lungs. Visualization of a cystic structure, the gallbladder, in the right chest has been a useful ancillary finding used to confirm this diagnosis.

The mortality associated with CDH is extremely high (generally considered >75%) and even higher among those fetuses with other malformations.[30, 33] The mortality associated with a CDH detected in the fetus is higher than that reported postnatally. Despite the most valiant efforts at surgical correction postnatally, the prognosis appears to be most closely related to the presence of associated malformations, the volume of herniated bowel contents, and the timing of the herniation. Thus, larger hernias and those that occur earliest in gestation carry the worst prognoses.[33, 35] Although it would be useful to estimate the size of the defect in the fetus, it has not been possible to precisely predict the size of the defect. This is because the defect

itself is difficult to observe and quantitate and the volume of herniated viscera is difficult to quantitate. Large hernias are generally judged by the degree of mediastinal shift and the presence of dilated bowel loops (including stomach) within the chest. Unfortunately, as mentioned previously, the degree of pulmonary hypoplasia cannot currently be established by the antepartum sonographic appearance of lung volume or compression. Outcome does seem to be influenced by the age at which the defect is detected, which is probably a reflection of the size and severity of the malformation. Poorer survival has been reported in fetuses in whom the sonographic diagnosis is made before 25 weeks' gestation (17%), compared with fetuses diagnosed after 25 weeks' gestation (40%).[32] Survival is improved further (48%) in the latter group if all fetuses with associated malformations are excluded.[32] Polyhydramnios is commonly associated with this defect. Some investigators have suggested that the presence of polyhydramnios is a poor prognostic indicator[33]; however, others have not confirmed this prognostic association.[32]

In addition to pulmonary hypoplasia, an important cause of perinatal mortality in these infants is persistent fetal circulation.[33, 37] Both pulmonary hypoplasia and persistent fetal circulation are presumed to result from persistent and severe lung compression in intrauterine life. Sonographic features associated with a poor outcome in fetuses with CDH include the presence of a persistently dilated stomach in the chest and left-sided heart underdevelopment. Cardiac ventricular disproportion as demonstrated by a reduced left-to-right ventricular size is a good, but not perfect, "predictor" of poor outcome.[32] Left-sided heart underdevelopment is associated with left-sided CDH (similar to right-sided heart underdevelopment in association with a right-sided CDH) and is likely related to sequelae of direct compression on the heart.

Because of the extremely poor prognosis, in a number of fetuses with CDH surgical repair of the defect has been attempted by way of hysterotomy. Thus far, survival has not been greatly improved but too few fetal surgeries for CDH have been performed at the time of this writing to draw meaningful conclusions.

Sonographically, CDH may be confused with other intrathoracic fetal abnormalities, such as CCAM, bronchogenic cysts, or extralobar sequestration. However, normal upper fetal abdominal anatomy would be expected in the other lesions.

CONGENITAL CYSTIC ADENOMATOID MALFORMATION

Congenital cystic adenomatoid malformation is a rare pulmonary lesion that can be diagnosed prenatally by ultrasonography.[38–44] These lesions tend to be large, bulky, and noncompressible. Large CCAMs can displace mediastinal structures with compression of the heart and inferior vena cava. Like CDH, a CCAM may be associated with fetal hydrops, maternal polyhydramnios, and pulmonary hypoplasia. The prenatal diagnosis can be helpful in planning both the site of delivery and the immediate postnatal care, as well as in counseling the parents about the outcome.

Congenital cystic adenomatoid malformation is a hamartomatous pulmonary lesion.[45–48] It is typically unilateral and usually involves one lobe or segment, although, on rare occasions, it may be bilateral or a single whole lung may be involved.[49] Most CCAMs communicate with the normal tracheobronchial tree. It is thought that they may become obstructed postnatally with air trapping due to the absence of cartilaginous bronchi within the lesion.[50] Furthermore, some investigators have suggested that fluid produced in the CCAM may contribute to polyhydramnios in some cases. Stocker and associates described the pathologic appearance of lesions as macrocystic, medium-sized cystic, and solid (Fig. 15–12).[45] Associated renal and chromosomal anomalies have been reported but have not been confirmed by all investigators.[51, 52] Chromosomal analysis as well as careful fetal survey is recommended when this lesion is suspected.

Relatively few cases have been described prenatally. The sonographic appearance has ranged from a multicystic mass to a solid pulmonary lesion with mass effect and mediastinal shift (Figs. 15–13 through 15–16). The prenatal sonographic findings and outcome were described in 12 cases by Adzick and colleagues.[39] Among these cases, two general categories of lesions

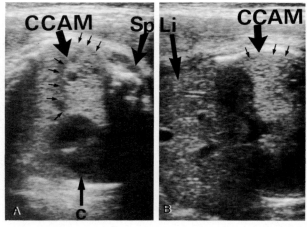

Figure 15–13. *A* and *B.* Congenital cyst adenomatoid malformation. Echogenic mass lesion with scattered cysts in the right fetal chest (CCAM), with displacement of the heart (c) to the left. Sp, spine; Li, liver.

emerged: (1) those that appeared microcystic and (2) those that appeared macrocystic on sonography. In that series, fetuses with solid-appearing lesions had a poorer outcome than those with macrocystic forms. Histologically, the lesions that appear solid contain many small cysts. They are thought to appear solid secondary to the numerous reflections from interfaces of the myriad tiny cysts (similar to infantile polycystic kidney disease). As with all space-occupying chest lesions, the prognosis of a fetus with CCAM appears to be adversely affected by fetal hydrops, polyhydramnios, or lesions of large volume.[39] Although associated fetal hydrops carries a poor prognosis in these fetuses, it is interesting to note that the majority of patients with isolated CCAM who survive after delivery will be asymptomatic during the neonatal period. In these

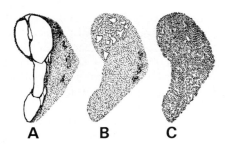

Figure 15–12. The three types of congenital cyst adenomatoid malformation of the lung as described by Stocker and colleagues.[45] *A.* Type 1 lesions have large cysts of variable sizes. *B.* Type 2 lesions have smaller cysts. *C.* Type 3 lesions appear solid owing to reflections from numerous adenomatoid structures along with scattered, thin-walled structures similar to bronchioles. (From Stocker JT, Madewell JE, Drake RM: Congenital cystic adenomatoid malformation of the lung. Hum Pathol 8:155, 1977.)

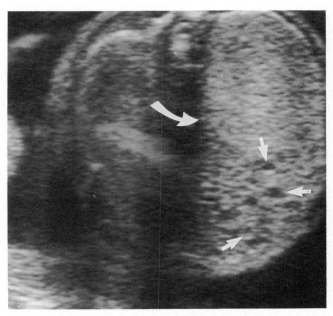

Figure 15–14. Echogenic lung mass (*curved arrow*) with small cysts (*small arrows*) characteristic of congenital cystic adenomatoid malformation.

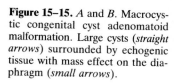

Figure 15–15. *A* and *B*. Macrocystic congenital cyst adenomatoid malformation. Large cysts (*straight arrows*) surrounded by echogenic tissue with mass effect on the diaphragm (*small arrows*).

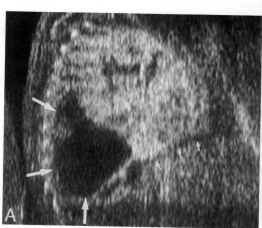
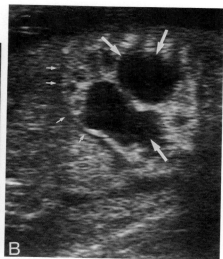

cases, the lesions are amenable to surgical correction and the infant stands a good chance of survival.[47] In some cases, macrocystic lesions in the fetus have been drained percutaneously but fluid often reaccumulates.[39, 53] When large and associated with hydrops, these lesions have also been successfully resected in the fetus (in utero).[54]

It is now well documented that occasionally these large, bulky lesions may regress in utero without intervention.[50, 55] MacGillivray and associates reported a series of nine large pulmonary lesions (three CCAMs and six sequestrations) observed prenatally that spontaneously decreased in size or disappeared during gestation.[56] Thus, immediate intervention is less warranted when a large fetal chest mass is first observed (unless it is accompanied by hydrops) because we cannot predict which lesions will spontaneously regress. There is no known recurrence risk for future pregnancies. The differential diagnosis includes pulmonary sequestration, bronchogenic cyst, bronchial atresia, and neurenteric cyst.

PULMONARY SEQUESTRATION, BRONCHOGENIC CYSTS, AND BRONCHIAL/TRACHEAL ATRESIA

Although the exact etiology of these abnormalities is unknown, pulmonary sequestrations probably represent bronchopulmonary foregut abnormalities.[48] Sequestrations are characterized by lack of communication with the normal bronchial tree. The lesions have been divided into extralobar and intralobar forms, and although the former is least common overall (25%), extralobar sequestration is the most common form found in neonates and nearly the only form that has been detected prenatally.[43, 57–59] The extralobar lesion consists of a mass of ectopic pulmonary tissue that is enveloped by its own pleura. This lung tissue receives its arterial supply ectopically, usually from the descending aorta, and its venous drainage is to systemic (inferior vena cava, azygous, or portal veins) rather than pulmonary veins (Fig. 15–17).[60, 61] Sequestrations occur

Figure 15–16. Congenital cyst adenomatoid malformation. *A*. Transverse image demonstrating homogeneous, solid-appearing pulmonary lesion (*curved arrows*) displacing the heart (C) to the right. *B*. Oblique coronal view demonstrating mass effect of malformation (*curved arrows*), with bowing of the diaphragm (*straight arrows*). C, heart; h, head.

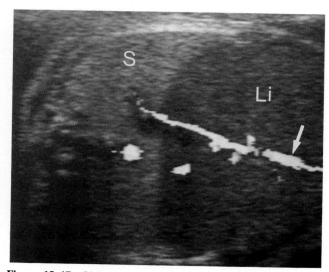

Figure 15–17. Oblique coronal image of sequestration (S) with venous drainage below the diaphragm to the left portal vein (*arrow*). Li, liver.

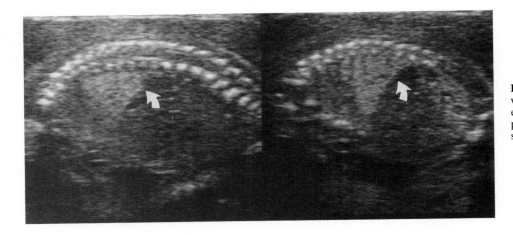

Figure 15–18. Dual image of fetus with left lower lobe, wedge-shaped, echogenic mass (*curved arrow*) proven to be an extralobar pulmonary sequestration.

most commonly on the left (90%) in the posterior and basal segments. Occasionally, sequestered lobes are found outside the thoracic cavity.[62] Subdiaphragmatic lesions (which account for 2.5% of bronchopulmonary foregut malformations) have been observed prenatally with ultrasound evaluation.[63, 64] The extralobar form is associated with other anomalies, including foregut abnormalities and CDH in 58% of cases.[48, 62, 65] The latter association may obscure the extralobar sequestration and account for the fact that this form of sequestration has only rarely been diagnosed prenatally. Alternatively, intralobar sequestration may be acquired lesions, thus explaining their notable scarcity in the fetal literature. Karyotype abnormalities do not seem to be increased.

Sonographically, a pulmonary sequestration appears as a well-circumscribed, uniformly echogenic mass in the fetal thorax (Fig. 15–18).[43, 57–59] Like CCAM and CDH, they, too, have been associated with fetal hydrops and maternal polyhydramnios that is presumed secondary to mass effect and compression of the fetal esophagus or mediastinum and heart. Although these lesions may be similar to CDH, they are distinguished by the normal intra-abdominal anatomy associated with pulmonary sequestration. In addition, color Doppler flow imaging has been used to detect the feeding systemic artery in the fetus (which has been traced from the descending aorta to lower lobe mass) (Fig. 15–19).[66] This important observation is worthy of the time required to find a small vessel because it distinguishes a pulmonary sequestration from a CCAM, lobar emphysema, or CDH.

Bronchogenic cysts are uncommon congenital anomalies that result from an abnormal development in the budding or branching of the tracheobronchial tree, probably between the 26th and 40th day of fetal life, when the most active tracheobronchial development is occurring.[67] They also represent foregut abnormalities and result from abnormal budding of the ventral diverticulum of the foregut.[48, 67] Recall that the respiratory tract and the esophagus are derived from the primitive foregut: the esophagus from the posterior aspect and the tracheobronchial tree from the anterior. Therefore, posterior mediastinal neurenteric cysts occur as an anomaly of the posterior (dorsal) aspect of the foregut and notochord and, as expected, are asso-

ciated with spinal anomalies. Abnormal development in the *middle* of the foregut is believed to result in esophageal duplications, and abnormal budding of the anterior diverticulum of the foregut results in bronchial cysts, most of which occur in the mediastinum, with a minority in the pulmonary parenchyma.[48] Bronchogenic cysts are not usually associated with other congenital anomalies.[48, 68] They may enlarge in infancy and cause respiratory distress. Their presence in the fetus is suggested by mediastinal shift and bronchial obstruction. In one reported case, a small bronchogenic cyst caused bronchial obstruction of the left lung in the fetus. The enlarged, echogenic, obstructed lung, not the bronchogenic cyst, was the abnormality detected prenatally on the sonogram.[69] Very few cases have been detected antenatally, but those that have were seen as unilocular or multilocular cystic masses in the fetal chest.[43] Mediastinal cysts tend to compress the trachea.

Congenital bronchial atresia is another unusual pulmonary anomaly that rarely has been described on

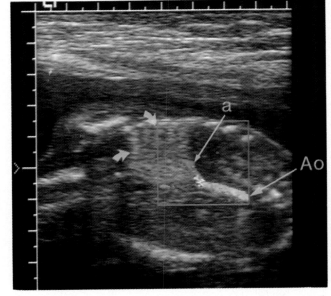

Figure 15–19. Color Doppler scan is helpful in detecting the ectopic vascular (a) supply to a fetal pulmonary sequestration (*curved arrows*), thus confirming the diagnosis. Ao, aorta.

Figure 15–20. Laryngeal/tracheal atresia. *A.* Transverse axial image demonstrates the enlarged echogenic lungs bilaterally. The differential diagnosis of the two round fluid-filled structures (*arrows*) includes dilated fluid-filled bronchi, dilated pulmonary arteries, pulmonary/bronchogenic cysts. C, heart. *B.* Coronal image of the same fetus. The symmetric dilated fluid-filled bronchi can be observed (*arrows*). Color Doppler scan showed no flow in these structures, confirming the diagnosis of tracheal atresia. Curved arrow indicates ascites.

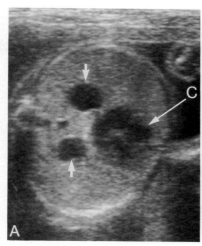
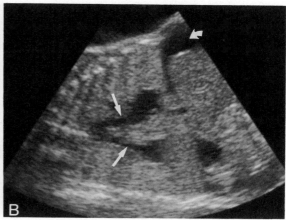

prenatal sonography as an echogenic pulmonary mass lesion.[70] The cause is unknown, but the lesion is characterized by a *focal* obliteration of a segment of the bronchial lumen and occurs most commonly in the left upper lobe. Other relatively common sites are the right upper middle lobes. This lesion rarely occurs in the lower lobe[48] and in this way might be distinguished from extralobar pulmonary sequestration or CDH.

Both fetal tracheal and laryngeal atresia have been observed prenatally. If the trachea or larynx is atretic or completely obstructed, the fluid secreted by the lungs cannot be expelled. The distended lungs appear hyperechogenic, and the bronchi become dilated by the trapped fluid. Histologically, these lungs are not hypoplastic but normal or hyperplastic. Fetal ascites is usually associated, perhaps secondary to venous compression of the mediastinal vessels and heart, by the enlarged lungs. Mortality in fetuses in whom these lesions have been detected prenatally has been 100% (Fig. 15–20).[71, 72]

PLEURAL EFFUSION

Fluid in the pleural space of the fetus is abnormal at any gestational age. Pleural effusions may occur in the fetus as an isolated abnormality or in association with more serious conditions, such as the multiple causes of immune or nonimmune hydrops fetalis, chest mass, or posterior urethral valves associated with urinary ascites. In cases of nonimmune hydrops fetalis, prognosis is usually poor,[73–75] and these serous effusions represent only a single manifestation of a more serious underlying dysfunction (cardiac anomaly, lymphangiectasia, intrauterine infection, Turner syndrome, chromosomal anomaly, and similar defects). If the fetus is believed to have immune hydrops fetalis, current therapy is directed toward intrauterine transfusion or prompt delivery, depending on the gestational age.[76] Primary pleural effusions are generally chylous and, when unassociated with hydrops, carry a much more optimistic fetal prognosis. This is generally poorer than the prognosis of the neonate whose chylous effusion is discovered after birth. Overall mortality in

the fetus approaches 50%,[77, 78] with death after birth due to pulmonary hypoplasia, hydrops, and prematurity. Bilateral effusions, diagnosis before 33 weeks, and hydrops are all associated with poorer outcome (Table 15–2).[78, 79] On the contrary, the *absence* of hydrops predicted 100% survival in Longaker and coworkers' series of 32 fetuses with hydrothorax. Spontaneous resolution of the pleural fluid is associated with near 100% survival.[78]

Sonographically, pleural effusions appear as anechoic fluid collections in the fetal chest that usually conform to the normal chest and diaphragmatic contour (Fig. 15–21) but, when large enough, may be associated with bulging of the chest and flattening or inversion of the diaphragm (Figs. 15–22 and 15–23).[75] Although chylous effusions in the feeding infant or adult typically appear whitish and have been described as milky, if a chylous effusion in the fetus is aspirated, the fluid is generally clear and straw colored. This fluid does not contain chylomicrons—the fetus is "fasting." These effusions are therefore indistinguishable based on the sonographic appearance from serous effusions

Table 15–2. FETAL PLEURAL EFFUSIONS: PROGNOSTIC INDICATORS

Characteristic	% Survival
Age at diagnosis	
< 33 wk	43
≥ 33 wk	80
Age at delivery	
< 35 wk	30
≥ 35 wk	79
Spontaneous resolution	
Yes	100
No	52
Hydrops	
Yes	52
No	100
Bilateral	
Yes	52
No	100*

*Without mediastinal shift.
From Longaker MT, Laberge J-M, Dansereau J, et al: Primary hydrothorax: Natural history and management. J Pediatr Surg 24:573, 1989.

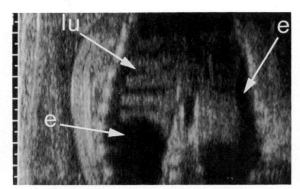

Figure 15–21. Fetal pleural effusions (e) may conform to the normal chest contour, with slight compression of the lung parenchyma (lu). This appearance is not reliable for predicting future pulmonary function.

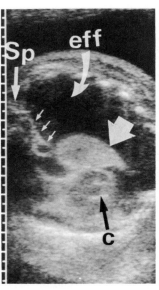

Figure 15–23. Fetal pleural effusion. Transverse image of the fetal thorax demonstrates bowing of the mediastinum. Large arrow indicates lung. Sp, spine; eff, effusion; c, heart.

of hydrops fetalis.[80–84] Aspirated chylous fetal effusions generally show a large number of lymphocytes. Sonographic features suggestive of fetal chylothorax include the following:

1. The pleural effusion occurs as an isolated finding.
2. The size of the effusion is disproportionately large compared with other effusions, if present.
3. The effusion occurs first as an isolated finding and is later followed by the development of other features associated with hydrops fetalis, such as ascites and integumentary edema.

Chylothorax is the most frequent cause of isolated pleural effusion leading to respiratory distress in the neonate.[81, 82] The importance of this diagnosis is underscored by the fact that respiratory distress of the neonate associated with pleural effusions has a 15% to 25% mortality.[83, 84] The etiology is unknown.[81–85] It is

more common in males and is usually unilateral, although a small fraction will be bilateral.[82] Prenatal sonographic findings have been reported in a number of cases.[77–80, 86] In the most severe cases, these effusions

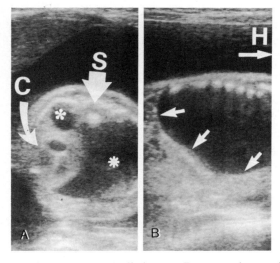

Figure 15–22. Fetal pleural effusion. *A.* Transverse image of the fetal thorax. Largely unilateral effusion (*asterisks*). The heart (C) is shifted. S, spine. *B.* The diaphragm was bowed by the mass effect of this large fetal effusion (*arrows*). This effusion was drained and redrained following catheter failure in utero at 30 and 32 menstrual weeks. The fetus was born approximately 2 weeks later and did not require ventilatory assistance. H, head.

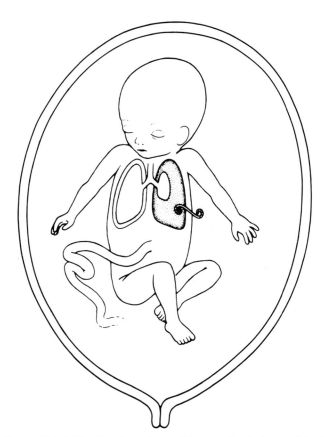

Figure 15–24. Pigtail catheter inserted in utero for drainage of fetal pleural effusion. (From Longaker MT, Laberge J-M, Dansereau J, et al: Primary fetal hydrothorax: Natural history and management. J Pediatr Surg 24:573, 1989.)

have been associated with mediastinal shift, fetal hydrops, and maternal polyhydramnios.[76, 83] In some cases, drainage of large effusions in utero have been performed in an attempt either to relieve mediastinal shift believed to be the cause of hydrops or to allow for better lung expansion and growth in utero (Fig. 15–24).[80, 83] In addition, in utero thoracentesis can be performed just before delivery to improve ventilation in the immediate postpartum period.[86] Postnatally, these effusions are treated with chest tube drainage for days to weeks; and in a series of cases diagnosed at birth, the condition eventually resolved with normal outcome in almost all.[81, 85]

References

1. Moore KL: Development of body cavities, primitive mesenteries, and the diaphragm. In: The Developing Human: Clinically Oriented Embryology, 4th ed. Philadelphia, WB Saunders, 1988.
2. Jeanty P, Romero R, Hobbins JC: Fetal pericardial fluid: A normal finding in the second half of gestation. Am J Obstet Gynecol 149:529, 1984.
3. Yagel S, Hurwitz A: Fetal pericardial fluid. (Letter) Am J Obstet Gynecol 152:721, 1985.
4. Jeanty P, Romero R, Hobbins JC: Vascular anatomy of the fetus. J Ultrasound Med 3:113, 1984.
5. Cooper C, Mahony BS, Bowie JD, et al: Ultrasound evaluation of the normal fetal upper airway and esophagus. J Ultrasound Med 4:343, 1985.
6. Hislop AA, Wigglesworth JS, Desai R: Alveolar development in the human fetus and infant. Early Hum Dev 13:1, 1986.
7. Fewell JE, Ching Lee CHU, Kitterman JA: Effects of phrenic nerve section on the respiratory system of fetal lambs. J Appl Physiol 51:293, 1981.
8. Harrison MR, Bressack MA, Churg AM, et al: Correction of congenital diaphragmatic hernia in utero: II. Simulated correction permits fetal lung growth with survival at birth. Surgery 88:260, 1980.
9. Ohlsson A, Fong KW, Rose TH, Moore DC: Prenatal sonographic diagnosis of Pena-Shokeir syndrome type I, or fetal akinesia deformation sequence. Am J Med Genet 25:59, 1988.
10. Alcorn D, Adamson TM, Lambert TF, et al: Morphologic effects of chronic tracheal ligation and drainage in the fetal lamb. J Anat 123:649, 1977.
11. Fewell JE, Hislop AA, Kitterman JA, Johnstone P: Effect of tracheostomy on lung development in fetal lambs. J Appl Physiol 55:1103, 1983.
12. Hislop A, Hey E, Reid L: The lung in congenital bilateral renal agenesis of dysplasia. Arch Dis Child 54:32, 1979.
13. Nicolini U, Fisk NM, Rodeck CH, et al: Low amniotic pressure in oligohydramnios: Is this the cause of pulmonary hypoplasia? Am J Obstet Gynecol 161:1098, 1989.
14. Silver MM, Thurston WA, Patrick JE: Perinatal pulmonary hypoplasia due to laryngeal atresia. Hum Pathol 19:110, 1988.
15. Scurry JP, Adamson TM, Cussen LJ: Fetal lung growth in laryngeal atresia and tracheal agenesis. Austr Paediatr 25:47, 1989.
16. Fried AM, Loh FK, Umer MA, et al: Echogenicity of fetal lung: Relation to fetal age and maturity. AJR 145:591, 1985.
17. Gayea PD, Grant DC, Doubilet PM, et al: Prediction of fetal lung maturity: Inaccuracy of study using conventional ultrasound instruments. Radiology 155:473, 1985.
18. Birnholz JC, Farrell EE: Fetal lung development: Compressibility as a measure of maturity. Radiology 154:495, 1985.
19. Nimrod C, Davies D, Stanislaw W, et al: Ultrasound prediction of pulmonary hypoplasia. Obstet Gynecol 68:495, 1986.
20. Devore GR, Horenstein J, Platt LD: Fetal echocardiography: Assessment of cardiothoracic disproportion: A new technique for the diagnosis of thoracic hypoplasia. Am J Obstet Gynecol 155:1066, 1986.
21. Songster GS, Gray DL, Crane JP: Prenatal prediction of lethal pulmonary hypoplasia using ultrasonic fetal chest circumference. Obstet Gynecol 73:261, 1989.
22. Chitkara U, Rosenberg J, Chervenak FA, et al: Prenatal sonographic assessment of the fetal thorax: Normal values. Am J Obstet Gynecol 156:1069, 1987.
23. D'Alton M, Mercer B, Riddick E, Dudley D: Serial thoracic versus abdominal circumference ratios for the prediction of pulmonary hypoplasia in premature rupture of the membranes remote from term. Am J Obstet Gynecol 166:658, 1992.
24. Vintzileos AM, Campbell WA, Rodis JF, et al: Comparison of six different ultrasonographic methods for predicting lethal fetal pulmonary hypoplasia. Am J Obstet Gynecol 161:606, 1989.
25. Roberts AB, Mitchell JM: Direct ultrasonographic measurement of fetal lung length in normal pregnancies and pregnancies complicated by prolonged rupture of membranes. Am J Obstet Gynecol 163:1560, 1990.
26. Schumacher RE, Farrell PM: Congenital diaphragmatic hernia: A major remaining challenge in neonatal respiratory care. Perinatol Neonatol 9:29, 1985.
27. Wenstrom KD, Weiner CP, Hanson JW: A five-year statewide experience with congenital diaphragmatic hernia. Am J Obstet Gynecol 165:838, 1991.
28. Greenwood RD, Rosenthal A, Nadas AS: Cardiovascular abnormalities associated with congenital diaphragmatic hernia. Pediatrics 57:92, 1976.
29. David TJ, Illingsworth CA: Diaphragmatic hernia in the southwest of England. J Med Genet 13:253, 1976.
30. Nakayama DK, Harrison MR, Chinn DH, et al: Prenatal diagnosis and natural history of the fetus with a congenital diaphragmatic hernia: Initial clinical experience. J Pediatr Surg 20:118, 1985.
31. Puri P, Gorman F: Lethal nonpulmonary anomalies associated with congenital surgery. J Pediatr Surg 19:29, 1984.
32. Sharland GK, Lockhart SM, Heward AJ, Allan D: Prognosis in fetal diaphragmatic hernia. Am J Obstet Gynecol 166:9, 1992.
33. Harrison MR, Adzick NS, Nakayama DK, et al: Fetal diaphragmatic hernia: Fatal but fixable. Semin Perinatol 9:103, 1985.
34. Farrant P: The antenatal diagnosis of oesophageal atresia by ultrasound. Br J Radiol 53:1202, 1980.
35. Harrison MR, Golbus MS, Filly RA: Congenital diaphragmatic hernia. In: The Unborn Patient, pp 237–276. Orlando, FL, Grune & Stratton, 1984.
36. Gilsanz V, Emons D, Hansmann M, et al: Hydrothorax, ascites, and right diaphragmatic hernia. Radiology 158:243, 1986.
37. Harrison MR, Bjordal RI, Landmark F, et al: Congenital diaphragmatic hernia: The hidden mortality. J Pediatr Surg 13:227, 1979.
38. Vintzileos AM, Campbell WA, Nochimson DJ: Antenatal evaluation and management of ultrasonically detected fetal anomalies. Obstet Gynecol 69:640, 1987.
39. Adzick NS, Harrison MR, Glick PL, et al: Fetal cystic adenomatoid malformation: Prenatal diagnosis and natural history. J Pediatr Surg 20:483, 1985.
40. Johnson JA, Rumack CM, Johnson ML, et al: Cystic adenomatoid malformation: Antenatal demonstration. AJR 142:483, 1984.
41. Pezzuti RT, Isler RJ: Antenatal ultrasound detection of cystic adenomatoid malformation of lung: Report of a case and review of the recent literature. J Clin Ultrasound 11:342, 1983.
42. Graham D, Winn K, Dex W, et al: Prenatal diagnosis of cystic adenomatoid malformation of the lung. J Ultrasound Med 1:9, 1982.
43. Mayden KL, Tortora M, Chervenak F: The antenatal sonographic detection of lung masses. Am J Obstet Gynecol 143:349, 1984.
44. Miller RK, Sieber WK, Yunis EJ: Congenital adenomatoid malformation of the lung: A report of 17 cases and a review of the literature. Pathol Annu 1:387, 1980.
45. Stocker JT, Madewell JE, Drake RM: Congenital cystic adenomatoid malformation of the lung. Hum Pathol 8:155, 1977.
46. Van Dijk C, Wagenvoort CA: The various types of congenital adenomatoid malformations of the lung. J Pathol 110:131, 1973.
47. Wolf SA, Hertzler JH, Philippart AL: Cystic adenomatoid dysplasia of the lung. J Pediatr Surg 15:925, 1980.
48. Fraser RG, Pare JAP: Pulmonary abnormalities of developmental origin. In Pare PD, Fraser RS, Genereux GP (eds): Diagnosis

of Diseases of the Chest, 3rd ed, pp 695–773. Philadelphia, WB Saunders, 1989.

49. Morcos SF, Lobb MO: The antenatal diagnosis by ultrasonography of type III congenital cystic adenomatoid malformation of the lung. Br J Obstet Gynaecol 93:1002, 1986.

50. Fine C, Adzick NS, Doubilet PM: Decreasing size of a congenital cystic adenomatoid malformation in utero. J Ultrasound Med 7:405, 1988.

51. Bale PM: Congenital cystic malformation of the lung. Am J Clin Pathol 71:411, 1979.

52. Oster AG, Fortune DW: Congenital cystic adenomatoid malformation of the lung. Am J Clin Pathol 70:595, 1978.

53. Clark SL, Vitale DJ, Minton SD, et al: Successful fetal therapy for cystic adenomatoid malformation associated with second trimester hydrops. Am J Obstet Gynecol 157:284, 1987.

54. Harrison MR, Adzick NS, Jennings R, et al: Antenatal intervention for congenital cystic adenomatoid malformation. Lancet 336:965, 1990.

55. Saltzman DH, Adzick NS, Benacerraf BR: Fetal cystic adenomatoid malformation of the lung: Apparent improvement in utero. Obstet Gynecol 71:1000, 1988.

56. MacGillivray TE, Adzick S, Goldstein RB, Harrison MR: Disappearing fetal lung lesions. J Pediatr Surg, in press.

57. Thomas CS, Leopold GR, Hilton S, et al: Fetal hydrops associated with extralobar sequestration. J Ultrasound Med 5:668, 1986.

58. Mariona F, McAplin C, Zador I, et al: Sonographic detection of fetal extrathoracic pulmonary sequestration. J Ultrasound Med 5:283, 1986.

59. Romero R, Chervenak FA, Kotzen J, et al: Antenatal sonographic findings of extralobar pulmonary sequestration. J Ultrasound Med 1:131, 1982.

60. Buntain WL, Woolley MM, Mahour GH, et al: Pulmonary sequestration in children: A twenty-five year experience. Surgery 81:413, 1977.

61. Levine MM, Nudel DB, Gootman N, et al: Pulmonary sequestration causing congestive heart failure in infancy: A report of two cases and review of the literature. Ann Thorac Surg 34:581, 1981.

62. Savic B, Birtel FJ, Tholen W, et al: Lung sequestration: Report of seven cases and review of 540 published cases. Thorax 34:96, 1979.

63. Davies RP, Ford WDA, Lequesne GW, Orell SR: Ultrasonic detection of subdiaphragmatic pulmonary sequestration in utero and postnatal diagnosis by fine-needle aspiration biopsy. J Ultrasound Med 8:47, 1989.

64. Weinbaum PJ, Bors-Koefoed R, Green KW, Prenatt L: Antenatal sonographic findings in a case of intra-abdominal pulmonary sequestration. Obstet Gynecol 73:860, 1989.

65. DeParedes CG, Pierce WS, Johnson DG, et al: Pulmonary sequestration in infants and children: A 20-year experience and review of the literature. J Pediatr Surg 5:136, 1970.

66. West MS, Donaldson JS, Shkolnik A: Pulmonary sequestration: Diagnosis by ultrasound. J Ultrasound Med 8:125, 1989.

67. Pare JAP, Fraser RG: Synopsis of Diseases of the Chest, pp 239–242. Philadelphia, WB Saunders, 1983.

68. Dumontier C, Graviss ER, Silberstein MJ, et al: Bronchogenic cysts in children. Clin Radiol 36:431, 1985.

69. Young G, L'Heureux PR, Krueckeberg ST, Swanson DA: Mediastinal bronchogenic cyst: Prenatal sonographic diagnosis. AJR 152:125, 1989.

70. McAlister WH, Wright JR, Crane JP: Main-stem bronchial atresia: Intrauterine sonographic diagnosis. AJR 148:364, 1987.

71. Dolkart LA, Reimers FT, Wertheimer IS, Wilson BO: Prenatal diagnosis of laryngeal atresia. J Ultrasound Med 11:496, 1992.

72. Watson WJ, Thorp JM Jr, Miller RC, et al: Prenatal diagnosis of laryngeal atresia. Am J Obstet Gynecol 163:1456, 1990.

73. Harrison MR, Golbus MS, Filly RA: Management of the fetus with nonimmune hydrops. In: The Unborn Patient, pp 193–216. Orlando, FL, Grune & Stratton, 1984.

74. Hutchinson AA, Drew JH, Yu VYH, et al: Nonimmunologic hydrops fetalis: A review of 61 cases. Obstet Gynecol 59:347, 1982.

75. Mahony BS, Filly RA, Callen PW, et al: Severe non-immune hydrops fetalis: Sonographic evaluation. Radiology 151:757, 1984.

76. Frigoletto FD, Greene MF, Benacerraf BR: Ultrasonographic fetal surveillance in the management of the isoimmunized pregnancy. N Engl J Med 315:430, 1986.

77. Weber AM, Philipson EH: Fetal pleural effusion: A review and meta-analysis for prognostic indicators. Obstet Gynecol 79:281, 1992.

78. Longaker MT, Laberge J-M, Dansereau J, et al: Primary fetal hydrothorax: Natural history and management. J Pediatr Surg 24:573, 1989.

79. Estroff JA, Parad RB, Frigoletto FD Jr, Benacerraf BR: The natural history of isolated fetal hydrothorax. Ultrasound Obstet Gynecol 2:162, 1992.

80. Benacerraf BR, Frigoletto FD: Mid-trimester fetal thoracentesis. J Clin Ultrasound 13:202, 1985.

81. Vain NE, Swarner OW, Cha CC: Neonatal chylothorax: A report and discussion of nine consecutive cases. J Pediatr Surg 15:261, 1980.

82. Chernick V, Reed MH: Pneumothorax and chylothorax in the neonatal period. J Pediatr 76:624, 1970.

83. Petres RE, Redwine FO, Cruikshank DP: Congenital bilateral chylothorax: Antepartum diagnosis and successful intrauterine surgical management. JAMA 248:1360, 1982.

84. Lange IR, Manning FA: Antenatal diagnosis of congenital pleural effusion. Am J Obstet Gynecol 140:839, 1981.

85. Brodman RF: Congenital chylothorax. NY State J Med 75:553, 1975.

86. Seeds JW, Bowes WA: Results of treatment of severe fetal hydrothorax with bilateral pleuroamniotic catheters. Obstet Gynecol 68:577, 1986.

CHAPTER 16

■■■■■ ## Ultrasound Evaluation of the Fetal Abdomen

RUTH B. GOLDSTEIN, M.D.

By the second trimester, most of the fetal abdominal organs are large enough to have attained their normal adult position and structure. Viscera, including the liver, gallbladder, spleen, stomach, and kidneys, may be easily identified on ultrasound evaluation. The fetal abdomen, however, differs from that of the adult in several ways:

1. The umbilical arteries and veins provide important anatomic landmarks for fetal abdominal anatomy and measurements.

2. A conduit between portal veins and systemic veins, the ductus venosus is patent and may be visualized on the fetal sonogram (Figs. 16–1 through 16–3).

3. The proportions of the fetal body differ from those of the adult in that the size of the fetal abdomen is relatively larger compared with body length, and the liver occupies a relatively larger volume of the abdomen in the fetus.[1]

4. The fetal pelvic cavity is relatively small and, thus, structures such as the urinary bladder, ovaries, and uterus tend to lie almost completely in the abdominal cavity. The filled fetal bladder is, therefore, not confined to the pelvis; and ovarian cysts, when they occur in the fetus, frequently are found in the fetal abdominal cavity or flanks.

5. The apron of the greater omentum is relatively small, contains relatively little fat, and remains unfused in the fetus. Fetal ascites may therefore separate the omental leaves.[2]

THE ABDOMEN IN THE EMBRYO: THE FIRST TRIMESTER

The yolk sac is often the first embryonic structure observed sonographically within the gestational sac. The yolk sac is connected to the primitive gut by a focal constriction known as the yolk stalk. The dorsal part of the yolk sac is incorporated into the primitive gut, and the remaining yolk sac (secondary yolk sac) and stalk detach from the developing midgut loop by the end of the eighth menstrual week (Fig. 16–4).[3] The yolk sac detected on the sonogram is almost always the secondary yolk sac.

It appears as a tiny anechoic round structure with an echogenic rim that becomes visible on transabdominal sonography by 5 to 6 menstrual weeks and on endovaginal sonography by the end of the fifth menstrual week. At this time it is still attached to the midgut. The secondary yolk sac lies outside the amniotic sac within the chorionic cavity. Because the yolk sac is often observed before the embryo can be visualized, the presence of two yolk sacs may be the earliest indication of monochorionic twins.

The yolk sac increases in size to approximately 5 mm at about 11 weeks, and thereafter it decreases in size (see Chapter 6).[4, 5] While the yolk sac gradually involutes it may remain visible on sonograms until 14 to 15 menstrual weeks, at which time the chorioamniotic membranes fuse and obliterate the distinct "chorionic" cavity that houses the yolk sac.[6] An abnormally small or large yolk sac in the first trimester has been associated with poor pregnancy outcome, but the wide variability of yolk sac size at each gestational age limits its predictive value.

On occasion, remnants of the intra-abdominal yolk stalk (also known as the omphalomesenteric or vitelline duct) persist and result in a diverticulum near the terminal ileum, a Meckel diverticulum, present in approximately 2% of adults.[7] Meckel diverticula have not been observed on antenatal sonograms, but complications resulting from their rupture (i.e., meconium peritonitis) have been observed in the fetus. Remnants of the omphalomesenteric duct may be observed as cysts within the umbilical cord (Fig. 16–5). These cysts, historically observed in the second and third trimesters, have usually been seen in fetuses with abdominal wall defects and chromosomal abnormalities.[8, 9] With the improved resolution of available equipment, umbilical cord cysts can rarely be seen in the first trimester, but in the few reported cases, first-trimester cord cysts do not seem to be associated with fetal defects. Umbilical cord cysts were observed in eight first-trimester fetuses described by Skibo and coworkers[10]; among five fetuses

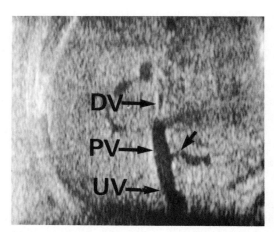

Figure 16–1. The umbilical vein (UV) as it becomes the left portal vein (PV). The branch vessel (*arrow*) distinguishes this vessel (PV) from the umbilical vein. DV, ductus venosus.

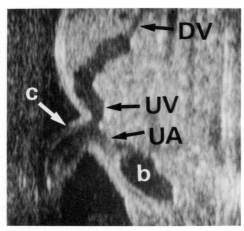

Figure 16–2. Umbilical vein (UV). c, umbilical cord; b, bladder; UA, umbilical artery; DV, ductus venosus.

followed to term all were normal, and of the eight cysts detected all disappeared by the 12th week. The precise origin of these early cysts is not known, but this small study indicates that an excellent outcome is likely.

The allantois is a small structure in the human fetus, and although it is not identified on the sonogram, it gives rise to other anatomic structures, defects of which may be observed on the sonogram. The allantois forms as a caudal outpouching of the yolk sac at day 16 (approximately 4 menstrual weeks).[3] Its function is quite limited in human fetuses, but primitive blood formation occurs in its wall in early embryonic development, and the umbilical arteries and veins are derived from the vessels of the allantois. The extraembryonic portion of the allantois degenerates during the second fetal month. Remnants of the allantois may result in cysts (allantoic cysts) that usually occur between the vessels in the umbilical cord, most commonly near the insertion of the cord in the ventral abdominal wall. Omphalomesenteric duct cysts and allantoic cysts in the cord are sonographically indistinguishable (see Fig. 16–5). The intraembryonic allantois connects the apex of the fetal bladder to the umbilicus. As the bladder enlarges, the allantois involutes and gives rise to the urachus, a midline structure located between the umbilical arteries. The urachus in turn involutes, giving rise to the median umbilical ligament, a fibrous cord of tissue between the bladder apex and umbilicus. Patent areas along this remnant result in urachal cysts or sinuses. Although these nonoccluded urachal segments are commonly found in autopsy specimens, they usually are not clinically detected in the adult unless they become infected.[11] Patencies of the urachus (urachal sinuses or diverticula) have been observed in the fetus, usually in association with bladder outlet obstruction, prune-belly syndrome, or partial bladder exstrophy.[12, 13]

The umbilical cord forms during the first 5 weeks of gestation (7 menstrual weeks) as a fusion of the omphalomesenteric (yolk stalk) and allantoic ducts. The umbilical cord acquires its epithelial lining as a result of the enlargement of the amniotic cavity and the resultant envelopment of the cord by amniotic membrane (see Fig. 16–4).[3]

The intestines, growing at a faster rate than the abdomen, herniate into the proximal umbilical cord at approximately 9 menstrual weeks and remain there until approximately the middle of the 12th menstrual week.[7, 14] Sonographically, this physiologic cord herniation may be visualized as a bulge or thickening within the cord near the fetal abdomen (Fig. 16–6).[15] While in the base of the umbilical cord, the midgut loop grows and rotates 90° on the axis of the superior mesenteric artery. When the loops of bowel return to the fetal abdomen, they rotate another 180° in a counterclockwise direction, completing the normal rotation of the bowel.[7] The umbilical cord insertion into the ventral abdominal wall is an important sonographic anatomic landmark because scrutiny of this area will reveal the most common congenital ventral abdominal wall defects (omphalocele, gastroschisis, limb–body wall complex) (see Chapter 17). Despite the fact that pathologic defects of the fetal ventral abdominal wall can be observed at earlier gestational ages with high-resolution endovaginal sonography, distinction between a physiologic bowel herniation and a pathologic defect cannot always be made in the first trimester. For example, during 220 well-dated pregnancies scanned transabdominally, Green and colleagues[5] reported that some bowel was noted to remain outside of the abdomen at 12 weeks in 20% of fetuses. Therefore, unless the "bulge" in the umbilical cord insertion is large and clearly pathologic, the diagnosis of ventral abdominal wall defects should be deferred until at least 14 menstrual weeks, after which the normal migration of midgut back into the abdomen is certain.[15, 16]

The vessels of the umbilical cord may be followed with real-time sonography as they enter the abdomen and travel toward the liver and iliac arteries (Fig. 16–7). The single thin-walled umbilical vein may be followed cephalad from the cord insertion to the left portal vein (Fig. 16–8). The umbilical vein has no branches in the liver; therefore, if branching structures are identified associated with a vein near the ligamentum teres, it is the left portal vein (possibly the umbilical portion of the left portal vein), not the umbilical vein. The diameter of the fetal intra-abdominal umbilical vein increases linearly from approximately 3 mm at 15 menstrual weeks to 8 mm at term.[17]

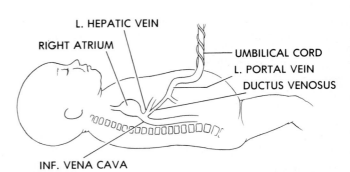

Figure 16–3. Schematic representation of the course of the umbilical vein.

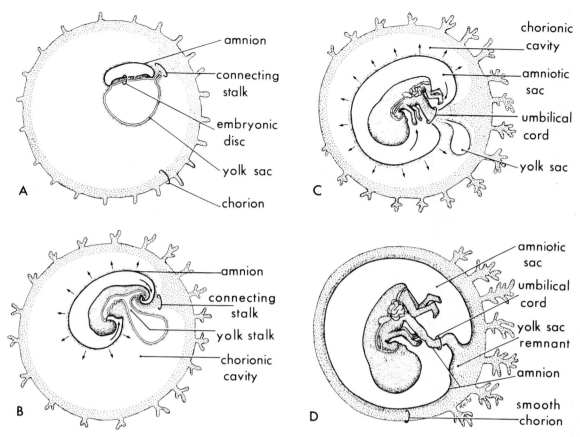

Figure 16–4. Development of the umbilical cord. As the amniotic cavity enlarges, its membrane envelops the cord, forming the epithelial lining of the cord. (From Moore KL: The Developing Human: Clinically Oriented Embryology, 4th ed. Philadelphia, WB Saunders, 1988.)

Varicosity of the umbilical vein is characterized by focal dilatation, usually in the intra-amniotic portion. Mahony and coworkers described a series of nine fetuses with isolated intra-abdominal umbilical vein vein varix (Fig. 16–9), among whom four (44%) died in utero before 30 weeks.[17] The umbilical vein may also enlarge in some abnormal fetuses in whom the cause of the fetal compromise is known (i.e., chorioangiomas or immune hydrops fetalis). Unfortunately, measurements of umbilical vein diameter are neither sufficiently reliable nor predictive to be effective in predicting or excluding significant distress in fetuses with these conditions.[18, 19] From the left portal vein, umbilical blood flows either through the ductus venosus to systemic veins (inferior vena cava or left hepatic vein) bypassing the liver or through the portal sinus to the right portal vein, perfusing the fetal liver (see Figs. 16–1 through 16–3). The ductus venosus, which has the structure of a muscular vein,[1] in this way forms the conduit between the portal system and systemic veins. Sonographically, the ductus venosus appears as a thin

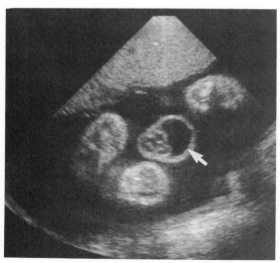

Figure 16–5. Allantoic cyst (*arrow*).

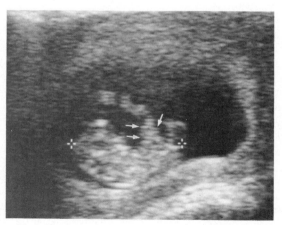

Figure 16–6. Physiologic umbilical hernia. A bulge in the cord at the insertion site (*arrows*) is a normal finding before 13 menstrual weeks. Cursors, crown-rump length measurement.

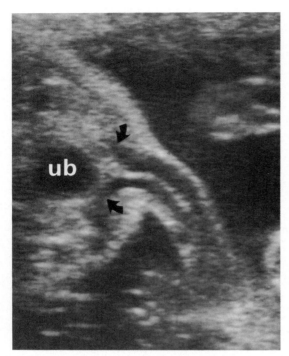

Figure 16–7. The umbilical cord insertion demonstrates the proximity of the distal umbilical arteries (*arrows*) to the wall of the urinary bladder (ub).

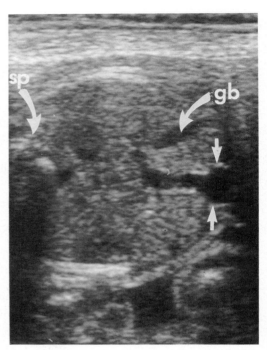

Figure 16–9. Umbilical vein varix (*straight arrows*). gb, gallbladder; sp, spine.

intrahepatic channel with echogenic walls. It lies within the two layers of the lesser omentum (hepatogastric ligament), in a groove between the left lobe and the caudate lobe (fissure for the ligamentum venosum), and thus becomes an anatomic landmark for both the hepatogastric ligament and caudate lobe of the liver (Fig. 16–10). Although 40% to 60% of umbilical venous flow passes into the liver through the portal veins, the remainder passes directly to the cava through this fetal conduit.[20] The ductus venosus is patent during

fetal life and remains so until shortly after birth, when transformation of the ductus into the ligamentum venosum occurs (beginning in the second week after birth).[1]

The two umbilical arteries may be followed caudad from the cord insertion, in their normal path adjacent to the fetal bladder, to the internal iliac arteries (see Fig. 16–7). Post partum, most of the intra-abdominal umbilical arteries become the medial umbilical ligaments and proximally they become the superior vesical arteries in the adult.[1]

Uncommonly, a congenital anatomic variation occurs in which there is persistence of the right umbilical vein that normally becomes obliterated early in development. Persistent right umbilical vein may replace the normal left umbilical vein or be supernumerary,[21] but, in either case, this anomaly is associated with numerous and occasionally lethal malformations. This fetal malformation is easily recognized on the sonogram by the appearance of the intrahepatic portion of the umbilical vein lateral to the gallbladder (Fig. 16–11).

THE FETAL ABDOMEN IN THE SECOND AND THIRD TRIMESTERS

An enormous amount of information about the normal and abnormal fetal abdomen in the second and third trimesters can be gleaned during the sonogram with currently available real-time equipment. The liver, gallbladder, and spleen are detected as distinct structures in nearly every normal fetus by the mid second trimester and can be assessed for size, echotexture, and morphology. Important malformations of the hol-

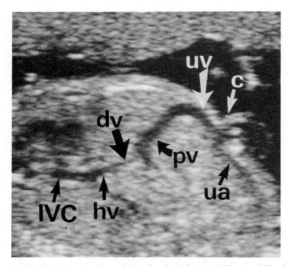

Figure 16–8. Sagittal view of the fetal abdomen. The umbilical vein (uv) courses cephalad to the left portal vein (pv). The ductus venosus (dv) is a narrow channel that connects the left portal vein to the left hepatic vein (hv) or inferior vena cava (IVC). c, umbilical cord insertion; ua, umbilical artery.

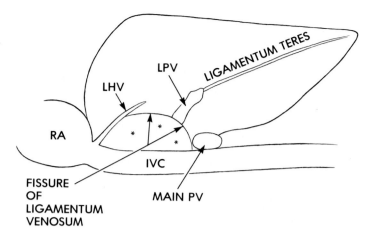

Figure 16–10. Schematic diagram of the sagittal hepatic venous anatomy, through the plane of the left hepatic vein. From the left portal vein (LPV), the ductus venosus travels in the fissure of the ligamentum venosum to the left hepatic vein (LHV) or inferior vena cava (IVC). In this plane, the liver dorsal to the fissure is the caudate lobe (*asterisk*). RA, right atrium.

low gastrointestinal tract also have distinctive appearances that allow for their sonographic detection in the fetus.

THE HEPATOBILIARY SYSTEM AND SPLEEN

The fetal liver is relatively large, accounting for approximately 10% of the total weight of the fetus at 11 menstrual weeks and 5% of the total weight at term. It is the site of most hematopoiesis in the fetus between the 8th and 14th menstrual weeks, and bile formation by hepatic cells begins at the end of the first trimester (approximately 14 menstrual weeks).[7]

Many of the adult anatomic relationships of the liver and its lobes may be depicted even in the small fetus. The hepatic veins can often be traced to their confluence at the intrahepatic vena cava (Fig. 16–12). The right and left hepatic lobes are distinguished by the separating landmarks of the main lobar fissure, middle hepatic vein, and gallbladder. The left hepatic lobe and caudate lobe are separated by the hepatogastric ligament, through which courses the ductus venosus.

A few, but significant, abnormalities of the liver have been observed in the fetus with sonography.

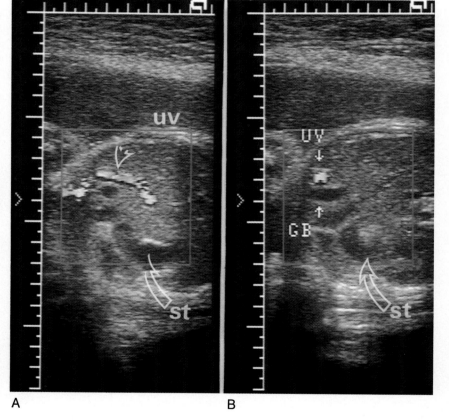

Figure 16–11. Persistent right umbilical vein. *A* and *B*. Color Doppler scans show the right umbilical vein (uv) to the right of the gallbladder (GB). st, stomach.

A   B

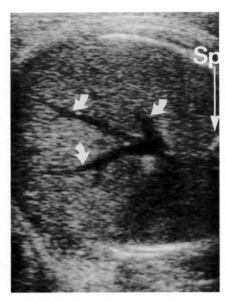

Figure 16–12. Hepatic veins and their confluence. Arrows indicate right, middle, and left hepatic veins. Sp, spine.

Observations have been essentially limited to hepatic calcifications and space-occupying lesions. Fetal hepatic calcifications may be due to tumor, vascular insult, or infection. In some cases, the cause of hepatic calcifications cannot be determined. Diffuse and branching calcifications in the fetal liver have been observed in association with ischemic hepatic infarcts; the mechanism is unknown but presumed to be secondary to an intrauterine vascular insult.[22] Scattered calcifications within the liver may be seen in the setting of intrauterine infection with *Toxoplasma* and herpes simplex virus. The examiner should look for associated ascites and for calcification in the brain and spleen if infection is suspected. Other considerations for fetal hepatic calcifications might include calcified portal vein thromboemboli[23, 24]; these findings have been described in neonates and stillborns but not in the living fetus. In some cases, the etiology of these calcifications is never uncovered, but it has been noted that when they are isolated or there is no morphologic or serologic evidence of fetal infection or mass lesion, fetal hepatic calcification may be completely benign and the fetal outcome can be excellent.[25]

Fetal hepatic neoplasms, also uncommon, include hepatic teratoma, adenoma, hepatoblastoma, hemangioendothelioma, hemangioma, and hamartoma or, rarely, metastases from neuroblastoma.[26, 27] Solid fetal liver lesions are extremely rare. A solitary liver adenoma was detected as a focal hypoechoic solid lesion in a term fetus by Marks and coworkers.[28] Solid echogenic metastases from an adrenal neuroblastoma have also been reported.[29] Hepatoblastoma is the most common malignant hepatic neoplasm discovered in the neonatal period but has not been described in the fetus.[30] Hemangioendothelioma is the most common symptomatic vascular liver tumor of infancy.[31] Few lesions have been diagnosed prenatally, but hepatic hemangioendothelioma has been reported as the cause of nonimmune hydrops in one fetus.[32] In the latter case, the lesion appeared cystic and solid, and pulsed Doppler imaging was used to confirm its vascular nature prenatally. Apparently these lesions can also regress spontaneously.[33] Hepatic hemangioma, which is usually a solid lesion, may appear quite cystic on sonograms and may appropriately be considered in the differential diagnosis of a cystic liver mass in the fetus.

Rarely, a fetal liver cyst is detected during routine scanning. The two major categories of cystic disease of the liver seen in infancy and childhood are nonparasitic hepatic cysts and mesenchymal hamartomas.[34] Both of these entities are believed to represent developmental abnormalities, and both have been detected in the fetus with sonography. The majority of solitary cysts probably results from a focal developmental interruption of the biliary tree of unknown cause.[35] The diagnosis of a solitary nonparasitic cyst of the liver in the fetus was reported by Chung.[36] Hepatic mesenchymal hamartoma, histologically similar to a lymphangioma, has also been described in the fetus as a large multiloculated cystic fetal liver mass.[37] Mesenchymal hepatic hamartomas, however, are usually discovered in the first year of life; fatalities have been attributed to treatment complications or other causes, rather than to the lesion itself.

Diffuse cystic diseases of the liver may occur in association with cysts of other organs, including the kidneys, pancreas, and lungs, but these have not been reported prenatally. Although most fetuses with autosomal recessive polycystic kidney disease also have biliary ductular ectasia or hepatic fibrosis, liver abnormalities are generally not observed sonographically until later in childhood. Davies and associates,[38] however, reported a case of an infant with infantile polycystic kidney disease in whom saccular dilation of intrahepatic bile ducts was detected within the first 3 days of life. This early detection suggests the associated cystic liver disease may be a potentially detectable abnormality in the fetus.[38]

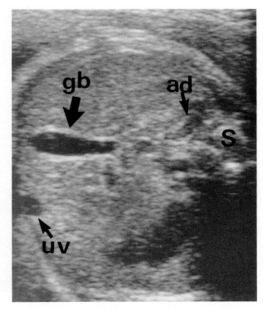

Figure 16–13. The fetal adrenal gland (ad), spine (S), gallbladder (gb), and umbilical vein (uv) are visualized.

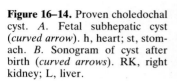
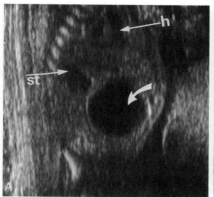
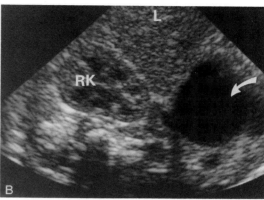

Figure 16–14. Proven choledochal cyst. *A.* Fetal subhepatic cyst (*curved arrow*). h, heart; st, stomach. *B.* Sonogram of cyst after birth (*curved arrows*). RK, right kidney; L, liver.

The gallbladder forms as a caudal part of the hepatic diverticulum at approximately 7 menstrual weeks.[7] In my experience, the gallbladder is sonographically visible in almost all fetuses after 20 weeks. Despite its small size, it is readily detected by virtue of the intrinsic contrast between it and the surrounding liver parenchyma. Both the gallbladder and portal/umbilical vein appear as oblong fluid-filled structures on the transverse view of the fetal abdomen through the liver. The gallbladder, however, should be distinguished by its location to the right of the portal/umbilical vein and as an oblong, more oval structure than the "tubular" intrahepatic umbilical vein (Fig. 16–13). It has been suggested that the gallbladder plays a passive role in fetal life, since it is most commonly observed filled after 20 gestational weeks of age and has not been demonstrated to contract in response to a maternal fatty meal.[39]

Abnormalities of the fetal biliary tree that have been detected using sonography include choledochal cysts (Fig. 16–14) and fetal cholelithiasis (Fig. 16–15).[40–43]

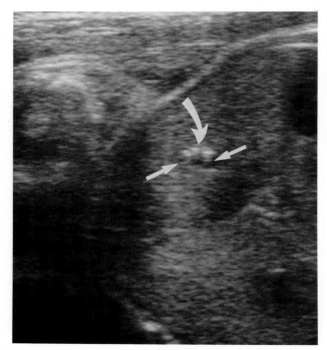

Figure 16–15. Fetal gallstones. Straight arrows indicate gallbladder. Curved arrow indicates intraluminal gallstones.

Choledochal cysts are uncommon abnormalities and clinically present most often in the second and third decades of life.[44] Although several morphologic forms occur, the most common is type I, or a cystic dilatation of the common bile duct. This abnormality has been detected uncommonly in the fetus, seen as early as 25 menstrual weeks, but in most cases prenatal diagnoses have been made in the third trimester.[40] Because choledochal cysts may be associated with intermittent biliary obstruction and severe biliary cirrhosis, early diagnosis is important and surgical resection is considered optimal therapy.

On prenatal sonography, a choledochal cyst appears in the right upper quadrant (see Fig. 16–14). Differential diagnosis includes hepatic or omental cyst, kidney cyst or hydronephrotic renal pelvis, or dilated bowel loop. Recall that because of the small fetal pelvis ovarian cysts can move to the upper abdomen as well and, especially if the fetus is female, ovarian cyst should be considered in the differential diagnosis of a fetal abdominal cyst. The likelihood that the cystic lesion is a choledochal cyst is greater if the location is subhepatic and intraperitoneal, if the morphology does not change with observed peristalsis of the fetal bowel, and, lastly, if tubular structures (i.e., bile ducts) are identified entering and leaving the cyst.[40, 41]

Cholelithiasis is uncommon in children and has been observed in utero (see Fig. 16–15).[42] Most investigators believe that the presence of fetal gallstones does not alter fetal prognosis. In most cases, the gallstones seem to resolve spontaneously in utero or asymptomatically in the childhood period. Neither the etiology of fetal gallstone formation nor the predisposing factors are known. The largest series of fetal gallstones was reported by Brown and colleagues,[45] who described findings in 26 fetuses in whom gallbladder sludge or stones were observed in the third trimester. In 53% of those with follow-up, the findings resolved asymptomatically. In 3 fetuses, the findings persisted into childhood but the children remained asymptomatic.

Biliary atresia, a sclerosing process of both intrahepatic and extrahepatic bile ducts, is a life-threatening abnormality in the neonate. Although this process is often associated with nonvisualization of the gallbladder on neonatal sonography, this disease has not been detected prenatally. The etiology of biliary atresia (congenital versus acquired) remains unknown and controversial, but many believe this to be an acquired

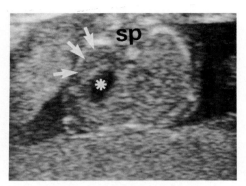

Figure 16–16. The fetal spleen is indicated by arrows and is located behind the fluid-filled stomach (*asterisk*). sp, spine.

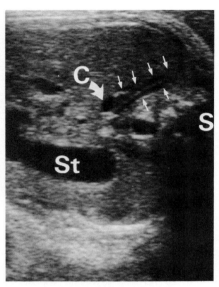

Figure 16–17. The fetal adrenal gland is indicated by small arrows. Note that it "kisses" the inferior vena cava (C), a useful anatomic relationship. S, spine; St, stomach.

disease, possibly related to viral infection.[46–50] It has not been described in stillborns and is unlikely to be detected on prenatal sonography.

The spleen can be identified in virtually all fetuses at between 18 and 40 menstrual weeks (Fig. 16–16).[51] It increases in size during gestation.[52, 53] Splenic enlargement has been associated with rhesus immunization disease, premature rupture of the membranes, and cytomegalovirus infections.[54] In the fetus, the echotexture of the normal spleen is homogeneous: it is of similar echogenicity to the kidney and slightly less echogenic than the liver.[55] Congenital cysts rarely occur in the spleen, are believed to represent endothelial inclusion cysts, and have been observed in the fetus.[56] The spleen is not easy to visualize but, with effort, can be detected in most second- and third-trimester fetuses. If the spleen is absent, especially when fetal heart block and/or complex congenital diseases are associated, the polysplenia/asplenia syndrome should be considered. Chitayat and coworkers[57] described absence of the spleen in two fetuses with heart block and congenital heart disease who were shown to have the polysplenic syndrome. Autopsy confirmed the absence of a single spleen but showed many small splenic nodules within the abdomen that were not seen prenatally.

The kidneys may be identified in the expected location in the flanks and will be sonographically visible in 90% of patients at 17 to 22 gestational weeks of age.[58] The flanks are relatively shallow in the fetus, and thus the anterior surface of the kidneys project more anteriorly in the fetus than in the adult (see Chapter 18).

The fetal adrenal glands are relatively large in the third trimester and at birth are 20 times their relative adult size.[59, 60] Because of their large size and typical sonographic morphology, they are readily visualized in the third trimester of pregnancy. It is estimated that at least one gland may be identified in 90% of fetuses more than 27 gestational weeks of age.[61] The relatively thick outer zone of the fetal adrenal is hypoechoic and presumed to represent a combination of the inner fetal zone of the adrenal cortex (from which neonatal adrenal hemorrhages originate) and an outer thin "permanent" cortex. The fetal zone comprises approximately 80% of the bulk of the fetal adrenal gland before birth[61] but atrophies and disappears within 3 to 12 postnatal months.[60] The echogenic inner zone of the

fetal adrenal gland is presumed to represent the fetal adrenal medulla (Figs. 16–17 and 16–18). Human chorionic gonadotropin contributes to adrenal growth in the first half of pregnancy; thereafter, adrenocorticotropic hormone controls the fetal adrenal. This may, in part, explain the smaller adrenals sometimes noted in anencephalic fetuses who lack a well-developed hypothalamic-pituitary axis.[61, 62] The adrenal glands are so prominent in the normal fetus that they have been confused for renal parenchyma when one or both kidneys are absent (i.e., renal agenesis) or ectopically located. Interestingly, unlike the situation in the adult,

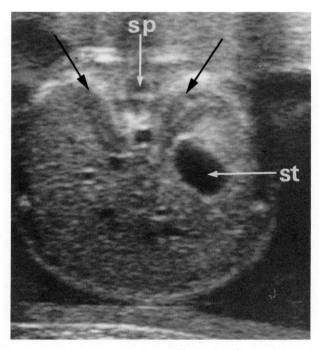

Figure 16–18. The adrenal glands (*black arrows*) are often quite conspicuous in the fetus. st, stomach; sp, spine.

the left adrenal is usually imaged superior to the upper pole of the left kidney in fetal life and apparently moves to its normal position (more anterior and medial to the left kidney) in early childhood.[63] The morphology of the adrenal may provide a clue to the diagnosis of renal agenesis. In this setting, because the adrenal is not "capping" the kidney, the adrenal becomes flattened and, on the left, appears to "lie down" on the aorta, described as the "lying down adrenal" of renal agenesis.[64] Other abnormalities in the fetal adrenal gland are rarely detected, but adrenal neuroblastoma, cysts, and hemorrhages have been observed prenatally.[65–67] I have observed autopsy-proven bilateral adrenal hemorrhages in one fetus later proven to have Beckwith-Wiedemann syndrome. The hemorrhages appeared as large perinephric fluid collections in association with normal-appearing kidneys. "Simple" adrenal cysts detected prenatally in two fetuses disappeared uneventfully by 6 weeks of postnatal age in otherwise normal neonates.[67]

It is unusual to visualize the fetal pancreas by virtue of its morphology alone because of the paucity of retroperitoneal fat in the fetal abdomen and the similar echotexture compared with surrounding structures. Visualization of the fetal pancreas may be accomplished, however, with special care and attention to the associated anatomic landmarks of the superior mesenteric artery and vein in the fetus. The head of the pancreas is relatively larger than its body in the neonate, as compared with the adult.[1]

THE HOLLOW GASTROINTESTINAL TRACT IN THE FETUS: NORMAL DEVELOPMENT

The esophagus, trachea, and stomach originate from the foregut. The esophagus becomes anatomically separate from the trachea in the sixth and seventh menstrual weeks. The normal fetal esophagus is collapsed and not usually visualized sonographically (Fig. 16–19). The stomach assumes its adult shape and position at approximately 9 to 10 menstrual weeks.[14, 62] Swallowing is possible at 12 to 13 weeks, and by 13 to 16 weeks the fetus is swallowing enough to detect a fluid-filled stomach on the sonogram. The volume of amniotic fluid swallowed increases dramatically with age (from 7 mL/d at 16 menstrual weeks to 400 to 750 mL/d at term).[1, 3, 68–70] The stomach, like all fetal organs, grows as gestation progresses; and this, in conjunction with increasing volumes of swallowed fluid, results in a fairly predictable increase in the size of the imaged stomach with gestational age.[71] Sonographically, the stomach "bubble" appears as an anechoic crescent-shaped structure in the left hemiabdomen (see Fig. 16–17) and is often visualized in the same transverse axial image in which the abdominal circumference is measured. Importantly, a fluid-filled stomach can be detected in nearly all normal fetuses after 18 weeks. Its absence should strongly raise suspicion for a fetal abnormality (see section on the absent stomach). Among 995 fetuses scanned after 11 weeks, Pretorius and colleagues[72] reported that the stomach was visualized in 98%.[72] Furthermore, among fetuses in whom

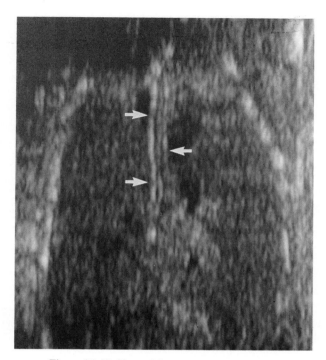

Figure 16–19. Normal fetal esophagus (*arrows*).

the stomach was not visualized, 55% had an abnormal outcome; and if the stomach was nonvisualized after 19 weeks, the outcome was abnormal in all cases. These results underscore the importance of imaging a fluid-filled stomach in all second- and third-trimester fetal sonograms, as recommended by the American Institute of Ultrasound in Medicine and the American College of Radiology.[73]

Movement of the gastric musculature begins in approximately the fourth to fifth month of gestation. In the second trimester, this, in combination with increased swallowing, results in the delivery of increased amniotic fluid volume distally into the small bowel and colon where fluid and nutrients are reabsorbed.[14] As a result of developmental changes, as well as the increasing volume of swallowed fluid delivered to the bowel, the appearances of small bowel and colon in the distal gastrointestinal tract also change in a fairly predictable pattern during gestation. Zilianti and Fernandez[74] have correlated these changing patterns with gestational age. After the 15th to 16th menstrual week, meconium begins to accumulate in the distal part of the small intestine as a combination of desquamated cells, bile pigments, and mucoproteins.[75] The term *meconium*, derived from *mekonion* (Gk., meaning "poppy"), was named by Aristotle, who believed that meconium kept the fetus asleep in utero.[14] Early in the second trimester, the meconium-filled small bowel is often observed as somewhat echogenic and can appear masslike (fetal abdominal pseudomasses) (Fig. 16–20).[14, 76, 77] This appearance is believed to reflect collapsed loops of small bowel. Echogenic bowel has also been reported in association with cystic fibrosis (see later).[78] As more swallowed amniotic fluid is delivered distally, these echogenic areas give rise to more typical and readily identifiable sonolucent, fluid-filled loops of small bowel

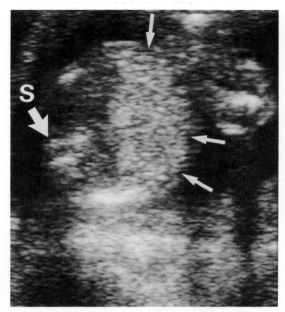

Figure 16–20. Early in gestation, collapsed fetal small bowel may appear as an echogenic mass (pseudomass) (*arrows*). S, spine.

(Fig. 16–21).[76, 77] Active small bowel peristalsis, which first occurs early in the second trimester,[14] is commonly noted in these fluid-filled loops during real-time sonography after 26 to 30 menstrual weeks.[79]

Sonographically, the colon is first identified at the end of the second trimester and, if sought, can be visualized in most fetuses after 28 menstrual weeks.[74, 79]

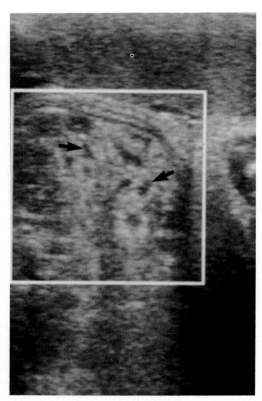

Figure 16–21. Normal fluid-filled small bowel (*arrows*) becomes visible later in gestation as more swallowed amniotic fluid is delivered distally.

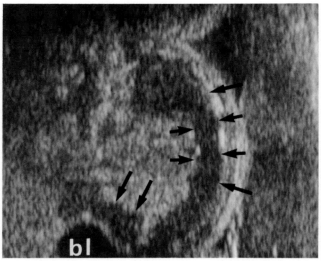

Figure 16–22. Normal fetal colon (*arrows*). Low-level echoes (meconium) are seen within this tubular structure, in the flanks and pelvis. bl, urinary bladder.

The colon appears as a long tubular hypoechoic structure with well-defined walls, located in the flanks and upper abdomen (Fig. 16–22). Low-level echoes secondary to meconium can usually be detected within its lumen (see Fig. 16–22). Unlike the small bowel, the colon does not usually exhibit active peristalsis that is sonographically detectable in the fetus but acts as a reservoir for the meconium propelled from by the small bowel.[79] As a result, the normal colonic diameter increases linearly during gestation (Fig. 16–23).[79]

SONOGRAPHICALLY DETECTABLE ABNORMALITIES IN THE FETAL ABDOMEN

Stomach

GASTRIC PSEUDOMASSES

Although the fetal stomach is readily visualized as a homogeneous fluid-filled structure in the left upper

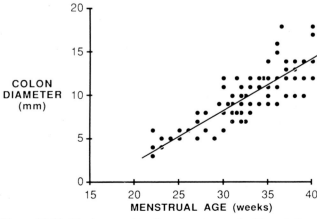

Figure 16–23. Maximum colon diameter compared with gestational age. (From Nyberg DA, Mack LA, et al: Fetal bowel: Normal sonographic findings. J Ultrasound Med 6:3, 1987.)

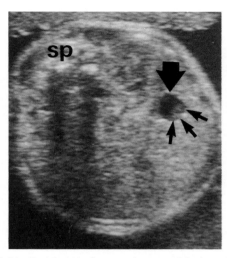

Figure 16–24. Gastric pseudomass. A transaxial view of the fetal abdomen demonstrates that the stomach (*large arrow*) is fluid filled and contains a small mass of medium echoes (*small arrows*) presumed to represent swallowed "debris." sp, spine.

quadrant, occasionally a discrete, intraluminal, echogenic "mass" is observed (Figs. 16–24 and 16–25). Although the etiology of these gastric pseudomasses is unknown, they are presumed to result from aggregates of swallowed cells and debris, before coordinated and active gastric peristalsis has developed. We have observed debris in normal fetuses in the third trimester. Swallowed blood can also produce this appearance in fetuses who have had intraperitoneal (i.e., inadvertent intrabowel) transfusions or as a result of swallowed blood in those cases following intra-amniotic hemorrhage.

ABSENT STOMACH

Because the stomach can be visualized in nearly all second- and third-trimester pregnancies,[72] nonvisuali-

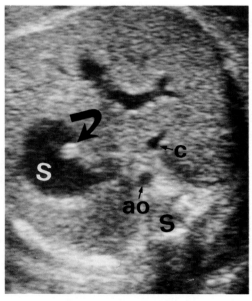

Figure 16–25. Gastric pseudomass. In this case, the echogenic focus (*curved arrow*) along the lesser curvature of the fetal stomach may represent swallowed debris or the incisura angularis. S (*white*), stomach; ao, aorta; c, inferior vena cava; S (*black*), spine.

Table 16–1. CAUSES OF ABSENT STOMACH

Mechanical obstruction
 Esophageal atresia
 Chest mass
Facial clefts
Depressed swallowing
 Central nervous system abnormalities
 Neuromotor syndrome (i.e., Pena-Shokeir and arthrogryposis)
 "Sick fetuses" (hydrops, infection)
Oligohydramnios
Ectopic (congenital diaphragmatic hernia)

zation should be considered pathologic until proven otherwise. A number of fetal abnormalities may be associated with a small or absent stomach (Table 16–1): mechanical obstructions (esophageal atresia, chest masses); physical defects that impair normal swallowing (facial clefts); syndromes in which normal fetal behavior, including swallowing, is depressed (severe central nervous system anomalies, neuromotor syndromes, hydrops, infection); oligohydramnios (less fluid to swallow); and congenital diaphragmatic hernia (abnormally positioned stomach). Therefore, if a fluid-filled stomach is not detected in a fetus of equal to or more than 18 weeks' gestation, a careful survey for features characteristic of these potential abnormalities is warranted. In some normal fetuses, repeat examination will demonstrate a normally filled stomach (Fig. 16–26).

Esophageal atresia occurs in 1 in 2500 live births and is the major morphologic defect considered when the stomach is absent.[80] The causative insult is unknown but probably occurs very early in development (approximately 6 menstrual weeks). Sonographically, esophageal atresia is suspected when the fluid-filled stomach is absent and features suggestive of an alternate diagnosis, such as oligohydramnios or significant depressed fetal behavior, are not present. Five types of esophageal atresia occur, but the most common form (approximately 90%) involves esophageal atresia and fistula to a distal segment of the bronchial tree (Fig. 16–27). It follows then that because fluid can enter the stomach through a fistula in most affected fetuses, a fluid-filled stomach may be present despite the presence of esophageal atresia, thus obscuring the diagnosis. In many cases, even if a fistula is present, the distal passage of fluid is impeded sufficiently to result in a poorly filled small or absent fetal stomach on the sonogram. Because a fistula is commonly associated with esophageal atresia, absent stomach is an insensitive indicator of esophageal atresia. In fact, the fluid-filled stomach is sonographically absent in less than 50% of affected fetuses. Polyhydramnios results from impaired reabsorption of swallowed fluid and is often associated with esophageal atresia, but it usually does not develop until the third trimester. Absent stomach and polyhydramnios are very suggestive for the diagnosis of esophageal atresia, but this combination is observed in only approximately one third of fetuses with esophageal atresia.[72, 81–83] Sonographic visualization of the proximal esophageal pouch has been described,[84] but this is an extremely difficult observation to make, and, therefore, visualization of the

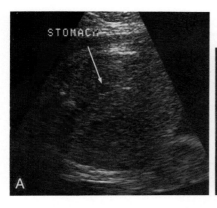
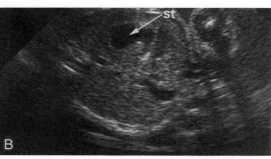

Figure 16–26. Small stomach (*A*) reverted to normal-appearing stomach (*B*) when the fetus was reexamined 1 week later. st, stomach.

esophageal "pouch" is not necessary for the sonographic diagnosis. Fetuses with a tracheoesophageal fistula often have associated anomalies (50% to 70%), including vertebral, anal, cardiac, renal, and limb anomalies (VACTERL), and many (up to 40%) of the affected fetuses are also growth retarded. In addition, 20% of fetuses with esophageal atresia with or without fistula will be chromosomally abnormal (most commonly, trisomy 18). This contrasts to neonatal series in which only 3% to 4% of affected neonates have abnormal karyotypes.

This is a difficult diagnostic area for sonologists because it is often not possible to make the prenatal diagnosis of tracheoesophageal fistula with certainty. If the diagnosis is suspected, however, a careful anatomic survey and a karyotype analysis of the fetus are warranted. Prognosis of fetuses and neonates with tracheoesophageal fistula is related to the presence of

associated anomalies, birthweight, and development or respiratory complications. Even if the diagnosis cannot be made with certainty before birth, prenatal suggestion of this anomaly will be a useful warning to the pediatrician to, at the minimum, probe the neonate's esophagus before beginning feedings.

Congenital diaphragmatic hernia, because it most commonly occurs on the left, with stomach herniated into the chest, also results in a nondetectable fluid-filled stomach in the expected location in the fetal abdomen. This may be distinguished from esophageal atresia by virtue of the intrathoracic abnormalities (mainly mediastinal shift) that accompany congenital diaphragmatic hernia (see Chapter 15).

In my practice, the most common cause for a small or poorly visualized fetal stomach is oligohydramnios (Fig. 16–28), probably due to the paucity of fluid available for swallowing. This strongly contrasts to the situation in which esophageal atresia without fistula is present, in which polyhydramnios would be the likely accompaniment. Fetuses who are severely distressed (i.e., infected), or whose overall motor function is severely depressed, may also demonstrate a small or absent stomach, likely due to depressed swallowing. This can occur in syndromes such as the Pena-Shokeir syndrome and arthrogryposis. In most of these cases, increased amniotic fluid volume or frank polyhydramnios will be associated. Thus, fetal tone and movement are important observations that may help the examiner distinguish fetuses with esophageal atresia from fetuses with neuromotor diseases.

ESOPHAGEAL ATRESIA TRACHEOESOPHAGEAL FISTULA

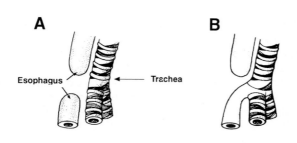

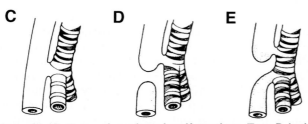

Figure 16–27. Types of esophageal malformations. Type B is the most common. (From Nyberg DA: Intra-abdominal abnormalities. In Nyberg DA, Mahony BS, Pretorius DH [eds]: Diagnostic Ultrasound of Fetal Anomalies: Text and Atlas. Chicago, Year Book Medical Publishers, 1990.)

Dilated Stomach and Duodenum: The "Double Bubble"

Duodenal atresia is the most common type of fetal small bowel atresia, occurring in 1 in 10,000 live births.[85] Most investigators believe that the atresia results from failure of recanalization of the duodenum, which normally occurs at about 10 menstrual weeks.[7, 86–89] Sonographic findings suggestive of duodenal atresia are extremely important because of the frequent concurrent morphologic abnormalities (nearly 50%) found in association with duodenal atresia (gut malrotations, tracheoesophageal fistula, hepatobiliary and pancreatic duct anomalies), including 30% who have trisomy 21 and 20% to 30% with congenital heart disease.[86, 90–92] Duodenal atresia is associated with

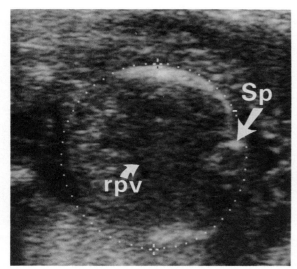

Figure 16–28. Absent or poorly visualized stomach in association with oligohydramnios. Transverse view of the fetal abdomen. The fluid-filled stomach is poorly visualized. Sp, spine; rpv, right portal vein.

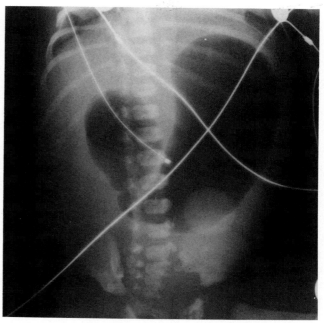

Figure 16–30. Radiograph of a neonate with duodenal atresia: double-bubble sign.

polyhydramnios in 45% of reported cases[85] and with symmetric growth retardation in 50%.[93]

Sonographic signs of fetal duodenal obstruction are a dilated stomach and proximal duodenum (Figs. 16–29 and 16–30), often accompanied by polyhydramnios. A persistently fluid-filled duodenum in the fetus is virtually always abnormal and, when observed, should strongly raise suspicion of duodenal obstruction, even in the absence of polyhydramnios. Unfortunately, like esophageal atresia, the sonographic diagnosis is an important one but usually not possible until after 24 menstrual weeks.[85, 94] There are many causes of double bubble in the fetus (duodenal atresia, duodenal stenosis, annular pancreas, obstructing Ladd's bands, volvulus, or intestinal duplications), but most fetuses with prenatally observed duodenal obstruction prove to have duodenal atresia.

The site of obstruction in duodenal atresia typically is near the ampulla in the descending duodenum, and atresia of the bile duct may also be present. Duodenal stenosis that typically involves the third or fourth segment of the duodenum is less often associated with other morphologic chromosomal abnormalities and may be secondary to an early ischemic event.[7] The

overall mortality rate of neonates with duodenal atresia is high (36%), but associated anomalies are the leading cause of death, underscoring the importance of karyotype analysis and a detailed fetal survey when fetal duodenal obstruction is suspected.[90]

Small Bowel Distal to the Duodenum

After 27 weeks, peristalsis of normal small bowel is increasingly observed. Studies of normal fetuses suggest that the diameters of small bowel and colon steadily increase as gestation progresses; the normal small bowel lumen diameter is less than or equal to 6 mm and the colon lumen is less than or equal to 23 mm.[79, 95]

The presence of a number of dilated loops of bowel, or a single loop in the lower abdomen, discontinuous with the stomach suggests a fetal small bowel obstruction (Figs. 16–31 and 16–32). The most common causes

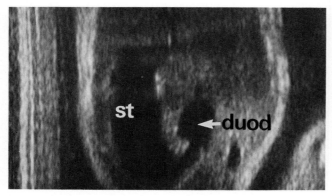

Figure 16–29. Double-bubble sign suggests fetal duodenal obstruction. st, stomach; duod, dilated duodenal bulb.

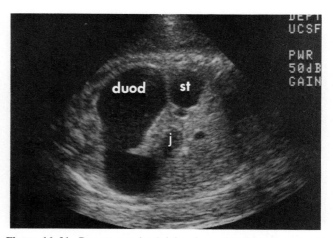

Figure 16–31. Proven proximal jejunal atresia. Dilated stomach, duodenum, and proximal jejunum were observed prenatally in association with polyhydramnios. st, stomach; duod, duodenum; j, jejunum.

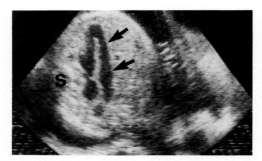

Figure 16–32. Midgut volvulus. The overall appearance of these "isolated" fluid-filled proximal bowel loops (*arrows*) did not change configuration during real-time imaging. S, spine.

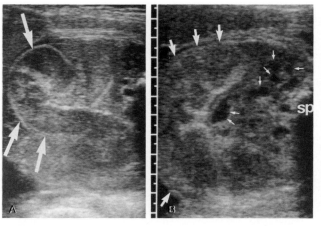

Figure 16–34. Meconium ileus in association with cystic fibrosis. The appearance of the dilated ileum was misinterpreted as colon. After birth the neonate was found to have a microcolon. *A.* Dilated loop of small bowel, low in the anterior abdomen, appears similar to the sigmoid colon (*large arrows*). *B.* Dilated, meconium-filled loop of bowel in the anterior midabdomen simulates the appearance of the transverse colon (*larger arrows*), in contrast to the smaller fluid-filled loops in the central abdomen, more typical of small bowel (*small arrows*). sp, spine.

of fetal small bowel dilatation and obstruction are atresias, volvulus, malrotation, peritoneal bands, and cystic fibrosis. The dilated bowel loops may be observed as an isolated finding or occur in association with ascites, meconium peritonitis, or other morphologic defects.

Jejunoileal atresias are slightly more common than duodenal atresias, occurring in 1 in 3000 to 5000 births. The most common sites of atresia are at the proximal jejunum and distal ileum (Fig. 16–33), with each accounting for approximately one third of small bowel atresias. Most believe that they are sporadic, acquired defects that result from a vascular insult and/or ischemia during development. In keeping with this theory, neither extraintestinal abnormalities (less than 10%) nor karyotype abnormalities are usually present in association with jejunoileal atresias. A specific cause of the atresia (e.g., volvulus, malrotation, gastroschisis) is found postnatally in only approximately one fourth of neonates. Polyhydramnios often accompanies fetal small bowel obstructions but usually does not develop until the third trimester. As a general rule, the more distal the obstruction, the less severe the polyhydramnios, and the later it will develop. The diagnosis is suggested on the sonogram when fluid-filled loops of small bowel are abnormally dilated, although the exact site and cause of obstruction is usually difficult to determine until after birth.

Meconium ileus is a unique form of small bowel obstruction that results from impaction of abnormally thick meconium in the distal ileum and is nearly always associated with cystic fibrosis, a recessive disorder that affects 1 in 2200 white births. Meconium ileus, therefore, is an important exception to the rule that fetal small bowel obstructions tend not to be associated with other important abnormalities. Characteristically, the ileum is dilated and distended with meconium and the colon is small and empty (microcolon). Meconium ileus has been difficult to accurately diagnose in utero because the ileum may not become significantly distended until quite late in gestation or the diagnosis may be missed because the distended ileum is confused with a dilated colon (Fig. 16–34).[96] Fetuses with cystic fibrosis may also have small bowel atresias with or without meconium ileus. A number of other observations in the fetal abdomen have also been associated with cystic fibrosis, most notably meconium peritonitis, pseudocysts, and "echogenic bowel."

ECHOGENIC ABDOMINAL MASSES

As mentioned earlier, echogenic masses in the fetal abdomen have been reported as a normal variant or in association with fetal pathologies such as small bowel atresia or volvulus, fetal viral infection, chromosomal abnormalities, and cystic fibrosis (Fig. 16–35). The described "echogenic masses" are believed to represent small bowel loops with impacted meconium, and the specific significance of this observation has been debated. Dicke and Crane[78] observed extremely echogenic bowel (echogenicity ≥ bone) in 30 of 12,776 fetuses (0.2%) scanned in their prenatal diagnostic center. Significantly, 4 of these 30 (13.3%) fetuses were later found to have cystic fibrosis. These results suggest that if extremely echogenic bowel is detected

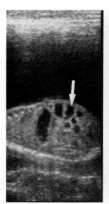 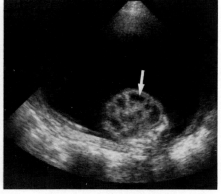

Figure 16–33. Distal jejunal atresia. Abnormal, fluid-filled bowel loops (*arrows*). More loops are visualized than are expected with duodenal atresia. Marked polyhydramnios was also present.

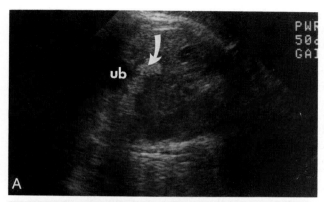

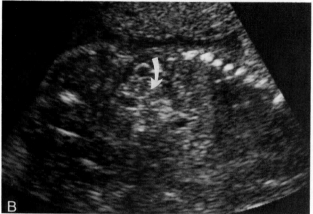

Figure 16–35. *A* and *B*. Two fetuses with cystic fibrosis and prenatally observed echogenic bowel (*curved arrows*). ub, urinary bladder.

also be warranted. Although all of these observations are important, the finding of echogenic fetal bowel should be interpreted with great caution. Recall that (1) the echogenicity of the bowel may be altered depending on the frequency of the transducer, (2) there is variability in the way different observers interpret bowel echogenicity, and (3) fetal bowel may be interpreted as more echogenic than normal by many examiners even though it is not quite as echogenic as bone. It should be emphasized that slightly echogenic bowel is fairly commonly seen as a normal variant before 20 weeks.[76] Furthermore, echogenic colon is an apparently benign finding near term.[99]

Although the most common causes of dilated fetal bowel obstructions distal to the duodenum are small bowel atresia(s), volvulus, and malrotation, cystic fibrosis is also an important consideration in fetuses with dilated bowel. Among 15 consecutive fetuses with dilated bowel (distal to the duodenum) examined between 17 and 40 weeks, and reported by Estroff and coworkers, 5 (33%) ultimately were proven to have cystic fibrosis.[100] In the latter study, the sonographic appearance of bowel dilatation in fetuses with cystic fibrosis was indistinguishable from the appearance of the bowel when dilatation was due to other causes. These results also support the recommendation for parental cystic fibrosis carrier testing when fetal bowel dilatation is detected.

Meconium peritonitis (see section on calcification in the abdomen) has been observed in fetuses and neonates with cystic fibrosis, as well as those with other causes of bowel perforation (Fig. 16–36). The peritonitis occurs secondary to an in utero bowel perforation. The extruded meconium incites a chemical peritonitis that calcifies 10 or more days after the peritoneal spillage. Fetal prognosis associated with meconium peritonitis is variable and most closely linked to the underlying cause of the bowel perforation and the presence of associated abnormalities. Although 15% of children with cystic fibrosis have meconium peritonitis (10% to 25% have intestinal atresias), cystic fibrosis is the cause of meconium peritonitis in less than 10% of fetuses. Among 26 cases of meconium peritonitis reviewed by one author, only two infants

in the second trimester, parental carrier testing for cystic fibrosis (approximately 80% sensitive for carrier status) is warranted.[97] Furthermore, Scioscia and coworkers[98] reported abnormal karyotypes in 6 of 22 fetuses (5 with trisomy 21 and 1 with trisomy 18) with a prospective sonographic diagnosis of echogenic bowel (subjectively determined to be more echogenic than normal),[98] although none had cystic fibrosis. In 4 of the 6 chromosomally abnormal fetuses, the echogenic bowel defects were observed. Their study suggests that karyotype testing in fetuses with echogenic bowel may

Figure 16–36. Calcification in association with meconium peritonitis. *A*. Transverse image of the fetal abdomen demonstrates ascites (a) and peritoneal calcifications (ca). S, spine. *B*. Sagittal image of the same fetus. Note calcification (ca) with shadowing secondary to meconium peritonitis.

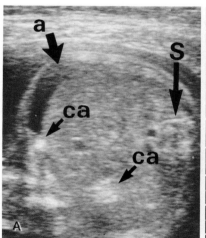
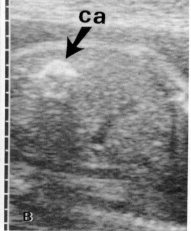

(8%) had cystic fibrosis and, interestingly, neither of these fetuses demonstrated peritoneal calcifications on prenatal sonograms.[101] These data suggest that cystic fibrosis is more likely when small bowel dilatation (as opposed to meconium peritonitis) is observed in the fetus. Nevertheless, when meconium peritonitis is detected, the risk of cystic fibrosis is definitely increased, especially if there is a positive family history,[102] and parental carrier testing for cystic fibrosis may be appropriate.

Megacystis microcolon intestinal hypoperistalsis syndrome is a rare, usually lethal, anomaly that occurs mostly in females (80%) and is believed to be inherited as an autosomal recessive trait.[103] Characteristic features include an enlarged, unobstructed urinary bladder, small bowel dilatation, and malrotated microcolon. Polyhydramnios is common in the third trimester,[104] but the bowel dilatation is usually not detected until late in the third trimester. Therefore, this diagnosis should be considered when both bowel dilatation and an enlarged bladder are detected near term.

Another rare form of fetal bowel dysfunction, congenital chloridorrhea, has been detected prenatally by bowel dilatation.[105] It is inherited as an autosomal recessive trait and results from impaired active transport of chloride from the distal ileum and colon, resulting in profuse chloride diarrhea in the infant.[106, 107] The diagnosis has been suggested on prenatal sonography by the presence of dilated, fluid-filled loops of bowel undergoing active peristalsis in a fetus known to be at risk for the disease.[106, 107] Of all causes of small bowel obstruction or dilation, however, congenital chloridorrhea is one of the rarest and should really only be seriously considered in a fetus known to be at risk for the disease.

The Fetal Colon and Anorectal Malformations

The true function of the colon in utero is unknown. Histologically, some features suggest that the fetal colon may be involved in processes such as water absorption or secretion,[14] but from an imaging perspective, the colon merely acts as a reservoir for the accumulating meconium in the fetus. Meconium normally does not pass the rectal folds or anal sphincter in fetal life unless the fetus is distressed late in gestation. Although some investigators have related stress-induced fetal meconium passage to cord compression[108] or fetal hypoxia,[109] others have suggested that the passage of meconium may be a normal physiologic event, reflecting increasing fetal maturity.[110] Regardless, meconium staining of the amniotic fluid appears to occur exclusively in relatively mature fetuses. Matthews and Warshaw[111] correlated meconium staining of the amniotic fluid with gestational age. Over 98% of the infants born with evidence of meconium-stained amniotic fluid were at least 37 menstrual weeks old, and infants born at less than 34 weeks do not demonstrate meconium staining in the amniotic fluid.[111] Because the innervation of the intestine develops in a craniocaudal direction some suggest that the less developed and possibly less reactive colonic gastrointestinal motility may account for this difference.[111]

A number of congenital anomalies of the colon occur, but only a few have been diagnosed prenatally, including persistent cloaca, anorectal atresia,[112-114] and one report of fetal Hirschsprung disease.[79, 115]

Anorectal malformations occur in 1 in 5000 live births, along a spectrum ranging from the most severe developmental abnormality, persistent cloaca, to the mildest developmental abnormality, imperforate anus. These malformations may occur as isolated findings, but more commonly a variety of concurrent anomalies is present (more than 70%), most notably those of the VACTERL association or the caudal regression syndrome. Anorectal malformations are a complex group of anomalies that basically result from some element of either abnormal descent of the urorectal septum and/or faulty division of the cloaca by the urorectal septum. Anorectal atresias can be simplified into "high" (supralevator) lesions that terminate above the levator sling and "low" (infralevator) lesions that terminate below it, although this distinction is difficult to make in the fetus. High lesions are more common and more likely to be associated with genitourinary malformations, as well as vesicoenteric and enteroenteric fistulas (Fig. 16–37). The latter may be suggested by bizarre pelvic cystic masses, dilated bowel, and enterolithiasis on sonograms of the fetus. Enterolithiasis appears as flocculent, brightly echogenic intraluminal material, believed to result from the mixture of urine and meconium that occurs secondary to the colovesicle fistulas.

On occasion, anorectal atresia is suggested by dilatation of bowel in the lower abdomen of the fetus.[112, 113] Harris and coworkers[112] reviewed prenatal sonographic findings in 12 proven cases of anorectal atresia and found evidence of a peculiar focal bowel dilatation in the pelvis or lower abdomen suggestive of low colonic obstruction in 5 of the 12 cases (42%). Although the numbers are small, it appears that features suggestive of colonic obstruction may, indeed, be present on prenatal sonograms. The sensitivity of sonographic detection of colonic obstruction appears to be directly related to gestational age and, in previous reports, the distal colonic obstructions were more obvious as the fetuses approached term.

It is somewhat surprising that anorectal atresia causes any detectable dilatation of the fetal colon since the fetus does not normally pass meconium in utero. When dilatation is present, some have speculated that it occurs secondary to a colovesicle fistula. Others speculate that some fluid is normally passed through the anus during fetal life; and because anal atresia prevents this passage, colonic dilatation results. Findings suggestive of an anorectal malformation are important, however, not only to expedite early prenatal surgical correction but also to alert the sonographer and perinatologist to search for the commonly associated fetal VACTERL defects. Other diagnoses to be considered when these observations are made, but probably less likely, are the meconium plug syndrome and Hirschsprung disease.[79, 115]

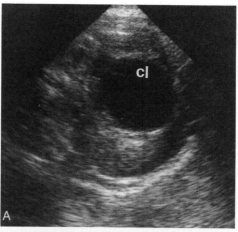

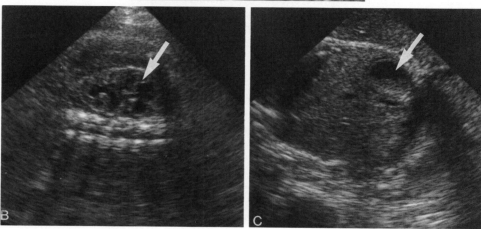

Figure 16–37. Persistent cloaca. *A.* Large cystic mass in pelvis (*arrow*) represents the persistent cloaca (cl). *B.* Same fetus with associated hydronephrosis (*arrow*). *C.* Crystalline matter or "debris" in bowel loop (*arrow*) is due to enteric "vesicle" fistula.

Persistent cloaca is a rare malformation (1 in 40,000 to 50,000 neonates) that is almost always found in phenotypic females. The abdominal wall is intact in this malformation, distinguishing it from cloacal exstrophy. In persistent cloaca, the genital and intestinal tracts converge into a common outflow structure and there is a single perineal opening that serves as the outlet for urine, feces, and genital secretions. The cloacal malformation is believed to result from failure of the urorectal septum to join the cloacal membrane during the fourth to sixth weeks of embryonic life, resulting in a persistent communication between the urogenital sinus and rectum. The cloacal membrane covering the perineum will not rupture unless joined by the urorectal septum, and normal perineal openings will not develop. In addition, normal mesonephric and paramesonephric duct development is altered. As a result, associated abnormalities of the lower urinary tract (reflux, ureteral ectopia, bladder and urethral duplications), genital tract (uterine and vaginal duplications and atresias), and kidneys (agenesis, obstruction, horseshoe kidney) are common. Spinal anomalies, including tethered spinal cord, sacral agenesis, spina bifida, and segmentation anomalies are also commonly associated.

Sonographically, a septated or bilobed cystic pelvic mass is often observed in the fetus. In many cases, this represents a dilated vagina and/or uterus, although dilated rectum can apparently also produce such an appearance. The distinction between the bladder and vagina may be difficult, even postnatally. Interestingly, esophageal atresia has been reported in 10% of neonates with persistent cloaca.

Although the anomalies involved in persistent cloaca are complex, increasing success has been reported with childhood repairs of persistent cloaca. With early diversion of the fecal stream, death is very rare. The diagnosis should be considered if a bizarre bilobed cystic mass is detected in the lower fetal abdomen, especially if there are associated lower spinal malformations.

In approximately 6% of third-trimester fetuses, the meconium-filled rectosigmoid may appear as a "presacral mass." Although other diagnostic considerations for a mass of this type might include sacrococcygeal teratoma (1 in 40,000 livebirths), presacral meningocele, rectal duplication, or anorectal atresia, the frequency with which this normal variant is observed compels the examiner to consider this normal variant as the most likely diagnosis if the amniotic fluid volume is normal and no other morphologic anomalies can be detected. This presacral "pseudomass" can be confirmed by observing its continuity with the colon during real-time scanning, in addition to the visualization of a normal bladder, kidneys, and caudal spine.

ASCITES

True ascites in the fetal abdomen is always abnormal. Intraperitoneal fluid is most readily identified in the peritoneal recesses of the subhepatic space, the flanks, and the lower abdominal cavity or pelvis. In fetuses, because of the small size of the pelvis, fluid is only rarely seen in the rectovesical recess, unlike free intraperitoneal fluid in the adult. Furthermore, ascites fluid often collects between the two leaves of unfused omentum,[2] resulting in a cystlike appearance in the abdomen (Fig. 16–38).

When fetal ascites is associated with hydrops fetalis, pleural effusions and pericardial effusion, integumentary edema will often be observed. In cases of nonimmune hydrops, the prognosis is poor. Fetal ascites may also occur without other serous effusions, and, in these cases, in utero bowel perforation (atresias, volvulus, stenoses, cystic fibrosis) or urinary ascites secondary to bladder or forniceal rupture should be considered. The prognosis in cases of bowel obstruction may be quite good if there are no other malformations, but a poor outcome has been reported in fetuses with ascites due to bladder rupture.[116]

Ascites is always abnormal in the fetus, and thus the implications for fetal prognosis and intervention may be quite significant for both mother and fetus. It is therefore important to avoid false-positive diagnoses of fetal ascites. Familiarity with a potential pitfall, "pseudoascites," may be helpful. A thin rim of lucent tissue observed along the anterior surface of the fetal abdominal cavity just beneath the skin is often confused for fetal peritoneal fluid. This lucency is produced by the hypoechoic anterior abdominal musculature (internal oblique, external oblique, and transverse muscles) (Fig. 16–39)[117] but can be distinguished from true ascites through the following observations:

1. Owing to the insertion of the oblique muscles into the ribs, this lucent rim "fades" posterolaterally and is not visualized between the dorsal ribs and liver.

2. True ascites generally insinuates itself between the bony rib cage and viscera (both liver and spleen) and can be confirmed by its presence in the peritoneal recesses of the fetal subhepatic space, flanks, and between bowel loops, whereas pseudoascites cannot.

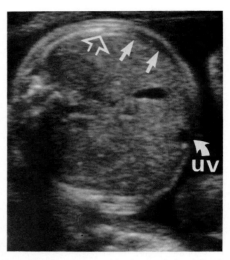

Figure 16–39. "Pseudoascites." The hypoechoic abdominal musculature (*arrows*) "fades" along the interface with the ribs (*open arrow*). Also note that the hypoechoic pseudoascites does not outline the umbilical vein (uv).

3. Ascites frequently outlines the falciform ligament and umbilical vein, but pseudoascites does not.

CALCIFICATIONS IN THE ABDOMEN

If calcifications are parenchymal or are associated with a solid abdominal mass, then neuroblastoma, fetal teratoma, hamartoma, and viral infection should be considered.[22–24] When brightly echogenic foci that are not within an organ and do not appear intraluminal are observed in the fetal abdomen, they are likely to be peritoneal, and meconium peritonitis is the favored diagnosis. The latter is a sterile chemical peritonitis resulting from in utero intestinal perforation, nearly always involving the small intestine (see Fig. 16–36). The bowel perforations that cause meconium peritonitis are believed to occur after the onset of gastric movement and bowel peristalsis, and in some instances they have occurred as early as 24 weeks of life (the mean menstrual age at diagnosis is 29.5 weeks).[118] If the extruded meconium becomes encysted and/or calcified, a meconium pseudocyst develops.[119] In half of cases, an identifiable underlying bowel abnormality, most commonly volvulus, atresia, intussusception, or meconium ileus, is detected; but in many cases the source of the perforation is not uncovered postnatally and the defect heals spontaneously.[120]

The most common sonographic findings are peritoneal calcifications, ascites, dilated bowel, and polyhydramnios. Sonographically, calcifications are distributed on the peritoneal surfaces. The location of the calcifications should be cautiously distinguished from intraluminal (i.e., colonic) or intraparenchymal (i.e., intrahepatic) calcifications. In male fetuses, because of the patent processus vaginalis, these calcifications may extend into the scrotal sac (Fig. 16–40).[121] Owing to the small size of the calcifications, acoustic shadowing from the intraperitoneal calcifications may be difficult to demonstrate sonographically. It has been noted that the calcifications of meconium peritonitis are not seen

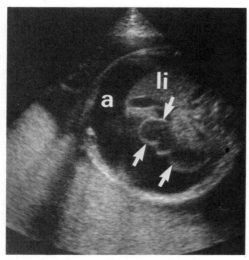

Figure 16–38. Fetal ascites. Fluid has accumulated between the unfused omental sheets (*arrows*). a, ascites; li, liver.

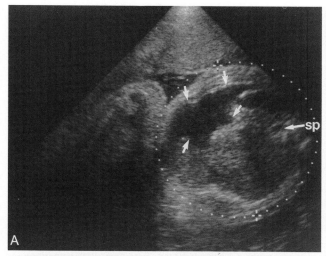

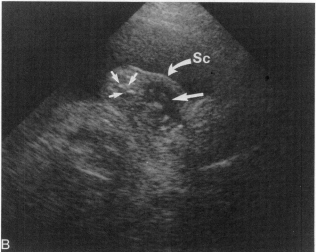

Figure 16–40. Fetus with meconium peritonitis resulting from in utero perforation of Meckel diverticulum. *A.* Loculated ascites (*straight arrows*) suggests meconium pseudocyst. sp, spine. *B.* Scrotum (Sc) is enlarged by a hydrocele (*large arrow*) that contains a number of bright echoes (*small arrows*), suggesting meconium peritonitis/hydrocele.

until at least 10 days after the peritoneal spillage; and thus, if the fetus is scanned after perforation but before this interval, ascites may be the only finding.[122]

Although ascites, meconium pseudocyst formation, and bowel dilatation appear ominous on the sonogram, it is important to recall that small bowel perforations and atresias are less likely to be associated with other extraintestinal anomalies than proximal (i.e., esophageal) or very distal (i.e., rectal) gut atresias. Furthermore, these lesions are successfully repaired postnatally in most neonates.

As sonographic resolution has improved, tiny, relatively inconspicuous, brightly echogenic foci (presumed to be calcifications) have been observed in a number of otherwise normal-appearing fetuses (Fig. 16–41). To determine the prognosis of these seemingly benign findings, my colleagues and I reviewed the outcome of 20 fetuses with peritoneal calcifications.[123] Seventy percent of these fetuses survived. Among the six fetuses with oligohydramnios, all had either bowel dilatation

or ascites in addition to the calcifications. Among these six fetuses, there were no survivors (five of these six pregnancies were terminated and the sixth neonate died). In four, peritoneal calcifications were associated with bowel abnormalities and/or ascites but amniotic fluid volume was normal or increased. All of the latter four fetuses had isolated small bowel obstructions that were successfully surgically corrected postnatally. Among 10 fetuses in whom the peritoneal calcifications were an isolated finding (no bowel or other morphologic abnormality; normal amniotic fluid volume), all but 1 were normal at 28 months. Few had been tested for cystic fibrosis, but none was diagnosed with the disease at the time of follow-up. We therefore concluded that when they are an isolated finding, tiny, relatively inconspicuous peritoneal calcifications are associated with an excellent fetal outcome.

ABDOMINAL CYSTS

Cysts are occasionally discovered in the fetal abdomen during routine prenatal sonography and are virtually never malignant. The largest fetal abdominal "cysts" I have encountered in my practice have originated from the urinary system and represent dilated renal pelves or perinephric urinomas. Determining the site of origin of the abdominal cysts is not always possible; one rule that has been helpful and reliable for determining the renal origin of the cyst is that if the cyst touches the fetal spine, it is most likely renal in origin. Other cystic structures may pose greater diagnostic difficulty. If the cyst is lower in the abdomen and the fetus is female, ovarian cyst should be considered. Recall, however, that ovarian cysts may "wander" in the fetus and can be visualized quite "high" in the abdominal cavity (Fig. 16–42). Some ovarian cysts have achieved such great size (up to 11 cm in diameter)

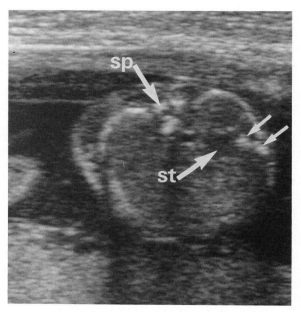

Figure 16–41. Small, inconspicuous bright echoes (*small arrows*) adjacent to the stomach (st) in this otherwise normal fetus are suggestive of intraperitoneal calcification. sp, spine.

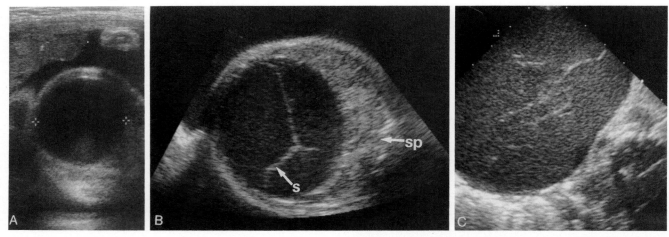

Figure 16–42. Fetal ovarian cyst. *A.* Large unilocular cyst (*cursors*) in female fetal abdomen. *B.* Same fetus 3 weeks later. Interval appearance of septations (s) and internal echoes strongly suggest torsion and hemorrhage. sp, spine. *C.* Neonatal scan. Large cyst with septations and internal echoes. This cyst (and ovary) was removed. Pathologic diagnosis was ovarian cyst and torsion.

that they have extended from the pelvis to the liver, impressing upon the diaphragm and thorax.[124, 125] They may be simple, without internal echoes, or contain septations. Although they may be complicated by torsion or hemorrhage,[126] fetal ovarian cysts are nearly always benign.[127] Meizner and colleagues[128] reported findings in 15 fetuses in whom ovarian cysts were detected prenatally (in 8 fetuses before 28 weeks' gestation). If the cysts were untorsed in utero, they were observed as simple cysts and all disappeared within 6 months of postnatal life. In 6 fetuses, the cysts demonstrated fluid levels and internal echoes. All of these fetuses had their cysts surgically removed in the early neonatal period, and all were benign. Fetal ovarian cysts may be unilateral or bilateral and have been associated with polyhydramnios in 10% of cases. They are believed to result from excessive stimulation by both placental and maternal hormones.[129, 130] Some have been shown to be follicular, and others have nonspecific cyst linings. Ovarian cysts have been reported in association with fetal hypothyroidism.[131] Theca lutein cysts are believed to result from elevated circulating human chorionic gonadotropin levels and have been associated with diabetes in pregnancy.[132] Small follicular cysts, although common in fetal autopsy specimens (33%), are generally too small to be seen on sonograms of the fetus.[133]

The differential diagnosis of fetal abdominal cyst should include mesenteric cyst, gut duplication, choledochal and urachal cysts, and cystic teratoma, as well as cysts of renal origin. Choledochal cysts, as described previously, generally appear in the right upper quadrant near the expected location of the common bile duct. Urachal cysts occur near the ventral apex of the bladder wall and tend to be associated with the ventral abdominal wall. Cysts of renal origin tend to be located more dorsally and in close proximity to the spine. Occasionally, a dilated ureter may be confused with colon or vice versa.

Mesenteric cysts, on the other hand, are thought to be lymphatic and have been reported to occur most commonly in the mesentery of the small bowel.[134, 135]

There is some confusion regarding the nomenclature of a lymphangioma and mesenteric cyst. Although the two may be distinguished histologically using current electron micrographic techniques, these distinctions have not always been drawn in the literature. Takiff and colleagues, in a study of surgical cases including children and adults, found lymphangiomas to be rare, more frequently multilocular, larger, more commonly symptomatic, and usually occurring in children.[136] Alternatively, mesenteric cysts in this series appeared to be more common, smaller, more localized to the omentum, asymptomatic, unilocular, and most often occurring in adults. Mesenteric cysts, when discovered in childhood, are reported to be uniformly benign.[137] Regardless, mesenteric cysts or lymphangiomas are extremely rare lesions.

References

1. Creline ES: Functional Anatomy of the Newborn, pp 47–69. New Haven, Yale University Press, 1973.
2. Gross BH, Callen PW, Filly RA: Ultrasound appearance of the fetal greater omentum. J Ultrasound Med 1:67, 1982.
3. Moore KL: The placenta and fetal membranes. In: The Developing Human: Clinically Oriented Embryology, 4th ed. Philadelphia, WB Saunders, 1988.
4. Crooji MJ, Westhuis M, Schoemaker J, Exalto N: Ultrasonographic measurement of the yolk sac. Br J Obstet Gynaecol 89:931, 1982.
5. Green JJ, Hobbins JC: Abdominal ultrasound examination of the first trimester fetus. Am J Obstet Gynecol 159:165, 1988.
6. Lyons EA, Levi CS: Ultrasound in the first trimester of pregnancy. In Callen PW (ed): Ultrasonography in Obstetrics and Gynecology, pp 10–11. Philadelphia, WB Saunders, 1983.
7. Moore KL: The digestive system. In: The Developing Human: Clinically Oriented Embryology, 4th ed. Philadelphia, WB Saunders, 1988.
8. Jauniaux E, Donner C, Thomas C, et al: Umbilical cord pseudocyst in trisomy 18. Prenat Diagn 8:557, 1988.
9. Fink IJ, Filly RA: Omphalocele associated with umbilical cord allantoic cyst: Sonographic evaluation in utero. Radiology 149:473, 1983.
10. Skibo LK, Lyons ER, Levi CS: First trimester umbilical cord cysts. Radiology 182:719, 1992.
11. Moore KL: The urogenital system. In: The Developing Human:

Clinically Oriented Embryology, 4th ed. Philadelphia, WB Saunders, 1988.

12. Currarino G: The genitourinary tract. In Silverman FN (ed): Caffey's Pediatric X-Ray Diagnosis, 8th ed, vol II, pp. 1671–1672. Chicago, Year Book Medical Publishers, 1985.

13. Ney C, Friedenberg RM: Radiographic Atlas of the Genitourinary System, pp 1359–1360. Philadelphia, JB Lippincott, 1981.

14. Grand RI, Watkins JB, Torti FM: Development of the human gastrointestinal tract. Gastroenterology 70:790, 1976.

15. Cyr DR, Mack LA, Schoenecker SA, et al: Bowel migration in the normal fetus: US detection. Radiology 161:119, 1986.

16. Schmidt W, Yarkoni S, Crelin ES, et al: Sonographic visualization of physiologic anterior abdominal wall hernia in the first trimester. Obstet Gynecol 69:911, 1987.

17. Mahony BS, McGahan P, Nyberg DA, Reisner DP: Varix of the fetal intra-abdominal umbilical vein: Comparison with normal. J Ultrasound Med 11:73, 1992.

18. Harman CR: Specialized applications of obstetrical ultrasound: Management of the alloimmunized pregnancy. Semin Perinatol 9:184, 1985.

19. Witter FR, Graham D: The utility of ultrasonically measured umbilical vein diameters in isoimmunized pregnancies. Am J Obstet Gynecol 146:225, 1983.

20. Rudolph AM: Hepatic and ductus venosus blood flows during fetal life. Hepatology 3:254, 1983.

21. Jeanty P: Persistent right umbilical vein: An ominous prenatal finding? Radiology 177:735, 1990.

22. Nguyen DL, Leonard JC: Ischemic hepatic necrosis: A cause of fetal liver calcification. AJR 147:596, 1986.

23. Blanc WA, Berdon WE, Baker DH, et al: Calcified portal vein thromboemboli in newborn and stillborn infants. Radiology 88:287, 1967.

24. Friedman AP, Hally JO, Boyer B, Looper R: Calcified portal vein thromboemboli in infants: Radiography and sonography. Radiology 140:381.

25. Hill LM: Sonographic detection of fetal gastrointestinal anomalies. Ultrasound Q 1:35, 1988.

26. Krandel K, Williams CH: Ultrasound case report of hepatic teratoma in newborns. J Clin Ultrasound 12:98, 1984.

27. Namakoto SK, Dreilinger A, Dattel B, et al: The sonographic appearance of hepatic hemangiomas in utero. J Ultrasound Med 2:239, 1983.

28. Marks F, Thomas P, Lustig I, et al: In utero sonographic description of a fetal liver adenoma. J Ultrasound Med 9:119, 1990.

29. Liyanage IS, Katoch D: Ultrasonic prenatal diagnosis of liver metastases from adrenal neuroblastoma. J Clin Ultrasound 20:401, 1992.

30. Ishak KG, Glunz PR: Hepatoblastoma and hepatocellular carcinoma in infancy and childhood: Report of 47 cases. Cancer 20:396, 1967.

31. Dachman AH, Lichtenstein JE, Friedman AC, Hartman DS: Infantile hemangioendothelioma of the liver: A radiologic-pathologic clinical correlation. AJR 140:1091, 1983.

32. Gonen R, Fong K, Chiasson DA: Prenatal sonographic diagnosis of hepatic hemangioendothelioma with secondary nonimmune hydrops fetalis. Obstet Gynecol 73:485, 1989.

33. Horgan GJ, King DL, Taylor KJW: Sonographic detection of prenatal liver mass. J Clin Gastroenterol 6:277, 1984.

34. Edmonson HA: Differential diagnosis of tumors and tumor-like lesions of the liver in infancy and childhood. Am J Dis Child 91:168, 1956.

35. Longmire WP, Mandrola SA, Gordon HE: Congenital cystic disease of the liver and biliary system. Ann Surg 174:711, 1971.

36. Chung WM: Antenatal detection of hepatic cyst. J Clin Ultrasound 14:217, 1986.

37. Foucar E, Wilhamson RA, Yiu-Chin V, et al: Mesenchymal hamartoma of the liver identified by fetal sonography. AJR 140:970, 1981.

38. Davies CH, Stringer DA, Whyte H, et al: Congenital hepatic fibrosis with saccular dilatation of intrahepatic bile ducts and infantile polycystic kidney disease. Pediatr Radiol 16:302, 1986.

39. Jouppila P, Heikkinen J, Kirkinen P: Contractibility of maternal and fetal gallbladder: An ultrasonic study. J Clin Ultrasound 13:461, 1985.

40. Elrad H, Mayden KL, Ahart S, et al: Prenatal ultrasound diagnosis of choledochal cyst. J Ultrasound Med 4:553, 1985.

41. Frank JL, Hill MC, Chirathivat S, et al: Antenatal observation of a choledochal cyst by sonography. AJR 137:166, 1981.

42. Beretsky I, Lankin DH: Diagnosis of fetal cholelithiasis using real-time high-resolution imaging employing digital detection. J Ultrasound Med 2:381, 1983.

43. Dewbury KC, Aluwihare M, Birch SJ, et al: Prenatal ultrasound demonstration of a choledochal cyst. Br J Radiol 53:906, 1980.

44. Yamaguchi M: Congenital choledochal cyst. Am J Surg 140:653, 1980.

45. Brown DL, Teele RL, Doubilet PM, et al: Echogenic material in the fetal gallbladder: Sonographic and clinical observations. Radiology 182:73, 1992.

46. Lilly JR: Choledochal cyst and "correctable" biliary atresia. J Pediatr Surg 20:299, 1985.

47. Kamath KR: Abnormalities of the biliary tree. Clin Gastroenterol 15:157, 1986.

48. Andrews HG, Zwiren GT, Caplan DB, et al: Biliary atresia: An evolving perspective. South Med J 79:581, 1986.

49. Moore TC, Hyman PE: Extrahepatic biliary atresia in one human leukocyte antigen identical twin. Pediatrics 76:604, 1985.

50. Green D, Carroll BA: Ultrasonography in the jaundiced infant: A new approach. J Ultrasound Med 5:323, 1986.

51. Schmidt W, Yarkoni S, Jeanty P, et al: Sonographic measurements of the fetal spleen: Clinical implications. J Ultrasound Med 4:667, 1985.

52. Potter EL: Pathology of the Fetus and Infant, p 14. Chicago, Year Book Medical Publishers, 1961.

53. Gruenwald P, Minh HN: Evaluation of body and organ weights in perinatal pathology. Am J Clin Pathol 34:247, 1960.

54. Eliezer S, Feldman E, Ehud W, et al: Fetal splenomegaly, ultrasound diagnosis of cytomegalovirus infection: A case report. J Clin Ultrasound 12:520, 1984.

55. Mittlestaedt CA: Ultrasound of the spleen. Semin Ultrasound 2:233, 1981.

56. Lichman JP, Miller EI: Prenatal ultrasonic diagnosis of splenic cyst. J Ultrasound Med 7:637, 1988.

57. Chitayat D, Lao A, Wilson RD, et al: Prenatal diagnosis of asplenia/polysplenia syndrome. Am J Obstet Gynecol 158:1085, 1988.

58. Lawson TL, Foley WD, Berland L, et al: Ultrasonic evaluation of fetal kidneys. Radiology 138:153, 1981.

59. Netter NH: Endocrine System and Selected Metabolic Diseases, pp 77–81. Summit, NJ, CIBA, 1965.

60. Robbins SL, Cotran RS: Pathologic Basis of Diseases, 2nd ed, pp 1387–1388. Philadelphia, WB Saunders, 1979.

61. Rosenberg ER, Bowie JD, Andreotti RF, et al: Sonographic evaluation of fetal adrenal glands. AJR 139:1145, 1982.

62. Villee DB: The development of steroidogenesis. Am J Med 53:533, 1972.

63. Co CS, Filly RA: Normal fetal adrenal gland location. (Letter to the editor) J Ultrasound Med 5:117, 1986.

64. Hoffman CH, Filly RA, Callen PW. The lying down adrenal sign: A sonographic indicator of renal agenesis or ectopia in fetuses and neonates. J Ultrasound Med 11:533, 1992.

65. Giulian BB, Chang CCN, Yoss BS: Prenatal ultrasonographic diagnosis of fetal adrenal neuroblastoma. J Clin Ultrasound 14:225, 1986.

66. Gotoh T, Adachi Y, Nounaka O, et al: Adrenal hemorrhage in the newborn with evidence of bleeding in utero. J Urol 141:1145, 1989.

67. Morganti VJ, Anderson NG: Simple adrenal cysts in fetus, resolving spontaneously in neonate. J Ultrasound Med 10:521, 1991.

68. Pritchard JA: Fetal swallowing and amniotic fluid volume. Obstet Gynecol 28:606, 1966.

69. Kimura RE, Warshaw JB: Intrauterine development of gastrointestinal tract function. In Lebenthal E (ed): Textbook of Gastroenterology and Nutrition in Infancy, vol I, pp 39–46. New York, Raven Press, 1981.

70. Abramovich DR: Fetal factors influencing the volume and composition of liquor amnii. J Obstet Gynaecol Br Commonw 77:865, 1970.

71. Goldstein I, Reece A, Yarkone S, et al: Growth of the fetal stomach in normal pregnancies. Obstet Gynecol 70:741, 1987.
72. Pretorius DH, Gosink BB, Clautice-Engle T, et al: Sonographic evaluation of the fetal stomach: Significance of nonvisualization. AJR 151:987, 1988.
73. AIUM: Guidelines for performance of the antepartum obstetric ultrasound examination. J Ultrasound Med 10:576, 1991.
74. Zilianti M, Fernandez A: Correlation of ultrasonic images of fetal intestine with gestational age and fetal maturity. Obstet Gynecol 62:569, 1983.
75. Bustamante S, Koldovsky O: Synopsis of development of the main morphological structures of the human gastrointestinal tract. In Lebenthal E (ed): Textbook of Gastroenterology and Nutrition in Infancy, pp 49–55. New York, Raven Press, 1981.
76. Fakhry J, Reiser M, Shapiro LR, et al: Increased echogenicity in the lower fetal abdomen: A common normal variant in the second trimester. J Ultrasound Med 5:489, 1986.
77. Manco LG, Nunan FA, Sohnen H, et al: Fetal small bowel simulating abdominal mass at sonography. J Clin Ultrasound 14:404, 1986.
78. Dicke JM, Crane JP: Sonographically detected hyperechoic fetal bowel: Significance and implications for pregnancy management. Obstet Gynecol 80:778, 1992.
79. Nyberg DA, Mack LA, Patten RM, et al: Fetal bowel, normal sonographic findings. J Ultrasound Med 6:3, 1987.
80. Moore KL: The respiratory system. In: The Developing Human: Clinically Oriented Embryology, 4th ed. Philadelphia, WB Saunders, 1988.
81. Pretorius DH, Meier PR, Johnson ML: Diagnosis of esophageal atresia in utero. J Ultrasound Med 2:475, 1983.
82. Duenhoelter JH, Santos-Ramos R, Rosenfeld CR, et al: Prenatal diagnosis of gastrointestinal tract obstruction. Obstet Gynecol 47:618, 1976.
83. Jassani MN, Gauderer MWL, Fanaroff AA, et al: A perinatal approach to the diagnosis and management of gastrointestinal malformations. Obstet Gynecol 59:33, 1982.
84. Eyheremendy E, Fister M: Antenatal real-time diagnosis of esophageal atresia. J Clin Ultrasound 11:395, 1983.
85. Nelson LH, Clark CE, Fishburne JI, et al: Value of serial sonography in the in utero detection of duodenal atresia. Obstet Gynecol 59:657, 1982.
86. Loveday BJ, Barr JA, Atkens J: The intrauterine demonstration of duodenal atresia by ultrasound. Br J Radiol 48:1031, 1975.
87. Weinberg B, Diakoumalis EE: Three complex cases of foregut atresia: Prenatal sonographic diagnosis with radiographic correlation. J Clin Ultrasound 13:481, 1985.
88. Touloukian RJ: Intestinal atresia. Clin Perinatol 5:3, 1978.
89. Kirkpatrick JA, Wagner ML, Pilling GP: A complex of anomalies associated with tracheoesophageal fistula and esophageal atresia. AᵀR 95:208, 1965.
90. Boychuk RB, Lyons EA, Goodhard TK: Duodenal atresia diagnosed by ultrasound. Radiology 127:500, 1978.
91. Zimmerman HB: Prenatal demonstration of gastric and duodenal obstruction by ultrasound. J Can Assoc Radiol 29:138, 1978.
92. Lees RF, Alford BA, Brenbridge NAG, et al: Sonographic appearance of duodenal atresia in utero. AJR 131:701, 1978.
93. Grivan DP, Stephens GA: Congential intrinsic duodenal obstruction: A twenty-year review of its surgical management and consequences. J Pediatr Surg 9:833, 1974.
94. Bovicelli L, Rizzo N, Orsini LF, et al: Prenatal diganosis and management of fetal gastrointestinal abnormalities. Semin Perinatol 7:109, 1983.
95. Parulekar SG: Sonography of normal fetal bowel. J Ultrasound Med 10:211, 1991.
96. Goldstein RB, Filly RA: Diagnosis of meconium ileus in utero. J Ultrasound Med 6:663, 1987.
97. Elias S, Annas GJ, Simpson JL: Carrier screening for cystic fibrosis: Implications for obstetric and gynecology practice. Am J Obstet Gynecol 164:1077, 1991.
98. Scioscia AL, Pretorius DH, Budorick NE, et al: Second-trimester echogenic bowel and chromosomal abnormalities. Am J Obstet Gynecol 167:889, 1992.
99. Paulson EK, Hertzberg BS: Hyperechoic meconium in the third trimester fetus: An uncommon normal variant. J Ultrasound Med 10:677, 1991.
100. Estroff JA, Parad RB, Benacerraf BR: Prevalence of cystic fibrosis in fetuses with dilated bowel. Radiology 183:677, 1992.
101. Foster MA, Nyberg DA, Mahony BS, et al: Meconium peritonitis: Prenatal sonographic findings and their clinical significance. Radiology 165:661, 1987.
102. Brugman S, Bjelland JC: Cancer of the mouth. Ariz Med 35:802, 1978.
103. Winter RM, Knowles SA: Megacystis-microcolon-intestinal hypoperistalsis syndrome: Confirmation of autosomal recessive inheritance. J Med Genet 23:360, 1986.
104. Srtamm E, King G, Thickman D: Megacystis-microcolon-intestinal hypoperistalsis syndrome: Prenatal identification in siblings and review of the literature. J Ultrasound Med 10:599, 1991.
105. Patel PJ, Kolawole TM, Ba'Aqueel HS, Al-Jisi N: Antenatal sonographic findings of congenital chloride diarrhea. J Clin Ultrasound 17:115, 1989.
106. Groli C, Zucca S, Cesaretti A: Congenital chloridorrhea: Antenatal ultrasonographic appearance. J Clin Ultrasound 14:293, 1986.
107. Kirkinen P, Jouppila P: Prenatal ultrasonic findings in congenital chloride diarrhoea. Prenat Diagn 4:457, 1984.
108. Hon EH: The foetal heart rate. In Carey HM (ed): Modern Trends in Human Reproductive Physiology, p 245. London, Butterworth, 1963.
109. Saling E, Schneider D: Biochemical supervision of the foetus during labour. J Obstet Gynaecol Br Commonw 74:799, 1967.
110. Fenton AN, Steer CM: Fetal distress. Am J Obstet Gynecol 83:354, 1962.
111. Matthews TC, Warshaw JB: Relevance of the gestational age distribution of meconium passage in utero. Pediatrics 64:30, 1979.
112. Harris RD, Nyberg DA, Mack LA, Weinberger E: Anorectal atresia: Prenatal sonographic diagnosis. AJR 149:395, 1987.
113. Miller SF, Angtuaco TL, Quirk G, Hairston K: Anorectal atresia presenting as an abdominopelvic mass. J Ultrasound Med 9:669, 1990.
114. Bean WJ, Calonje MA, Aprill CN, Geshner J: Anal atresia: A prenatal ultrasound diagnosis. J Clin Ultrasound 6:111, 1978.
115. Vermesh M, Mayden KL, Confino E, et al: Prenatal sonographic diagnosis of Hirschsprung's disease. J Ultrasound Med 5:37, 1986.
116. Mahony BS, Callen PW, Filly RA: Fetal urethral obstruction: US evaluation. Radiology 157:221, 1985.
117. Hashimoto BE, Filly RA, Callen PW: Fetal pseudoascites: Further anatomic observations. J Ultrasound Med 5:151, 1986.
118. Dillard JP, Edwards DU, Leopold GR: Meconium peritonitis masquerading as fetal hydrops. J Ultrasound Med 6:49, 1987.
119. McGahan JP, Hanson F: Meconium peritonitis with accompanying pseudocyst: Prenatal sonographic diagnosis. Radiology 148:125, 1983.
120. Farouhar E: Meconium peritonitis: Pathology, evolution and diagnosis. Am J Clin Pathol 78:208, 1982.
121. Heydenrych JJ, Marcus PB: Meconium granuloma of the tunica vaginalis. J Urol 115:596, 1976.
122. Martin L: Meconium peritonitis. In Ravitch MM, Welch Kl. Benson CD, et al (eds): Pediatric Surgery, 3rd ed, vol II, pp 952–955. Chicago, Year Book Medical Publishers 1979.
123. Chaffey MH, Goldstein RB, Russell SA, Goldbus M: Prenatally observed abdominal calcifications: Fetal prognosis. In prepation.
124. Suita S, Ikeda K, Koyamagi T, et al: Neonatal ovarian cyst diagnosed antenatally: Report of two patients. J Clin Ultrasound 12:517, 1984.
125. Landrum B, Ogburn PL, Feinberg S, et al: Intrauterine aspiration of a large fetal ovarian cyst. Obstet Gynecol 68:11S, 1986.
126. Preziosi P, Fariello G, Moiorana A, et al: Antenatal sonographic diagnosis of complicated ovarian cysts. J Clin Ultrasound 14:196, 1986.
127. Tabsh KM: Antenatal sonographic appearance of a fetal ovarian cyst. J Ultrasound Med 1:329, 1982.
128. Meizner I, Levy A, Katz M, et al: Fetal ovarian cysts: Prenatal

ultrasonographic detection and postnatal evaluation and treatment. Am J Obstet Gynecol 164:874, 1991.

129. Pryse-Davies J, Dewhurst CJ: The development of the ovary and the uterus in the foetus, newborn and infant: Morphological and enzyme histochemical study. J Pathol 103:5, 1971.

130. Evers JL, Rolland R: Primary hypothyroidism and ovarian activity: Evidence for an overlap in the synthesis of pituitary glycoproteins. Br J Obstet Gynaecol 88:195, 1981.

131. Jafri SZH, Bree RL, Silver TM, et al: Fetal ovarian cysts: Sonographic detection and association with hypothyroidism. Radiology 150:809, 1984.

132. Nguyen KT, Reid RL, Sauerbrei E: Antenatal sonographic detection of a fetal theca lutein cyst: A clue to maternal diabetes mellitus. J Ultrasound Med 5:665, 1986.

133. DeSa DJ: Follicular ovarian cysts in stillbirths and neonates. Arch Dis Child 50:45, 1975.

134. Haller JO, Schneider M, Kassner EG, et al: Sonographic evaluation of mesenteric and omental masses in children. AJR 130:269, 1978.

135. Girdany BR: The abdomen and gastrointestinal tract. In Silverman FN (ed): Caffey's Pediatric X-Ray Diagnosis, 8th ed, vol II, pp 1398–1399. Chicago, Year Book Medical Publishers, 1985.

136. Takiff H, Calabria R, Yin L, et al: Mesenteric cysts and intraabdominal cystic lymphangiomas. Arch Surg 120:1266, 1985.

137. Kurtz RI, Heimann TM, Beck AR, et al: Mesenteric and retroperitoneal cysts. Ann Surg 203:109, 1986.

CHAPTER 17

Ultrasound Evaluation of Fetal Abdominal Wall Defects

LUÍS FLÁVIO GONÇALVES, M.D.
PHILIPPE JEANTY, M.D., Ph.D.

EMBRYOGENESIS

Abdominal Wall Development

By the end of the fifth week of menstrual age, the embryo is a flat disk consisting of three layers: ectoderm, mesoderm, and endoderm (Fig. 17–1). During the sixth week of menstrual age, through a process called *folding,* this flat embryo transforms itself into a cylindrical shape. Folding happens at the cranial, caudal, and lateral ends of the embryo at the same time (Figs. 17–2 and 17–3) and is a crucial step in the closure of the abdominal wall.

When the embryo folds at the cranial end, the base of the yolk sac is partially incorporated as the foregut, which will develop later as the pharynx and its derivatives, lower respiratory system, esophagus, stomach, duodenum (proximal to the opening of the bile duct), liver, pancreas, gallbladder, and biliary duct system. Growth of the developing neural tube causes the embryo to fold at the caudal end, incorporating part of the yolk sac as the hindgut, which in turn dilates to form the cloaca. It also causes the connecting stalk, previously located at the tail, to move to the ventral surface of the embryo, incorporating the allantois into the umbilical cord. The derivatives of the hindgut are the distal part of the transverse colon, the descending colon, the sigmoid colon, the rectum, the superior portion of the anal canal, the epithelium of the urinary bladder, and most of the urethra. Folding at the sides of the embryo (see Fig. 17–3) will ultimately lead to the formation of the lateral and anterior abdominal wall. The lateral body wall, or somatopleure, progressively folds toward the median plane on both sides. The midgut is the primordium of the small intestines (including most of the duodenum), cecum, vermiform appendix, ascending colon, and the right half to two thirds of the transverse colon. The connection of the yolk sac and body stalk will form the umbilical cord at the ventral region of the embryo. Further expansion of the amniotic cavity will cover the umbilical cord by the amnion.[1]

Fusion of the myotomes at the midline begins during the seventh week of menstrual age and is complete by the eighth week.[2] The junction of the body stalk and the somatopleure containing muscle primordia can be observed from this stage on. However, the paraumbilical region remains indistinguishable from the tissue of the umbilical cord. A clear differentiation will only arise during the 11th week, when the fetal period begins. The rectus abdominis muscles are still separated from the body stalk by a ring of highly cellular mesoderm that appears to be continuous with the posterior rectus sheath. Thereafter, the already formed abdominal musculature gradually approaches the median plane.[2]

Vascularization of the Primitive Abdominal Wall

Three afferent venous systems drain the blood of the early embryo to the sinus venosus (Figs. 17–4 and 17–5): (1) the umbilical veins drain the placenta, body

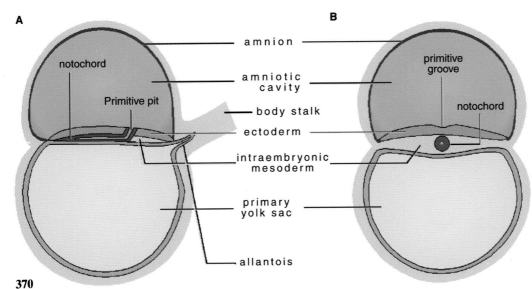

A   **B**

amnion

notochord

amniotic cavity

Primitive pit

primitive groove

notochord

body stalk

ectoderm

intraembryonic mesoderm

primary yolk sac

allantois

Figure 17–1. Fifth week of menstrual age. The embryo is a flat disk, consisting of ectoderm, mesoderm, and endoderm. *A.* Sagittal view. Observe the insertion of the body stalk at the caudal pole of the embryo. *B.* Coronal view.

Figure 17–2. Sixth week of menstrual age. Folding of the embryo as viewed from the sagittal plane. Observe the change of the body stalk position in relation to the embryo. Also, part of the yolk sac is incorporated by the embryo as the foregut, midgut, and hindgut. By the end of the process, the distal part of the yolk sac will be called the secondary yolk and will connect to the embryo through the vitelline duct. The secondary yolk sac is visualized on ultrasound evaluation as a round anechoic structure that migrates away from the embryo toward the placenta and finally disappears as gestational age progresses. *A.* Six weeks. *B.* Six weeks and 2 days. *C.* Six weeks and 4 days. *D.* Six weeks and 6 days.

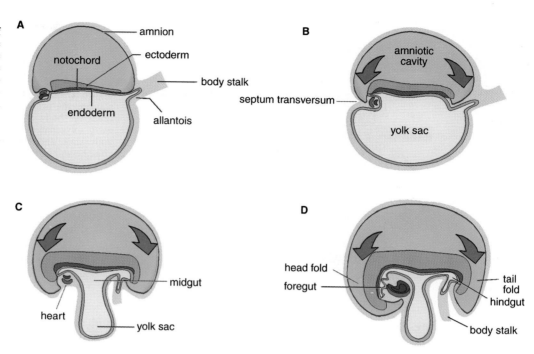

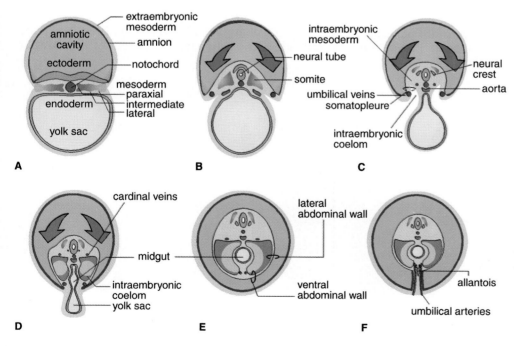

Figure 17–3. Folding of the embryo as viewed from the coronal plane. Note the presence of the right and left umbilical veins close to the junction of the somatopleure with the amnion. *A.* End of the fifth week. *B.* Beginning of the sixth week. *C.* Six weeks and 2 days. *D.* Six weeks and 4 days. *E.* Six weeks and 6 days. *F.* Coronal section at the level of the body stalk showing components of the umbilical cord at this stage: two umbilical veins, two umbilical arteries, and the allantois.

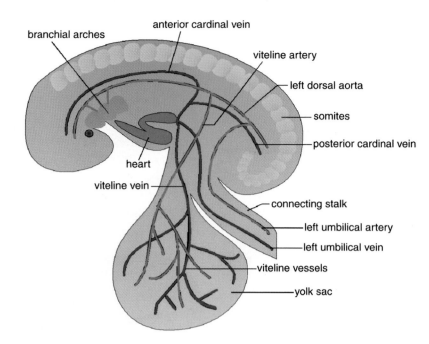

Figure 17–4. Sagittal view of the 6-week embryo showing the primitive circulation: the cardinal veins drain the body of the embryo, the umbilical veins carry oxygenated blood from the placenta to the body stalk and evolving abdominal wall, and the vitelline veins drain the yolk sac.

stalk, and evolving abdominal wall; (2) the vitelline or omphalomesenteric veins drain the yolk sac; and (3) the cranial and caudal cardinal veins drain the body of the embryo.

The umbilical veins originate from a capillary network at the junction of the most lateral regions of the embryo with the amnion and yolk sac. They drain the placenta, the body stalk, and the evolving abdominal wall. Between 6 and 7 weeks' gestation, both veins remain at the junction of the body stalk with the somatopleure and drain the lower body wall, chorionic villi, and developing upper limb buds. They empty in the sinus venosus, laterally to the hepatocardinal veins. The hepatocardinal veins drain the tubular gut and the

yolk sac through the vitelline veins. During the seventh week, rerouting of blood takes place (Fig. 17–6). The hepatic bud enlarges, and a progressive atrophy of the entire right umbilical vein along with its communication with the omphalomesenteric veins occurs. The proximal portion of the left umbilical vein between the subhepatic portion and the common cardinal vein also atrophies. The nutritive function of the umbilical veins with respect to the developing abdominal wall is replaced by branches of the aorta. The venous blood drainage is taken over by the thoracoepigastric vein and branches of the caudal cardinal vein.[2]

The omphalomesenteric arteries are branches of the embryonic aorta. After rearrangement of the vascular

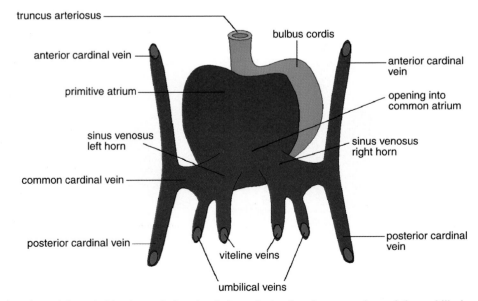

Figure 17–5. Posterior view of the primitive heart during the sixth week showing the connections of the umbilical, cardinal, and vitelline veins with the sinus venosus.

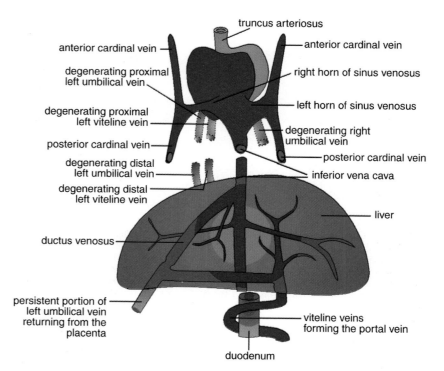

Figure 17–6. Rerouting of blood during the seventh week. The enlargement of the liver kinks the right umbilical vein and the right omphalomesenteric artery, which results in their occlusion. At the same time, the proximal portion of the left umbilical vein reconnects to the portal vein and the left vitelline vein atrophies. After rearrangement of the vascular connections, the left omphalomesenteric artery persists, becoming the superior mesenteric artery.

connections, only the right omphalomesenteric artery persists, becoming the superior mesenteric artery. The distal portion follows the omphalomesenteric duct through the umbilical ring, supplying the yolk sac.[3]

Umbilical Herniation

Umbilical herniation takes place during the eighth week of development. The midgut extends to the extraembryonic coelom in the proximal portion of the umbilical cord. Because of the massive liver and kidneys, the midgut grows faster than the abdominal cavity at this stage of gestation and herniates. The midgut, before herniation, is a U-shaped loop of gut having just a cranial and a caudal limb nourished by the superior mesenteric artery, oriented in a perpendicular plane to a sagittal section passing through the median axis of the embryo. Its cranial limb grows fast and will form the small intestine. The caudal limb does not change much and will form the cecum, vermiform appendix, descending colon, and one half to two thirds of the transverse colon. While it herniates through the umbilical cord, it rotates 90° clockwise around the axis of the superior mesenteric artery.

The return of the intestines to the abdominal cavity occurs at the 12th week of menstrual age; this is called reduction. The order of returning is as follows: the small intestines return first, then the large intestine rotates 180° clockwise. Considering both herniation and reduction, the intestines undergo a total of 270° of rotation. It is likely that reduction happens for the same reasons as herniation. Thus, enlargement of the abdominal cavity together with a relative decrease in the size of liver and kidneys is the possible explanation for this process.[1, 4] Timor-Tritsch and colleagues studying 61 embryos or fetuses between 7 and 12 weeks of gestational age with endovaginal ultrasonography were unable to demonstrate ventral herniation in any fetuses after 12 completed weeks.[5]

GASTROSCHISIS

Synonyms

Other names for this disorder include paraomphalocele, laparoschisis, abdominoschisis, and embryonal ruptured omphalocele.[2]

Definition

Gastroschisis is a right paraumbilical defect involving all layers of the abdominal wall, usually measuring from 2 to 4 cm (Fig. 17–7). The small bowel always eviscerates through the defect and is, by definition, nonrotated and lacking secondary fixation to the posterior abdominal wall. Skin is rarely interposed between the defect and the umbilical cord.[2] The loops of bowel are never covered by a membrane; hence, they are directly exposed to the amniotic fluid. α-Fetoprotein levels are markedly elevated. The loops usually develop a fibrous coating and are matted together. Other organs that may eviscerate are the large bowel (often), the stomach, portions of the genitourinary system (occasionally), and the liver (very rarely).[6, 7] The location of the defect on the left side has been reported but is rare.[7, 8]

Prevalence

Gastroschisis occurs in 1.75 to 2.5 in 10,000 live births.[2, 9] Although the vast majority of cases are sporadic, a few cases of familial occurrence have been

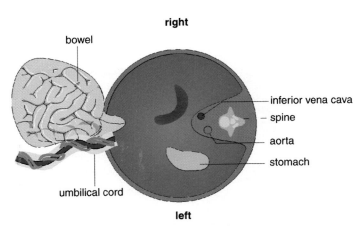

Figure 17–7. Gastroschisis. Drawing of a transverse section through the fetal abdomen in gastroschisis. Observe the bowel herniating through a right paraumbilical defect of the abdominal wall. This defect may be due to the local ischemia that results from the occlusion of the right umbilical vein and the right omphalomesenteric artery. Also, note the normal insertion of the cord to the left of the loops. The intestines are not covered by a membrane in this condition.

reported.[1, 9, 10] A male preponderance is often observed.[8]

Pathogenesis

Three theories have been suggested to explain the pathogenesis of gastroschisis: (1) abnormal involution of the umbilical vein[2]; (2) intravascular accident of the omphalomesenteric artery[3]; and (3) early intrauterine rupture of an omphalocele with complete resorption of the sac.[10]

According to deVries,[2] either premature atrophy or persistence of the right umbilical vein could explain the localized right paraumbilical defect found in gastroschisis. If premature atrophy happens before the establishment of collateral circulation from the aorta, localized ischemia at the junction of the somatopleure with the body stalk will follow. Persistence of the right umbilical vein, on the other hand, could impair the development of collateral circulation from the aorta, leading to infarction of the surrounding tissues by the time the right umbilical vein atrophies. Whatever is the mechanism, mesenchymal damage would impair skin formation at the ischemic site, since differentiation of the epidermis depends on the integrity of the mesoblast. The small bowel would then prolapse through the paraumbilical defect, rupturing the somatopleure before umbilical herniation. It would continue to grow in the amniotic cavity rather than in the intraembryonic coelom. Since the intestine rotates 270° during the normal umbilical herniation and reduction, tethering at the level of the defect would explain why the intestine is nonrotated in gastroschisis.

A second theory states that gastroschisis is the result of an intravascular accident of the omphalomesenteric artery.[3] The basis for this assumption is that the majority of the defects associated with gastroschisis involve the absence or disruption of a structure in which

clinical and experimental evidence support a vascular accident as the underlying process (e.g., nonduodenal intestinal atresia, "apple peel bowel" in jejunal atresia, porencephaly, unilateral absence of a kidney, and gallbladder atresia). Since the distal portion of the right omphalomesenteric artery supplies the right portion of the umbilical ring, the hypothesis claims that its disruption would lead to infarction, necrosis of the base of the cord, and herniation of gut through the infarcted area.[3] However, studies of chicken and human embryos between 6 and 30 weeks' gestation performed by Tibboel and colleagues failed to demonstrate the ischemic changes mentioned earlier.[8]

Rupture of a small omphalocele and transformation into "gastroschisis" has been observed in utero.[11] This supports the idea that some gastroschisis could represent simply a ruptured omphalocele occurring at some time after folding of the somatic components of the anterior abdominal wall but before the fusion of the umbilical ring.[10, 11] However, the increased incidence of associated malformations in omphalocele, including aneuploidy, fails to support this theory.

The fibrous coating of the bowel in gastroschisis is probably due to direct exposure to fetal urine in the amniotic fluid. Support for this hypothesis comes from a study in chicken and human embryos demonstrating the following: (1) in the chicken embryo the development of the fibrous coating coincided with changes in the amniotic and allantoic fluid composition that consisted in a drop in osmolality and sodium concentration and a rise in potassium, urea, and creatinine concentrations; (2) in the human embryo a significant rise in potassium, urea, and creatinine concentrations and a drop in osmolality and sodium concentrations occur after 30 weeks of gestation; and (3) no fetuses before 30 weeks' gestation developed the fibrous coating, whereas all fetuses after 33 weeks' gestation did so.[8]

Hypoperistalsis and intestinal atresia are related to ischemic damage to the bowel occurring at a late stage of development. Progressive compression of the developing bowel protruding through a relatively small abdominal wall defect would explain this and the edematous aspect.[8] Hypoperistalsis could also be a consequence of the fibrous coating itself.[12]

Associated Anomalies

Gastroschisis has a lower incidence of associated anomalies than does omphalocele, ranging from 7% to 30%.[3] Two anomalies are obviously associated: (1) malrotation and (2) absent secondary fixation of the bowel to the dorsal abdominal wall. Other anomalies related to the herniation (ischemia due to kinking of vessels and jejunal and multiple atresia) or to the chemical irritation by the amniotic fluid are difficult to detect. Peristaltic activity is decreased or absent and may not return for weeks or months after surgery, requiring parenteral nutrition. Anomalies not directly related to the defect are less common than in omphalocele and include anencephaly, cleft lip and palate, atrial septal defect, ectopia cordis, diaphragmatic hernia, scoliosis, syndactyly, and amniotic band.[13-15] Growth retardation is not as prevalent as it is for omphalocele, but prematurity is common.

Diagnosis

Gastroschisis is found either serendipitously or because of elevated maternal serum α-fetoprotein levels.[16] The diagnosis can be made before 20 weeks[17] and was correctly made with endovaginal sonography as early as 12 weeks.[18]

The striking feature in the fetus presenting with gastroschisis is the multiple loops of bowel floating freely in the amniotic fluid. Since herniated bowel can be seen in conditions other than gastroschisis, a careful approach should lead to the diagnosis. When scanning a fetus suspected of having gastroschisis, one should try to answer the following questions:

1. *What organs can be identified outside the abdomen?* In gastroschisis, only the small and large intestine are commonly herniated. Bowel can be identified by the characteristic sonographic pattern and peristalsis (Fig. 17-8A). Occasionally the stomach, gallbladder, uterus, adnexa, and urinary bladder may be found, too. However, when the older literature reports herniation of organs other than small or large bowel, one should suspect that some cases of body stalk anomaly have been mistaken for gastroschisis.[19]

2. *Is there a membrane covering the herniated structures?* The loops are *not* contained by a membrane; therefore, their edges are irregular.

3. *Where is the umbilical cord inserted?* In virtually all cases, the defect is on the right of the umbilical cord and just a few left-sided lesions have been described.[20] Hence, the umbilical cord is normally inserted and to the left of the defect (see Fig. 17-8B).

4. *Is ascites present?* Since there is no membrane, ascites is not present in the abdominal cavity.

5. *Are there associated anomalies of other organs and systems?* Gastroschisis is usually not associated with anomalies of other organs and systems, as opposed to omphalocele, amniotic band syndrome, and body stalk anomaly.

6. *Are there additional signs?* Because of the emptying of the abdominal cavity, some structures such as the bladder and the stomach can be found abnormally close to each other. Bowel perforation can be suspected by the presence of calcifications and an intramesenteric, extra-abdominal pseudocyst.[20]

Although the diagnosis appears relatively straightforward, the identification of the herniated loops of bowel may not always be easy, and cases have been missed in spite of careful prenatal scans.

Differential Diagnosis

The usual differential diagnosis is with omphalocele, but with current equipment the differentiation should not be a problem. Other abdominal wall defects (such as bladder exstrophy,[21] body stalk anomalies,[20] or amniotic band syndrome) may resemble gastroschisis. There are reports of gastroschisis resulting from in utero rupture of omphaloceles.[11] When the liver is intra-abdominal the diagnosis of omphalocele is less obvious and the natural tendency is to classify the lesion as being a gastroschisis. These ruptures must be truly exceptional if they really exist, and they more likely represent an artifact of delivery (either vaginal or abdominal). An old notion of early versus perinatal gastroschisis sometimes is mentioned.[2] Some probably represent ruptured omphalocele, missed diagnosis, and potentially a few genuine cases, although, here again, the condition must be quite unusual. Blood clots around the cord (either from placenta abruptio[19] or traumatic amniocentesis) may result in an appearance similar to that of gastroschisis.

Prognosis

Since gastroschisis is usually not associated with other congenital or chromosomal anomalies, it carries a much better prognosis. Possible causes of death in this group would include sepsis, surgical complications, and low birth weight.[8] These fetuses seem to get the most benefit from early prenatal diagnosis since they can be prospectively followed for intrauterine growth

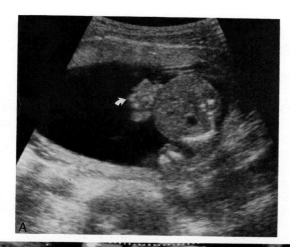

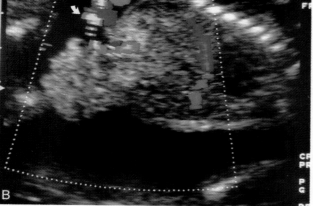

Figure 17-8. Gastroschisis. *A.* Transverse section through the fetal abdomen demonstrating multiple loops of bowel adjacent to the anterior abdominal wall *(arrow)*. *B.* A similar section in another fetus, showing the insertion of the umbilical cord *(arrow)* on the left side of the gastroschisis.

retardation and obstruction of the gastrointestinal tract, as well as delivery in a tertiary care center with an available pediatric surgeon. Because of improvements in surgical technique and in parenteral nutrition in the past 2 decades, the survival rate is 80% to 90%. In uncomplicated cases delivered in a tertiary care center, the survival rate can approach 100%. The size of the defect[22] or the length between the diagnosis and delivery does not influence the prognosis; thus, early delivery does not appear indicated. The thickening and distention of loops of bowel[7, 23] and extracorporeal liver[24] are associated with a poor outcome.

Recurrence Risk

Recurrence is not expected, although it occasionally occurs, and occurrence in twins has been reported.[25]

Management

The follow-up of the fetus with gastroschisis involves screening for intrauterine growth retardation and signs of bowel obstruction, bowel wall thickening, and perforation (Fig. 17–9). Bowel obstruction happens inside or outside the abdominal cavity and appears sonographically as dilation of the loops, which may look like multiple cysts. Polyhydramnios may follow gastrointestinal obstruction. Calcifications on the surface of extra-abdominal bowel and intramesenteric extra-abdominal pseudocyst are signs of bowel perforation (Fig. 17–10).[26] Since the incidence of chromosomal anomalies in fetuses with gastroschisis is not greater than that for the general population, fetal karyotyping is not recommended.

Although it appears rational to deliver these fetuses by cesarean section to prevent bowel injury, this is controversial in the literature. Some authors are skeptical about the benefits, while others strongly recommend primary cesarean section at 36 weeks when lung maturity has been documented. Trauma to the bowel can also occur during cesarean section. Studies that have compared the outcome of fetuses delivered in either way did not demonstrate any benefit from either technique; however, the comparison was made only on mortality and not morbidity, which would be a more sensitive indicator. Signs of obstruction, bowel wall thickening, and perforation might help to select fetuses who would benefit from early abdominal delivery. Surgical resection of necrotic bowel with a one- or two-stage closure (depending on the compression of the diaphragm) should be performed immediately after birth.

OMPHALOCELE

Definition

Omphalocele (also known as exomphalos) is a defect of the anterior abdominal wall in which there is extrusion of the abdominal contents into the base of the umbilical cord. The herniated mass is covered by the parietal peritoneum. After 10 weeks' gestation, amnion and Wharton's jelly also cover the omphalocele. The umbilical cord inserts onto the sac rather than in the abdominal wall as in gastroschisis (Fig. 17–11).[9] The size of the defect depends on the amount and type of viscera herniated into the amniotic sac.[9]

Prevalence

The incidence of omphalocele is higher than gastroschisis, occurring in 2.5 in 10,000 births. The sex ratio is 1:1.[9]

Pathogenesis

The etiology is unknown. Two theories have been proposed to explain the embryology of omphaloceles: (1) failure of the bowel to return to the abdomen and (2) defective enclosing growth of the lateral folds, which normally grow and surround the abdominal contents during the fifth to sixth week.

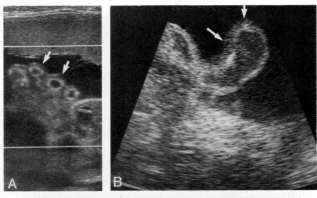

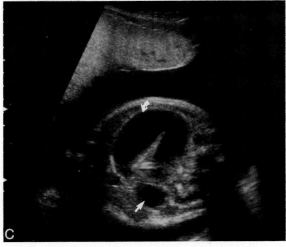

Figure 17–9. Gastroschisis. *A* and *B*. Multiple loops of abnormal bowel floating in the amniotic fluid. The walls are markedly thickened *(arrows)*, and in real time, no peristalsis could be observed.

C. Transverse section through the fetal abdomen showing a normal stomach *(arrow)* and distended bowel *(curved arrow)* in a fetus with gastroschisis and intestinal obstruction.

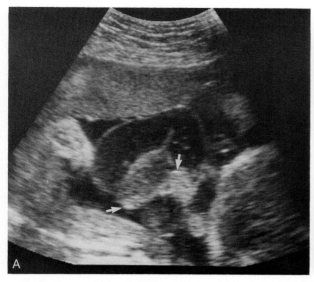
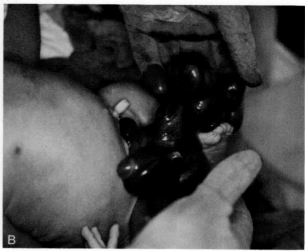

Figure 17–10. Gastroschisis. *A.* Dilated loops of bowel outside the abdominal wall with multiple calcifications on the external surface *(arrows)*, indicating perforation.

B. Neonatal aspect. Observe the fibrous coating, the meconium plugs identified as calcifications, and the appearance of the loops matted together.

Associated Anomalies

Omphalocele is associated with other anomalies in 50% to 70% of cases.[6, 24, 27–30] In prenatal studies, at least 50% of the fetuses have associated anomalies.[22] Chromosome anomalies occur in 40% to 60%[27, 31–34] and are predominantly due to trisomies (18, 13, and 21) and Turner, Klinefelter, and triploidy syndromes. When abnormal amniotic fluid volumes are present (oligohydramnios or polyhydramnios)[35] or when the omphalocele contains only bowel, the association with chromosomal anomalies is significantly more common.[36] Fifty percent of the associated anomalies affect the heart (e.g., ventricular and atrial septal defects, tetralogy of Fallot, pulmonary artery stenosis, pulmonary hypoplasia, double outlet right ventricle, coarctation of the aorta, bicuspid aortic valve, transposition of the great vessels).[31, 37, 38] The association between omphalocele and ectopia cordis is discussed later (see section on pentalogy of Cantrell).

Other reported anomalies occur in 40% of the fetuses and include clubfeet, neural tube defects, microcephaly, cloacal exstrophy, imperforate anus, ureteropelvic junction obstruction, diaphragmatic hernia, cleft lip, Beckwith-Wiedemann syndrome, single umbilical artery, allantoic cyst, and chorioangioma of the placenta.[38, 39] The association between omphalocele and cloacal exstrophy is discussed later.

Gastrointestinal anomalies (diaphragmatic hernia, intestinal duplications and atresias, ascites, absent gallbladder, tracheoesophageal fistula, and imperforate anus) occur in 40% of fetuses.[40] Malrotation is the rule. Numerous other anomalies, such as cystic hygroma, micrognathia, scoliosis, hemivertebra, meningomyelocele, campomelic dwarfism, facial clefts, cleft lip, clubfeet, syndactyly, and other digital anomalies, can be present in 10% to 30% of fetuses. Furthermore, immaturity and prematurity are superimposed in most fetuses.

right

amnion + peritoneum

liver

spine

umbilical cord

left

Figure 17–11. Omphalocele. Drawing of a transverse section through the fetal abdomen showing herniation of the liver through a large abdominal wall defect, covered by peritoneum and amnion. The umbilical cord inserts into the defect rather than in the abdominal wall.

Diagnosis

The anomaly is usually detected during routine examination or in the investigation for elevated α-fetoprotein levels. A weak band of acetylcholinesterase can also be detected on chromatography.[22] This is probably related to the proximity of nerve termination with amniotic fluid.

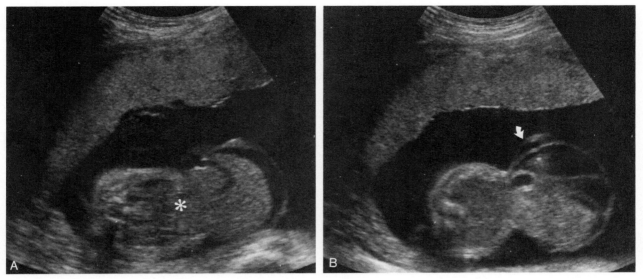

Figure 17–12. Large omphalocele. *A.* The liver herniates through the defect *(asterisk). B.* Observe herniation of the stomach and bowel together with the liver. Also of note is the ascites. In all cases the defect is covered by a membrane and the umbilical cord *(arrow)* inserts into the defect, rather than into the abdominal wall.

The diagnosis of omphalocele is made by the demonstration of an anterior midline mass of the abdominal wall. This mass contains the herniated viscera (e.g., bowel, stomach, liver) and has a smooth surface, since it is contained in the peritoneal-amniotic membrane. The membrane is not always visible,[22] but with improved resolution this is rarely a problem. The umbilical cord enters the omphalocele, and the umbilical vein can be seen within the mass. Ascites is commonly present (Figs. 17–12 and 17–13).

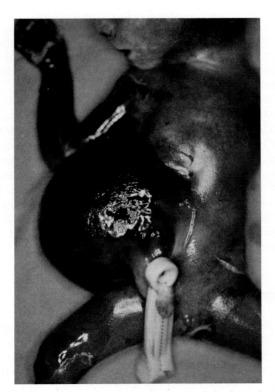

Figure 17–13. Omphalocele. Postnatal aspect of the fetus shown in Figure 17–12*B.*

The physiologic herniation of bowel in the first trimester has been described at the beginning of this chapter. When the omphalocele is greater than the abdomen, one can probably make the diagnosis in the first trimester[41]; otherwise, a repeat scan after 12 weeks is indicated.[42] The size of the omphalocele is best quantified by measuring the ratio of the transverse diameter of the omphalocele over the transverse diameter of the abdomen. When the ratio of the omphalocele to abdomen transverse diameter is less than 60%, it usually only contains bowel, not liver. The relative size of the omphalocele to abdomen may decrease during pregnancy.[14]

Differential Diagnosis

Pseudo-omphalocele may occur in oligohydramnios or other causes of lateral compression of the lower thorax.[19, 43] When the ribs are pressed medially the abdomen assumes an hourglass shape. The condition is easily recognized, however, since omphaloceles are uncharacteristically associated with oligohydramnios. A small pseudo-omphalocele has also been described in polyhydramnios,[44] but this case is clearly exceptional.

Gastroschisis is the commonly questioned differential diagnosis. In fact, the only common finding between the two anomalies is that they both present with an anterior abdominal mass. Gastroschisis is not covered by a membrane and thus has a ragged edge; they are right sided, the umbilical vein enters the abdomen on their left, and they almost never contain the liver. A potential problem is the spontaneous rupture of the membrane of omphalocele, making the omphalocele resemble a gastroschisis.[11, 45] This complication, however, has been reported so rarely that it is of little practical significance[37] and probably represents trauma at delivery.

Beckwith-Wiedemann syndrome, pentalogy of Cantrell, and cloacal exstrophy are discussed in separate sections.

Prognosis

Stillbirth is common among fetuses with omphalocele.[34] Neonatal death is highly correlated with associated anomalies detected by ultrasound evaluation,[32, 35] with death occurring in virtually all fetuses whose anomalies are not benign ones. Conversely, when the defect is not associated with major anomalies the prognosis is good. Oligohydramnios and polyhydramnios have a pejorative prognosis. The size of the omphalocele, which influences the surgical procedure and the postoperative morbidity, does not appear to affect the mortality: if the neonate makes it to surgery without major associated anomalies, it usually can be treated. The presence of ascites is mentioned in various studies to represent[35] or not represent[22] a significant risk factor for fetal death.

Severe associated anomalies are responsible for 80% to 100% of the deaths; sepsis and surgical complications are responsible for 0% to 13%, while low birthweight is responsible for 10%. Excluding terminations of pregnancy, over 50% of the fetuses will die. The recurrence risk is quoted to be less than 1%.[46]

Management

The ultrasound diagnosis of an omphalocele prompts a full search for associated anomalies, including a fetal echocardiogram and a karyotype. If associated anomalies are detected before viability, the choice of pregnancy termination can be offered. After viability, in the presence of associated malformations and consequent lethal outcome, an operative delivery for fetal reasons should be avoided. Fetuses without major associated anomalies should be delivered in a tertiary care center.[47]

BECKWITH-WIEDEMANN SYNDROME

Synonyms

Synonyms include Beckwith syndrome, EMG syndrome, exomphalos-macroglossia-gigantism syndrome, macroglossia-omphalocele-visceromegaly syndrome, visceromegaly-umbilical hernia-macroglossia, and Wiedemann-Beckwith syndrome.

Definition

Beckwith-Wiedemann syndrome is a group of disorders having in common the coexistence of an omphalocele, macroglossia, and visceromegaly.

Prevalence

Eighty-five percent of the cases are sporadic.[9] The syndrome has an autosomal dominant pattern of inheritance with variable transmission.[48] In over 90% of the cases, the affected parent is the mother.

Pathogenesis

Placental endocrine dysfunction leading to increased levels of growth hormone and insulinlike growth factors would cause the visceromegaly. Early visceromegaly may predispose to omphalocele, malrotation anomalies, and diaphragmatic herniation.[9]

Associated Anomalies

Trisomy 11p has been associated with the Beckwith-Wiedemann syndrome. Other inconstant anomalies include horizontal ear lobe crease, visceromegaly, pancreatic hyperplasia, cardiac malformations and cardiomegaly, polyhydramnios, placental enlargement[49] with chorioangiomas,[50] clitoromegaly, renal cysts or enlargement,[51, 52] and renal tumors (Wilms tumors).[53]

Diagnosis

The most common features are omphalocele (75%), macroglossia (97%),[54] gigantism (32%) or hemihypertrophy, hepatosplenomegaly (32%), nephromegaly (23%), and cardiac anomalies (15%). Four percent of the omphaloceles are associated with the Beckwith-Wiedemann syndrome.

In a pregnancy at risk for the syndrome, any of the anomalies listed earlier should be sought. In one case prospectively studied, an omphalocele was not detected at 13 weeks but was present at 18 weeks.[55] Most often, however, the syndrome will be detected because of the discovery of an omphalocele. Macroglossia is easily recognizable in either a coronal anterior section through the lips and nose or in a facial profile (Fig. 17–14). The tongue size is normal if the tip remains behind an imaginary line drawn from the upper to the lower gum in the facial profile during most of the scan.[56] When abnormal, the tongue clearly protrudes from the open mouth.[49, 56] The characteristic thin groove of the ear lobe, although discrete, is potentially detectable by a tangential section of the ear lobe. The association of polyhydramnios and a large fetus, especially in the presence of very large kidneys, should also suggest the diagnosis.[57]

Differential Diagnosis

Beckwith-Wiedemann syndrome should be considered in the differential diagnosis whenever omphalocele, macroglossia, or other visceromegaly associated with the syndrome are observed.

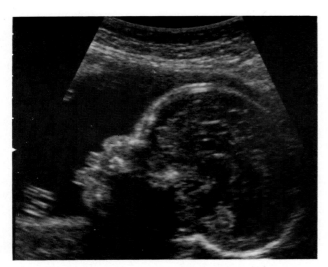

Figure 17–14. Macroglossia. Midsagittal scan of the fetal head demonstrating protrusion of the tongue through an imaginary line drawn from the upper to the lower gum.

Recurrence Risk

The recurrence risk in an apparent sporadic disease is difficult to estimate, and the couple should be counseled to have ultrasound examination early in future pregnancies.

Prognosis

These neonates have a poor prognosis as a result of metabolic complications (hypoglycemia) and suffocation because of the macroglossia. Intubation at birth is thus recommended. Furthermore, these neonates are at risk to develop malignant tumors (nephroblastoma, adrenal tumors). However, if they survive early childhood, they have relatively normal intelligence.

Management

The diagnosis of Beckwith-Wiedemann syndrome should prompt a chromosomal evaluation. Before viability, the option for pregnancy termination can be offered. If the patient decides to continue with the pregnancy, the management is similar as for an omphalocele. During delivery, the presence of the pediatrician is mandatory owing to the risk of hypoglycemia and to the possibility that intubation may be required. If the macroglossia persists, partial glossectomy may be indicated.

PENTALOGY OF CANTRELL

Synonyms

Other names of pentalogy of Cantrell include Cantrell-Haller-Ravitch syndrome, Cantrell pentalogy, pentalogy syndrome, peritoneopericardial diaphragmatic hernia, and thoracoabdominal ectopia cordis.[9]

Definition

The pentalogy of Cantrell is the association of two major defects: an omphalocele and an ectopic heart. The three other anomalies are consequential to the former two; they represent a defect of the structures interposed between the heart and the omphalocele: the lower sternum, the anterior diaphragm, and the diaphragmatic pericardium.

Prevalence

The male-to-female ratio is 1:1. The syndrome is very rare, and only about 50 cases have been reported in the literature.[9]

Pathogenesis

The defect is believed to result from defective lateral mesoderm folds around 28 to 32 days of menstrual age. The transverse septum of the diaphragm does not form, and the ventromedial migration of the upper abdominal paired mesodermal folds fails to occur.

Associated Anomalies

The syndrome has been reported in monozygotic twins.[58] Variants, including the association of an ectopia cordis with a gastroschisis, have also been reported.[23] Vertebral deformities are common. The most prevalent associated cardiac anomalies include atrial septal defect (50%), ventricular septal defect (20%), and tetralogy of Fallot (10%).[9, 59] Noncardiac anomalies include trisomies 13 and 18, Turner syndrome, craniofacial anomalies (cephalocele, cleft lip, microphthalmia, low-set ears), kyphoscoliosis, clinodactyly, two-vessel cord, and ascites.[60, 61]

Diagnosis

The ultrasound examination reveals the association of an omphalocele and an ectopic heart (Fig. 17–15). The ectopic heart may be entirely out of the chest or simply bulge through a defective sternum. Pleural and pericardial effusions are common. The abdominal wall defect ranges from diastasis of the rectal muscles with the heart palpable beneath a hyperpigmented skin covering to huge omphaloceles containing bowel, liver, and the cardiac apex covered by a translucent membrane.[9] The diagnosis has been made as early as the 17th week[62] and could probably be made even earlier.

Differential Diagnosis

The differential diagnosis includes isolated ectopia cordis, body stalk anomaly, and amniotic band syndrome.

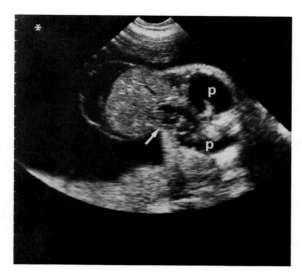

Figure 17–15. Pentalogy of Cantrell. Transverse scan demonstrating a large omphalocele, herniation of the heart *(arrow)*, and bilateral pleural effusions (p).

Prognosis

The prognosis will depend on the severity of the anomalies. Complications include rupture of viscera during delivery, sepsis, cyanosis, congestive heart failure, cardiorespiratory difficulty, and cardiac compression. Many patients have undergone repair of what seemed to be a simple omphalocele and were found later to have pentalogy of Cantrell. Most of the cases detected prenatally had a fatal outcome (Fig. 17–16).[60, 63] For the severe forms, the prognosis is very

poor, since the reduction of the heart in the chest causes kinking of the great vessels. Recurrence has not been described.

Management

Once the diagnosis is established, a fetal karyotype should be obtained and a complete search for associated anomalies performed. Before viability, the option of pregnancy termination can be offered. If the patient chooses to continue the pregnancy, there is no evidence that cesarean section can improve the outcome.[56] After delivery, correction of the abdominal, diaphragmatic, pericardial, and sternal defects can be attempted at the same time.[63]

CLOACAL EXSTROPHY

Synonyms

Other names for cloacal exstrophy include OEIS (omphalocele, exstrophy, imperforate anus, spina bifida) complex, exstrophy of cloaca sequence, and exstrophia splanchnica.

Definition

Cloacal exstrophy is the rare association of an omphalocele, exstrophy of the bladder, imperforate anus, and spinal defects such as meningomyelocele.[64]

Prevalence

The prevalence is 0.05 in 10,000 births.[65]

Pathogenesis

Cloacal exstrophy is due to nondevelopment of the urorectal septum and consequent failure of separation of the urogenital sinus from the rectum. Concomitantly, the mesodermal proliferation forming the infraumbilical abdominal wall and genital tubercle fails to develop.[66]

Associated Anomalies

Other associated anomalies include multicystic kidney dysplasia, hydronephrosis, undescended testicles, lower limb anomalies (clubfoot, abnormal angle of the iliac wings), hypoplastic chest, diaphragmatic hernia, hydrocephaly, meningocele, and two-vessel cord.[67] Besides an elevated α-fetoprotein level, the acetylcholinesterase level is increased, but not to the levels usually found in open neural tube defects.

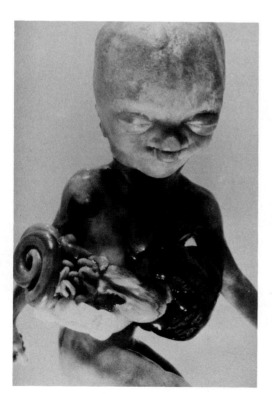

Figure 17–16. Pentalogy of Cantrell. Postnatal aspect.

Diagnosis

Because of the multiple defects affecting the integrity of skin coverage, the fetuses will often present with markedly elevated α-fetoprotein levels (over 10 multiples of mean). The hemibladders are on either side of the intestines.

On ultrasound evaluation, the image is similar to that of bladder exstrophy: a large infraumbilical defect that extends to the pelvis[68] and an irregular anterior mass (Fig. 17–17). A posterior anomalous component (meningomyelocele) may be present. The bladder cannot be visualized since the urine is excreted directly from the ureters into the amniotic fluid.[65] A single umbilical artery, ascites, vertebral anomalies, and clubfoot should also be sought. Severe luxation of the legs may be present. In boys, the penis is divided and duplicated. Color Doppler imaging aids in the localization of the bladder by demonstrating the umbilical arteries in the lower fetal abdomen.[65]

Differential Diagnosis

The differential diagnosis should include amniotic band syndrome, sacrococcygeal teratoma, and body stalk anomaly when the cord is not seen. Three cases described in the literature as cloacal exstrophy probably represent body stalk anomalies.[69]

Prognosis

Because of the severity of the anomalies the defect may be fatal, but in milder forms corrective surgery can be offered.[70]

Management

Before viability, the option of pregnancy termination can be offered. After viability, standard obstetric management should not be altered for this condition.

AMNIOTIC BAND SYNDROME

Synonyms

Synonyms include ADAM complex (amniotic deformities, adhesion, mutilation), amniotic band sequence, amniotic disruption complex, annular grooves, congenital amputation, congenital constricting bands, Streeter bands, transverse terminal defects of limb,[9] aberrant tissue bands, amniochorionic mesoblastic fibrous strings, and amniotic bands.[71]

Definition

Amniotic band syndrome is a set of congenital malformations ranging from minor constriction rings and lymphedema of the digits to complex and bizarre multiple congenital anomalies that are attributed to amniotic bands that stick, entangle, and disrupt fetal parts.

Prevalence

The prevalence of amniotic band syndrome among live births is estimated to be around 7.8 in 10,000.[9] For spontaneous abortions, it can be as high as 178 in 10,000.[72] It affects males and females in the same proportion.

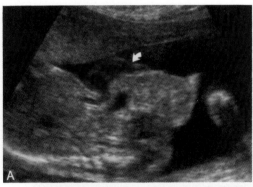
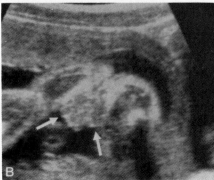
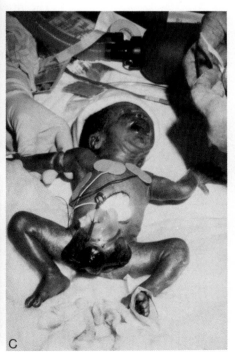

Figure 17–17. Exstrophy of the cloaca sequence. *A.* Longitudinal scan of the lower abdomen demonstrates an irregular protruding mass that contains bladder and bowel. The umbilical cord *(arrow)* inserts above the mass. *B.* Scan demonstrating abnormal genitalia. *C.* Postnatal aspect. (From Erb R, Jaffe R, Braren V, et al: Exstrophy of the cloaca sequence. Fetus 2:7515, 1992.)

Pathogenesis

The etiology is unknown. There have been reports associating amniotic band syndrome with maternal trauma, oophorectomy during pregnancy,[73] intrauterine contraceptive device,[74] and amniocentesis,[75–77] but these are clearly a minority. There are case reports in families with connective tissue disorders (Ehler-Danlos syndrome).[78] Since 17 of the 18 cases of amniotic band syndrome in twins that have been published in the literature were in monozygotic twins, and since monozygotic twinning is theorized to be the result of a teratogenic stimulus, a teratogenic insult might be implicated as causing the disorder.[79, 80]

Two theories have been suggested to try to explain the mechanism of the fetal malformations in amniotic band syndrome.

Endogenous Theory. For many years, the defects associated with amniotic band syndrome were believed to result from focal developmental errors in the formation of limb connective tissue.[81]

Exogenous Theory. Torpin[82] studied 400 cases of amniotic band syndrome. According to him, rupture of the amnion but without rupture of the chorion would lead to transient oligohydramnios due to loss of amniotic fluid through the initially permeable chorion. The fetus would pass from the amniotic to the chorionic cavity through the defect. The contact of the fetus with "sticky" mesoderm from the chorionic surface of the amnion would lead to entanglement of the fetal parts and skin abrasions. Entanglement of the fetal parts would cause constriction rings and amputations, whereas skin abrasions would lead to disruption defects such as cephaloceles. Furthermore, swallowing of the bands would cause asymmetric clefts on the face.[52, 82, 83]

Lockwood and colleagues[79, 80] contest the exogenous theory based on clinical and experimental evidence. Among the clinical evidence against the exogenous theory are the high prevalence of internal visceral anomalies and anomalies not readily explainable by the amniotic disruption sequence as proposed by Torpin (Table 17–1), cases of amniotic band syndrome with a histologically normal and intact amniotic lining, and the frequent finding of disruptive defects in fetuses not in contact with bands. Experiments injecting vasoactive substances in rats have reproduced external and internal features of amniotic band syndrome without disruption of the amnion.[84, 85] Furthermore, histologic evidence supports that hemorrhages precede limb constrictions, amputations, clefts, and clubfoot in the rat model.[58] The pathogenesis would involve damage of the mesenchymal and endothelial cells of the superficial vessels of the embryo and the amnion, disruption of epiblastic cells and secondary limb amputation, constriction bands, encephaloceles, syndactyly, clubfoot, and clubbed hands.[86] Amniotic band formation would be a late and secondary event analogous to adhesion formation.

Associated Anomalies

The following anomalies are associated with amniotic band syndrome.[39, 48, 52, 53, 87–89]

Table 17–1. ANOMALIES ASSOCIATED WITH AMNIOTIC BAND SYNDROME

Explainable by Exogenous Theory	Lacking Explanation by Exogenous Theory
Scalp adhesions	Holoprosencephaly
Skull defects	Cerebellar dysplasia
Asymmetric facial clefts	Absent olfactory bulbs
Eye disruptions	Anophthalmia
Abdominal wall disruptions	Hypertelorism
Syndactyly	Small foramen magnum
Amputation	Migrational defects
Clubfeet	Heterotopic brain
Constriction rings	Cardiac anomalies
Hip dislocation	Tracheoesophageal fistula
Sacral rotation	Renal agenesis
	Accessory spleens
	Gallbladder agenesis
	Malrotation of the gut
	Single umbilical artery
	Internal genital malformation
	Anal atresia
	Simian crease

- *Limbs:* constriction rings of limbs or digits, lymphedema, amputation of limbs or digits (Fig. 17–18*F*), pseudosyndactyly (pseudosyndactyly originates at the distal portion of the digits, whereas syndactyly includes the base of the digits), abnormal dermal ridge patterns, simian crease, clubfeet
- *Cranium:* multiple and asymmetric encephaloceles (see Fig. 17–18*A* and *F*), anencephaly
- *Face:* cleft lip, cleft palate, nasal deformities, asymmetric microphthalmos, incomplete or absent cranial calcifications (see Fig. 17–18*C*)
- *Thorax:* thoracic rib clefting
- *Spine:* scoliosis
- *Abdominal wall:* gastroschisis, omphalocele, bladder exstrophy (see Figs. 17–18*D* through *F*)
- *Perineum:* Ambiguous genitalia, imperforate anus

Diagnosis

The most common finding in amniotic band syndrome is constriction rings of the fingers and toes.[90] Seventy-seven percent of the fetuses present with multiple anomalies.[58] The association of the abnormalities described earlier should be regarded as strong evidence and immediately raise the suspicion of amniotic band syndrome. The further visualization of the amniotic bands attaching to a fetus with restriction of motion is diagnostic of the condition, precluding the need for fetal karyotyping (see Fig. 17–18*B*).[58, 61] We advise the reader that the visualization of amniotic bands or sheets in the absence of fetal deformities should by no means lead to the diagnosis of amniotic band syndrome, since several types of membranes may be seen in normal pregnancies.[61] The diagnosis is confirmed at autopsy by the demonstration of chronic rupture of the chorion in histologic sections of the placenta.

Differential Diagnosis

Amniotic folds are recognized by prenatal ultrasonography as reflecting membranes with a free edge in

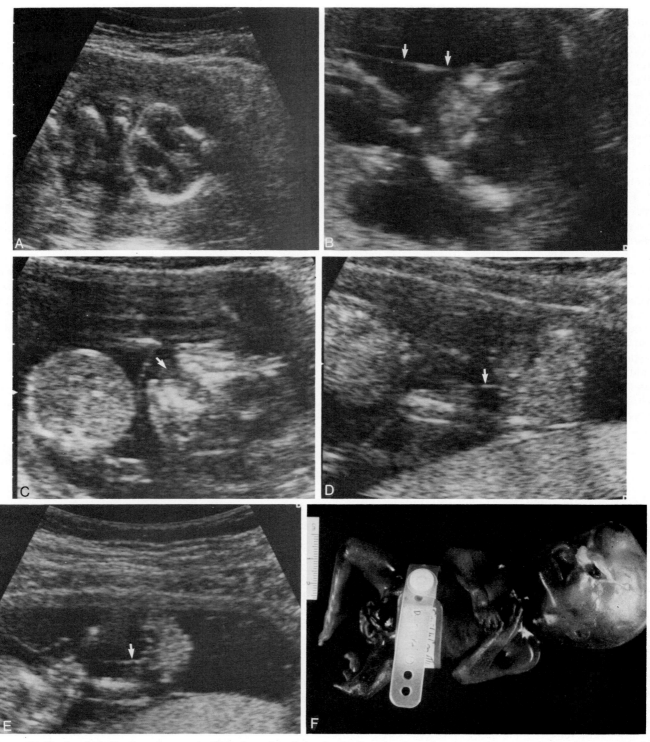

Figure 17–18. Amniotic band syndrome. *A.* Right frontal cephalocele. *B.* Strands of amnion *(arrows)* are attached and move with the forehead. *C.* Large facial cleft *(arrow).* *D* and *E.* Amniotic bands *(arrows)* attach to the lower abdomen and disrupt it. *F.* Postnatal aspect. Observe the amputation of the left lower leg, the lower abdominal wall disruption, the facial cleft toward the left eye, and the right frontal cephalocele. (From Gonçalves LF, Jeanty P: Amniotic band syndrome. Fetus 2:6588, p 1–6, 1992.)

the amniotic fluid. They have been reported in patients who had instrumentation of the uterine cavity resulting in intrauterine scars or adhesions. Randel and colleagues[91] hypothesize that the "adhesions resulting from such instrumentation and stretching across the endometrial cavity could cause the amnion and chorion to grow around the scar."[91] The membrane is thick, with two layers of amnion and two layers of chorion. It has a free edge and does not attach to the fetus, so the fetus can move independently of the membrane. The fetus is morphologically normal.

Short umbilical cord syndrome (limb–body wall complex) refers to a complex set of disruptive abnormalities having in common the failure of closure of the ventral body wall. Although some of the features are similar from those of the amniotic band syndrome, there are distinctive characteristics: marked scoliosis, evisceration of abdominal contents into the extraembryonic coelom, and a shortened umbilical cord.[92]

Recurrence Risk

Most of the cases are sporadic, with no recurrence in siblings or children of affected adults.[48] However, there are some reports of amniotic band syndrome among families with collagen disorders, more specifically Ehler-Danlos syndrome.[51]

Prognosis

The prognosis varies depending on the associated anomalies. It can be quite good for infants with only minor constriction rings and lymphedema of the digits. Children with amputations of the limbs may require reconstructive plastic surgery and prosthesis. Good results have been reported in the literature using Ombredanne's two-stage operation or serial excision and repair with Z-plasties.[93, 94] There is normal life expectancy in these cases. The severe forms of the syndrome with multiple associated anomalies are fatal.[48, 58]

Management

The prenatal management of amniotic band syndrome will depend largely on the type and extent of malformations. Minor and isolated constriction rings are unlikely to be diagnosed prenatally. The same is not true for the fetuses affected with multiple congenital abnormalities, which is sometimes incompatible with life. Hence, the approach to counseling will vary from case to case, depending on the extension of the diagnosed anomalies. For the severe forms, before viability, the option for pregnancy termination can be offered.

SHORT UMBILICAL CORD SYNDROME

Synonyms

Synonyms for this disorder include limb–body wall complex, cyllosomas, and body stalk anomaly.

Definition

Short umbilical cord syndrome refers to a complex set of disruptive abnormalities having in common the failure of closure of the ventral body wall. The disorder is characterized by a short or absent umbilical cord and disruption of the lateral body wall, spine, limbs, face, and cranium, isolated or in combination.[95, 96]

Prevalence

The prevalence of short umbilical cord syndrome is unknown.

Pathogenesis

It is hypothesized that alterations in blood flow lead to disruption and incomplete development of embryonic tissue due to hemorrhagic necrosis and anoxia during the fourth through sixth week of development. A large spectrum of defects would result from vascular damage to the developing embryo and are associated with adhesion to the amnion and persistence of the extraembryonic coelom.[97]

Diagnosis

The most common defects are a short or absent umbilical cord, scoliosis (77%) (Fig. 17–19), and lateral thoracoabdominoschisis (three times more frequent on the left side) (64%) (Fig. 17–20). Limb abnormalities are very common and include clubfoot, oligodactyly, arthrogryposis, decreased muscle mass, absence of limbs, single forearm or lower leg bone, pseudosyndactyly, split hand and foot, radial and ulnar hypoplasia, rotational defects, and preaxial polydactyly (Fig. 17–21). Midfacial clefts associated with encephalocele, exencephaly, and holocranium occur in 40%. Because of the large body wall defects, gross evisceration of the heart, liver, bowel, and other viscera occurs. Amniotic bands can be present in 40% of the cases as a consequence of early vascular disruption.[65] α-Fetoprotein levels are markedly elevated, and the karyotype is normal.[68, 69]

The association of these malformations usually results in a grotesque mass composed of membranes and organs that, in addition to the oligohydramnios, may be very hard to evaluate sonographically. Amnioinfusion can be a helpful diagnostic tool in these cases.

Differential Diagnosis

The main differential diagnoses are amniotic band syndrome, omphalocele, and gastroschisis.

Prognosis

The condition is fatal.

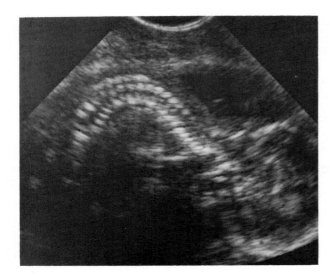

Figure 17–19. Severe scoliosis in a fetus with the short umbilical cord syndrome (limb–body wall complex).

Figure 17–20. Short umbilical cord syndrome. Sagittal scan of the fetal thorax, abdomen, and pelvis demonstrating thoracoabdominal wall disruption with herniation of the abdominal contents and heart. Observe the complete loss of anatomic landmarks in this condition.

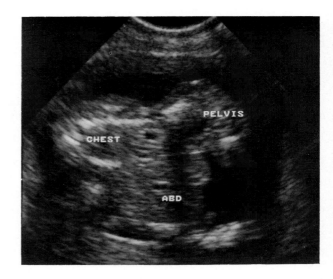

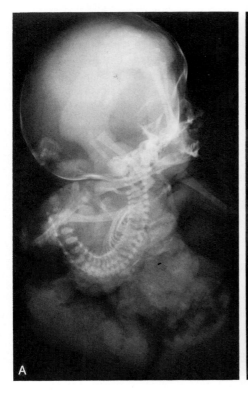

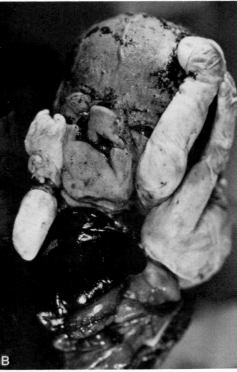

Figure 17–21. Short umbilical cord syndrome. *A.* Postnatal radiograph demonstrating massive disarrangement of the fetal structures. Observe the severe scoliosis, the bizarre displacement of the limbs toward the cranium, and the evisceration of the abdominal and thoracic structures. *B.* Postnatal aspect.

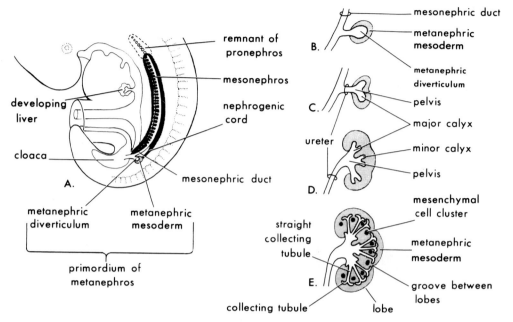

Figure 18–2. *A.* Sketch of a lateral view of a 5-week embryo, showing the primordium of the metanephros or permanent kidney. *B* through *E.* Sketches showing successive stages in the development of the metanephric diverticulum or ureteric bud (fifth to eighth weeks) into the ureter, renal pelvis, calyces, and collecting tubules. The renal lobes, shown in *E* are still visible in the kidneys of the neonates. (From Moore KL [ed]: The Developing Human: Clinically Oriented Embryology, 4th ed. Philadelphia, WB Saunders, 1988.)

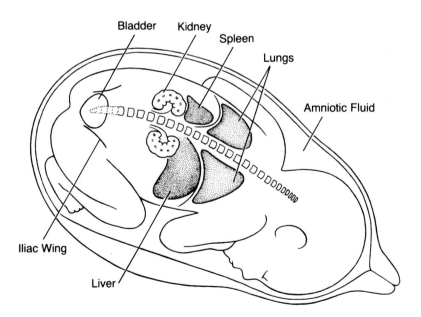

Figure 18–3. Normal renal function permits adequate amniotic fluid volume and normal lung development. The normal kidney spans four to five vertebrae in length, even in utero, when its proportions approximate those of the adult.

Table 18–1. AMNIOTIC FLUID INDEX VALUES (mm) CORRELATED WITH MENSTRUAL AGE IN NORMAL PREGNANCIES

	Amniotic Fluid Index Percentile Values				
Week	2.5th	5th	50th	95th	97.5th
16	73	79	121	185	201
17	77	83	127	194	211
18	80	87	133	202	220
19	83	90	137	207	225
20	86	93	141	212	230
21	88	95	143	214	233
22	89	97	145	216	235
23	90	98	146	218	237
24	90	98	147	219	238
25	89	97	147	221	240
26	89	97	147	223	242
27	85	95	146	226	245
28	86	94	146	228	249
29	84	92	145	231	254
30	82	90	145	234	258
31	79	88	144	238	263
32	77	86	144	242	269
33	74	83	143	245	274
34	72	81	142	248	278
35	70	79	140	249	279
36	68	77	138	249	279
37	66	75	135	244	275
38	65	73	132	239	269
39	64	72	127	226	255
40	63	71	123	214	240
41	63	70	116	194	216
42	63	69	110	175	192

Modified from Moore TR, Cayle JE: The amniotic fluid index in normal human pregnancy. Am J Obstet Gynecol 162:1168, 1990.

becomes apparent.[13] The hypoechoic fetal renal pyramids orient in anterior and posterior rows, in a configuration corresponding to the calyces around the central sinus (Fig. 18–5). The relative hypoechoic intensity of the renal pyramids contrasts to the echotexture of the normal fetal renal cortex, which usually approximates or may even be slightly greater than that of the surrounding tissues. Identification of the characteristic configuration of the pyramids in anterior and posterior rows permits positive identification of the kidney and avoids any potential confusion between renal pyramids and parenchymal cysts.

Standard measurements for renal circumference, volume, thickness, width, and length have been reported as a function of menstrual age (Table 18–2).[14–17] These measurements increase throughout gestation and correspond with those of renal size obtained on stillborn fetuses postnatally. Renal length and anteroposterior diameter represent the technically easiest measurements of renal size to obtain. A good rule of thumb is that the menstrual age in weeks approximates the normal fetal kidney length in millimeters or twice the anteroposterior diameter in millimeters. Significant deviation from this pattern enables antenatal detection of renal enlargement. Diminution in renal size may be more difficult to detect because the exact renal border may be hard to discern.

Nondilated fetal ureters are not routinely visualized. However, sonography readily identifies a dilated ureter. A useful guideline in identification of the fetal urinary tract and differentiation between it and other abdominal structures is the following: an abdominal structure or mass that touches the fetal spine most likely originates within the retroperitoneal urinary tract. This rule holds true in correct identification of ureters, kidneys, and abnormal perirenal masses (urinomas). One should beware of the normal hypoechoic psoas muscle that touches the spine and may occasionally mimic a distended ureter. Observation of its characteristic location and triangular configuration should avoid any confusion with a distended ureter.

Shortly after the commencement of fetal urine production, on ultrasound evaluation fluid can be seen within the fetal urinary bladder. The normal bladder has a very thin or virtually invisible wall and occupies an anterior midline position within the fetal pelvis. When distended, the urinary bladder becomes spherical or elliptical. Changes in volume over time differentiate the urinary bladder from other cystic pelvic structures. Visualization of filling and emptying of the fetal bladder confirms that the fetus produces urine but does not indicate the quality of urine produced. The internal iliac arteries course around the lateral margins of the urinary bladder on their path toward the umbilicus and assist in definitive identification of the urinary bladder (Fig. 18–6).

The nondilated urethra is difficult to detect in fe-

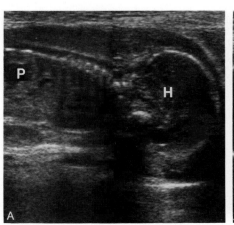
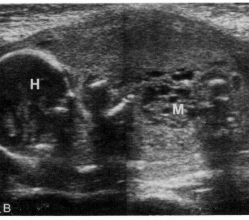

Figure 18–4. *A* and *B*. Dual longitudinal scans of the uterus in two separate pregnancies show fetal crowding and severe oligohydramnios. This should alert the sonologist to search for causes for decreased urine excretion into the amniotic cavity. One fetus had bilateral multicystic dysplastic kidneys, and the other had urethral level obstruction. H, fetal head; P, dilated renal pelvis; M, multicystic dysplastic kidney.

Figure 18–5. Transverse *(A)* and sagittal *(B)* sonograms of the fetal kidney at 37 weeks' gestation show the hypoechoic pyramids arranged in anterior and posterior rows *(arrows)*. This constitutes positive identification of the kidneys. Broad arrow indicates the spine.

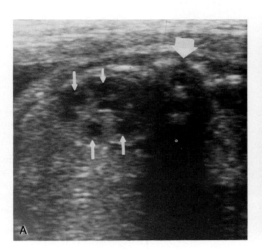
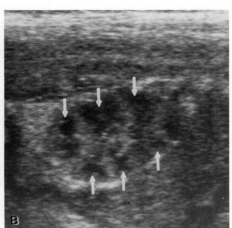

Table 18–2. NORMAL FETAL RENAL DIMENSIONS (mm) CORRELATED WITH MENSTRUAL AGE

Age (weeks)	Kidney Thickness (mm)			Kidney Width (mm)			Kidney Length (mm)			Kidney Volume (cm³)		
	5th	50th	95th	5th	50th	95th	5th	50th	95th	5th	50th	95th
16	2	6	10	6	10	13	7	13	18		0.4	2.6
17	3	7	11	6	10	14	10	15	20		0.6	2.8
18	4	8	12	6	10	14	12	17	22		0.7	2.9
19	5	9	13	7	10	14	14	19	24		0.9	3.1
20	6	10	13	7	11	15	15	21	26		1.1	3.3
21	6	10	14	8	12	15	17	22	28		1.4	3.6
22	7	11	15	8	12	16	19	24	29		1.7	3.9
23	8	12	16	9	13	17	21	26	31		2.1	4.3
24	9	13	17	10	14	18	22	28	33	0.3	2.5	4.7
25	10	14	18	11	15	19	24	29	34	0.8	3.0	5.2
26	11	15	19	12	16	19	25	31	36	1.3	3.5	5.7
27	11	15	19	12	16	20	27	32	37	1.9	4.1	6.3
28	12	16	20	13	17	21	28	33	38	2.5	4.7	6.9
29	13	17	21	14	18	22	29	35	40	3.2	5.4	7.6
30	14	18	22	15	19	23	31	36	41	3.9	6.1	8.3
31	14	18	22	16	20	24	32	37	42	4.6	6.8	9.0
32	15	19	23	17	20	24	33	38	43	5.4	7.5	9.7
33	16	20	23	17	21	25	34	39	44	6.1	8.3	10.5
34	16	20	24	18	22	26	35	40	45	6.8	9.0	11.2
35	17	21	25	18	22	26	35	41	46	7.4	9.6	11.8
36	17	21	25	19	23	27	36	41	47	8.1	10.2	12.4
37	18	22	26	19	23	27	37	42	47	8.6	10.8	13.0
38	18	22	26	19	23	27	37	43	48	9.0	11.2	13.4
39	19	23	27	19	23	27	38	43	48	9.4	11.6	13.8
40	19	23	27	19	23	27	38	44	49	9.6	11.8	14.0

From Romero R, Pilu G, Jeanty P, et al: Prenatal Diagnosis of Congenital Anomalies. East Norwalk, CT, Appleton & Lange, 1989.

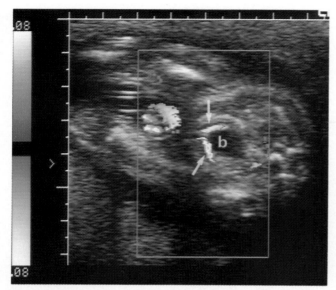

Figure 18–6. The internal iliac arteries *(arrows)* course adjacent to the urinary bladder (b) and provide convincing evidence for identification of the bladder.

Table 18–3. COMMON GENITOURINARY ABNORMALITIES EVIDENT ON PRENATAL SONOGRAMS

Absent or malformed/mispositioned kidneys
    Renal agenesis or severe hypoplasia (unilateral or bilateral)
    Crossed renal ectopia
    Pelvic kidney
    Horseshoe kidney
Abnormal urinary bladder
    Bladder or cloacal exstrophy
    Enterovesicle fistula
    Patent urachus
    Obstructed bladder (dilated, hypertrophied, dystrophic calcification)
Urinary tract dilation
    Urethral level obstruction or megacystis
    Ureterovesicle junction obstruction and megaureter
    Ureteropelvic junction obstruction
Renal cystic disease
    Multicystic dysplastic kidney disease
    Obstructive cystic renal dysplasia
    Autosomal recessive (infantile) polycystic kidney disease
    Autosomal dominant (adult) polycystic kidney disease
    Syndromes associated with renal cysts
Renal tumors
Genital and gynecologic abnormalities
    Ambiguous genitalia
    Hydrocolpos
    Ovarian cyst
    Scrotal inguinal hernia

males, and in males it is imaged at a time when the penis is flaccid but appears as an echogenic line extending the length of an erect penis. After 20 menstrual weeks, the pulsating dorsal arteries of the penis can occasionally be seen. Sonography may also detect streaming of urine into the amniotic fluid during voiding (Fig. 18–7).

URINARY TRACT ABNORMALITIES

Congenital malformations of the urinary tract occur with high frequency, probably because of the complicated embryologic development of this organ system. The sonographer plays a crucial role in the evaluation of the fetal urinary tract by detecting, localizing, and characterizing the severity of anomalies in an attempt to predict prognosis and to optimize perinatal management.[18–21] A limited range of urinary tract anomalies manifest in utero (Table 18–3).

A systematic approach to the abnormal urinary tract will most often permit accurate prenatal diagnosis and assessment of prognosis. This approach includes (1) assessment of the appropriateness of amniotic fluid volume, (2) localization and characterization of urinary tract abnormalities, and (3) search for associated abnormalities. Oligohydramnios during the second trimester, either from decreased urinary production or decreased egress of urine into the amniotic fluid, carries a very poor prognosis.[9] Conversely, normal amniotic fluid volume in the setting of a urinary tract abnormality typically signifies a good prognosis, although the urinary tract finding warrants follow-up.[22] Polyhydramnios in association with a urinary tract anomaly characteristically occurs with a mesoblastic nephroma or with associated abnormalities of the central nervous system or gastrointestinal tract.[3, 23] Occasionally and paradoxically, polyhydramnios may occur with incom-

plete obstruction at the level of the ureteropelvic junction, which presumably impairs the renal concentrating ability and leads to increased renal output.[24] Isolated mesoblastic nephroma or ureteropelvic junction obstruction has a good prognosis; the prognosis for cases with concomitant abnormalities varies depending on the associated findings.

Localization and characterization of urinary tract abnormalities often permits accurate prediction of diagnosis and, occasionally, of prognosis regarding fetal genitourinary anomalies. This assessment involves the following parameters:

1. *Are the kidneys and bladder identified?* If the kidneys are not visible in the renal fossae, are they in the pelvis or is the contralateral kidney of abnormal size or shape?

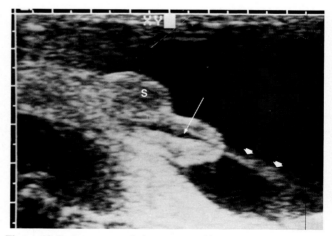

Figure 18–7. Sonogram of the scrotum (s) and penis shows fetal urination *(arrowheads)* into the amniotic fluid. u, fetal penile urethra.

2. *Is the urinary tract dilated?* If so, to what degree and what portions are dilated?

3. *Are renal cysts present or are the kidneys abnormally echogenic?*

4. *Are the genitourinary abnormalities unilateral or bilateral, and are they symmetric or asymmetric?*

Unilateral disease occurs at or proximal to the ureteral bud and has a good prognosis. Bilateral but asymmetric disease implies either involvement at the level of the cloaca (urethral level) or asymmetric ureteral bud abnormality with obstruction or reflux. Bilateral symmetric disease often heralds a genetic abnormality (autosomal recessive polycystic kidney disease) or other severe abnormalities involving both ureteral bud systems (bilateral multicystic dysplastic kidney or renal agenesis).

Prenatal detection of a genitourinary anomaly may indicate the presence of concomitant abnormalities, a syndrome, or chromosome abnormality and warrants a search for associated anomalies. As examples, bilateral renal cystic disease with encephalocele indicates the presence of the Meckel-Gruber syndrome and a 25% autosomal recessive recurrence risk,[25] renal cysts in a short-limbed dwarf with a small thorax strongly suggests the presence of asphyxiating thoracic dysplasia (Jeune syndrome),[26] and renal anomalies may herald the presence of the VACTERL association (*v*ertebral, *a*nal, *c*ardiac, *t*rachoesophageal, *r*enal and *l*imb) abnormalities.

Absent Visualization of Kidneys

Absence of visualization of one or both kidneys (not secondary to inopportune fetal positioning) most commonly signifies the presence of bilateral renal agenesis or severe hypoplasia, pelvic kidney, unilateral renal agenesis, or crossed fused ectopia.[27]

BILATERAL RENAL AGENESIS OR SEVERE HYPOPLASIA

Absence of ureteral bud formation occurs in approximately 1 in 4000 births and causes bilateral renal agenesis and death from pulmonary hypoplasia.[28, 29] The lack of urine production results in severe oligohydramnios and absence of a demonstrable urinary bladder, the only constant sonographic features of this uniformly fatal entity (Fig. 18–8). A small midline urachal diverticulum may mimic the bladder, but its lack of filling and emptying distinguishes it from the bladder. Identification of a normal bladder excludes this diagnosis. Nonvisualization of the bladder is more significant than apparent visualization of the kidneys because, in renal agenesis, the adrenal glands may assume an oval or reniform shape or bowel in the renal fossae may simulate kidneys (Fig. 18–9).[30, 31] The most reliable feature that discriminates a kidney from bowel or an adrenal gland is identification of hypoechoic medullary pyramids. Bilateral severe renal hypoplasia exhibits a similar clinical course and similar sonographic features to that of renal agenesis, although the small kidneys may be identified.

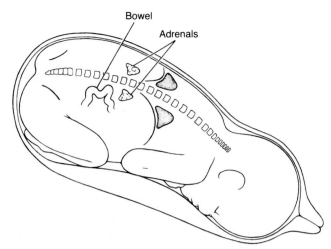

Figure 18–8. Bilateral renal agenesis or severe hypoplasia results in severe oligohydramnios, pulmonary hypoplasia, Potter facies, and contractures. Bowel or adrenals in the renal fossa should not be mistaken for kidneys.

Although the fetal kidneys begin to produce urine after the 10th week of gestation, they do not become a major source of urine production until the 14th to 16th week. Oligohydramnios may occur in pregnancies with bilateral renal agenesis as early as the 14th week of gestation, but a normal amount of amniotic fluid at 10 to 14 weeks of gestation does not exclude the diagnosis of bilateral renal agenesis.[3]

Bilateral renal agenesis correlates with an increased incidence of numerous concomitant fetal anomalies involving the cardiovascular (14%) and musculoskeletal (40%, especially sirenomelia) systems.[32] Central nervous system and gastrointestinal anomalies have also been reported. Ten percent of cases with multicystic dysplastic kidney have the lethal combination of contralateral renal agenesis.

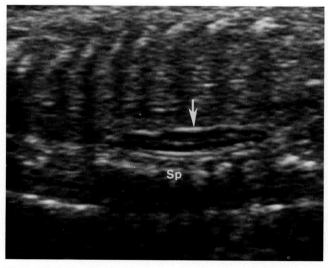

Figure 18–9. In the absence of a kidney in the renal fossa, the adrenal gland *(arrow)* may assume an oval or elongated shape and should not be mistaken for a kidney. Bowel within the renal fossa may also mimic the kidney. Sp, fetal spine on this parasagittal scan of the renal fossa.

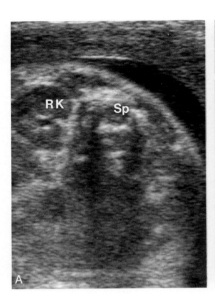
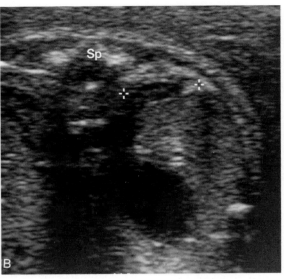

Figure 18–10. *A.* In this fetus with unilateral renal agenesis, the transverse scan at the level of the lumbar spine shows the right kidney (RK) but not the left kidney. *B.* A transverse scan slightly higher shows the left adrenal gland *(cursors)* within the left renal fossa. Sp, spine.

UNILATERAL RENAL AGENESIS

The incidence of unilateral renal agenesis has not been definitively determined, but it probably occurs 4 to 20 times more commonly than does bilateral renal agenesis.[29] It may be a difficult diagnosis to confirm prenatally because the adrenal or bowel in the renal fossa may simulate the kidney, but newer ultrasound technology often permits accurate diagnosis.[27] Unlike bilateral renal agenesis, fetuses with unilateral renal agenesis would be expected to have a normal amount of amniotic fluid, fill their bladder normally, and have a good prognosis (Fig. 18–10). The contralateral kidney tends to be abnormally large because of compensatory hypertrophy.[27] This entity may also be associated with concomitant genitourinary anomalies.[33]

CROSSED RENAL ECTOPIA, PELVIC KIDNEY, AND HORSESHOE KIDNEY

Crossed renal ectopia occurs in approximately 1 in 7000 births and may mimic unilateral renal agenesis on the prenatal sonogram.[34] The ectopic kidney in crossed fused ectopia is abnormally large and bilobed. Renal ectopia may result in obstructive uropathy or reflux and may occur in conjunction with other cardiovascular or gastrointestinal abnormalities.

Pelvic kidney may also mimic unilateral renal agenesis, but the ectopic kidney may be identified adjacent to the bladder or iliac wing (Fig. 18–11).[35] It occurs in approximately 1 in 1200 autopsies. Pelvic kidney may be associated with concomitant skeletal, cardiovascular, gastrointestinal, and gynecologic abnormalities.

Horseshoe kidney occurs in 1 in 400 persons and results from fusion of the upper or lower poles of the kidneys between 7 and 9 weeks of gestation. Despite its prevalence, it is rarely reported prenatally, presumably because it produces subtle findings.[36, 37] The kidneys may be malrotated, and the bridge of renal tissue connecting the kidneys may be visualized. In stillborn fetuses, horseshoe kidney frequently occurs in associ-

ation with other more serious anomalies. In the absence of associated anomalies, increased morbidity after birth may result from renal calculi, infections, and hydronephrosis.

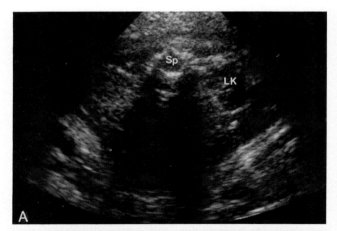
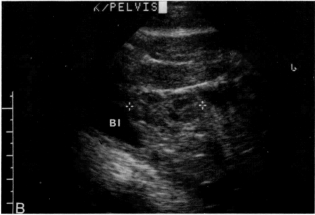

Figure 18–11. *A.* Transverse scan shows a normal left kidney (LK) but empty right renal fossa. *B.* A right pelvic kidney *(cursors)* adjacent to the bladder was confirmed with oblique scan through the right fetal pelvis. Bl, bladder; SP, spine.

The Urinary Bladder

The fetus normally fills and partially or completely empties the urinary bladder approximately every 25 minutes (range, 7 to 43 minutes) throughout gestation.[38] At 20 weeks' gestation the fetal urine production and maximum bladder volume have a mean value of 5 mL/h and 1 mL, respectively. These mean values increase with advancing gestation such that at 41 menstrual weeks the fetus produces 56 mL/h of urine and the maximum bladder volume increases to 36 mL.[38] Small-for-gestational age fetuses significantly decrease their urine production rate relative to appropriate-for-gestational age fetuses and the decreased urine production correlates with the degree of fetal hypoxemia and the degree of fetal smallness.[39, 40]

The urinary bladder is visualized in approximately 94% of fetuses after 14 menstrual weeks.[41] According to Clautice-Engle and colleagues,[41] nonvisualization of the bladder with an otherwise normal sonogram probably is not clinically significant and requires no follow-up. Conversely, nonvisualization of the urinary bladder in the setting of oligohydramnios indicates strong evidence for bilateral severe renal abnormality with decreased urine production. Therefore, if the bladder is not seen in the setting of oligohydramnios, the examination should be carried out for 60 to 90 minutes before stating its absence.

Although nonvisualization of the normal urinary bladder with normal amniotic fluid volume may be clinically insignificant, this constellation of findings may also occur with bladder or cloacal exstrophy as well as other abnormalities that alter the appearance of the bladder.[42–48] Bladder exstrophy results in eversion and exteriorization of the pelvic viscera on the abdominal surface (Fig. 18–12). This occurs in approximately 1 in 25,000 to 40,000 births. Cloacal exstrophy is a rarer (1 in 200,000 births) and more complex disorder in which intestinal mucosa separates two exstrophied hemibladders. Calcifications or debris within the urinary bladder may produce a confusing appearance of the bladder but constitutes strong evidence for an enterovesical fistula (Fig. 18–13).[49] A patent urachus results in complete or partial communication between the bladder and anterior abdominal wall at the umbilicus, and a urachal cyst may resemble a distended or abnormally shaped bladder (Fig. 18–14).

Urinary Tract Dilation

Dilation of the urinary tract frequently, but not necessarily, signifies obstruction.[50–53] Conversely, a fetus can have obstructive uropathy in the absence of urinary tract dilatation.[54, 55] Nevertheless, measurements of the anteroposterior diameter of the fetal renal pelvis and of the kidney and assessment of the degree of caliectasis may provide important clinical information that permits early and effective postnatal management.

A renal pelvic diameter measuring less than 5 mm occurs commonly and may be clinically insignificant, but this remains in debate (Fig. 18–15).[56] Spectral or color Doppler imaging may be useful to distinguish

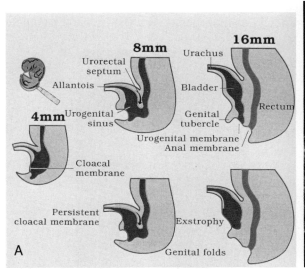

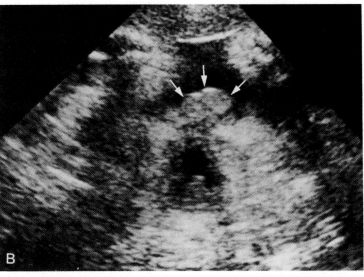

Figure 18–12. *A.* Normal embryology *(upper drawings)* and development of bladder exstrophy *(lower drawings).* In the 4-mm embryo, the entoderm tube has reached the ectoderm and the region of fusion is called the cloacal membrane. In the normal 8-mm embryo *(top),* the urorectal septum separated the hindgut posteriorly from the anterior allantois and urogenital sinus. In the embryo with bladder exstrophy *(lower drawing),* the persistent cloacal membrane prevents the normal movement of mesoderm and the genital folds meet below the membrane. In the 16-mm embryo, the separation between the bladder and rectum is complete. In the affected fetus, the anterior wall of the bladder is only composed of the persistent cloacal membrane. When it ruptures, the bladder becomes exposed. (From Erb RE, Jeanty P: Bladder exstrophy. Fetus 1:4, 1991.) *B.* Bladder exstrophy at 28 weeks' gestation showed heaped-up mucosa *(arrows)* on the anterior surface of the lower abdominal wall, presumably trapping a small amount of fluid within the exteriorized bladder. (From Nyberg DA, Mahony BS, Pretorius DH: Diagnostic Ultrasound of Fetal Anomalies: Text and Atlas. Chicago, Year Book Medical Publishers, 1990.)

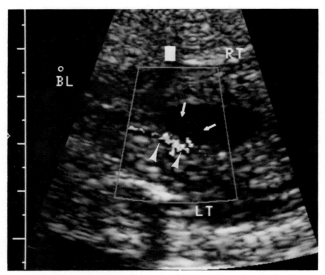

Figure 18–13. Doppler *(arrowheads)* study showed the internal iliac artery coursing adjacent to the urinary bladder in this fetus with severe oligohydramnios at 19 weeks' gestation. A small amount of low-level echogenic debris was present in the bladder *(arrow)*, and meconium was aspirated from the fetal bladder in this fetus with anal atresia and enterovesical fistula.

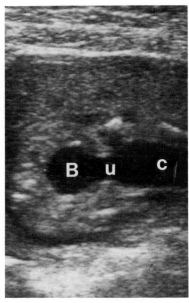

Figure 18–14. The urinary bladder (B) communicated with a patent urachus (u) and urachal cyst (c) in this fetus on this transverse sonogram of the lower abdomen.

normal hilar vessels from the renal pelvis.[57] A pelvic diameter of 5 to 9 mm and a pelvic-to-kidney diameter ratio of less than 50% in the absence of rounded calyces has been reported rarely to progress or to require postnatal management (Tables 18–4 and 18–5).[50, 51] For example, Grignon and coworkers reported that only 1 of 29 similarly affected fetuses had a mild ureteropelvic junction obstruction and did not require postnatal therapy.[51] Rounded calyces, on the other hand, have been reported to indicate significant hydronephrosis, even when the renal pelvic-to-kidney ratio is less than 50%.[24] Similarly, a renal pelvic diameter of more than 10 mm and a renal pelvic-to-kidney diameter ratio of 50% represents significant pelviectasis that rarely regresses, often progresses, and frequently requires postnatal surgical management.[51, 58, 59]

In an evaluation of 63 fetuses with pelviectasis not caused by bladder outlet obstruction, Corteville and colleagues[60] analyzed data regarding degrees of pelviectasis at different stages of gestation and reported a higher percentage of newborns requiring postnatal corrective urinary tract surgery or showing evidence of renal compromise (Tables 18–6 through 18–8).[60] For example, in Table 18–6 it shows that if only a renal pelvic anteroposterior diameter of greater than or equal to 10 mm is considered abnormal at less than 24 weeks, then 68% of fetuses with congenital hydronephrosis would be misdiagnosed but that if the threshold is decreased to 4 mm then no fetuses with congenital hydronephrosis would be missed. Similarly, Table 18–7 indicates that a ratio of the anteroposterior diameters of the renal pelvis and kidney exceeding 50% before 24 weeks would fail to detect 60% of fetuses with congenital hydronephrosis but that decreasing the threshold ratio to 28% would increase the sensitivity to 90% to 100%. Table 18–8 suggests that if the anteroposterior renal pelvic diameter measures 4 to 6

mm before 24 weeks, 41% of fetuses will have congenital hydronephrosis at birth and that the risk for clinically significant renal compromise increases to 72% to 73% if the renal pelvis measures more than 10 mm before 33 weeks and to 59% after 33 weeks.

Therefore, Corteville and colleagues[60] recommend (1) follow-up ultrasound evaluation in 3 to 4 weeks if an anteroposterior diameter of the renal pelvis is greater than or equal to 4 mm before 33 weeks or greater than or equal to 7 mm after 33 weeks and (2) postnatal follow-up after neonatal rehydration if the renal pelvic dilation persists on the prenatal examina-

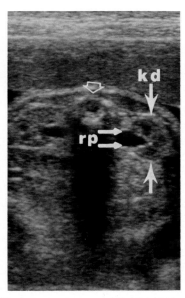

Figure 18–15. Transverse sonogram of the fetal kidneys in the third trimester shows bilateral fluid-filled renal pelves measuring 5 to 9 mm in anteroposterior diameter with a pelvic diameter/kidney diameter of less than 50%. Open arrow indicates spine. rp, renal pelvis, kd, kidney diameter.

Table 18–4. GRADING OF DEGREES OF FETAL HYDRONEPHROSIS AFTER 20 MENSTRUAL WEEKS

Grade	Size of Renal Pelvis	Calyceal Dilatation
I	<10 mm	Physiologic
II	10–15 mm	Normal calyces
III	>15 mm	Slight dilatation
IV	>15 mm	Moderate dilatation
V	>15 mm	Severe dilatation

Modified from Grignon A, Filion R, Filiatrault D, et al: Urinary tract dilatation in utero: Classification and clinical applications. Radiology 160:645–647, 1986.

Table 18–5. POSTNATAL OUTCOME OF 92 KIDNEYS WITH SUGGESTED HYDRONEPHROSIS AFTER 20 MENSTRUAL WEEKS CORRELATED WITH THE GRADE OF PELVOCALIECTASIS

Prenatal Grade	Postnatal Outcome			No. of Kidneys
	Normal	Medical Management	Surgical Management	
I	97%	3%	0	29
II	48%	13%	39%	31
III	13%	25%	62%	16
IV	0	0	100%	14
V	0	0	100%	2

Modified from Grignon A, Filion R, Filiatrault D, et al: Urinary tract dilatation in utero: Classification and clinical applications. Radiology 160:645–647, 1986.

tions. Although their recommendations would lead to a high false-positive rate (i.e., abnormal ultrasound evaluation but no congenital hydronephrosis), the thresholds would yield a high sensitivity and, therefore, minimize the number of fetuses misinterpreted as having renal pelvic dilatation.

Benacerraf and coworkers[61] report a possible association between mild fetal pelviectasis and Down syndrome. In their retrospective review of 44 fetuses with Down syndrome, 25% had mild pelviectasis (defined as renal pelvis anteroposterior diameter of 4 mm or greater at 15 to 20 weeks, 5 mm or greater between 20 and 30 weeks and 7 mm or greater between 30 and 40 weeks). During a 1-year prospective evaluation, 2.8% of all fetuses had mild pelviectasis and 7 of 210 (3.3%) fetuses with mild pelviectasis (6 to 8 mm anteroposterior diameter of the renal pelvis at 24 to 35 weeks) had Down syndrome.

When prenatal sonography demonstrates unequivocal pelvocaliectasis, a normal neonatal ultrasound evaluation in the first 48 hours after birth should not alter this assessment. Confirmation of in utero findings at 5 to 7 days post partum avoids the confusion introduced by the dehydration typically present in the first 48 hours after birth.[62] Although urinary tract dilatation may occur with reflux, nonobstructive megacystis, or megacalyces, it almost always implies an intrinsic genitourinary abnormality. Hydrocolpos or other pelvic masses (e.g., intrapelvic sacrococcygeal teratoma) represent rare causes for urinary tract obstruction and dilatation.[63]

Among fetuses with obstructive uropathy, several sonographic criteria permit assessment of fetal renal function in utero and may assist in selection of fetuses who may potentially benefit from prenatal surgery.[4] In fetuses with obstructive uropathy, detection of cortical cysts or intense cortical echogenicity indicates cystic renal dysplasia and correlates with poor renal function, but not all dysplastic kidneys have sonographically visible cysts or increased cortical echogenicity (see Table 18–6).

Physiologic means of assessing the fetal renal function require interventive procedures, most commonly through catheterization of the fetal bladder and determination of fetal urine electrolytes (Fig. 18–16). The predominant utility of measuring fetal urine electrolytes is in the exclusion of those fetuses with markedly hypertonic urine from those who might benefit from in utero diversion of a urinary tract obstruction.[65] Urinary sodium concentration less than 100 mEq/L, chloride concentration less than 90 mEq/L, and osmolarity less than 210 mOsm/L are prognostic factors reported to correlate with good postnatal renal function.[66, 67] although Elder and coworkers[68] reported five cases in which the fetal urinary electrolytes were not predictive of ultimate renal function. Evans and associates[69] suggest that a single determination of fetal urine biochemistry may be insufficient to declare the presence of irreversible renal damage and that improvement (or its lack) in urine biochemistry may be more representative of ultimate outcome. In addition, Nicolaides and colleagues[70] reported that decreasing urinary sodium values and increasing creatinine concentration with advancing gestation indicates matura-

Table 18–6. ANTEROPOSTERIOR DIAMETER OF THE FETAL RENAL PELVIS AT DIFFERENT STAGES OF GESTATION CORRELATED WITH THE RISK OF POSTNATAL CONGENITAL HYDRONEPHROSIS

Anteroposterior Pelvic Diameter (mm)	14–23 wk		24–32 wk		33–42 wk	
	Sensitivity (%)	False-Positive Rate (%)	Sensitivity (%)	False-Positive Rate (%)	Sensitivity (%)	False-Positive Rate (%)
≥4	100	55	100	42	100	24
≥7	61	35	91	34	100	21
≥10	32	18	74	14	82	18

From Corteville JE, Gray DL, Crane JP: Congenital hydronephrosis: Correlation of fetal ultrasonographic findings with infant outcome. Am J Obstet Gynecol 165:384, 1991.

Table 18–7. RATIO BETWEEN THE ANTEROPOSTERIOR DIAMETER OF THE FETAL RENAL PELVIS TO KIDNEY AT DIFFERENT STAGES OF PREGNANCY CORRELATED WITH THE RISK OF POSTNATAL CONGENITAL HYDRONEPHROSIS

Anteroposterior Diameter, Pelvis/Kidney Ratio	14–22 wk		23–32 wk		33–42 wk	
	Sensitivity (%)	*False-Positive Rate* (%)	*Sensitivity* (%)	*False-Positive Rate* (%)	*Sensitivity* (%)	*False-Positive Rate* (%)
>0.28	100	50	90	37	91	20
>0.30	92	48	88	33	84	20
>0.40	64	47	69	15	68	21
>0.50	40	47	52	8	50	15

From Corteville JE, Gray DL, Crane JP: Congenital hydronephrosis: Correlation of fetal ultrasonographic findings with infant outcome. Am J Obstet Gynecol 165:384, 1991.

tion of fetal renal function and correlates with a good prognosis.

Urethral Level Obstruction

Distal urinary tract obstruction, most commonly from posterior urethral valves, produces a variable and often insidious clinical presentation.[71] Nevertheless, antenatal diagnosis followed by prompt postnatal therapy improves the outcome in many cases, and some fetuses may benefit from in utero diversion of the obstructed urinary tract.[20, 72]

Urethral level obstruction produces a broad spectrum of sonographic features antenatally, but the cardinal signs include persistent dilatation of the urinary bladder and proximal urethra and thickening of the bladder wall (Figs. 18–17 through 18–20).[71, 73] Documentation of the dilated proximal urethra, which resembles a keyhole extending from the bladder toward the fetal perineum, constitutes convincing (but not always demonstrable) evidence of urethral obstruction.

A dilated urinary bladder fills the true pelvis (and frequently extends into the false pelvis and abdomen) and does not empty during the course of the examination. This has been reported in association with bladder outlet obstruction as early as 11 menstrual weeks.[74] Conversely, Silver and coworkers[75] report a fetus with posterior urethral valves who had a normal ultrasound evaluation at 24 menstrual weeks but a dilated bladder, oligohydramnios, and increased renal

echogenicity at 28 menstrual weeks. Rarely the dilated bladder may prolapse through the perineum (Fig. 18–21). Since the normal urinary bladder wall is almost imperceptibly thin, a pathologically thickened bladder wall has a finite thickness of more than approximately 2 mm. In fetuses with urethral obstruction but a nondilated bladder, the bladder wall characteristically thickens to 10 to 15 mm (see Fig. 18–20).

When considering the diagnosis of urethral level obstruction, the sonographer should examine the fetal perineum to determine the sex. Documentation of male external genitalia provides strong evidence that the urethral level obstruction results from posterior urethral valves. If male genitalia cannot be documented in fetuses with massive distention of the urinary bladder, one must consider caudal regression anomaly, urethral atresia, or megacystis intestinal hypoperistalsis syndrome. Each of these occurs in either gender, but the latter occurs more commonly in females. In such cases, and in fetuses with posterior urethral valves, the urethral level obstruction may dilate the bladder to the point that it distends the fetal abdomen and elevates the hemidiaphragms and may contribute to the lax abdominal musculature characteristic of the prune-belly syndrome.

Other features indicative of fetal urinary tract obstruction, such as oligohydramnios, ureterectasis, and caliectasis, assist in the diagnosis of obstructive uropathy. Their absence should not preclude the diagnosis, however, since they do not occur uniformly. Oligohydramnios occurs in approximately 50% of fetuses with

Table 18–8. ANTEROPOSTERIOR DIAMETER OF THE FETAL RENAL PELVIS AT DIFFERENT STAGES OF GESTATION CORRELATED WITH SUBSEQUENT CONGENITAL HYDRONEPHROSIS CONFIRMED POSTNATALLY AND WITH POSTNATAL URINARY TRACT CORRECTIVE SURGERY OR RENAL COMPROMISE

Anteroposterior Pelvic Diameter (mm)	14–23 wk		24–32 wk		33–42 wk	
	CH (%)	*S/C* (%)	*CH* (%)	*S/C* (%)	*CH* (%)	*S/C* (%)
<3	0	0	0	0	0	0
4–6	41	19	38	13	0	0
7–9	53	40	33	6	67	50
>10	82	73	86	72	82	59

CH, Congenital hydronephrosis confirmed postnatally; S/C, postnatal surgery and/or evidence of renal compromise.
From Corteville JE, Gray DL, Crane JP: Congenital hydronephrosis: Correlation of fetal ultrasonographic findings with infant outcome. Am J Obstet Gynecol 165:384, 1991.

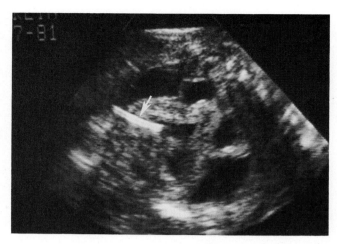

Figure 18–16. In the setting of fetal urinary tract obstruction, catheterization of the fetal bladder may decompress the bladder and provide useful information regarding renal function. Arrow indicates catheter extending into the decompressed bladder.

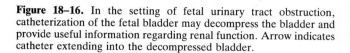
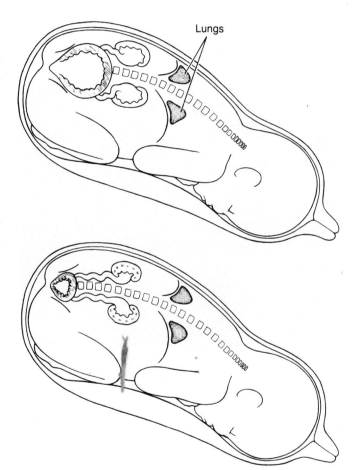

Figure 18–17. Although the sonographic features of urethral level obstruction vary, the cardinal signs include a thick-walled, dilated bladder and a dilated proximal urethra. The degree of pelvocaliectasis, ureterectasis, and megacystis varies and may be mild. Oligohydramnios, when present, leads to pulmonary hypoplasia and a poor prognosis.

Figure 18–18. Representative sonograms of urethral level obstruction. *A.* Dilated, trabeculated urinary bladder with a dilated proximal urethra. *B.* Nondilated but thick-walled bladder with severe bilateral pelvocaliectasis. Each case exhibits oligohydramnios. bl, bladder; pu, proximal urethra; t, trabeculations; p, pelvocaliectasis, S, spine.

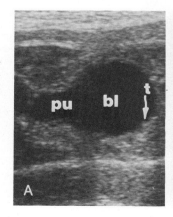
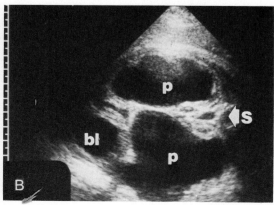

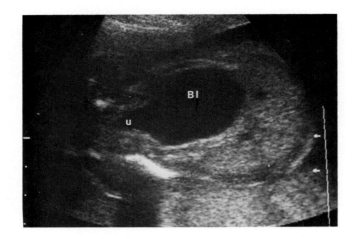

Figure 18–19. The dilated proximal urethra (u) and urinary bladder (Bl) form the shape of a keyhole characteristic of urethral level obstruction.

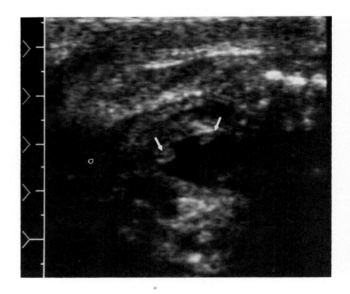

Figure 18–20. The urinary bladder in this fetus with urethral level obstruction is trabeculated *(arrows)* but not dilated.

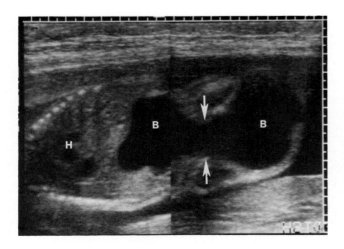

Figure 18–21. The longitudinal dual-image scan demonstrates an unusual case with dilatation of the urinary bladder and prolapse of the bladder through the perineum. Arrows indicate the expected level of the perineum. B, bladder; H, heart. (From Nyberg DA, Mahony BS, Pretorius DH: Diagnostic Ultrasound of Fetal Anomalies: Text and Atlas. Chicago, Year Book Medical Publishers, 1990.)

urethral level obstruction, whereas only 40% of affected fetuses have associated pyelocaliectasis or ureterectasis. Several observations explain the apparent discrepancy between urinary tract obstruction and absence of oligohydramnios, ureterectasis, or caliectasis. Because egress of urine from the bladder may potentially occur, except in the presence of urethral atresia, lack of oligohydramnios does not preclude the diagnosis of urethral obstruction. Caliectasis and proximal ureterectasis may be absent because urethral obstruction most prominently affects the organs most proximal to the site of obstruction (i.e., the bladder and distal ureters), probably from reflux of urine under high pressure from the hypertrophied bladder into the ureters. Furthermore, in 10% to 20% of fetuses with urethral obstruction, the urinary bladder may spontaneously decompress through rupture of the urinary tract or development of a paranephric pseudocyst.[64, 76] Finally, diminution or cessation of urine production may result from renal dysplasia caused by increased intraluminal pressure within the urinary tract during nephrogenesis.[77]

Just as absence of urinary tract dilatation does not preclude an obstructive uropathy, its presence does not necessarily imply obstruction. In a rare case of massive vesicoureteral reflux without obstruction, for example, the bladder may appear persistently dilated because it empties but rapidly refills with refluxed urine.[53] Nevertheless, even in the absence of one or two of the cardinal signs of urethral level obstruction, the sonographer can frequently diagnose fetal urethral obstruction confidently, especially in the presence of a constellation of findings including oligohydramnios and evidence of spontaneous urinary tract decompression (perirenal urinoma, urinary ascites, or dystrophic peritoneal calcification). Often, these associated features dominate the sonographic findings, and occasionally one must resort to percutaneous antegrade pyelography to confirm the diagnosis (Table 18–9).

Oligohydramnios represents a poor prognostic sign in urethral obstruction, probably because it leads to pulmonary hypoplasia.[78] Approximately 95% of fetuses with urethral level obstruction and oligohydramnios will not survive the neonatal period.[71] Conversely, one may predict a good prognosis for fetuses with obstructive uropathy but with a normal amount of amniotic fluid.[22] Other sonographic signs, such as lack of caliectasis or a large amount of ascites and dystrophic calcifications, also indicate a poor prognosis.[71] Lack of caliectasis in the absence of urinary tract decompres-

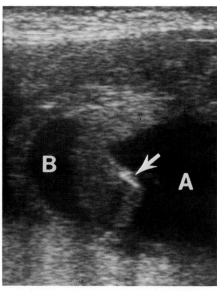

Figure 18–22. Fetal urinary ascites (A) and fluid within the bladder (B) delineate the thickened bladder wall with a focus of dystrophic calcification *(arrow)* at the site of prior bladder perforation in this fetus with urethral level obstruction. (From Mahony BS, Callen PW, Filly RA: Fetal urethral obstruction: US evaluation. Radiology 157:221–224, 1985.)

sion suggests the presence of renal dysplasia, resulting in diminution of urine production. A large amount of urinary ascites from spontaneous urinary tract decompression is also a poor prognostic indicator, perhaps secondary to elevation of the fetal diaphragms, which may contribute to the pulmonary hypoplasia. Occasionally, the sonographer may detect dystrophic bladder wall calcification at the site of bladder perforation; this finding also correlates with a poor prognosis for survival beyond the neonatal period, probably because it indicates previous high pressure within the urinary tract that may lead to dysplasia (Fig. 18–22).

In urethral level obstruction, oligohydramnios probably represents the overriding feature that indicates a poor prognosis, as it does in any circumstance, especially during the second trimester of pregnancy. The absence of caliectasis or the presence of a large amount of ascites or dystrophic calcification lends corroborative evidence for a poor prognosis.

Ureterovesical Junction Obstruction

Duplication of the renal collecting system occurs in up to 4% of the population and represents the most common major genitourinary anomaly (Fig. 18–23).[79, 80] In ureteral duplication, presumably from anomalous initial division of the ureteral bud, the upper pole moiety characteristically obstructs, whereas the lower pole moiety refluxes (Fig. 18–24). Because prenatal detection of hydronephrosis of the upper pole of a duplex collecting system permits the use of prophylactic antibiotics initiated at birth and continued until surgical correction, this decreases the proportion of affected neonates who subsequently present with urinary tract infection and urosepsis.[81]

Table 18–9. OBSTRUCTIVE UROPATHY: MANIFESTATIONS THAT MAY DOMINATE THE PICTURE IN UTERO

Oligohydramnios
Cystic dysplasia
Urinary tract rupture
    Urinary ascites—small, moderate, large
    Paranephric urinoma
    Dystrophic calcification
Massively dilated bladder
Pelvocaliectasis/ureterectasis

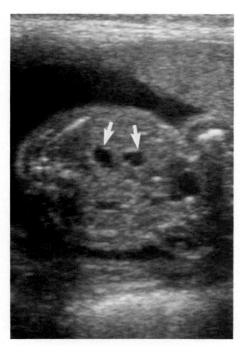

Figure 18–23. The fetal kidney at 25 weeks' gestation is abnormally elongated (4.3 cm) with duplication of mildly dilated renal pelvis and collecting structures *(arrows)* but no other focal mass effect or cortical echotectural abnormality.

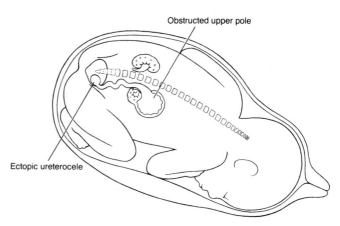

Figure 18–24. An ectopic ureterocele typically produces an obstructed upper pole moiety.

Documentation of the dilated upper pole moiety with a normal lower pole intrarenal collecting system represents the key feature that permits accurate sonographic diagnosis of an obstructed duplex collecting system (Figs. 18–25 through 18–27). The dilated upper renal pole moiety may enlarge to the point that it displaces the nondilated lower pole of the kidney inferiorly and laterally. The associated thin-walled and fluid-filled ectopic ureterocele within the bladder may be very difficult to detect in utero, as is visualization of two distant ureters and collecting systems. Often, however, the dilated ureter (either from reflux or from obstruction) presents as a serpentine fluid-filled structure that may mimic bowel. Documentation that the structure touches the fetal spine, originates from the renal pelvis, and extends into a retrovesicular position

without debris distinguishes a dilated ureter from fluid-filled bowel. Ectopic ureterocele occurs bilaterally in approximately 15% of cases. The amniotic fluid volume should be appropriate unless the obstruction is severe bilaterally.

Unlike ureterectasis associated with a duplex collecting system, which frequently requires postnatal surgery, primary megaureter represents a benign congenital anomaly that typically requires no therapy (Fig. 18–28).[82] Localized dysfunction of the distal ureter produces predominant distal ureteral dilatation not associated with obstruction, reflux, or bladder dysfunction. Proximal dilatation of the renal collecting structures occurs only rarely. Documentation that the dilated ureter arises symmetrically from the kidney should avoid confusion between this entity and the more common duplex collecting system.

Ureteropelvic Junction Obstruction

Obstruction frequently occurs at the level of the ureteropelvic junction, the site of the first bifurcation of the ureteral bud (Figs. 18–29 and 18–30). This represents the most common cause of neonatal hydronephrosis.[83] Since 85% to 90% of affected neonates

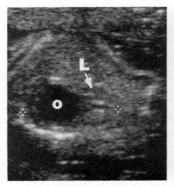
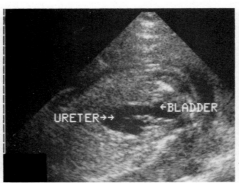
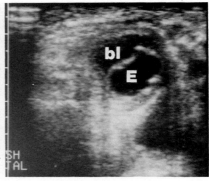

Figure 18–25. Representative scans show an ectopic ureterocele within the bladder and ureterectasis leading to the obstructed upper pole moiety. Note that the obstructed upper pole resembles a solitary cyst, but its thick rind is continuous with and displaces the parenchyma of the lower pole inferiorly. The ureterocele and ureterectasis frequently are not evident. bl, bladder; E, ectopic ureterocele; o, obstructed upper pole moiety; L, displaced lower pole moiety. (Courtesy of Jack H. Hirsch, M.D., Swedish Hospital Medical Center, Seattle, WA.)

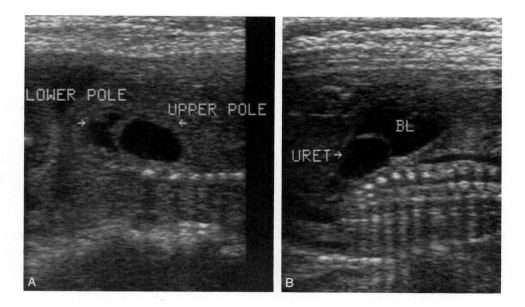

Figure 18–26. *A* and *B*. A moderately dilated upper pole moiety and an ectopic ureterocele (URET) within the urinary bladder (BL) were identified in this fetus, but the ureter was not dilated at the time of the examination.

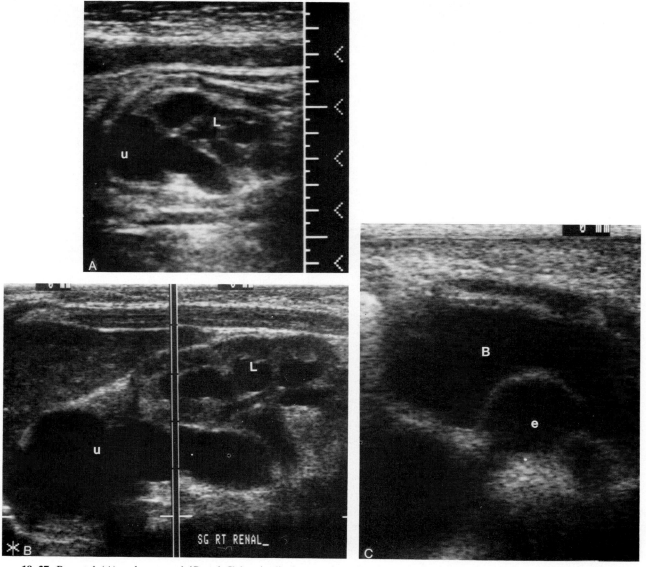

Figure 18–27. Prenatal *(A)* and postnatal *(B* and *C)* longitudinal scans show the characteristic features of a duplex collecting system with a severely dilated upper pole moiety (u) that displaces a moderately dilated lower pole (L) moiety inferiorly. Postnatal scans showed the ectopic ureterocele (e) within the bladder (B). (From Nyberg DA, Mahony BS, Pretorius DH: Diagnostic Ultrasound of Fetal Anomalies: Text and Atlas. Chicago, Year Book Medical Publishers, 1990.)

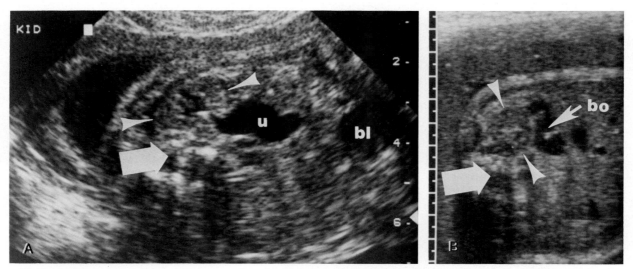

Figure 18–28. *A,* Primary megaureter at 26 menstrual weeks shows a normal-sized bladder with no dilatation of the distal ureter but with fusiform dilatation of the ureter proximally. There is no pelvocaliectasis, and the amniotic fluid volume is normal. *B.* A fluid-filled segment of bowel should not be confused with a dilated ureter. Unlike the ureter, bowel typically does not touch the fetal spine, cannot be traced to the renal pelvis, and frequently coexists with polyhydramnios. Arrowheads indicate the kidney, and the wide arrow indicates the spine. bl, bladder; u, ureter; bo, bowel.

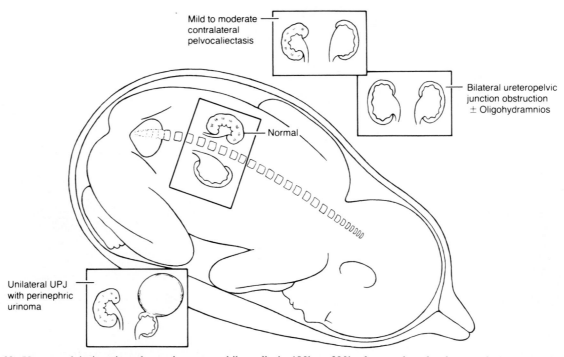

Figure 18–29. Ureteropelvic junction obstruction occurs bilaterally in 10% to 30% of cases, but the degree of obstruction is usually not symmetric. If severe, it can cause extreme thinning of the renal parenchyma, or the kidney may rupture, resulting in a urinoma.

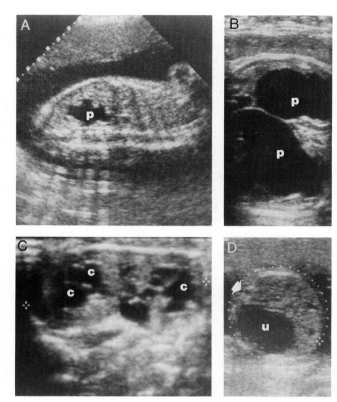

Figure 18–30. The degree of dilatation in ureteropelvic junction obstruction varies. In *A* there is moderate unilateral pelvocaliectasis, but in *B* only a thin rim of tissue surrounds the markedly dilated renal pelves bilaterally. Occasionally, stenosis of the pelves and infundibula *(C)* produces dilatation predominantly of the calyces. Urinary tract obstruction may lead to rupture and formation of a perinephric urinoma *(D)*, a unilocular paraspinous fluid-filled mass. Arrow indicates the spine. p, renal pelves; c, calyces; u, urinoma.

may appear entirely normal on physical examination, prenatal detection of ureteropelvic junction obstruction permits early therapy of a correctable lesion that may otherwise remain unrecognized for years.[84]

In unilateral ureteropelvic junction obstruction, the renal pelvis, infundibula, and calyces are dilated, and the pelvic-to-kidney diameter ratio is greater than 50% (Fig. 18–31). In more severe cases of ureteropelvic junction obstruction, one visualizes only a single fluid-filled structure representing the dilated renal pelvis with a thin rim of surrounding parenchyma. In dramatic cases, the renal pelvis may dilate to create a giant abdominal cyst without recognizable parenchyma. It may distend the abdomen and compress the thorax.[85] In ureteropelvic junction obstruction, the nondilated ureters are not visible. In rare instances, the renal pelvis and infundibula may be stenotic, such that only the calyces dilate (see Fig. 18–30C).[86] The nonobstructed contralateral kidney produces a normal amount of amniotic fluid, and the urinary bladder fills and empties normally, even if the degree of obstruction causes renal dysplasia of the ipsilateral kidney. In cases with ureteropelvic junction obstruction, the degree of dilatation rarely progresses in utero and frequently exceeds that observed postnatally, presumably because of circulating maternal hormones that relax smooth muscle.[87] This discrepancy should not preclude the antenatal diagnosis.

Unilateral ureteropelvic junction obstruction may be associated with contralateral multicystic dysplasia or renal agenesis, both of which may produce profound oligohydramnios. Bilateral ureteropelvic junction obstruction occurs in 10% to 30% of cases (see Fig. 18–30B).[87] Fortunately, involvement is usually asymmetric and severe obstruction rarely occurs. Although cases with severe bilateral ureteropelvic junction obstruction may result in oligohydramnios and an empty urinary bladder, milder forms are unlikely to be fatal.[87] Ureteropelvic junction obstruction may paradoxically result in polyhydramnios in up to 25% of cases.[87] Visualization of a paranephric urinoma from rupture of the collecting system correlates with severe obstruction and a low probability of residual renal function (Fig. 18–32). A paranephric urinoma appears as a large unilocular cystic flank mass that touches the fetal spine.[76]

Renal Cysts

Most fetuses with renal cysts have either multicystic dysplastic kidney disease (Potter type II) or obstructive uropathy resulting in renal cystic dysplasia (Potter type IV). However, numerous other syndromes and diseases may also produce renal cysts.[88] Therefore, detection of renal cysts warrants careful search for associated anom-

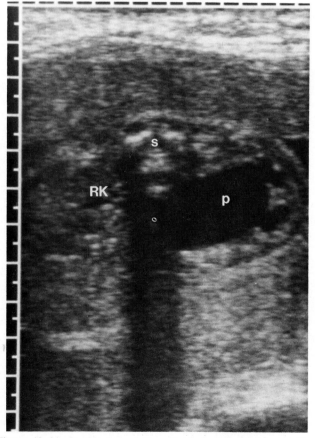

Figure 18–31. In this fetus with unilateral ureteropelvic junction obstruction the left renal pelvis (p) measures approximately 2.2 cm in anteroposterior diameter and the calyces are rounded. The right kidney (RK) is normal on this transverse image. S, spine.

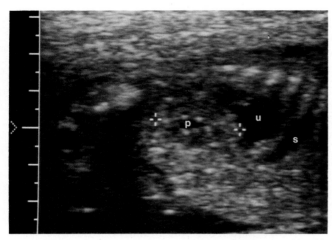

Figure 18–32. The renal pelvis (p) is only minimally dilated in this fetus following formation of a small urinoma (u) extending partially around the upper pole of the left kidney inferior to the stomach (s). Other scans showed a normal adrenal gland. Cursors indicate kidney.

alies, especially in the absence of features indicative of urinary tract obstruction.

Renal dysplasia results from anomalous differentiation of metanephric tissue and implies irreversible renal damage.[89, 90] The functional capacity of an affected kidney depends on the extent and severity of the dysplasia. Disorganized epithelial structures and abundant fibrous tissue characterize renal dysplasia histologically; cortical cysts frequently, but not necessarily, occur in renal dysplasia and represent the key feature to search for sonographically.

Approximately 90% of dysplastic kidneys result from urinary tract obstruction during nephrogenesis. The severity of obstruction as well as the patterns of dysplasia correspond with the site of obstruction.[90] Bernstein classifies renal dysplasia into four major groups: (1) multicystic dysplasia, usually caused by ureteropelvic atresia; (2) focal and segmental cystic dysplasia, typically resulting from obstruction or atresia of one of the ureters leading from a duplex kidney; (3) cystic dysplasia associated with nonatretic urinary tract obstruction, most commonly from posterior urethral valves; and (4) heredofamilial cystic dysplasia.[89] Only the relatively uncommon heredofamilial cystic dysplasia results from nonobstructive causes.

MULTICYSTIC DYSPLASTIC KIDNEY

Multicystic dysplastic kidney (MCDK) disease probably occurs during embryogenesis, resulting from atresia of the ureteral bud system at the level of the upper third of the ureter, with concomitant atresia of the renal pelvis and infundibula. Rarely, segmental atresia of the proximal third of the ureter without atresia of the renal pelvis and infundibula produces the hydronephrotic type of MCDK.[91] Ureteral atresia of a duplex kidney causes segmental MCDK involving the collecting system supplied by the atretic ureter.[92] The ureteral atresia in MCDK prevents the metanephric blastema from inducing formation of nephrons, such that an MCDK characteristically has no normal renal paren-

chyma proximal to the atretic ureter. The collecting tubules distributed randomly throughout the anomalous kidney become cystically enlarged to variable degrees, without macroscopic intercommunications. Since the drastic reduction in nephron formation is seldom absolute, an MCDK may exhibit some (usually very minimal) residual urine formation. For practical purposes, however, an MCDK represents a functionless kidney.[93]

The sonographic appearance of an MCDK correlates well with the pathologic appearance (Figs. 18–33 and 18–34).[94] The renal pelvis and the ureter are usually atretic and not visible. Occasionally, however, the renal pelvis may be dilated in cases with isolated ureteral atresia. Multicystic dysplasia typically visualizes as a paraspinous flank mass, characterized by numerous cysts of variable sizes without identifiable communication or anatomic arrangement (Figs. 18–35 and 18–36). The large cysts frequently distort the contour of the mass, and no normal renal parenchyma exists. Any tissue resembling possible renal parenchyma localizes as small islands of echogenic material interspersed between these cysts.

An MCDK may change markedly in size and appearance as gestation progresses.[93] The MCDK and its cysts may undergo progressive enlargement or diminution or may initially enlarge, then decrease later in pregnancy. Minimal residual capacity for glomerular filtration explains this variable appearance of the MCDK. As progressive fibrosis of nephrons occurs, the MCDK ceases to grow and then involutes.

Once the sonographer has confirmed the diagnosis of MCDK, assessment of the contralateral kidney assumes primary importance, since the MCDK produces little filtrate and no urine that reaches the amniotic fluid. Contralateral renal anomalies occur in approximately 40% of fetuses with an MCDK.[95] If overlying fetal parts obscure the contralateral renal region, an appropriate amount of amniotic fluid and normal emptying and filling of the fetal urinary bladder imply normal contralateral renal function. Profound oligohydramnios and absence of fetal urinary bladder filling, on the other hand, imply lethal fetal renal disease, which occurs in 30% of fetuses with an MCDK, from either bilateral multicystic dysplasia (20%) or contralateral renal agenesis (10%). Oligohydramnios may occur with bilateral MCKD as early as 12 menstrual weeks, even before the renal abnormalities are evident.[96] Typical multicystic flank masses are usually readily visible after approximately 16 menstrual weeks in MCKD. When only a unilateral MCDK is visible, the sonographer can infer the diagnosis of contralateral renal agenesis or severe hypoplasia in the setting of profound oligohydramnios with absence of urinary bladder filling. Approximately 10% of patients with a unilateral MCDK have contralateral hydronephrosis, usually from obstruction at the ureteropelvic junction. In such cases, the degree of obstruction determines the amount of amniotic fluid, since the obstructed kidney is the only potentially functional one. For this reason, one must obtain close follow-up of the contralateral kidney to watch for progression of

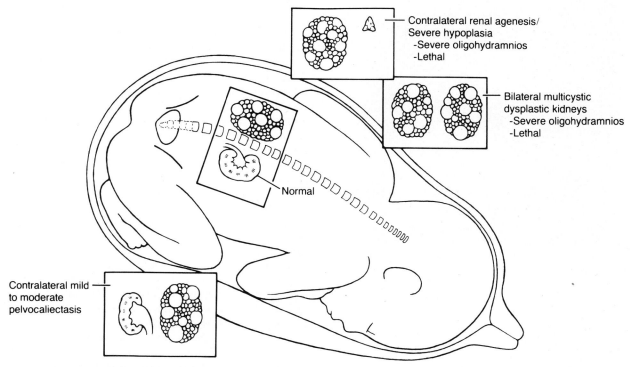

Figure 18–33. The multicystic dysplastic kidney is essentially nonfunctional. Attention must be focused on the contralateral kidney since it is the only potentially functional kidney.

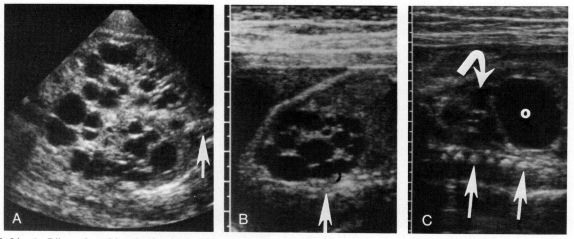

Figure 18–34. *A*. Bilateral multicystic dysplastic kidneys cause profound oligohydramnios and multiple cysts of varying sizes without demonstrable communication or anatomic arrangement. This is a lethal entity. *B*. Unilateral disease with a normal amount of amniotic fluid presumes a functioning contralateral kidney that must be followed closely. In this case, the renal contour is relatively preserved. *C*. Segmental disease occurs with atresia of one of the ureters leading from a duplex kidney. Straight arrows indicate spine, and curved arrow indicates multicystic dysplastic lower pole of duplex kidney. o, obstructed upper pole moiety.

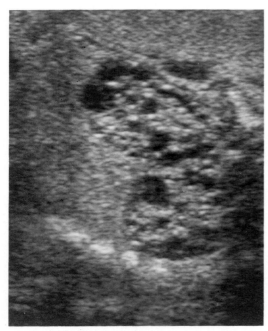

Figure 18–35. Numerous small bilateral cysts mixed with several larger cysts and no normal renal parenchyma in the setting of anhydramnios indicate bilateral multicystic dysplastic kidneys.

dilatation or diminution of amniotic fluid that might necessitate interventive measures. Minimal contralateral renal pelvic distention occurs with approximately the same frequency as in fetuses without an MCDK and usually lacks clinical significance.[95]

Since MCDK and hydronephrosis constitute the two most common causes of a neonatal (and presumably fetal) abdominal mass and because their potential function and perinatal management differ dramatically, distinction between these two entities is critical.[97] In cases with mild pelvocaliectasis or a typical MCDK, this distinction is elementary. Differentiation between the atypical cases of the hydronephrotic form of MCDK and cases of hydronephrosis with predominant caliceal dilatation, but without multicystic dysplasia, may be much more difficult.[86, 98] The latter maintains the reniform contour, with renal parenchyma arranged at the periphery of the dilated calyces that are of uniform size, communicate with each other centrally, and align in anterior and posterior rows.

OBSTRUCTIVE CYSTIC RENAL DYSPLASIA

Experiments in fetal lambs demonstrate that urethral obstruction in the first half of gestation produces renal dysplasia.[77, 99] The dysplasia associated with urinary tract obstruction represents irreversible renal damage that probably results from elevated pressures within the developing nephron system.[90] In humans, cystic renal dysplasia occurs most frequently with urethral level obstruction but may also occur with obstruction at the level of the ureteropelvic junction (Fig. 18–37). Although the severity of renal dysplasia varies, extensive renal dysplasia correlates with drastically reduced renal functional capacity. For this reason, sonographic

detection of cystic renal dysplasia in a fetus with urinary tract obstruction provides useful prognostic information regarding renal function.

Among fetal kidneys with obstructive uropathy, sonographic demonstration of cortical cysts effectively indicates the presence of cystic renal dysplasia as early as 21 menstrual weeks (Fig. 18–38).[64] Since not all dysplastic kidneys have cysts or the cysts may be smaller than sonographic resolution capabilities, one cannot accurately predict the absence of dysplasia when cortical cysts are not visible. Dysplastic kidneys tend to exhibit greatly increased echogenicity relative to surrounding fetal structures, presumably from the abundant fibrous tissue (Fig. 18–39). Assessment of renal echogenicity is quite subjective, however, and not all echogenic kidneys are dysplastic. Furthermore, one cannot predict the absence of dysplasia with normal renal echogenicity in obstructive uropathy; therefore, it offers only limited predictive value for dysplasia.[64, 100] Aspiration and catheter measurement of fetal urine provide corroborative quantitative information about fetal renal function. One can predict a poor prognosis for a fetus with bilateral obstructive uropathy and decreased output of isotonic urine.[65–70]

Just as the differentiation between MCDK and hydronephrosis may be difficult, the distinction between an MCDK and cystic renal dysplasia associated with urinary tract obstruction (but not urethral atresia) may also be difficult, especially in the absence of hydronephrosis. As delineated previously, however, documentation of one of several of the cardinal signs of urethral level obstruction (the most common cause of cystic renal dysplasia) assists in this distinction. Furthermore, in MCDK, only small islands of tissue localize between predominant cysts, whereas in cystic dysplasia from urinary tract obstruction, recognizable parenchyma surrounds the relatively small cysts. In addition, cystic dysplasia from distal urinary tract obstruction frequently involves both kidneys but bilateral MCDK disease occurs in only 20% of cases. Obstruction at the

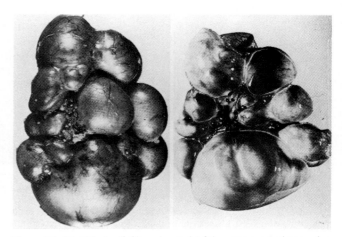

Figure 18–36. Whole *(left)* and cut *(right)* autopsy specimen of a multicystic dysplastic kidney demonstrate the absence of normal renal parenchyma and numerous variably sized cysts without detectable intercommunication. (From Zerres K, Volpel M-C, Weif H: Cystic kidneys: Genetics, pathologic anatomy, clinical picture and prenatal diagnosis. Hum Genet 68:104, 1984.)

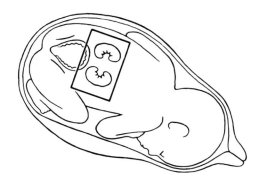

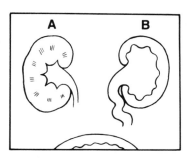

A. Normal
B. Thinned, normal
   echogenicity:
   no cysts

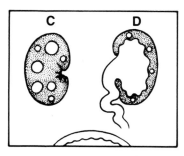

C. Increased
   echogenicity with
   cysts — dysplasia
D. Thinned, increased
   echogenicity with
   cysts — dysplasia

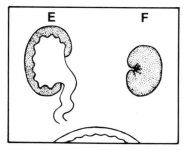

E. Thinned, increased
   echogenicity:
   no cysts—probable
   dysplasia
F. Small, increased
   echogenicity:
   no cysts—probable
   dysplasia

Figure 18–37. Urinary tract obstruction produces a varied response from the kidneys. *A.* The kidney may remain normal in urethral obstruction, without reflux. *B.* Pelvocaliectasis may attenuate the parenchymal thickness. *C.* The kidney may suffer cystic dysplasia (parenchymal cysts), become fibrotic (increased echogenicity), and cease to function (lack of pelvocaliectasis). *D.* Alternatively, it may undergo cystic dysplasia with parenchymal cysts and increased echogenicity but continue to have pelvocaliectasis and a thinned parenchyma. If no cysts are visible, but the parenchyma is of greatly increased echogenicity, either with *(E)* or without *(F)* pelvocaliectasis, dysplasia is probably, but not invariably, present.

Figure 18–38. *A* and *B.* Urethral level obstruction with renal dysplasia shows severe oligohydramnios, a massively dilated bladder (BL) with a mildly thick-walled bladder wall *(open arrows)*, and a distended proximal urethra *(arrow)*, as well as dilated ureters (u). The kidney *(black arrows)* is intensely echogenic without dilatation. (From Mahony BS, Callen PW, Filly RA: Fetal urethral obstruction: US evaluation. Radiology 157:221–224, 1985.)

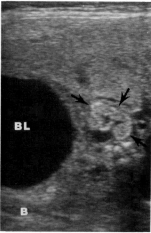

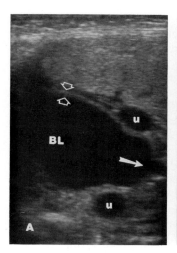

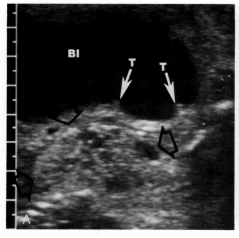

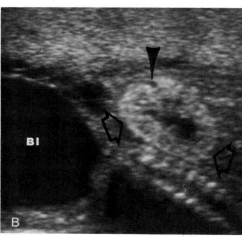

Figure 18–39. *A* and *B.* This case of urethral level obstruction produced bilateral renal cysts indicative of cystic dysplasia and irreversible damage. The number of parenchymal cysts in each kidney varies markedly. Greatly increased renal echogenicity provides corroborative but nondiagnostic information regarding dysplasia. Open arrows indicate kidneys, and arrowhead indicates parenchymal cyst (the contralateral kidney has numerous parenchymal cysts). T, trabeculations of bladder wall; Bl, bladder.

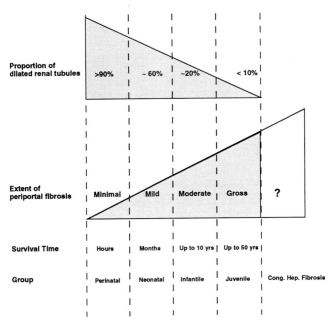

Proportion of dilated renal tubules	>90%	~ 60%	~20%	< 10%	
Extent of periportal fibrosis	Minimal	Mild	Moderate	Gross	?
Survival Time	Hours	Months	Up to 10 yrs	Up to 50 yrs	
Group	Perinatal	Neonatal	Infantile	Juvenile	Cong. Hep. Fibrosis

Figure 18–40. The manifestations of autosomal recessive polycystic kidney disease vary markedly from severe early renal disease with minimal hepatic fibrosis but early death to minimal renal disease with marked hepatic fibrosis and longer survival. (From Zerres K, Volpel M-C, Weif H: Cystic kidneys: Genetics, pathologic anatomy, clinical picture and prenatal diagnosis. Hum Genet 68:104, 1984.)

level of the ureteropelvic junction may result in cystic renal dysplasia that would typically be unilateral.[64, 87] The distinction between MCDK disease and cystic dysplasia from urinary tract obstruction, although helpful in terms of diagnosis, may be somewhat artificial in terms of prognosis, since in either case, the affected kidney typically maintains only minimal functional capacity.

Autosomal Recessive (Infantile) Polycystic Kidney Disease. Bilateral medullary ectasia, producing innumerable 1- to 2-mm cysts of nonobstructive renal collecting tubules, occurs in autosomal recessive (infantile) polycystic kidney disease.[5] Although this entity may be visible pathologically as early as 48 to 50 days of gestation, it expresses variably, depending on the degree of renal involvement,[101–103] the severity of which correlates inversely with proliferation of bile ducts and hepatic fibrosis (Fig. 18–40.) Severely affected fetuses and neonates have a very high mortality rate, usually from pulmonary hypoplasia secondary to oligohydramnios from diminished renal function.

The diagnosis of autosomal recessive (infantile) polycystic kidney disease can be made as early as 16 menstrual weeks on the basis of oligohydramnios and characteristic renal abnormalities seen on the prenatal sonogram, especially when the sonogram is performed because of a familial risk for the disorder (Figs. 18–41 and 18–42). This entity typically causes bilaterally enlarged fetal kidneys that maintain their reniform shape but exhibit increased echogenicity. Early in pregnancy, the renal cortex may appear echogenic, whereas the medullae appear echopenic. Later in pregnancy, the pattern reverses, and a peripheral rim of hypoechoic renal cortex surrounds the echogenic me-

dullae. Diminished renal function usually produces nondilated renal pelves, ureters, and bladder, with a decreased amount of amniotic fluid. Although the numerous tiny cysts are usually smaller than the limit of sonographic resolution, the multiple interfaces produced by these cysts result in the characteristic diffusely increased renal echogenicity. Newer technology now often permits visualization of innumerable 1- to 2-mm cysts scattered throughout symmetrically enlarged kidneys. The enlarged kidneys may lead to dystocia.[102]

When bilaterally enlarged and very echogenic kidneys occur in a fetus at risk for autosomal recessive (infantile) polycystic kidney disease, one can strongly suspect the diagnosis of recurrence. However, biologic variability of this disease may prevent accurate diagnosis in all cases, and a normal sonogram of a fetus at risk for autosomal recessive (infantile) polycystic kidney disease does not ensure absence of this genetic disease.[102–104] Usually, but not always, the sonogram shows evidence for recurrence by approximately 24 menstrual weeks. In the absence of a genetic risk for this entity, sonographic visualization of enlarged fetal kidneys most likely indicates autosomal recessive polycystic kidney disease. Other very rare possibilities that the sonographer could conceivably confuse with autosomal recessive polycystic kidney disease include bilateral renal tumors, medullary sponge kidney, bilateral nephroblastomatosis, Finnish nephrosis, medullary cystic disease, or congenital metabolic diseases (i.e., glycogen storage disease or tyrosinosis).[105, 106] Oligohydramnios and absence of urine within the urinary bladder would favor autosomal recessive (infantile) polycystic kidney disease over all of these other rare entities.

Autosomal Dominant (Adult) Polycystic Kidney Disease. Although autosomal dominant (adult) polycystic kidney disease has been reported as early as the end of the second trimester of pregnancy, the kidneys may be normal in appearance in the mid second trimester and become abnormal on serial examinations.[3] The disease may be suspected when cystic and echogenic fetal kidneys but normal amniotic fluid occur in a pregnancy when there is a family history of the

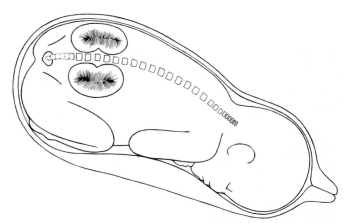

Figure 18–41. Autosomal recessive (infantile) polycystic kidney disease produces enlarged, echogenic kidneys, often with oligohydramnios.

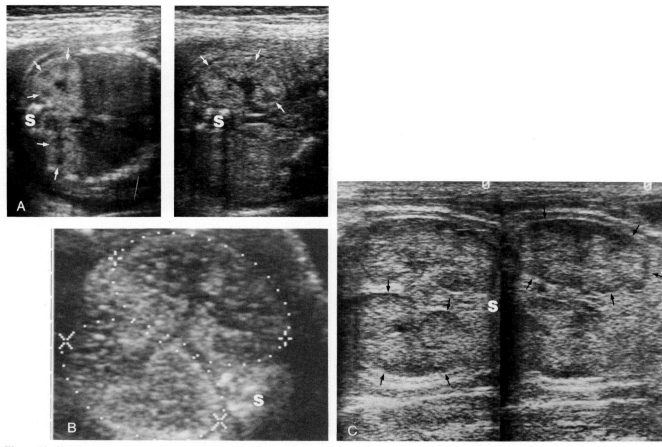

Figure 18–42. These sonograms demonstrate the variable appearance of autosomal recessive polycystic kidney disease in utero. *A.* Typically, the kidneys are enlarged and echogenic. *B.* Technology occasionally permits visualization of the numerous 1- to 2-mm cysts as early as 16 menstrual weeks. *C.* Later in pregnancy, a peripheral sonolucent rim may become evident. Small arrows or dotted outlines indicate kidneys. S, spine.

disorder. Chorionic villus sampling using a highly polymorphic probe genetically linked to the locus of the mutant gene for adult polycystic kidney disease has been reported in prenatal diagnosis.

HEREDOFAMILIAL CYSTIC DYSPLASIA

Numerous additional rare inherited syndromes may produce cystic dysplasia from nonobstructive causes (Table 18–10).[89] Detection of the multiple renal cysts with the features associated with each syndrome, especially in the setting of familial risk for recurrence, permits confident prenatal diagnosis (Fig. 18–43). Meckel-Gruber syndrome, for example, is a fatal entity that recurs in an autosomal recessive manner (25% recurrence risk for subsequent pregnancies). Characteristic features, the presence of at least two of which enables definitive diagnosis, include (1) bilateral nonobstructive MCDK disease (95% of cases), (2) occipital encephalocele (80% of cases), and (3) postaxial polydactyly (75% of cases).[25, 107] In a fetus with a familial risk for Meckel-Gruber syndrome, the sonographer must focus on these regions to search for recurrence. Conversely, detection of an occipital encephalocele or of multiple bilateral cysts in the absence of a positive family history mandates careful search for other features indicative of the syndrome.

Jeune syndrome (asphyxiating thoracic dystrophy) or short-rib polydactyly syndrome may also manifest prenatally with nonobstructive cystic renal dysplasia (see Chapter 13 on ultrasound evaluation of the fetal musculoskeletal system). Visualization of multiple

Table 18–10. REPRESENTATIVE SYNDROMES ASSOCIATED WITH FETAL CYSTIC KIDNEYS

Syndrome	Frequency of Renal Cystic Involvement
Meckel syndrome	Nearly always
Ivemar syndrome	Always
Retinal-renal dysplasia syndromes	Always
Asphyxiating thoracic dysplasia	Frequent
Zellweger syndrome	Frequent
Ehlers-Danlos syndrome	Frequent
Laurence-Moon-Bardet-Biedl syndrome	Frequent
Kaufman-McKusick syndrome	Frequent
Von Hippel-Lindau syndrome	Frequent
Fryns syndrome	Frequent
Branchio-oto-renal syndrome	Frequent
VACTERL association	50%
Trisomy 13	33%
Trisomy 18	10%

Modified from Zerres K, Volpel M-C, Weif H: Cystic kidneys: Genetics, pathologic anatomy, clinical picture and prenatal diagnosis. Hum Genet 68:104, 1984.

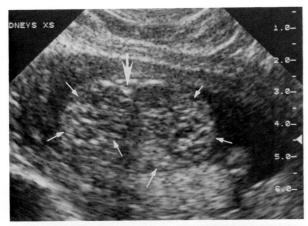

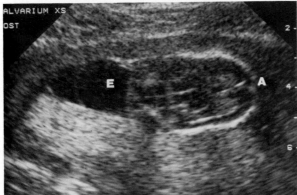

Figure 18–43. Multiple small renal cysts in conjunction with an encephalocele imply Meckel-Gruber syndrome. Small arrows indicate kidneys; large arrow indicates spine, E, encephalocele; A, anterior. (Courtesy of Robert A. Schor, MD, Swedish Hospital Medical Center, Seattle, WA.)

renal cysts in a fetus with a familial risk for Jeune syndrome or short-rib polydactyly syndrome and with shortened extremities, a noticeably small thorax, and polydactyly provides convincing evidence for recurrence.

Renal cysts may also indicate the presence of a severe chromosome abnormality. Approximately 33% of fetuses with trisomy 13 and 10% of fetuses with trisomy 18 have renal cysts. Affected fetuses often have additional anatomic abnormalities. Therefore, detection of renal cysts, especially in the absence of urinary tract obstruction, warrants a careful search for associated anomalies suggestive of trisomy and consideration for prenatal karyotyping.

Renal Tumors

Congenital renal tumors occur only rarely. Mesoblastic nephroma represents the most common congenital renal neoplasm (Figs. 18–44 and 18–45).[21] It is a solitary hamartoma with a usually benign course. Although rare reports of recurrence after nephrectomy exist, curative therapy usually consists of nephrectomy alone. Prenatal detection of a mesoblastic nephroma, therefore, should not necessitate preterm delivery.

Nevertheless mesoblastic nephroma frequently coexists with polyhydramnios, which may contribute to premature labor. The reason for a clear association between mesoblastic nephroma and polyhydramnios remains unclear.

Mesoblastic nephroma visualizes as a large, solitary, predominantly solid, retroperitoneal mass arising from and not separable from adjacent normal kidney. It does not have a well-defined capsule and may contain cystic areas. Its predominantly solid texture distinguishes mesoblastic nephroma from an unusual case of ureteropelvic junction obstruction with polyhydramnios. Although its sonographic appearance resembles a Wilms tumor, the age of presentation provides an important differentiating factor. Whereas mesoblastic nephroma is the most common congenital renal neoplasm, Wilms tumor is exceptionally rare in the neonate. Identification of a predominantly solid fetal renal mass in the presence of polyhydramnios provides convincing evidence for a mesoblastic nephroma.

FETAL GENDER

Determination of fetal gender is by no means a trivial matter. Attempts to document fetal gender in utero serve numerous purposes, especially during the second trimester of pregnancy.[108] Gender determination among fetuses at risk for severe X-linked disorders assumes paramount importance since unequivocal identification of a female fetus excludes the possibility of the disorder. Documentation of different genders in twin pregnancy permits accurate assessment of dizygosity, which precludes the possibility of twin transfusion syndrome, cord entanglement, or conjoined twins.[109] It also confirms that both sacs have been sampled in amniocentesis. In cases with discrepant sonographic and amniocentesis data, sonography may detect an intersex state. Even without amniocentesis data, careful analysis of the fetal perineum may detect ambiguous genitalia (Fig. 18–46). Furthermore, whether verbalized or not, determination of fetal gender constitutes one of the prime expectations the parents have during their sonogram. The physician's duty of full disclosure and the parent's right to know may create a complicated ethical and moral problem.[108]

Accurate sonographic assessment of fetal gender requires adequate perineal visualization to permit unequivocal distinction between the labia and scrotum. Only documentation of testicles within the scrotum provides 100% reliability in gender assessment, but this is not possible in utero until 28 to 34 menstrual weeks.[110] Unfortunately, inopportune fetal positioning precludes perineal visualization in approximately 30% of fetuses, especially before 24 menstrual weeks.[108, 110] Even after adequate perineal visualization, sonography incorrectly assigns fetal gender in approximately 3% of cases.[108] The sonographer should bear in mind this small but definite error rate and avoid using sonography as the sole method for gender determination.

Antenatal sonography usually visualizes the ovaries, uterus, and vagina only when these organs enlarge and

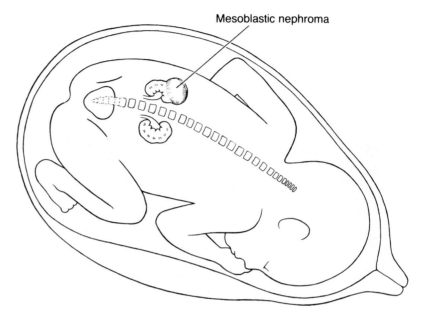

Figure 18–44. A mesoblastic nephroma is a solitary, predominantly solid, benign renal tumor associated with polyhydramnios.

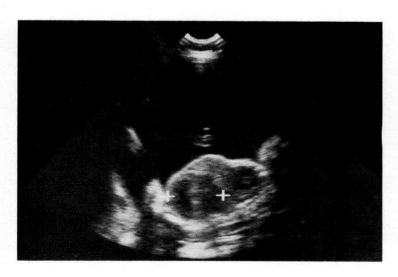

Figure 18–45. Mesoblastic nephroma creates a large solid renal mass *(cursors)* in this fetus at 34 weeks' gestation with polyhydramnios. (From Guilian BB: Prenatal ultrasonographic diagnosis of fetal renal tumors. Radiology 152:69, 1984.)

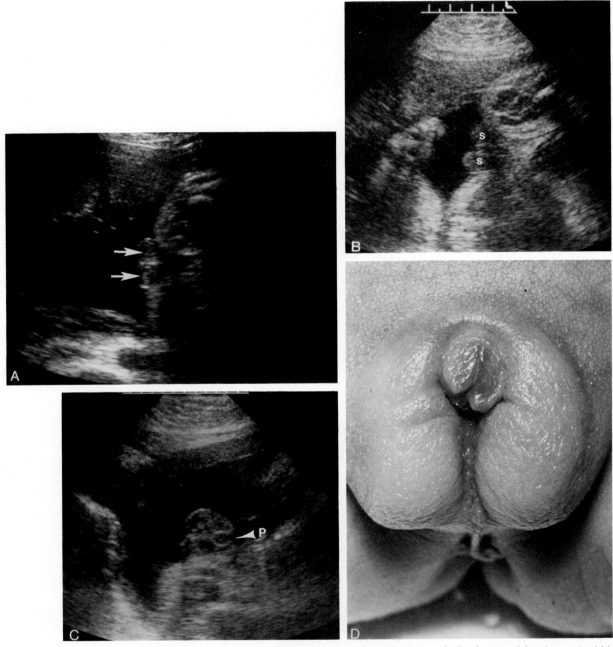

Figure 18–46. *A* through *C.* Sonograms of the perineum of this male fetus with ambiguous genitalia show testicles *(arrows)* within bifid scrotum (s) with phallus (P) resembling clitoris. *D.* The postnatal photograph illustrates the prenatal findings of the genotypic male.

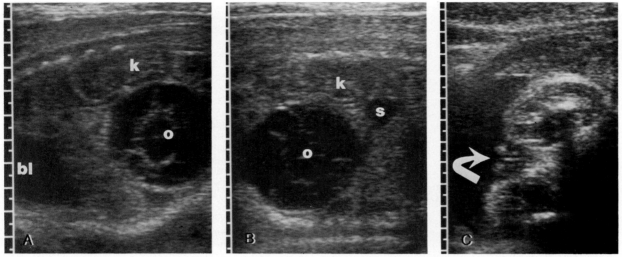

Figure 18–47. *A* through *C*. Visualization of a multiseptated lower abdominal mass separate from the kidneys (k), bladder (bl) and stomach (s) in a female fetus provides strong evidence of an enlarged ovarian cyst. Curved arrow indicates labia. o, ovary.

produce a pelvic mass. Hydrometrocolpos, for example, produces a hypoechoic mass posterior to the bladder, extending to the abdomen in female fetuses with vaginal obstruction.[63] In approximately 55% of patients, the hydrometrocolpos compresses the urinary tract and causes hydronephrosis or hydroureter.[63] Ovarian cysts, on the other hand, typically do not compress the urinary tract but may obstruct the small bowel.[111, 112] Documentation that the ovarian cyst is separate from the normal urinary tract assists in the diagnosis but does not differentiate it from an enteric duplication, a mesenteric cyst, or a urachal cyst. However, duplication cysts tend to be more tubular and urachal cysts extend to the umbilicus. In a female fetus, a multiseptated intra-abdominal cystic mass strongly suggests ovarian cysts, especially if bilateral (Fig. 18–47). Fetal ovarian cysts probably result from maternal hormonal stimulation and are characteristically benign but may be associated with hypothyroidism.[111] Furthermore, large but benign ovarian cysts may cause dystocia and require prompt perinatal surgical management, since they may lead to torsion, rupture, or intestinal obstruction.[113]

References

1. American Institute of Ultrasound in Medicine: Guidelines for performance of the Antepartum Obstetrical Ultrasound Examination, 1991. J Ultrasound Med 10:577, 1991.
2. American College of Obstetricians and Gynecologists: Technical Bulletin No. 116. Washington, DC, May 1988.
3. Grannum PA: The genitourinary tract. In Nyberg DA, Mahony BS, Pretorius DH (eds): Diagnostic Ultrasound of Fetal Anomalies: Text and Atlas. Chicago, Year Book Medical Publishers, 1990.
4. Moore KL: The urinary system. In: The Developing Human: Clinically Oriented Embryology, 4th ed. Philadelphia, WB Saunders, 1988.
5. Mellins HZ: Cystic dilatations of the upper urinary tract: A radiologist's development model. Radiology 153:291, 1984.
6. Abramovich DR: The volume of amniotic fluid and its regulating factors. In Fairweather DVI, Eskes TKA (eds): Amniotic Fluid Research and Clinical Application, 2nd ed, pp 31–49. Amsterdam, Excerpta Medica, 1978.
7. Hill LM: Abnormalities of amniotic fluid. In Nyberg DA, Mahony BS, Pretorius DH (eds): Diagnostic Ultrasound of Fetal Anomalies: Text and Atlas. Chicago, Year Book Medical Publishers, 1990.
8. Moore TR, Cayle JE: The amniotic fluid index in normal human pregnancy. Am J Obstet Gynecol 162:1168, 1990.
9. Barss VA, Benacerraf BR, Frigoletto FD: Second trimester oligohydramnios, a predictor of poor fetal outcome. Obstet Gynecol 64:608, 1984.
10. Bronshtein M, Kushnir O, Ben-Rafael Z, et al: Transvaginal sonographic measurement of fetal kidneys in the first trimester of pregnancy. J Clin Ultrasound 18:299, 1990.
11. Lawson TL, Foley WD, Berland LL, et al: Ultrasonic evaluation of fetal kidneys: Analysis of normal size and frequency of visualization as related to stage of pregnancy. Radiology 138:153, 1981.
12. Patriquin H, Lefaivre J-F, Lafortune M, et al: Fetal lobation: An anatomo-ultrasonographic correlation. J Ultrasound Med 9:191, 1990.
13. Bowie JD, Rosenberg ER, Andreotti MD, et al: The changing sonographic appearance of fetal kidneys during pregnancy. J Ultrasound Med 2:505, 1983.
14. Bertagnoli L, Lalatta F, Gallicchio MD, et al: Quantitative characterization of the growth of the fetal kidney. J Clin Ultrasound 11:349, 1983.
15. Cohen HL, Cooper J, Eisenberg P, et al: Normal length of fetal kidneys: Sonographic study in 397 obstetric patients. AJR 157:545, 1991.
16. Romero R, Pilu G, Jeanty P, et al: Prenatal Diagnosis of Congenital Anomalies. East Norwalk, CT, Appleton & Lange, 1989.
17. Sampaio FJB, Aranao AHM: Study of the fetal kidney length growth during the second and third trimester of gestation. Eur Urol 17:62, 1990.
18. Mandell J, Blyth BR, Peters CA, et al: Structural genitourinary defects detected in utero. Radiology 178:193, 1991.
19. Callan NA, Blakemore K, Park J, et al: Fetal genitourinary tract anomalies: Evaluation, operative correction and follow-up. Obstet Gynecol 75:67, 1990.
20. Schwoebel MG, Sacher P, Bucher HU, et al: Prenatal diagnosis improves the prognosis in children with obstructive uropathy. J Pediatr Surg 19:187, 1984.
21. Guys JM, Borella F, Monfort G: Ureteropelvic junction obstructions: Prenatal diagnosis and neonatal surgery in 47 cases. J Pediatr Surg 23:156, 1988.
22. Hellstrom WJG, Kogan BA, Jeffrey RB, et al: The natural history of prenatal hydronephrosis with normal amounts of amniotic fluid. J Urol 132:947, 1984.

23. Guilian BB: Prenatal ultrasonographic diagnosis of fetal renal tumors. Radiology 152:69, 1984.

24. Giersson RT, Ricketts NEM, Taylor DJ, et al: Prenatal appearance of a mesoblastic nephroma associated with polyhydramnios. J Clin Ultrasound 12:488, 1985.

25. Nyberg DA, Hallesy D, Mahony BS, et al: Meckel-Gruber syndrome: Importance of prenatal diagnosis. J Ultrasound Med 9:691, 1990.

26. Mahony BS: The Extremities. In Nyberg DA, Mahony BS, Pretorius DH (eds): Diagnostic Ultrasound of Fetal Anomalies: Text and Atlas. Chicago, Year Book Medical Publishers, 1990.

27. Jeanty P, Romero R, Kepple D, et al: Prenatal diagnoses in unilateral empty renal fossa. J Ultrasound Med 9:651, 1990.

28. Dubbins PA, Kurtz AB, Wapner RJ, et al: Renal agenesis: Spectrum of in utero findings. J Clin Ultrasound 9:189, 1981.

29. Romero R, Cullen M, Crannum P, et al: Antenatal diagnosis of renal anomalies with ultrasound: III. Bilateral renal agenesis. Am J Obstet Gynecol 151:38, 1985.

30. Krebs CA, Adcock D: Postnatal sonographic evaluation of bilateral renal agenesis with filling of the renal fossa by the adrenal glands. J Diagn Med Sonogr 1:43, 1990.

31. Austin CW, Brown JM, Friday RO: Unilateral renal agenesis presenting as a pseudomass in utero. J Ultrasound Med 3:177, 1984.

32. Wilson RD, Baird PA: Renal agenesis in British Columbia. Am J Med Genet 21:153, 1985.

33. Trigaux J-P, Van Beers B, Belchambre F: Male genital tract malformations associated with ipsilateral renal agenesis: Sonographic findings. J Clin Ultrasound 19:3, 1991.

34. Greenblatt AM, Beretsky I, Lankin DH, et al: In utero diagnosis of crossed renal ectopia using high-resolution real-time ultrasound. J Ultrasound Med 4:105, 1985.

35. Hill LM, Peterson CS: Antenatal diagnosis of fetal pelvic kidneys. J Ultrasound Med 6:393, 1987.

36. King KL, Kofinas AD, Simon NV, et al: Antenatal ultrasound diagnosis of fetal horseshoe kidney. J Ultrasound Med 10:643, 1991.

37. Sherer DM, Cullen JBH, Thompson HO, et al: Prenatal sonographic findings associated with a fetal horseshoe kidney. J Ultrasound Med 9:477, 1990.

38. Rabinowitz R, Peters MT, Vya S, et al: Measurement of fetal urine production in normal pregnancy by real-time ultrasonography. Am J Obstet Gynecol 161:1264, 1989.

39. Nicolaides KH, Peters MT, Vyas S, et al: Relation of rate of urine production to oxygen tension in small-for-gestational-age fetuses. Am J Obstet Gynecol 162:387, 1990.

40. Groome LJ, Owen J, Neely CL, et al: Oligohydramnios: Antepartum fetal urine production and intrapartum fetal distress. Am J Obstet Gynecol 165:1077, 1991.

41. Clautice-Engle T, Pretorius DH, Budorick NE: Significance of nonvisualization of the fetal urinary bladder. J Ultrasound Med 10:615, 1991.

42. Nyberg DA, Mack LA: Abdominal wall defects. In Nyberg DA, Mahony BS, Pretorius DH (eds): Diagnostic Ultrasound of Fetal Anomalies: Text and Atlas. Chicago, Year Book Medical Publishers, 1990.

43. Barth RAD, Filly RA, Sondheimer FK: Prenatal sonographic findings in bladder exstrophy. J Ultrasound Med 9:359, 1990.

44. Petrikovsky BM, Walzak MP, D'Addario PF: Fetal cloacal anomalies: Prenatal sonographic findings and differential diagnosis. Obstet Gynecol 72:464, 1988.

45. Wood BP: Cloacal malformations and exstrophy syndromes. Radiology 177:326, 1990.

46. Jaramillo D, Lebowitz RL, Hendren WH: The cloacal malformation: Radiologic findings and imaging recommendations. Radiology 177:441, 1990.

47. Hill LM, Kislak S, Belfar HL: The sonographic diagnosis of urachal cysts in utero. J Clin Ultrasound 18:434, 1990.

48. Frazier HA, Guerrieri JP, Thomas RL, et al: The detection of a patent urachus and allantoic cyst of the umbilical cord on prenatal ultrasonography. J Ultrasound Med 11:117, 1992.

49. Hill LM, Rivello D, Martin JG: Intraluminal bladder calcifications: An antenatal sign of an enterovesical fistula. Obstet Gynecol 76:500, 1990.

50. Arger PH, Coleman BG, Mintz MC, et al: Routine fetal genitourinary tract screening. Radiology 156:485, 1985.

51. Grignon A, Filion R, Filiatrault D, et al: Urinary tract dilatation in utero: Classification and clinical applications. Radiology 160:645, 1986.

52. Blane CE, Koff SA, Baverman RA, et al: Nonobstructive hydronephrosis: Sonographic recognition and therapeutic implications. Radiology 147:95, 1983.

53. Reuter KL, Lebowitz RL: Massive vesicoureteral reflux mimicking posterior urethral valves in a fetus. J Clin Ultrasound 13:584, 1985.

54. Mahony BS, Callen PW, Filly RA: Fetal urethral obstruction: US evaluation. Radiology 157:221, 1985.

55. Glazer GM, Filly RA, Callen PW: The varied sonographic appearance of the urinary tract in the fetus and newborn with urethral obstruction. Radiology 144:563, 1982.

56. Hoddick WK, Filly RA, Mahony BS, Callen PW: Minimal fetal renal pyelectasis. J Ultrasound Med 4:85, 1985.

57. Betz BW, Hertzberg BS, Carroll BA, et al: Mild fetal renal pelviectasis: Differentiation from hilar vasculature using color Doppler sonography. J Ultrasound Med 10:243, 1991.

58. Ghidini A, Sirtori M, Vergani P, et al: Uteropelvic junction obstruction in utero and ex utero. Obstet Gynecol 75:805, 1990.

59. Ransley PG, Dhillon HK, Gordon I, et al: The postnatal management of hydronephrosis diagnosed by prenatal ultrasound. J Urol 144(2):584, 1990.

60. Corteville JE, Gray DL, Crane JP: Congenital hydronephrosis: Correlation of fetal ultrasonographic findings with infant outcome. Am J Obstet Gynecol 165:384, 1991.

61. Benacerraf BR, Mandell J, Estroff JA, et al: Fetal pyelectasis: A possible association with Down syndrome. Obstet Gynecol 76:58, 1990.

62. Laing FC, Burke VD, Wing VW, et al: Postpartum evaluation of fetal hydronephrosis: Optimal timing for follow-up sonography. Radiology 152:423, 1984.

63. Davis GH, Wapner RJ, Kurtz AB, et al: Antenatal diagnosis of hydrometrocolpos by ultrasound examination. J Ultrasound Med 3:371, 1984.

64. Mahony BS, Filly RA, Callen PW: Fetal renal dysplasia: Sonographic evaluation. Radiology 152:143, 1984.

65. Fries MH, Norton ME, Goldberg JD, et al: Renal function after in-utero intervention for obstructive uropathy. Am J Obstet Gynecol, in press.

66. Crombleholme TM, Harrison MR, Golbus MS, et al: Fetal intervention in obstructive uropathy: Prognostic indicators and efficacy of intervention. Am J Obstet Gynecol 162:1239, 1990.

67. Glick PL, Harrison MR, Golbus MS, et al: Management of the fetus with congenital hydronephrosis: II. Prognostic criteria and selection for treatment. J Pediatr Surg 20:376, 1985.

68. Elder JS, O'Grady JP, Ashmead G, et al: Evaluation of fetal renal function: Unreliability of fetal urinary electrolytes. J Urol 144(2):574, 1990.

69. Evans MI, Sacks AJ, Johnson MP, et al: Sequential invasive assessment of fetal renal function and the intrauterine treatment of fetal obstructive uropathies. Obstet Gynecol 77:545, 1991.

70. Nicolaides KH, Cheng HH, Snijders RJM, et al: Fetal urine biochemistry in the assessment of obstructive uropathy. Am J. Obstet Gynecol 166:932, 1992.

71. Mahony BS, Callen PW, Filly RA: Fetal urethral obstruction: US evaluation. Radiology 157:221, 1985.

72. Glick PL, Harrison MR, Adzick NS, et al: Correction of congenital hydronephrosis in utero: IV. In utero decompression prevents renal dysplasia. J Pediatr Surg 19:649, 1984.

73. Hayden SA, Russ PD, Pretorius DH, et al: Posterior urethral obstruction: Prenatal sonographic findings and clinical outcome in fourteen cases. J Ultrasound Med 7:371, 1988.

74. Stiller RJ: Early ultrasonic appearance of fetal bladder outlet obstruction. Am J Obstet Gynecol 160:584, 1989.

75. Silver RK, MacGreegor SN, Cook WA, et al: Fetal posterior urethral valve syndrome: A prospective application of antenatal prognostic criteria. Obstet Gynecol 76:951, 1990.

76. Callen PW, Bolding D, Filly RA, et al: Ultrasonographic evaluation of fetal paranephric pseudocysts. J Ultrasound Med 2:309, 1983.

77. Beck AD: The effect of intrauterine urinary obstruction upon the development of the fetal kidney. J Urol 105:784, 1971.

78. Thomas IT, Smith DW: Oligohydramnios: Cause of the non-

renal features of Potter's syndrome, including pulmonary hypoplasia. J Pediatr 84:811, 1974.

79. Jeffery RB, Laing FC, Wing VW, et al: Sonography of the fetal duplex kidney. Radiology 153:123, 1984.

80. Montana MA, Cyr DR, Lenke RR, et al: Sonographic detection of fetal ureteral obstruction. AJR 145:595, 1985.

81. Winters WD, Lebowitz RL: Importance of prenatal detection of hydronephrosis of the upper pole. AJR 155:125, 1990.

82. Dunn V, Glasier CM: Ultrasonographic antenatal demonstration of primary megaureters. J Ultrasound Med 4:101, 1985.

83. Lebowitz RL, Griscomb NT: Neonatal hydronephrosis—146 cases. Radiol Clin North Am 15:49, 1971.

84. Grignon A, Filiatrault D, Homsy Y, et al: Ureteropelvic junction stenosis: Antenatal ultrasonographic diagnosis, postnatal investigation, and follow-up. Radiology 160:649, 1986.

85. Jaffe R, Abramowicz J, Fejgin M, et al: Giant fetal abdominal cyst: Ultrasonic diagnosis and management. J Ultrasound Med 6:45, 1987.

86. Lycaya J, Enriquez G, Delgado R, et al: Infundibulopelvic stenosis in children. AJR 142:471, 1984.

87. Kleiner B, Callen PW, Filly RA: Sonographic analysis of the fetus with ureteropelvic junction obstruction. AJR 148:359, 1987.

88. Zerres K, Volpel M-C, Weif H: Cystic kidneys: Genetics, pathologic anatomy, clinical picture and prenatal diagnosis. Hum Genet 68:104, 1984.

89. Bernstein J: A classification of renal cysts. In Gardner KD (ed): Cystic Diseases of the Kidney, pp 7–30. New York, John Wiley & Sons, 1976.

90. Bernstein J: The morphogenesis of renal parenchymal maldevelopment (renal dysplasia). Pediatr Clin North Am 18:395, 1971.

91. Felson B, Cussen LJ: The hydronephrotic type of unilateral congenital multicystic disease of the kidney. Semin Roentgenol 10:113, 1975.

92. Diard F, LeDosseur P, Cadier L, et al: Multicystic dysplasia in the upper component of the complete duplex kidney. Pediatr Radiol 14:310, 1984.

93. Hashimoto BE, Filly RA, Callen PW: Multicystic dysplastic kidney in utero: Changing appearance on US. Radiology 159:107, 1986.

94. Stack KJ, Koff SA, Silver TM: Ultrasonic features of multicystic dysplastic kidney: Expanded criteria. Radiology 143:217, 1982.

95. Kleiner B, Filly RA, Mack L, et al: Multicystic dysplastic kidney: Observations of contralateral disease in the fetal population. Radiology 161:27, 1986.

96. Stiller RJ, Pinto M, Heller C, et al: Oligohydramnios associated with bilateral multicystic dysplastic kidneys: Prenatal diagnosis at 15 weeks' gestation. J Clin Ultrasound 16:436, 1988.

97. Sanders RC, Hartman DS: The sonographic distinction between neonatal muticystic kidney and hydronephrosis. Radiology 151:621, 1984.

98. Garcia CJ, Taylor KJW, Weiss RM: Congenital megacalyces: Ultrasound appearance. J Ultrasound Med 6:163, 1987.

99. Glick PL, Harrison MR, Noall RA, et al: Correction of congenital hydronephrosis in utero: III. Early mid-trimester ureteral obstruction produces renal dysplasia. J Pediatr Surg 18:681, 1983.

100. Estroff JA, Mandell J, Benacerraf BR: Increased renal parenchymal echogenicity in the fetus: Importance and clinical outcome. Radiology 181:135, 1991.

101. Vinaixa F, Gotzens VJ, Tejedo-Mateu A: Tubular gigantism of the kidney in a 41 mm, Streeter's 23rd horizon, human fetus with a comparative study of renal structures in normal human fetuses at a similar stage of development. Eur Urol 10:331, 1984.

102. Mahony BS, Callen PW, Filly RA, et al: Progression of infantile polycystic kidney disease in early pregnancy. J Ultrasound Med 3:277, 1984.

103. Luthy DA, Hirsch JH: Infantile polycystic kidney disease: Observations from attempts at prenatal diagnosis. Am J Med Genet 20:505, 1985.

104. Barth RA, Guillot AP, Capeless EL, et al: Prenatal diagnosis of autosomal recessive polycystic kidney disease: Variable outcome within one family. Am J Obstet Gynecol 166:560, 1992.

105. Ambrosino MM, Hernanz-Schulman M, Horii SC, et al: Prenatal diagnosis of nephroblastomatosis in two siblings. J Ultrasound Med 9:49, 1990.

106. Moore BS, Pretorius DH, Scioscia AL, et al: Sonographic findings in a fetus with congenital nephrotic syndrome of the Finnish type. J Ultrasound Med 11:113, 1992.

107. Pardes JG, Engel IA, Blomquist K, et al: Ultrasonography of intrauterine Meckel's syndrome. J Ultrasound Med 3:33, 1984.

108. Elejalde BR, de Elejalde MM, Heitman T: Visualization of the fetal genitalia by ultrasonography: A review of the literature and analysis of its accuracy and ethical implications. J Ultrasound Med 4:633, 1985.

109. Mahony BS, Filly RA, Callen PW: Amnionicity and chroinicity in twin pregnancies: Prediction using ultrasound. Radiology 155:205, 1985.

110. Birnholz JC: Determination of fetal sex. N Engl J Med 309:942, 1983.

111. Jafrie SZH, Bree RL, Silver TM, et al: Fetal ovarian cysts: Sonographic detection and association with hypothyroidism. Radiology 150:809, 1984.

112. Holzgreve W, Winde B, Willital GH, et al: Prenatal diagnosis and perinatal management of a fetal ovarian cyst. Prenat Diagn 5:155, 1985.

113. Sherer DM, Shah YG, Eggers PC, et al: Prenatal sonographic diagnosis and subsequent management of fetal adnexal torsion. J Ultrasound Med 9:161, 1990.

114. Meizner I, Levy A, Katz M, et al: Prenatal ultrasonographic diagnosis of fetal scrotal inguinal hernia. Am J Obstet Gynecol 166:907, 1992.

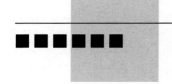

CHAPTER 19

Ultrasound Evaluation of Hydrops Fetalis

DARYL H. CHINN, M.D.

Hydrops fetalis is the condition characterized by excessive fluid accumulation within fetal extravascular compartments and body cavities. This serious condition, which presents as varying degrees of fetal anasarca, ascites, pericardial effusion, pleural effusion, placental edema, and polyhydramnios, was first described nearly 100 years ago by Ballantyne.[1] In 1939, Levine and coworkers discovered that maternal sensitization to a fetal blood group antigen played a major role in the development of hydrops fetalis.[2] In 1940, Landsteiner and Weiner discovered the sensitizing antigen, the Rh factor.[3] In 1943, Potter identified a subgroup of hydrops fetalis in which maternal Rh sensitization was not present.[4] With these observations, hydrops fetalis was characterized into those cases caused by an immunologic response, immune hydrops fetalis, and those cases not caused by an immunologic response, nonimmune hydrops fetalis.

IMMUNE HYDROPS FETALIS

Pathogenesis

The pathogenesis of immune hydrops fetalis is initiated by the presence of maternal serum IgG antibody against one of the fetal red blood cell antigens. A maternal serum antibody to a red blood cell develops if the mother is exposed to red blood cell antigens different from her own. Typically, this occurs during the release of fetal red blood cells into the maternal blood circulation at parturition of a preceding pregnancy. Maternal sensitization can also result from other causes of fetal-maternal hemorrhage, as might occur with placental abruption, amniocentesis, therapeutic abortion, spontaneous abortion, and placental intravillous hemorrhage. Blood transfusion may also provide an opportunity for maternal sensitization.

In the sensitized mother, maternal IgG crosses the placental-fetal barrier and enters the fetal circulation. If the fetal red blood cells are antigenic to the maternal IgG, then the IgG antibodies bind to the red blood cell membranes and induce fetal hemolysis. If significant, fetal hemolytic anemia occurs.

The following pathophysiologic interactions are generally accepted to contribute to the development of immune hydrops fetalis.

Fetal anemia stimulates extramedullary hematopoiesis. Hematopoietic and fibroblastic tissues replace normal liver and splenic tissue. Hepatosplenomegaly

develops. Normal hepatic protein synthesis is impaired. Portal venous hypertension occurs and leads to fetal ascites. Umbilical venous hypertension develops and results in placental edema and placental enlargement. Impaired placental diffusion of maternal amino acids, combined with decreased fetal hepatic protein synthesis, results in fetal hypoproteinemia.[5, 6]

The fetus responds to the anemia by increasing cardiac output. If this adaptation is insufficient to maintain fetal tissue oxygenation, then hypoxemia and acidosis occurs. This results in capillary dilatation and increased capillary permeability (Fig. 19–1).

It is likely that these complex interactions of hypoproteinemia, increased venous hydrostatic pressure, and increased capillary permeability combine in the development of excess fluid accumulation within fetal extravascular compartments and body cavities, the hallmark of hydrops fetalis.

The previously described interactions are complex and inconstant. For example, the relationship of fetal hematocrit and immune hydrops fetalis is not constant. Some fetuses are hydropic with hemoglobin levels greater than 7 g/dL, and some fetuses are not hydropic with hemoglobin levels less than 3 g/dL.[7] Anemia-induced high-output cardiac failure likely plays a role, and yet the blood volume in fetuses and neonates with immune hydrops fetalis is reported to be normal.[8, 9] Isolated severe fetal hypoproteinemia, as present with hypoalbuminemia and congenital nephrotic syndrome, does not always cause fetal hydrops.

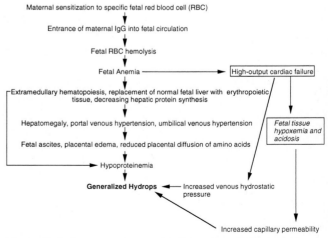

Figure 19–1. Sequence of events leading to immune hydrops fetalis.

Clinical Background

The Rh factor was determined to be the (D) antigen in the Rh blood group system. The Rh (D) antigen initially accounted for 98% of all fetuses with immune hydrops fetalis.[10]

In the United States, 15% of whites and 8% of blacks are Rh (D) antigen negative (commonly termed *Rh negative*).[11] Hence the potential for immune hydrops fetalis existed predominately in situations when an Rh (D) antigen–negative mother, who had been sensitized to the Rh (D) antigen, was pregnant with an Rh (D) antigen–positive fetus.

The so-called atypical blood group antigens such as c and E of the Rh system, K and k of the Kell system, and Fy[a] of the Duffy system have less frequently been the cause of severe immune hydrops fetalis (Table 19–1).[10] Rare instances of severe immune hydrops fetalis have been described with ABO blood type incompatibility as well.[12]

Prophylaxis against Rh (D) sensitization has significantly altered the clinical impact of immune hydrops fetalis. Rh (D) immunoglobulin (Rhogam) is now given to the Rh (D) antigen–negative woman at the time of potentially sensitizing events. Then if Rh (D) antigen–positive red blood cells enter the woman's circulation, they are removed by the Rh (D) immunoglobulin before their recognition by the woman's immune system. This thereby prevents the sensitization of the woman at risk.

Table 19–1. ANTIBODIES CAUSING HEMOLYTIC DISEASE

Blood Group System	Antigens Related to Hemolytic Disease	Severity of Hemolytic Disease
Rh	D	Mild to severe
	C	Mild to moderate
	c	Mild to severe
	E	Mild to severe
	e	Mild to moderate
Lewis		Not a proved cause of hemolytic disease
Ii		Not a proved cause of hemolytic disease
Kell	K	Mild to severe with hydrops
	k	Mild to severe
Duffy	FY[a]	Mild to severe with hydrops
	FY[b]	Not a proved cause of hemolytic disease
Kidd	JK[a]	Mild to severe
	JK[b]	Mild to severe
MNSs	M	Mild to severe
	N	Mild
	S	Mild to severe
	s	Mild to severe
Lutheran	Lu[a]	Mild
	Lu[b]	Mild
Diego	Di[a]	Mild to severe
	Di[b]	Mild to severe
Xg	Xg[a]	Mild
P	PP$_1$pk (Tj[a])	Mild to severe
Public antigens	YT[a]	Moderate to severe
	YT[b]	Mild
	Lan	Mild
	EN[a]	Moderate
	Ge	Mild
	JR[a]	Mild
	CO[a]	Severe
Private antigens	COa[1-b]	Mild
	Batty	Mild
	Becker	Mild
	Berrens	Mild
	Biles	Moderate
	Evans	Mild
	Gonzales	Mild
	Good	Severe
	Heibel	Moderate
	Hunt	Mild
	Jobbins	Mild
	Radin	Moderate
	Rm	Mild
	Ven	Mild
	Wright[a]	Severe
	Wright[b]	Mild
	Zd	Moderate

Modified from Weinstein L: Irregular antibodies causing hemolytic disease of the newborn: A continuing problem. Clin Obstet Gynecol 25:321, 1982.

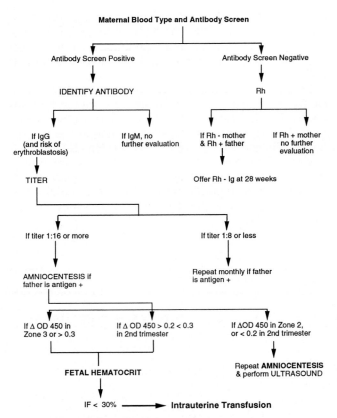

Figure 19–2. Management scheme for Rh isoimmunization. (Modified from Parer JT: Severe Rh isoimmunization: Current methods of in utero diagnosis and treatment. Am J Obstet Gynecol 158:1323, 1988.)

With prophylaxis, the incidence of Rh (D) sensitization, which had initially accounted for 98% of sensitized pregnancies, has decreased such that the Rh (D) antigen sensitization now accounts for 55% of sensitized pregnancies.[13] Sensitization to atypical red blood cell antigens then accounts for the other cases of maternal sensitization.

General guidelines for the management of the Rh (−) pregnancy is noted schematically in Figure 19–2.

Despite the existence of effective prophylaxis against Rh (D) antigen sensitization, the eradication of Rh (D) isoimmunization will not occur because of several factors, including a failure to determine all mothers' blood type, errors in determining blood type, failure to administer Rhogam, and failure to administer an adequate amount of Rhogam in the presence of severe fetal-maternal hemorrhage.

All pregnancies are routinely screened with the indirect Coombs test for the presence of red blood cell antibodies in maternal serum. If red blood cell antibodies are present, they are identified and quantified. The father will be tested for the corresponding antigen; and if this antigen is present in the father, the fetus is considered at risk for the blood type antigenic to the maternal red blood cell antibodies. In addition, the fetus of that pregnancy is considered at risk for fetal hemolysis and immune hydrops fetalis.

If antibody levels in the mother are at or above a critical level, frequently stated to be 1:16 (note that the "critical level" varies between laboratories), then Parer[14] recommends amniocentesis to determine the Δ OD 450 of the amniotic fluid.

The Δ OD 450 is the spectrophotometric optical density of amniotic fluid at 450 nm wavelength of light, when compared with normal amniotic fluid optical density at 450 nm wavelength of light. This measurement is an indirect measurement of the bilirubin concentration in the amniotic fluid. The bilirubin level reflects the severity of fetal hemolysis.

The Δ OD 450 is then analyzed with the aid of a Liley chart to determine the risk of severe fetal anemia. The Liley charts established normal values of Δ OD 450 from 27 to 40 weeks' gestation. Based on the Δ OD 450, pregnancies were classified into level 1, level 2, and level 3, which were indicators of the risk of severe fetal anemia and immune hydrops fetalis. In the third trimester, if the Δ OD 450 was in level 3, then direct evaluation of fetal blood through a cordocentesis (percutaneous umbilical cord puncture) is recommended to determine the fetal hematocrit. In the third trimester, a pregnancy in level 2 will be followed by repeat amniocentesis and ultrasound evaluation.

The need to assess fetuses before 27 weeks led to various extrapolations of the Liley data into the second trimester (Fig. 19–3).

The utility of the extrapolated Liley charts to predict the severe fetal anemia in fetuses of less than 27 weeks' gestation has been the subject of considerable debate. Parer[14] recommends cordocentesis if the Δ OD 450 value is greater than 0.2 in the second trimester.[14] Those fetuses at risk who do not require cordocentesis are followed by repeat ultrasound examination and Δ OD 450 measurements at 1 to 3 week intervals.

Others believe that the Liley charts are severely limited in the second trimester in their ability to predict severe fetal anemia.[11, 13, 15] Nicholaides and coworkers[15] have shown poor correlation between fetal hematocrit and Δ OD 450 values during the second trimester. Because of this, some centers recommend direct cordocentesis in the second trimester of all pregnancies at risk for fetal hemolytic anemia.[11, 13] This more aggressive approach has not been adopted by all investigators, given the 1% to 2% mortality of cordocentesis and given the increased risks of further maternal sensitization with the iatrogenic fetal-maternal hemorrhage resulting from cordocentesis.[16]

Within this framework, ultrasonography has an extremely valuable role. During the second trimester, when the Liley charts are of uncertain value, the absence of ultrasound evidence of hydrops fetalis is reassuring to many practitioners and supports follow-up amniocentesis rather than proceeding with cordocentesis.

Similarly, if ultrasound assessment demonstrates evidence of immune hydrops fetalis, cordocentesis will be necessary. If cordocentesis is required, ultrasound guidance of the aspirating needle is essential. If an intrauterine transfusion into the fetal vasculature or fetal peritoneal cavity is required because of fetal

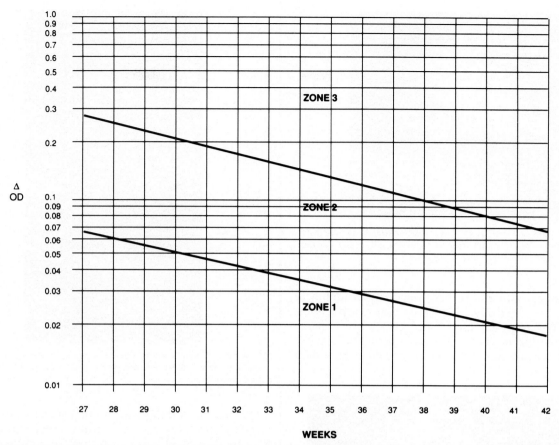

Figure 19–3. Modified Liley graph used to depict degrees of sensitization. (Modified from Liley AW: Liquor amnii analysis in management of pregnancy complicated by rhesus sensitization. Am J Obstet Gynecol 82:1359, 1961.)

anemia or fetal immune hydrops, ultrasound guidance is necessary. Ultrasonography is also used to evaluate the postprocedural status of the fetus to determine the effectiveness of therapy.

The guidelines noted earlier are for Rh (D)–sensitized pregnancies. Pregnancies sensitized to atypical red blood cell antigens known to cause moderate to severe hemolytic anemia are managed by amniotic fluid Δ OD 450 analysis, since the indirect Coombs titers with these antibodies can be unpredictable in detecting fetal anemia.[17]

In addition to ultrasound imaging and Δ OD 450 amniotic fluid evaluation, the evaluation of the fetus by a biophysical profile and with nonstress tests has been advocated as an early sign of fetal anemia.[18]

Until recently, the goal of many centers was to deliver the fetus at risk as soon as fetal lung maturity was established. However, recently the goal of a term fetal delivery has been advocated by Weiner and colleagues,[19] who believe that the more mature fetus is better able to metabolize bilirubin and thus avoid the deleterious effects of hyperbilirubinemia.

Ultrasound Features of Immune Hydrops Fetalis

Since the Liley charts are unable to identify all fetuses experiencing severe hemolytic anemia, and since many laboratories are unwilling to subject all fetuses at risk for severe anemia to cordocentesis to determine fetal hematocrit, most laboratories rely on ultrasound evaluation to identify the decompensating severely anemic fetus.

Additionally, since it is known that the prognosis of treated severely anemic hydropic fetuses is not as good as the prognosis of treated severely anemic nonhydropic fetuses,[19] there is a persistent effort to identify the earliest sonographic feature of incipient immune hydrops fetalis before the development of frank hydrops. Frank hydrops is defined as a fetus with subcutaneous edema and serous effusions, either pericardial effusion, pleural effusions, or ascites. Severe fetal anemia is defined as a fetal hematocrit of less than 30%.[13] In a series of fetuses with sonographic evidence of frank immune hydrops, all had hematocrits of 15% or less.[20]

On review of the pathophysiologic events leading to immune hydrops fetalis listed in Figure 19–1, one would anticipate that ultrasound evaluation would display a number of these morphologic manifestations.

Serous effusions, such as ascites, pericardial effusion, or pleural effusion are hallmark features of frank immune hydrops fetalis. Consistent with our understanding of pathophysiology, ascites is one of the early signs of frank immune hydrops.[20, 21] Small amounts of ascites can be detected as triangular sonolucent regions outlining adjacent bowel loops (Fig. 19–4) or as sono-

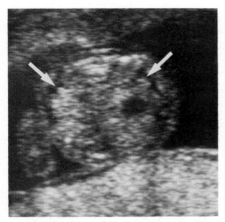

Figure 19–4. Transverse axial view of a fetal abdomen demonstrates a small amount of ascites, appearing as angular sonolucency *(arrows)* interposed between echogenic bowel loops.

lucent regions outlining the intra-abdominal umbilical vein (Figs. 19–5 through 19–7). At times, a phenomenon known as pseudoascites can create the appearance of sonolucent fluid within the peritoneal cavity. This entity always lies at the periphery of the abdomen

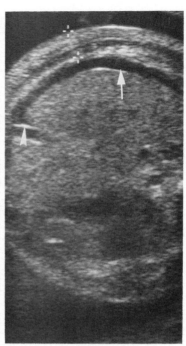

Figure 19–6. Small amount of ascites *(arrow)* outlining one wall of the umbilical vein *(arrowhead).* Note cursor marks indicating subcutaneous edema.

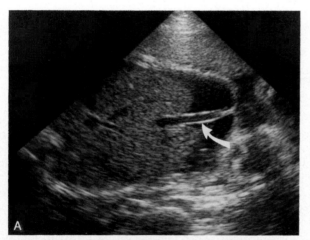

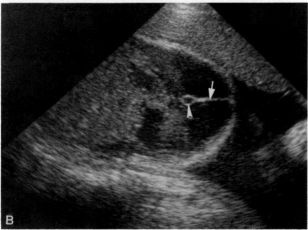

Figure 19–5. *A.* Oblique axial view of fetal abdomen with sonolucent ascites outlining the umbilical vein *(curved arrow). B.* Oblique coronal view of fetal abdomen with umbilical vein seen "end-on" *(arrowhead),* supported by the falciform ligament *(arrow)* surrounded by sonolucent ascites.

and does not outline the umbilical vein nor does it interpose itself between adjacent bowel loops (Fig. 19–8). Pseudoascites can also outline the periphery of the retroperitoneum, an observation that offers another clue that the sonolucency does not represent intraperitoneal ascites.[22]

Pericardial effusion has been proposed by DeVore and colleagues as the earliest sign of immune hydrops fetalis. In a small series, using M-mode ultrasonography, they identified pericardial effusion before the development of ascites, pleural effusion, or anasarca.[23] Small volumes of pericardial fluid have been reported as a normal finding after 20 weeks' gestation.[24] Hence, a sonolucent ring of pericardial fluid of at least 2 mm is necessary to determine that the fluid collection is abnormal.[25] Both two-dimensional and M-mode ultrasonography are useful in documenting the pathologic effusion.

The diagnosis of fetal pleural effusions is sought by searching for sonolucency outlining the contours of the fetal thorax. On occasion, ascites can herniate through a diaphragmatic hiatus and mimic a pleural effusion.

Subcutaneous edema is a hallmark of frank immune hydrops fetalis and is considered abnormal when measuring more than 5 mm. Measurements of this type, however, are quite subjective, and the observation of a small amount of skin edema is extremely difficult. Skin edema is considered to be a late sign of frank immune hydrops fetalis (Fig. 19–9).[26]

Since fetal intrahepatic extramedullary hematopoiesis is an early compensating response to fetal anemia, one predicts that fetal hepatomegaly would be an early sign of immune hydrops fetalis. Attempts to quantify fetal liver length versus abdominal circumference, abdominal circumference ratios, and intraperitoneal vol-

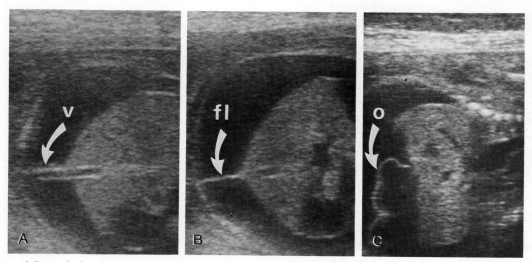

Figure 19–7. Potentially confusing structures in the presence of a large amount of fetal ascites. *A.* Ascites outlining the umbilical vein (v). *B.* Ascites outlining the falciform ligament (fl). *C.* Fluid in the greater and lesser peritoneal cavities, separated by the omentum (o).

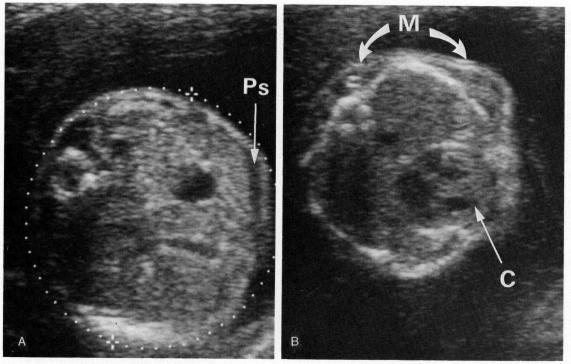

Figure 19–8. Pitfalls in sonographic diagnosis of hydrops fetalis. *A.* Pseudoascites (Ps). *B.* Pseudo–body wall edema. M, normal fetal musculature; C, cardiac structures.

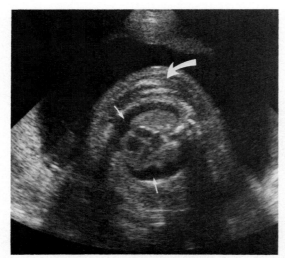

Figure 19–9. Transverse axial view of the fetal thorax. Bilateral pleural effusions *(small arrows)* outline the fetal lungs and heart. Note also the subcutaneous edema *(curved arrow)*.

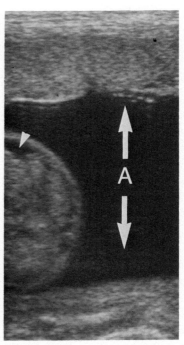

Figure 19–10. Longitudinal sonogram demonstrating polyhydramnios (A) and fetal ascites *(arrowhead)* in a fetus with hydrops fetalis. There also were pleural effusions and a pericardial effusion. The relatively normal appearance of the placenta may be misleading owing to the thinning effect of the increased amniotic fluid volume.

umes have not been successful.[15, 26, 27] However, longitudinal measurements of the right hepatic lobe when compared with normal values have been correlated with fetal hemoglobin levels and fetal reticulocyte count.[28] Therefore, there is cautious optimism that the fetal liver length measurement will be of value.

Polyhydramnios, the excess of amniotic fluid, is frequently identified in the fetus with frank immune hydrops. Furthermore, polyhydramnios is frequently the first sonographic abnormality in severely anemic fetuses before the onset of frank immune hydrops. In one series, 6 of 10 fetuses scanned serially displayed polyhydramnios as the earliest abnormal sonographic feature. In the fetuses with polyhydramnios, their hematocrit was 26% or less.[20] As discussed elsewhere (see Chapter 22), polyhydramnios can be defined meaningfully both quantitatively or qualitatively (Fig. 19–10). It is noteworthy that occasionally severely anemic hydropic fetuses will demonstrate oligohydramnios rather than polyhydramnios.

Placental thickness is defined as abnormal when greater than 4 cm.[29] This measurement, however, varies with gestational age and with the amount of amniotic fluid. Using the 4-cm threshold, abnormal placental thickening can occur before frank hydrops (Fig. 19–11). This measurement is not as sensitive as polyhydramnios in the identification of the nonhydropic anemic fetus.[20] Qualitatively, placental edema has been described as being ground glass in appearance with disappearance of the chorionic plate, buckling of the fetal surface, and loss of cotyledon formation.[30] However, the qualitative identification of early placental edema is extremely difficult owing to the subjectivity of the observations.

Given the better prognosis of transfused severely anemic nonhydropic fetuses compared with the prognosis of transfused hydropic fetuses, ultrasound features of severe anemia, before the onset of frank hydrops, are sought.

The umbilical vein diameter has been proposed as an early sign of impending immune hydrops fetalis.[31, 32]

However, subsequent studies have contradicted this observation.[20, 33, 34] Recently, Doppler waveform analysis has been advanced as a sign of fetal anemia. Theoretically, with the onset of hemolytic anemia, the fetus would respond by increasing cardiac output. This would result in a velocity increase within the umbilical

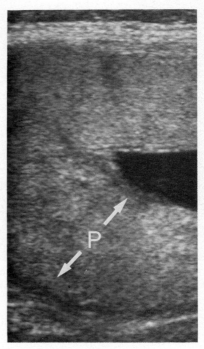

Figure 19–11. Longitudinal sonogram demonstrating markedly enlarged and edematous placenta (P).

vein and fetal descending aorta. Yet, this initial enthusiasm has not been substantiated in follow-up studies.[35]

In summary, the sonographic features of frank immune hydrops include subcutaneous edema and serous effusions. Both ascites and pericardial effusion have been described as early features of frank hydrops. Subcutaneous edema is a late feature of frank hydrops fetalis. In an attempt to identify the severely anemic fetus before the development of frank hydrops fetalis, features of incipient hydrops have been defined. Significantly, polyhydramnios and/or placental thickening can indicate incipient hydrops fetalis.

Prognosis of Immune-Mediated Fetal Hemolytic Anemia

Owing to the advances in the understanding, prophylaxis, diagnosis, and treatment of fetal hemolytic anemia, the impact of fetal hemolytic disease has been significantly reduced. With the proper use of Rh (D) immune globulin, there has been a fourfold reduction in the sensitization of the Rh-negative woman.[36] Additionally, Weiner and associates report the survival rates in fetuses undergoing intrauterine transfusions in sensitized pregnancies of up to 100% for nonhydropic fetuses, 85% in hydropic fetuses, and 96% survival overall.[19]

This progressive improvement in the survival of fetuses requiring transfusion with fetal immune hemolytic disease is illustrated in Figure 19–12. Although this improvement is due to many factors, ultrasonography has played a major contribution in this progress through its ability to detect severe anemia in the fetus by virtue of the sonographic signs of incipient and frank immune hydrops. Additionally, advancements in

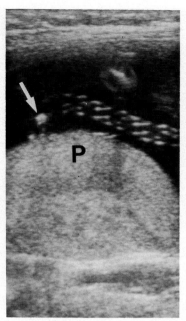

Figure 19–13. Cordocentesis needle *(arrow)* entering the umbilical vessel at the cord insertion site. P, placenta.

diagnostic and therapeutic techniques such as amniocentesis and cordocentesis have relied on the ultrasound technique (Figs. 19–13 through 19–15).

NONIMMUNE HYDROPS FETALIS

In 1943, Potter[4] described a clinical entity that affected non–Rh-sensitized pregnancies and was characterized by fetal anasarca, placental edema, and, often, fetal serous effusions. Potter recognized that this entity, since termed *nonimmune hydrops fetalis,* did not represent a specific disease but rather a late manifestation of many severe diseases. When Potter first described nonimmune hydrops fetalis, this entity represented less than 20% of all cases of hydrops fetalis; however, since the advent of effective prophylaxis against Rh (D) sensitization, the relative frequency of nonimmune hydrops fetalis has risen to 90%.[26]

Depending on the clinical series and patient referral patterns, the incidence of nonimmune hydrops fetalis has been reported to range from 1 in 1600 to 1 in 7000.[37] In a highly selected series performed at a major referral center the incidence of nonimmune hydrops fetalis was 1 in 165.[38] The mortality rate of nonimmune hydrops fetalis ranges from 50% to 98%, depending on the patient mix and the causes of nonimmune hydrops fetalis in the reported series.[37, 39–44]

Unlike the situation with immune hydrops fetalis, there are no sensitive laboratory tests to screen all pregnancies at risk for nonimmune hydrops fetalis. Ultrasound evaluation, if performed in the second and third trimester, will detect nearly all cases. Unfortunately, approximately 30% of pregnancies with nonimmune hydrops fetalis are clinically uneventful and ultrasonography in these cases is not performed.[44] Even

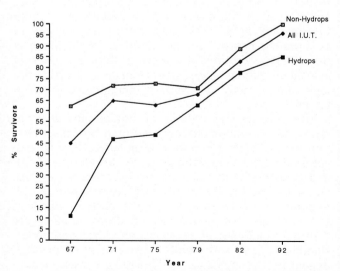

Figure 19–12. Line graphs of the percentage of surviving fetuses undergoing first intrauterine transfusion (I.U.T.) for nonhydropic disease, all stages of disease, and hydrops. (From Harmon CR, Manning FA, Bowman JM, Lange JR: Severe RH disease: Poor outcome is not inevitable. Am J Obstet Gynecol 145:823, 1983; and Weiner CP, Williamson RA, Weinstrom KD: Management of fetal hemolytic disease by cordocentesis: II. Outcome of treatment. Am J Obstet Gynecol 165:1302, 1991.)

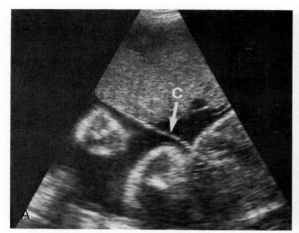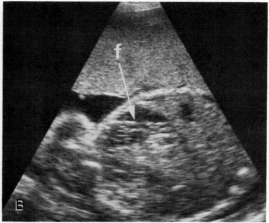

Figure 19–14. Intraperitoneal blood transfusion in a fetus with immune hydrops fetalis. *A.* Catheter (c) traversing the amniotic fluid and entering the fetal peritoneal cavity. *B.* Intraperitoneal bubbles and fluid (f) following intraperitoneal transfusion.

when routine ultrasound assessment is not performed, the identification of a pregnancy complication often leads to an ultrasound examination. In most series, polyhydramnios is the most frequent maternal complication, presenting as a size–date discrepancy. Polyhydramnios occurs in 50% to 75% of patients with nonimmune hydrops fetalis.[40, 44] Pregnancy induced hypertension occurs in 15% to 46% of patients.[37, 44] Maternal anemia occurs in 7% to 45%, depending on the definition of anemia and on the demographics of the particular study.[40, 45] Maternal hypoalbuminemia occurs in 7% to 67%. Other less frequent maternal complications include urinary tract infections, antepartum hemorrhage, and gestational diabetes mellitus.[40, 44] Clinical evidence of fetal arrhythmia was reported in 15% of one series of pregnancies with nonimmune hydrops fetalis.[41]

Etiology

The etiologies of nonimmune hydrops are extremely numerous. Table 19–2 is a list of conditions associated

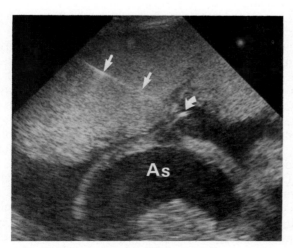

Figure 19–15. Intravascular transfusion in a fetus with immune hydrops fetalis. Note the needle *(straight arrows)* traversing the thickened placenta and entering the umbilical cord *(curved arrow).* As, ascites.

with nonimmune hydrops fetalis.[46] Our knowledge of which conditions listed in Table 19–2 are truly causative of nonimmune hydrops fetalis is extremely limited. For instance, homozygous α-thalassemia causes nonimmune hydrops fetalis through its precipitation of severe fetal anemia, initiating the pathophysiologic cascade similar to immune hydrops fetalis (see Fig. 19–1). Homozygous α-thalassemia is clearly etiologic in the development of nonimmune hydrops fetalis. On the contrary, pulmonary hypoplasia, which is listed in many tables as etiologic in the development of nonimmune hydrops fetalis is rather, in most cases, a consequence of this condition. The pleural effusions that frequently accompany nonimmune hydrops fetalis do not permit proper development of the fetal lungs, and pulmonary hypoplasia results.[41]

Although homozygous α-thalassemia and fetal pulmonary hypoplasia are clear-cut examples of a cause and a result of nonimmune hydrops fetalis, an attempt to separate Table 19–2 into causes and results of nonimmune hydrops fetalis would be problematic at this point. Additionally, likely a third category of associated entities exists that are neither directly etiologic nor directly a result of nonimmune hydrops fetalis.

The sonographic criteria of nonimmune hydrops fetalis differs among authors, and therefore case selection varies.[42, 47] Furthermore, as noted earlier, investigators differ in their willingness to consider an identified abnormality as causative of nonimmune hydrops, and subsequently the number of cases considered idiopathic in etiology varies. In the past, as many as 50% of cases of nonimmune hydrops fetalis were considered idiopathic; however, with improved understanding of this entity and improvements in prenatal diagnosis, the incidence of idiopathic causes of nonimmune hydrops fetalis has been reduced to approximately 15%.[48, 49] It is inevitable that with further advances, additional etiologies of and associations with nonimmune hydrops fetalis will be described. Although it is beyond the scope of this chapter to discuss each entity listed in Table 19–2, a few general comments are warranted.

Table 19–2. CONDITIONS ASSOCIATED WITH NONIMMUNE HYDROPS FETALIS

Categories	Individual Conditions	Categories	Individual Conditions
Cardiovascular	Tachyarrhythmia Complex dysrhythmia Congenital heart block Anatomic defects (atrial septal defect, ventricular septal defect, hypoplastic left heart, pulmonary valve insufficiency, subaortic stenosis, aortic valve stenosis, subaortic stenosis, atrioventricular canal defect with mitral regurgitation, single ventricle, tetralogy of Fallot, premature closure of the foramen ovale or of the ductus arteriosus, subendocardial fibroelastosis, dextrocardia in combination with pulmonic stenosis, Ebstein anomaly) Calcified aortic valve Coronary artery embolus Cardiomyopathy Myocarditis (coxsackievirus or cytomegalovirus) Atrial hemangioma Intracardial rhabdomyoma Endocardial teratoma	Respiratory Gastrointestinal Liver	Diaphragmatic hernia Cystic adenoma of the lung Pulmonary lymphangiectasia Hamartoma of the lung Mediastinal teratoma Pulmonary hypoplasia Hemangioma of the lung Extralobar pulmonary sequestration Jejunal atresia Midgut volvulus Malrotation of the intestines Duplication of the intestinal tract Meconium peritonitis Hepatic calcifications Hepatic fibrosis Cholestasis Polycystic disease of the liver Biliary atresia Hepatic vascular malformations/ hemangioma Familial cirrhosis Lysozymal storage disease (Gaucher disease)
Chromosomal	Down syndrome (trisomy 21) Other trisomies Turner syndrome XX/XY mosaicism Triploidy	Maternal	Severe diabetes mellitus Severe anemia Hypoproteinemia Theca lutein cysts
Malformation syndromes	Thanatophoric dwarfism Arthrogryposis multiplex congenita Asphyxiating thoracic dystrophy Hypophosphatasia Osteogenesis imperfecta Achondrogenesis Saldino-Noonan syndrome Neu-Laxova syndrome Francois syndrome, type 3 Recessive cystic hygroma Pena-Shokier syndrome, type 1 Osteopetrosis Myotonic dystrophy Multiple pterygium syndrome Opitz-Frias syndrome	Placenta–umbilical cord	Chorioangioma Chorionic vein thrombosis Fetal-maternal transfusion Placental and umbilical vein thrombosis Umbilical cord torsion True cord knots Angiomyxoma of the umbilical cord Aneurysm of the umbilical artery Placental endovasculitis
Twin pregnancy Hematologic	Twin transfusion syndrome α-Thalassemia Arteriovenous shunts (e.g., large vascular tumors) Fetal Kasabach-Merritt syndrome In utero closed space hemorrhage Vena cava, portal vein, or femoral obstruction, renal vein (e.g., thrombosis) Erythrocyte enzymopathy (G6PD deficiency) Hemophilia A	Medications Infections	Antepartum indomethacin (taken to stop premature labor, causing fetal ductus closure and secondary nonimmune hydrops fetalis) Cytomegalovirus Toxoplasmosis Syphilis Congenital hepatitis Herpes simplex type I Rubella Leptospirosis Chagas disease Parvovirus B19
Genitourinary	Urethral stenosis or atresia Posterior urethral valves Bladder neck obstruction Spontaneous bladder perforation Congenital nephrosis (Finnish type) Neurogenic bladder with reflux Ureterocele Prune-belly syndrome	Miscellaneous	Congenital lymphedema Congenital hydrothorax or chylothorax Polysplenia syndrome Congenital neuroblastoma Tuberous sclerosis Torsion of an ovarian cyst Fetal trauma Sacrococcygeal teratoma Congenital leukemia Wilms tumor

Modified from Holzgreve W, Holzgreve B, Curry JR: Nonimmune hydrops fetalis: Diagnosis and management. Semin Perinatol 9:52, 1985.

Major causes of nonimmune hydrops fetalis among North American and northern European populations are cardiac structural abnormalities and cardiac arrhythmias, accounting for 20% to 76% of cases, depending on the series.[24, 50] Details of the cardiac evaluation are discussed in detail in Chapter 14. Fetal cardiac arrhythmias must be specifically considered in all cases of nonimmune hydrops fetalis, since this may be amenable to in utero therapy.

Chromosomal abnormalities account for 14% of cases of nonimmune hydrops fetalis.[51] The most common aneuploidies associated with nonimmune hydrops fetalis are trisomy 21, trisomy 18, triploidy, and Turner syndrome (45 XO).

It is noteworthy that severe subcutaneous edema, so-called lymphangiectasia, and cystic hygromas are frequently associated with Turner syndrome. This association is briefly discussed later in this chapter.

In North America, hematologic disorders account for 10% of cases of nonimmune hydrops fetalis.[51] Homozygous α-thalassemia is the major hematologic cause of nonimmune hydrops fetalis.

In Taiwan, homozygous α-thalassemia accounts for 57% of cases of nonimmune hydrops fetalis. In homozygous α-thalassemia, Bart's hemoglobin is found. Because Bart's hemoglobin binds oxygen avidly, it is incapable of oxygen transport and therefore α-thalassemia is uniformly fatal for the fetus.[52] If fetuses with α-thalassemia are allowed to advance to the third trimester, the mother is placed at high risk for the development of preeclampsia and microcytic anemia. Because of its uniform fetal lethality and high risk to the mother in the third trimester, the detection of α-thalassemia in the second trimester is important so that termination of the pregnancy can be offered to the parents.[34] The diagnosis of α-thalassemia relies on a hemoglobin electrophoresis performed on fetal blood acquired by cordocentesis.[52]

Because of the diverse associations with nonimmune hydrops fetalis, knowledge of the pathophysiology of most cases is limited. It is appealing to classify the etiologies of nonimmune hydrops fetalis by their speculated pathologic mechanisms based on our knowledge of neonatal pathophysiology. Hence in Table 19–3, the pathophysiologic mechanisms of increased intravascular hydrostatic pressure, decreased plasma oncotic pressure, increased capillary permeability, and obstruction of lymphatic flow are listed with examples of corresponding etiologies.

Diagnostic Evaluation

Ultrasound evaluation is the primary means of identifying the hydropic fetus. Once identified, immune hydrops fetalis can be excluded by the indirect Coombs test, which, in the case of nonimmune hydrops fetalis, would demonstrate the absence of IgG antibodies to red blood cells in the maternal serum. Further testing of the pregnancy affected by nonimmune hydrops is included in Table 19–4. These tests are organized in levels of diagnostic invasiveness.

Table 19–3. CLASSIFICATION OF HYDROPS FETALIS BASED ON SPECULATIVE PATHOPHYSIOLOGIC MECHANISMS

Increased intravascular hydrostatic pressure (due to hemodynamic disturbances)
  Primary myocardial failure
    Arrhythmia (e.g., paroxysmal atrial tachycardia, familial heart block)
    Severe anemia (e.g., G6PD deficiency, α-thalassemia)
    Twin transfusion syndrome
    Myocarditis (e.g., coxsackievirus, TORCH parvovirus)
    Cardiac malformation
  High-output failure
    Parabiotic syndrome
    Arteriovenous shunt
  Obstruction of venous return
    Congenital neoplasm/other space-occupying lesions (e.g., neuroblastoma, retroperitoneal fibrosis, vena caval thrombosis)
Decreased plasma oncotic pressure
  Decreased albumin formation (e.g., congenital cirrhosis, hepatitis)
  Increased albumin excretion (e.g., congenital nephrotic syndrome of Finnish type)
Increased capillary permeability
  Anoxia (e.g., congenital infection, placental edema)
Obstruction of lymph flow (e.g., Turner syndrome)

From Im SS, Rizos N, Joutsi P, et al: Nonimmunologic hydrops fetalis. Am J Obstet Gynecol 148:566, 1984.

Maternal blood tests for complete blood cell count and hemoglobin electrophoresis can give evidence for α-thalassemia. Blood chemistry evaluations can yield evidence for fetal red blood cell enzyme deficiency. The Kleihauer-Betke test may yield evidence for significant fetal-maternal hemorrhage. Serologic evaluation can yield evidence for maternal-fetal infections. The glucose tolerance test may indicate maternal diabetes mellitus.

Ultrasonography is the most significant noninvasive means for evaluating the pregnancy to identify major causes of nonimmune hydrops.

Amniocentesis is of benefit for determining fetal karyotype with amniocyte culture. Additionally, microbiologic cultures of the amniotic fluid provide evidence of fetal infection. α-Fetoprotein can be measured for evidence of congenital nephrosis. Specific metabolic tests can be performed for glycogen storage diseases, and restriction endonuclease tests can be performed for α-thalassemia.

A more invasive technique involves aspiration of fetal blood by cordocentesis. This permits rapid karyotype evaluation and specific fetal metabolic tests. Immunologic, hematologic, and microbiologic evaluation of the fetal blood can be performed for the diagnosis of various chemical, infectious, and hematologic disorders (Fig. 19–16).

Sonographic Evaluation

The sonographic identification of the fetus with nonimmune hydrops is conceptually identical to the

Table 19–4. DIAGNOSTIC STEPS IN THE PRENATAL EVALUATION OF NONIMMUNE HYDROPS FETALIS

Levels of Diagnostic Invasiveness	Diagnostic Test	Possible Etiology
Maternal Noninvasive	Complete blood cell count and indices	Hematologic disorders
	Hemoglobin electrophoresis	α-Thalassemia
	Blood chemistry (e.g., maternal G6PD, pyruvate kinase carrier status)	Possibility of fetal red blood cell enzyme deficiency
	Betke-Kleihauer stain	Fetal-maternal transfusion
	Viral titers (coxsackievirus, parvovirus)	Fetal infection
	Syphilis (VDRL) and TORCH titers	
	Ultrasonography	Assessment of nonimmune hydrops fetalis and its progression, exclusion of multiple pregnancy and congenital malformations
	Fetal echocardiography	Congenital heart defects
		Rhythm disturbances of the fetal heart
	Oral glucose tolerance test	Maternal diabetes mellitus
Amniocentesis	Fetal karyotype	Chromosomal abnormalities
	Amniotic fluid culture	Cytomegalovirus
	α-Fetoprotein	Congenital nephrosis, sacrococcygeal teratoma
	Specific metabolic tests	Gaucher, Tay-Sachs, GM_1 gangliosidosis, etc.
	Restriction endonuclease tests	α-Thalassemia
Fetal blood aspiration	Rapid karyotype and metabolic tests	Chromosomal or metabolic abnormalities
	Hemoglobin chain analysis	Thalassemias
	Fetal plasma analysis for specific IgM	Intrauterine infection
	Fetal plasma albumin	Hypoalbuminemia
	Complete blood cell count	Fetal anemia

From Holzgreve W, Holzgreve B, Curry JR: Nonimmune hydrops fetalis: Diagnosis and management. Semin Perinatol 9:52, 1985.

identification of immune hydrops fetalis discussed previously. The sonographer searches for the classic findings of skin thickening greater than 5 mm, placental enlargement greater than 4 cm, ascites, pericardial effusion, pleural effusion, and polyhydramnios. In some studies, ascites alone is considered diagnostic of nonimmune hydrops fetalis.[47] Other studies are purposely skewed to severe nonimmune hydrops fetalis, requiring serous effusion in two body cavities or serous effusion in one body cavity in addition to anasarca for the diagnosis.[42] This lack of precision leads to variation in the cases included in a series of nonimmune hydrops fetalis. Furthermore, variations in the assigned significance of skin thickening (i.e., whether secondary to maternal diabetes or redundant integument in dwarfism) will affect whether a fetus and the associated findings are included in a series of nonimmune hydrops fetalis.

Although it is true that ascites can be seen in the hydropic state and may be the initial sign of impending decompensation into frank nonimmune hydrops fetalis, when it occurs alone it is most often from a local rather than a generalized condition. As an isolated finding, ascites has often been associated with urinary and intestinal tract obstruction.[54] Fetuses displaying only ascites, unassociated with generalized hydrops, have a better prognosis and should be considered separately. Those fetuses with isolated ascites require careful follow-up to exclude the development of generalized hydrops (Figs. 19–17 and 19–18). I believe that the diagnosis of nonimmune hydrops fetalis should be made only when there are either serous effusions in two body cavities or serous effusion in one cavity in addition to anasarca (Figs. 19–19 through 19–21). With

these criteria, when the diagnosis of nonimmune hydrops is made, the poor prognosis reported to the parents is likely to be realistic.

Pleural effusion can be diagnosed when fluid is demonstrated in the supradiaphragmatic location within the thorax. This appearance, however, can be mimicked by ascites that is present in a diaphragmatic hernia. Several studies have concluded that pulmonary hypoplasia is a major cause of death in fetuses with nonimmune hydrops fetalis.[40, 43] It has been proposed that the pleural effusions that frequently accompany nonimmune hydrops fetalis are responsible for the pulmonary hypoplasia. Therefore, attempts have been made to ameliorate the development of pulmonary hypoplasia by aspirating the fetal pleural effusions. One study that reviewed the literature concludes that prenatal therapy for pleural effusion is recommended when accompanied by hydrops fetalis, particularly at a gestational age of less than 32 weeks.[55] Another study suggests that the occurrence of pleural effusions in hydrops is most frequently associated with fetuses not experiencing anemia.[56]

Placental thickening greater than 4 cm is considered abnormal; however, in the presence of polyhydramnios, abnormal placental thickness may be present with measurements less than 4 cm. The placental thickening appears to correlate with disorders having abnormal umbilical blood flow, such as fetal anemia.[56] Placental thickening is also associated with fetal cardiac abnormalities.[42]

Polyhydramnios is identified in up to 75% of fetuses with nonimmune hydrops.[41] It may play a role in the development of prematurity among fetuses with nonimmune hydrops (95% delivered at less than 37 weeks'

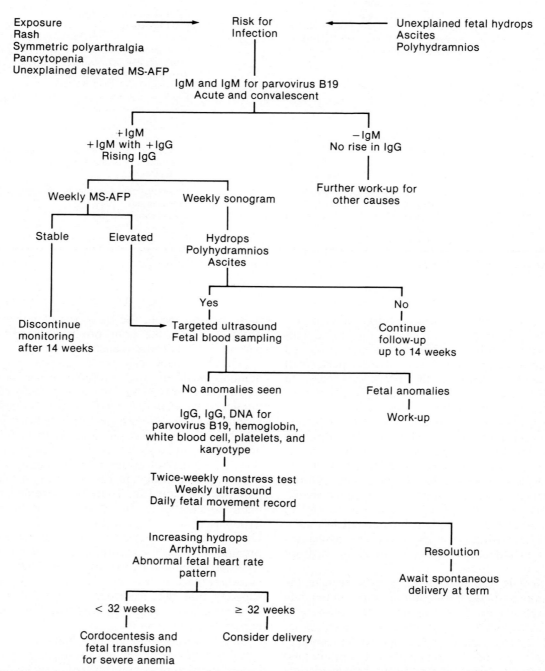

Figure 19–16. Diagnostic evaluation in the fetus with suspected parvovirus infection. (From Sheikh AF, Ernest M, O'Shea M: Long-term outcome in fetal hydrops from parvovirus B19 infection. Am J Obstet Gynecol 167:337, 1992.)

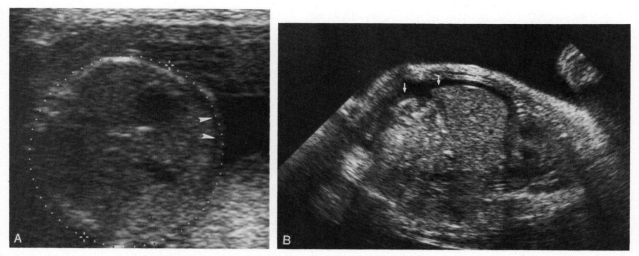

Figure 19–17. Development of nonimmune hydrops due to severe fetomaternal hemorrhage. *A.* Transverse view of fetal abdomen before onset of hydrops. Note pseudoascites *(arrowheads). B.* Sagittal view of fetus after development of nonimmune hydrops. Note the sonolucent ascites *(arrows)* outlining the bowel and liver. Note subcutaneous edema.

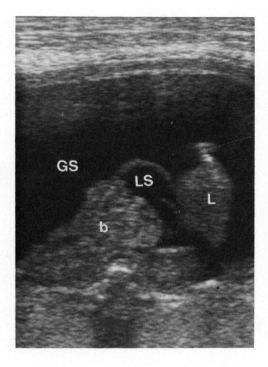

Figure 19–18. Sagittal view of fetal abdomen. Massive amount of ascites is present in the greater sac (GS) and lesser sac (LS). Note the absence of amniotic fluid. L, liver; b, bowel.

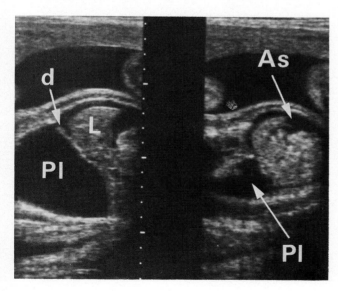

Figure 19–19. Sagittal images of the chest and abdomen, depicting a large pleural effusion (Pl) and ascites (As). d, diaphragm; L, liver.

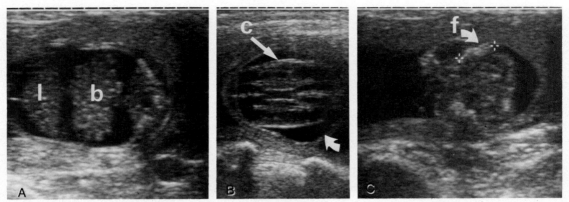

Figure 19–20. Severe nonimmune hydrops fetalis in hypophosphatasia dwarfism. *A.* Coronal view of the fetal abdomen, displaying ascites surrounding the liver (l) and bowel (b). *B.* Transverse axial images of the fetal head, depicting massive scalp edema *(arrow).* Note the poorly mineralized calvaria (c) due to hypophosphatasia. *C.* Short, poorly mineralized femur (f).

gestation).[37] Oligohydramnios associated with nonimmune hydrops has a very poor prognosis. It is seen not infrequently with homozygous α-thalassemia[52] and with severe lymphangiectasia.

The definition of skin thickening is skin that is greater than 5 mm of thickness. In one series, the finding of marked skin thickening was more commonly seen in fetuses without anemia when compared with those fetuses with anemia.[56]

Fetuses with generalized skin thickening (anasarca) or severe lymphatic dysplasia (diffuse lymphangiectasia) have an extremely poor prognosis (Figs. 19–22 through 19–24). It is important to distinguish these fetuses with generalized skin thickening from the fetus with localized skin thickening.

Cystic hygroma is a type of localized skin thickening usually occurring in the neck (Figs. 19–25 and 19–26). Cystic hygromas are seen in over one third of fetuses with nonimmune hydrops fetalis,[38] and it is hypothesized that abnormal lymphatic development causes these lesions. They are frequently associated with Turner syndrome. Cystic hygromas do not invariably progress to diffuse lymphangiectasia. On the contrary, in one series of fetuses with first- and second-trimester cystic hygromas, the cystic hygromas completely re-

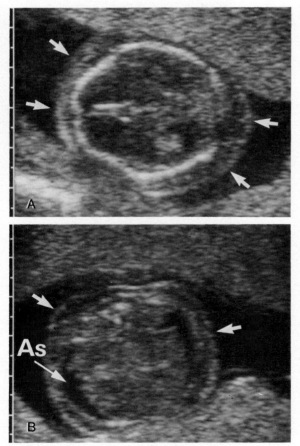

Figure 19–21. *A.* Transverse axial images of the fetal head, demonstrating scalp edema *(arrows).* *B.* Transverse axial images of the upper abdomen, demonstrating integumentary edema *(arrows)* and a rim of ascites (As).

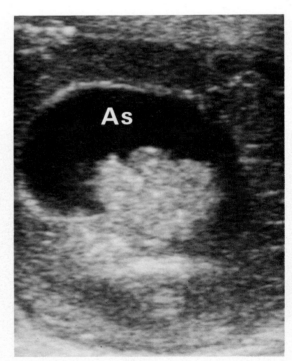

Figure 19–22. Transverse view of fetal abdomen in diffuse lymphangiectasia. Note ascites (As), marked subcutaneous edema, and oligohydramnios.

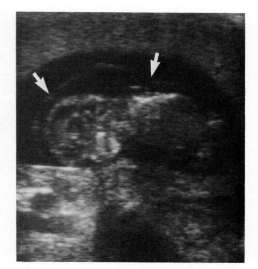

Figure 19–23. Nonimmune hydrops fetalis secondary to generalized lymphangiectasia. Longitudinal scan in a fetus of 11 to 12 menstrual weeks. Note the severe integumentary edema *(arrows)*. This should be differentiated from the amnion.

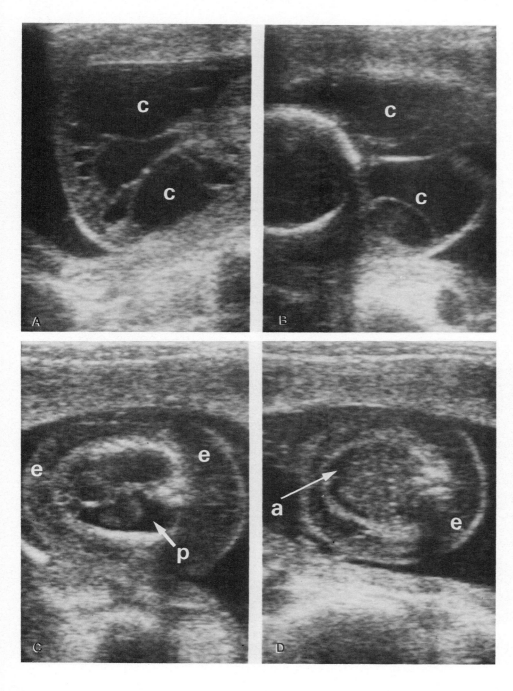

Figure 19–24. *A* and *B*. Diffuse lymphangiectasia. Large cystic hygromas (c) in *(A)* nuchal and *(B)* occipital regions. *C*. Transverse axial view of the fetal thorax, demonstrating integumentary edema (e) and pleural effusions (p). *D*. Transverse axial view of the fetal abdomen, demonstrating integumentary edema (e) and a thin rim of ascites (a).

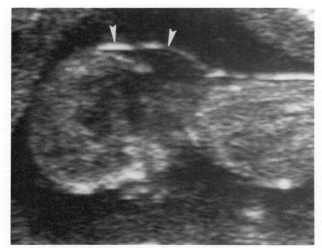

Figure 19–25. Sagittal view of small nuchal cystic hygroma *(arrowheads)*.

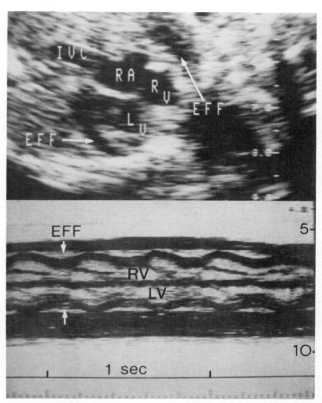

Figure 19–27. Pericardial effusion. Two-dimensional and M-mode ultrasound evaluation of fetus with a pericardial effusion (EFF). IVC, inferior vena cava; RA, right atrium; RV, right ventricle; LV, left ventricle.

solved in 37% of the fetuses, of which all were completely normal at birth.[57]

Pericardial effusion defined as at least a 2-mm hypoechogenic cardiac rim is necessary to substantiate that the pericardial fluid collection is abnormal.[25] DeVore[58] reported that isolated pericardial effusion was one of the earliest sonographic findings of hydrops in fetuses with cardiac anomalies. This observation has been supported by Shenker and colleagues,[59] who noted that in a series of fetuses with pericardial effusion, fetal heart failure was the predominant cause (Figs. 19–27 and 19–28). The major causes of heart failure in that series were tachyarrhythmias, congenital heart disease, and twin transfusion syndrome.

In addition to identifying the hydropic status of the fetus, ultrasonography can identify associated fetal structural abnormalities in 25% to 40% of cases.[37, 41] Since nearly every organ of the fetus may display an abnormality that has been associated with nonimmune hydrops fetalis, careful systematic sonographic evalu-

ation is required. Special attention must be given to the cardiovascular system, owing to the high frequency of structural abnormalities and arrhythmias.

The use of ultrasound in directing fetal intervention

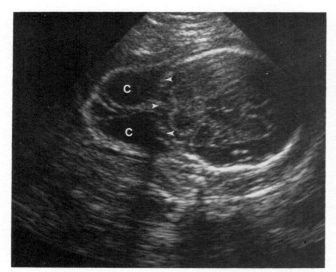

Figure 19–26. Transverse view of a large septated nuchal cystic hygroma (c). Note the intact calvarium *(arrowheads)*, which distinguishes this entity from an encephalocele.

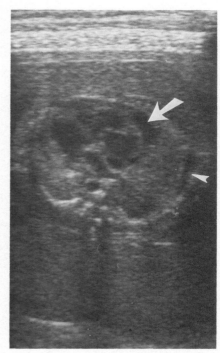

Figure 19–28. Nonimmune hydrops in congenital heart block. Heart rate is 47 beats per minute. Note the pericardial effusion *(large arrow)* and pleural effusion *(arrowhead)*.

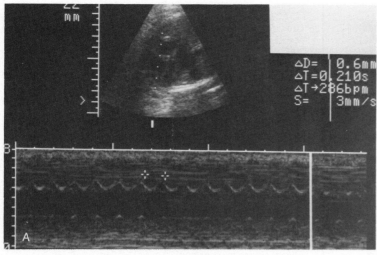
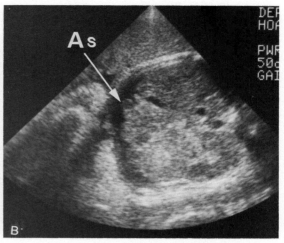

Figure 19–29. Nonimmune hydrops fetalis in a fetus with supraventricular tachycardia. *A.* Four-chamber heart view of M-mode sonogram demonstrating tachyarrhythmia with a heart rate equal to 286 beats per minute. *B.* Transverse view of the fetal abdomen, showing ascites (As).

will likely play a greater role. In addition to ultrasound guidance of cordocentesis, this modality plays a significant role in the guidance of other fetal interventive therapy, such as fetal pleural effusion aspiration and drainage. Ultrasound guidance of intrauterine transfusions in fetal nonimmune anemia has been reported.[60] Ultrasound monitoring of the fetus following therapy is valuable.

Prognosis

In general, the prognosis of nonimmune hydrops fetalis is poor. The mortality rate ranges from 50% to 98%.[39–40] The sonographic identification of a fetal structural abnormality in a fetus with nonimmune hydrops indicates a perinatal risk of mortality approaching 100%.[37, 41, 61] Generalized lymphangiectasia is nearly always fatal.[62] A major exception, however, is nonimmune hydrops fetalis associated with fetal arrhythmias. Cardiac fetal arrhythmias are among the most treatable causes of nonimmune hydrops fetalis (Fig. 19–29).

Two series evaluated the utility of sonographic findings to predict the fetal outcome. Based on the collective experience with immune hydrops fetalis, one would anticipate a worse prognosis in nonimmune hydrops in those fetuses displaying anasarca and large serous effusions. However, in these two analyses of sonographic features, the prognosis could not be predicted.[42, 47] These analyses, however, were based on a single observation. Serial sonographic evaluations of the fetus with nonimmune hydrops fetalis remain useful to identify improvement or worsening of the fetal pathophysiologic state. Despite the dismal clinical outcome of fetuses with nonimmune hydrops fetalis, it is useful to keep in mind several instances of spontaneous resolution of sonographically severe nonimmune hydrops fetalis.[63–66]

Although nonimmune hydrops fetalis remains poorly understood, a few generalizations concerning the utility of ultrasonography can be made:

1. Ultrasonography is the pivotal examination in identifying nonimmune hydrops fetalis.

2. A sonographically demonstrated structural fetal anomaly in the setting of nonimmune hydrops implies a very poor prognosis. Generalized congenital lymphangiectasia is nearly always fatal.

3. The cardiovascular system is the most frequent organ system affected in identifiable causes of nonimmune hydrops fetalis among North American and Northern European populations. Arrhythmias are among the fetal anomalies that are most amenable to therapy.

4. Knowledge of the etiology of nonimmune hydrops fetalis and the fetal karyotype in fetuses with nonimmune hydrops will determine whether aggressive management is warranted.

Thus, sonography plays a pivotal role in the diagnosis and management of the hydropic fetus.

References

1. Ballantyne JW: The Disease of the Fetus. Edinburgh, Oliver & Boyd, 1982. Cited in Potter EL: Universal edema of the fetus unassociated with erythroblastosis. Am J Obstet Gynecol 46:130, 1943.
2. Levine P, Burnham L, Katzin EM, Vogel P: The role of isoimmunization in the pathogenesis of erythroblastosis fetalis. Am J Obstet Gynecol 42:925, 1941.
3. Landsteiner K, Weiner AS: Agglutinable factor in human blood recognized by immune sera for rhesus blood. Proc Soc Exp Biol Med 43:223, 1940.
4. Potter EL: Universal edema of the fetus unassociated with erythroblastosis. Am J Obstet Gynecol 46:130, 1943.
5. James LS: Shock in the newborn in relation to hydrops. Ann Obstet Ginecol Med Perinat 92:599, 1971.
6. Barnes SE: Hydrops fetalis. Mol Aspect Med 1:244, 1977.
7. Bowman JM: The management of Rh-isoimmunization. Obstet Gynecol 52:1, 1978.
8. Nicolaides KH, Clewell WH, Rodeck CA: Measurement of human fetoplacental blood volume in erythroblastosis fetalis. Am J Obstet Gynecol 157:50, 1987.
9. Phibbs RH, Johnson P, Tooley WH: Cardiorespiratory status of erythroblastotic newborn infants: II. Blood volume, hematocrit,

and serum albumin concentration in relation to hydrops fetalis. Pediatrics 53:13, 1974.

10. Frigoletto FD, Umansky I: Erythroblastosis fetalis: Identification, management, and prevention. Clin Perinatol 6:321, 1979.

11. Reece EA, Copel JA, Scioscia AL: Diagnostic fetal umbilical blood sampling in the management of isoimmunization. Am J Obstet Gynecol 159:1057, 1988.

12. Sherer DM, Abramowicz JS, Ryan RM: Severe fetal hydrops resulting from ABO incompatibility. Obstet Gynecol 78:898, 1991.

13. Weiner CP, Williamson RA, Wenstrom KD: Management of fetal hemolytic disease by cordocentesis: I. Prediction of fetal anemia. Am J Obstet Gynecol 165:546, 1991.

14. Parer JT: Severe Rh isoimmunization: Current methods of in utero diagnosis and treatment. Am J Obstet Gynecol 158:1323, 1988.

15. Nicolaides KH, Rodeck CH, Bibashan RS, Kemp JR: Have Liley charts outlived their usefulness? Am J Obstet Gynecol 155:90, 1986.

16. Spinnato JA, Ralston KK, Greenwell ER: Amniotic fluid bilirubin and fetal hemolytic disease. Am J Obstet Gynecol 165:1030, 1991.

17. American College of Obstetricians and Gynecologists: Management of isoimmunization in pregnancy. Technical Bulletin No. 90. Washington, DC, 1986.

18. Lowe TW, Leveno KJ, Quirk JB, et al. Sinusoidal fetal heart rate pattern after intrauterine transfusion. Obstet Gynecol 64:215, 1984.

19. Weiner CP, Williamson RA, Weinstrom KD: Management of fetal hemolytic disease by cordocentesis: II. Outcome of treatment. Am J Obstet Gynecol 165:1302, 1991.

20. Chitkara U, Wilkins I, Lynch L: The role of sonography in assessing severity of fetal anemia in Rh- and Kell-isoimmunized pregnancies. Obstet Gynecol 71:393, 1988.

21. Benacerraf BR, Frigoletto FD: Sonographic sign for the detection of early fetal ascites in the management of severe isoimmune disease without intrauterine transfusion. Am J Obstet Gynecol 152:1039, 1985.

22. Hashimoto BE, Filly RA, Callen PW: Fetal pseudoascites: Further anatomic observations. J Ultrasound Med 5:151, 1986.

23. DeVore G, Donnerstein R, Kleinman C, et al: Fetal echocardiography: II. The diagnosis and significance of a pericardial effusion in the fetus using real-time directed M-mode ultrasound. Am J Obstet Gynecol 144:693, 1982.

24. Jeanty P, Romero R, Hobbins JG: Fetal pericardial fluid: A normal finding of the second half of gestation. Am J Obstet Gynecol 149:529, 1984.

25. Shenker L, Reed K, Anderson CF: Fetal pericardial effusion. Am J Obstet Gynecol 160:1505,1989.

26. Warsof SL, Nicolaides KH, Rodeck C: Immune and nonimmune hydrops. Clin Obstet Gynecol 29:533, 1986.

27. Vintzileos A, Campbell WA, Storlazzi E, et al: Fetal liver ultrasound measurements in isoimmunized pregnancies. Obstet Gynecol 68:162, 1986.

28. Roberts AB, Mitchell JM, Pattison NS: Fetal lung length in normal and isoimmunized pregnancies. Am J Obstet Gynecol 161:42, 1989.

29. Hoddick WK, Mahony BS, Callen PW, Filly RA: Placental thickness. J Ultrasound Med 4:479, 1985.

30. Harman CR, Manning FA, Bowman JM, Lange IR: Severe Rh disease: Poor outcome is not inevitable. Am J Obstet Gynecol 145:823, 1983.

31. DeVore G, Mayden K, Tortora M, et al: Dilation of the fetal umbilical vein in rhesus hemolytic anemia: A predictor of severe disease. Am J Obstet Gynecol 141:464, 1981.

32. Mayden K: The umbilical vein diameter in Rh isoimmunization. Med Ultrasound 4:119, 1980.

33. Witter FR, Graham D: The utility of ultrasonically measured umbilical vein diameters in isoimmunized pregnancies. Am J Obstet Gynecol 146:225, 1983.

34. Reece EA, Gabriella S, Abdulla M, et al: Reassessment of the utility of fetal umbilical vein diameter in the management of isoimmunization. Am J Obstet Gynecol 159:937, 1988.

35. Copel JA, Grannum PA, Green JJ, et al. Pulsed Doppler flow-velocity waveforms in the prediction of fetal hematocrit of the

36. Bowman JM: Suppression of Rh-isoimmunization. Obstet Gynecol 52:385, 1978.

37. IM SS, Rizos N, Joutsi P, et al: Nonimmunologic hydrops fetalis. Am J Obstet Gynecol 148:566, 1984.

38. Santolaya J, Alley D, Jaffe R, et al: Antenatal classification of hydrops fetalis. Obstet Gynecol 79:256, 1992.

39. Etches PC, Lemmons JA: Nonimmune hydrops fetalis: Report of 22 cases including three siblings. Pediatrics 64:326, 1979.

40. Hutchison A, Drew JA, Yu V, et al: Nonimmunologic hydrops fetalis: A review of 61 cases. Obstet Gynecol 59:247, 1982.

41. Castillo RA, DeVope LD, Hadi HA, et al: Nonimmune hydrops fetalis: Clinical experience and factors related to poor outcome. Am J Obstet Gynecol 155:812, 1986.

42. Mahony BS, Filly RA, Callen PW, et al: Severe nonimmune hydrops fetalis: Sonographic evaluation. Radiology 151:757, 1984.

43. Watson J, Campbell S: Antenatal evaluation and management in nonimmune hydrops fetalis. Obstet Gynecol 67:589, 1986.

44. Graves GR, Baskett TF: Nonimmune hydrops fetalis: Antenatal diagnosis and management. Am J Obstet Gynecol 148:563, 1984.

45. Brown B: The ultrasonographic features of nonimmune hydrops fetalis: A study of 30 successive patients. J Can Assoc Radiol 37:164, 1986.

46. Holzgreve W, Holzgreve B, Curry JR: Nonimmune hydrops fetalis: Diagnosis and management. Semin Perinatol 9:52, 1985.

47. Fleischer AC, Killam AP, Boehm FH, et al: Hydrops fetalis: Sonographic evaluation and clinical implications. Radiology 141:163, 1981.

48. Buttino L: Idiopathic non-immune hydrops: A common entity (Letter to the editor). Am J Obstet Gynecol 152:606, 1985.

49. Jauniaux E, Maldergem LV, De Munta C: Nonimmune hydrops fetalis associated with genetic abnormalities. Obstet Gynecol 75:585, 1990.

50. Kleinman C, Donnerstein, DeVore G, et al: Fetal echocardiography for evaluation of in utero congestive heart failure. N Engl J Med 306:568, 1982.

51. Holzgreve W, Curry CJR, Golbus MS, et al: Investigation of nonimmune hydrops fetalis. Am J Obstet Gynecol 150:805, 1984.

52. Hseih FJ, Chang FM, Ko TM, Chen HU: Percutaneous ultrasound-guided fetal blood sampling in management of nonimmune hydrops fetalis. Am J Obstet Gynecol 157:44, 1987.

53. Guy G, Coady DJ, Jansen V, et al: D-Thalassemia hydrops fetalis: Clinical and ultrasonographic considerations. Am J Obstet Gynecol 153:500, 1985.

54. Hadlock FP, Deter RL, Garcia-Pratt J, et al: Fetal ascites not associated with Rh incompatibility: Recognition and management with sonography. AJR 134:1225, 1980.

55. Weber AM, Philipson EH: Fetal pleural effusion: A review and meta-analysis for prognostic indicators. Obstet Gynecol 79:281, 1992.

56. Saltzman DH, Frigoletto FD, Harlow BL, et al: Sonographic evaluation of hydrops fetalis. Obstet Gynecol 74:106, 1989.

57. Bronshtein M, Rottem S, Yoffe N, et al: First-trimester and early second-trimester diagnosis of nuchal cystic hygroma by transvaginal sonography: Diverse prognosis of the septated from the non-septated lesion. Am J Obstet Gynecol 161:78, 1989.

58. DeVore G: The prenatal diagnosis of congenital heart disease: A practical approach for the actual sonographer. J Clin Ultrasound 13:229, 1985.

59. Shenker L, Reed KL, Anderson CF, et al: Fetal pericardial effusion. Am J Obstet Gynecol 160:1505, 1989.

60. Cardwell MS: Successful treatment of hydrops fetalis caused by fetomaternal hemorrhage: A case report. Am J Obstet Gynecol 158:131, 1988.

61. Vintzileos A, Campbell WA, Nochimson DJ, Weinbaum PJ: Antenatal evaluation and management of ultrasonically detected fetal anomalies. Obstet Gynecol 69:640, 1987.

62. Weingast GR, Hopper KD, Gottesfeld SA, et al: Congenital lymphangiectasis with fetal cystic hygroma: Report of two cases with co-existent Down's syndrome. J Clin Ultrasound 16:663, 1988.

63. Humphrey W, Magoon M, O'Shaughnessy R: Severe nonim-

mune hydrops secondary to parvovirus B-19 infection: Spontaneous reversal in utero and survival of a term infant. Obstet Gynecol 78:900, 1991.

64. Mostello DJ, Bofinger MK, Siddigi T: Spontaneous resolution of fetal cystic hygroma and hydrops in Turner's syndrome. Obstet Gynecol 73:862, 1989.

65. Robertson L, Ott A, Mack L, Brown Z: Sonographically documented disappearance of non-immune hydrops fetalis associated with maternal hypertension. West J Med 143:382, 1985.

66. Shapiro T, Scharf M: Spontaneous intrauterine remission of hydrops fetalis in one identical twin: Sonographic diagnosis. J Clin Ultrasound 13:427, 1985.

CHAPTER 20

Ultrasound Evaluation of the Placenta and Umbilical Cord

RONALD R. TOWNSEND, M.D.

Examination of the placenta is an important part of every obstetric sonogram. It becomes of critical importance when there is any clinical indication of placental pathology, for example, in the setting of vaginal bleeding. Examination of the placenta and associated membranes can also give important diagnostic clues when fetal structural or growth abnormalities are questioned. Chorionicity and amnionicity of twin pregnancies can frequently be identified with this examination, providing important prognostic information.

The umbilical cord can also be readily examined with standard commercially available ultrasound equipment. Identification of a single umbilical artery increases the risk of fetal anomalies and should lead to a thorough evaluation for such anomalies. Examination of the cord is also particularly important in twin pregnancies. The ability to image the cord facilitates some invasive procedures, including umbilical venous blood sampling and in utero transfusion.

In this chapter, the normal development and sonographic appearances of the placenta and associated membranes are first discussed. Sonographic features of developmental and acquired placental abnormalities are then reviewed. Finally, normal and abnormal sonographic findings of the umbilical cord are discussed.

PLACENTAL DEVELOPMENT

The placenta functions as the primary site of nutrient and gas exchange between the fetal and maternal circulations. This function depends on the proper placental development from tissues derived from both the mother *(decidua)* and fetus *(chorion)*. The endometrial lining of the uterus develops into the decidual layers illustrated in Figure 20–1 under hormonal influence and the effects of the implanted blastocyst. The decidua basalis underlies the implantation site of the blastocyst and will subsequently interface with fetal chorionic tissues to form the placenta. The decidua capsularis overlies the implanted blastocyst and exists as a layer of tissue between the fetal chorionic tissues and the uterine cavity. The decidualized endometrium along the remainder of the inner surface of the uterus is known as the decidua parietalis (or decidua vera) (see Fig. 20–1).

In the process of blastocyst implantation in the uterus, fetally derived trophoblastic tissue invades the decidualized endometrium. In a complex series of events, trophoblastic and mesenchymal tissue (together

referred to as chorion) interact with maternally derived decidua to form a network of villi and sinusoidal spaces allowing close approximation of fetal and maternal circulations. This development at first proceeds around the entire surface of the gestational sac, involving chorion with decidua capsularis as well as basalis. Subsequently, however, the villi formed along the surface of the gestational sac opposite the implantation site (involving the decidua capsularis) atrophy. This part of the chorion is then referred to as the chorion laeve. The chorion at the base of the implantation site (interacting with the decidua basalis) is then known as the chorion frondosum, which will continue to develop into the definitive placenta (see Fig. 20–1). In the mid and late first trimester, the site of the chorion frondosum can be visualized sonographically as an area of apparent thickening in the echogenic decidualized endometrium (Fig. 20–2). A much more detailed discussion of placental development is available in the texts by Fox[1] or Benirschke and Kaufmann.[2]

The fully developed placenta has a discoid shape and a weight approximately one sixth that of the fetus.[2] From the maternal surface the placenta can be seen to consist of approximately 20 lobes of various size.[3]

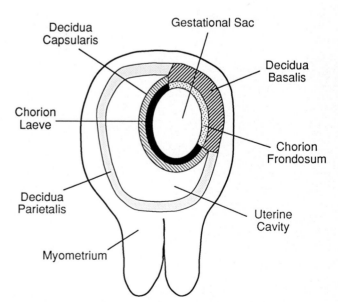

Figure 20–1. Diagram of the decidua and chorion associated with a first-trimester gestational sac. The chorion frondosum is the precursor of the placenta.

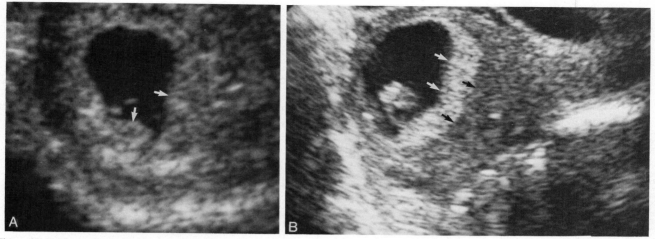

Figure 20–2. The early placenta. *A.* Focal thickening of the echogenic tissue (decidua plus chorion frondosum) at the margin of the gestational sac *(arrows)* indicates the site of the developing placenta (7.5 weeks menstrual age). *B.* The placenta *(white arrows)* is sharply defined from the subjacent hypoechoic myometrium *(black arrows)* in this 11-week gestation.

SONOGRAPHY OF THE NORMAL PLACENTA

Throughout pregnancy, the placenta is detectable as a relatively echogenic discoid mass of tissue, distinct from the hypoechoic subjacent myometrium (see Figs. 20–2 and 20–3). The margin of the placenta with the myometrium may be sharply defined by a network of vascular channels at the placental-myometrial junction referred to as the subplacental complex.[4, 5] Recognition of the interface of the placenta with the hypoechoic subjacent tissues is important to avoid false localizations of placentas. Near-field reverberation artifacts may mimic an anterior placenta, but the hypoechoic subplacental complex is not visualized deep to the pseudoplacenta in this situation. Focal myometrial

contractions or fibroids can also mimic masses of placental tissue.

The normal placenta increases in volume through gestation. It is possible to measure placental volume,[6] but the technique is cumbersome and, therefore, not commonly used clinically. The thickness of the placenta, however, can be readily measured sonographically. Hoddick and associates[7] evaluated placental thickness throughout gestation (Fig. 20–4). Measurement obtained at the mid placenta, perpendicular to the plane of the placenta, results in a mean thickness in millimeters approximately equal to the menstrual age in weeks. The thickness of a normal placenta rarely exceeds 4 cm, and no patient had a placenta thicker than 4 cm in the study by Hoddick and associates.[7] It should be noted that placentas with relatively small

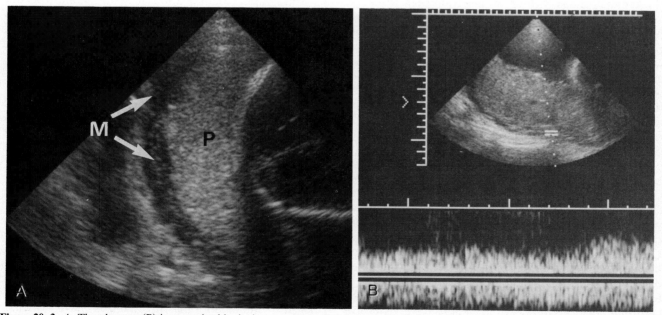

Figure 20–3. *A.* The placenta (P) is recognized by its increased echogenicity compared with the less echogenic myometrium (M). *B.* Doppler venous flow study. The poor echogenicity of the region adjacent to the placenta is in large part due to veins at the junction of the decidua basalis and myometrium.

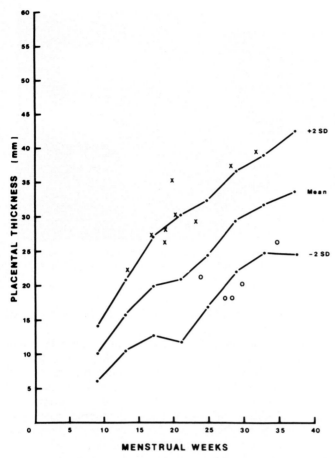

Figure 20–4. Relationship of placental thickness to menstrual age. The mean thickness of the placenta in millimeters is approximately equal to the menstrual age in weeks. (From Hoddick WK, Mahony BS, Callen PW, Filly RA: Placental thickness. J Ultrasound Med 4:479, 1985.)

myometrial insertion sites will tend to be somewhat thicker than those with broad insertion sites.

Calcium deposition occurs normally in the placenta.[3] Macroscopic areas of calcification become visible pathologically and sonographically in the third trimester. These macroscopic calcifications appear sonographically as bright intraplacental echoes, with or without acoustic shadowing.[8] Calcium may be deposited primarily along the basal plate of the placenta and along septa separating placental lobes. More than 50% of placentas show some sonographic evidence of calcification after 33 weeks.[9]

Some authors have found it useful to assign placentas a numerical grade (0 to III) based on the appearance of calcification within the placenta (Fig. 20–5).[8] If this classification is used, grade 0 is assigned to placentas without any visible calcification and with a smooth chorionic plate on the fetal surface of the placenta. Grade I placentas have scattered bright echoes reflecting scattered calcifications. Grade II indicates increased basal echogenicities and commalike echogenicities extending into the placenta from indentations of the chorionic plate. Grade III placentas have extensive basal echogenicity, and the curvilinear echogenicities extending from the chorionic plate reach the basal plate (Fig. 20–6). It was initially suggested that a grade III placenta was a reliable sign of fetal lung maturity,[8] but this has not proved to be definitive (see the discussion of sonography of fetal lung maturity in Chapter 21).

The homogeneous echotexture of the placenta may also normally be interrupted by hypoechoic or anechoic vascular spaces. These are described in the subsequent discussion of focal placental masses.

THE PLACENTA AND MEMBRANES IN TWIN GESTATIONS

The sonographic appearance of the placenta(s) and associated membranes can be used to differentiate twin pregnancies into groups of differing prognoses.[10] This sonographic analysis has become an important factor in the management of such patients and should be part of every obstetric sonogram performed in a multiple gestation.

A dizygotic pregnancy results from the development of two fertilized eggs (commonly referred to as fraternal twinning). With dizygotic twins, the development is as intuitively expected with the simultaneous development of two complete and separate but adjacent intrauterine pregnancies. The dizygotic pregnancy is, then, diamniotic (two amniotic sacs) and dichorionic (two chorions or two placentas).

Monozygotic (identical) twins result from division of a single fertilized egg. Depending on the time at which this division occurs, monozygotic twins may be either dichorionic (two placentas) or monochorionic (one placenta). Monochorionic/monozygotic twins may be either diamniotic (two amniotic sacs) or monoamniotic (one amniotic sac). Figure 20–7 illustrates the variable placentation in monozygotic twins, depending on the time at which division occurs.

Sonographic identification of two separate placental sites confirms that a twin pregnancy is dichorionic/diamniotic. These twins have the best overall prognosis among multiple gestations. If two placentas are not visualized, the pregnancy may still be dichorionic because two adjacent placentas may abut each other and appear as one.

Visualization of a membrane separating twin fetuses allows diagnosis of a diamniotic gestation, but the gestation may be either monochorionic or dichorionic if only one placental site is visualized. The sonographic appearance of the membrane may help in making this discrimination.[11, 12] The membrane separating gestational sacs consists of two layers of amnion in monochorionic/diamniotic pregnancies and two layers of chorion plus two layers of amnion in dichorionic/diamniotic pregnancies. Sonographic detection of a "thick" membrane suggests dichorionic/diamniotic gestation (Fig. 20–8), while detection of a "thin" membrane (Fig. 20–9) suggests monochorionic/diamniotic gestation. This distinction is important clinically because monochorionic pregnancies have vascular communications between the two gestations while dichorionic pregnancies do not. These vascular commu-

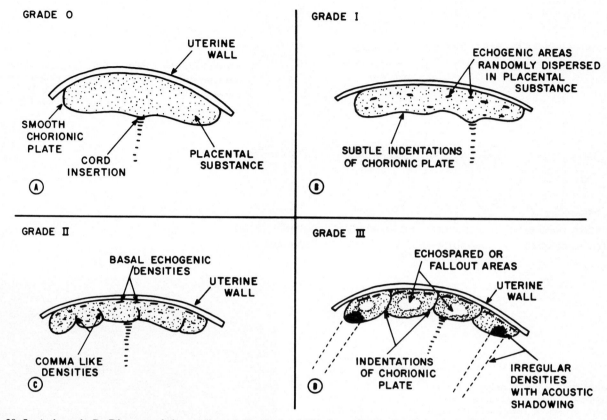

GRADE 0

UTERINE WALL

SMOOTH CHORIONIC PLATE

CORD INSERTION

PLACENTAL SUBSTANCE

Ⓐ

GRADE I

ECHOGENIC AREAS RANDOMLY DISPERSED IN PLACENTAL SUBSTANCE

SUBTLE INDENTATIONS OF CHORIONIC PLATE

Ⓑ

GRADE II

BASAL ECHOGENIC DENSITIES

UTERINE WALL

COMMA LIKE DENSITIES

Ⓒ

GRADE III

ECHOSPARED OR FALLOUT AREAS

UTERINE WALL

INDENTATIONS OF CHORIONIC PLATE

IRREGULAR DENSITIES WITH ACOUSTIC SHADOWING

Ⓓ

Figure 20–5. *A* through *D*. Diagram of the grading of placental calcifications. (From Grannum PAT, Berkowitz RL, Hobbins JC: The ultrasonic changes in the maturing placenta and their relation to fetal pulmonic maturity. Am J Obstet Gynecol 133:915, 1979.)

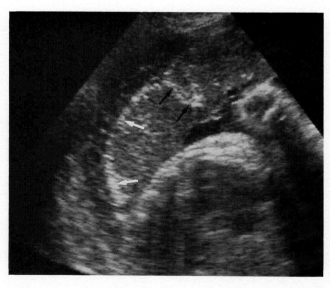

Figure 20–6. Grade III placenta with calcification along the base *(white arrows)* and interlobular septa *(black arrows)*.

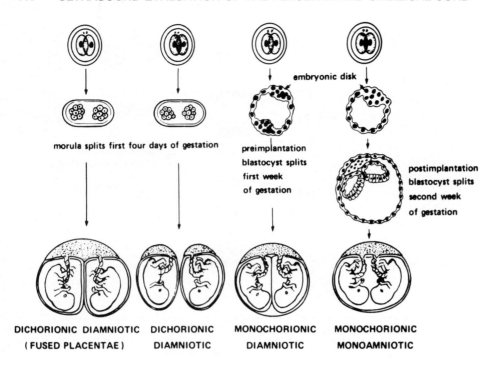

embryonic disk

morula splits first four days of gestation

preimplantation
blastocyst splits
first week
of gestation

postimplantation
blastocyst splits
second week
of gestation

Figure 20–7. Diagram of the development and placentation of monozygotic twins. (From Fox H: Pathology of the Placenta. Philadelphia, WB Saunders, 1978.)

DICHORIONIC DIAMNIOTIC
(FUSED PLACENTAE)

DICHORIONIC
DIAMNIOTIC

MONOCHORIONIC
DIAMNIOTIC

MONOCHORIONIC
MONOAMNIOTIC

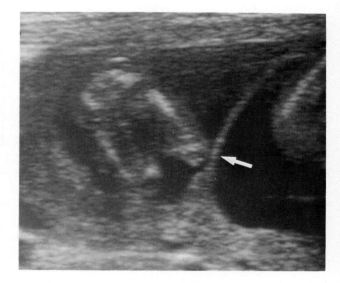

Figure 20–8. "Thick" membrane *(arrow)* in a dichorionic twin gestation at 15 weeks. The membrane was readily visible over its entire course. (From Townsend RR, Simpson GF, Filly RA: Membrane thickness in ultrasound prediction of chorionicity of twin gestations. J Ultrasound Med 7:327, 1988.)

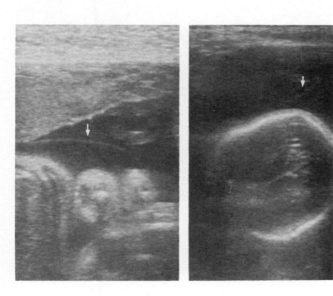

Figure 20–9. "Thin" membrane in two monochorionic/diamniotic gestations at 29 and 30 weeks. The membrane *(arrows)* was visualized in several short isolated segments in each case. (From Townsend RR, Simpson GF, Filly RA: Membrane thickness in ultrasound prediction of chorionicity of twin gestations. J Ultrasound Med 7:327, 1988.)

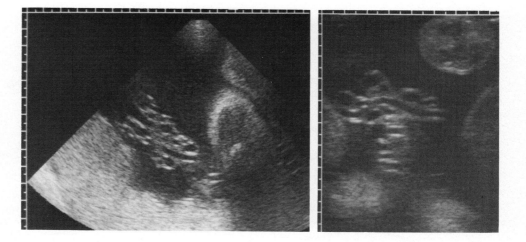

Figure 20–10. Entangled umbilical cords in monoamniotic twins. Images show entangled umbilical cords in two different twin pregnancies. In both cases the cords could be followed into this location from each fetus. (From Townsend RR, Filly RA: Sonography of nonconjoined monoamniotic twin pregnancies. J Ultrasound Med 7:665, 1988.)

nications make monochorionic pregnancies at risk for twin transfusion syndrome and for disseminated intravascular coagulation of a surviving twin following the death of one twin.

Lack of sonographic visualization of a membrane does not accurately predict monoamniotic gestation, because the thin membrane may be missed for technical reasons.[10–12] If the umbilical cords associated with the two fetuses are seen to entangle, a diagnosis of monoamniocity can safely be made (Fig. 20–10).[13, 14] This is important, since monoamniotic twins have an approximately 50% mortality due to knotting of the umbilical cords.

ABNORMALITIES OF PLACENTAL SHAPE

Developmental abnormalities of the placenta may result in shapes distinct from the usual discoid placenta. Normally, the placenta develops where chorionic villi interfacing with decidua basalis proliferate. Chorionic villi around the remainder of the gestational sac normally atrophy. Diffuse failure of this atrophy results in development of a thin layer of placenta covering nearly the entire surface of the uterine cavity and is referred to as *placenta membranacea*. This has been detected sonographically.[15] Focal failure of this atrophy may result in development of a focus of placental tissue separate from the main body of the placenta. This tissue is referred to as a *succenturiate,* or accessory, lobe of the placenta. This accessory lobe can be identified sonographically (Fig. 20–11).[16] It is important to identify and report the existence of an accessory lobe, because of the risk of postpartum bleeding and infection if it is not delivered along with the main body of the placenta. Rupture of the vessels connecting the main placenta to the accessory lobe can also lead to significant bleeding during labor and delivery.[16]

Placenta extrachorialis is an anomaly in which the chorionic plate of the placenta, from which the villi develop, is smaller than the basal plate (Fig. 20–12).[17] The interface between the fetal membranes and placenta may remain flat, referred to as a *circummarginate placenta*. This has no clinical significance.[17] If the margin is raised, often with a rolled edge, the condition is termed *circumvallate placenta*. This diagnosis has

been reported sonographically, with visualization of an infolding of fetal membranes and placenta on the fetal surface of the placenta (Fig. 20–13).[18] Circumvallate placenta is significant, being associated in various reports with vaginal bleeding, preterm labor, and possibly increased fetal mortality.[17, 18]

ABNORMAL PLACENTAL POSITION— PLACENTA PREVIA

The placenta may develop anywhere along the endometrial surface of the uterus, related to the site of

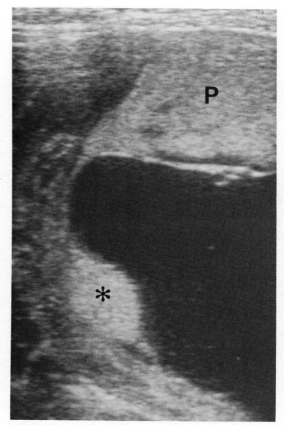

Figure 20–11. Succenturiate lobe of the placenta. The major portion of the placenta lies anteriorly (P). A small island of placental tissue *(asterisk)* is seen to lie in the fundus posteriorly.

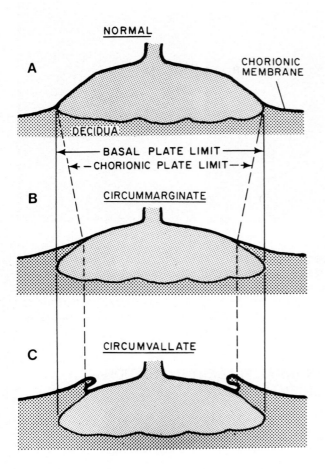

Figure 20–12. Diagram comparing extrachorial placentas with the normal placenta. *A.* Normal placenta. The transition of membranous to villous chorion is at the placental edge. *B.* Circummarginate placenta. The transition of membranous to villous chorion occurs central to the edge of the placenta, but the chorionic surface remains smooth. *C.* Circumvallate placenta. Appearance is as in *B* except for folding of the chorionic membrane. (From Spirt BA, Kagan EH: Sonography of the placenta. Semin Ultrasound 1:293, 1980.)

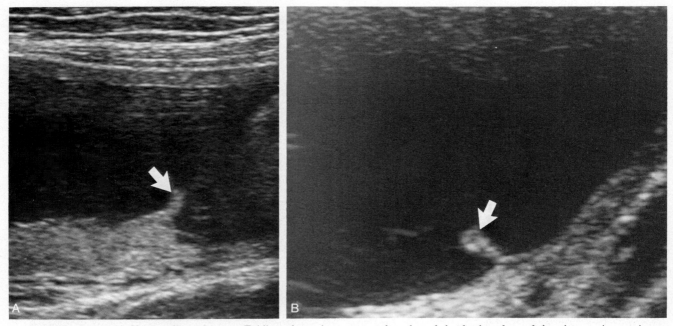

Figure 20–13. *A* and *B*. Circumvallate placenta. Folding of membranes near the edge of the fetal surface of the placenta is seen in two patients *(white arrows)*. Compare with Figure 20–12C.

blastocyst implantation. If the placenta implants over the internal cervical os (placenta previa), disastrous consequences can occur. Clinically, painless vaginal bleeding is the hallmark of placenta previa. This usually occurs in the third trimester but can occur as early as 20 weeks' gestation.[19] Massive vaginal bleeding can result in maternal and fetal death with attempted vaginal delivery in the presence of placenta previa. Cesarean section is required in patients with true complete placenta previa. There is an increased incidence of transverse fetal lie in the presence of placenta previa.

Although palpation of the placenta by vaginal examination has been the gold standard for diagnosis and categorization of placenta previa, ultrasonography has become the standard method for placental localization. Clinically, localization of the placenta is important not just if there is a question of previa but also if invasive procedures are contemplated for which knowledge of the position of the placenta may affect the way the procedure is performed. This includes contemplated cesarean section, amniocentesis, or other percutaneous procedures (e.g., umbilical venous sampling or in utero transfusion). A comment regarding placental position and presence or absence of previa should be part of every second or third trimester obstetric ultrasound report.

Various forms of placenta previa are recognized based on the exact relationship of the placenta to the internal cervical os (Fig. 20–14). A complete placenta previa is one in which the placenta is implanted on both sides of the internal cervical os, bridging the os. A central or symmetric complete previa is one in which the placenta is centered over the internal cervical os (Fig. 20–15). An asymmetric complete previa may have a large part of the placenta implanted on one side of the cervical os, but there is some attachment on the contralateral side. A partial placenta previa is one in which the placenta is implanted on only one side of

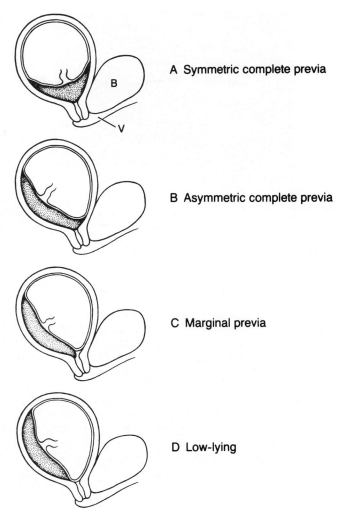

A Symmetric complete previa

B Asymmetric complete previa

C Marginal previa

D Low-lying

Figure 20–14. *A* through *D*. Classification of placental location in placenta previa. (From Nyberg DA, Callen PW: Ultrasound Evaluation of the Placenta. In Callen PW [ed.]: Ultrasonography in Obstetrics and Gynecology, 2nd ed, pp 297–322, Philadelphia, WB Saunders, 1988.)

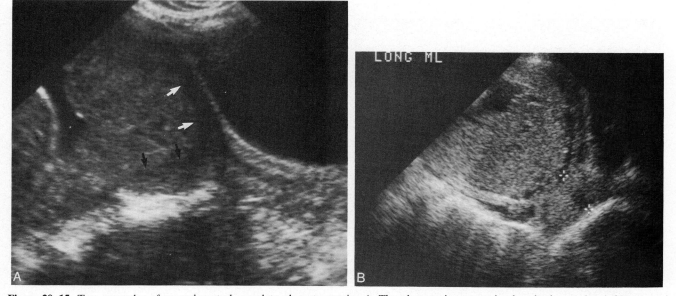

Figure 20–15. Two examples of proved central complete placenta previa. *A*. The placenta is seen to implant both anterior *(white arrows)* and posterior *(black arrows)* to the internal cervical os. There was no change in the appearance with bladder emptying. *B*. The placenta is centered over the area of the internal cervical os *(cursors)*.

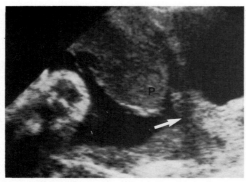

Figure 20–16. A partial anterior placenta previa (P) is seen next to the internal cervical os *(arrow)*. This diagnosis, made at 26 weeks, was confirmed at cesarean section performed because of persistent vaginal bleeding. (From Townsend RR, Laing FC, Nyberg DA, et al: Technical factors responsible for "placental migration": Sonographic assessment. Radiology 160:105–108, 1986.)

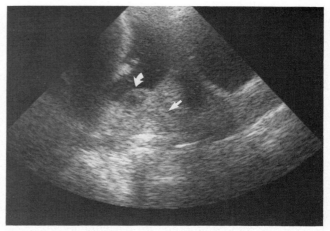

Figure 20–18. Marginal placenta previa with a prominent vein *(curved arrow)* at edge of placenta. The vein abuts the internal cervical os. Straight arrow indicates cervical canal.

the internal cervical os but partially covers it (Fig. 20–16). A marginal placenta previa ends at the margin of the cervical os without covering it (Fig. 20–17). Veins at the edge of the placenta may be related to bleeding if they abut the cervical os (Fig. 20–18).

Ultrasound cannot always reliably distinguish marginal from partial placenta previas and they are commonly grouped together. A placenta that is low lying but not a previa (extending close to, but not abutting, the internal cervical os) may still be significant. Bleeding complications, while not as frequent or severe as with previa, are more common in these gestations than are those with placentas farther from the internal cervical os.[20]

Placenta previa is observed in approximately 0.5% of pregnancies at the time of delivery.[19] Ultrasonography has proved to have a high sensitivity in detecting such abnormally low placentas but may result in a large number of false-positive diagnoses of this condi-

tion, particularly early in pregnancy. Early sonographic reports suggested that placenta previa is very common in the second trimester and was observed in up to 45% of patients.[21] The cause of this discrepancy appears to be multifactorial and will be explored below.

Attention to detail is essential in the sonographic diagnosis of placenta previa. Because of the potential disastrous consequences of missing a diagnosis of placenta previa, it is important not to underdiagnose this condition. On the other hand, a large number of false-positive diagnoses may result in unnecessary hospitalizations and cesarean sections. The goal of sonography, therefore, should be to maximize sensitivity for diagnosing placenta previa while minimizing false-positive diagnoses.

If the internal cervical os can be visualized at sonography and seen to be free of overlying placenta, placenta previa can reliably be excluded. If the internal os cannot be visualized, but the placenta is identified and is seen to end above the area of the os, placenta previa is unlikely but not definitively excluded. This is because of the possible existence of an accessory lobe of placenta at the cervical os. The initial sonographic approach to image the cervical os is generally made transabdominally in longitudinal projection with a full urinary bladder as a window to the lower uterus. If the initial image demonstrates placenta at the os, suggesting placenta previa, then several technical factors need to be considered before making that diagnosis.

An overly distended urinary bladder may compress the anterior myometrium of the lower uterus against the posterior myometrium, resulting in the apparent localization of the internal cervical os several centimeters proximal to its true location (Fig. 20–19).[22–24] A placenta that is low in position may then mimic a previa (Fig. 20–20). If the apparent length of the cervical canal is greater than approximately 3.5 cm it is likely that the cervix is being artificially lengthened related to bladder volume. Reimaging the patient after partial emptying of the bladder may allow placenta previa to be excluded.

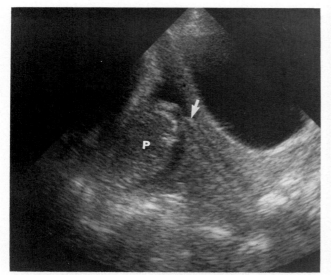

Figure 20–17. Marginal placenta previa. The end of this posterior placenta (P) is adjacent to the internal cervical os *(white arrow)*.

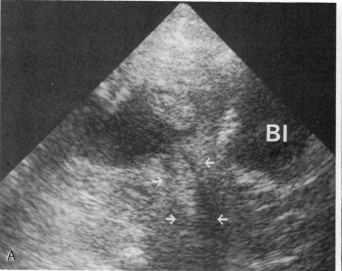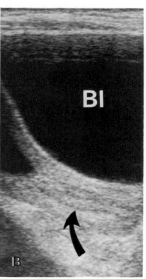

Figure 20–19. *A.* Normal cervical canal. Longitudinal scans demonstrate a normal cervical canal *(arrows)*, which is in a nearly vertical orientation because of an empty urinary bladder (Bl). *B.* With a full urinary bladder (Bl), the cervical canal *(arrow)* is in a more horizontal orientation. Also note that the cervical canal and lower uterine segment are artificially lengthened from compression by a distended urinary bladder.

Another common problem that may result in false-positive diagnosis of placenta previa is alteration of the anatomy of the lower uterus related to myometrial contraction (Fig. 20–21).[24, 25] The contraction may result in myometrial thickening, mimicking placenta. Alternatively, the contraction may lift the edge of the placenta against the cervical os, mimicking previa. If the myometrium appears to be thicker than approximately 1.5 cm, contraction should be considered and examination repeated after an appropriate delay, with 30 minutes usually being adequate.[24]

Even with attention to these considerations a large number of second-trimester sonographic diagnoses of placenta previa will be false positive. Townsend and coworkers[24] found that 72% of second-trimester diagnoses of placenta previa proved to be false positive. In their retrospective review, two thirds of the false-positive diagnoses could be explained by technical factors, including overly distended urinary bladders and contractions. However, no technical explanation could be found for one third of the false-positive diagnoses (Fig. 20–22). Importantly, no false-positive diagnoses of complete placenta previa were encountered. If attention is paid to technical considerations, it is unlikely that a second trimester diagnosis of complete previa, especially central complete previa, will prove to be in error (Fig. 20–23). However, most early diagnoses of marginal previa will be false positive (93%).[24]

Second-trimester false-positive diagnoses of placenta previa were attributed in early studies to "placental migration."[26] It is extremely unlikely that the placenta ever actually disrupts and re-forms its uterine attachment. The apparent motion appears to be a result of differential growth rates between the lower uterine segment and the placenta (Fig. 20–24). Relatively rapid growth of the myometrium just above the level of the cervix may make a placenta that initially appeared to be close to the cervical os several centimeters above the os at subsequent evaluation.

If difficulty is encountered in imaging the area of the internal cervical os with conventional transabdominal imaging with a full bladder, several alternative techniques are available to assist in making or excluding a diagnosis of placenta previa. Placement of the patient in the Trendelenburg position with use of gentle traction on the fetal head may allow visualization of the internal cervical os despite cephalic presentation with low position of the head.[27] One group of investigators has suggested that optimal images of the lower uterine segment may be obtained transabdominally with a completely empty urinary bladder.[25, 28] However, technical difficulties related to refractive shadowing at the

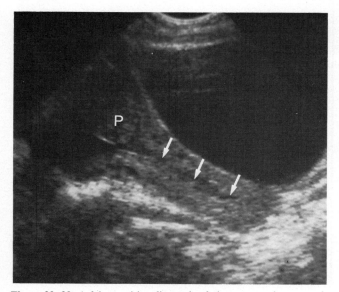

Figure 20–20. A false-positive diagnosis of placenta previa was made in this case owing to an overly distended urinary bladder, which resulted in elongation of the cervix to 7 cm. Arrows indicate artificially elongated endocervical canal. P, placenta. (From Townsend RR, Laing FC, Nyberg DA, et al: Technical factors responsible for "placental migration": Sonographic assessment. Radiology 160:105–108, 1986.)

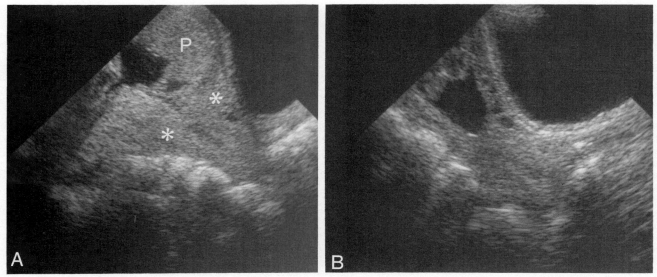

Figure 20–21. Myometrial contraction resulting in false-positive diagnosis of placenta previa. *A.* Lower uterine segment contraction of anterior and posterior uterine walls *(asterisks)* gives a false impression of placenta previa. P, placenta. *B.* Subsequent scan demonstrates resolution of the contraction.

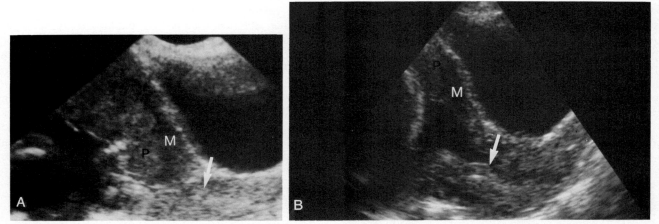

Figure 20–22. Second-trimester false-positive diagnosis of partial placenta previa without clear technical explanation. Arrow indicates internal cervical os. P, placenta; M, myometrium. *A.* Placenta is visible adjacent to the internal cervical os in the mid second trimester. *B.* Follow-up sonogram during the third trimester shows no evidence of placenta previa. For explanation, see Figure 20–24. (From Townsend RR, Laing FC, Nyberg DA, et al: Technical factors responsible for "placental migration": Sonographic assessment. Radiology 160:105–108, 1986.)

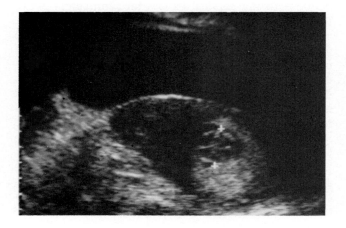

Figure 20–23. Early diagnosis of central placenta previa. A diagnosis of placenta previa was made at 13 weeks (as seen on this longitudinal image) and confirmed at cesarean section. Even a very early diagnosis of central complete placenta previa is unlikely to be false positive. (From Townsend RR, Laing FC, Nyberg DA, et al: Technical factors responsible for "placental migration": Sonographic assessment. Radiology 160:105–108, 1986.)

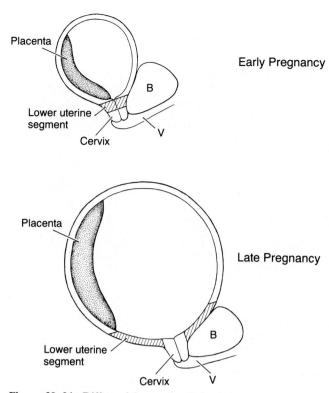

Figure 20–24. Differential growth of the lower uterine segment during pregnancy, explaining placental "migration." B, bladder; V, vagina. (From Nyberg DA, Callen PW: Ultrasound Evaluation of the Placenta. In Callen PW [ed.]: Ultrasonography in Obstetrics and Gynecology, 2nd ed, pp 297–322, Philadelphia, WB Saunders, 1988.)

bladder–uterine interface, acoustic shadowing from the pubic bones, and so on limit this technique, and it has not gained wide acceptance.

More recently, the ability to visualize the relationship of the placenta to the internal os with endovaginal scanning in cases of questioned placenta previa has been explored. Leerentveld and colleagues[29] evaluated 100 patients suspected of having placenta previa with this technique. They found a positive predictive value of 93% when placenta previa was diagnosed, much higher than with transabdominal technique. They had two false-negative examinations: sonographic diagnoses of low lying placentas that proved to be previas. Importantly, they found no evidence of aggravation of vaginal bleeding by the examination. The theoretical possibility of dislodging clots and causing significant bleeding with the endovaginal transducer has limited the willingness of some to attempt this examination. Although a real risk has not been documented with vaginal transducers, bleeding is a well-recognized complication of manual examination of the cervix in the attempt to clinically evaluate placenta previa.[19]

Another alternative technique to image the lower uterus and cervix is transperineal sonography.[30, 31] The examination is performed with a 3.5-MHz sector transducer positioned directly on the perineum, over the labia minora (Figs. 20–25 and 20–26). Hertzberg and colleagues[31] reported the application of this technique in the third trimester in cases of possible placenta previa. The internal cervical os and lower edge of the placenta can be well visualized (Fig. 20–27). Hertzberg

and colleagues found a positive predictive value of 90% and a negative predictive value of 100% for diagnosis of placenta previa by transperineal scanning. This examination is readily performed with the same transducer commonly used to image the fetus transabdominally and can rapidly visualize the internal cervical os in cases when that is not possible transabdominally.

Magnetic resonance imaging has also been performed to evaluate patients with possible placenta previa.[32, 33] With the availability of the newer sonographic techniques discussed earlier, this should hardly ever be necessary.

PLACENTA ACCRETA, INCRETA, PERCRETA

Placenta accreta is an abnormal adherence of the placenta to the underlying uterine wall. This has been attributed to complete or partial absence of the decidua basalis underlying the placenta, resulting in the placental villi adhering to the myometrium.[17] If the placental villi are attached to, but do not invade, the myome-

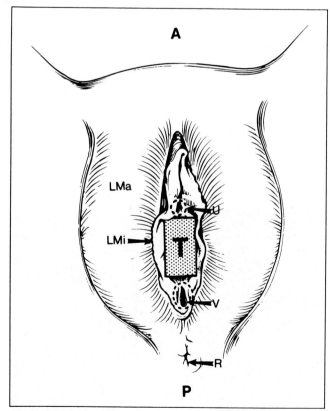

Figure 20–25. Diagram of perineum shows location of transducer (T) during transperineal sonography. The transducer is applied directly over the labia minora (LMi) in a sagittal plane just posterior to the urethra (U). Transducer location and angle are adjusted under sonographic control to optimize visualization of the cervix. A, anterior; LMa, labia majora; V, vaginal orifice; R, rectal orifice; P, posterior. (From Hertzberg BS, Bowie JD, Weber TM, et al: Sonography of the cervix during the third trimester of pregnancy: Value of the transperineal approach. AJR 157:73, 1991).

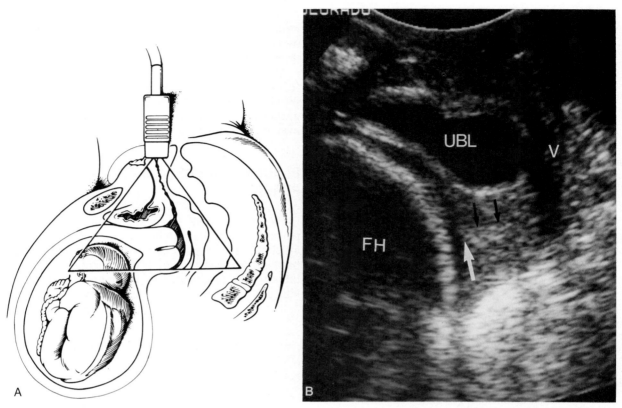

Figure 20–26. Transperineal sonography. *A.* Sagittal illustration of a gravid uterus in a supine patient with the transducer positioned on the perineum reveals the typical scanning plane obtained during transperineal sonography. *B.* Sagittal transperineal image of the pelvis. The internal cervical os is well seen *(white arrow),* and there is clearly no placenta at the os. Black arrows indicate cervical canal. FH, fetal head; UBL, urinary bladder; V, vagina. (A, from Hertzberg BS, Bowie JD, Weber TM, et al: Sonography of the cervix during the third trimester of pregnancy: Value of the transperineal approach. AJR 157:73, 1991.)

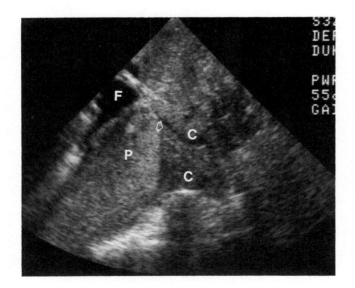

Figure 20–27. Complete placenta previa diagnosed by transperineal sonography. The sonogram shows placental tissue (P) covering the entire cervical os *(open arrow).* F, amniotic fluid; C, cervix. (From Hertzberg BS, Bowie JD, Carroll BA, et al: Diagnosis of placenta previa during the third trimester: Role of transperineal sonography. AJR 159:83, 1992.)

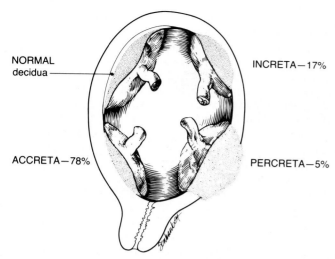

Figure 20–28. Differences between normal decidualization and placenta accreta, increta, and percreta. (From Benedetti TJ: Obstetric hemorrhage. In Gabbe SG, Niebyl JR, Simpson JL [eds]: Obstetrics: Normal and Problem Pregnancies. Churchill Livingstone, New York, 1986.)

trium, the condition is termed *placenta accreta* (Fig. 20–28). If the villi invade the myometrium, the condition is referred to as *placenta increta,* and if the villi penetrate completely through the myometrium to the serosal surface of the uterus, the term *placenta percreta* is applied. The term placenta accreta is commonly used as a generic term to refer to all three of these conditions together. The reported incidence of placenta accreta is extremely variable, ranging from less than 1 in 70,000 to approximately 1 in 500.[34] One factor contributing to this variability is the extent of pathologic proof required before this diagnosis is made.[17] It has been argued that the incidence of placenta accreta may be increasing.[35] Placenta accreta is much more common than are the more invasive conditions. In one reported series of 40 patients, 78% had placenta accreta, 17% had placenta increta, and 5% had placenta percreta.[34] Placenta accreta is more common in multiparous females, especially those with previous cesarean section. It is thought that implantation of the placenta over a scar is an important predisposing condition. There is a high association with placenta previa, which has similar predisposing factors.[36, 37]

The morbidity of placenta accreta is related to the fact that it may be difficult or impossible to completely extract the placenta after delivery. Severe bleeding may result, and there is increased risk of postpartum infection related to retained placental fragments. Hysterectomy is frequently required, especially with placenta increta or percreta. Placenta percreta may result in invasion of adjacent organs, especially the bladder.

The sonographic diagnosis of placenta accreta is difficult. Lack of visualization of a hypoechoic myometrium subjacent to the placenta may suggest the diagnosis (Fig. 20–29).[36–38] With placenta percreta, ultrasound evaluation may detect tissue extension into adjacent organs, especially the urinary bladder. The sonographic diagnosis of placenta accreta is more readily made with anterior placentas, related to better

visualization of the placental-myometrial interface at this location. Two recent reports described increased numbers of sonolucent placental masses (vascular spaces) in patients with placenta accreta.[36, 37]

Finberg and Williams[37] have reported sonographic findings of placenta accreta in a prospective study. Although placenta accreta is rare, these investigators selected a population of pregnancies with a combination of history of cesarean section, placenta previa, and placenta located along the lower anterior uterine wall as a high risk group for this condition. Their sonographic criteria for diagnosis of placenta accreta (collectively, including increta and percreta) were (1) absence or severe thinning of the hypoechoic myometrium between the placenta and the uterine serosa–bladder wall; (2) thinning, irregularity, or disruption of the linear hyperechoic uterine serosa–bladder wall complex; and (3) extension of tissue of placental echogenicity beyond the uterine serosa.[37] They made true positive diagnoses in 14 of 18 patients and true negative diagnoses in 15 of 16 patients. Thus, in high-risk patients, accurate prospective sonographic diagnosis of placenta accreta may be possible.

PLACENTAL ABRUPTION AND HEMATOMA

The normal placenta separates from the underlying myometrium at the time of delivery. Placental abruption has been defined as premature separation of a normally implanted placenta.[39] Classically, this is associated with pain and vaginal bleeding. There can be devastating consequences to the mother and fetus. However, there is a wide spectrum of clinical, pathologic, and sonographic findings related to hematomas associated with a normally implanted placenta. These conditions, focusing particularly on the role of sonog-

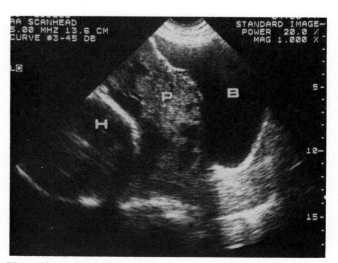

Figure 20–29. Sagittal middle sonogram of the lower uterine segment at 35 to 37 weeks' gestation reveals partial placenta previa and the absence of the hypoechoic zone peripheral to the placenta (P), which abuts the dome of the bladder (B). Invasion of the bladder wall is suspected from this view and was confirmed surgically. H, fetal head. (From Hoffman-Tretin JC, Koenigsberg M, Rabin A, Anyaegbunam A: Placenta accreta: Additional sonographic observations. J Ultrasound Med 11:29, 1992.)

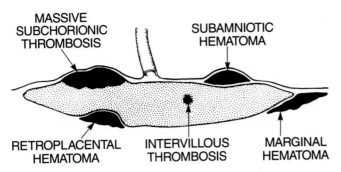

MASSIVE
SUBCHORIONIC
THROMBOSIS

SUBAMNIOTIC
HEMATOMA

RETROPLACENTAL
HEMATOMA

INTERVILLOUS
THROMBOSIS

MARGINAL
HEMATOMA

Figure 20–30. Sites of hemorrhage in and around the placenta, which have been described pathologically. (From Fox H: Pathology of the Placenta. London, WB Saunders, 1978.)

raphy, are discussed below. Evaluation of bleeding related to the abnormally implanted placenta (placenta previa) has been discussed previously.

Pathologically, several varieties of hematoma related to the placenta have been described (Fig. 20–30). Although pathologic analysis may provide the definitive diagnosis, ultrasonography has the advantage of evaluating the placenta and the hematoma present during fetal life and may allow prognostication as well as follow-up evaluation during the pregnancy.

The clinical picture accompanying placental hemorrhage is extremely variable, related to the site of bleeding, size of the hematoma, gestational age, chronicity of the bleeding, and the underlying disease process. With severe abruption the classic clinical picture consists of severe pain, which may be described as tearing, knifelike, and unremitting.[19] External bleeding may be moderate or may not be present. The fetus is frequently stillborn. Shock and consumptive coagulopathy may be expected.[19] With mild abruption there may be no symptoms other than painless vaginal bleeding, mimicking placenta previa. The nature of the pathology and sonographic findings may vary dramatically with these different clinical presentations. However, it has been pointed out that clinical abruption and pathologic demonstration of premature separation of the placenta do not always coincide, but that the outlook for the infant is worse when the two do coincide.[40]

Retroplacental hematoma separates the basal plate of the placenta from the uterine wall (Fig. 20–31). This type of hematoma has been reported pathologically in approximately 4.5% of all placentas.[41] This is much higher than the clinical incidence of abruption (approximately 1%[42]), and most small retroplacental hematomas are asymptomatic.[41] However, larger hematomas may have devastating consequences. The presence of this hematoma results in placental infarction by separation of placental villi from the maternal blood vessels. If the hematoma involves more than 30% to 40% of the maternal surface of the placenta then there will likely be significant hypoxia to the fetus.[41] This may result in fetal growth retardation or death. Retroplacental bleeding appears to be related to hemorrhage from spiral arteries.[3] The cause of this bleeding is not known in many cases, but maternal

hypertension is commonly a factor. It can be seen with abdominal trauma and it is commonly associated with preeclampsia. Retroplacental hematoma may complicate cocaine abuse, presumably related to the hypertensive and vasoconstrictive effects of cocaine.[43]

Marginal hematomas are seen at the periphery of the placenta and commonly elevate the edge of the placenta slightly (see Fig. 20–31). The hematoma extends away from the placenta in a subchorionic position. In some situations the subchorionic hematoma may be seen in a site remote from the placenta and is presumed to have originated from bleeding at the margin of the placenta. This type of hematoma is thought to be related to bleeding from veins at the margin of the placenta.[41] This low pressure bleeding is generally associated with fewer sequelae than arterial retroplacental hemorrhage but may be significant. The etiology of this condition is frequently unknown, but the associated pathologic finding of decidual necrosis at the placental margin has been associated with maternal cigarette smoking.[44]

Reports of the usefulness of sonography in diagnosis of hematomas related to abruption have been variable. Hurd and colleagues[45] reviewed 59 cases of pathologically proven placental abruption and found ultrasonography useful only in excluding placenta previa. In only one case was a subchorionic hematoma identified on ultrasound evaluation. The presence of a normal ultrasound study certainly does not exclude the possibility of placental abruption. It has been pointed out that the ultrasound examination may be negative despite bleeding if all of the blood leaves the uterus through the cervical canal without a sonographically detectable hematoma accumulation.[46]

However, with attention to detail and high-resolution ultrasound equipment, ultrasonography can detect hematomas in many patients and provide useful prognostic information. Retroplacental hematoma may be

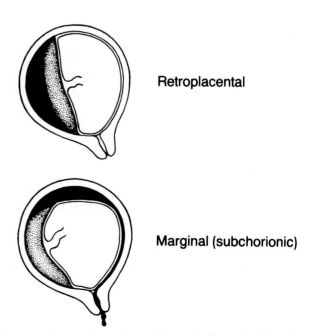

Retroplacental

Marginal (subchorionic)

Figure 20–31. Locations of retroplacental and marginal abruptions.

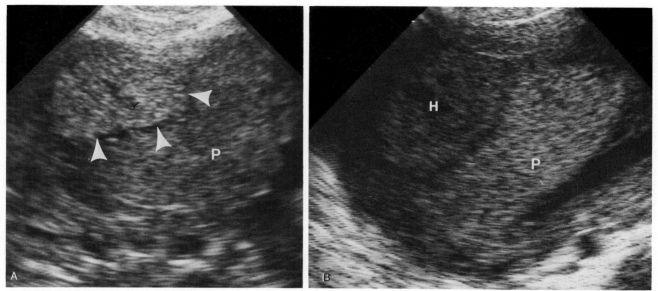

Figure 20–32. *A.* Retroplacental hematoma. Initial sonogram at 25 weeks' gestation demonstrates a large hyperechoic hematoma *(arrowheads)* beneath the placenta (P). *B.* Repeat sonogram 1 week later shows that the hematoma (H) has become hypoechoic relative to the placenta (P). There was subsequent fetal death. (From Hurd WW, Miodovinik M, Hertzberg V, Lavin JP: Selective management of abruptio placentae: A prospective study. Obstet Gynecol 61:467, 1983.)

detected as an area of hypoechoic material (blood) separating the placenta from the underlying myometrium. However, the appearance varies with the age of the hematoma (Fig. 20–32).[47–49] An acute hematoma may be echogenic and isoechoic with the overlying placenta (Fig. 20–33). It may only be detectable as an apparent area of thickening within the placenta (Fig. 20–34).[48] As time goes by, the hematoma is expected to evolve into a more heterogeneous collection as the blood lyses. The hematoma commonly becomes hypoechoic in 1 to 2 weeks.[49] A retroplacental contraction may mimic a hematoma sonographically (Fig. 20–35). A heterogeneous hematoma may mimic a retroplacental fibroid (Fig. 20–36). The size of the visualized hematoma may correlate negatively with prognosis. Nyberg and colleagues[50] found a significant relationship between the percentage of the surface of the placenta elevated by a retroplacental hematoma and fetal mortality. If 50% or more of the placental surface was involved there was a 75% mortality. If less than 20% of the surface of the placenta was involved, there was only a 13% mortality. They also found a correlation between overall volume of detected hematoma and mortality, with mortality more common with a volume greater than 60 mL.[50]

Subchorionic hematomas (Fig. 20–37) (generally associated with marginal separations of the placenta) have been associated with lower fetal mortality than retroplacental hematomas.[50] Indeed, Fox states that "a marginal hematoma is of no consequence as far as the fetus is concerned."[41] However, some sonographic studies have shown significance to the finding of subchorionic hematoma. Goldstein and colleagues[51] evaluated 50 patients with vaginal bleeding between 9 and 16 weeks of gestation and found that in the absence of sonographic evidence of a subchorionic hematoma,

100% of the pregnancies progressed to term.[51] In cases in which subchorionic blood was visualized sonographically, only 80% survived to term. Sauerbrei and Pham[52] evaluated 30 patients with vaginal bleeding at between 10 and 20 weeks' gestation and identified marginal separation of the placenta and subchorionic hematoma in 60% of these patients. They found that larger hematoma volumes were associated with poor pregnancy outcomes (including abortion, stillbirth, and preterm birth). Hematoma volumes of less than 60 mL tended to have a favorable outcome.[52]

Preplacental hematomas (also termed *massive subchorial thrombosis* or *Breus' mole*) are much less common than retroplacental or marginal hematomas. These hematomas appear as a mass extending from the anterior placental surface bulging into the amniotic cavity.[53] The etiology of this type of hematoma is

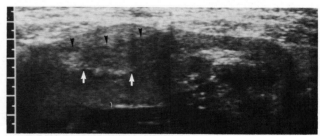

Figure 20–33. Retroplacental hematoma. The patient presented with vaginal bleeding, pelvic pain, and a low hematocrit after cocaine abuse. Sonogram shows a large retroplacental hematoma that involves more than 50% of the placental surface. Arrows mark the interface of the hematoma with the posterior surface of the placenta, and arrowheads mark the indistinct margins of the hematoma with the myometrium. (From Townsend RR, Laing FC, Jeffrey RB: Placental abruption associated with cocaine abuse. AJR 150:1339, 1988.)

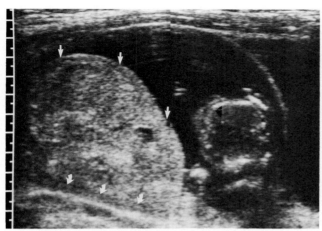

Figure 20–34. Placental abruption with isoechoic hematoma. The sonogram shows a large hematoma that is isoechoic with the placenta and that has no distinct margin with the placenta. Straight arrows mark the anterior surface of the placenta, and curved arrows mark the posterior extent of the hematoma at the myometrium. (From Townsend RR, Laing FC, Jeffrey RB: Placental abruption associated with cocaine abuse. AJR 150:1339, 1988.)

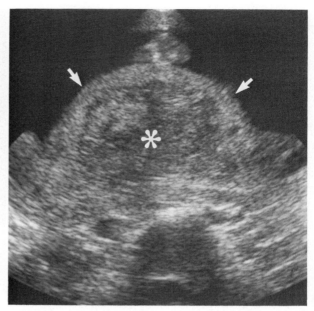

Figure 20–36. Large retroplacental hematoma. A large hematoma of heterogeneous echotexture *(asterisk)* is seen behind a posterior placenta *(arrows)*. This hematoma could easily be mistaken for a myoma or contraction.

uncertain. Prognosis is not well defined, but fetal death may result. A single sonographic report described an apparently thickened placenta due to isoechoic subchorionic thrombosis. It increased in size over many weeks.[54] Subamniotic hemorrhages are also seen on

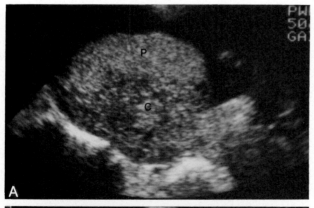

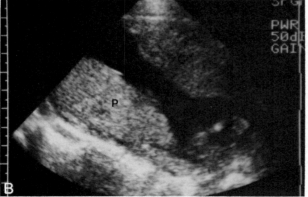

Figure 20–35. Contraction mimicking retroplacental hematoma. *A.* The placenta (P) is elevated by a heterogeneous mass (C) suggestive of hematoma. The patient had no vaginal bleeding. *B.* Thirty minutes later the "hematoma" has resolved and a new contraction is seen anteriorly. P, placenta; C, contraction.

the anterior surface of the placenta and are likely related to rupture of fetal vessels on the placental surface.[55] It is unlikely that they would be distinguishable sonographically from other preplacental hematomas.

Intraplacental hematomas may be seen as focal masses of varying echogenicity within the placenta, often related to infarct if there is an underlying abruption. These abnormalities are discussed further later with focal placental masses. Large amounts of intraplacental hematoma may be associated with massive retroplacental hematoma dissecting into the placenta and/or associated large hemorrhagic areas of infarction.

DIFFUSE PLACENTAL ABNORMALITY

Diffusely thickened placentas are seen with conditions causing edema or inflammation of the placenta (Fig. 20–38). These include hydrops (multiple causes), viral infections, and diabetes. Pseudothickening of the placenta may be seen with abruption if the retroplacental or intraplacental hematoma has the same echotexture as the placenta.[48] With current high-resolution equipment this is less likely to be a problem than in the past. Detection of a thick placenta should lead to a careful search of the fetus for signs of infection or hydrops.[56]

The placenta may appear to be thinned in cases of polyhydramnios[7] or in cases of preeclampsia.[41]

FOCAL PLACENTAL MASSES

Focal sonolucent masses in the placenta are commonly identified (Fig. 20–39). Spirt and associates[57]

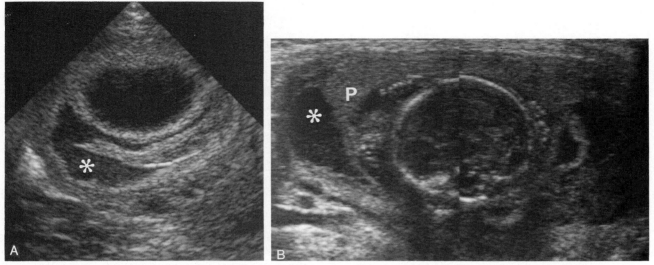

Figure 20–37. Subchorionic hematoma. *A.* Subchorionic hematoma *(asterisk)* contains some internal echoes and lifts the edge of this early placenta. *B.* Three months later the hematoma persists *(asterisk)* with fewer internal echoes. P, placenta.

identified subchorionic sonolucent areas in 10% to 15% of obstetric sonograms in 1978. They are more commonly recognized with the improved resolution of ultrasound equipment in common use today. These subchorionic sonolucencies have been attributed to areas of subchorionic fibrin deposition, hematoma, or cystic degeneration, none of which appears to be clinically significant.[57, 58] It is common to visualize, at real-time sonography, slowly moving echoes in subchorionic lucencies, likely related to liquefication of hematoma or fibrin deposit and communication with the venous spaces of the placenta.

Intraplacental sonolucencies, at any depth within the placental tissue, may also be seen with intervillous thrombosis (Fig. 20–40).[59, 60] Pathologically, this has

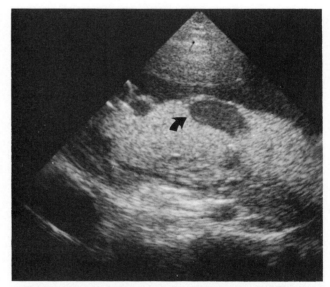

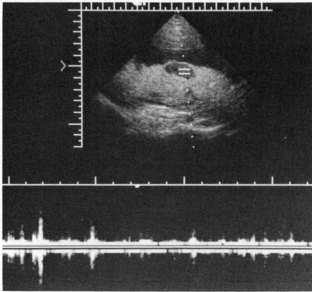

Figure 20–39. Subchorionic "lakes." Sonogram at 25 weeks' gestation, performed for fetal age determination, shows a subchorionic fluid collection *(arrow)*. Doppler evaluation reveals flow within the collection.

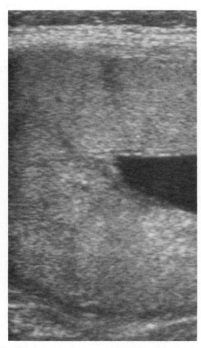

Figure 20–38. Thickened placenta. This fundal placenta was thickened (6.0 cm thick at 28 weeks' gestation), related to fetal hydrops.

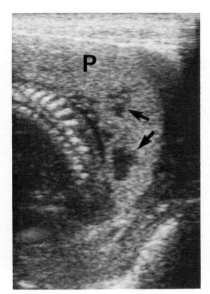

Figure 20–40. Intervillous thrombi. Sonogram performed at 18 menstrual weeks because of an elevated maternal serum α-fetoprotein level, demonstrates several prominent sonolucencies *(arrows)* within the placenta (P), representing intervillous thrombi.

been defined as "a villous free nodular focus of coagulated blood in the intervillous space" and is seen in 36% of placentas.[41] Sonographically, these hypoechoic masses have been reported to vary from less than 1 cm in diameter to 2 × 8 × 10 cm.[59] Although these masses generally appear not to be significant, Hoogland and colleagues[60] suggested that they may be related to Rh isoimmunization in pregnancies at risk, related to mixing of maternal and fetal blood in these spaces. The association of these sonolucent spaces with elevated maternal serum α-fetoprotein also suggests that they may be a site of mixing of maternal and fetal blood.[61] Javert and colleagues[62] suggest mixing of fetal and maternal blood as the primary cause of intervillous hematoma.

Hypoechoic placental masses may also be seen with prominent maternal venous lakes.[63] Flow may be evident within these spaces at real-time examination. Septal cysts are also commonly detected pathologically (11% to 20% of placentas)[41] and likely cause some of the sonographically detected hypoechoic or anechoic masses.

In general, focal sonolucent placental masses are unlikely to be clinically significant. Even multiple subchorionic lucencies covering 50% of the placental surface have not proved to be significant.[58] When there are numerous hypoechoic masses within the substance of the placenta, several diagnostic entities should be considered. Diffuse intraparenchymal sonolucent lesions may be seen with hydatidiform mole or hydropic swelling of the placenta.[57] As noted earlier, it has recently been suggested that multiple sonolucencies may be more commonly present in association with placenta accreta.[36, 37] One reason that placental hypoechoic areas have largely proved not to be significant is that the most common significant focal placental lesion, an infarct, is generally not detected sonograph-

ically.[64] Infarcts may occasionally be identified with ultrasound evaluation, however, particularly if there has been associated hemorrhage[64] (Fig. 20–41).

Solid placental masses are relatively uncommon. The most common of these is the hemangioma, which is also referred to as chorangioma. Clinically significant hemangiomas are uncommon, but small hemangiomas are evident on careful pathologic examination in about 1% of placentas.[41] These are most commonly single but may be multiple. Large hemangiomas produce symptoms as a result of the large amount of blood shunting through them, bypassing the normal placenta. This can result in polyhydramnios, bleeding, preterm labor, fetal hydrops, growth retardation, and fetal death.[41]

Large hemangiomas most commonly protrude from the fetal surface of the placenta, but they can be anywhere in the placenta.[41] Sonographically, a solid echogenic mass may be detected (Fig. 20–42).[65-67] Smaller hemangiomas may be more isoechoic with the placenta and difficult to detect sonographically. Placental chorangiomas have been associated with elevated amniotic fluid α-fetoprotein levels.[68]

A rare cause of a solid placental mass or masses is metastatic disease, which is reported most commonly from melanoma or carcinoma of the breast or lung.[41] Placental teratomas are large complex masses but are extremely rare.

UMBILICAL CORD

The umbilical cord serves as an essential conduit for oxygen and nutrients between mother and fetus. It is often ignored, but it is easily seen on sonographic evaluation since it is surrounded by amniotic fluid.

The normal umbilical cord is between 54 and 61 cm long,[69] but because of its tortuous course its length cannot be readily determined sonographically. An ab-

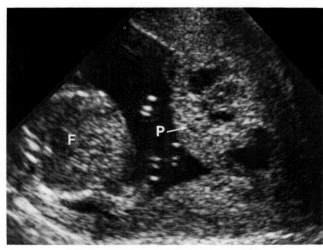

Figure 20–41. Placental infarcts. Sonogram from a 20-year-old patient with long-standing systemic lupus erythematosus demonstrates confluent sonolucencies through the placenta (P) at 19 weeks' gestation, representing multiple infarcts. Intrauterine fetal death occurred 3 weeks after the sonogram. F, fetus.

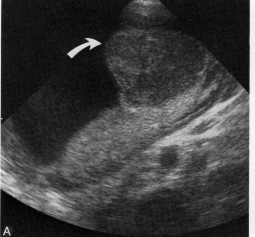
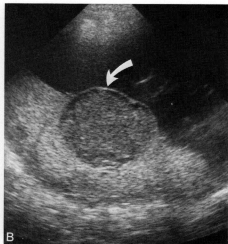

Figure 20-42. Two examples of chorangioma. *A* and *B*. A solid mass *(curved arrow)* protrudes into the amniotic cavity from the placenta.

normally short cord (less than 32 cm) may not be mechanically compatible with vaginal delivery and an abnormally long cord (greater than 100 cm) may predispose to knotting, torsion, and prolapse.[69]

The umbilical cord normally inserts near the center of the placenta. Both placental and fetal cord insertions are generally well visualized sonographically (Fig. 20-43), but at any one point visualization may be difficult or impossible owing to fetal position. The normal cord consists of three vessels (two arteries and one vein) bathed in Wharton's jelly. The cord is surrounded by amnion. The normal diameter of the cord is 1 to 2 cm.[70] However, sonographic detection of a large diameter (≥ 3 cm) cord is not always abnormal (Fig. 20-44).[71] The normal vascular complement of the cord can be confirmed with images perpendicular to the length of the cord (Fig. 20-45). Color Doppler imaging may be helpful in identifying the number of cord vessels (Fig. 20-46). A spiral configuration of the vessels is commonly detected in longitudinal images (Fig. 20-47).

The most commonly detected abnormality of the umbilical cord is the presence of only a single umbilical artery (two-vessel cord). This has been reported in 0.2% to 1.1% of deliveries or 2.7% to 12% of perinatal autopsies.[69] The higher incidence in autopsy studies is the result of a high frequency of anomalies in fetuses with only one umbilical artery. This abnormality can be readily diagnosed with sonography (Fig. 20-48). When only a single artery is present, it is larger than usual and may approach the size of the umbilical vein. If technical difficulty is encountered in attempting to image the cord, the umbilical arteries may be visualized

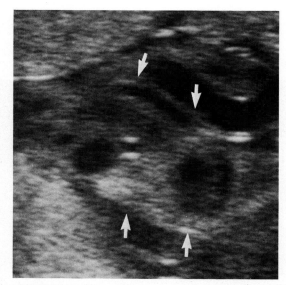

Figure 20-43. Placental cord insertion site. The site of umbilical cord insertion into this anterior placenta is well seen *(arrow)*.

Figure 20-44. Normal large umbilical cord. An abundance of Wharton's jelly results in a large umbilical cord *(arrows)*.

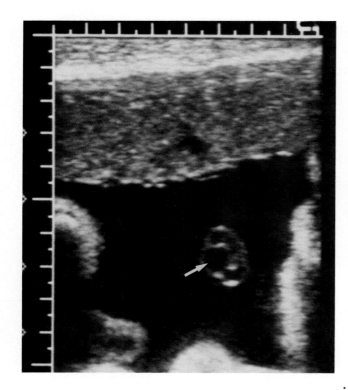

Figure 20–45. Normal three-vessel umbilical cord. This image was obtained perpendicular to the length of the umbilical cord and shows the normal umbilical vein *(arrow)* and two adjacent umbilical arteries.

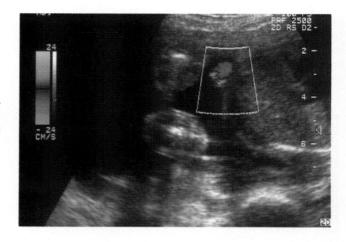

Figure 20–46. Normal three-vessel umbilical cord confirmed by color Doppler sonography. The single vein *(blue)* and two arteries *(red)* are readily detected in this image nearly perpendicular to the length of the cord.

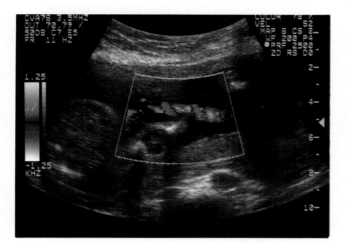

Figure 20–47. Spiral configuration of the umbilical arteries (not individually resolved on this color Doppler image) and umbilical vein seen on longitudinal sonogram of the umbilical cord.

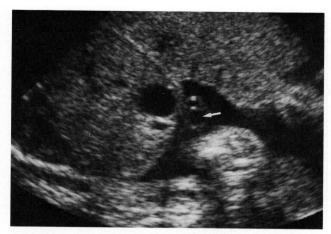

Figure 20–48. Single umbilical artery. This image obtained perpendicular to the length of the umbilical cord shows the normal umbilical vein *(arrow)* and only a single adjacent umbilical artery.

and counted at the cord insertion into the fetus, coursing caudally and laterally around the bladder into the fetal pelvis. Jeanty[72] described a curve in the distal fetal abdominal aorta toward the common iliac artery on the side of a single patent umbilical artery. It has been pointed out that the two umbilical arteries may normally communicate or fuse at the placental end of the cord, so that this condition may be overdiagnosed if images are taken only at that location.[69]

The sonographic detection of a single umbilical artery should prompt a thorough evaluation of the fetus for associated abnormalities. The frequency of associated abnormalities has been variably reported but is 25% to 50% in most studies.[69] The malformations are not limited to any one fetal organ system and may be either minor or multiple and lethal. Chromosome abnormalities may be present in cases with single umbilical artery and another fetal malformation.[73] In

one sonographic study, 50% of fetuses with a single umbilical artery had another anomaly identified.[74] These were minor in 3 of 15 and major in 12 of 15 fetuses. Major anomalies included cardiac defects, holoprosencephaly, skeletal dysplasia, hydrocephalus, omphalocele, hydrothorax, large cisterna magna, and diaphragmatic hernia. Six of the fetuses with major anomalies had chromosomal abnormalities. Importantly, none of the sonographically normal fetuses had a significant abnormality detected after birth. The investigators concluded that sonographic detection of a single umbilical artery, in the absence of additional anomalies, should not alter obstetric management.[74] The sonographic identification of a single umbilical artery certainly should prompt a thorough evaluation for associated anomalies. If none are identified in experienced hands (and this should be expected at least 50% of the time), then the outlook should generally be favorable.

More than three vessels in the umbilical cord may occasionally be seen. Additional vessels detected pathologically may be very small,[69] and this may account for the lack of sonographic reports of supernumerary cord vessels. Conjoined twins may have one or two cords and anomalous (increased or decreased) numbers of vessels in the cords.[75]

While variations in umbilical vein number are relatively uncommon, sonographic findings of altered umbilical vein size have been reported.[76-78] Mahony and colleagues identified dilatation of the intra-abdominal portion of the umbilical vein (umbilical vein varix) in nine fetuses, four of whom subsequently died (Fig. 20–49).[76] Estrof and Benacerraf reported good outcome for five fetuses with the same condition, although their diagnoses were generally made later in gestation.[77] Sonographic identification of ectasia of the umbilical vein in the cord was reported by Vesce and colleagues,[78] who noted fetal distress when thrombus developed. Thrombosis of a normal-sized umbilical

Figure 20–49. Umbilical vein varix. *A* and *B.* Two fetuses demonstrate dilatation of the intra-abdominal component of the umbilical vein *(arrows)*. Bl, urinary bladder.

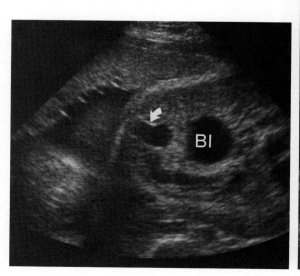

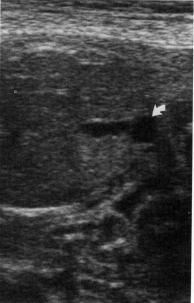

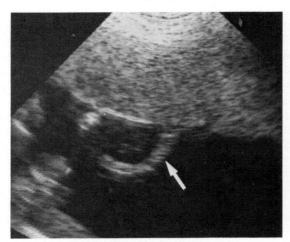

Figure 20–50. Umbilical vein thrombosis *(arrow)* in a dead fetus. (From Abrams SL, Callen PW, Filly RA: Umbilical vein thrombosis: Sonographic detection in utero. J Ultrasound Med 4:283, 1985.)

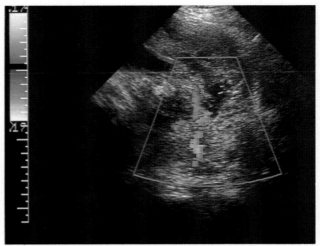

Figure 20–51. Vasa previa. The intramembranous vessels at the cervical os are more readily detected with color Doppler ultrasound imaging.

vein is seen with fetal death (Fig. 20–50),[79] but is not always fatal.[69] Umbilical cord hematoma outside the confines of the umbilical vein may also be detected sonographically.[80, 81] This may occur spontaneously or as a complication of amniocentesis or umbilical venipuncture.

Although the umbilical cord normally inserts into the central area of the placenta, eccentric insertions are common and not significant.[69] Insertion into the margin of the placenta ("battledore placenta") may be associated with neonatal asphyxia, but this is controversial.[69] In 1.0% to 1.6% of deliveries the cord inserts not into the placenta but into the attached membranes (velamentous insertion).[69] A small minority of these pregnancies may be complicated by hemorrhage related to tearing of these unprotected vessels, especially

during labor and delivery. When the intramembranous vessels course across the cervical os the condition is known as *vasa previa,* and devastating hemorrhage may result. The diagnosis of vasa previa may be made with ultrasound[82] and is facilitated with color Doppler studies (Fig. 20–51).[83, 84]

Focal umbilical cord masses are relatively uncommon but readily detected sonographically. A localized deposition of Wharton's jelly may result in an insignificant but sonographically evident umbilical cord mass.[85] Hematomas have been mentioned earlier and are of variable echogenicity depending on the age of the hematoma. A cystic mass of the umbilical cord may represent an allantoic cyst, amniotic inclusion cyst, or omphalomesenteric duct cyst (Fig. 20–52).[86] In five

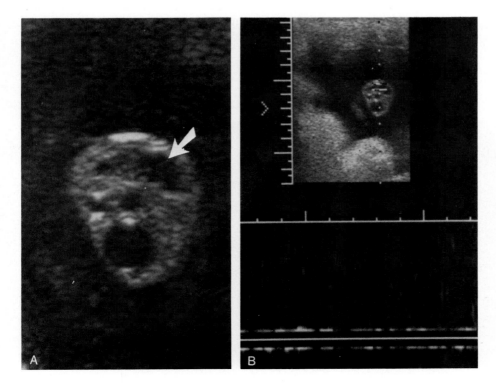

Figure 20–52. Umbilical cord cyst. *A.* An image perpendicular to the length of the umbilical cord demonstrates a hypoechoic structure *(arrow)* in addition to the normal complement of two arteries and one vein. *B.* Doppler evaluation confirmed absence of flow in this cyst.

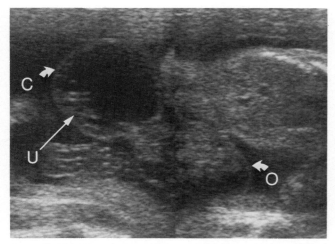

Figure 20–53. Allantoic cyst. A large cyst (C) is seen in the umbilical cord (U) of this fetus with an omphalocele (O).

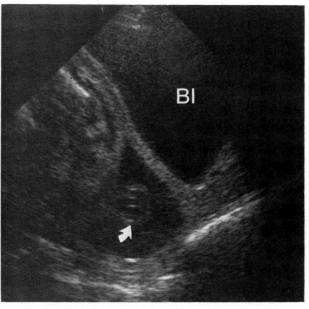

Figure 20–55. Prolapsed umbilical cord. Longitudinal sonogram at 30 weeks' gestation, performed for preterm labor, demonstrates the umbilical cord *(arrow)* prolapsed below the fetus into a dilated cervix. Bl, urinary bladder.

fetuses with ultrasound evidence of an umbilical cord cyst identified in the first trimester by Skibo and colleagues,[86] the cysts subsequently resolved and the fetus and cord were normal at birth. Cysts identified in the second or third trimester may also be insignificant,[87] but Fink and Filly[88] reported the association of umbilical cord allantoic cysts with omphalocele in three patients (Fig. 20–53). It would appear prudent to examine the fetal abdominal wall carefully for evidence of an omphalocele when an umbilical cord cyst is detected. An echogenic or complex mass of the umbilical cord may represent a hemangioma, also known as an angiomyxoma.[69, 89–91] This may be associated with elevated α-fetoprotein levels[89, 91] and can be associated with umbilical cord edema, fetal hydrops, and hemorrhage.

As would be expected with a long cordlike structure, mechanical problems can result in vascular compromise to the fetus and distress or death. True knots can occur within a single cord or involving both cords in a monochorionic/monoamniotic twin pregnancy. Normal redundancy of the cord may mimic a knot, however (Fig. 20–54). Observation of mere entanglement of two cords in a twin pregnancy confirms that it is monoamniotic, but care should be used to avoid overdiagnosis of significant knots (see Fig. 20–11).[14] Umbilical cord torsion can also compromise fetal blood supply and result in death, but I am unaware of its diagnosis sonographically. A stricture of the umbilical cord can also result in vascular compromise.

If the umbilical cord prolapses below the presenting fetal part during labor, the outcome may be disastrous. Cord compression compromises circulation to the fetus. Sonographic diagnosis of cord prolapse with grayscale[92] or duplex Doppler imaging[93] has been reported (Fig. 20–55).

References

1. Fox H: Pathology of the Placenta, pp 1–37. London, WB Saunders, 1978.
2. Benirschke K, Kaufmann P: Pathology of the Human Placenta, 2nd ed, pp 1–79. New York, Springer-Verlag, 1990.
3. Wigglesworth JS: Perinatal Pathology, pp 48–83. Philadelphia, WB Saunders, 1984.
4. Callen PW, Filly RA: The placental-subplacental complex: A specific indicator of placental position on ultrasound. J Clin Ultrasound 8:21, 1980.
5. Marx M, Casola G, Scheible W, Deutch A: The subplacental complex: Further sonographic observations. J Ultrasound Med 4:459, 1985.
6. Wolf H, Oosting H, Treffers PE: Placental volume measurement by ultrasonography: Evaluation of the method. Am J Obstet Gynecol 156:1191, 1987.
7. Hoddick WK, Mahony BS, Callen PW, Filly RA: Placental thickness. J Ultrasound Med 4:479, 1985.
8. Grannum PAT, Berkowitz RL, Hobbins JC: The ultrasonic

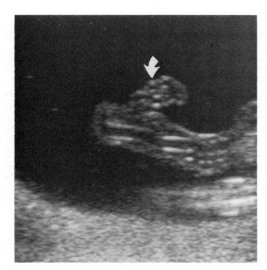

Figure 20–54. False cord knot. Although a true knot of the umbilical cord is potentially life threatening, a false knot is not significant. Here, an extra loop of umbilical vessel *(arrow)* gives the appearance of a knot.

changes in the maturing placenta and their relation to fetal pulmonic maturity. Am J Obstet Gynecol 133:915, 1979.

9. Spirt BA, Cohen WN, Weinstein HM: The incidence of placental calcification in normal pregnancies. Radiology 142:707, 1982.

10. Mahony BS, Filly RA, Callen PW: Amnionicity and chorionicity in twin pregnancies: Prediction using ultrasound. Radiology 155:205, 1985.

11. Hertzberg BS, Kurtz AB, Choi HY, et al: Significance of membrane thickness in the sonographic evaluation of twin gestations. AJR 148:151, 1987.

12. Townsend RR, Simpson GF, Filly RA: Membrane thickness in ultrasound prediction of chorionicity of twin gestations. J Ultrasound Med 7:327, 1988.

13. Nyberg DA, Filly RA, Golbus MS, Stephens JD: Entangled umbilical cords: A sign of monoamniotic twins. J Ultrasound Med 3:29, 1984.

14. Townsend RR, Filly RA: Sonography of nonconjoined monoamniotic twin pregnancies. J Ultrasound Med 7:665, 1988.

15. Hurley VA, Beischer NA: Placenta membranacea: Case reports. Br J Obstet Gynecol 94:798, 1987.

16. Jeanty P, Kirkpatrick C, Verhoogen C, Struyven J: The succenturiate placenta. J Ultrasound Med 2:9, 1983.

17. Fox H: Pathology of the Placenta, pp 50–72. London, WB Saunders, 1978.

18. Bey M, Dott A, Miller JM Jr: The sonographic diagnosis of circumvallate placenta. Obstet Gynecol 78:515, 1991.

19. Goplerud CP: Bleeding in late pregnancy. In Danforth DN (ed): Obstetrics and Gynecology, 5th ed, pp 433–445. Philadelphia, JB Lippincott, 1986.

20. Gillieson MS, Winer-Muram HT, Muram D: Low-lying placenta. Radiology 144:577, 1982.

21. Wexler P, Gottesfeld KR: Early diagnosis of placenta previa. Obstet Gynecol 54:231, 1979.

22. Bowie JD, Rochester D, Cadkin AV, et al: Accuracy of placental localization by ultrasound. Radiology 128:177, 1978.

23. Zemlyn S: The effect of the urinary bladder in obstetrical sonography. Radiology 128:169, 1978.

24. Townsend RR, Laing FC, Nyberg DA, et al: Technical factors responsible for "placental migration": Sonographic assessment. Radiology 160:105, 1986.

25. Artis AA, Bowie JD, Rosenberg ER, Rauch RF: The fallacy of placental migration: Effect of sonographic techniques. AJR 144:79, 1985.

26. King DL: Placental migration demonstrated by ultrasonography. Radiology 109:167, 1973.

27. Jeffrey RB, Laing FC: Sonography of the low-lying placenta: Value of Trendelenburg and traction scans. AJR 137:547, 1981.

28. Bowie JD, Andreotti RF, Rosenberg ER: Sonographic appearance of the uterine cervix in pregnancy: The vertical cervix. AJR 140:737, 1983.

29. Leerentveld RA, Gilberts ECAM, Arnold MJCWJ, Wladimiroff JW: Accuracy and safety of transvaginal sonographic placental localization. Obstet Gynecol 76:759, 1990.

30. Hertzberg BS, Bowie JD, Weber TM, et al: Sonography of the cervix during the third trimester of pregnancy: Value of the transperineal approach. AJR 157:73, 1991.

31. Hertzberg BS, Bowie JD, Carroll BA, et al: Diagnosis of placenta previa during the third trimester: Role of transperineal sonography. AJR 159:83, 1992.

32. Powell MC, Buckley J, Price H, et al: Magnetic resonance imaging and placenta previa. Am J Obstet Gynecol 154:565, 1986.

33. Kay HH, Spritzer CE: Preliminary experience with magnetic resonance imaging in patients with third-trimester bleeding. Obstet Gynecol 78:424, 1991.

34. Breen JL, Neubecker R, Gregori CA, Franklin JE Jr: Placenta accreta, increta, and percreta: A survey of 40 cases. Obstet Gynecol 49:43, 1977.

35. Read JA, Cotton DB, Miller FC: Placenta accreta: Changing clinical aspects and outcome. Obstet Gynecol 56:31, 1980.

36. Hoffman-Tretin JC, Koenigsberg M, Rabin A, Anyaegbunam A: Placenta accreta: Additional sonographic observations. J Ultrasound Med 11:29, 1992.

37. Finberg HJ, Williams JW: Placenta accreta: Prospective sonographic diagnosis in patients with placenta previa and prior cesarean section. J Ultrasound Med 11:333, 1992.

38. Pasto ME, Kurtz AB, Rifkin MD, et al: Ultrasonographic findings in placenta increta. J Ultrasound Med 2:155, 1983.

39. Sexton LI, Hertig AT, Reid DE, et al: Premature separation of the normally implanted placenta: A clinicopathological study of 476 cases. Am J Obstet Gynecol 59:13, 1950.

40. Gruenwald P, Levin H, Yousem H: Abruption and premature separation of the placenta: The clinical and the pathologic entity. Am J Obstet Gynecol 102:604, 1968.

41. Fox H: Pathology of the Placenta, pp 95–148. London, WB Saunders, 1978.

42. Hibbard BM, Jeffcoate TNA: Abruptio placentae. Obstet Gynecol 27:155, 1966.

43. Townsend RR, Laing FC, Jeffrey RB: Placental abruption associated with cocaine abuse. AJR 150:1339, 1988.

44. Naeye RL, Harkness WL, Utts J: Abruptio placentae and perinatal death: A prospective study. Am J Obstet Gynecol 128:740, 1977.

45. Hurd WW, Miodovnik M, Hertzberg V, Lavin JP: Selective management of abruptio placentae: A prospective study. Obstet Gynecol 61:467, 1983.

46. Sprit BA, Kagan EH, Rozanski RM: Abruptio placentae: Sonographic and pathologic correlation. AJR 133:877, 1979.

47. McGahan JP, Phillips HE, Reid MH, Oi RH: Sonographic spectrum of retroplacental hemorrhage. Radiology 142:481, 1982.

48. Mintz MC, Kurtz AB, Arenson R, et al: Abruptio placentae: Apparent thickening of the placenta caused by hyperechoic retroplacental clot. J Ultrasound Med 5:411, 1986.

49. Nyberg DA, Cyr DR, Mack LA, et al: Sonographic spectrum of placental abruption. AJR 148:161, 1987.

50. Nyberg DA, Mack LA, Benedetti TJ, et al: Placental abruption and placental hemorrhage: Correlation of sonographic findings with fetal outcome. Radiology 164:357, 1987.

51. Goldstein SR, Subramanyam BR, Raghavendra BN, et al: Subchorionic bleeding in threatened abortion: Sonographic findings and significance. AJR 141:975, 1983.

52. Sauerbrei EE, Pham DH: Placental abruption and subchorionic hemorrhage in the first half of pregnancy: US appearance and clinical outcome. Radiology 160:109, 1986.

53. Shanklin DR, Scott JS: Massive subchorial thrombohaematoma (Breus' mole). Br J Obstet Gynecol 82:476, 1975.

54. Olah KS, Gee H, Rushton I, Fowlie A: Massive subchorionic thrombohaematoma presenting as a placental tumour. Case report. Br J Obstet Gynecol 94, 995, 1987.

55. deSa DJ: Rupture of fetal vessels on placental surface. Arch Dis Child 46:495, 1971.

56. Drose JA, Dennis MA, Thickman D: Infection in utero: US findings in 19 cases. Radiology 178:369, 1991.

57. Spirt BA, Kagan EH, Rozanski RM: Sonolucent areas in the placenta: Sonographic and pathologic correlation. AJR 131:961, 1978.

58. Katz VL, Blanchard GF, Watson WJ, et al: The clinical implications of subchorionic placental lucencies. Am J Obstet Gynecol 164:99, 1991.

59. Sprit BA, Gordon LP, Kagan EH: Intervillous thrombosis: Sonographic and pathologic correlation. Radiology 147:197, 1983.

60. Hoogland HJ, de Haan J, Vooys GP: Ultrasonographic diagnosis of intervillous thrombosis related to Rh isoimmunization. Gynecol Obstet Invest 10:237, 1979.

61. Perkes EA, Baim RS, Goodman KJ, Macri JN: Second-trimester placental changes associated with elevated maternal serum alpha-fetoprotein. Am J Obstet Gynecol 144:935, 1982.

62. Javert CT, Reiss C: The origin and significance of macroscopic intervillous coagulation hematomas (red infarcts) of the human placenta. Surg Gynecol Obstet 94:257, 1952.

63. Cooperberg PL, Wright VJ, Carpenter CW: Ultrasonographic demonstration of a placental maternal lake. J Clin Ultrasound 7:62, 1979.

64. Harris RD, Simpson WA, Pet LR, et al: Placental hypoechoic-anechoic areas and infarction: Sonographic-pathologic correlation. Radiology 176:75, 1990.

65. Sprit BA, Gordon L, Cohen WN, Yambao T: Antenatal diagnosis of chorioangioma of the placenta. AJR 135:1273, 1980.

66. O'Malley BP, Toi A, deSa DJ, Williams GL: Ultrasound appearances of placental chorioangioma. Radiology 138:159, 1981.

67. Rodan BA, Bean WJ: Chorioangioma of the placenta causing intrauterine fetal demise. J Ultrasound Med 2:95, 1983.
68. Willard DA, Moeschler JB: Placental chorioangioma: A rare cause of elevated amniotic fluid alpha-fetoprotein. J Ultrasound Med 5:221, 1986.
69. Fox H: Pathology of the Placenta, pp 426–457. London, WB Saunders, 1978.
70. Rushton DI: Pathology of the Placenta. In Wigglesworth JS, Singer DB (eds): Textbook of Fetal and Perinatal Pathology, pp 161–219. Boston, Blackwell Scientific Publishers, 1991.
71. Casola G, Scheible W, Leopold GR: Large umbilical cord: A normal finding in some fetuses. Radiology 156:181, 1985.
72. Jeanty P: Fetal and funicular vascular anomalies: Identification with prenatal US. Radiology 173:367, 1989.
73. Byrne J, Blanc WA: Malformations and chromosome anomalies in spontaneously aborted fetuses with single umbilical artery. Am J Obstet Gynecol 151:340, 1985.
74. Nyberg DA, Mahony BS, Luthy D, Kapur R: Single umbilical artery: Prenatal detection of concurrent anomalies. J Ultrasound Med 10:247, 1991.
75. Benirschke K, Kaufmann P: Pathology of the Human Placenta, 2nd ed, pp 711–715. New York, Springer-Verlag, 1990.
76. Mahony BS, McGahan JP, Nyberg DA, Reisner DP: Varix of the fetal intra-abdominal umbilical vein: Comparison with normal. J Ultrasound Med 11:73, 1992.
77. Estroff JA, Benacerraf BR: Fetal umbilical vein varix: Sonographic appearance and postnatal outcome. J Ultrasound Med 11:69, 1992.
78. Vesce F, Guerrini P, Perri G, et al: Ultrasonographic diagnosis of ectasia of the umbilical vein. J Clin Ultrasound 15:346, 1987.
79. Abrams SL, Callen PW, Filly RA: Umbilical vein thrombosis: Sonographic detection in utero. J Ultrasound Med 4:283, 1985.
80. Sutro WH, Tuck SM, Loesevitz A, et al: Prenatal observation of umbilical cord hematoma. AJR 142:801, 1984.
81. Keckstein G, Tschurtz S, Schneider V, et al: Umbilical cord haematoma as a complication of intrauterine intravascular blood transfusion. Prenat Diagn 10:59, 1990.
82. Gianopoulos J, Carver T, Tomich PG, et al: Diagnosis of vasa previa with ultrasonography. Obstet Gynecol 69:488, 1987.
83. Nelson LH, Melone PJ, King M: Diagnosis of vasa previa with transvaginal and color flow Doppler ultrasound. Obstet Gynecol 76:506, 1990.
84. Hsieh F-J, Chen H-F, Ko T-M, et al: Antenatal diagnosis of vasa previa by color-flow mapping. J Ultrasound Med 10:397, 1991.
85. Ramanathan K, Epstein S, Yaghoobian J: Localized deposition of Wharton's jelly: Sonographic findings. J Ultrasound Med 5:339, 1986.
86. Skibo LK, Lyons EA, Levi CS: First-trimester umbilical cord cysts. Radiology 182:719, 1992.
87. Sachs L, Fourcroy JL, Wenzel DJ, et al: Prenatal detection of umbilical cord allantoic cyst. Radiology 145:445, 1982.
88. Fink IJ, Filly RA: Omphalocele associated with umbilical cord allantoic cyst: Sonographic evaluation in utero. Radiology 149:473, 1983.
89. Pollack MS, Bound LM: Hemangioma of the umbilical cord: Sonographic appearance. J Ultrasound Med 8:163, 1989.
90. Ghidini A, Romero R, Eisen RN, et al: Umbilical cord hemangioma: Prenatal identification and review of the literature. J Ultrasound Med 9:297, 1990.
91. Jauniaux E, Moscoso G, Chitty L, et al: An angiomyxoma involving the whole length of the umbilical cord: Prenatal diagnosis by ultrasonography. J Ultrasound Med 9:419, 1990.
92. Hales ED, Westney LS: Sonography of occult cord prolapse. J Clin Ultrasound 12:283, 1984.
93. Johnson RL, Anderson JC, Irsik RD, Goodlin RC: Duplex ultrasound diagnosis of umbilical cord prolapse. J Clin Ultrasound 15:282, 1987.

CHAPTER 21

Sonographic Prediction of Fetal Lung Maturity

FRANK P. HADLOCK, M.D.

Normal fetal lung development is a sequential process that involves several phases. The important alveolar phase generally begins at the 24th menstrual week and extends into postnatal life. During this time, the alveolar cells secrete phospholipids (surfactant) that play a key role in the functional integrity of the fetal lung at delivery. If these phospholipids are not present in sufficient quantities at birth, the fetal alveoli will collapse and the fetus will receive inadequate oxygenation. This form of respiratory embarrassment is called respiratory distress syndrome (RDS) or, more specifically, hyaline membrane disease. This condition usually affects fetuses that are born prematurely.

There are two major clinical situations in which it is useful to have an accurate assessment of fetal lung maturity in utero, since both may result in RDS secondary to premature delivery. One is the preterm patient who is at high risk of imminent delivery secondary to premature labor or in whom early delivery is mandated by maternal or fetal indications (e.g., a 34-week pregnancy with severe preeclampsia and growth retardation). The second category is the otherwise uncomplicated pregnancy with unknown dates in which a cesarean delivery is necessary. Assessment of fetal lung maturity in the former category is less critical, since maternal or fetal factors may dictate immediate delivery regardless of the fetal lung's status. In the latter case, however, knowledge of fetal lung maturity is necessary to avoid iatrogenic RDS due to unnecessary premature delivery.[1]

In such cases, fetal lung maturity can be accurately assessed by biochemical analysis of amniotic fluid samples obtained through amniocentesis.[2] Amniocentesis performed with ultrasound guidance is usually a benign procedure,[3] but it carries the potential for serious complications, such as premature separation of the placenta, premature rupture of membranes, premature labor, fetal or maternal bleeding, and even fetal death. Because of these possible complications, efforts have been made to use prenatal diagnostic ultrasonography as a means of evaluating fetal lung maturity. The purpose of this chapter is to determine what role, if any, ultrasonography can play in predicting fetal lung maturity in utero.

BIOCHEMICAL MARKERS

In 1971, Gluck and Kulovich[2] demonstrated that the relationship between the surface-active phospholipids in amniotic fluid could be used to evaluate the maturity of the human fetal lung. They demonstrated that in random pregnancies, both normal and abnormal, when the lecithin/sphingomyelin (LS) ratio was 2 or greater, there was an absence of RDS at birth, irrespective of age and weight.[4] They also noted that certain maternal conditions, such as diabetes mellitus (classes A to C) and Rh incompatibility, may cause a delay in fetal lung maturation, whereas other maternal conditions, such as chronic hypertension or severe diabetes mellitus (classes D, F, R), may actually accelerate the development of fetal lung maturity in utero.[4, 5]

Refinements in the evaluation of amniotic fluid phospholipids for determination of fetal lung maturity have resulted in a complete fetal *lung profile,*[5] which consists of the LS ratio, as well as percentages of disaturated (acetone-precipitated) lecithin, phosphatidylinositol, and phosphatidylglycerol. The relative changes in the concentration of these phospholipids in amniotic fluid over time can be seen in Figure 21–1. One should note that in normal pregnancies the fetal lung is generally not mature before 34 weeks but is mature after 37 weeks. From 34 to 37 weeks there is a transitional phase in which varying degrees of fetal lung maturity can be expected. Subsequent clinical experience has indicated that the lung profile predicts fetal lung maturity more accurately than it does immaturity; that is, there is a virtual absence of RDS in fetuses with a mature lung profile whereas some fetuses with an immature lung profile will not develop RDS at delivery. Because of the ability of the mature lung profile to predict fetal lung maturity, it serves as a "gold standard" against which sonographic predictors of fetal lung maturity can be judged.

SONOGRAPHIC PREDICTORS

Theoretical Considerations

If one were to design a study for evaluation of an ultrasound marker of fetal lung maturity, it would be important to test the marker in a large series of patients in the third trimester of pregnancy. Ideally, all patients would be scanned at weekly intervals from the 28th week, and cesarean delivery would be done on the day the marker is first identified, regardless of menstrual age. However, in view of the increased perinatal morbidity and mortality associated with premature (< 37 weeks) delivery, such a study would be both unethical and clinically unjustifiable.[1]

Because of these constraints, the design of any

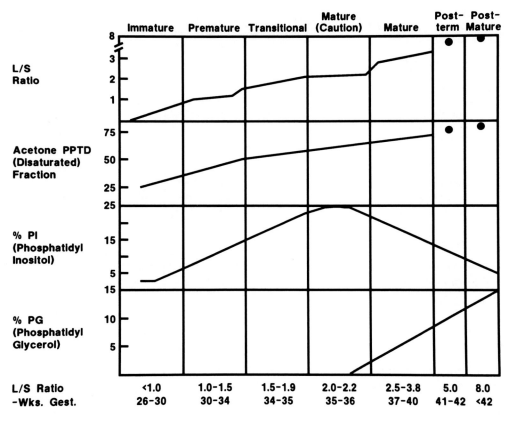

Figure 21–1. This "lung profile" form identifies the stages of maturational development of the fetal lung through amniotic fluid analysis. (From Kulovich MV, Hallman MB, Gluck L: The lung profile: I. Normal pregnancy. Am J Obstet Gynecol 135:57, 1979. Copyright 1979, Regents of the University of California.)

sonographic study for predicting fetal lung maturity will be limited in two major respects. First, although it is relatively easy to obtain a large sample of *term* patients who have undergone amniocentesis before cesarean delivery, it is virtually impossible to obtain a correspondingly large sample of *preterm* uncomplicated pregnancies, since there is no clinical indication for amniocentesis in this group. Thus, not only is the preterm population invariably smaller than the term population, but virtually all amniocenteses in the preterm period will be in patients with maternal or fetal complications that are known to accelerate fetal lung maturity (e.g., premature labor, ruptured membranes, maternal hypertension or toxemia, fetal growth retardation, nongestational diabetes mellitus, and steroid therapy). The results from the biochemical testing in this population will thus be skewed in favor of fetal lung maturity in comparison with a corresponding preterm control group.[1]

Second, since a sonographic study with development of RDS as an endpoint would not be ethical, one must evaluate sonographic markers of fetal lung maturity in terms of their ability to predict a mature biochemical lung profile. Based on reports to date,[1] the combination of an LS ratio equal to or greater than 2 and a PG concentration of at least 0.02% should predict fetal lung maturity in all nondiabetic patients, regardless of menstrual age. When the LS ratio is less than 2 and PG is absent, or present in a concentration less than 0.02% in the amniotic fluid, a high percentage of cases of fetal RDS can be expected after immediate cesarean delivery in an uncomplicated nondiabetic pregnancy.

The exact percentage of such fetuses in which RDS would develop if delivered immediately is not known, but it would relate in large part to the actual menstrual age at the time of delivery. Based on the available data,[4, 6–9] the risk of RDS in such patients between 35 and 37 weeks would be 20% to 40%, whereas deliveries between 32 and 35 weeks would carry a risk of 40% to 85%. These risks are clearly unacceptable when the timing of cesarean delivery is elective.

Biparietal Diameter

Early reports by Goldstein and associates[10] and Spellacy and colleagues[11] suggested that use of a biparietal diameter (BPD) equal to or greater than 9.0 cm resulted in an unacceptably high false-positive rate (27% to 30%) in predicting fetal lung maturity as judged by an LS ratio greater than 2. Strassner and coworkers[12] subsequently confirmed this finding and demonstrated that in the presence of an immature LS ratio, a BPD equal to or greater than 9.0 cm provided no significant information on the presence or absence of PG in the amniotic fluid. Harman,[13] in a study of 235 third-trimester patients, demonstrated that a BPD of at least 9.0 cm correlated with a mature LS ratio in only 79% of cases, whereas a BPD less than 9.0 cm was associated with a mature LS ratio in 80% of cases. My colleagues and I found quite similar results (Table 21–1).[1, 10–18]

Hayashi and colleagues,[14] Golde and associates,[15] and Petrucha and coworkers[16] focused on the presence

Table 21–1. RELATION BETWEEN BIPARIETAL DIAMETER AND FETAL LUNG MATURITY

Author	No.	Age*	BPD (cm)	Index of Lung Maturity	False Positive (%)
Goldstein et al[10]	61	NG	≥9.0	LS ≥ 2	29.5
Spellacy et al[11]	84	NG	≥9.0	LS ≥ 2	27.3
	84	NG	≥9.3	LS ≥ 2	14.3
Strassner et al[12]	83	NG	≥9.0	LS ≥ 2	10.7
	55	NG	≥9.0	PG +	31.0
Harman et al[13]	108	NG	≥9.0	LS ≥ 2	21.3
Hayashi et al[14]	91	>38 wk	≥9.3	RDS	0.0
Golde et al[15]	92	NG	≥9.2	RDS	0.0
	57	NG	≥9.2	LS ≥ 2; PG +	7.0
Petrucha et al[16]	124	NG	≥9.2	RDS	0.0
Newton et al[17]	100	NG	≥9.2	LS ≥ 2	17.0
			≥9.2	OD650 ≥ 0.15	19.0
			≥9.2	LS ≥ 2; OD ≥ 0.15	9.0
Golde et al[18]	200	≈38 wk	≥9.2	RDS	0.5
Hadlock et al[1]	105	≥37 wk	≥9.3	LS ≥ 2; PG +	9.5
	7	<37 wk	≥9.3	LS ≥ 2; PG +	85.6

RDS, respiratory distress syndrome; PG +, phosphatidylglycerol of at least 0.02%; LS, lecithin/sphingomyelin ratio; NG, not given; OD, optical density.

False positive (%) is the number of fetuses, predicted to have mature lungs by biparietal diameter, who actually had immature lungs on the basis of the index of lung maturity used.

*Age is the menstrual age at the time of study.

or absence of hyaline membrane disease at delivery as a standard against which to judge the prediction of fetal lung maturity. They suggested that a BPD greater than 9.2 cm is adequate evidence of fetal lung maturity in the absence of maternal diabetes mellitus. In Hayashi's sample population,[14] the menstrual age at the time of the sonogram was thought to be at least 38 menstrual weeks, an age known to be associated with fetal lung maturity, irrespective of the BPD.[1, 4] Golde[15] and Petrucha[16] concluded that a BPD of at least 9.2 cm had 100% predictive power for fetal lung maturity, but these studies were limited by failure to indicate the menstrual ages of the fetuses studied and by inclusion of patients with maternal and fetal problems known to be associated with accelerated fetal lung maturity. The importance of the age distribution of the fetal population tested is indicated in Figure 21–2. For example, if one evaluates only fetuses in the white zone (> 37 weeks), one would expect a virtual absence of RDS at delivery based on the well-known relation between fetal lung maturity and menstrual age.[4] However, if the sample of fetuses with a BPD equal to or greater than 9.3 cm included only the group in the gray zone (< 37 weeks), a high incidence of RDS would be expected, increasing as menstrual age decreases.[1, 4, 6–9]

In another work by Golde and coworkers,[18] an effort was made to evaluate a BPD equal to or greater than 9.2 cm as a predictor of fetal lung maturity. The fetuses of their nondiabetic patient population were thought to be at least 38 weeks of gestational age based on the last menstrual period; RDS developed in only one fetus with a BPD equal to or greater than 9.2 cm when delivery was within 1 week of the ultrasound examination. Predictably, in this infant, the dates were incorrect; the actual fetal age based on neonatal examination was 34 weeks. It is meaningless to further test a BPD equal to or greater than 9.2 cm (or any sonographic marker) as a predictor of fetal lung maturity in fetuses known to be at least 38 menstrual

weeks of age, since it is age and not the BPD measurement that determines fetal lung maturity in such cases.[1] In my opinion, there is no BPD measurement above which one can be certain that the fetus has mature lungs.

Evaluation of Placental Maturity

In the original study by Grannum and colleagues (Fig. 21–3),[19] a grade III placenta was associated with

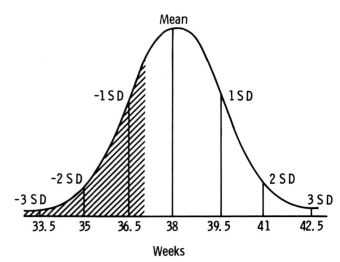

Figure 21–2. A normal bell-shaped curve that would be anticipated for the frequency distribution of menstrual ages for a biparietal diameter of 9.3 cm in an unselected fetal population. Approximately 24% of these fetuses would be less than 37 menstrual weeks (*shaded area*), and 14% of this group would be less than 35 menstrual weeks. Given the well-known relation between fetal lung maturity and advancing menstrual age, substantial differences would be expected if a biparietal diameter of 9.3 cm or greater was used to predict lung maturity in a study population limited to either the white area (greater than 37 weeks) or the shaded area (less than 37 weeks). (From Hadlock FP, Irwin JF, Roecker E, et al: Ultrasound prediction of fetal lung maturity. Radiology 155:469–472, 1985.)

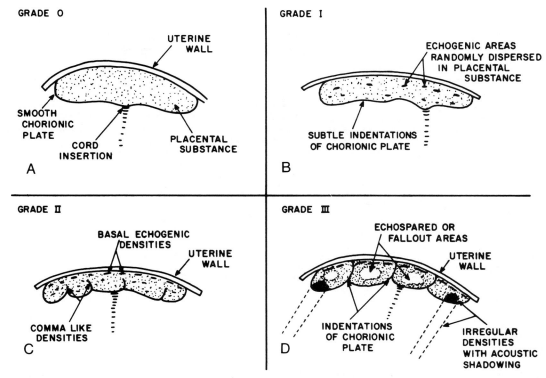

Figure 21–3. Sonographic characteristics used to determine the stage of "maturation" of the placenta. A grade III represents the most mature placenta. (From Grannum PA, Berkowitz RL, Hobbins JC: The ultrasonic changes in the maturing placenta and their relation to fetal pulmonic maturity. Am J Obstet Gynecol 133:915, 1979.)

fetal lung maturity (as assessed by the LS ratio) in 100% of cases. A subsequent study[20] confirmed this finding, but the data on the menstrual ages of the fetuses and on maternal fetal complications that might accelerate lung maturity were inadequate; thus, one could not deduce how accurate a grade III placenta would be in predicting lung maturity in an uncomplicated population undergoing cesarean delivery at varying menstrual ages. Several case reports that followed indicated that a grade III placenta could be associated with biochemical fetal lung immaturity as well as RDS, and, not surprisingly, these concerned fetuses delivered preterm by cesarean section.[21, 22] In several studies, representing 349 cases with grade III placentas, it has been shown that a grade III placenta has less than 100% predictive power for fetal lung maturity (Table 21–2).[1, 13, 19, 20, 23–28] Moreover, the effect of menstrual age demonstrated for the BPD has also been seen in these studies. For example, in the work of Kazzi and colleagues,[26] a grade III placenta had 100% predictive power for fetal lung maturity when seen after 38 weeks, whereas the predictive power for the presence of PG before 38 weeks was only 15.8%. Such an age effect has also been demonstrated in the studies by Tabsh[27] and Hills and associates,[28] and my colleagues and I confirmed this in our study (see Table 21–2).[1] Subsequent to our study, a nondiabetic mother was delivered of a 32-week fetus with a florid case of RDS seen in the presence of a grade III placenta. As with the BPD, knowing that a grade III placenta is associated with fetal lung maturity after 38 weeks is of limited clinical usefulness, since fetuses delivered after 38 weeks with-

out grade III placentas also have fetal lung maturity.[1]

In 1985, Destro and colleagues[29] reported data from what is, in my opinion, the definitive evaluation of the relation between placental grade and fetal lung maturity in the preterm fetus. These investigators evaluated 32 normal pregnant women between 29 and 33 menstrual weeks for determination of placental grade by ultrasonography, with simultaneous biochemical evaluation of fetal lung maturity by LS ratio and Clements' foam stability test. A grade I placenta was observed in 10 cases, and in this group there was only one mature LS ratio, which was in a patient at 33 menstrual weeks. A grade II placenta was observed in the remaining 22 cases, and again only one mature LS ratio was seen, occurring in a patient at 33 menstrual weeks. No patients with a grade III placenta were identified in this group. These authors concluded that placental grading is of no value in evaluating pulmonary maturity of the fetus before 34 weeks.

Fetal Epiphyseal Ossification Centers

Chinn and colleagues[30] and Mahony and associates[31, 32] demonstrated that sonographically visible lower extremity epiphyseal ossification centers in the distal femur and proximal tibia can be useful in the evaluation of fetal age and lung maturity by ultrasonography (Figs. 21–4 and 21–5). They demonstrated that sonographically visible distal femoral epiphyses indicated a menstrual age of at least 33 weeks with 95% accuracy and that the presence of the proximal

Table 21–2. RELATION BETWEEN PLACENTA GRADE III AND FETAL LUNG MATURITY

Author	No.	Age*	Index of Fetal Lung Maturity	False Positive (%)
Grannum et al[19]	23	>35 wk	LS ≥ 2.0	0.0
Petrucha et al[20]	15	>37 wk	LS ≥ 2.0	0.0
	15	>37 wk	RDS	0.0
	13	>37 wk	PG +	8.0
Quinlan et al[23]	12	NG	LS ≥ 2.0	41.7
Harman et al[13]	130	30–44 wk	LS ≥ 2.0	7.0
	100	30–44 wk	PG +	25.0
Clair et al[24]	13	Near term	LS ≥ 2.0	7.7
Ragozzino et al[25]	12	>37 wk	LS ≥ 3.0	8.0
	12	>37 wk	RDS	0.0
Kazzi et al[26]	61	>38 wk	LS ≥ 2.0	0.0
	61	>38 wk	PG +	0.0
	19	<38 wk	LS ≥ 2.0	21.0
	19	<38 wk	PG +	84.2
	19	<38 wk	RDS	15.8
Tabsh[27]	68	>37 wk	LS ≥ 2.0	5.9
	7	<37 wk	LS ≥ 2.0	28.6
Hills et al[28]	17	>37 wk	LS ≥ 2.0	0.0
	10	<37 wk	LS ≥ 2.0	50.0
Hadlock et al[1]	51	>37 wk	LS ≥ 2.0: PG +	5.9
	2	<37 wk	LS ≥ 2.0: PG +	100.0

RDS, respiratory distress syndrome; PG +, phosphatidylglycerol of at least 0.02%; LS, lecithin/sphingomyelin ratio.
False positive (%) is the number of fetuses, predicted to be mature by placental grading, who actually had immature lungs on the basis of the index of lung maturity used.
*Age is the menstrual age at the time of study.

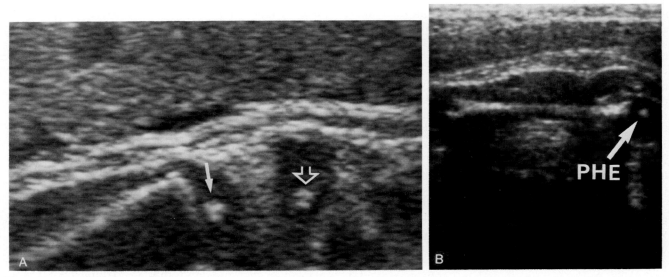

Figure 21–4. *A,* Typical sonographic appearance of the distal femoral epiphysis *(open arrow)* and proximal tibial epiphysis *(closed arrow)* in a 36-week fetus. *B,* Sonographic appearance of the proximal humeral epiphysis (PHE). (Courtesy of Barry S. Mahony, M.D.)

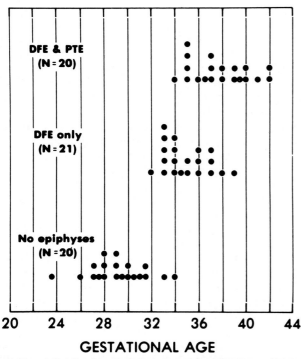

**DFE & PTE
(N = 20)**

**DFE only
(N = 21)**

**No epiphyses
(N = 20)**

20   24   28   32   36   40   44

GESTATIONAL AGE
WHEN AT LEAST 2 OF 3 PARAMETERS AGREE

N = 61

Figure 21–5. The appearance of the distal femoral epiphysis (DFE) and proximal tibial epiphysis (PTE) in a small series of patients in whom gestational age was confirmed by at least two parameters. (From Chinn DH, Bolding DB, Callen PW, et al: Ultrasonographic identification of fetal lower extremity epiphyseal ossification centers. Radiology 147:815–818, 1983.)

tibial epiphyses indicated a menstrual age of at least 35 weeks with 95% accuracy (see Fig. 21–5). Shortly thereafter, several investigators evaluated the presence of such ossification centers as indicators of fetal lung maturity. Gentili and coworkers[33] evaluated 51 normal pregnancies between 31 and 38 weeks and found a mature LS ratio in every case in which the distal femoral epiphyseal ossification center was equal to or greater than 6 mm in diameter. In the same year, Tabsh[34] evaluated 133 nondiabetic patients and demonstrated a mature LS ratio in 100% of cases in which the proximal tibial epiphysis was greater than 5 mm in diameter; he also noted that when a distal femoral epiphysis measured more than 5 mm in diameter, a mature LS ratio was present in 95% of the cases. In 1986, Mahony and coworkers[32] demonstrated that 100% of the fetuses studied had a mature fetal lung profile when the combined diameters of the distal femoral epiphyses and proximal tibial epiphyses were greater than 11 mm. They also noted that when there was less than a 1 mm difference in the size of the distal femoral and proximal tibial epiphyses, similar results were obtained. In addition, Mahony demonstrated that 100% of fetuses studied had a mature lung profile when there were sonographically visible proximal humeral epiphyses.

What can be concluded from these studies about the use of epiphyseal ossification centers in predicting fetal lung maturity? Certainly, when one looks at the relation between the appearance time of these ossification centers and menstrual age, it is not surprising that they correlate relatively well with the presence of mature fetal lungs. In my opinion, the size of the distal femoral epiphysis should never be used alone as a predictor of fetal lung maturity. In addition, the presence of a proximal tibial epiphysis greater than 5 mm in diameter should be viewed with some suspicion, since, as indicated in the work of Tabsh,[34] epiphyses of this size can be seen as early as 35 menstrual weeks, a time in pregnancy when most, but not all, fetuses can be expected to have mature lungs.[4] The work of Mahony and coworkers[32] regarding the proximal humeral epiphyses is more provocative, because this marker generally occurs at approximately 38 weeks or thereafter, a point in pregnancy when virtually all fetuses can be expected to have mature lungs.[4] As Mahony cautions, however, great care must be used in the demonstration of the proximal humeral epiphyses, since other reflective structures (e.g., synovium or capsule) in this area may be mistaken for the proximal humeral epiphyses. Furthermore, it should be noted that although the presence of the proximal humeral epiphyses may be an indication of fetal lung maturity, failure to demonstrate them does not necessarily imply immature fetal lungs; Mahony[32] noted that the predictive value of the proximal humeral epiphyses' absence with immature amniocentesis was only 24%.

Sonographically Detected Free-Floating Particles in Amniotic Fluid

In 1978, Bree[35] reported sonographic identification of reflective material in the amniotic fluid that he believed was fetal vernix, and he theorized that this material may be a marker of fetal maturity. In 1983, however, Parulekar[36] demonstrated that free-floating particles (FFP) may be seen in amniotic fluid as early as mid second trimester and concluded that they have no pathologic significance. Khaleghian,[37] on the other hand, in the same year, reported echogenic material in the amniotic fluid in the second trimester, which he considered a sign of fetal distress. Although there was some controversy about the significance of this material, there was no question that it could be identified using modern ultrasound equipment.

In 1985, Gross and coworkers[38] noted that the turbidity of amniotic fluid was related to the LS ratio in a positive way; that is, the proportion of mature LS ratio values in their study increased with increasing turbidity of the amniotic fluid. This prompted a second study in which the relationship between fetal lung maturity and the presence of FFP in amniotic fluid were evaluated. (This study used a strict definition of FFP, defined as multiple linear densities between 1 and 5 mm in length, suspended, but gradually settling, in the amniotic fluid. It was noted that fetal movement causes a swirling of these particles, giving the appearance of a blizzard.) In a study of 135 patients between 34 and 42 weeks' gestation, FFPs were present in 39 patients and absent in 96. When FFPs were present, the LS ratio was uniformly mature; however, when they were absent, the LS ratio was mature in 74% of patients.[38] A secondary finding in this study was that of increased FFP in association with large-for-gestational-age infants.

Gross and coworkers[38] concluded that the presence of FFP on real-time ultrasonography at greater than 38 weeks' gestation can serve to confirm fetal maturity. Surely such a limited conclusion warrants caution in the use of FFP as a predictor of fetal lung maturity. In my experience, there have been fetuses with FFP in amniotic fluid who had immature lung profiles at amniocentesis, and I therefore caution against the use of this finding in evaluation of fetal lung maturity. This is particularly true since large-for-gestational-age infants, who are perhaps at greatest risk for iatrogenic prematurity, more commonly have FFP than normal or small infants of the same age.

Tissue Characterization of Fetal Lung

Because of the potential complications of amniocentesis and in part because of the failure of other sonographic methods in predicting fetal lung maturity, several authors[39–45] have attempted this estimation by direct sonographic evaluation of the fetal lung. This approach, which has considerable theoretical appeal, was first evaluated by Thieme and associates,[45] and later by Benson and colleagues,[39] Morris,[44] and Cayea and coworkers.[42] Thieme had noted that the developing alveolus can be thought of as a hollow sphere of tissue filled with fluid, the walls of which become thinner with maturity. Thus, the ratio of the volume of the central cavity containing fluid to the total volume of the sphere increases with maturity. Thieme[45] hypothesized that ultrasonography should be able to detect an increase in fluid content by demonstrating enhanced through-transmission of sound in the fetal lungs. Cayea and coworkers further theorized that the reflectivity (echogenicity) of the fetal lung should increase with maturity because of the increased number of acoustic interfaces provided by the increased number of alveoli.[42]

Clinical research aimed at determining the utility of direct fetal lung evaluation has taken several forms. Benson and associates,[39] recognizing that much of the information present in the radiofrequency signal is discarded during the formation of clinical sonographic images, theorized that analysis of the entire radiofrequency signal may yield sufficient data to distinguish between mature and immature fetal tissue. In their study, definite differences between mature and immature tissue were demonstrated for both fetal lung and the placenta, but correlations with objective predictors of the functional maturity of the fetal lung, such as the biochemical lung profile, were not provided; thus, the clinical utility of these data is not known at this time.[39]

In 1984, Morris[44] used a more subjective approach for sonographic evaluation of fetal lung maturity. Morris described a liver/lung ratio based on the observed reflectivity pattern in these two organs, considering the fetal lung to be mature when its reflectivity was greater than that of the fetal liver (Fig. 21–6). In a small group of patients, there was excellent correlation between a mature liver/lung ratio and a mature biochemical lung profile. Morris concluded that the liver/lung ratio alone (or in combination with vernix in the amniotic fluid and a mature placenta) correlates very well with a mature LS ratio but cautioned that confirmation of these results in a large prospective study is needed. At the present time, no such study has been forthcoming.[44]

In 1985, Cayea and associates[42] evaluated subjective sonographic signs of fetal lung maturity using conventional ultrasound instrumentation. They evaluated the fetal lung/liver ratio, in terms of both echogenicity and texture, as well as through-transmission of sound by the fetal lung. In a group of 81 patients, these authors demonstrated no correlation between these sonographic indices of fetal lung maturity in comparison with objective standards, such as the LS ratio, or specific measurements of phosphatidylcholine. In 1985, Fried and coworkers[43] evaluated fetal lung echogenicity (see Fig. 21–6) in predicting fetal lung maturity as determined by the LS ratio and phosphatidylglycerol concentration obtained by amniocentesis. No clinically applicable relation was established in their study. In the same year, Birnholz and Farrell[40] evaluated lung compressibility noted on real-time sonograms and concluded that increased compressibility correlates rather well with lung maturity.

It is clear from the foregoing that the results of predicting fetal lung maturity by direct sonographic evaluation have been mixed. Carson and coworkers[41] have also been active in the investigation of the fetal lung by ultrasonography, and they urge caution in drawing negative conclusions too early from preliminary studies. They note that technical problems can drastically affect experimental outcomes in such studies and have urged that future research in this area be done using consistent techniques, with regard to both experimental design and instrumentation. Until further research has been completed, however, one must conclude that this approach for predicting fetal lung maturity should not form the basis of clinical decision-making in obstetrics.

A Multiple Parameter Scoring System

In 1986, at the annual meeting of the American Institute of Ultrasound in Medicine, Salman and Quetel[46] described preliminary results from an ongoing study in which multiple observations and measurements were used to assess fetal lung maturity. In their scoring system, which is described in detail in Table 21–3, a score of 5 or greater out of a possible total of 10 indicated fetal lung maturity in their initial study group of 104 patients. This approach has considerable theoretical appeal because it takes into account many sonographic parameters that, when used alone, have been demonstrated to have some relation to fetal lung maturity. To gain wide acceptance, however, this sys-

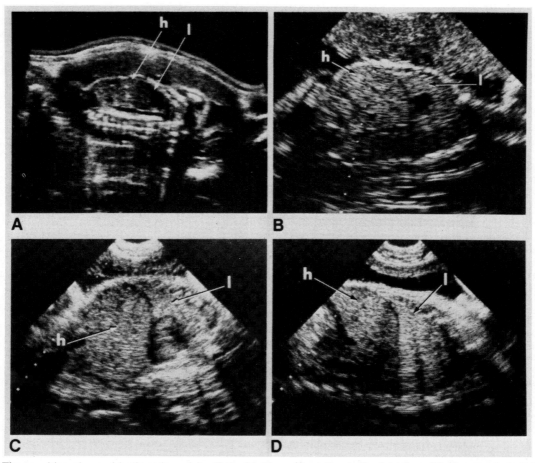

Figure 21–6. The transition observed in the echogenicity of the fetal lung (l) relative to the fetal liver (h). Some authors believe that fetal lung maturity can be assured when the fetal lung is more echogenic than the fetal liver, as noted in *D*. (From Fried AM, Loh FK, Umer MA, et al: Echogenicity of fetal lung: Relation to fetal age maturity. AJR 145:591, 1985.)

Table 21–3. A COMPOSITE SCORING SYSTEM FOR FETAL LUNG MATURITY

Ultrasound Measurements and Observations	Lung Maturity Score
Composite age (by BPD, HC, AC, FL) (Hadlock et al[47])	
<35 wk	0
35–37 wk	1
>37 wk	2
Placenta grade (Grannum et al[19])	
0–I	0
II	1
III	2
Fetal bowel pattern (Zilianti and Fernandez[48])	
Stages 1–2	0
Stage 3	1
Stage 4	2
Lung/liver ratio (Morris[44])	
<1	0
1	1
>1	2
Distal femoral epiphysis (Chinn et al[30])	
Absent	0
Slitlike	1
Globular	2

BPD, biparietal diameter; HC, head circumference; AC, abdominal circumference; FL, femoral length.

From Salman F, Quetel T: Sonographic scoring of fetal pulmonary maturity. J Ultrasound Med 5(Suppl):145, 1985.

tem must have its positive and negative predictive values evaluated in a large prospective study of series of patients throughout the third trimester age range.

At present, primarily because of the small number of fetuses studied and the possible effect of their ages on the results, no sonographic finding in the third trimester of pregnancy can be considered unequivocal evidence of fetal lung maturity. The presence of the proximal humeral epiphyses may prove to be the exception, but further evaluation of this finding will be necessary. The use of a combination of findings, as described by Salman and Quetel,[46] is a rational approach that also may prove sufficiently accurate to obviate the need for amniocentesis; it, too, will require further evaluation by other investigators before it can be used routinely in clinical practice.

Ultrasonography, at present, is best used in one of the following ways: (1) in nondiabetic patients who present early in pregnancy, sonographic documentation of the fetal age allows elective delivery after 38 menstrual weeks with virtually no risk of RDS, and (2) in patients who present late in pregnancy with no validation of menstrual dates, ultrasonography can be used to guide amniocentesis for determination of lung maturity by the fetal lung profile. In the future, however, some composite scoring system, such as that reported by Salman and Quetel,[46] may allow the prediction of functional maturity of the fetal lungs by prenatal ultrasonography.

References

1. Hadlock FP, Irwin JF, Roecker E, et al: Ultrasound prediction of fetal lung maturity. Radiology 155:469, 1985.
2. Gluck L, Kulovich MV, Borer RD, et al: Diagnosis of the respiratory distress syndrome by amniocentesis. Am J Obstet Gynecol 109:440, 1971.
3. Williamson RA, Varner MW, Grant SS: Reduction in amniocentesis risk using a real-time needle guide procedure. Obstet Gynecol 65:751, 1985.
4. Gluck L, Kulovich MV: Lecithin-spingomyelin ratios in amniotic fluid in normal and abnormal pregnancy. Am J Obstet Gyhnecol 115:539, 1973.
5. Kulovich MV, Hallman MB, Gluck L: The lung profile: I. Normal pregnancy. Am J Obstet Gynecol 135:57, 1979.
6. Collaborative Group on Antenatal Steroid Therapy: Effect of antenatal dexamethasone administration on the prevention of respiratory distress syndrome. Am J Obstet Gynecol 141:276, 1981.
7. Donald IR, Freeman RK, Goebelsmann U, et al: Clinical experience with the amniotic fluid lecithin-sphingomyelin ratio: I. Antenatal prediction of pulmonary maturity. Am J Obstet Gynecol 115:547, 1973.
8. MacKenna J, Hodson CA, Brame RG: Clinical utility of fetal lung maturity profile. Obstet Gynecol 57:493, 1981.
9. Whittle MJ, Wilson AI, Whitefield CR, et al: Amniotic fluid phosphatidylglycerol and the lecithin/sphingomyelin ration in the assessment of fetal lung maturity. Br J Obstet Gynaecol 89:727, 1982.
10. Goldstein P, Gershenson D, Hobbins JC: Fetal bi-parietal diameter as a predictor of a mature lecithin/sphingomyelin ratio. Obstet Gynecol 48:667, 1976.
11. Spellacy WN, Gelman SR, Wood SD, et al: Comparison of fetal maturity evaluation with ultrasonic biparietal diameter and amniotic fluid lecithin-sphingomyelin ratio. Obstet Gynecol 51:109, 1978.
12. Strassner HT, Platt LD, Whittle M: Amniotic fluid phosphatidylglycerol and real-time ultrasonic cephalometry. Am J Obstet Gynecol 135:804, 1979.
13. Harman CR, Manning FA, Sterns E, et al: The correlation of ultrasonic placental grading and fetal pulmonary maturation in five hundred sixty-three pregnancies. Am J Obstet Gynecol 143:941, 1982.
14. Hayashi RH, Berry JL, Castillo S: Use of ultrasound biparietal diameter in timing of repeat cesarean section. Obstet Gynecol 57:325, 1981.
15. Golde SH, Petrucha R, Meade KW, et al: Fetal lung maturity: The adjunctive use of ultrasound. Am J Obstet Gynecol 142:445, 1982.
16. Petrucha RA, Golde SH, Platt LD: The use of ultrasound in the prediction of fetal pulmonary maturity. Obstet Gynecol 144:931, 1982.
17. Newton ER, Cetrulo CL, Kosa DJ: Biparietal diameter as a predictor of fetal lung maturity. J Reprod Med 28:480, 1983.
18. Golde SH, Tahilramaney MP, Platt LD: Use of ultrasound to predict fetal lung maturity in 247 consecutive elective cesarean deliveries. J Reprod Med 29:9, 1984.
19. Grannum PAT, Berkowitz RL, Hobbins JC: The ultrasonic changes in the maturing placenta and their relation to fetal pulmonic maturity. Am J Obstet Gynecol 133:915, 1979.
20. Petrucha RA, Golde ST, Platt LD: Real-time ultrasound of the placenta in assessment of fetal pulmonic maturity. Am J Obstet Gynecol 142:463, 1982.
21. Gast MJ, Ott W: Failure of ultrasonic placental grading to predict severe respiratory distress in a neonate. Am J Obstet Gynecol 145:464, 1983.
22. Kollitz J, Dattel BJ, Key TC, et al: Acute respiratory distress syndrome in an infant with grade III placental changes. J Ultrasound Med 1:205, 1982.
23. Quinlan RW, Cruz AC, Buhi WC, et al: Changes in placental ultrasonic appearance: I. Incidence of grade III changes in the placenta in correlation to fetal pulmonary maturity. Am J Obstet Gynecol 144:468, 1982.
24. Clair MR, Rosenberg ET, Tempkin D, et al: Placental grading in the complicated or high risk pregnancy. J Ultrasound Med 2:297, 1983.
25. Ragozzino MW, Hill LM, Breckle R, et al: The relationship of placental grade by ultrasound to markers of fetal lung maturity. Radiology 148:805, 1983.
26. Kazzi GM, Gross TL, Rosen MG, et al: The relationship of placental grade, fetal lung maturity, and neonatal outcome in normal and complicated pregnancies. Am J Obstet Gynecol 148:54, 1984.
27. Tabsh KM: Correlation of real-time ultrasonic placental grading with amniotic fluid lecithin/sphingomyelin ratio. Am J Obstet Gynecol 145:504, 1983.
28. Hills D, Tuck S, Irwin GAL: The unreliability of placental gradings as an indicator of lung maturity in the pre-term fetus. Presented to the Society for Perinatal Obstetricians Annual Meeting. San Antonio, Texas, 1984.
29. Destro F, Calcagnile F, Ceccarello P: Placental grade and pulmonary maturity in premature fetuses. J Clin Ultrasound 13:637, 1985.
30. Chinn DH, Bolding DB, Callen PW, et al: Ultrasonographic identification of fetal lower extremity epiphyseal ossification centers. Radiology 147:815, 1983.
31. Mahony BS, Callen PW, Filly RA: The distal femoral epiphyseal ossification center in the assessment of third trimester age: Sonographic identification and measurement. Radiology 155:201, 1985.
32. Mahony BS, Bowie JD, Killiam AP, et al: Epiphyseal ossification centers in the assessment of fetal maturity: Sonographic correlation with the amniocentesis lung profile. Radiology 159:521, 1986.
33. Gentili P, Trasimeni A, Giorlandino C: Fetal ossification centers as predictors of gestational age in normal and abnormal pregnancies. J Ultrasound Med 3:193, 1984.
34. Tabsh KM: Correlation of ultrasonic epiphyseal centers and the lecithin-sphingomyelin ratio. Obstet Gynecol 64:92, 1984.
35. Bree RL: Sonographic identification of fetal vernix in amniotic fluid. J Clin Ultrasound 6:269, 1978.
36. Paruekar SG: Ultrasonographic demonstration of floating particles in amniotic fluid. J Ultrasound Med 2:107, 1983.
37. Khaleghian R: Echogenic amniotic fluid in the second trimester: A new sign of fetal distress. J Clin Ultrasound 11:498, 1983.
38. Gross TL, Wolfson RN, Kuhnert PM, et al: Sonographically detected free floating particles in amniotic fluid predict a mature lecithin-sphingomyelin ratio. J Clin Ultrasound 13:405, 1985.
39. Benson DM, Waldroup LD, Kurtz AB, et al: Ultrasonic tissue characterization of fetal lung, liver, and placenta for the purpose of assessing fetal maturity. J Ultrasound Med 2:489, 1983.
40. Birnholz JC, Farrell EE: Fetal lung development: Compressibility as a measure of maturity. Radiology 157:495, 1985.
41. Carson PL, Meyer CR, Bowerman RA: Predictions of fetal lung maturity with ultrasound. Radiology 155:533, 1985.
42. Cayea PD, Grant DC, Doublet PM, et al: Prediction of fetal lung maturity: Inaccuracy of study using conventional ultrasound instruments. Radiology 155:473, 1985.
43. Fried AM, Loh FK, Umer MA, et al: Echogenicity of fetal lung: Relation to fetal age maturity. AJR 145:591, 1985.
44. Morris SE: Ultrasound: A predictor of fetal lung maturity. Med Ultrasound 8:1, 1984.
45. Thieme GA, Banjavic RA, Johnson ML, et al: Sonographic identification of lung maturation in the fetal lamb. Invest Radiol 18:18, 1983.
46. Salman F, Quetel T: Sonographic scoring of fetal pulmonic maturity. J Ultrasound Med 5(suppl):145, 1985.
47. Hadlock FP, Deter RL, Harrist RB, et al: Estimating fetal age: Computer-assisted analysis of multiple fetal growth parameters. Radiology 152:497, 1984.
48. Zilianti M, Fernandez S: Correlation of ultrasonic images of fetal intestine with gestational age and fetal maturity. Obstet Gynecol 62:569, 1983.

CHAPTER 22

■■■■■■ Ultrasound Evaluation of Amniotic Fluid

PETER M. DOUBILET, M.D., Ph.D.
CAROL B. BENSON, M.D.

Amniotic fluid plays a major role in fetal growth and development. Abnormalities of fluid volume can interfere directly with fetal development, causing structural anomalies such as pulmonary hypoplasia. Abnormal amount or appearance of the fluid may also be an indirect sign of an underlying disorder, such as fetal hypoxia, neural tube defect, or gastrointestinal obstruction. Sonographic evaluation of the amniotic fluid can, thus, aid in the diagnosis of fetal structural anomalies and fetal compromise and can help guide pregnancy management decisions.

Our goal in this review is to summarize the physiology of amniotic fluid production and consumption and to discuss the sonographic evaluation of amniotic fluid. Because of the pivotal role of amniotic fluid in fetal development, we touch on many aspects of obstetric ultrasound, including abnormalities of fetal structure, growth, and state, focusing on the relationship of these entities to amniotic fluid volume and composition.

PHYSIOLOGY

Amniotic fluid surrounds and protects the fetus in the amniotic cavity. It provides a cushion against the constricting confines of the gravid uterus, allowing the fetus room for movement and growth and protecting it from external trauma. The space around the fetus is necessary for the normal development and maturation of fetal lungs. It also promotes normal development of limbs by permitting periodic extension, thus preventing joint contractures. The fluid bathing the fetus helps maintain the fetal body temperature and plays a part in the homeostasis of fluid and electrolytes.[1]

The mechanisms of amniotic fluid production and consumption, and the composition and volume of amniotic fluid, depend on gestational age. During the first trimester, the major source of amniotic fluid is the amniotic membrane, a thin membrane lined by a single layer of epithelial cells. Water crosses the membrane freely with no active transport mechanism, so that the production of fluid in the amniotic cavity is most likely accomplished by active transport of electrolytes and other solutes by the amnion, with passive diffusion of water following in response to osmotic pressure changes.[2-4] The amnion may also synthesize proteins for secretion into the amniotic cavity.[5]

During the latter half of the first trimester and the early second trimester, as the fetus and placenta differentiate, develop, and grow, other pathways for amniotic fluid production and consumption come into play. These include movement of fluid across the chorion frondosum and fetal skin, fetal urine output, and fetal swallowing and gastrointestinal absorption (Fig. 22–1). The chorion frondosum, the portion of the chorion that develops into the fetal portion of the placenta, is a site at which water is exchanged freely between fetal blood and amniotic fluid across the amnion.[1-5] Fetal skin is permeable to water and some solutes, permitting direct exchange between the fetus and amniotic fluid until keratinization occurs at 24 to 26 weeks' gestation.[2-5]

Fetal urine production and swallowing both begin at 8 to 11 weeks' gestation and become the major pathways for amniotic fluid production and consumption from the mid second trimester onward. At 25 weeks the fetus produces approximately 100 mL of urine daily, with production increasing to about 600 mL/d by term and then declining somewhat after 40 weeks. Fetal swallowing leads to amniotic fluid consumption, as the swallowed fluid is absorbed by the fetal gastrointestinal tract. The volume of fluid swallowed increases with gestational age to 200 to 500 mL/d by term.[2-5]

The fetal respiratory system may also provide a mechanism for production and consumption of amniotic fluid, although the exact contribution of this system is unknown. Fluid may be absorbed or excreted across the alveolar capillaries or trachea.[1-4] There may be a net flow of fluid from the fetus across the respiratory tract into the amniotic fluid.[3, 4] Some exchange of alveolar fluid with amniotic fluid does occur, as manifested by increasing concentrations of fetal pulmonary phospholipids in the amniotic fluid as pregnancy progresses.[6]

As the mechanisms for amniotic fluid production change during the course of pregnancy, the composition of the fluid changes concomitantly. In the first and early second trimesters, fluid production primarily involves passive flow of water across membranes or fetal skin, so that the amniotic fluid is similar in composition and osmolality to maternal and fetal serum. Thereafter, amniotic fluid becomes increasingly similar to fetal urine, which itself changes in nature as the fetus develops. Like fetal urine, amniotic fluid becomes increasingly hypotonic with respect to maternal and fetal serum from the mid second trimester onward. Sodium and chloride concentrations decrease, and urea and creatinine concentrations increase.[3-5]

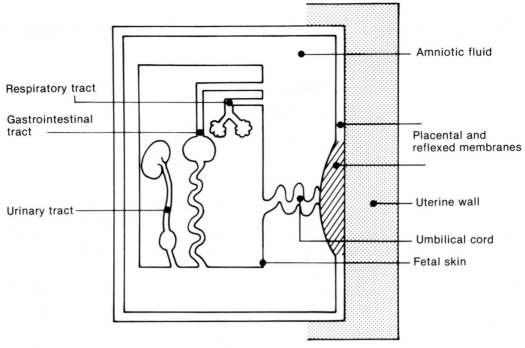

Figure 22–1. The major fetal and maternal anatomic structures involved in the formation and reabsorption of amniotic fluid. (From Wallenburg HCS: The amniotic fluid. J Perinatal Med 5:193, 1977.)

The total volume of amniotic fluid increases throughout gestation until 38 to 40 weeks, after which it decreases. At the end of the first trimester, normal fluid volume is approximately 60 mL, with a range of 35 to 100 mL. By 16 weeks, the mean amniotic fluid volume is approximately 200 mL, with a range for normal of 125 to 300 mL. At term it measures approximately 900 mL, with a wide normal range of 500 to 1200 mL. Fluid around the post-term fetus declines to 250 to 500 mL as the pregnancy proceeds.[3–5, 7]

In addition to its relationship with gestational age, fluid volume also correlates with fetal and placental weight.[7] In particular, fetuses that are small-for-gestational age tend to have decreased amniotic fluid, while those that are large-for-gestational age tend to have increased fluid volumes.[8–13]

Maternal factors play a small role in modulating amniotic fluid. Amniotic fluid volume correlates with maternal plasma volume, a relationship that is mediated predominantly by the fetus. Fluid is exchanged freely between maternal and fetal sera across the highly permeable placenta. Alterations in maternal hydration lead to changes in net movement of fluid into or from the fetus. This, in turn, affects fetal urine production and, hence, amniotic fluid volume.[3] Increased maternal hydration leads to increased fetal hydration, increased fetal urine output, and increased amniotic fluid volume.[14, 15] Maternal dehydration is associated with oligohydramnios that returns to normal following rehydration of the mother.

Amniotic fluid provides a reservoir for homeostasis of fetal hydration. Fetuses with excess water transfer fluid to the amniotic space, while dehydrated fetuses can conserve water by swallowing more amniotic fluid, absorbing more water across the gastrointestinal tract, and reducing urine production.[3]

DISORDERS OF AMNIOTIC FLUID VOLUME

Polyhydramnios

Polyhydramnios (sometimes called hydramnios) is defined as amniotic fluid volume above the normal range for gestational age or, by some authors, as a fluid volume above 1500 to 2000 mL in the third trimester.[1, 4, 16] It may be caused by a variety of fetal or maternal disorders or may be idiopathic (Table 22–1).[16–22] Most fetal causes are the result of decreased fluid consumption through the gastrointestinal tract. In particular, any fetal anomaly that impairs swallowing (e.g., anencephaly, facial tumor) or that prevents swallowed fluid from contacting the absorptive surface of the small intestine (e.g., duodenal atresia) may cause polyhydramnios.

Diabetes mellitus is associated with an increased frequency of polyhydramnios and represents the most common maternal cause of elevated amniotic fluid volume. Polyhydramnios is especially frequent when the diabetes is poorly controlled. The underlying mechanism is unknown, and, in particular, no relationship has been found between polyhydramnios and fetal urine production rate in diabetic mothers.[23]

The majority of cases of polyhydramnios are mild or moderate in severity and are idiopathic. When the polyhydramnios is severe, an underlying fetal cause is likely. When all cases of polyhydramnios are considered, approximately 20% are due to fetal causes (the

Table 22–1. CAUSES OF POLYHYDRAMNIOS

Cause	Postulated Mechanism
Fetal Causes	**Idiopathic**
Central nervous system lesions: Neural tube defects (encephalocele, meningomyelocele, hydrancephaly, holoprosencephaly)	Fetal swallowing neurologically impaired Polyuria due to lack of antidiuretic hormone Transudation through meninges
Gastrointestinal lesions:	Decreased gastrointestinal tract absorption
Esophageal atresia, duodenal atresia/obstruction, proximal small bowel atresia/obstruction	
Thorax/diaphragm lesions:	Decreased lung absorption
Cystic adenomatoid malformation, diaphragmatic hernia, congenital chylothorax, mediastinal mass	Esophageal compression
Miscellaneous:	
Thanatophoric and other short-limbed dwarfs, facial tumors, cleft lip/palate, cystic hygroma, nonimmune fetal hydrops	
Maternal Causes	
Diabetes mellitus (poorly controlled)	
Isoimmunization (e.g., Rh incompatibility)	

majority of which are central nervous system or gastrointestinal anomalies), 20% are due to maternal causes, and 60% are idiopathic.[16–21] Among the subset of cases with severe polyhydramnios, approximately 75% are caused by a fetal abnormality and the remainder are due to maternal causes or are idiopathic.[22] The practical implication is that when a careful fetal survey reveals no abnormality in the setting of mildly increased fluid, a confident diagnosis of idiopathic polyhydramnios can be made; but when polyhydramnios is severe and no fetal anomaly is seen, repeat examination or referral to a tertiary center should be strongly considered.

Increased amniotic fluid volume produces uterine stretching and enlargement that may lead to preterm labor, as well as a variety of other maternal symptoms. The enlarged uterus itself may be painful. It can also compress adjacent organs, resulting in edema from inferior vena cava compression, oliguria from ureteral compression, and dyspnea from diaphragmatic elevation. These complications are more likely to occur when the polyhydramnios develops acutely than in the setting of chronic polyhydramnios.[24]

When the patient is symptomatic, early delivery may be indicated. If the fetus cannot be delivered safely, treatment of polyhydramnios may be undertaken through amniocentesis or medical therapy. Therapeutic amniocentesis may be considered for polyhydramnios of any etiology, while medical therapy is mainly applicable in cases of severe idiopathic polyhydramnios. Therapeutic amniocentesis reduces the fluid volume immediately, although reaccumulation is usually rapid, making repeated procedures necessary. No more than 1 to 2 liters should be removed at a time, since excessive decompression may lead to placental separation. Indomethacin, a prostaglandin synthetase inhibitor, can be given orally to the mother as a medical treatment for polyhydramnios (Fig. 22–2).[25–27] Indomethacin most likely reduces fluid volume by decreasing fetal urine production. Complications of this therapy include fetal renal shutdown and premature closure of the ductus arteriosus. Close sonographic surveillance

is recommended, including Doppler assessment of blood flow through the ductus arteriosus.[26–28]

Oligohydramnios

Amniotic fluid volume that is abnormally low for gestational age is termed *oligohydramnios*. Oligohydramnios with intact membranes may be caused by a variety of conditions in which fetal urine output is low (Table 22–2). These include a number of urinary tract anomalies, especially bilateral renal agenesis and posterior urethral valves (Fig. 22–3). The prognosis in fetuses with posterior urethral valves is closely related to the presence and severity of oligohydramnios: the lower the fluid volume, the worse the prognosis.[29, 30] Infantile polycystic kidney disease causes oligohydramnios when renal failure occurs prenatally.[31, 32]

Intrauterine growth retardation, particularly that resulting from placental insufficiency, is associated with oligohydramnios. Placental insufficiency produces fetal hypoxia, which in turn leads to reflex redistribution of fetal blood flow away from the kidneys and toward the brain, resulting in oligohydramnios from decreased urine production.[33, 34] Oligohydramnios may also occur in post-term pregnancy, as a result of decreased fetal urine production.[35]

Prolonged severe oligohydramnios, particularly that beginning in the second trimester, may lead to a constellation of fetal abnormalities due primarily to pressure on the fetus by the uterine wall. These include pulmonary hypoplasia, abnormal facies (flattened nose, low-set ears, recessed chin), and limb positional abnormalities (clubfeet, contractures, hip dislocation). The most serious of these is pulmonary hypoplasia, which may be fatal shortly after birth. Pulmonary hypoplasia in the presence of oligohydramnios may also be due to a loss of the normal stenting of the fetal lung from an egress of fluid from the lungs into the low-pressure amniotic space. This constellation of pulmonary, facial, and orthopedic abnormalities is referred to as Potter syndrome when it occurs in the

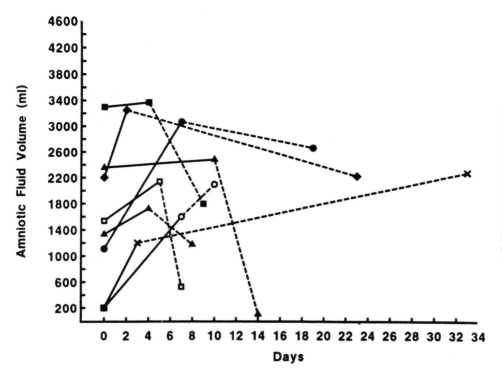

Figure 22–2. Amniotic fluid volumes in patients not taking indomethacin *(solid lines)* and taking indomethacin *(dashed lines)*. The first value for each patient is the residual volume after amniocentesis. (From Kirshon B, Mari G, Moise KJ Jr: Indomethacin therapy in the treatment of symptomatic polyhydramnios. Reprinted with permission from the American College of Obstetricians and Gynecologists [Obstetrics and Gynecology, 1990, 75:202].)

Table 22–2. CAUSES OF OLIGOHYDRAMNIOS

Cause	Postulated Mechanism
Fetal urinary tract anomalies	Decreased urine output
Bilateral renal agenesis	
Posterior urethral valves	
Infantile polycystic kidney disease	
Bilateral multicystic dysplastic kidneys	
Intrauterine growth retardation	Decreased fetal renal blood flow leading to decreased urine production
Post-term pregnancy	Decreased urine output
Ruptured membranes	Fluid leakage

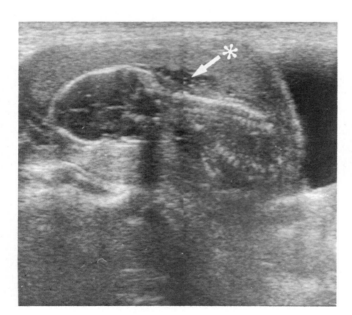

Figure 22–3. Sonogram of a fetus with renal agenesis. Virtually no amniotic fluid is seen. The only relatively anechoic space is occupied by the umbilical cord *(asterisk)*.

setting of bilateral renal agenesis.[36] The term *Potter sequence* has been applied to the same findings resulting from other causes of prolonged severe oligohydramnios.

Umbilical cord compression, which can cause fetal asphyxia, is another potential complication of oligohydramnios. The cord normally floats freely in the amniotic fluid, but with diminished fluid it may be squeezed between the fetus and the uterine wall. Cord accidents from oligohydramnios may be an important factor in the high morbidity and mortality of post-term fetuses.[37]

Treatment of oligohydramnios can be achieved by infusion of a saline solution into the amniotic cavity. Although amnioinfusion does not treat the underlying cause of the oligohydramnios, it can potentially relieve or prevent cord compression. Some studies of amnioinfusion suggest a beneficial effect, including a lower incidence of variable decelerations in fetal heart rate patterns, but the results are not uniformly positive. Further studies are needed to evaluate this procedure.[38–41]

SONOGRAPHIC ASSESSMENT OF AMNIOTIC FLUID VOLUME

Methods of Assessment

Assessment of amniotic fluid volume should be a component of every obstetric sonogram, particularly in the second and third trimesters.[42] In the usual clinical setting, the goal is to classify the fluid as normal, polyhydramnios, or oligohydramnios, rather than to measure the actual fluid volume. Several methods have been proposed for sonographic assessment of amniotic fluid volume. These include subjective assessment, measurement of the single deepest pocket, amniotic fluid index, planimetric measurement of total intra-uterine volume, and a variety of mathematical formulae.

Subjective Assessment. Subjective assessment of amniotic fluid volume is accomplished by real-time scanning through the entire uterus and observing the amount of fluid in the gestational sac surrounding the fetus (Fig. 22–4).[1, 11, 43–46] The fluid volume is subjectively classified as normal, high, or low for the gestational age. Fluid volume may be further subclassified using categories such as moderate or severe oligohydramnios or polyhydramnios.

This approach is quick and efficient and takes into account gestational age–related variation in fluid volume. This method, however, may be unreliable in the hands of an inexperienced operator. Furthermore, the basis for classifying fluid as normal, high, or low is difficult to document on hard copy. This can pose problems when the operator is not the person who renders the final interpretation of the scan or when the fluid volume is followed over repeated scans.

Single-Deepest-Pocket Measurement. Assessment of amniotic fluid volume using the single-deepest-pocket method involves measuring the maximum vertical depth of any amniotic fluid pocket (Fig. 22–5). A measurement below 1 to 2 cm is considered to represent oligohydramnios, and one above 8 cm represents polyhydramnios (Fig. 22–6).[8, 9, 12, 45]

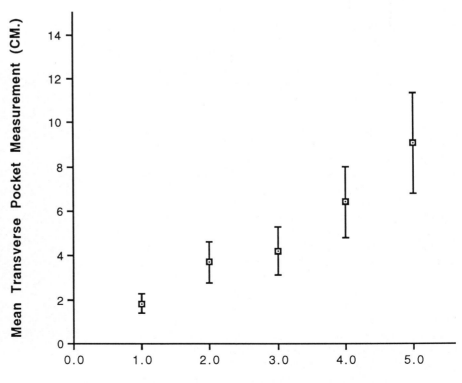

Figure 22–4. Mean of transverse measurements of the largest amniotic fluid pocket versus subjectively judged amniotic fluid volume (AFV). There is a good correlation between amniotic fluid volume estimates judged with pocket measurements and estimates judged subjectively. 1.0, oligohydramnios (little to no amniotic fluid, virtually no pocket free of umbilical cord, crowding of small parts); 2.0, somewhat decreased amniotic fluid (not frank oligohydramnios, but subjectively less than expected amniotic fluid volume for gestational age); 3.0, normal (good fluid–fetal interface, especially about small parts, with fetus filling the anteroposterior diameter of the uterus); 4.0, somewhat increased (more fluid than expected around small parts, slight interface of fluid between fetus and uterine wall); 5.0, frank polyhydramnios (fetus does not fill the uterine cavity in the anteroposterior dimension and much more than expected fluid around both the fetal trunk and small parts). (From Goldstein RB, Filly RA: Sonographic estimation of amniotic fluid volume. J Ultrasound Med 7:363, 1988.)

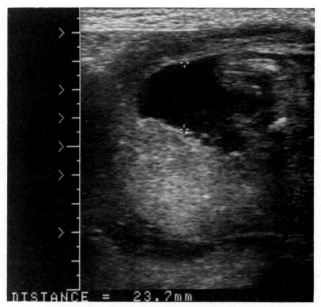

Figure 22–5. Normal amniotic fluid volume assessed by measurement of the largest single pocket of fluid. In this 22-week gestation, the largest vertical pocket of amniotic fluid, devoid of umbilical cord, is 24 mm.

This method is simple and straightforward but has little mathematical validity or rationale. The volume of a simple shape, such as a sphere or cube, is directly related to, and can be calculated from, a single measurement. In contrast, the volume of a highly irregular shape, such as that occupied by amniotic fluid, cannot be calculated from, or even accurately approximated by, one measurement. In addition, the single-deepest-pocket measurement can vary considerably if the fetus changes position. Furthermore, measurement of a deep but thin "pancake"-shaped collection between the fetal legs or alongside the fetus may yield a normal value even in the presence of severe oligohydramnios. Finally, variation in amniotic fluid volume with gestational age is not taken into account if a lower limit of 1 to 2 cm and an upper limit of 8 cm is used for all ages.

Four-Quadrant Amniotic Fluid Index. The amniotic fluid index is determined by dividing the uterus into four quadrants by sagittal and transverse lines through the umbilicus and summing the vertical dimensions of the deepest pocket in each quadrant (Fig. 22–7; Table 22–3). When the sum results in a value below 5 cm, it is considered to signify oligohydramnios and one above 18 to 20 cm, polyhydramnios.[47–50]

This approach is fairly quick and gives a better assessment of amniotic fluid volume than does the single-deepest-pocket measurement, because the sum of four measurements will always correlate more closely with volume than will a single measurement. However, since the measurement of the deepest pocket in each quadrant bears little relationship to the amount of amniotic fluid in that quadrant, their sum will not accurately reflect the overall fluid volume. Furthermore, changes in fetal position and gestational age variation in fluid volume represent limitations for the four-quadrant amniotic fluid index, as they do for the single-deepest-pocket measurement.

Planimetric Measurement of Total Intrauterine Volume. Total intrauterine volume can be estimated by obtaining multiple scans through the uterus at regular intervals. The intrauterine area is determined on each scan and multiplied by the width of the interval. These values are summed to yield the total intrauterine volume.[51–55]

The approach is slow and cumbersome, requiring tracing the uterine outline on each scan to compute the area. An articulated arm is needed to ensure that proper scan planes are obtained. The result of this time-consuming calculation is not the amniotic fluid volume itself, but rather the sum of amniotic fluid, fetal, and placental volumes.

Mathematical Formulae for Volume Calculation. A variety of formulae using sonographic measurements to approximate total intrauterine volume,[56] total intrauterine volume minus fetal and placental volumes,[57] and volume of the largest pocket[58] have been proposed. However, all these approaches make the assumption that the uterus (or fetus, placenta, or deepest pocket) conforms to a regular shape, such as a prolate ellipsoid. Unfortunately, such assumptions are oversimplifications that can lead to substantial inaccuracy.[54]

Given these five proposed methods for amniotic fluid volume assessment, which approach should be used in clinical practice? Unfortunately, the medical literature provides no substantive basis for choosing among these methods based on their accuracies or reproducibilities. None of the commonly employed approaches for amniotic fluid volume assessment has been tested against a reliable "gold standard" for amniotic fluid volume, such as the dye-dilution method.[57, 59] Although the single-deepest-pocket method has been compared with the subjective assessment approach[45] and with the am-

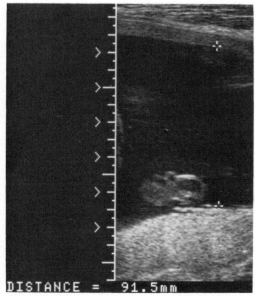

Figure 22–6. Sonogram of a fetus with polyhydramnios due to gastrointestinal tract obstruction. A pocket of amniotic fluid larger than 8 cm is seen.

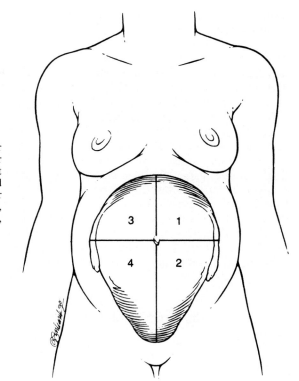

Figure 22–7. Diagram of the division of the uterus into four equal quadrants for determination of the amniotic fluid index. With the ultrasound transducer perpendicular to the table the vertical depth of the largest amniotic fluid pocket that is free of umbilical cord in each quadrant is measured. It should be noted that some examiners measure the pockets in millimeters and total the four quadrants while others measure the pockets in centimeters. (From Gabbe SG, Niebyl JR, Simpson JL [eds.]: Obstetrics: Normal and Problem Pregnancies, 2nd ed. Churchill Livingstone, New York, 1991.)

Table 22–3. AMNIOTIC FLUID INDEX VALUES IN NORMAL PREGNANCY

| | Amniotic Fluid Index Percentile Values | | | | | |
Week	2.5th	5th	50th	95th	97.5th	n
16	73	79	121	185	201	32
17	77	83	127	194	211	26
18	80	87	133	202	220	17
19	83	90	137	207	225	14
20	86	93	141	212	230	25
21	88	95	143	214	233	14
22	89	97	145	216	235	14
23	90	98	146	218	237	14
24	90	98	147	219	238	23
25	89	97	147	221	240	12
26	89	97	147	223	242	11
27	85	95	146	226	245	17
28	86	94	146	228	249	25
29	84	92	145	231	254	12
30	82	90	145	234	258	17
31	79	88	144	238	263	26
32	77	86	144	242	269	25
33	74	83	143	245	274	30
34	72	81	142	248	278	31
35	70	79	140	249	279	27
36	68	77	138	249	279	39
37	66	75	135	244	275	36
38	65	73	132	239	269	27
39	64	72	127	226	255	12
40	63	71	123	214	240	64
41	63	70	116	194	216	162
42	63	69	110	175	192	30

Note: Amniotic fluid index values are obtained by measuring the vertical depth of the largest clear amniotic fluid pocket in each of four equal uterine quadrants. The values from each quadrant are measured in millimeters and added together.

From Moore TR, Cayle JE: The amniotic fluid index in normal human pregnancy. Am J Obstet Gynecol 162:1168, 1990.

niotic fluid index,[60] neither comparison was based on an independent "gold standard."

The reproducibilities of subjective assessment of amniotic fluid volume, single-deepest-pocket measurement, and amniotic fluid index have all been evaluated. The intraobserver and interobserver variabilities for all of these methods are low and are too similar to provide a basis for choosing among them.[45, 48, 50]

In the absence of any solid evidence favoring one approach, we recommend that an experienced sonographer or sonologist rely on subjective assessment of fluid volume, especially in a setting where the person rendering the final interpretation has the opportunity to perform real-time scanning. The four-quadrant amniotic fluid index is a reasonable choice for those with little experience at obstetric ultrasound evaluation or in a facility where the person interpreting the scan has little or no involvement in real-time scanning.

Use of Amniotic Fluid Volume in Fetal Diagnosis

DIAGNOSIS OF INTRAUTERINE GROWTH RETARDATION

Numerous studies have examined whether the presence of oligohydramnios, as determined by various methods of sonographic assessment, can serve as a reliable diagnostic criterion for intrauterine growth retardation (IUGR).[11, 12, 43, 56, 61–63] The results of these studies have been mixed, with some suggesting that oligohydramnios is a useful diagnostic criterion for IUGR and others finding it to be a poor predictor of IUGR.

In a statistical analysis of the pooled published data on proposed sonographic criteria for IUGR, we found that oligohydramnios is not a reliable predictor of IUGR. When total intrauterine volume is low, the likelihood of the fetus being growth retarded is no more than 25%. In the presence of oligohydramnios diagnosed either subjectively or through the 1 cm deepest-pocket rule, the chance of IUGR is 55%. Like other individual sonographic criteria for IUGR, therefore, the presence of oligohydramnios does not permit a confident diagnosis of IUGR.[64]

In subsequent studies, we have found that the subjectively assessed amniotic fluid volume can be used in conjunction with two other parameters—estimated fetal weight and maternal blood pressure status—to accurately diagnose or exclude IUGR. In particular, when there is both oligohydramnios (with intact membranes) and a low estimated weight percentile, IUGR can be diagnosed with confidence, especially in a hypertensive mother. The accuracy of these three parameters in combination is superior to that achieved by any single-parameter approach to diagnosing IUGR.[65, 66]

DIAGNOSIS OF FETAL COMPROMISE

Multiple studies have demonstrated that pregnancies with oligohydramnios are at increased risk for perinatal morbidity, including fetal distress in labor, low Apgar scores, and meconium staining.[46, 49, 67–70] Oligohydramnios is also associated with an elevated perinatal mortality rate.[46, 71] These higher rates of unfavorable pregnancy outcome occur whether the oligohydramnios is diagnosed subjectively,[46] through the single-deepest-pocket measurement,[67, 68, 70, 71] or using the amniotic fluid index.[49] The poor outcome associated with oligohydramnios results in some cases from the underlying cause of the low fluid and in other cases from cord accidents.

Because of the association between oligohydramnios and poor pregnancy outcome, some authors have suggested that fluid volume may be useful to guide decisions concerning the timing of delivery in certain high-risk pregnancies, such as post-term patients[72, 73] and those with preterm rupture of the membranes.[74, 75]

A better approach than using the fluid volume on its own to diagnose fetal compromise is to employ it as a component of the multiparameter biophysical profile.[33, 76] In the biophysical profile scoring system, the amniotic fluid volume is used as a marker of chronic fetal asphyxia, in combination with four other acute indicators of asphyxia: (1) fetal body movements, (2) tone, (3) breathing movements, and (4) heart rate reactivity. The score that encompasses these five parameters has been shown to correlate with perinatal morbidity and mortality[76, 77] and to have a very low false-negative rate, in that the rate of fetal death within 1 week of a normal biophysical profile score is exceedingly low.[78] Most importantly, a management scheme in which the biophysical profile score influences the timing of delivery appears to lower perinatal mortality in high-risk fetuses.[79–81]

LOW FLUID IN THE FIRST TRIMESTER

While the term *oligohydramnios* is usually applied in the second and third trimesters, low fluid volume in the first trimester (as evidenced by small sac size) is a predictor of poor fetal outcome. In one study, 94% (15 of 16) mothers of living fetuses with small sac size in the first trimester went on to have spontaneous abortions.[82]

ECHOGENICITY

Normal amniotic fluid is anechoic throughout the first trimester. In second- and third-trimester pregnancies, small particles are often observed sonographically within the amniotic fluid, either dependent or suspended, swirling within the fluid when the fetus or mother moves. The frequency with which such particles are seen increases as pregnancy progresses, from approximately 50% in the latter half of the second trimester to virtually all cases after 35 weeks.[83] The density of the visualized particles also tends to increase. When the density of particles is high, the fluid becomes homogeneously hyperechoic (Fig. 22–8), similar in echogenicity to the fetal liver. In such cases, the anechoic umbilical cord stands out prominently and the fetal stomach may be difficult to identify because of the echogenic swallowed fluid within it.[84]

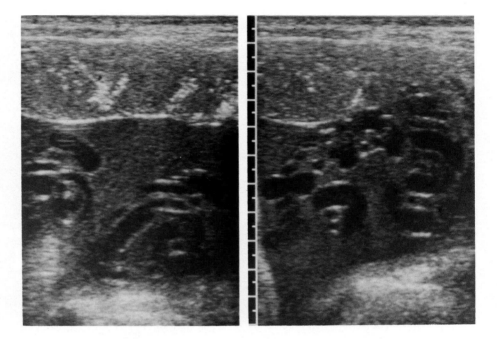

Figure 22–8. Two images of the amniotic fluid in a third-trimester gestation. Highly echogenic fluid is seen surrounding the umbilical cord.

The particles visualized sonographically may represent vernix caseosa, blood, or meconium. Vernix is desquamated fetal epithelial cells and sebaceous material produced by the fetal skin. Intra-amniotic blood may arise from spontaneous bleeding or may occur as a result of amniocentesis or other interventional procedure. Meconium may be passed from the fetus into the amniotic fluid.

Vernix, blood, and meconium in the amniotic fluid may all have the same sonographic appearance.[83–87] When particles are visualized in the amniotic fluid before 15 weeks, they are most often due to blood. In the first and second trimester, markedly hyperechoic fluid is highly unusual and suggests massive intra-amniotic bleeding. In our experience, this unusual finding is seen predominantly in women with coagulation disorders or an anticoagulation therapy.[88] In the third trimester, intra-amniotic particles are due to vernix in the large majority of cases. Regardless of their density, the finding has little, if any, clinical significance in the latter part of pregnancy.

Amniotic fluid echogenicity has been suggested as a means for predicting fetal lung maturity. When fluid is anechoic, the lungs are highly likely to be immature, while 53% of fetuses with hyperechoic fluid have mature lungs.[89] This relationship, however, between increasing fluid echogenicity and lung maturity is largely due to their common association with gestational age. Amniotic fluid echogenicity on its own is an unreliable indicator of fetal lung maturity, providing little if any additional information over and above that provided by the gestational age.

Twin Gestation

Amniotic fluid volume assessment in multiple gestation can often be quite difficult. In dizygotic gesta-

tions in which each gestation resides within its own amniotic sac, the subjective assessment of amniotic fluid volume or largest single pocket of amniotic fluid must be utilized, since the four-quadrant amniotic fluid index is meaningless. In addition to the subjective assessment of fluid surrounding the fetus, we like to obtain views of the fluid seen on either side of the dividing amniotic membrane. Normal pockets of fluid on either side of the membrane are reassuring. In dizygotic gestations, assuming that IUGR has not occurred, it is our experience that the most common error is to overestimate amniotic fluid volume.

In cases of monozygotic monochorionic gestations two additional problems present with amniotic fluid volume assessment. Cases of monoamniotic pregnancy will make it virtually impossible to determine fluid volume for an individual twin. Although in one sense this is problematic, in most cases, adequacy of amniotic fluid volume as it relates to normal fetal lung and limb development as well as overall dramatically increased amniotic fluid can still be assessed.

The second problem in monochorionic twin gestations is the twin transfusion or "stuck twin" syndrome. In approximately one third of cases of monochorionic twin gestations there is a marked disparity of amniotic fluid volumes in each amniotic sac.[90–93] One of the twins is in a polyhydramniotic sac and may be hydropic, and the other is in an oligohydramniotic sac and may be growth retarded. The mortality for such pregnancies is said to be as high as 100%.[91, 94] Although the pathophysiology is still being debated the most common explanation is that one twin is believed to donate blood to the other twin through placental vascular anastomoses.[95, 96] The donor twin becomes growth retarded and the recipient fetus becomes hydropic in a polyhydramniotic sac.

The high mortality of this condition has resulted in a number of therapeutic attempts to alleviate this

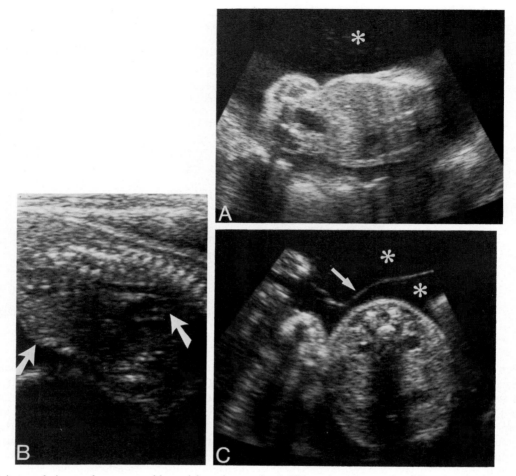

Figure 22–9. Twin-transfusion syndrome treated by serial amniocentesis. *A.* This patient presented at 24 weeks' gestation large for dates. A sonogram revealed marked polyhydramnios in one amniotic sac *(asterisk)*. *B.* The remaining twin *(arrows)* was "stuck" to the anterior uterine wall enshrouded by the amniotic membrane in an oligohydramniotic sac. *C.* After therapeutic amniocentesis of the polyhydramniotic sac, the fluid normalized in both sacs *(asterisks)* and the growth of the "stuck twin" improved. The dividing amniotic membrane is now visible *(arrow)*. Of incidental note is bilateral fetal pyelectasis.

condition varying from feticide to hysterotomy.[97, 98] In the past 5 years it has been recognized that in a number of cases in which therapeutic amniocentesis was performed in the polyhydramniotic twin, the fluid and growth around the stuck twin normalized after removal of excess fluid. There subsequently have been a number of reports confirming this finding.[99, 100] Procedurally, serial amniocenteses are required with removal of fluid varying from 200 to 5000 mL (Fig. 22–9).[100] Although the explanation for this dramatic improvement is not known, there is no question that this procedure is often quite successful.

References

1. Graham D, Sanders RC: Amniotic fluid. Semin Roentgenol 17:210, 1982.
2. Seeds AE: Current concepts of amniotic fluid dynamics. Am J Obstet Gynecol 138:575, 1980.
3. Brace RA, Wolf EJ: Normal amniotic fluid volume changes throughout pregnancy. Am J Obstet Gynecol 161:382, 1989.
4. Moore PT, Mencini RA, Spitz HB: Sonographic diagnosis of hydramnios and oligohydramnios. Semin Ultrasound CT MR 5:157, 1984.
5. Wallenburg HCS: The amniotic fluid: I. Water and electrolyte homeostasis. J Perinat Med 5:193, 1977.
6. Hallman M, Kulovich M, Kirkpatrick E, et al: Phosphatidylinositol and phosphatidylglycerol in amniotic fluid. Am J Obstet Gynecol 125:613, 1976.
7. Queenan JT, Thompson W, Whitfield CR, Shah SI: Amniotic fluid volumes in normal pregnancies. Am J Obstet Gynecol 114:34, 1972.
8. Chamberlain PF, Manning FA, Morrison I, et al: Ultrasound evaluation of amniotic fluid volume: I. The relationship of marginal and decreased fluid volumes to perinatal outcome. Am J Obstet Gynecol 150:245, 1984.
9. Chamberlain PF, Manning FA, Morrison I, et al: Ultrasound evaluation of amniotic fluid volume: II. The relationship of increased fluid volume to perinatal outcome. Am J Obstet Gynecol 150:250, 1984.
10. Varma TR, Bateman S, Patel RH, et al: The relationship of increased amniotic fluid volume to perinatal outcome. Int J Gynecol Obstet 27:327, 1988.
11. Philipson EH, Sokol RJ, Williams T: Oligohydramnios: Clinical associations and predictive value for intrauterine growth retardation. Am J Obstet Gynecol 146:271, 1983.
12. Manning FA, Hill LM, Platt LD: Qualitative amniotic fluid

volume determination by ultrasound: Antepartum detection of intrauterine growth retardation. Am J Obstet Gynecol 139:254, 1981.

13. Benson CB, Coughlin BF, Doubilet PM: Amniotic fluid volume in large-for-gestational-age fetuses of nondiabetic mothers. J Ultrasound Med 10:149, 1991.

14. Powers DR, Brace RA: Fetal cardiovascular and fluid responses to maternal volume loading with lactated Ringer's or hypotonic solution. Am J Obstet Gynecol 165:1504, 1991.

15. Goodlin RC, Anderson JC, gallagher TF: Relationship between amniotic fluid volume and maternal plasma volume expansion. Am J Obstet Gynecol 146:505, 1983.

16. Wallenburg HCS, Wladimiroff JW: The amniotic fluid: II. Polyhydramnios and oligohydramnios. J Perinat Med 6:233, 1977.

17. Hobbins JC, Grannum PAT, Berkowitz RL, et al: Ultrasound in the diagnosis of congenital abnormalities. Am J Obstet Gynecol 134:331, 1979.

18. Alexander ES, Spitz HB, Clark RA: Sonography of polyhydramnios. AJR 138:343, 1982.

19. Quinlan RW, Cruz AC, Martin M: Hydramnios: Ultrasound diagnosis and its impact on perinatal management and pregnancy outcome. Am J Obstet Gynecol 145:306, 1983.

20. Sivit CJ, Hill MC, Larsen JW, Lande IM: Second-trimester polyhydramnios: Evaluation with US. Radiology 165:467, 1987.

21. Hill LM, Breckle R, Thomas ML, Fries JK: Polyhydramnios: Ultrasonically detected prevalence and neonatal outcome. Obstet Gynecol 69:21, 1987.

22. Barkin SZ, Pretorius DH, Beckett MK, et al: Severe polyhydramnios: Incidence of anomalies. AJR 148:155, 1987.

23. van Otterlo LC, Wladimiroff JW, Wallenburg HCS: Relationship between fetal urine production and amniotic fluid volume in normal pregnancy and pregnancy complicated by diabetes. Br J Obstet Gynaecol 84:205, 1977.

24. Pritchard JA, MacDonald PC, Gant NF: William's Obstetrics, 17th ed, p 463. East Norwalk, CT, Appleton-Century-Crofts, 1990.

25. Cabrol D, Landesman R, Muller J, et al: Treatment of polyhydramnios with prostaglandin synthetase inhibitor (indomethacin). Am J Obstet Gynecol 157:422, 1987.

26. Mamopoulos M, Assimakopoulos E, Reece EA, et al: Maternal indomethacin therapy in the treatment of polyhydramnios. Am J Obstet Gynecol 162:1225, 1990.

27. Kirshon B, Mari G, Moise KJ: Indomethacin therapy in the treatment of symptomatic polyhydramnios. Obstet Gynecol 75:202, 1990.

28. Moise KJ, Huhta JC, Fharif BS: Indomethacin in the treatment of preterm labor: Effects on the fetal ductus arteriosus. N Engl J Med 319:327, 1988.

29. Mahony BS, Callen PW, Filly RA: Fetal urethral obstruction: US evaluation. Radiology 157:221, 1985.

30. Golbus MS, Filly RA, Callen PW, et al: Fetal urinary tract obstruction: Management and selection for treatment. Semin Perinatol 9:91, 1985.

31. Mahony BS, Callen PW, Filly RA, Golbus MS: Progression of infantile polycystic kidney disease in early pregnancy. J Ultrasound Med 3:277, 1984.

32. Romero R, Cullen M, Jeanty P, et al: The diagnosis of congenital renal anomalies by ultrasound: II. Infantile polycystic kidney disease. Am J Obstet Gynecol 150:259, 1984.

33. Manning FA: The use of sonography in the evaluation of the high-risk pregnancy. Radiol Clin North Am 28:205, 1990.

34. Cohn HE, Sacks GT, Hermann MA, Rudolph AM: Cardiovascular responses to hypoxemia and acidemia in fetal limbs. Am J Obstet Gynecol 120:817, 1974.

35. Trimmer KJ, Leveno KJ, Peters MT, Kelly MA: Observations on the cause of oligohydramnios in prolonged pregnancy. Am J Obstet Gynecol 163:1900, 1990.

36. Potter EL: Bilateral absence of kidneys and ureters: A report of 50 cases. Obstet Gynecol 25:3, 1965.

37. Leveno KJ, Quirk JG, Cunningham FG, et al: Prolonged pregnancy: I. Observations concerning the causes of fetal distress. Am J Obstet Gynecol 150:465, 1984.

38. Imanaka M, Ogita S, Sugawa T: Saline solution amnioinfusion for oligohydramnios after premature rupture of the membranes: A preliminary report. Am J Obstet Gynecol 161:102, 1989.

39. Strong TH, Hetzler G, Sarno AP, Paul RH: Prophylactic intrapartum amnioinfusion: A randomized clinical trial. Am J Obstet Gynecol 162:1370, 1990.

40. Owen J, Henson BV, Hauth JC: A prospective randomized study of saline solution amnioinfusion. Am J Obstet Gynecol 162:1146, 1990.

41. Nageotte MP, Bertucci L, Towers CV, et al: Prophylactic amnioinfusion in pregnancies complicated by oligohydramnios: A prospective study. Obstet Gynecol 77:677, 1991.

42. Standards and Guidelines for the Performance of the Antepartum Obstetrical Examination. Bethesda, MD, American Institute of Ultrasound in Medicine, 1990.

43. Hill LM, Breckle R, Wolfgram KR, O'Brien PC: Oligohydramnios: Ultrasonically detected incidence and subsequent fetal outcome. Am J Obstet Gynecol 147:407, 1983.

44. Sivit CJ, Hill MC, Larsen JW, et al: The sonographic evaluation of fetal anomalies in oligohydramnios between 16 and 30 weeks' gestation. AJR 146:1277, 1986.

45. Goldstein RB, Filly RA: Sonographic estimation of amniotic fluid volume: Subjective assessment versus pocket measurements. J Ultrasound Med 7:363, 1988.

46. Moore TR, Longo J, Leopold GR, et al: The reliability and predictive value of an amniotic fluid scoring system in severe second-trimester oligohydramnios. Obstet Gynecol 73:739, 1989.

47. Phelan JP, Smith CV, Broussard P, Small M: Amniotic fluid volume assessment with the four-quadrant technique at 36–42 weeks' gestation. J Reprod Med 32:540, 1987.

48. Rutherford SE, Smith CV, Phelan FP, et al: Four-quadrant assessment of amniotic fluid volume: Interobserver and intraobserver variation. J Reprod Med 32:587, 1987.

49. Rutherford SE, Phelan JP, Smith CV, Jacobs N: The four-quadrant assessment of amniotic fluid volume: An adjunct to antepartum fetal heart rate testing. Obstet Gynecol 70:353, 1987.

50. Moore TR, Cayle JE: The amniotic fluid index in normal human pregnancy. Am J Obstet Gynecol 162:1168, 1990.

51. Jones TB, Price RR, Gibbs SJ: Volumetric determination of placental and uterine growth relationships from B-mode ultrasound by serial area-volume determinations. Invest Radiol 16:101, 1981.

52. Geirsson RT, Christie AD, Patel N: Ultrasound volume measurements comparing a prolate ellipsoid method with a parallel planimetric area method against a known volume. J Clin Ultrasound 10:329, 1982.

53. Geirsson RT, Patel NB, Christie AD: In-vivo accuracy of ultrasound measurements of intrauterine volume in pregnancy. Br J Obstet Gynecol 91:37, 1984.

54. Kurtz AB, Shaw WM, Kurtz RJ, et al: The inaccuracy of total uterine volume measurements: Sources of error and a proposed solution. J Ultrasound Med 3:289, 1984.

55. Kurtz AB, Kurtz RJ, Rifkin MD, et al: Total uterine volume: A new graph and its clinical applications. J Ultrasound Med 3:299, 1984.

56. Gohari P, Berkowitz RL, Hobbins JC: Prediction of intrauterine growth retardation by determination of total intrauterine volume. Am J Obstet Gynecol 127:255, 1977.

57. Schiff E, Ben-Baruch G, Kushnir O, Mashiach S: Standardized measurement of amniotic fluid volume by correlation of sonography with dye dilution technique. Obstet Gynecol 76:44, 1990.

58. Hashimoto B, Filly RA, Belden C, et al: Objective method of diagnosing oligohydramnios in postterm pregnancies. J Ultrasound Med 6:81, 1987.

59. Gadd RL: The volume of the liquor amnii in normal and abnormal pregnancies. J Obstet Gynaecol Br Commonw 73:11, 1966.

60. Moore TR: Superiority of the four-quadrant sum over the single-deepest-pocket technique in ultrasonographic identification of abnormal amniotic fluid volumes. Am J Obstet Gynecol 163:762, 1990.

61. Levine SC, Filly RA, Creasy RK: Identification of fetal growth retardation by ultrasonographic estimation of total intrauterine volume. J Clin Ultrasound 7:21, 1979.

62. Chinn DH, Filly RA, Callen PW: Prediction of intrauterine growth retardation by sonographic estimation of total intrauterine volume. J Clin Ultrasound 9:175, 1981.

63. Hoddick WK, Callen PW, Filly RA, Creasy RK: Ultrasonographic determination of qualitative amniotic fluid volume in intrauterine growth retardation: Reassessment of the 1 cm rule. Am J Obstet Gynecol 149:758, 1984.

64. Benson CB, Doubilet PM, Saltzman DH: Intrauterine growth retardation: Predictive value of ultrasound criteria for antenatal diagnosis. Radiology 160:415, 1986.

65. Benson CB, Boswell SB, Brown DL, et al: Improved prediction of intrauterine growth retardation using multiple parameters. Radiology 168:7, 1988.

66. Benson CB, Belville JS, Lentini JF, Doubilet PM: Intrauterine growth retardation: Diagnosis based on multiple parameters—a prospective study. Radiology 177:499, 1990.

67. Bochner CJ, Medearis AL, Davis J, et al: Antepartum predictors of fetal distress in postterm pregnancy. Am J Obstet Gynecol 157:353, 1987.

68. Eden RD, Seifert LS, Kodack LD, et al: A modified biophysical profile for antenatal fetal surveillance. Obstet Gynecol 71:365, 1988.

69. Manning FA, Morrison I, Harman CR, Menticoglou SM: The abnormal fetal biophysical profile score: V. Predictive accuracy according to score composition. Am J Obstet Gynecol 162:918, 1990.

70. Mercer LJ, Brown LG, Petres RE, Messer RH: A survey of pregnancies complicated by decreased amniotic fluid. Am J Obstet Gynecol 149:355, 1984.

71. Barss VA, Benacerraf BR, Frigoletto FD Jr: Second trimester oligohydramnios, a predictor of poor fetal outcome. Obstet Gynecol 64:608, 1984.

72. Crowley P, O'Herlihy C, Boylan P: The value of ultrasound measurement of amniotic fluid volume in the management of prolonged pregnancies. Br J Obstet Gynecol 91:444, 1984.

73. Phelan JP, Platt LD, Yeh S-Y, et al: The role of ultrasound assessment of amniotic fluid volume in the management of the postdate pregnancy. Am J Obstet Gynecol 151:304, 1985.

74. Gonick B, Bottoms SF, Cotton DB: Amniotic fluid volume as risk factor in preterm premature rupture of the membranes. Obstet Gynecol 65:456, 1985.

75. Vintzileos AM, Campbell WA, Nochimson DJ, Weinbaum PJ: Degree of oligohydramnios and pregnancy outcome in patients with premature rupture of the membranes. Obstet Gynecol 66:162, 1985.

76. Manning FA, Platt LD, Sipos L: Antepartum fetal evaluation: Development of a fetal biophysical profile. Am J Obstet Gynecol 136:787, 1980.

77. Manning FA, Harman CR, Morrison I, et al: Fetal assessment based on fetal biophysical profile scoring: IV. An analysis of perinatal morbidity and mortality. Am J Obstet Gynecol 162:703, 1990.

78. Manning FA, Morrison I, Harman CR, et al: Fetal assessment based on fetal biophysical profile scoring: Experience in 19,221 referred high-risk pregnancies: II. An analysis of false-negative fetal deaths. Am J Obstet Gynecol 157:880, 1987.

79. Manning FA, Morrison I, Lange IR, et al: Fetal assessment based on fetal biophysical profile scoring: Experience in 12,620 referred high-risk pregnancies: I. Perinatal mortality by frequency and etiology. Am J Obstet Gynecol 151:343, 1985.

80. Platt LD, Paul RH, Phelan J, et al: Fifteen years of experience with antepartum fetal testing. Am J Obstet Gynecol 156:1509, 1987.

81. Basket TF, Allen AC, Gray JH, et al: Fetal biophysical profile and perinatal death. Obstet Gynecol 70:357, 1987.

82. Bromley B, Harlow BL, Laboda LA, Benacerraf BR: Small sac size in the first trimester: A predictor of poor fetal outcome. Radiology 178:375, 1991.

83. Parulekar SG: Ultrasonographic demonstration of floating particles in amniotic fluid. J Ultrasound Med 2:107, 1983.

84. Hill LM, Breckle R: Vernix in amniotic fluid: Sonographic detection. Radiology 158:80, 1986.

85. Benacerraf BR, Gatter MA, Ginsburgh F: Ultrasound diagnosis of meconium-stained amniotic fluid. Am J Obstet Gynecol 149:570, 1984.

86. Devore GR, Platt LD: Ultrasound appearance of particulate matter in amniotic cavity: Vernix or meconium? J Clin Ultrasound 14:229, 1986.

87. Sherer DM, Abramowicz JS, Smith SA, Woods J Jr: Sonographically homogeneous echogenic amniotic fluid in detecting meconium-stained amniotic fluid. Obstet Gynecol 78:819, 1991.

88. Saltzman DH, Benson CB, Lavery MJ, Jones TB: Echogenic amniotic fluid secondary to heparin therapy. J Diagn Med Sonogr 1:155, 1985.

89. Helewa M, Harman C: Amniotic fluid particles: Are they related to a mature amniotic fluid phospholipid profile? Obstet Gynecol 74:893, 1989.

90. Mahony BS, Filly RA, Callen PW: Amnionicity and chorionicity in twin pregnancies: Prediction using ultrasound. Radiology 155:205, 1985.

91. Chescheir NC, Seeds JW: Polyhydramnios and oligohydramnios in twin gestations. Obstet Gynecol 71:882, 1988.

92. Patten RM, Mack LA, Harvey D, et al: Disparity of amniotic fluid volume and fetal size: Problem of the stuck twin—US studies. Radiology 172:153, 1989.

93. Arvis P, Roze JM, Priou G, et al: Acute hydramnios with twin pregnancy. J Gynecol Obst Biol Reprod (Paris) 12:283, 1983.

94. Weir PE, Raten G, Beisher N: Acute polyhydramnios: A complication of monozygous twin pregnancy. Br J Obstet Gynecol 86:848, 1979.

95. Robertson EG, Neer KJ: Placental injection studies in twin gestation. Am J Obstet Gynecol 147:170, 1983.

96. Sekiya S, Hafez ESE: Physiomorphology of twin transfusion: A study of 86 twin gestations. Obstet Gynecol 50:288, 1977.

97. Wittmann BK, Farquharson DF, Thomas WDS, et al: The role of feticide in the management of severe twin transfusion. Am J Obstet Gynecol 155:1023, 1986.

98. Bernirschke K, Kim CK: Multiple pregnancy. N Engl J Med 288:1276, 1986.

99. Mahony BS, Petty CN, Nyberg DA, et al: The "stuck twin" phenomenon: Ultrasonographic findings, pregnancy outcome, and management with serial amniocentesis. Am J Obstet Gynecol 163:1513, 1990.

100. Elliott JP, Urig MA, Clewell WH: Aggressive therapeutic amniocentesis for treatment of twin transfusion syndrome. Obstet Gynecol 77:537, 1991.

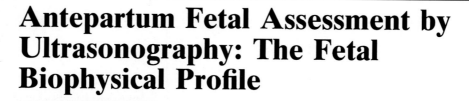

CHAPTER 23

Antepartum Fetal Assessment by Ultrasonography: The Fetal Biophysical Profile

ANTHONY M. VINTZILEOS, M.D.
WINSTON A. CAMPBELL, M.D.
JOHN F. RODIS, M.D.

Since the introduction of electronic fetal heart rate monitoring, the nonstress test (NST) and the contraction stress test (CST) have been the most frequently used methods for antepartum detection of fetal asphyxia (Figs. 23–1 and 23–2). The major disadvantage, however, of these two tests is that in both the only information used to derive a judgment about fetal health is the fetal heart rate. As a result, both tests are associated with low false-negative rates (<1% to 2.7%) but also with very high false-positive rates (50% to >75%).[1-5] The low false-negative rates and high false-positive rates indicate that the NST and CST are reasonable tools to detect the healthy (nonasphyxiated) fetus at the time of testing; however, they are of limited value in detecting the unhealthy (asphyxiated) fetus. In addition, performance of CST is contraindicated in many high-risk situations such as premature rupture of the membranes (PROM), multiple gestations, vaginal bleeding, or preterm labor.

With the introduction of real-time ultrasonography it became possible to evaluate multiple fetal biophysical activities other than fetal heart rate and fetal heart rate activity, thus making possible a more detailed and direct examination of the fetus. To circumvent the high false-positive rates of NST or CST, several investigators have incorporated fetal body movements, fetal breathing movements, fetal tone, amniotic fluid volume, and even placental grading to improve the diagnostic accuracy of antepartum fetal asphyxia (Figs. 23–3 and 23–4). Manning and colleagues[6] were the first to report on the use of five fetal biophysical variables to predict perinatal outcome.[7] These investigators introduced the use of the scoring system in which each biophysical activity or component was scored as 0 (when abnormal) or 2 (when normal). The biophysical variables used were the NST, fetal breathing movements, fetal body movements, fetal tone, and amniotic fluid volume. This scoring system is illustrated in Table 23–1. Another scoring system, which was proposed by Vintzileos and coworkers in 1983,[7] included placental grading as one of the biophysical variables and is shown in Table 23–2. In both systems the fetal evaluation starts with the performance of the NST. After the NST, a real-time ultrasound evaluation is undertaken to observe and quantitate the fetal biophysical components. The examination is ended when each of the

Table 23–1. FETAL BIOPHYSICAL PROFILE SCORING

Variable	Score 2	Score 0
Fetal breathing movements	The presence of at least 30 seconds of sustained fetal breathing movements in 30 minutes of observation	Less than 30 seconds of fetal breathing movements in 30 minutes
Fetal movements	Three or more gross body movements in 30 minutes of observation. Simultaneous limb and trunk movements are counted as a single movement	Two or less gross body movements in 30 minutes of observation
Fetal tone	At least one episode of motion of a limb from a position of flexion to extension and a rapid return to flexion	Fetus in a position of semi- or full-limb extension with no return to flexion with movement. Absence of fetal movement is counted as absent tone
Fetal reactivity	The presence of two or more fetal heart rate accelerations of at least 15 beats per minute and lasting at least 15 seconds and associated with fetal movement in 40 minutes	No acceleration or less than two accelerations of the fetal heart rate in 40 minutes of observation
Qualitative amniotic fluid volume	A pocket of amniotic fluid that measures at least 1 cm in two perpendicular planes	Largest pocket of amniotic fluid measures <1 cm in two perpendicular planes
Maximal score	10	
Minimal score		0

From Manning FA, Platt LD, Sipos L: Antepartum fetal evaluation: Development of a fetal biophysical profile score. Am J Obstet Gynecol 136:787, 1980.

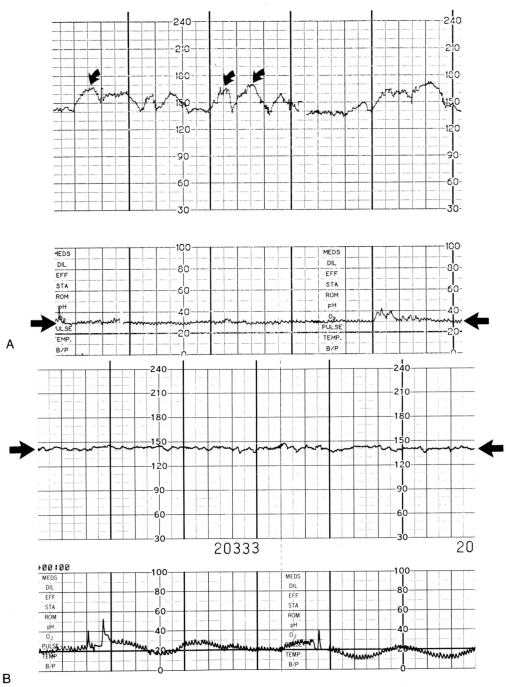

Figure 23–1. *A.* Reactive nonstress test. Fetal heart rate accelerations (*curved arrows*) of at least 15 beats per minute lasting 15 seconds or longer are readily identified in this patient. Arrows indicate uterine activity. *B.* Nonreactive nonstress test. Lack of fetal heart rate acceleration (*arrows*). This pattern could indicate the effect of fetal sleep, medications, or hypoxia.

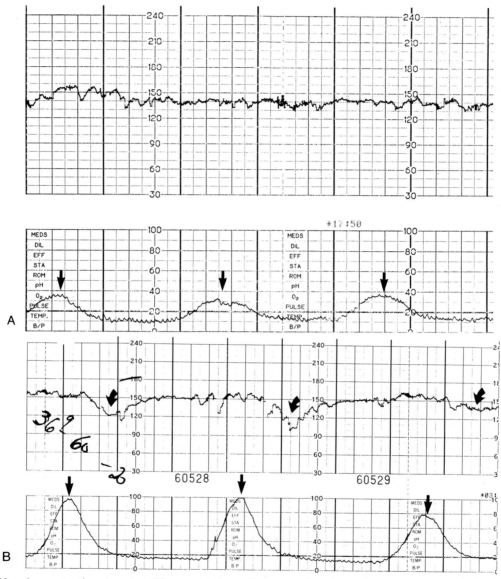

Figure 23–2. *A.* Negative contraction stress test. There are three uterine contractions (*arrows*) within a 10-minute period, none of which is associated with fetal heart rate decelerations. This indicates fetal well-being. *B.* Positive contraction stress test. Each contraction (*arrows*) is associated with fetal heart rate decelerations (*curved arrows*), indicating fetal hypoxia due to uteroplacental insufficiency.

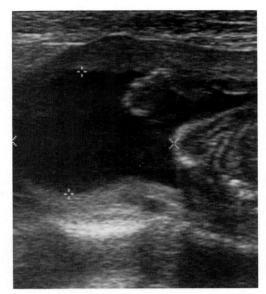

Figure 23–3. Sonogram demonstrating amniotic fluid measurement as part of the biophysical profile. The amniotic fluid pocket is measured in two perpendicular planes.

biophysical components meets normal criteria or 30 minutes of real-time ultrasonography have elapsed. In both scoring systems, fetal biophysical scores of 8 or more are associated with good perinatal outcome. However, scores of less than 8 need to be followed up by further testing or delivery. The presence of oligohydramnios is compatible with an abnormal assessment regardless of the normality or abnormality of the other components. It should be emphasized, however, that work from our institution, as well as from other investigators, has suggested that the most crucial information of the biophysical profile assessment is not the score per se.[8–10] What is most important is understand-

Table 23–2. CRITERIA FOR SCORING BIOPHYSICAL VARIABLES*

Nonstress Test

Score 2 (NST 2): 5 or more fetal heart rate accelerations of at least 15 beats per minute in amplitude and at least 15 seconds' duration associated with fetal movements in a 20-minute period.

Score 1 (NST 1): 2 to 4 accelerations of at least 15 beats per minute in amplitude and at least 15 seconds' duration associated with fetal movements in a 20-minute period.

Score 0 (NST 0): 1 or fewer accelerations in a 20-minute period.

Fetal Movements

Score 2 (FM 2): At least 3 gross (trunk and limbs) episodes of fetal movements within 30 minutes. Simultaneous limb and trunk movements were counted as a single movement.

Score 1 (FM 1): 1 or 2 fetal movements within 30 minutes.

Score 0 (FM 0): Absence of fetal movements within 30 minutes.

Fetal Breathing Movements

Score 2 (FBM 2): At least 1 episode of fetal breathing of at least 60 seconds' duration within a 30-minute observation period.

Score 1 (FBM 1): At least 1 episode of fetal breathing lasting 30 to 60 seconds within 30 minutes.

Score 0 (FBM 0): Absence of fetal breathing or breathing lasting less than 30 seconds within 30 minutes.

Fetal Tone

Score 2 (FT 2): At least 1 episode of extension of extremities with return to position of flexion and also one episode of extension of spine with return to position of flexion.

Score 1 (FT 1): At least 1 episode of extension of extremities with return to position of flexion or 1 episode of extension of spine with return to flexion.

Score 0 (FT 0): Extremities in extension. Fetal movements not followed by return to flexion. Open hand.

Amniotic Fluid Volume

Score 2 (AF 2): Fluid evident throughout the uterine cavity; a pocket that measures 2 cm or more in vertical diameter.

Score 1 (AF 1): A pocket that measures less than 2 cm but more than 1 cm in vertical diameter.

Score 0 (AF 0): Crowding of fetal small parts; largest pocket less than 1 cm in vertical diameter.

Placental Grading

Score 2 (PL 2): Placental grading 0, 1, or 2

Score 1 (PL 1): Placenta posterior difficult to evaluate

Score 0 (PL 0): Placental grading 3

---

*Maximal score 12; minimal score 0.

From Vintzileos AM, Campbell WA, Ingardia CJ, et al: The fetal biophysical profile and its predictive value. Reprinted with permission from The American College of Obstetricians and Gynecologists (Obstetrics and Gynecology, 1983, 62:271).

ing the different significance of each biophysical variable, or combination of variables, to predict or rule out fetal compromise. In this chapter we briefly discuss the basic physiology and pathophysiology of the components of the fetal biophysical profile, the contribution of each component or combination of components in predicting fetal asphyxia (gradual hypoxia concept), and the clinical applications of this testing method in high-risk patients with intact as well as ruptured membranes.

BASIC PHYSIOLOGY AND PATHOPHYSIOLOGY OF THE INDIVIDUAL BIOPHYSICAL COMPONENTS

The fetal biophysical profile is a combination of acute and chronic markers. The fetal heart rate reac-

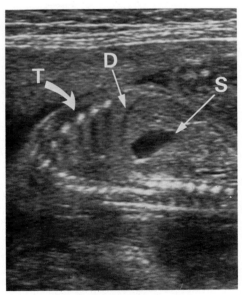

Figure 23–4. Longitudinal sonogram of a fetus demonstrating the recommended plane of section for evaluating fetal breathing movements. Downward movement of the fetal diaphragm (D) and abdomen and an inward, rocking motion of the fetal thorax (T) can be seen when fetal breathing is present. S, stomach.

Table 23–3. FETAL CENTRAL NERVOUS SYSTEM CENTERS

Test	Center			
Fetal tone	Cortex (subcortical area ?)			↑
Fetal movements	Cortex-nuclei			
Fetal breathing movement	Ventral surface of the fourth ventricle	Embryogenesis		Hypoxia
Nonstress test	Posterior hypothalamus, medulla	↓		

From Vintzileos AM, Campbell WA, Ingardia CJ, et al: The fetal biophysical profile and its predictive value. Reprinted with permission from The American College of Obstetricians and Gynecologists (Obstetrics and Gynecology, 1983, 62:271).

tivity, fetal breathing movements, fetal movements, and fetal tone are the acute markers. Amniotic fluid volume and placental grading have been considered chronic markers. The acute markers are biophysical activities that are initiated and controlled by different fetal central nervous system (CNS) centers (Table 23–3).[7] These CNS centers are developed at different times during fetal life. For instance, the CNS center that initiates and regulates fetal tone is the earliest to function at 7.5 to 8.5 weeks' gestation. The fetal body movement center starts functioning at approximately 9 weeks' gestation, the fetal breathing movement center after 21 weeks' gestation, and the fetal heart rate reactivity center by the end of the second or early third trimester. An interesting observation by Vintzileos and coworkers[8, 9] and others[10] is that the biophysical activities that appear first during fetal life are the last to disappear during fetal asphyxia (gradual hypoxia concept). There are convincing data from the University of Connecticut Health Center,[8, 9] as well as from other institutions,[10] that during in utero hypoxia and acidosis the first biophysical activities to become compromised are fetal heart rate reactivity and fetal breathing movements. In advanced fetal hypoxia and acidosis, fetal body movements and fetal tone are also absent.[8–10] The degree of fetal hypoxia and acidosis required for the fetal biophysical activities to become compromised has been such that fetal heart rate activity and fetal breathing movements are abolished at pH (umbilical cord artery pH) levels lower than 7.20. pH values between 7.10 and 7.20 are associated with compromised fetal body movements and tone, whereas pH values lower than 7.10 are associated with absent body movements and tone.[8] These observations imply that biophysical activities (acute markers of the fetal biophysical profile) do not have the same weight in predicting fetal asphyxia, and therefore the assignment of an arbitrary score, as used in biophysical scoring methods, comes into question. Later in this chapter the data regarding the relationship between fetal biophysical activities and fetal acid–base status at the time of testing are discussed in detail. From the clinical point of view it should be emphasized that the gradual hypoxia concept, which suggests different degrees of sensitivity to hypoxia and acidosis, should be kept in mind when interpreting fetal biophysical assessment data.[11] The presence of a given biophysical activity during real-time observation suggests that the fetal CNS center that controls the activity is functioning properly and therefore CNS hypoxia is ruled out. The absence of biophysical activity, however, cannot always be attrib-

uted to fetal hypoxia and acidosis. Fetal hypoxia and acidosis should be a diagnosis of exclusion and factors such as normal periodicity and maternal administration of depressant medications, sedatives, and drugs should be ruled out first. In the absence of any other explanation the presence of diminished biophysical activities should raise suspicion for fetal asphyxia or infection.

The chronic markers of the fetal condition (amniotic fluid volume and placental grading) are not altered by acute hypoxic changes. The presence of oligohydramnios is considered to be the result of chronic fetal distress and reflects the presence of fetal hypoxia of long duration, which is associated with redistribution of the fetal cardiac output away from nonvital organs such as the kidney. Renal hypoperfusion will result in decreased urinary output and oligohydramnios. The presence of oligohydramnios constitutes an abnormal biophysical assessment because there is high risk for cord compression and in utero death. There have been several studies demonstrating a strong association between reduced amniotic fluid and increased frequency of adverse perinatal outcome.[6, 7, 12, 13] In Chamberlain and colleagues' study[12] it was found that patients with normal amniotic fluid volume (largest pocket between 2 and 8 cm) had a perinatal mortality rate of 1.97 per 1000. However, patients with marginal amniotic fluid volume (largest pocket, 1 to 2 cm) and severe oligohydramnios (largest pocket < 1 cm) had perinatal mortality rates of 37.7 per 1000 and 109.4 per 1000, respectively. At the University of Connecticut Health Center placental grading has been included as part of the biophysical profile because our experience has shown that grade 3 placentas are associated with an increased incidence of abnormal fetal heart rate patterns (44.4%) and abruptio placentae (14.8%) during labor.[7]

At this point it should be emphasized that in addition to diurnal variation, short-term periodicity, maternal drug administration, fetal asphyxia, and infection, the variation of individual biophysical components also depends on the gestational age. With the use of the scoring criteria of Vintzileos and coworkers (see Table 23–2), the changes in frequency of the individual biophysical components are described along with biophysical scoring of the healthy fetus from 25 to 44 weeks' gestation (Table 23–4).[14] The frequency of reactive NSTs was significantly increased after 32 weeks as compared with earlier gestations. Fetal breathing and amniotic fluid volume were found to be decreased after 40 weeks as compared with earlier gestations. Grade 3 placentas appear after 32 weeks. Fetal move-

Table 23–4. FREQUENCY OF INDIVIDUAL BIOPHYSICAL VARIABLES AND BIOPHYSICAL SCORING OF 8 OR MORE IN PREGNANCIES WITH INTACT MEMBRANES

Biophysical Variable	Gestation (wk) and Total Number = 951 (% of the Total No.)								
	25–28 No. = 61 (6.4)	P Value	29–32 No. = 192 (20.1)	P Value	33–36 No. = 347 (36.4)	P Value	37–40 No. = 257 (27.0)	P Value	41–44 No. = 94 (9.8)
NST-2	22 (36.0)	NS	82 (42.7)	<0.01	223 (64.2)	NS	188 (73.1)	NS	77 (81.9)
NST-1	19 (31.1)	NS	68 (35.4)	<0.01	86 (24.7)	NS	44 (17.1)	NS	9 (9.5)
NST-0	20 (32.7)	NS	42 (21.8)	<0.01	38 (10.9)	NS	25 (9.7)	NS	8 (8.5)
FBM-2	36 (59.0)	NS	143 (74.4)	NS	264 (76.0)	NS	181 (70.4)	<0.05	52 (55.3)
FBM-1	4 (6.5)	NS	15 (7.8)	NS	31 (8.9)	NS	20 (7.7)	NS	6 (6.3)
FBM-0	21 (34.4)	NS	34 (17.7)	NS	52 (14.9)	NS	56 (21.7)	<0.05	36 (38.3)
FM-2	61 (100)	NS	188 (97.9)	NS	331 (95.3)	NS	242 (94.1)	NS	86 (91.4)
FM-1	0	NS	4 (2.0)	NS	14 (4.0)	NS	12 (4.6)	NS	5 (5.3)
FM-0	0	NS	0	NS	2 (0.5)	NS	3 (1.1)	NS	3 (3.1)
FT-2	61 (100.0)	NS	182 (94.7)	NS	324 (93.3)	NS	232 (90.2)	NS	79 (84.0)
FT-1	0	NS	9 (4.6)	NS	21 (6.0)	NS	24 (9.3)	NS	12 (12.7)
FT-0	0	NS	1 (0.5)	NS	2 (0.5)	NS	1 (0.4)	NS	3 (3.1)
AF-2	58 (95.0)	NS	189 (98.4)	NS	331 (95.3)	NS	231 (89.8)	<0.01	70 (74.4)
AF-1	1 (1.6)	NS	3 (1.5)	NS	11 (3.1)	NS	22 (8.5)	<0.01	16 (17.0)
AF-0	2 (3.2)	NS	0	NS	5 (1.4)	NS	4 (1.5)	<0.01	8 (8.5)
PL-2	61 (100.0)	NS	189 (98.4)	NS	321 (92.5)	NS	212 (82.4)	<0.01	64 (68.0)
PL-1	0	NS	3 (1.5)	NS	12 (3.4)	NS	10 (3.8)	<0.01	13 (13.8)
PL-0	0	NS	0	<0.05	14 (4.0)	<0.01	35 (13.6)	<0.01	17 (18.0)
Total score 8 or more	61 (100)	NS	186 (96.8)	NS	341 (98.2)	NS	249 (96.8)	NS	83 (88.2)

NST, nonstress test; FBM, fetal breathing movements; FM, fetal movements, FT, fetal tone; AF, amniotic fluid volume; PL, placental grading; NS, not significant.

From Vintzileos AM, Feinstein SJ, Lodeiro JG, et al: Fetal biophysical profile and the effect of premature rupture of the membranes. Reprinted with permission from The American College of Obstetricians and Gynecologists (Obstetrics and Gynecology, 1986, 67:818).

ments and fetal tone were not influenced by gestational age. Several other investigators have also studied the relationship between fetal biophysical data and gestational age with similar findings. Baskett, by using the scoring criteria of Manning and colleagues (see Table 23–1), studied 5582 fetuses (11,012 biophysical profiles) with similar findings.[15] The number of reactive NSTs at 34 to 41 weeks was significantly higher when compared with earlier gestations. The NST, fetal breathing movements, fetal tone, and amniotic fluid were more likely to be abnormal in 42 to 44 weeks as compared with 37 to 41-week gestations. In the study of Vintzileos and coworkers,[14] as well as the study by Baskett,[15] although many of the individual biophysical components were found to change throughout gestation, the frequency of reassuring biophysical scores (8 or greater) was not altered by gestational age. The effect of PROM on the fetal biophysical components throughout gestation has also been investigated by Vintzileos and coworkers.[14] Biophysical profiles were determined from 25 to 44 weeks in patients with intact membranes (see Table 23–4) and compared with profiles of patients with PROM of comparable gestational ages (Table 23–5). Both groups had good perinatal outcome, suggesting the presence of a healthy fetus during the biophysical assessment. Table 23–5 shows the frequency of individual biophysical components in patients with PROM. Patients with PROM were found to have greater amounts of amniotic fluid volume after 32 weeks and more grade 3 placentas after 40 weeks as compared with earlier gestations. However, the frequency of reactive NSTs, fetal breathing, fetal movement, and fetal tone was not altered at any point throughout gestation in patients with PROM. In studying the effect of PROM in the fetal biophysical com-

ponents it was found that PROM per se is associated with the following alterations in the biophysical components observed in most gestational age groups: increase in fetal heart rate reactivity (Fig. 23–5); decrease in fetal breathing movements (Fig. 23–6); decrease in amniotic fluid volume (Fig. 23–7); and no change in fetal body movements, fetal tone, and overall biophysical score. The alterations in fetal biophysical activities by the presence of PROM throughout gestation are essential to understand to apply properly biophysical assessment data in evaluating high-risk patients with ruptured membranes.

CLINICAL EXPERIENCE BY USING THE FETAL BIOPHYSICAL PROFILE AS MEANS OF EVALUATING HIGH-RISK PREGNANCIES WITH INTACT MEMBRANES

Manning and colleagues, in 1980, first reported on the fetal biophysical profile score on 216 high-risk patients who had weekly biophysical scores but were managed on the basis of the NST results only.[6] There was a significant relationship between a low biophysical score and abnormal perinatal outcome as reflected by low 5-minute Apgar scores, fetal distress in labor, and perinatal death rate. Having used the scoring system that is illustrated in Table 23–1, Manning and colleagues found that when the score was normal (10), the perinatal and fetal death rates were 0, whereas when the biophysical score was very abnormal (score 0) the perinatal and fetal death rates were 600 and 400 per 1000 population, respectively.[6] The same group reported reduction in the perinatal mortality in 1184

Table 23–5. FREQUENCY OF INDIVIDUAL BIOPHYSICAL VARIABLES AND BIOPHYSICAL SCORING OF 8 OR MORE IN PREGNANCIES WITH RUPTURED MEMBRANES

Biophysical Variable	Gestation (wk) and Total Number = 200 (% of the Total No.)								
	25–28 No. = 30 (15)	P Value	29–32 No. = 72 (36)	P Value	33–36 No. = 76 (38)	P Value	37–40 No. = 20 (10)	P Value	41–44 No. = 2 (1)
NST-2	17 (56.6)	NS	52 (72.2)	NS	56 (73.6)	NS	20 (100.0)	NS	2 (100.0)
NST-1	9 (30.0)	NS	10 (13.8)	NS	16 (21.0)	NS	0	NS	0
NST-0	4 (13.3)	NS	10 (13.8)	NS	4 (5.2)	NS	0	NS	0
FBM-2	10 (33.3)	NS	38 (52.7)	NS	49 (64.4)	NS	13 (65.0)	NS	2 (100.0)
FBM-1	1 (3.3)	NS	5 (6.9)	NS	8 (10.5)	NS	4 (20.0	NS	0
FBM-0	19 (63.3)	NS	29 (40.2)	NS	19 (25.0)	NS	3 (15.0)	NS	0
FM-2	30 (100)	NS	69 (95.8)	NS	73 (96.0)	NS	20 (100.0)	NS	2 (100.0)
FM-1	0	NS	3 (4.1)	NS	3 (3.9)	NS	0	NS	0
FM-0	0	NS	0	NS	0	NS	0	NS	0
FT-2	30 (100)	NS	69 (95.8)	NS	74 (97.3)	NS	20 (100.0	NS	2 (100.0)
FT-1	0	NS	3 (4.2)	NS	2 (2.6)	NS	0	NS	0
FT-0	0	NS	0	NS	0	NS	0	NS	0
AF-2	19 (63.3)	NS	46 (63.8)	<0.05	66 (86.8)	NS	16 (80.0)	NS	0
AF-1	5 (16.6)	NS	17 (23.6)	<0.05	7 (9.2)	NS	1 (5.0)	NS	0
AF-0	6 (20.0)	NS	9 (12.5)	<0.05	3 (3.9)	NS	3 (15.0)	NS	2 (100.0)
PL-2	29 (96.6)	NS	72 (100.0)	NS	71 (93.4)	NS	17 (85.0)	<0.05	0
PL-1	0	NS	0	NS	2 (2.6)	NS	0	NS	0
PL-0	1 (3.3)	NS	0	NS	3 (3.9)	NS	3 (15.0)	<0.5	2 (100.0)
Total score 8 or more	26 (86.6)	NS	70 (97.2)		75 (98.6)	NS	18 (90.0)	NS	2 (100.0)

NST, nonstress test; FBM, fetal breathing movements; FM, fetal movements, FT, fetal tone; AF, amniotic fluid volume; PL, placental grading; NS, not significant.

From Vintzileos AM, Feinstein SJ, Lodeiro JG, et al: Fetal biophysical profile and the effect of premature rupture of the membranes. Reprinted with permission from The American College of Obstetricians and Gynecologists (Obstetrics and Gynecology, 1986, 67:818).

high-risk patients who were managed based on the biophysical profile results to 5.06 per 1000.[16] During the same time period the perinatal mortality of the general population was 14.3 per 1000 and the predicted perinatal mortality for a similar high-risk population was 65 per 1000. Subsequently, the superiority of the biophysical score as compared with the NST alone was questioned by Platt and colleagues,[17] who performed fetal biophysical profiles on 283 patients. These patients were managed according to the NST results and had a perinatal mortality of 14 per 1000 (corrected perinatal mortality of 7 per 1000). Fetuses with a biophysical score of 8 or more had a perinatal mortality of 7.4 per 1000. A prospective comparison, however, between fetal biophysical profile score (375 patients) and NST (360 patients) subsequently showed that biophysical score was more accurate in predicting low Apgar scores.[18] In another study, Platt and colleagues conducted a randomized trial between one group of patients managed with NST (373 patients) and another managed with biophysical score results (279 patients).[19] The study showed that the biophysical profile group had better predictions in terms of perinatal mortality, fetal distress in labor, and intrauterine growth retardation. However, only the positive predictive value for overall abnormal outcome and the negative predictive value for intrauterine growth retardation were significantly improved by using the biophysical score. A

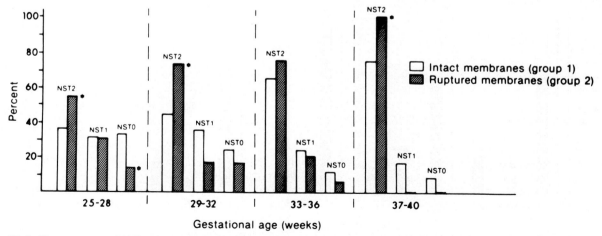

Figure 23–5. Nonstress test (NST) results throughout gestation in patients with intact versus ruptured membranes. Asterisk indicates significant difference, P < .05. (From Vintzileos AM, Feinstein SJ, Lodeiro JG, et al: Fetal biophysical profile and the effect of premature rupture of the membranes. Reprinted with permission from The American College of Obstetricians and Gynecologists [Obstetrics and Gynecology, 1986, 67:818]).

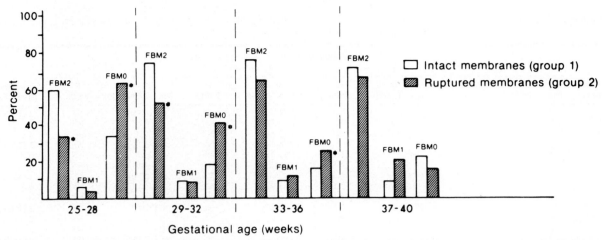

Figure 23–6. Incidence of fetal breathing movements (FBM) throughout gestation in patients with intact versus ruptured membranes. Asterisk indicates significant difference, $P < .05$. (From Vintzileos AM, Feinstein SJ, Lodeiro JG, et al: Fetal biophysical profile and the effect of premature rupture of the membranes. Reprinted with permission from The American College of Obstetricians and Gynecologists [Obstetrics and Gynecology, 1986, 67:818]).

reduction in the perinatal mortality rate of high-risk pregnancies by using the fetal biophysical score has been reported by Baskett and coworkers.[20] The perinatal mortality rate of patients managed by biophysical profiles was 9.2 per 1000, whereas the overall perinatal mortality at the University of Connecticut Health Center was 14.5 per 1000. Fetuses with normal biophysical scores had a perinatal mortality of 1 per 1000, and fetuses with very abnormal scores (0 to 4) had a perinatal mortality rate of 292 per 1000. In another study, Manning and colleagues further explored the use of the fetal biophysical profile in evaluating 12,620 high-risk patients.[21] There was a direct correlation between perinatal mortality and biophysical score. When the biophysical profile score was 8 or more the perinatal mortality was 0.652 per 1000 tests, and when the biophysical score was very abnormal (score 0) the perinatal mortality was 187 per 1000 tests. The corrected false-negative rate was 0.634 per 1000. In a subsequent study by the same authors reporting 19,221

high-risk pregnancies, it was found that the incidence of intrauterine death after a normal biophysical score (8 or more) was 0.726 per 1000.[22] The same false-negative rate (0.7 per 1000) was also reported by Baskett and colleagues, who used the biophysical score to manage 4184 high-risk pregnancies.[23] Baskett and colleagues found that normal biophysical scores (8 to 10) were associated with a perinatal mortality rate of 1 per 1000, intermediate scores (6) with perinatal mortality of 31.3 per 1000, and very abnormal scores (0 to 4) with perinatal mortality of 200 per 1000.

Manning and colleagues have specifically investigated the positive predictive value of the grossly abnormal score (0) by reporting 29 fetuses with biophysical scores of 0 found among 28,655 fetuses.[24] Almost half of these fetuses (48.3%) had a perinatal death. In utero death occurred as early as 30 minutes and as long as 11 days after the biophysical score of 0 was obtained. All fetuses with scores of 0 suffered perinatal morbidity as defined by the presence of fetal distress

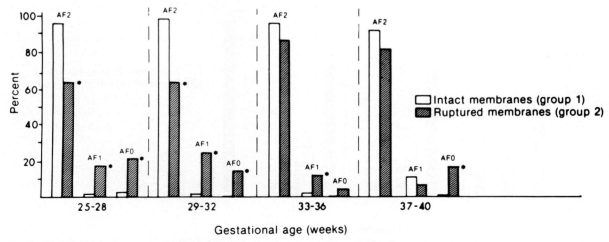

Figure 23–7. Incidence of qualitative amniotic fluid volume (AF) throughout gestation in patients with intact versus ruptured membranes. Asterisk indicates significant difference, $P < .05$. (From Vintzileos AM, Feinstein SJ, Lodeiro JG, et al: Fetal biophysical profile and the effect of premature rupture of the membranes. Reprinted with permission from The American College of Obstetricians and Gynecologists [Obstetrics and Gynecology, 1986, 67:818]).

in labor, 5 minute Apgar scores less than 7, umbilical vein pH less than 7.20, or admission to the neonatal intensive care unit for over 24 hours for reasons unrelated to prematurity. The main conclusion drawn is that some fetuses with grossly abnormal scores (scores 0) may survive after delivery and therefore inaction based on the assumption that the prognosis is dismal is not justified. The relationship between biophysical score and perinatal morbidity and mortality has been determined by Manning and colleagues in a study of 26,780 high-risk pregnancies.[25] The study showed an inverse linear correlation between biophysical profile score and perinatal morbidity. Manning and colleagues suggested that biophysical score may give some insight into the degree and extent of fetal compromise.

The practice of including only the ultrasound-monitored biophysical components (fetal breathing movements, fetal body movements, fetal tone, and amniotic fluid volume) without including the NST was initially reported by Manning and colleagues.[26] The NST was used only if one or more of the ultrasound components were abnormal. With this method the need for NST was reduced to only 2.7% of 2,712 tested patients without compromising perinatal morbidity or mortality. The practice of omitting the NST was subsequently challenged by Eden and coworkers, who found increased incidence of abnormal perinatal outcome in fetuses with variable decelerations during NST testing in spite of normal ultrasound-monitored biophysical components.[27] Mills and associates have proposed an alternative approach to fetal biophysical assessment.[28] After evaluating 500 high-risk pregnancies with 2038 biophysical profiles they concluded that if the fetal growth is normal no biophysical assessment is necessary, but in cases of abnormal fetal growth biweekly NSTs and ultrasound assessment of fetal growth every 2 weeks are needed. They reserve the use of the fetal biophysical profile only in cases with abnormal or equivocal NST results.

The use of the fetal biophysical profile score in specific high-risk conditions such as post dates, diabetes mellitus, and twin pregnancy has also been described.[29–31] Johnson and coworkers studied the use of fetal biophysical profile score in managing 307 postdate patients and found that normal biophysical score was associated with a higher rate of nonintervention and therefore spontaneous onset of labor, resulting in lower cesarean section rates (15% versus 42% for patients who underwent induction of labor).[29] Two hundred and thirty-eight diabetic pregnancies were also managed by the same group of investigators.[30] Fetuses with abnormal biophysical scores had higher rates of intensive care nursery admissions, cesarean section (50%), operative intervention, and neonatal morbidity. In evaluating twin high-risk pregnancies, Lodeiro and coworkers found the fetal biophysical profile score to be a useful tool.[31] The sensitivity, specificity, and positive and negative predictive values of the biophysical score in predicting fetal distress were 83.3%, 100%, 100%, and 97.7%, respectively.

RELATIONSHIP BETWEEN FETAL BIOPHYSICAL ACTIVITIES AND FETAL ASPHYXIA

Vintzileos and coworkers,[7] after reporting their initial experience with 150 high-risk pregnancies, were the first to question the wisdom of an arbitrary assignment of an equal score for each biophysical variable. Although the biophysical score was used for fetal evaluation, careful analysis of the fetal biophysical components of 11 hypoxic fetuses in that study suggested that each biophysical component has a different degree of accuracy and a different weight in predicting fetal compromise. It was observed that fetal heart rate and fetal breathing movements are the first biophysical activities to be abolished in fetuses with antepartum fetal distress. When in addition to fetal heart rate nonreactivity and absence of fetal breathing, fetal body movements and tone were compromised, the perinatal mortality rose to 100%. In a report by Manning and coworkers the use of an equal score for each biophysical component was also questioned.[32] Perinatal morbidity outcomes of 525 fetuses were studied and compared with the last abnormal biophysical score as a total score and also as score composition. Manning and coworkers found that the same biophysical scores do not have the same predictive accuracies but the score predictions depend on the combination of the individual biophysical components. In accordance with our own observations, fetal heart rate reactivity (NST), amniotic fluid volume and fetal breathing movements were the most powerful indicators of perinatal outcome. This finding is compatible with previous studies examining the relationship between fetal biophysical assessment and fetal acid-base status at the time of testing.[8–10]

The first report on the relationship between fetal biophysical profile results and fetal acid-base status at the time of testing was published by Vintzileos and coworkers.[8] One hundred and twenty-four women with high-risk pregnancies who underwent cesarean section before the onset of labor had a biophysical profile performed before the cesarean section. The results of the biophysical assessment were correlated with fetal acid-base status as determined by cord blood pH measurements. Figure 23–8 shows the correlation between biophysical score and cord arterial pH. A disturbing observation, however, was that 2% of fetuses with normal biophysical profile scores (8 or more) were acidemic (pH < 7.20) at the time of testing. Interestingly, both fetuses had biophysical scores of 8 because of nonreactive NST and no fetal breathing. Figure 23–9 shows the analysis according to the individual biophysical activities. The presence of reactive NST and/or fetal breathing (breathing lasting more than 30 seconds) rules out the presence of fetal acidemia. The frequency of acidemia in the group of fetuses with nonreactive NST and no breathing (groups 2, 3, and 4) depends on the presence or absence of fetal body movements and fetal tone. In fetuses with normal movements and tone, but nonreactive NST and no

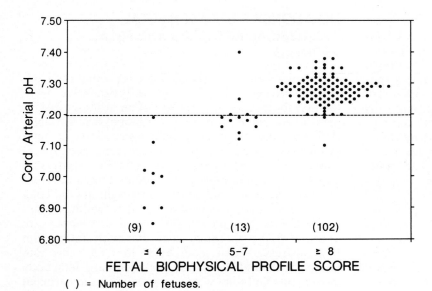

Figure 23–8. Relationship between the fetal biophysical profile score and cord arterial pH. (From Vintzileos AM, Gaffney SE, Salinger LM, et al: The relationship between fetal biophysical profile and cord pH in patients undergoing cesarean section before the onset of labor. Reprinted with permission from The American College of Obstetricians and Gynecologists [Obstetrics and Gynecology, 1987, 70:196]).

breathing, the incidence of acidemia was 59%. Fetuses with nonreactive NST, no breathing movements, and compromised body movements and tone had an incidence of acidemia of 75%. All fetuses with absence of all four biophysical activities were in the acidotic range. The study suggested that the fetal biophysical activities have different degrees of sensitivity to acidemia and also that careful analysis of the individual biophysical activities can give a clue as to the degree of fetal asphyxia. The fetal CNS centers that control fetal heart rate reactivity and fetal breathing are inhibited at pH values less than 7.20. Fetal body movements and fetal tone become compromised at pH values between 7.10 and 7.20, whereas movements and tone disappear at pH values less than 7.10.[8] The efficacy of each biophysical component alone and in combination to predict fetal acidemia is demonstrated in Table 23–6. The best accuracy was achieved by using a combination of "nonreactive NST and absent fetal breathing" as the

abnormal test. In a more recent study by Vintzileos and coworkers involving 62 patients undergoing cesarean section before the onset of labor, the fetal biophysical profile assessment and an umbilical artery systolic-to-diastolic (S/D) ratio were performed before delivery and umbilical cord blood gas measurements were obtained in all cases.[9, 33] Figures 23–10 through 23–14 demonstrate the different levels of cord arterial pH and blood gases at which the fetal biophysical activities are absent. It was observed that hypoxemia and acidemia are associated with nonreactive NST and no breathing, whereas advanced hypoxemia, acidemia, and hypercapnia are associated with loss of body movements and tone. A comparison between umbilical artery S/D ratio and fetal biophysical profile to detect fetal acidemia was also performed, and it was discovered that the NST had the best sensitivity (100%) and negative predictive value (100%).[33] The fetal biophysical profile had the best specificity (91%) and positive

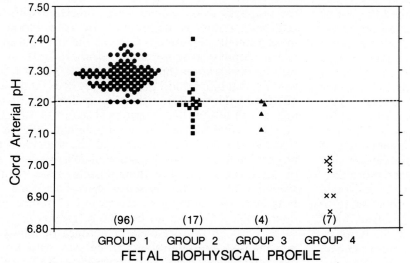

Figure 23–9. Relationship between the fetal biophysical activities (*acute markers*) and cord arterial pH. (From Vintzileos AM, Gaffney SE, Salinger LM, et al: The relationship between fetal biophysical profile and cord pH in patients undergoing cesarean section before the onset of labor. Reprinted with permission from The American College of Obstetricians and Gynecologists [Obstetrics and Gynecology, 1987, 70:196]).

Table 23–6. EFFICACY OF THE FETAL BIOPHYSICAL VARIABLES TO PREDICT FETAL ACIDEMIA

Biophysical Variable	Definition of the Abnormal Test	Sensitivity	Specificity	Positive Predictive Value	Negative Predictive Value
Biophysical score	≤7	90% (18/20)	96% (100/104)	82% (18/22)	98% (100/102)
Nonstress test, fetal breathing movements	Nonreactive NST and no breathing	100% (20/20)	92% (96/104)	71% (20/28)	100% (96/96)
Nonstress test	<1 acceleration in 20 minutes	100% (20/20)	76% (79/104)	44% (20/45)	100% (79/79)
Fetal breathing movements	<30 seconds	100% (20/20)	64% (67/104)	35% (20/57)	100% (67/67)
Fetal movements	<3	50% (10/20)	96% (100/104)	71% (10/14)	91% (100/100)
Fetal tone	Compromised or absent	45% (9/20)	100% (104/104)	100% (9/9)	90% (104/115)
Amniotic fluid	<1 cm	35% (7/20)	93% (97/104)	50% (7/14)	88% (97/100)
Amniotic fluid	<2 cm	45% (9/20)	86% (89/104)	38% (9/24)	89% (89/100)
Placental grading	Grade 3	5% (1/20)	94% (98/104)	14% (1/7)	84% (98/117)

Number of fetuses is indicated in parentheses.
From Manning FA, Morrison I, Harman CR, et al: Fetal assessment based on fetal biophysical profile scoring: Experience in 19,221 referred high risk pregnancies: II. An analysis of false-negative fetal deaths. Am J Obstet Gynecol 157:880, 1987.

predictive value (62%). The umbilical artery S/D ratio's sensitivity, specificity, and positive and negative predictive values were 66%, 42%, 16%, and 88%, respectively. The combination of S/D ratio and biophysical profile results did not improve diagnostic accuracy for fetal acidemia. The findings suggested that umbilical artery S/D ratio has no role in antepartum detection of fetal acidemia. Another study that examined the relationship between fetal biophysical profile results and cord blood gases obtained at funicentesis was reported by Ribbert and associates.[10] These investigators expressed their results in terms of delta pH differences (observed pH subtracted from the appropriate for gestational age mean pH). Fetal heart rate reactivity was found to be compromised by delta pH below −2 standard deviations (SD), the fetal breathing movements at delta pH values below −3 SD, and the fetal body movements and/or fetal tones were absent at delta pH values at or below −5 SD. The authors

also arrived at the conclusion that fetal acidemia in initial stages causes fetal heart rate nonreactivity and abolishes fetal breathing movements whereas body movements and tone are late manifestations of fetal asphyxia.

At the University of Connecticut Health Center fetal biophysical assessment relies on the analysis of the individual biophysical components rather than the score. Given the results of the aforementioned studies as well as the results of all the studies examining the relationship between fetal biophysical assessment and fetal acid-base status, we have adopted a protocol of fetal evaluation as illustrated in Figure 23–15. The fetal evaluation starts by performing an NST. The presence of fetal acidemia is ruled out when the NST is reactive. If, however, the NST is nonreactive for 40 minutes, real-time ultrasonography is undertaken. On detection

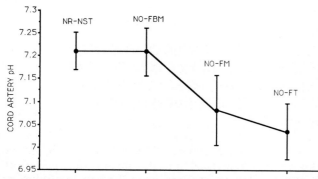

Figure 23–10. Relationship between cord artery pH and absent fetal biophysical activities. The pH tends to be lower in the absence of movements and/or tone as compared with nonreactive nonstress testing and/or absence of breathing. Results are expressed in means ±95% error bars. NR-NST, nonreactive nonstress test; NO-FBM, absent fetal breathing; NO-FM, absent fetal movements; NO-FT, absent fetal tone. (From Vintzileos AM, Fleming AD, Scorza WE, et al: Relationship between fetal biophysical activities and umbilical cord blood gases. Am J Obstet Gynecol 165:707, 1991.)

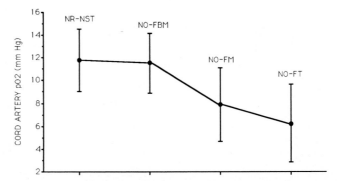

Figure 23–11. Relationship between cord artery PO_2 and absent fetal biophysical activities. The PO_2 tends to be lower in the absence of movements and/or tone as compared with nonreactive nonstress testing and/or absence of breathing. Results are expressed in millimeters of mercury (means ± 95% error bars). NR-NST, nonreactive nonstress test; NO-FBM, absent fetal breathing; NO-FM, absent fetal movements; NO-FT, absent fetal tone. (From Vintzileos AM, Fleming AD, Scorza WE, et al: Relationship between fetal biophysical activities and umbilical cord blood gases. Am J Obstet Gynecol 165:707, 1991.)

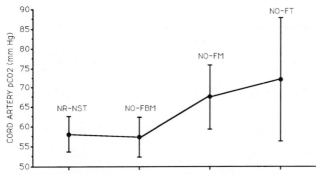

Figure 23–12. Relationship between cord artery P_{CO_2} and absent fetal biophysical activities. The P_{CO_2} tends to be higher in the absence of movements and/or tone as compared with nonreactive nonstress testing and/or absence of breathing. Results are expressed in millimeters of mercury (means ± 95% error bars). NR-NST, nonreactive nonstress test; NO-FBM, absent fetal breathing; NO-FM, absent fetal movements; NO-FT, absent fetal tone. (From Vintzileos AM, Fleming AD, Scorza WE, et al: Relationship between fetal biophysical activities and umbilical cord blood gases. Am J Obstet Gynecol 165:707, 1991.)

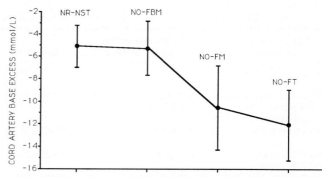

Figure 23–14. Relationship between cord artery base excess and absent fetal biophysical activities. The base excess tends to be lower in the absence of movements and/or tone as compared with non-reactive nonstress testing and/or absence of breathing. Results are expressed in millimoles per liter (means ± 95% error bars). NR-NST, nonreactive nonstress test; NO-FBM, absent fetal breathing; NO-FM, absent fetal movements; NO-FT, absent fetal tone. (From Vintzileos AM, Fleming AD, Scorza WE, et al: Relationship between fetal biophysical activities and umbilical cord blood gases. Am J Obstet Gynecol 165:707, 1991.)

of fetal breathing movements (lasting more than 30 seconds) the examination is ended since presence of fetal breathing is equally effective as a reactive NST in ruling out fetal acidemia. If during a 30-minute real-time observation, however, all biophysical activities are absent, prompt delivery is undertaken. If the NST is nonreactive and there are no detectable fetal breathing movements or breathing movements lasting less than 30 seconds, extended testing is undertaken to differentiate between fetal asphyxia and fetal sleep. The amniotic fluid volume is always evaluated regardless of the NST results. Oligohydramnios in a term or a near-term gestation is considered abnormal, and these patients are delivered to avoid cord accident and in utero death. In very preterm gestations with oligohydramnios, delivery or daily biophysical profiles are recommended. The use of umbilical artery velocimetry may help in the management of preterm high-risk fetuses when there is absent end-diastolic or reversed

flow indicating the need for delivery. It is our belief that Doppler velocimetry is still an investigational tool and that future studies may prove it to be useful in determining the frequency of fetal biophysical testing in cases with fetal growth retardation. However, many fetuses at risk (i.e., fetuses of diabetic mothers or post-date fetuses) do not suffer from reduced blood flow but from gas exchange disturbances at the trophoblastic membrane level; in these cases it is unlikely that umbilical artery velocimetry may be proven useful.

Our results by using this protocol in an 8-year period (1983–1991) were only two intrauterine deaths of structurally normal fetuses that occurred after a reassuring assessment. In addition, this protocol has decreased the testing time, increased the number of tested patients, and therefore has improved the efficacy of our unit. It is our belief that management on the basis of the total score rather than the individual biophysical components can result in misuse of this testing method. The most frequent errors in interpreting and applying fetal biophysical assessment data have been described in detail.[11]

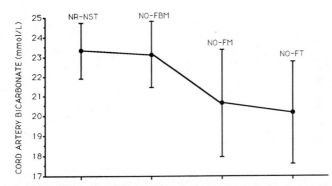

Figure 23–13. Relationship between cord artery bicarbonate level and absent fetal biophysical activities. The bicarbonate level tends to be lower in the absence of movements and/or tone as compared with nonreactive nonstress testing and/or absence of breathing. Results are expressed in millimoles per liter (means ± 95% error bars). NR-NST, nonreactive nonstress test; NO-FBM, absent fetal breathing; NO-FM, absent fetal movements; NO-FT, absent fetal tone. (From Vintzileos AM, Fleming AD, Scorza WE, et al: Relationship between fetal biophysical activities and umbilical cord blood gases. Am J Obstet Gynecol 165:707, 1991.)

CLINICAL USEFULNESS OF THE FETAL BIOPHYSICAL PROFILE IN DETECTING INTRA-AMNIOTIC INFECTION IN PATIENTS WITH PREMATURE RUPTURE OF THE MEMBRANES

After having established the effects of PROM on the fetal biophysical profile throughout gestation, Vintzileos and colleagues[14] were the first to publish an association between fetal biophysical assessment and intra-amniotic infection in this group of patients.[34] The initial study was observational, and the results from the biophysical assessment were not used for management. Patients with PROM were followed with frequent (every 1 to 3 days) biophysical profiles. None of the patients had any clinical signs of infection or labor

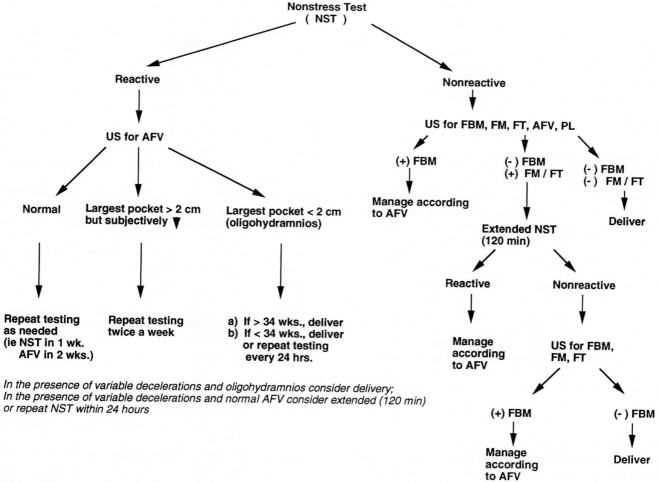

Figure 23–15. Protocol of antepartum fetal evaluation in pregnancies with intact membranes. US, ultrasound; AFV, amniotic fluid volume; FBM, fetal breathing movements; FM, fetal movements; FT, fetal tone; (+), present/normal; (−), absent/abnormal. (From Vintzileos AM, Gaffney SE, Salinger LM, et al: The relationships among the fetal biophysical profile, umbilical cord pH, and Apgar scores. Am J Obstet Gynecol 157:627, 1987.)

at the time of the ultrasound examinations. The last biophysical profile before delivery was correlated with the development of clinical infection (i.e., maternal chorioamnionitis, possible neonatal sepsis, and neonatal sepsis). When the interval between the last biophysical assessment and delivery was more than 24 hours there was not a strong correlation between abnormal assessment and development of infection outcome. However, when the interval between the last biophysical assessment and delivery was 24 hours or less, an abnormal biophysical profile was associated with an overall infection rate of 93.7%; on the other hand, a normal biophysical profile was associated with an overall infection rate of 2.7%. Although the development of clinical chorioamnionitis, without fetal or neonatal sepsis, was not necessarily associated with an abnormal biophysical profile, all fetuses in which possible neonatal sepsis or neonatal sepsis subsequently developed had an abnormal assessment 24 hours before delivery. An interesting observation was that the first manifestations of intra-amniotic infection included a nonreactive NST and absence of fetal breathing, whereas advanced infection (fetuses who subsequently developed neonatal sepsis) also had body movements

and tone compromised. The diminished biophysical activities were attributed to infection and not acidosis, since there were no cord pH differences between infected and noninfected cases. The association between abnormal biophysical assessment and intra-amniotic infection was subsequently confirmed by Goldstein and associates, who followed 41 patients with preterm PROM with daily biophysical profiles and weekly amniocenteses.[35] The authors found that fetal breathing of 30 seconds or more in duration ruled out the presence of intra-amniotic infection (negative amniotic fluid cultures in 100% of the cases). If there was extreme compromise of biophysical activities (i.e., fetal breathing absent or less than 30 seconds in duration and body movements lasting less than 50 seconds), there was intra-amniotic infection (positive amniotic fluid culture) in all cases. If, however, fetal breathing was abnormal (absent or less than 30 seconds) and the duration of body movements was normal (over 50 seconds in duration), approximately 64% of the patients had intra-amniotic infection. A subsequent report by Miller and colleagues on the use of an "ultrasonic" biophysical profile (without including the NST) on patients with PROM failed to demonstrate an association between clinical chorioamnionitis and abnormal biophysical assessment.[36] However, there were no cases with fetal or neonatal sepsis, and Miller and colleagues used as a gold standard the clinical diagnosis of chorioamnionitis that was not confirmed by appropriate placental pathology or cultures. Mercer and coworkers also reported a relationship between abnormal fetal biophysical assessment and infection outcome in patients with PROM.[37] The authors followed 139 women with preterm PROM with NSTs and biophysical profiles, and they found that nonreassuring biophysical assessment (nonreactive NST and abnormal biophysical profile) were associated with an increased frequency of clinical chorioamnionitis and neonatal sepsis. In a report by Roussis and coworkers each biophysical component alone and their combination ("modified" biophysical profile) were assessed in predicting infection outcome in 99 patients with PROM.[38] Roussis and coworkers found that absent fetal breathing or "modified" biophysical profile score less than or equal to 4 of 8 had the best sensitivities (93.8%) for predicting infection outcome. Absent fetal movement had the best specificity (100%), and a combination of absent fetal movement and absent breathing had the highest positive predictive value (100%). The overall test accuracy in predicting infection outcome was obtained by the combination of nonreactive NST and absent fetal breathing or a nonreactive NST and biophysical score less than or equal to 4 of 8. Roberts and coworkers conducted a comparison between quantitative fetal activity (sum of fetal breathing and fetal body movements) and the biophysical score (as scored by Manning and colleagues [see Table 23–1]) in predicting infection outcome in patients with PROM.[39] Although the sensitivity and positive and negative predictive values of the two methods were similar, abnormal total fetal activity (<10%) was found to have a better specificity (82%) as compared with the biophysical score (59%).

Reports involving the use of individual biophysical components to predict infection outcome in patients with PROM (i.e., NST alone,[40, 41] fetal breathing,[42] and quantitative amniotic fluid volume[13, 43]) have established the association between abnormal fetal behavior and intra-amniotic infection.

A comparison between transabdominal amniocentesis on admission for Gram stain and culture and daily biophysical profiles was done in 58 patients by Vintzileos and coworkers.[44] Amniocentesis results as well as abnormal biophysical profile results were used for patient management. Indications for delivery included positive amniotic fluid Gram stain, culture, mature lung profile, or abnormal biophysical assessment (score of ≤ 7 on two examinations 2 hours apart with nonreactive NST and no breathing). The results of the study showed that daily biophysical profiles were superior to amniocentesis in predicting infection outcome. To determine if pregnancy outcome is improved by acting on abnormal biophysical profile results, Vintzileos and coworkers[45] conducted a prospective study in 73 patients with preterm PROM. In this group of patients the biophysical profile results were used for management. The outcome of this group was compared with two other historic groups, one of which was managed without any invasive or fetal evaluation (control group) and the other was managed with amniocentesis alone (amniocentesis group). The results showed that the study group developed significantly fewer maternal and neonatal infections. Clinical amnionitis, possible neonatal sepsis, and neonatal sepsis occurred in 5.4%, 5.4%, and 1.4%, respectively, in the study group as compared with 25.5%, 13.6%, 13.5%, and 9.5%, respectively, in the control group. Neonatal sepsis was also less in the study group (1.3%) as compared with the group managed by amniocentesis (12.3%). Figure 23–16 represents the protocol currently used for management of preterm PROM at the University of Connecticut Health Center. This protocol is based on the individual biophysical components rather than on the total score (see Fig. 23–16).

Recent work by Vintzileos and coworkers has been directed toward the mechanism or mechanisms by which intra-amniotic infection causes diminished biophysical activities.[46] Of 53 patients with preterm PROM whose only indication for delivery was an abnormal biophysical assessment, only 5 of the 15 fetuses who

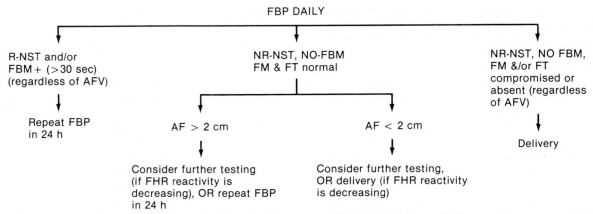

Figure 23–16. Protocol for management of premature rupture of the membranes. FBP, fetal biophysical profile; R-NST, reactive nonstress test; NR-NST, nonreactive nonstress test; FBM +, fetal breathing present; FM, fetal movements; FT, fetal tone; AFV, amniotic fluid volume; AF, amniotic fluid (largest vertical pocket); FHR, fetal heart rate.

subsequently developed neonatal sepsis were born acidemic. The remaining 10 septic neonates as well as all 17 with possible neonatal sepsis were born with normal cord blood pH values, suggesting that acidemia does not play a major role in diminishing the fetal biophysical activities in the setting of intra-amniotic infection. One speculation has been that increased prostaglandin production from phospholipase A2–producing bacteria, which cause chorioamnionitis, may cause hemodynamic changes of the fetal placental unit through vasoconstriction of the umbilical and chorionic vessels. Fleming and coworkers[47] tested this hypothesis by prospectively following patients with preterm PROM with daily biophysical profiles and daily umbilical artery S/D ratios. The study hypothesis was that if indeed there is increased production of prostaglandins with resultant placental vasoconstriction, the placental vascular resistance should be expected to be elevated in cases with intra-amniotic infection. The outcome used as an end point in this investigation was placental histologic evidence of infection. It was found that 2 to 7 days before delivery there are no differences in the biophysical assessment or S/D ratios regardless of the subsequent development of umbilical vasculitis. However, in the last examination, within 24 hours of delivery, fetuses with umbilical vasculitis had higher S/D ratios and lower biophysical scores as compared with the examinations of the previous days. Fetuses with intra-amniotic infection increased their average S/D ratio in the last examination within 24 hours of delivery, by approximately 30%. These human observations suggest that there is a simultaneous increase in placental vascular resistance and decrease in biophysical activities in fetuses with intra-amniotic infection. Thus, it is possible that in the absence of blood acidemia the hemodynamic changes associated with intra-amniotic infection may be causally related to the diminution of the biophysical activities. It still remains to be seen if serial umbilical artery S/D ratio studies would prove clinically useful in managing patients with preterm PROM.

References

1. Evertson LR, Gauthier RJ, Schifrin BS, et al: Antepartum fetal heart rate testing: I. Evolution of the nonstress test. Am J Obstet Gynecol 133:29, 1979.
2. Schifrin BS: The rationale of antepartum fetal heart rate monitoring. J Reprod Med 23:213, 1979.
3. Christie CB, Cudmore W: The oxytocin challenge test. Am J Obstet Gynecol 133:327, 1979.
4. Gauthier RJ, Evertson LR, Paul RH: Antepartum fetal heart rate testing: II. Intrapartum fetal heart rate testing and neonatal outcome following a positive contraction stress test. Am J Obstet Gynecol 133:34, 1979.
5. Ray M, Freeman R, Pine S, et al: Clinical experience with the oxytocin challenge test. Am J Obstet Gynecol 114:1, 1972.
6. Manning FA, Platt LD, Sipos L: Antepartum fetal evaluation: Development of a fetal biophysical profile score. Am J Obstet Gynecol 136:787, 1980.
7. Vintzileos AM, Campbell WA, Ingardia CJ, et al: The fetal biophysical profile and its predictive value. Obstet Gynecol 62:271, 1983.
8. Vintzileos AM, Gaffney SE, Salinger LM, et al: The relationship between fetal biophysical profile and cord pH in patients undergoing cesarean section before the onset of labor. Obstet Gynecol 70:196, 1987.
9. Vintzileos AM, Fleming AD, Scorza WE, et al: Relationship between fetal biophysical activities and umbilical cord blood gases. Am J Obstet Gynecol 165:707, 1991.
10. Ribbert LSM, Snijders RJM, Nicolaides KH, et al: Relationship of fetal biophysical profile and blood gas values at cordocentesis in severely growth-retarded fetuses. Am J Obstet Gynecol 163:569, 1990.
11. Vintzileos AM, Campbell WA, Nochimson DJ, et al: The use and misuse of the fetal biophysical profile. Am J Obstet Gynecol 156:527, 1987.
12. Chamberlain PFC, Manning FA, Morrison I, et al: Ultrasound evaluation of amniotic fluid volumes: I. The relationship of marginal and decreased amniotic fluid volumes to perinatal outcome. Am J Obstet Gynecol 150:245, 1984.
13. Vintzileos AM, Campbell WA, Nochimson DJ, et al: Degree of oligohydramnios and pregnancy outcome in patients with premature rupture of the membranes. Obstet Gynecol 66:162, 1985.
14. Vintzileos AM, Feinstein SJ, Lodeiro JG, et al: Fetal biophysical profile and the effect of premature rupture of the membranes. Obstet Gynecol 67:818, 1986.
15. Baskett TF: Gestational age and fetal biophysical assessment. Am J Obstet Gynecol 158:332, 1988.
16. Manning FA, Morrison I, Lange IR: Fetal biophysical profile scoring: A prospective study of 1,184 high-risk patients. Am J Obstet Gynecol 140:289, 1981.
17. Platt LD, Eglington GS, Sipos L, et al: Further experience with the fetal biophysical profile score. Obstet Gynecol 61:480, 1983.
18. Manning FA, Lange IR, Morrison I, et al: Fetal biophysical profile score and the nonstress test: A comparative trial. Obstet Gynecol 64:326, 1984.
19. Platt LD, Walla CA, Paul RH, et al: A prospective trial of fetal biophysical profile versus the nonstress test in the management of high risk pregnancies. Am J Obstet Gynecol 153:624, 1985.
20. Baskett TG, Gray JH, Prewett SJ, et al: Antepartum fetal assessment using a fetal biophysical profile score. Am J Obstet Gynecol 148:630, 1984.
21. Manning FA, Morrison I, Lange IR, et al: Fetal assessment based on fetal biophysical profile scoring: Experience in 12,620 referred high risk pregnancies: I. Perinatal morbidity by frequency and etiology. Am J Obstet Gynecol 151:343, 1985.
22. Manning FA, Morrison I, Harman CR, et al: Fetal assessment based on fetal biophysical profile scoring: Experience in 19,221 referred high risk pregnancies: II. An analysis of false-negative fetal deaths. Am J Obstet Gynecol 157:880, 1987.
23. Baskett TF, Allen AC, Gray JH, et al: Fetal biophysical profile and perinatal death. Obstet Gynecol 70:357, 1987.
24. Manning FA, Harman CR, Morrison I, et al: Fetal assessment based on fetal biophysical profile scoring: III. Positive predictive accuracy of the very abnormal test (biophysical profile score = 0). Am J Obstet Gynecol 162:398, 1990.
25. Manning FA, Harman CR, Morrison I, et al: Fetal assessment based on fetal biophysical profile scoring: IV. An analysis of perinatal morbidity and mortality. Am J Obstet Gynecol 162:703, 1990.
26. Manning FA, Morrison I, Lange IR, et al: Fetal biophysical profile scoring: Selective use of the nonstress test. Am J Obstet Gynecol 156:709, 1987.
27. Eden RD, Seifert LS, Kodack LD, et al: A modified biophysical profile for antenatal fetal surveillance. Obstet Gynecol 71:365, 1988.
28. Mills MS, James DK, Slade S: Two-tier approach to biophysical assessment of the fetus. Am J Obstet Gynecol 163:12, 1990.
29. Johnson JM, Harman CR, Lange IR, et al: Biophysical profile scoring in the management of postterm pregnancy: An analysis of 307 patients. Am J Obstet Gynecol 154:269, 1986.
30. Johnson JM, Lange IR, Harman CR, et al: Biophysical profile scoring in the management of the diabetic pregnancy. Obstet Gynecol 72:841, 1989.
31. Lodeiro JG, Vintzileos AM, Feinstein SJ, et al: Fetal biophysical profile in twin gestations. Obstet Gynecol 67:824, 1986.
32. Manning FA, Morrison I, Harman CR, et al: The abnormal fetal biophysical profile score: V. Predictive accuracy according to score composition. Am J Obstet Gynecol 162:918, 1990.
33. Vintzileos AM, Campbell WA, Rodis JF, et al: The relationship

between fetal biophysical assessment, umbilical artery velocimetry and fetal acidosis. Obstet Gynecol 77:622, 1991.

34. Vintzileos AM, Campbell WA, Nochimson DJ, et al: The fetal biophysical profile in patients with premature rupture of the membranes: An early predictor of fetal infection. Am J Obstet Gynecol 152:510, 1985.

35. Goldstein I, Romero R, Merrill S, et al: Fetal body and breathing movements as predictors of intraamniotic infection in preterm premature rupture of membranes. Am J Obstet Gynecol 159:363, 1988.

36. Miller JM, Kho MS, Brown HL, et al: Clinical chorioamnionitis is not predicted by an ultrasonic biophysical profile in patients with premature rupture of membranes. Obstet Gynecol 76:1051, 1990.

37. Mercer B, Moretti M, Shaver D, et al: Intensive antenatal testing for women with preterm premature rupture of the membranes. (Abstract No. 420). Presented before the 11th Annual Meeting of the Society of Perinatal Obstetricians, San Francisco, 1991.

38. Roussis P, Rosemond RL, Glass C, Boehm FH: Preterm premature rupture of membranes: Detection of infection. Am J Obstet Gynecol 165:1099, 1991.

39. Roberts AB, Goldstein I, Romero R, et al: Comparison of total fetal activity measurement with the biophysical profile in predicting intra-amniotic infection in preterm premature rupture of membranes. Ultrasound Obstet Gynecol 1:36, 1991.

40. Vintzileos AM, Campbell WA, Nochimson DJ, et al: The use of the nonstress test in patients with premature rupture of the membranes. Am J Obstet Gynecol 155:149, 1986.

41. Asrat T, Nageotte MP, Garite TJ, et al: Gram stain results from amniocentesis in patients with preterm premature rupture of membranes: Comparison of maternal and fetal characteristics. Am J Obstet Gynecol 163:887, 1990.

42. Vintzileos AM, Campbell WA, Nochimson DJ, et al: Fetal breathing as a predictor of infection in premature rupture of the membranes. Obstet Gynecol 67:813, 1986.

43. Goldstein I, Copel JA, Hobbins JC: Fetal behavior in preterm premature rupture of the membranes. Clin Perinatol 16:735, 1989.

44. Vintzileos AM, Campbell WA, Nochimson DJ, et al: Fetal biophysical profile versus amniocentesis in predicting infection in preterm premature rupture of the membranes. Obstet Gynecol 68:488, 1986.

45. Vintzileos AM, Bors-Koefoed R, Pelegano JF, et al: The use of fetal biophysical profile improves pregnancy outcome in premature rupture of the membranes. Am J Obstet Gynecol 157:236, 1987.

46. Vintzileos AM, Petrikovsky BM, Campbell WA, et al: Cord blood gases and abnormal fetal biophysical assessment in preterm premature rupture of the membranes. Am J Perinatol 8:155, 1991.

47. Fleming AD, Salafia CM, Vintzileos AM, et al: The relationships among umbilical artery velocimetry, fetal biophysical profile and placental inflammation in preterm premature rupture of the membranes. Am J Obstet Gynecol 164:38, 1991.

CHAPTER **24**

██████

Doppler Sonography in Obstetrics and Gynecology

ARTHUR C. FLEISCHER, M.D.
RUTH B. GOLDSTEIN, M.D.
JOSEPH P. BRUNER, M.D.
JOHN A. WORRELL, M.D.

The incorporation of Doppler-derived hemodynamic information into the standard anatomic sonographic assessment allows the additional evaluation of a variety of physiologic parameters in obstetrics and gynecology, previously out of reach to the sonologist and sonographer. Doppler sonography can provide useful and important information in a variety of gynecologic conditions, including ectopic pregnancy and ovarian masses. In obstetrics, Doppler velocimetry of the uteroplacental and fetoplacental circulation can be used to further investigate such complications of pregnancy as fetal growth retardation, other forms of fetal distress that result from fetal hypoxemia or asphyxia, fetal cardiac anomalies, and/or cord malformations. This chapter will serve as an overview to discuss and illustrate the many clinical applications of transabdominal and/or endovaginal continuous wave, pulsed wave duplex Doppler, or color Doppler sonography in obstetrics and gynecology.

THE DOPPLER EFFECT

The Doppler effect was described by Austrian physicist Johann Christian Doppler in 1842 to explain the appearance of "heavenly bodies." Simply put, the Doppler principle states that when energy is reflected from a moving boundary, the frequency of the reflected energy varies in relation to the velocity of the moving boundary. This change in frequency is known as the Doppler frequency shift and is related to velocity by the equation:

$$\Delta F = \frac{2F_0 V (\cos \theta)}{C} \quad or \quad V = \frac{F_r (C)}{2F_0 (\cos \theta)}$$

where F_0 is the frequency of the emitting source in cycles/s, V is the velocity of blood flow, cos θ is the cosine of the angle of insonation, C is the velocity of sound in tissue (1540 m/s), ΔF is the difference in frequency between the emitted and returning sound, and F_r is the returned frequency.

The Doppler principle was verified in 1845 by Dutch mathematician C. H. D. Buys Ballot, in a now famous experiment. One bugler playing middle C was placed aboard the newly introduced railroad engine and another stood on the station platform. Professor Ballot

and other observers noted that the pitch of a low note changed as a moving train passed through the station. Clinically, this principle is used to determine the velocity of blood flow in vessels. The frequency of sound reflected off moving blood cells is slightly altered from the sound emitted from the source (the transducer) in proportion to the velocity of the blood. This frequency shift can be determined by currently available technology and converted to velocity of blood flow if the beam's angle of insonation and other features in the above equation are known (Fig. 24–1).

INSTRUMENTATION

The sound source utilized for Doppler studies in human subjects is a piezoelectric crystal within the transducer that both transmits sound and receives the returning echo. A variety of devices utilize Doppler techniques for assessment of blood flow. These range from simple continuous wave devices to expensive color Doppler sonography equipment. Duplex Doppler equipment displays the real-time image simultaneously with pulsed wave Doppler waveforms. Color Doppler imaging translates mean velocities of flowing blood into a color display, the color of which reflects the direction of blood flow relative to the transducer. Color

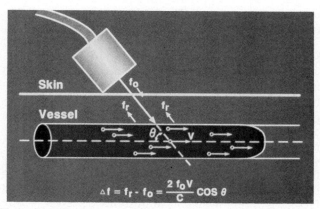

Figure 24–1. Doppler equation as shown in a diagram depicting the Doppler frequency shift in vessels relative to angle of interrogation. (From Lewis BD, James EM, Charboneau JW, et al: Current applications of color Doppler imaging in the abdomen and extremities. Radiographics 9:599–601, 1989.)

Doppler technology allows simultaneous imaging of a large field of view, displaying moving blood in all the vessels within the chosen area of interest. In this way, color Doppler images can provide a "road map" for the best sites to sample for spectral waveforms. The color assigned is arbitrary but, by convention, flow directed toward the transducer is usually displayed in red and that directed away in blue.

For any type of Doppler device, it is imperative that one consider the power emitted because this influences the exposure to the fetus. Continuous wave Doppler imaging uses ultrasound that is emitted continuously, and returning echoes are recorded from echoes at all depths. Thus, continuous wave Doppler devices provide information that is somewhat nonselective for the vessel interrogated. During duplex Doppler or color Doppler sonography, the sound waves are emitted as intermittent pulses, and depth information can be obtained based on the time interval between emitted and returning sound. With duplex Doppler sonography, relatively higher power output is required and, therefore, fetal exposure is generally higher. Color Doppler sonography, on the other hand, uses relatively low intensities. The Food and Drug Administration has set a limit at 94 mW/cm² (spatial peak temporal average) as the upper limit for intensity of Doppler imaging devices. For most color Doppler scanners, the intensities are in the 50- to 70-mW/cm² range. With the addition of duplex Doppler sonography, this increases to approximately 80 mW/cm². Many manufacturers provide a means for conveniently (i.e., a button on the console) diminishing the intensity to the range suggested by the Food and Drug Administration. Because color Doppler sonography expedites the visual localization of the vessel of interest for waveform analysis with duplex Doppler scanning, the use of color Doppler imaging serves indirectly to decrease the duration of the examination, and therefore the exposure of the fetus.

Duplex Doppler sonography in obstetrics and gynecology can be performed using either the transabdominal or endovaginal route. Both techniques necessitate rapid image processing from element to element. The transabdominal approach utilizes standard imaging transducers, whereas the endovaginal route necessitates the use of specially designed probes.

The ability to determine velocity is dependent on both the frequency shift and angle of insonation. If the vessels are large (> 3 mm), they can be visualized on the gray scale image and the angle of insonation can be determined and vessel diameter measured. This potentially allows the examiner to quantitate flow (in cubic centimeters per second). For precise measurements of flow, however, characteristics that influence velocity and flow in the vessel (i.e., parabolic or plug flow), in addition to the diameter of the vessel, should be known. Precise knowledge of all of these important factors is rarely available in obstetric settings. A true volume flow has been determined in the umbilical vein at the fetal abdominal insertion (± 10% to 15%) (see Fig. 24–1).[1]

However, because numerous sources of error exist in the determination of absolute flow (including the error associated with measuring the angle of insonation, the diameter of the vessel, and perhaps flow characteristics within a vessel), volume measurements have proven inaccurate and impractical in clinical use and are generally reserved for research centers.

In obstetrics, how best to assess clinically relevant alterations in maternal and fetal circulations with Doppler sonography is a complex and controversial issue. Because the vessels interrogated are often too small to measure accurately and too tortuous to determine the angle of insonation, three indices have been used by most investigators to quantitate velocities in systole *relative to* diastole (Fig. 24–2). The major benefit to the clinician of using these indices is that they are all independent of the angle of insonation (cos θ in both the numerator and denominator cancel out) and do not require a measurement of the diameter of the vessel. In clinical studies, vessels with relatively high diastolic flow velocities are believed to reflect a low downstream impedance to flow and those with low diastolic velocities reflect high impedance. In this way, all the most commonly used indices, *resistive index, systolic/diastolic ratio, and pulsatility index,* provide a semiquantitative assessment of impedance in the vessels interrogated. The systolic/diastolic ratio and resistive index, the simplest to use, are used most often in obstetrics. The latter indices, however, are associated with significant errors when end-diastolic velocity is zero or diastolic flow reversed. The pulsatility index

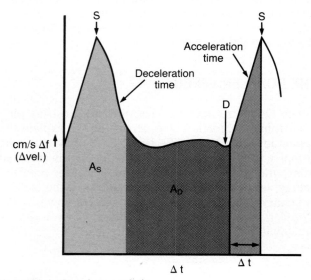

Figure 24–2. Waveform analysis.
Systolic/diastolic (S/D) = Maximum (max) systolic velocity ÷ minimum diastolic velocity
Resistive index (RI) = Maximum systolic velocity − diastolic velocity ÷ systolic velocity
Pulsatility index (PI) = Maximum systolic velocity − diastolic velocity ÷ mean velocity
Perfusion index (Per I) = Area under curve during systole ÷ area under curve during diastole
Acceleration time (ACC) = Time from initial systolic rise to peak (slope = rate)
Deceleration time (DCC) = Time from beginning of diastole to end diastole
Volume flow (cc/s) (Q) = Average velocity × lumen dimension

requires digitization of the entire waveform and is therefore least convenient.

Some work has been done to assess other features of the systolic portion and waveform such as acceleration time and upslope (see Fig. 24–2). However, because more sophisticated analysis of waveform characteristics does not improve the sensitivity and specificity, it provides no significant advantage over the previously mentioned, easier semiquantitative analyses.[2]

For assessment of intraparenchymal flow such as that within the ovary, the pulsability index is recommended since it better characterizes the waveform (see Fig. 24–2). New parameters such as the perfusion index are now being evaluated. For this index, the area under the curve, as determined by an integration function during systole, is divided by that of diastole.[3] This may potentially afford a means to better characterize actual parenchymal flow. Stenoses in major hilar vessels may produce a pulse reduced in overall amplitude and with delay in the upstroke, as reflected by an increase in the acceleration time.

The interobserver and intraobserver error for measurement of the systolic/diastolic ratio and other indices is relatively low and has been assessed in a variety of studies. When duplex Doppler sonography is used in obstetric studies, the interobserver and intraobserver error in measurement of the systolic/dystolic ratio is estimated at less than 10%.[4] For endovaginal color Doppler sonography, the coefficient of variation is also 7% to 10%.[5]

USE OF DOPPLER SONOGRAPHY IN OBSTETRICS FOR PREDICTION OF FETAL DISTRESS, GROWTH RETARDATION, AND HYPOXIA

One of the main goals of prenatal testing is to identify fetuses at increased risk for perinatal morbidity and mortality. Fetal hypoxia and asphyxia, often combined with intrauterine growth retardation (IUGR), is associated with significantly increased risk. Therefore, much of the interest in Doppler sonography has focused on its ability to identify the growth-retarded, hypoxic, and/or distressed fetus.

A number of investigators have demonstrated an association between abnormalities in maternal and fetal circulations and a variety of abnormal conditions in pregnancy. Abnormal Doppler waveforms are associated with growth retardation and/or fetal distress. The results of clinical studies have been conflicting, however, and especially among low-risk patients the positive predictive value of abnormal Doppler waveforms for IUGR has been disappointing (i.e., 20% to 40%). Because prenatal Doppler studies have not been proved to benefit pregnancy outcome, many investigators still consider obstetric Doppler velocimetry to be an investigational tool. If Doppler imaging has a role in obstetrics, the majority of data suggest that it may be more useful in the higher-risk population (Table 24–1)[6–15]; this technique is currently being used in practice at many centers as an adjunctive tool for

Table 24–1. STUDIES OF UMBILICAL ARTERY DOPPLER VELOCITIES AND FETAL OUTCOME

Source	No. at High Risk	Critria	Cutoff	Sensitivity	Specificity	Positive Predictive Value	Negative Predictive Value
Maulik et al., 1989[6]	350	IUGR 5' Apgar score <7 Arterial pH <7.25 Thick meconium Fetal distress Neonatal intensive care unit admission	3.0	79	93	83	91
Fleischer et al., 1985[7]	189/mix	IUGR	3.0	78	83	49	95
Schulman et al., 1989[8]	255/195	IUGR	3.0	65	91	43	96
Trudinger et al., 1985[9]	172/172	IUGR 5' Apgar score <7 Neonatal death	95%	64 62	77 79	55 63	83 78
Marsal, 1987[10]	142/142	IUGR	2 S/D	57	85	80	64
Arduini et al., 1987[11]	75/75	IUGR	1 S/D	61	73	50	81
Gaziano et al., 1988[12]	256/256	IUGR	4.0	79	66	79	96
Divon et al., 1988[13]	127/127	IUGR	>3.0	49	94	81	77
Berkowitz et al., 1988[14]	168/168	IUGR	3.0	45	89	58	86
Al-Ghazali et al., 1988[15]	300+ 71	IUGR	95%	72	87	82	79

Adapted from Maulik D, Yarlagadda P, Youngblood JP, Ciston P: The diagnostic efficacy of the umbilical arterial systolic/diastolic ratio as a screening tool: A prospective blinded study. Am J Obstet Gynecol 162:1518, 1990.

evaluation of fetuses known to be at increased perinatal risk (i.e., in fetuses with suspected IUGR, in hypertensive pregnant patients, in the setting of preeclampsia and/or poor prenatal care and nutrition).

Both the uterine and fetal circulations have been studied with Doppler sonography. The uterine artery first gives off branches at the level of the internal cervical os and then courses along the lateral aspect of the uterine body, where it is often sampled. The arcuate branch of the uterine artery can be sampled within the myometrium, and this, in part, reflects the (maternal) arterial blood supply to the placenta and intervillous space (Figs. 24–3 and 24–4). There is little diastolic flow in the uterine artery in the nongravid uterus. As normal gestation progresses, there is a progressive drop in impedance in the uterine artery through the second trimester, as evidenced by increased diastolic flow velocity with Doppler scanning. Thereafter, resistance remains stable. It should be emphasized that flow characteristics in the arcuate artery during pregnancy may vary depending on the site of placentation. For example, resistive indices are lower in placental than nonplacental sites (Fig. 24–5A and B). Therefore, an error may be introduced by sampling one area of the arterial supply that may not be representative of the entire circulation.

Abnormal waveform patterns in the uterine and/or arcuate arteries may be associated with maternal conditions that impair blood supply to the placenta and are associated with impaired fetal growth.[16] Pregnancy-induced hypertension is associated with inadequate physiologic change in the spiral arteries. Abnormal uterine/arcuate artery waveforms have been correlated with current or future development of maternal hypertension. In cases of pregnancy-induced hypertension, especially proteinuric pregnancy-induced hypertension, the resistance in the arcuate arteries may remain elevated. This is believed to reflect inadequate tropho-

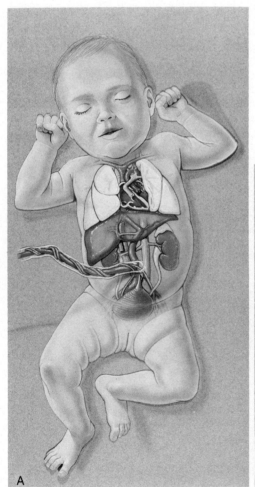
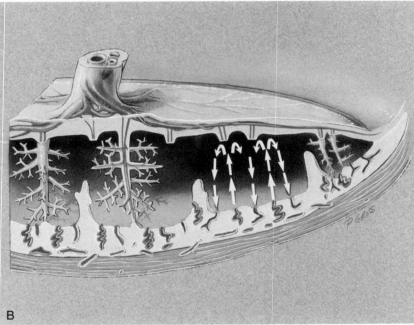

Figure 24–3. *A.* Oxygenated blood courses toward the fetus through the umbilical vein. Once within the liver, blood flows into the ductus venosus or portal sinus and empties into the inferior vena cava at the junction of the middle and left hepatic veins. Blood enters the heart through the right atrium. Blood then can pass into the right ventricle or cross the foramen ovale into the left atrium. Blood passing out of the left ventricle flows into the aorta, whereas blood coursing from the right ventricle can pass back into the aorta from the pulmonary arteries through the ductus arteriosus. Fetal tissues are supplied with oxygenated blood. *B.* Oxygenated blood courses through the spiral arteries in the decidua basalis/basal plate. The blood circulates around the chorionic villus unit. Oxygenated blood within the villus unit returns to the fetus by way of the umbilical vein. Deoxygenated blood is returned to the placenta by the paired umbilical arteries. *C.* Arterial and venous vessels within the myometrium/decidua at 8, 16, 20, 38, and 40 weeks of pregnancy. The relative thickness of the endometrium/decidua is compared, and the inner myometrium is shown to the left of each drawing. The arteries enlarge owing to trophoblastic infiltration of the muscular media. This configuration provides constant forward flow. The venous vessels are also distended.

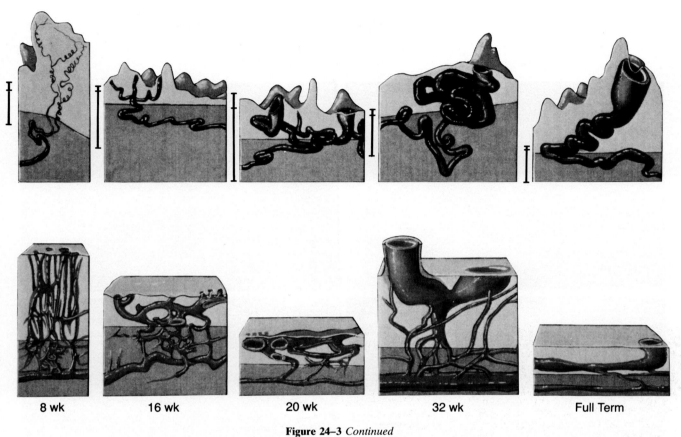

8 wk   16 wk   20 wk   32 wk   Full Term

Figure 24–3 *Continued*

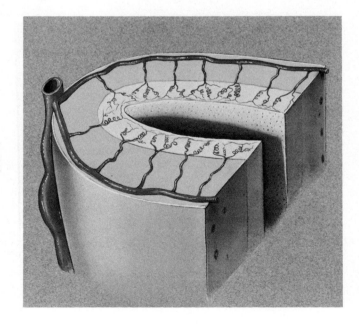

Figure 24–4. Uterine arterial circulation. The main uterine artery perforates the serosa and gives off the arcuates, which further branch into the radial arteries. The arcuate circulation is shown, as well as the spiral arteries, which course within the endometrium.

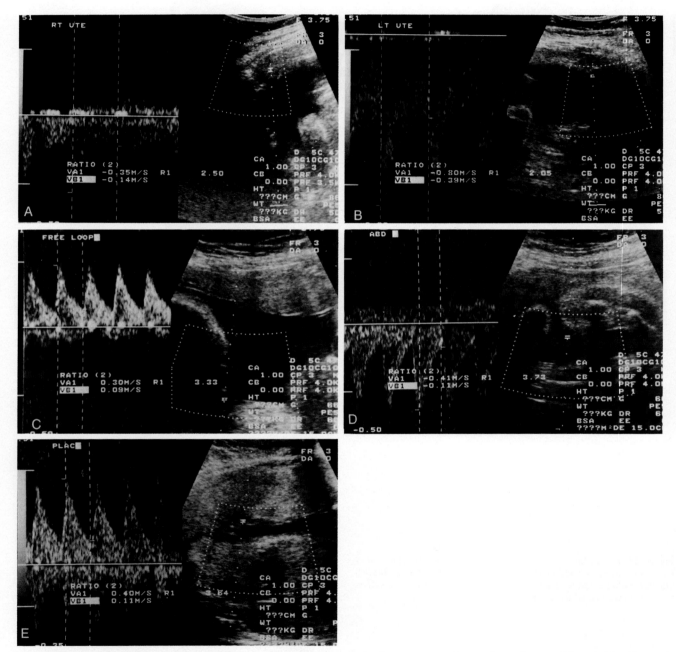

Figure 24–5. Normal duplex Doppler waveform. *A* and *B*. Differences in uterine artery waveforms when taken at different sides of uterus. *C*. Free loop of cord. *D*. Fetal abdomen insertion. *E*. Placental insertion.

blastic invasion of the spiral arteries and has been associated with IUGR. Independent of pregnancy-induced hypertension, abnormalities of uteroplacental waveforms have been observed in association with impaired fetal growth, although the results have been inconsistent. Currently, predictive values of uterine artery Doppler analysis for IUGR are too low to warrant use of Doppler sonography on the general obstetric populations.

The positive predictive values and sensitivities of uterine artery velocimetry for IUGR and/or fetal distress are generally poorer than the predictive values based on umbilical artery and Doppler examination of fetal vessels (see later). The clinical significance, and therefore the management of patients with an abnormal uteroplacental waveform in association with a normal umbilical artery waveform, remains unsettled. Perhaps determination of uteroplacental blood flow and actual flow of oxygenated blood in the umbilical vein to the fetus may be additional areas for refinement of the Doppler technique.[1]

Alterations in the fetoplacental circulation and specific fetal vessels reflect important hemodynamic modifications that occur in association with IUGR and fetal hypoxemia. The Doppler-detectable modifications in the fetal circulation associated with IUGR and fetal hypoxemia include increased resistance in the umbilical artery and fetal peripheral vessels (i.e., the descending thoracic artery), in association with decreased resistance in the fetal cerebral vessels. This pattern of hemodynamic alteration is believed to reflect the "brain-sparing" phenomenon described in experimental models of fetal hypoxia, in which fetuses that are rendered hypoxic preferentially perfuse the brain, heart, and adrenals at the expense of the integument and viscera, gut, and kidneys (Fig. 24–6).[17] Normal indices for the umbilical artery, descending aorta, internal carotid artery, middle cerebral artery, and fetal renal arteries have been established (see Fig. 24–6D and E).[18]

The following circulations have been most extensively studied:

1. Umbilical artery. The umbilical artery is one of the easiest targets to visualize, and umbilical artery Doppler waveforms have been studied most extensively. Normally, as gestation and trophoblastic invasion progress, there is a progressive increase in diastolic flow velocity in the umbilical artery, believed to reflect progressively decreasing placental resistance (see Figs. 24–3, 24–6D). The two most commonly used indices are the systolic/diastolic ratio and the pulsatility index. Clinical studies indicate that the resistive index, systolic/diastolic ratio, and pulsatility index are well correlated in normal pregnancies. In addition, when correlated against adverse perinatal events, both the systolic/diastolic ratio and pulsatility index have similar predictive values. Thus, many investigators use the simplest systolic/diastolic ratio.[2, 19] A systolic/diastolic ratio greater than 2 standard deviations above normal is considered abnormal. As a simpler approach, many consider a systolic/diastolic ratio greater than 3 in the umbilical artery after 30 weeks to be abnormal (see Fig. 24–6D).

Many physiologic factors can also affect the waveform, and the examiner should be aware of these. For example, the umbilical artery systolic/diastolic ratio will vary according to the site in the cord sampled[20]: highest resistances are recorded in the cord near the insertion into the fetal abdomen and lowest at the placental end of the cord (see Fig. 24–5C through E). Most prefer sampling the cord near the placenta or in a free-floating loop of cord. Fetal "breathing" and cardiac arrhymias may also influence cord indices (Fig. 24–7). With fetal breathing, the cardiac cycle length may be irregular, thus influencing the time for diastolic flow to fall to the baseline. If the heart rate is unusually slow (i.e., < 110 beats per minute), the longer cardiac cycles result in more time for diastolic flow velocity to fall to the baseline, artifactually increasing the ratio of systolic/diastolic flow velocity (Fig. 24–7).[21] Technical factors, including suboptimal insonation angle and improper gain settings, also influence systolic/diastolic calculations (Fig. 24–8).

2. Fetal internal carotid artery. The fetal internal carotid artery (as it enters the circle of Willis) or the middle cerebral artery (as it exits the circle of Willis) have been studied in the fetal cerebral circulation. The resistive indices tend to be slightly higher in the middle cerebral artery than the internal carotid artery. These vessels are studied at the base of the brain near the circle of Willis on axial view. Color Doppler sonography expedites the choice of sample volume by demonstrating flow in the vessels of the circle of Willis simultaneously (Fig. 24–9A). In normal fetuses there is little diastolic flow in these vessels, and the systolic/diastolic ratio is normally greater than 4 throughout (see Fig. 24–6E). The diastolic flow velocity increases slightly during gestation, resulting in some diminution of the systolic/diastolic ratio as a function of gestational age.

3. Fetal thoracic aorta. Most investigations of the fetal aorta have focused on the descending aorta, but this vessel has not been extensively studied. Doppler-measured resistances in the fetal aorta are believed to reflect blood flow to the fetal abdominal region and extremities. Approximately 55% of the blood in the fetal aorta enters the umbilical circulation, and the remainder supplies the viscera and lower part of the body.[12] The Doppler-measured resistance in the thoracic aorta normally increases gradually between 26 and 38 weeks.[13] Interobserver variability tends to be greater and reproducibility poorer than measurements of resistance in the umbilical artery or cerebral vessels. Recall also that aortic pulsatility is more dependent on cardiac contractility than on umbilical artery pulsatility. Nevertheless, absent end-diastolic velocity in the fetal descending aorta is a reliable observation and is always abnormal.

4. Fetal renal arteries. It is well known that diminished amniotic fluid is associated with IUGR and, with the use of Doppler velocimetry, the renal artery resistive index has also been shown to be increased in fetuses that are asymmetrically growth retarded.[24] Other fetal conditions that may affect renal blood flow include hydronephrosis and multicystic dysplastic kidney.[25, 26] Color Doppler sonography also expedites the choice of Doppler gate for waveform analysis (see

Text continued on page 514

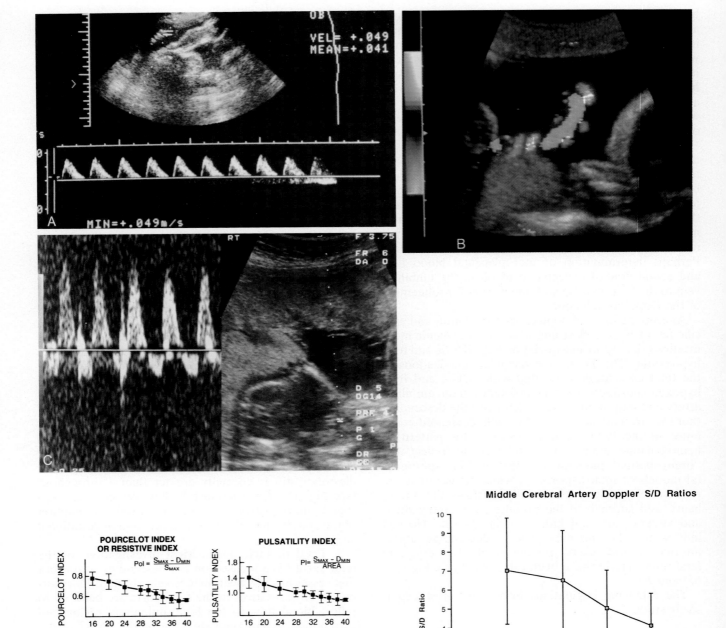

Figure 24–6. Doppler signs of fetal hypoxia. *A.* Absent diastolic flow. This 29-year-old mother was hypertensive. Estimated fetal weight was at the 10th percentile, but normal amniotic fluid quantity was noted. This examination at 32 weeks showed an extremely high impedance to flow in the umbilical artery, with absent end-diastolic flow. The mother was delivered of a 964-g neonate within hours of this examination. The neonate died 2 days later of complications of extreme prematurity. *B.* Twin pregnancy. Color Doppler study used to identify that the sample was taken at the cord insertion into the placenta of twin A. *C.* Reversed diastolic flow in twin B. This fetus died several hours after this study. *D.* Doppler waveform analysis of the fetal umbilical artery. With advancing gestation and increasing compliance of the placenta, there is a progressive decrease in the systolic/diastolic ratio, Pourcelot index (PoI), and pulsatility index (PI) of the umbilical artery that is a result of increased placental flow due to decreased resistance. *E.* Mean ± 2 SD of the middle cerebral artery systolic/diastolic ratio with respect to gestational age. (*D,* modified from Erskine RLA, Ritchie JWK: Umbilical artery blood flow characteristics in normal and growth retarded fetuses. Br J Obstet Gynecol 92:605, 1985; *E,* modified from Woo JSK, Liang ST, et al: Middle cerebral artery Doppler flow velocity. Reprinted with permission from The American College of Obstetricians and Gynecologists [Obstetrics and Gynecology, 1987, 70:613]).

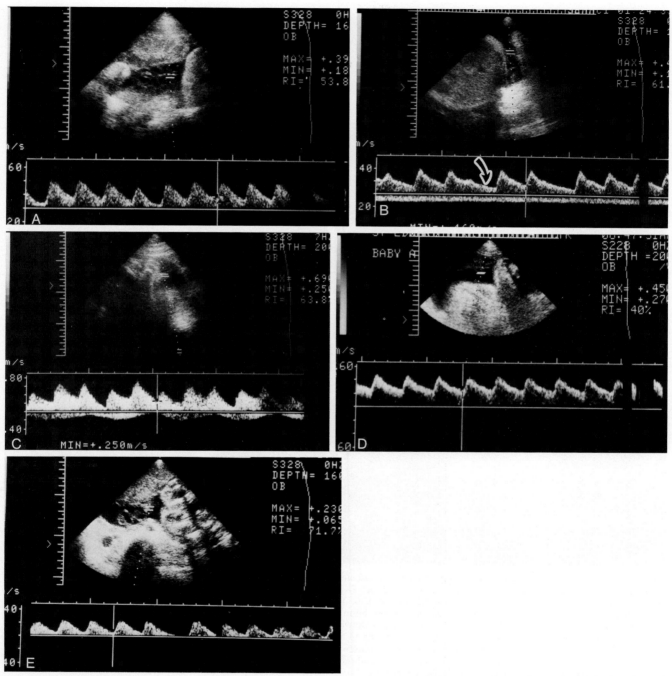

Figure 24–7. Intrinsic factors that affect Doppler assessment. *A.* This midcord Doppler sample taken in the third trimester was complicated by fetal breathing, which is causing the Doppler waveform to show a cyclic variance. This invalidates the resistive index (RI). *B.* The ventricular rate in this fetus is quite bradycardiac and measures approximately 60 beats per minute. There was a 2:1 block and atrioventricular canal defect in this fetus with Down syndrome. The effect of this severe bradycardia on the RI is illustrated (*arrow*), with near absence of the end-diastolic flow. Note the extra systole after the third normal systole. This is followed by an artificially depressed end-diastolic flow. The pattern is repeated after two more normal systoles. The accuracy of the RI is dependent on a regular cardiac rhythm and rate. *C.* This study shows the effect of fetal motion and breathing and also of venous contamination artifact. *D.* This G4P1Ab1 pregnancy was a complicated twin gestation. At 36 weeks, twin A had an estimated fetal weight greater than the 90th percentile and an RI of 40%. *E.* This is the twin of the fetus in *D,* also at 36 weeks. The RI is elevated at 0.7, and the estimated fetal weight was at the 31st percentile. Both neonates did well at birth, with a 20% difference in birth weight.

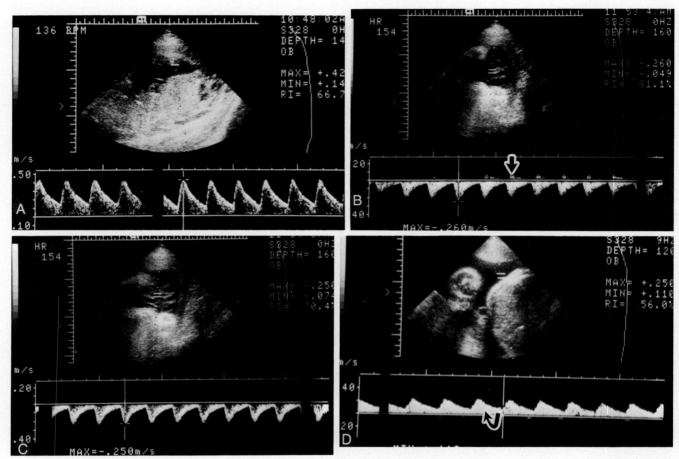

Figure 24–8. Technical factors that influence systolic/diastolic calculations. *A*. At placental insertion, resistive index (RI) = 0.67. *B*. At mid cord RI = 0.81. Note the aliasing (*arrow*) due to an ambiguous Doppler angle. *C*. This reading was taken 70 seconds later than that of *B*, with a better angle of insonation. The RI is still elevated at 0.70. The fetus was noted to be clinically growth retarded at birth. *D*. Third-trimester Doppler examination of the umbilical artery shows fill-in under the curve (*arrow*), which represents technical artifact from too much gain. RI is normal at 0.56. *E*. This is the same fetus as shown in *D* (*curved arrow*) within 90 seconds of *D*. Note the "cleaner" flow window from the improved technique. RI is still normal at 0.65. A normal neonate was subsequently delivered. *F*. This Doppler waveform is technically degraded by high gain settings and a low signal-to-noise ratio, making interpretation of the RI difficult. *G*. Normal flow window, but the RI is 0.73. This fetus is early in the second trimester, and this is a normal tracing. *H*. There is some filling in of the flow window and some venous contamination (*arrow*), but the RI is now normal at 0.5.

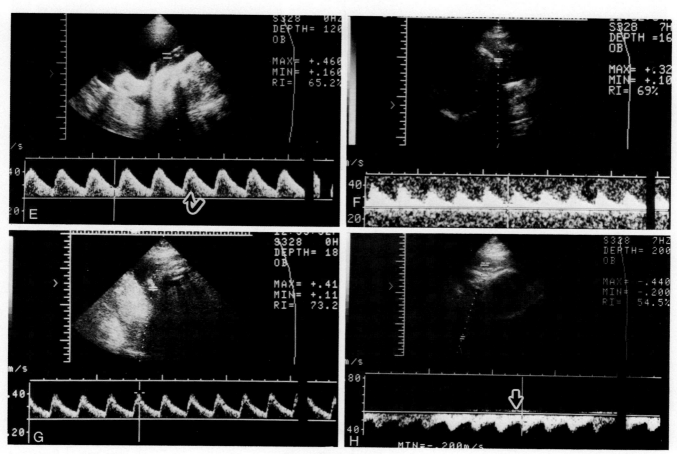

Figure 24–8 *Continued*

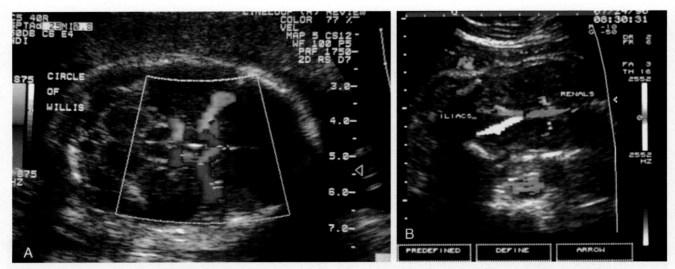

Figure 24–9. Relative perfusion. *A.* Doppler assessment of cerebral flow, determined by the waveform arising from the junction of the middle cerebral artery/internal carotid artery. *B.* Doppler assessment of somatic flow, determined from the infrarenal abdominal aorta.

Fig. 24–9*B*), but investigation with Doppler sonography of the fetal renal arteries is still quite preliminary. At this time, study of the renal arteries remains technically difficult, with lower predictive values for IUGR than those achieved with Doppler imaging of the umbilical artery or fetal vessels.

Of all vessels studied, abnormal resistivity in the umbilical artery has been studied most extensively as a predictor of IUGR.[27] In the laboratory, increased placental resistance has been produced experimentally by embolization of the terminal arteriolar branches in the placentae of fetal lambs with microspheres.[28, 29] Similarly, histologic studies have demonstrated a decrease in the number of small arteries from the terminal villi among small-for-gestational age fetuses who demonstrate increased umbilical artery resistance with

Doppler velocimetry.[30, 31] Clinical studies have also substantiated a statistically significant association between IUGR and abnormally increased resistance in the umbilical artery. However, the low predictive values of an abnormal test (i.e., 20% to 40%) in the general obstetric population have not been sufficient to be useful (Table 24–2).[7, 11, 13, 21, 30, 32–37] In fact, in a population with a relatively low prevalence of IUGR (i.e., < 20%), the systolic/diastolic ratio seems to be neither sensitive nor specific for the diagnosis (Table 24–3).[8]

In studying the efficacy of Doppler in obstetrics, both IUGR and fetal distress have been used as end points. A number of studies indicate that abnormal umbilical artery Doppler velocimetry seems to be somewhat better correlated with fetal distress and hypoxemia than with IUGR. As expected, the more

Table 24–2. PREDICTIVE VALUE OF FETAL BLOOD FLOW VELOCITY FOR FETAL GROWTH RETARDATION

Year	Series	Study Population			Study Protocol		Sensitivity (%)	Specificity (%)	Positive Predictive Value (%)	Negative Predictive Value (%)
		No.	SGA		Time of Observation	Index				
			n	%						
1986	Giles et al.[3]	42*	10	24	Final	S/D	100	88	71	100
1985	Fleischer et al.[7]	137*	23	16	3rd Tri.	S/D	78	83	49	95
1987	Mulders et al.[32]	48*	15	31	34 wk	S/D	53	88	66	80
1988	Divon et al.[13]	127*	45	35	3rd Tri.	S/D	49	94	81	77
1988	Berkowitz et al.[14]	168*	42	25	3rd Tri.	S/D	45	89	57	
1989	Dempster et al.[34]	205*	82	40	3rd Tri.	S/D	41	82	61	68
1987	Arduini et al.[11]	75*	23	31	26–28	PI	61	73	50	81
1989	Sijmons et al.[35]	400†	88	22	28 wk	PI	17	95	50	79
					34 wk	PI	22	94	53	81
1989	Beattie and Dornan[36]	2097†			28 wk	PI	28	89	11	97
					34 wk	PI	32	89	12	97
					38 wk	PI	31	86	9	97

S/D, Systolic/diastolic ratio; PI, pulsatile index; 3rd Tri., serial measures throughout third trimester.
*High-risk study population.
†Random study population.
From Low JA: The current status of maternal and fetal blood flow velocimetry. Am J Obstet Gynecol 164:1049, 1991.

Table 24–3. ABNORMAL UMBILICAL ARTERY WAVEFORMS AND INTRAUTERINE GROWTH RETARDATION (IUGR) IN A LOW-RISK POPULATION

| | Umbilical Artery S/D > 3 at 30 Weeks | | |
| | Disease State | | |
Test Result	IUGR Present	IUGR Absent	Total
Positive	15	20	35
Negative	8	212	220
Total	23	232	255

Other Test Criteria

Sensitivity	= 65%
Specificity	= 91%
Positive predictive value	= 43%
Negative predictive value	= 96%
Prevalence	= 9%

S/D, systolic/diastolic.

Adapted from Schulman H, Winter D, Farmakides G, et al: Pregnancy surveillance with Doppler velocimetry of uterine and umbilical arteries. Am J Obstet Gynecol 160:192, 1989.

abnormal the systolic/diastolic ratio, the more likely it will predict significant fetal compromise. Although slightly elevated umbilical artery systolic/diastolic ratios are only marginally predictive, absent or reversed diastolic flow in the umbilical artery in the third trimester is a more important and more ominous observation. Among 39 small-for-gestational age fetuses reported by Campbell and coworkers,[38] absent end-diastolic flow velocity was found in 22 and cordocentesis showed 21 of 22 to be hypoxemic and/or acidotic. In addition, clinical studies have shown that absent or reversed end diastolic flow velocity is associated with significantly increased risk for perinatal death (Table 24–4; see Figs. 24–6A and 24–10).[31, 39–41] Although the fetal and/or maternal conditions associated with absent diastolic flow are multifactorial, it has been well substantiated that this finding indicates significant fetal compromise regardless of its etiology.[42]

Some experimental studies have indicated that abnormal patterns of flow in specific fetal vessels are more closely correlated with fetal hypoxemia than waveforms in the umbilical artery. Thus, increased diastolic flow in the internal carotid artery is believed to reflect increased cerebral blood flow (i.e., "brain sparing") and this, in combination with increased resistance in the aorta, results in a cerebral to aortic systolic/diastolic ratio of less than 1, which is characteristic of chronic hypoxemia and IUGR.

Although small fetal size indicates increased fetal risk, it is known that small-for-gestational age fetuses are a heterogeneous group, and not all of them are hypoxemic or compromised. Investigators have attempted to use Doppler sonography to select the distressed or hypoxemic small-for-gestational age fetus among the group of small fetuses.[43] In a study of 120 small-for-gestational age fetuses, Arduini and Rizzo[18] found that the ratio of pulsatility of the fetal cerebral vessels (middle cerebral artery) and placental circulation (umbilical artery) offered the best predictive values for poor outcome. All cases of perinatal death

occurred in the subgroup with abnormal cerebral/umbilical artery pulsatility, and no mortality occurred in the group with a normal middle cerebral artery/umbilical artery ratio. Because 53% of small-for-gestational age fetuses in this study had a normal outcome, Arduini and Rizzo believed that these ratios helped distinguish the small, distressed fetuses from the small, relatively healthy ones.

Another method of assessing cerebral versus somatic flow is to correlate the maximum systolic flow of the fetal thoracic aorta to that of the fetal common carotid artery. This method has been used to assess the effect of maternal hyperoxygenation on the severely growth-retarded fetus.[44]

Currently, Doppler velocimetry is probably best used in obstetrics as an adjunctive test in prenatal monitoring. Because positive predictive values are not high enough to manage a pregnancy based solely on velocimetry data, Doppler sonography can be used to suggest the need for increased fetal surveillance. An abnormal Doppler result usually warrants such additional noninvasive testing as the biophysical profile and nonstress testing. The biophysical profile reflects oxygenation to the autonomic nervous system as evidenced by fetal breathing motion and tone, whereas an umbilical artery Doppler study is believed to reflect the integrity of placental perfusion. Both biophysical profile and umbilical artery fetal Doppler velocimetry aim to distinguish the truly growth-retarded fetus who is at risk for distress or death from the healthy but small-for-gestational age fetus. In some cases, the umbilical artery Doppler waveform may become abnormal before the development of an abnormal stress test but in the vast majority of significantly compromised fetuses both tests are abnormal. Biophysical profile testing has been more extensively studied than prenatal Doppler velocimetry. Further investigation will be needed before definite conclusions can be drawn about the significance of an isolated abnormal umbilical artery Doppler sonogram when the biophysical profile and nonstress test are normal.

FETAL CARDIAC AND UMBILICAL ARTERY ANOMALIES

Doppler sonography can be useful in evaluation of fetal cardiac anomalies as well as malformations of the

Table 24–4. ADVERSE OUTCOME ASSOCIATED WITH ABSENT OR REVERSED END-DIASTOLIC FLOW

Absent End-Diastolic Flow in 24 Fetuses*	Reversed End-Diastolic Flow in 12 Fetusus†
22/24 (91%) <5% birthweight	12/12 (100%) <10% birthweight
20/24 (83%) cesarean section	6/8 (75%) cesarean section
4/24 (16%) died	6/12 (50%) died
17 had normal fetal heart rate tracings	All had abnormal fetal heart rate tracings

*Data from Johnstone FD, Haddad NG, Hoskins P, et al: Umbilical artery Doppler flow velocity waveform: The outcome of pregnancies with absent end-diastolic flow. Eur J Obstet Gynecol 28:171, 1988.

†Data from Brar HS, Platt LD: Reverse end-diastolic flow velocity on umbilical artery velocimetry in high-risk pregnancies: An ominous finding with adverse pregnancy outcome. Am J Obstet Gynecol 159:559, 1988.

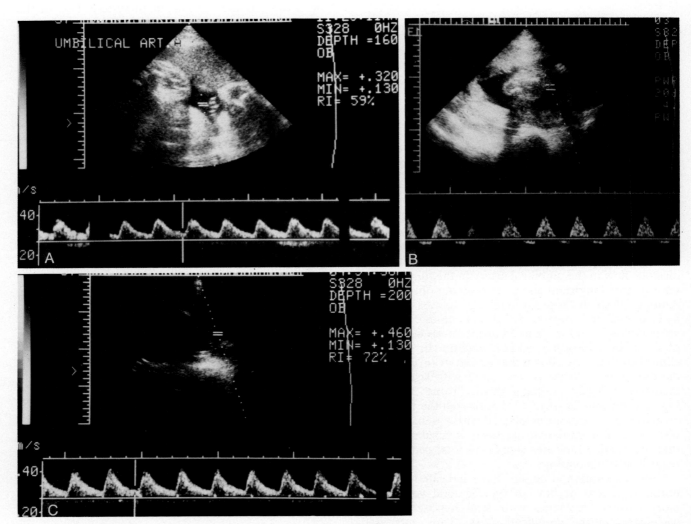

Figure 24–10. Intrauterine growth retardation. *A.* This 32-year-old G3P2Ab0 was first seen at 15 weeks and noted to have twins. One twin died at 25 weeks. The surviving twin was noted to have decreasing estimated fetal weights over the next several weeks. By 36 weeks, the estimated fetal weight was at the 17th percentile, with a biophysical profile score of 8/8. The resistive index (RI) at this point was 0.6. The fetus was judged to be growth retarded at birth but did well. *B.* This 29-week pregnancy was complicated by preeclampsia. At the time of this examination, the maternal blood pressure was 150/100 mm Hg. The Doppler examination of the umbilical cord flow showed reversed end-diastolic flow. The mother was immediately taken to a tertiary care center, where she had a seizure on admission. A 931-g baby neonate delivered with a 5-minute Apgar score of 6/9. Mother and neonate did well. *C.* This 24-year-old G5P3Ab0 mother was examined at 36 weeks. Amniotic fluid volume was normal, and the estimated fetal weight was at the 50th percentile. The RI was elevated at 0.72, but the mother was spontaneously delivered of a full-term, constitutionally small but otherwise normal neonate.

umbilical cord. Fetal cardiac malformations can be assessed using color Doppler sonography with frame-by-frame analysis of the stored cine loop. Ventriculo-septal defects, endocardial cushion defects, and hypoplastic heart syndromes can be clearly seen with color Doppler sonography.[45] Similarly, malformations of the outflow tracts can be determined (Fig. 24–11). Assess-

ment of flow in the ductus arteriosus can be serially performed in patients treated with indomethacin (which is known to cause premature closure of this structure). Umbilical cord malformations such as the absence of an umbilical artery (Fig. 24–12) may be associated with certain fetal anomalies (most commonly cardiac and genitourinary) in 15% to 20% of

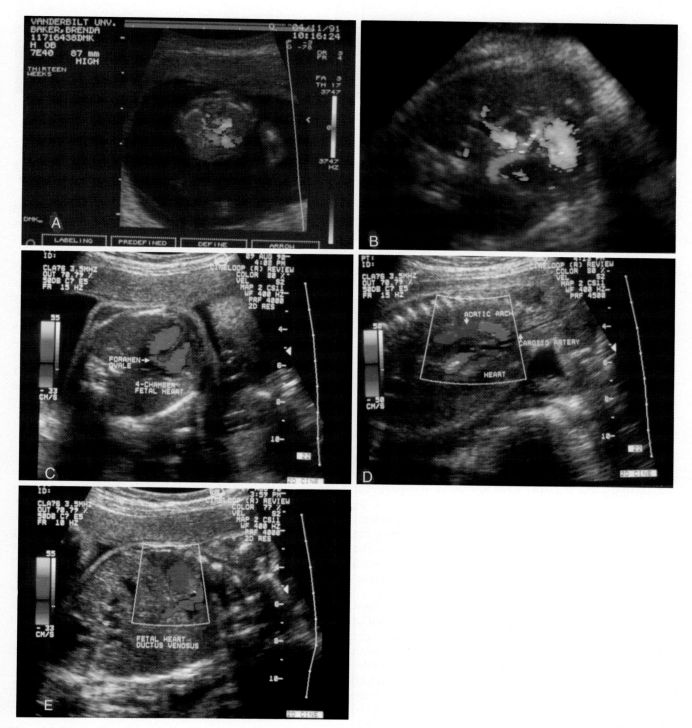

Figure 24–11. Normal and abnormal color Doppler sonography of the fetal heart. *A.* Ventricle/atria and foramen ovale. *B.* Ventricular septal defect. *C.* Foramen ovale. *D.* Normal aorta. *E.* Hypoplastic left heart in a 16-week fetus.

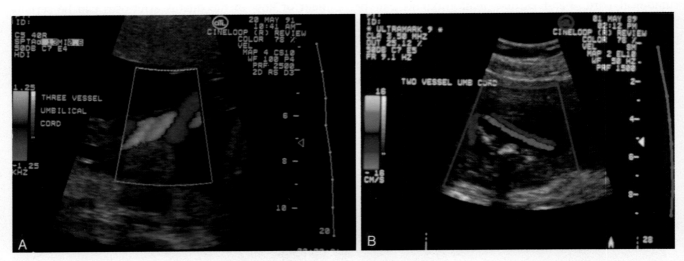

Figure 24–12. Color Doppler sonography of umbilical cord. *A.* Normal cord showing central vein and two arteries. *B.* Single artery cord.

cases. It is also seen more commonly in twin pregnancies. Cord entanglement or knots can also be diagnosed with color Doppler sonography.

PLACENTAL DISORDERS

Using color Doppler sonography, the presence of nuchal cord can be differentiated by a loop of cord adjacent to the fetal neck. Nuchal cords may be seen in up to one fourth of all pregnancies, although those with more than one loop are relatively rare (3%); detection of two or more should precipitate immediate notification of the obstetrician.

Color Doppler sonography affords detailed visualization of some of the vessels within the placenta (see Fig. 24–3).[46] Preliminary data suggest that spiral arteries and maternal veins can be differentiated from fetal vessels on the basis of their location within the placenta and waveform. Color Doppler imaging allows precise and expeditious assignment of a Doppler sample volume for assessment of flow, as well as an overall appreciation of placental and uterine flow. This has implications for patients with potential abruptio placentae or infarction, where there is lack of flow in the basal plate portion of the placenta. Intervillous thrombosis (probably the result of hemorrhages within the placenta, with development of a vascular pool in the intervillous space) may appear as hypoechoic areas on imaging, and slow flow can be demonstrated occasionally with color Doppler sonography.

Doppler studies may be used in twin-to-twin transfusion to assess flow dynamics in the umbilical cord of each fetus (Fig. 24–6B and C). In most cases, the recipient fetus has lower umbilical artery resistance than the donor.[47] The cord insertion of the smaller twin may be relatively eccentric in some cases, which may contribute to the cycle of underperfusion of the small twin and overperfusion of the larger twin. In the oligohydramniotic sac, the cord that is characteristically closely opposed to the donor twin's torso, as well as the eccentric cord insertion into the placenta, can be

better visualized with color Doppler sonography. Occasionally, the presence of a large communicating vessel within the monochorionic placenta may be observed (Fig. 24–13).

Color Doppler sonography can also detect cord vessels between the presenting part and the endocervical canal, the dangerous condition known as vasa previa (Fig. 24–14A and B).[48] This condition, which is potentially life threatening to both fetus and mother, occurs when an extra-amniotic or placental vessel is positioned between the fetal presenting part and the endocervical canal (see Fig. 24–14B). Abnormal invasion of the placental vessels into the myometrium in patients with placenta percreta, increta, or acreta can sometimes be detected with color Doppler sonography (see Fig. 24–14C). These patients usually have a history of previous cesarean section and often have a placenta previa.

EARLY PREGNANCY

Attempts have been made to use color Doppler sonography as a means to assess "viability" of early pregnancy by assessing flow within the choriodecidua. However, the absolute Doppler-derived values such as maximum systolic velocity seem to have little if any prognostic value (Fig. 24–15).[49, 50] Resistance in the small peritrophoblastic vessels is lower than other portions of the myometrium in first trimester intrauterine pregnancy. This focal change in resistivity is not appreciated in the decidual cast of an ectopic pregnancy. Occasionally, increased venous flow is seen before sloughing of decidua in abnormal pregnancies. Vascular lesions as well as invasive trophoblastic disease can be detected by color Doppler imaging.[51]

GYNECOLOGIC APPLICATIONS

For most gynecologic applications, endovaginal imaging is preferred due to the proximity of the probe to

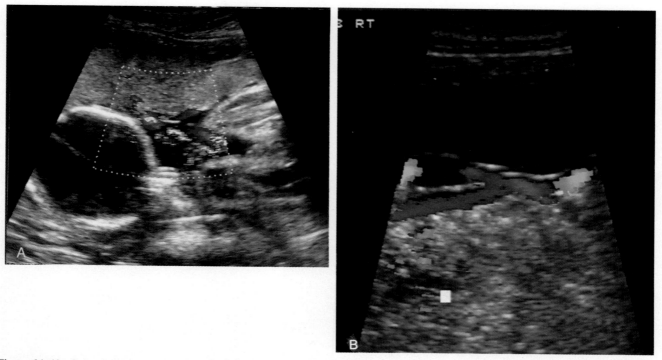

Figure 24–13. Color Doppler sonography of miscellaneous placental disorders. *A.* Twin-to-twin transfusion with both cords originating adjacent to each other. This predisposes to cord entanglement. *B.* Twin-to-twin transfusion with bridging veins.

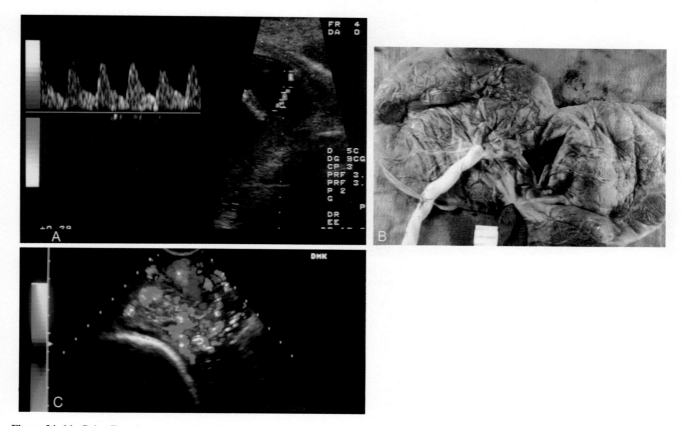

Figure 24–14. Color Doppler sonography of placental and related disorders. *A.* Vasa previa showing an artery crossing the area of internal cervical os. *B.* Specimen showing vessels curving area of internal cervical os. *C.* Endovaginal sonogram of placenta percreta showing vessels within the myometrium. (*A,* courtesy of Richard Rosemond, M.D.)

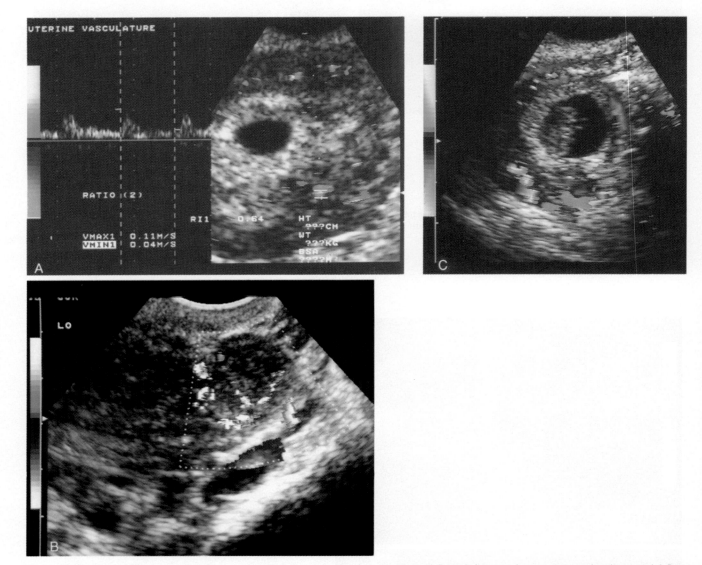

Figure 24–15. Endovaginal color Doppler sonography of early pregnancy. *A.* Normal 5-week intrauterine pregnancy showing arterial flow within the choriodecidua. *B.* Five-week unruptured ectopic pregnancy showing flow within tubal wall. *C.* Eight-week unruptured tubal ectopic pregnancy showing flow within tubal wall.

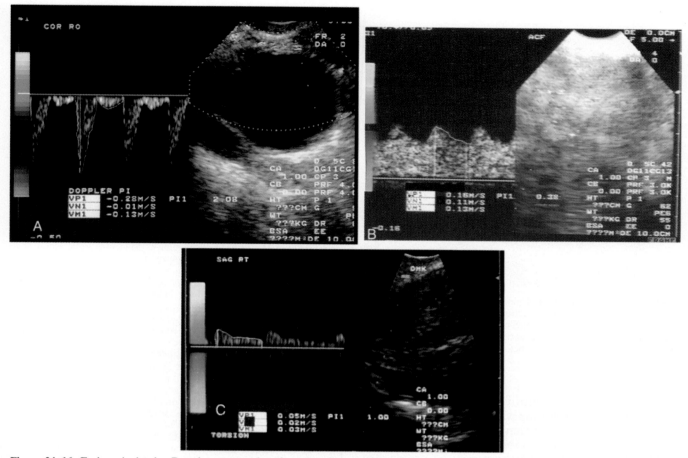

Figure 24–16. Endovaginal color Doppler sonography of ovarian mass and related disorders. *A.* Benign cystic ovarian mass showing high impedance flow. *B.* Malignant ovarian dysgerminoma showing low impedance flow. *C.* Torsed ovary showing minimal capsular flow.

the area of interest. Although endovaginal sonography affords detailed evaluation of the uterus and ovaries, in some women with large masses or masses located superior to the bladder dome, transabdominal sonography may be a better approach. The applications of color Doppler sonography include evaluation of ovarian masses and ectopic pregnancy (see Figs. 24–15*C* and 24–16), as well as assessment of uterine perfusion in patients with fibroids and endometrial disorders.

Uterine arterial flow arises from the hypogastric artery. The main uterine artery divides into an ascending branch that courses along the lateral aspect of the uterine corpus and, after penetrating the uterine serosa, forms an arcuate circulation with radial branches coursing toward the endometrium in a spokewheel pattern. The spiral arteries are the terminal arterial branches within the endometrium. A descending branch of the uterine artery supplies the upper vagina.

After the uterine artery reaches the cornua, an adnexal branch is given off to the ovary. The ovary has a dual blood supply, one from the adnexal branch of the uterine artery, the other directly off the abdominal aorta (Fig. 24–17). The main ovarian artery courses toward the ovary passing within the infundibulopelvic ligament. The intraovarian circulation is variable, with small arterioles supplying the ovarian parenchyma. The intraovarian arteries derive from the main ovarian artery and form an anastomosis from branches within the meso-ovarium.

The venous drainage of the uterus, tubes, and ovaries roughly parallels the arterial supply. The ovarian veins are usually no more than 5 mm in diameter if the valves are competent. The right ovarian vein drains into the inferior vena cava, whereas the left ovarian vein drains into the left renal vein.

For ovarian masses, neovascularity is required for tumor growth of more than 3 to 5 mm. Neovascularity associated with ovarian malignancies typically lacks a muscular media that results in sinusoid type spaces and increased diastolic flow. On endovaginal color and duplex Doppler studies, this is evidenced by low pulsatility index (see Fig. 24–16*A* and *B*).[52, 53] Besides being seen in malignancies, low pulsatility index is visible in inflammatory masses, metabolically "active" tumors, germ cell tumors, and corpus luteum cysts.

The diagnostic uses of endovaginal color and duplex Doppler sonography seem best applied to exclude malignancy since the reported negative predictive values range from 96% to 98% and the specificities are in the 90% range. On the other hand, not all masses with low pulsatility index will be malignancies since the positive predictive values have been reported in the range of 80% to 90%.[52, 53] Whether endovaginal color Doppler imaging can be used to accurately detect

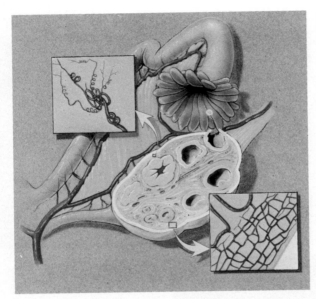

Figure 24–17. Ovarian arterial circulation. The ovary has a dual arterial blood supply from the adnexal branch of the uterine artery and the main ovarian artery, which courses in the infundibular pelvic ligament. Once these arteries penetrate the serosa, a vascular arcade is formed around developing follicles.

early stage tumor is controversial, but this technique seems to be very promising when used in the evaluation of women at risk for ovarian cancer.

In patients with ovarian torsion, a variety of findings related to the degree of torsion may be present (see Fig. 24–16C). In complete torsion, there is a lack of parenchymal blood flow early after torsion; but in partial torsion, only high resistance to flow can be seen, as evidenced by absent or reversed diastolic flow.

Other applications of endovaginal color Doppler sonography include improved detection of extrauterine vascularity associated with ectopic pregnancies, particularly those that may not be apparent as a morphologic abnormality on conventional endovaginal sonography; assessment of uterine blood flow in patients with fibroids who may consider medical treatment; and those with dilatation and curettage–proven or clinically suspected endometrial carcinoma.[54]

Endovaginal color Doppler sonography may be useful in evaluating which fibroid may be amenable to medical treatment, by displaying those that have an intact blood supply. It may also be helpful in evaluating women with thickened endometria, to decide which tumors may be invasive.[55]

References

1. Gill RW, Kossoff G, Warren PS, Garrett WJ: Umbilical venous flow in normal and complicated pregnancy. Ultrasound Med Biol 10:349, 1984.
2. Hoskins PR, Haddad NG, Johnstone FD, et al: The choice of index for umbilical artery Doppler waveforms. Ultrasound Med Biol 15:107, 1989.
3. Goswamy RK, Williams G, Steptoe DC: Decreased uterine perfusion: A cause of infertility. Hum Reprod 3:955, 1988.
4. Fleischer A, Reed G, Kepple D: Inter- and intra-observer error in duplex Doppler sonography in the third trimester. In preparation, 1992.
5. Bourne TH: Transvaginal color Doppler in gynecology. Ultrasound Obstet Gynecol 1:1, 1991.
6. Maulik D, Yarlagadda AP, Youngblood JP, Willoughby L: Components of variability of umbilical Doppler velocimetry—a prospective analysis. Am J Obstet Gynecol 160:1406, 1989.
7. Fleischer A, Schulman H, Farmakides G, et al: Umbilical artery velocity waveforms and intrauterine growth retardation. Am J Obstet Gynecol 151:502, 1985.
8. Schulman H, Winter D, Farmakides G, et al: Pregnancy surveillance with Doppler velocimetry of uterine and umbilical arteries. Am J Obstet Gynecol 160:192, 1989.
9. Trudinger BJ, Giles WB, Cook CM: Flow velocity waveforms in the maternal uteroplacental and fetal umbilical placental circulation. Am J Obstet Gynecol 152:155, 1985.
10. Marsal K: Ultrasound assessment of fetal circulation as a diagnostic test: A review. In Lipshitz J, Maloney J, Nimrod C, Carson G (eds): Perinatal Development of the Heart and Lung. pp 127–142. Ithaca, NY, Perinatology Press, 1987.
11. Arduini D, Rizzo G, Romanini C, Mancuso: Fetal blood flow velocity waveforms as predictors of growth retardation. Obstet Gynecol 70:7, 1987.
12. Gaziano E, Knox GE, Wager GP, et al: The predictability of the small-for-gestational-age infant by real-time ultrasound-derived measurements combined with pulsed Doppler umbilical artery velocimetry. Am J Obstet Gynecol 158:1431, 1988.
13. Divon MY, Guidetti DA, Braverman JJ, et al: Intrauterine growth retardation: A prospective study of the diagnostic value of real-time sonography combined with umbilical artery flow velocimetry. Obstet Gynecol 72:611, 1988.
14. Berkowitz GS, Chitkara U, Rosenberg J, et al: Sonographic estimation of fetal weight and Doppler analysis of umbilical artery velocimetry in the prediction of intrauterine growth retardation: A prospective study. Am J Obstet Gynecol 158:1149, 1988.
15. Al-Ghazali W, Chapman MG, Allan LD: Doppler assessment of the cardiac and uteroplacental circulation in normal and complicated pregnancies. Br J Obstet Gynaecol 95:575, 1988.
16. Fleischer A, Schulman H, Farmakides G, et al: Uterine artery Doppler velocimetry in pregnant women with hypertension. Am J Obstet Gynecol 154:806, 1986.
17. Peeters LLH, Sheldon RE, Jones MD, et al: Blood flow to fetal organs as a function of arterial oxygen content. Am J Obstet Gynecol 135:637, 1979.
18. Arduini D, Rizzo G: Normal values of pulsatility index from fetal vessels: A cross-sectional study on 1556 healthy fetuses. J Perinat Med 18:165, 1990.
19. Thompson RS, Trudinger BJ, Cook CM: A comparison of Doppler ultrasound waveform indices in the umbilical artery: I. Indices derived from the maximum velocity waveform; and II. Indices derived from mean velocity and first moment waveforms. Ultrasound Med Biol 12:835, 1986.
20. Kay HH, Carroll BA, Bowie JD, et al: Nonuniformity of fetal umbilical systolic/diastolic ratios as determined with duplex Doppler sonography. J Ultrasound Med 8:417, 1989.
21. Worrell JA, Fleischer AC, Drolshagen LF, et al: Duplex Doppler sonography of the umbilical arteries: Predictive value in IUGR and correlation with birth weight. Ultrasound Med Biol 17:207, 1991.
22. Eik-Nes SH, Marsel K, Brubbakk AO, et al: Ultrasound measurement of human fetus blood flow. J Biomed Engl 4:28, 1982.
23. Ferrazzi E, Gementi P, Bellotti M, et al: Doppler velocimetry: Critical analysis of umbilical, cerebral and aortic reference values. Eur J Obstet Gynaecol Reprod Biol 38:189, 1991.
24. Veille JC, Kanaan C: Duplex Doppler ultrasonographic evaluation of the fetal renal artery in normal and abnormal fetuses. Am J Obstet Gynecol 161:1502, 1989.
25. Gudmundsson S, Neerhof M, Weiner S, et al: Fetal hydronephrosis and renal artery blood velocity. Ultrasound Obstet Gynecol 1:413, 1991.
26. Kaminopetros P, Dykes EH, Nicolaides KH: Fetal renal artery blood velocimetry in multicystic kidney disease. Ultrasound Obstet Gynecol 1:410, 1991.
27. Groenenberg IAL, Baerts W, Hop WCJ, Wladimiroff JW: Relationship between fetal cardiac and extra-cardiac Doppler

flow velocity waveforms and neonatal outcome in intrauterine growth retardation. Early Hum Dev 26:185, 1991.

28. Trudinger BJ, Stevens D, Connelly A, et al: Umbilical artery flow velocity waveforms and placental resistance: The effects of embolization of the umbilical circulation. Am J Obstet Gynecol 157:1443, 1987.

29. Morrow RJ, Adamson SL, Bull SB, Ritchie JWK: Effect of placental embolization on the umbilical arterial waveform in fetal sheep. Am J Obstet Gynecol 161:1055, 1989.

30. Giles WB, Lingman G, Marsal K, Trudinger BJ: Fetal volume blood flow and umbilical artery flow velocity wave-form analysis: A comparison. Br J Obstet Gynaecol 93:461, 1986.

31. Rochelson B: The clinical significance of absent end-diastolic velocity in the umbilical artery waveforms. Clin Obstet Gynecol 32:692, 1989.

32. Mulders LG, Wijn PF, Jongsma HW, Hein PR: A comparative study of three indices of umbilical blood flow in relation to prediction of growth retardation. J Perinat Med 15:3, 1987.

33. Berkowitz GS, Mehalek KE, Chitkara U, et al: Doppler velocimetry in the prediction of adverse outcome in pregnancies at risk for intrauterine growth retardation. Obstet Gynecol 71:742, 1988.

34. Dempster J, Mires GJ, Patel N, Taylor DJ: Umbilical artery velocity waveforms: Poor association with small-for-gestational-age babies. Br J Obstet Gynaecol 96:692, 1989.

35. Sijmons EA, Reuwer PJ, van Beek E, Bruinse HW: The validity of screening for small-for-gestational-age and low-weight-for-length infants by Doppler ultrasound. Br J Obstet Gynaecol 96:557, 1989.

36. Beattie RB, Dornan JC: Antenatal screening for intrauterine growth retardation with umbilical artery Doppler ultrasonography. Br Med J 298:631, 1989.

37. Benson DB, Doubilet PM: Doppler criteria for intrauterine growth retardation: Predictive values. J Ultrasound Med 7:655, 1988.

38. Campbell S, Vyas S, Nicolaides KH: Doppler investigation of the fetal circulation. J Perinat Med 19:21, 1991.

39. Johnstone FD, Haddad NG, Hoskins P, et al: Umbilical artery Doppler flow velocity waveform: The outcome of pregnancies with absent end diastolic flow. Eur J Obstet Gynaecol 28:171, 1988.

40. Brar HS, Platt LD: Reverse end-diastolic flow velocity on umbilical artery velocimetry in high-risk pregnancies: An ominous finding with adverse pregnancy outcome. Am J Obstet Gynecol 159:559, 1988.

41. Yoon BH, Syn HC, Kim SW: The efficacy of Doppler umbilical artery velocimetry in identifying fetal acidosis. J Ultrasound Med 11:1, 1992.

42. Wenstrom KD, Weiner CP, Williamson RA: Diverse maternal and fetal pathology associated with absent diastolic flow in the umbilical artery of high-risk fetuses. Obstet Gynecol 77:374, 1991.

43. Arduini D, Rizzo G: Prediction of fetal outcome in small for gestational age fetuses: Comparison of Doppler measurements obtained from different fetal vessels. J Perinat Med 20:29, 1992.

44. Bilardo CM, Snijders RM, Campbell S, Nicolaides KH: Doppler study of the fetal circulation during long-term maternal hyperoxygenation for early onset intrauterine growth retardation. Ultrasound Obstet Gynecol 1:250, 1991.

45. McGahan JP, Choy M, Parrish MD, Brant WE: Sonographic spectrum of fetal cardiac hypoplasia. J Ultrasound Med 10:539, 1991.

46. Jauniaux E, Jurkovic D, Campbell S, et al: Investigation of placental circulations by color Doppler ultrasonography. Am J Obstet Gynecol 164:486, 1991.

47. Pretorius DH, Manchester D, Barkin S, et al: Doppler ultrasound of twin transfusion syndrome. J Ultrasound Med 7:117, 1988.

48. Hsieh FJ, Hsin-Fu C, Tsang-Ming K, et al: Antenatal diagnosis of vasa previa by color-flow mapping. J Ultrasound Med 10:397, 1991.

49. Kurjak A, Zalud I, Salihagic A, et al: Transvaginal color Doppler in the assessment of abnormal early pregnancy. J Perinat Med 19:155, 1991.

50. Arduini D, Rizzo G, Romanini C: Doppler ultrasonography in early pregnancy does not predict adverse pregnancy outcome. Ultrasound Obstet Gynecol 1:180, 1991.

51. Desai RK, Desberg AL: Diagnosis of gestational trophoblastic disease: Value of endovaginal color flow Doppler sonography. AJR 157:767, 1991.

52. Fleischer AC, Rodgers WH, Rao BK, et al: Assessment of ovarian tumor vascularity with transvaginal color Doppler sonography. J Ultrasound Med 10:563, 1991.

53. Kurjak A, Zalud I, Alfirevic Z: Evaluation of adnexal masses with transvaginal color ultrasound. J Ultrasound Med 10:295, 1991.

54. Alteri L, Cartier M, Emerson D, et al: Endovaginal color Doppler in early intrauterine pregnancy: Correlation with peak trophoblastic velocities, sac size, and hCG. (Abstract) Radiology 177:193, 1990.

55. Bourne TH, Whitehead MI, Campbell S, et al: Ultrasound screening for familial ovarian cancer. Gynecol Oncol 43:92, 1991.

ACKNOWLEDGMENTS

The authors acknowledge Paul Gross, M.S., for his superb artistic renditions. Alice Hammond is thanked for her typographical assistance and John Bobbit for his photography.

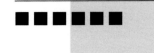

CHAPTER **25**

The Role of Computed Tomography and Magnetic Resonance Imaging in Obstetrics

VICKIE A. FELDSTEIN, M.D.
MARK J. POPOVICH, M.D.

Ultrasonography remains the primary imaging modality in the evaluation of the pregnant patient and fetus. This is because of its wide availability, low cost, lack of any known adverse effects, and excellent diagnostic capability. Other modalities, specifically computed tomography (CT) and magnetic resonance imaging (MRI), offer significant advantages for diagnostic visualization of maternal and fetal anatomy and pathology. For several clinically relevant applications, to be reviewed here, CT and MRI are important adjunctive studies, complementary to sonography.

COMPUTED TOMOGRAPHY

In current obstetric practice, the use of CT is limited, almost exclusively, to two indications: pelvimetry and amniography. Pelvimetry is performed to determine pelvic dimensions, particularly in cases of breech presentation when vaginal delivery is being considered. Presently, pelvimetry is the major single source of fetal radiation exposure. There is evidence of a low but real excess risk of childhood cancer associated with previous diagnostic radiation exposure in utero.[1, 2] In a review of 11 retrospective studies examining these data, the risk of childhood cancer was doubled with fetal irradiation exposure of 5 rads or less.[3] The International Commission on Radiologic Protection has recommended that the radiation dose to the fetus should not exceed 1 rad during a known pregnancy. It is agreed that every effort should be made to limit to a minimum the radiation that a fetus receives.

Computed Tomographic Pelvimetry

Computed tomographic pelvimetry has been shown to be as reliable as conventional radiographic pelvimetry and offers the important advantage of less radiation exposure.[4] The protocol for CT pelvimetry, as described by Federle and colleagues,[5] requires anteroposterior (AP) and lateral scout (digital) views and one transverse axial section through the fovea of the femoral heads (a landmark identified on the AP scout view) (Fig. 25–1). The AP and transverse diameters of the pelvic inlet are measured directly from the AP and

lateral scout views, using electronic calipers. The commonly used AP measurement (the obstetric or true conjugate) is measured from the sacral promontory to the posterosuperior margin of the pubic symphysis (normal $\geq$ 10 cm). The transverse pelvic inlet is the maximum distance between the arcuate lines of the iliac bones on either side (normal $\geq$ 11.5 cm). The interspinous diameter is the distance between the ischial spines, measured on the transverse axial CT image (normal $\geq$ 10.5 cm) (Table 25–1). Fetal radiation dose estimates for CT pelvimetry have been obtained using phantom measurements. With the use of low-exposure (40 mAs) technique, the maximal estimated dose to the fetus is approximately 0.23 rad.[6]

Computed Tomographic Amniography

Computed tomographic amniography is occasionally performed as a means of confirming monoamnionicity.[7, 8] This technique should be used only after extensive attempts to determine amnionicity have been performed by ultrasonography. Monoamnionicity can be excluded on ultrasound evaluation by demonstrating a membrane separating the fetuses, separate placental sites, different fetal sexes, or a "stuck twin." For CT amniography, ultrasonography is used to select a transverse plane of section and this location is marked. A single transverse axial precontrast CT scan may be obtained at this level. Under sonographic guidance, the amniotic sac is punctured and water-soluble iodinated contrast material is instilled. When a contrast agent with a concentration of approximately 300 mg of iodine per milliliter of solution is used, 1 mL per 100 mL of anticipated amniotic fluid volume provides adequate opacification. Typically, 8 to 10 mL of contrast agent is used in a third-trimester pregnancy with normal amniotic fluid volume. A post-contrast transverse

Table 25–1. NORMAL PELVIMETRIC MEASUREMENTS

Obstetric or true conjugate (anteroposterior diameter of pelvic inlet)	$\geq$10 cm
Transverse pelvic inlet	$\geq$11.5 cm
Interspinous diameter	$\geq$10.5 cm

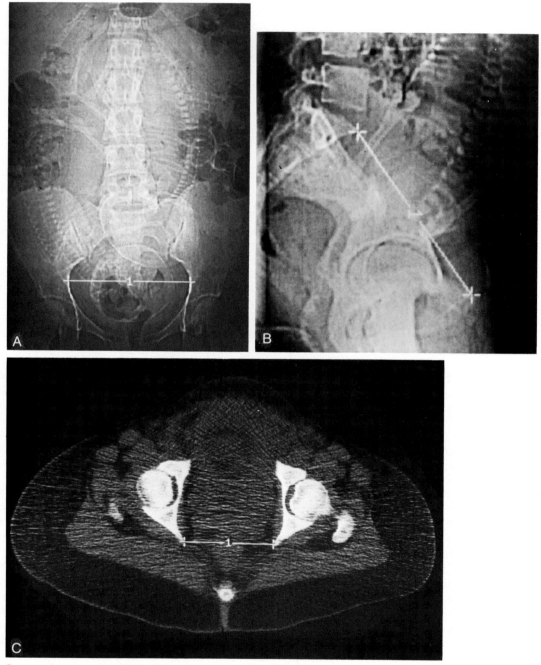

Figure 25–1. Computed tomography (CT) pelvimetry. *A.* Anteroposterior scout view demonstrating the transverse pelvic inlet, measured with electronic cursors. *B.* Lateral scout view demonstrating the obstetric conjugate measurement of the anteroposterior pelvic inlet. *C.* Transverse CT section through the ischial spines demonstrating the bispinous or transverse diameter.

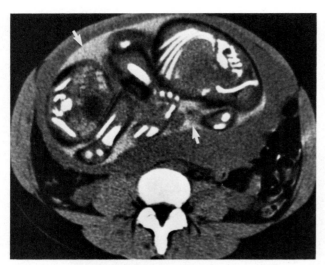

Figure 25–2. Computed tomography (CT) amniogram. Transverse CT section obtained following contrast instillation showing opacified amniotic fluid (*arrows*) completely surrounding both fetuses, confirming monoamnionicity.

axial CT scan at the same level is obtained (Fig. 25–2). Monoamnionicity is indicated by the presence of contrast material completely surrounding each twin, although rarely this appearance may be mimicked by a diamniotic pregnancy with a "stuck twin." Finberg and Clewell[9] have reported that the presence of contrast material within the gastrointestinal tract of both twins, after a delay of approximately 4 hours, is a reliable, unambiguous sign of monoamnionicity.

MAGNETIC RESONANCE IMAGING

Magnetic resonance is a relatively new, rapidly growing imaging modality that, like ultrasonography, offers several advantages. It, too, is noninvasive, involves no ionizing radiation, and provides images in multiple orthogonal planes. The physics of MRI are beyond the scope of this text. Simply put, multiple tissue parameters are used to generate contrast in MR images. Therefore, in addition to anatomic detail, MRI can provide tissue characterization information beyond that which may be detectable by ultrasonography. Furthermore, MRI allows clear fetal imaging in some situations in which ultrasonography may be difficult. These include maternal obesity, oligohydramnios, and overlying skeletal, fatty, or gas-filled maternal structures. The disadvantages of MRI include the greater expense, the relatively long imaging times, the conventional use of maternal (rather than fetal) oriented planes of section, and the image degradation secondary to maternal or fetal motion.

Much attention has been paid to the risks and potential fetal effects of MRI. At present, available experimental and clinical evidence indicates that MRI is safe for the fetus.[10–16] Biomedical investigation by means of bacteria or cell culture, in vivo studies, and clinical follow-up of patients has failed to identify any apparent deleterious effect.[11–15] Still, the National Radiological Protection Board has advised against imaging during the first trimester, the period of organogenesis, unless the patient is undergoing termination of the pregnancy.[16] Some institutions obtain written informed consent from patients that includes statements such as "there are no known or foreseeable hazards or risks associated with MRI, although there may be risks to you or your infant at a future time that are currently unforeseeable."

With these considerations in mind, appropriate clinical indications for MRI during pregnancy can be reviewed. MRI is best used as an adjunct when ultrasound information is insufficient, technically inadequate, or inconclusive. MRI is indicated following abnormal ultrasound results that need further characterization before management decisions, which may include surgery or early intervention, can be made. MRI may provide information regarding pelvimetric measurements or concomitant maternal conditions obviating the need for studies involving ionizing radiation.

In obstetric MRI, spin-echo and, more recently, fast-scanning techniques have proven most informative. These techniques require selection of imaging protocols that may be optimized to address the particular concerns of a given case. Spin-echo sequences involve the selection of pulse repetition time values (TR), of echo delay time values (TE), and of imaging planes. The sagittal view is preferred for the display of fetal anatomy, since the fetus is most commonly in longitudinal lie in either the cephalic or breech presentation. Likewise, questions of placental location or cervical anomalies can best be answered in this plane of section. Short TR and TE parameters (T1-weighted spin-echo images) allow for the best tissue contrast between the uterus and adjacent fat, between the placenta and amniotic fluid, and between amniotic fluid and subcutaneous adipose tissue of the fetus.[17] McCarthy and coworkers[18] report that spin-echo techniques with long repetition times (TR) and short-echo delays (TE) demonstrate the best anatomic detail, with optimum fetal tissue contrast and low background noise, and allow for acquisition of a large number of anatomic sections. Long TR, long TE sequences (T2-weighted images) are necessary for analysis of the maternal cervix and uterus.

Early obstetric MRI examinations were limited by image degradation from fetal and/or maternal motion, particularly when protocols prescribed relatively long imaging times. Reports describing intravenous administration of a benzodiazepine to the mother or intramuscular injection of pancuronium to the fetus to reduce fetal motion during MRI have been published.[19–21] However, this practice is not desirable for routine use, particularly with a technique that is otherwise noninvasive. Currently, these pharmacologic maneuvers are not standard procedure. Obstetric MRI is generally limited to the third trimester or to cases of oligohydramnios, settings in which fetal motion is restricted. In addition, new fast-scan techniques have drastically shortened imaging times, further reducing motion artifacts.

Magnetic Resonance Imaging Pelvimetry

Magnetic resonance imaging can be used to accurately determine traditional pelvimetric measurements. For MRI pelvimetry, T1-weighted midsaggital and transaxial images are obtained (Fig. 25–3). The previously described CT pelvimetric diameters and normal values apply, as well, to MRI. Advantages of MRI pelvimetry include the lack of ionizing radiation and the ability to examine maternal and fetal soft tissues and to assess fetal head and umbilical cord position. MRI pelvimetry has been shown to be an accurate technique with less than 1% instrument error in pelvic dimension measurements.[22]

Magnetic Resonance Imaging of Maternal Anatomy

Female pelvic anatomy is particularly well demonstrated by MRI. The MRI appearance of the normal gravid uterus and cervix vary, depending on the stage of pregnancy.[23, 24] These normal morphologic and physiologic changes are manifest as alterations in size and signal characteristics (Figs. 25–4 and 25–5).

Anomalous maternal pelvic anatomy, such as a gravid bicornuate uterus, is readily assessed with MRI.[25] Ultrasound visualization of deep maternal pelvic structures, such as the cervix in late pregnancy, may be obscured by the presenting fetal part and may be altered by the degree of bladder distention. MRI has the ability to clearly demonstrate, measure, and analyze cervical tissue properties. MRI can delineate internal changes of the cervix and can assess pathologic conditions including changes seen with premature labor (shortening of the cervical canal, dilatation of the lumen, effacement with loss of distinction of signal characteristics between epithelial and stromal layers) and with cervical incompetence.[26] Concomitant cervical disease, such as cervical cancer, is also readily seen with MRI.

Magnetic resonance imaging has been shown to be valuable in the evaluation of the nature and extent of pelvic masses in pregnant patients.[27, 28] The most common solid pelvic masses associated with pregnancy are uterine leiomyomas. Nondegenerative leiomyomas usually demonstrate medium signal intensity, often indistinguishable from adjacent myometrium, on T1-weighted scans and homogeneous low signal intensity on T2-weighted scans (Fig. 25–6). When degenerative, they have various and nonspecific MRI appearances. Their assessment is important since they may become acutely symptomatic during pregnancy, owing to hemorrhage or degeneration. If multiple, their size and location may influence obstetric decisions about route of delivery. In some cases, particularly with pedunculated, subserosal myomas, the ultrasound appearance can be confusing and difficult to differentiate from adnexal masses extrinsic to the uterus (Figs. 25–7 and 25–8). With MRI, improved lesion characterization and more accurate determination of the origin of a pelvic mass may be provided.

Magnetic resonance imaging can also be used in the assessment of nonuterine pelvic masses. The tissue characterization information afforded with MRI is perhaps best demonstrated in the evaluation of ovarian dermoids, another common pelvic mass lesion detected during pregnancy. MRI can depict characteristic tissue components of the mass, especially fat, based on variations in the pulse sequence parameters.

Pathologic processes unrelated to pregnancy and involving any part of the body can present special problems when they arise during pregnancy. Radiologic assessment is limited, given the desire to limit exposure to ionizing radiation. Evaluation of the abdomen and pelvis with ultrasonography may be hindered by anatomic distortion and the interposed gravid uterus and fetus. Furthermore, ultrasonography is inadequate in the investigation of the central nervous system, thoracic, or musculoskeletal processes. With MRI, maternal tumors in these sites can be readily displayed (Fig. 25–9). Appropriately selected sequences can provide images that delineate the location, nature, and extent of lesions and that demonstrate the anatomic relationships with adjacent structures. This is often necessary information in the preoperative evaluation of maternal conditions diagnosed during pregnancy that require surgical intervention. If a malignant neoplasm is diagnosed, MRI can be used for the staging workup.

Magnetic Resonance Imaging of Maternal-Fetal Structures

In most cases, placental location and architecture can be well visualized with ultrasonography. Transperineal ultrasound evaluation can be performed if transabdominal ultrasound evaluation is nondiagnostic. If, despite these maneuvers, visualization is insufficient, MRI can readily depict the position of the internal and external cervical os and their relationship to the placenta and to the presenting fetal part (Fig. 25–10). MRI has been shown to be useful and reliable in distinguishing a low-lying placenta from a placenta previa and a marginal from a complete placenta previa.[29]

Magnetic Resonance Imaging of Fetal Anatomy

Normal fetal anatomy is well displayed with MRI.[17, 18, 24, 30, 31] Various anatomic structures are optimally visualized with different pulse sequences. T1-weighted images (short TR, short TE) offer improved detail and contrast with less motion degradation compared with T2-weighted sequences. The recent development of fast spin-echo techniques allows acquistion of T2-weighted images of similar quality to standard T1-weighted images. With T1-weighted images, fluid with low solute content, such as amniotic fluid, exhibits low signal intensity and subcutaneous adipose tissue is of high signal intensity, providing valuable inherent con-

Text continued on page 532

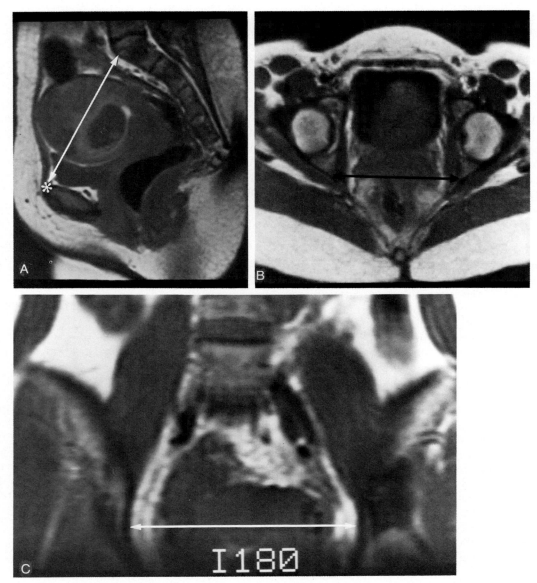

Figure 25–3. Magnetic resonance (MR) pelvimetry. *A.* Midline sagittal MR image demonstrating the anteroposterior pelvic inlet measurement. Asterisk indicates symphysis pubis. *B.* Transverse MR image through the lower pelvis showing the bispinous diameter measurement. *C.* Coronal MR image with measurement of the transverse pelvic inlet. Note that the cortical bone is signal void, maternal subcutaneous fat is bright, and fluid, in the amniotic cavity and in the maternal bladder, is dark on these T1-weighted images.

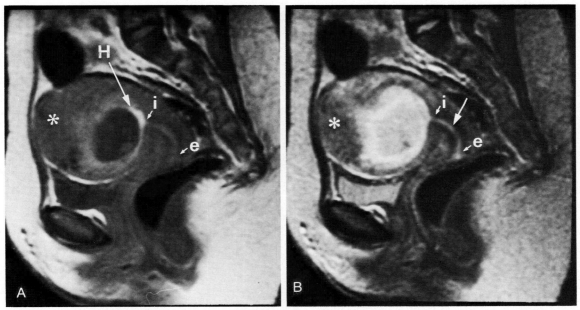

Figure 25–4. Midline sagittal MR scan of a gravid patient, in early pregnancy, showing morphology of the uterus and cervix. *A.* T1-weighted image. *B.* T2-weighted image. Arrow indicates endocervical canal. Asterisk indicates leiomyoma. H, subchorionic hematoma; i, internal cervical os; e, external cervical os.

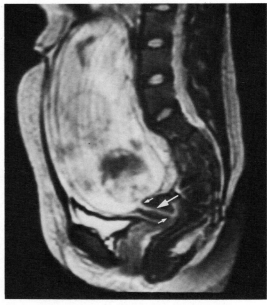

Figure 25–5. Midline sagittal T2-weighted MR image through a gravid uterus in second trimester. The endocervical canal (*large arrow*) and internal and external cervical os (*small arrows*) are clearly shown. The fetus is in cephalic presentation.

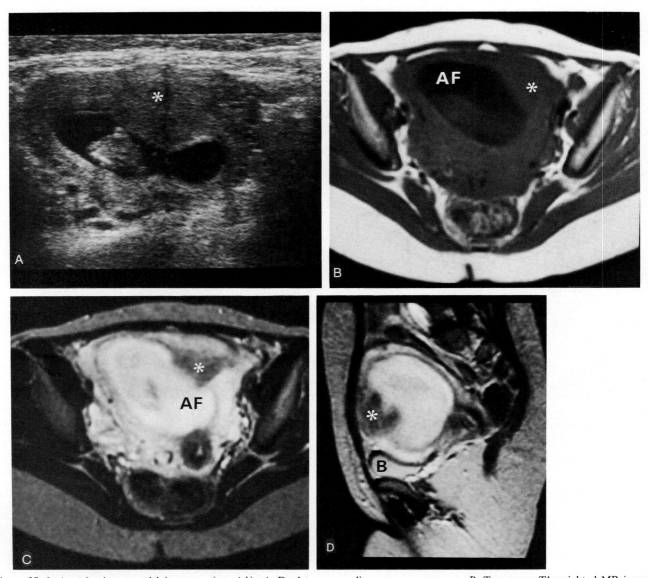

Figure 25–6. Anterior intramural leiomyoma (*asterisk*). *A.* Dual transverse linear-array sonogram. *B.* Transverse T1-weighted MR image. *C.* Transverse T2-weighted MR image. *D.* Sagittal T2-weighted MR image. The myoma demonstrates medium signal intensity, similar to adjacent myometrium, on T1-weighted scans and low signal intensity on T2-weighted scans. AF, amniotic fluid; B, maternal bladder.

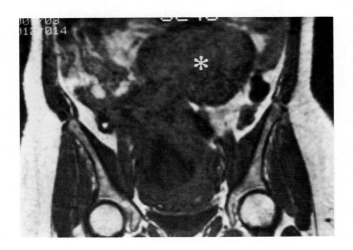

Figure 25–7. Coronal T1-weighted MR image showing a large pedunculated subserosal fundal leiomyoma (*asterisk*).

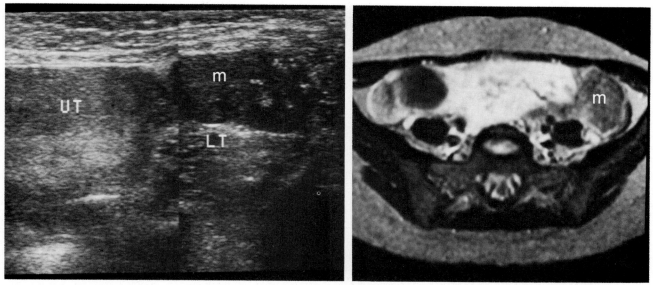

Figure 25–8. *A.* Transverse sonogram through the uterine fundus (UT) with adjacent solid left-sided mass (m) containing echogenic foci, suggestive of calcifications. LT, left. *B.* T2-weighted transverse MR image demonstrates that this mass (m) represents an exophytic leiomyoma arising from the left lateral aspect of the uterus. On ultrasound evaluation, it was difficult to distinguish this mass from an extrauterine adnexal lesion, such as an ovarian dermoid.

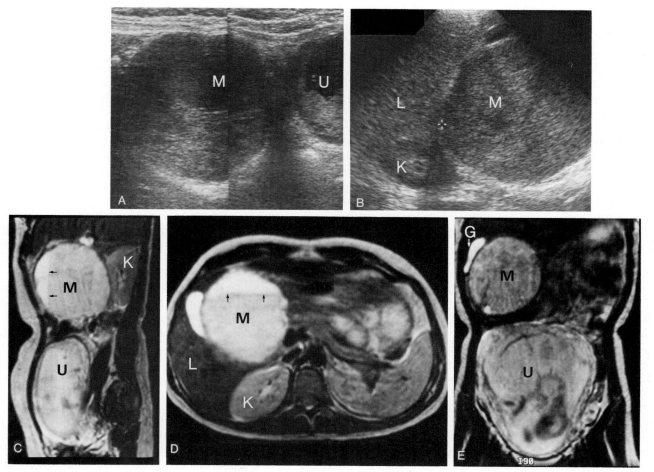

Figure 25–9. Large upper abdominal mass (solid and cystic papillary neoplasm of the pancreas) in a pregnant patient (gestational age 20 weeks). *A.* Longitudinal abdominal sonogram showing portion of the uterine fundus (U) adjacent to the mass (M). *B.* Transverse sonogram of maternal upper abdomen showing the relation of this mass (M) to the right kidney (K) and the liver (L). *C.* Right parasagittal T2-weighted MR image. *D.* Transverse T2-weighted MR image. *E.* Coronal T2-weighted MR image. The large mass demonstrates inhomogeneous signal intensity and is predominantly soft tissue with a fluid-fluid level (*arrows*). It is seen distinct from the gravid uterus (U) obsd from the maternal right kidney (K), liver (L), and gallbladder (G).

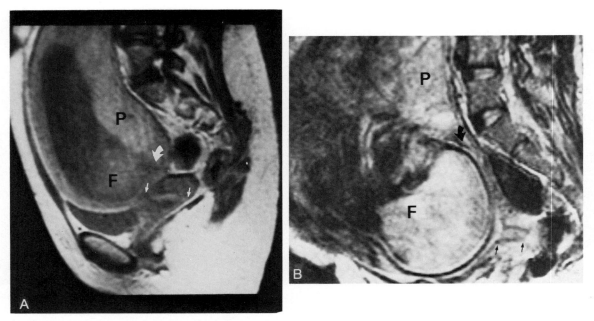

Figure 25–10. MR delineation of placental location, relative to internal cervical os, in two patients. *A.* Sagittal T1-weighted image at mid second trimester. *B.* Sagittal T2-weighted image in late third trimester. In the two cases shown, the cervix is well visualized and the internal and external cervical os (*small arrows*) are identified. The cervical length can easily be measured. In each, the fetus (F) is in cephalic presentation and the placenta (P) is located posteriorly. The inferior placental margin (*curved arrow*) is clearly distinct from the internal cervical os, thus excluding placenta previa.

trast. Fluid-filled fetal structures including the urinary bladder, stomach and gastrointestinal tract, and cerebral ventricles have signal characteristics similar to amniotic fluid or maternal urine with low signal intensity on T1-weighted images and increased signal intensity on longer TR, TE (T2-weighted) images. Flowing blood within the fetal heart chambers and blood vessels offers natural contrast as it appears as a signal void. Fetal lung and liver are of similar intermediate signal intensity on T1-weighted images but may be readily differentiated on T2-weighted images since the lungs have a longer T2 (due to contained fluid) and therefore exhibit higher signal intensity than the liver (Fig. 25–11).

Investigations of the clinical applications of MRI during pregnancy have shown its utility in demonstrating fetal structural anomalies.[32–35] MRI can confirm the presence of most gross fetal anomalies (88% in one series[34]) detected by ultrasonography in the second and third trimester. In many of these reports, MRI provided successful visualization without maternal sedation and, in some, despite the presence of oligohydramnios. Image interpretability was not significantly degraded by fetal motion.

The MRI appearances of a variety of fetal malformations have been described.[20, 32–34, 36–38] These include anomalies of the central nervous system (hydrocephalus, holoprosencephaly, anencephaly), ventral wall defects (omphalocele, gastroschisis), genitourinary abnormalities (hydronephrosis, ovarian cyst), and dysraphic malformations and spinal masses (meningocele, sacral teratoma) (Fig. 25–12). MRI has also proven useful in the evaluation of chest abnormalities, specifically in distinguishing herniated small bowel

loops of a congenital diaphragmatic hernia from an intrathoracic mass. MRI can confirm and occasionally refine sonographic diagnoses of fetal dysmorphologies, but it is not currently applied as the primary imaging modality.

Because of some of its unique properties in imaging fetal tissues and fluids, MRI may offer particular advantages in prenatal characterization and evaluation of fetal growth and organ development. Specifically, MRI has been considered in the evaluation of intrauterine growth retardation since fetal subcutaneous fat is easily visualized and can be roughly quantified by MRI (Fig. 25–13).[39–41] Other investigative pursuits include analysis of MR signal characteristics of amniotic fluid to estimate the concentration of meconium and potentially provide an indication of fetal distress.[42] It has been suggested, too, that MR signal characteristics of fetal lung tissue may reveal information regarding lung maturation and may eventually play a role as a noninvasive technique for quantification of fetal lung maturity.

Future Applications

Currently, MRI serves to complement difficult or equivocal ultrasound examinations. Its advantages include a larger field of view and multiplanar imaging of the whole maternal abdomen and pelvis. Clear anatomic relationships among maternal organs, uterus, fetus, and placenta can be demonstrated. New methods are actively being investigated to improve visualization, particularly of the fetus. These developments include fast-scan imaging techniques with shorter acquisition

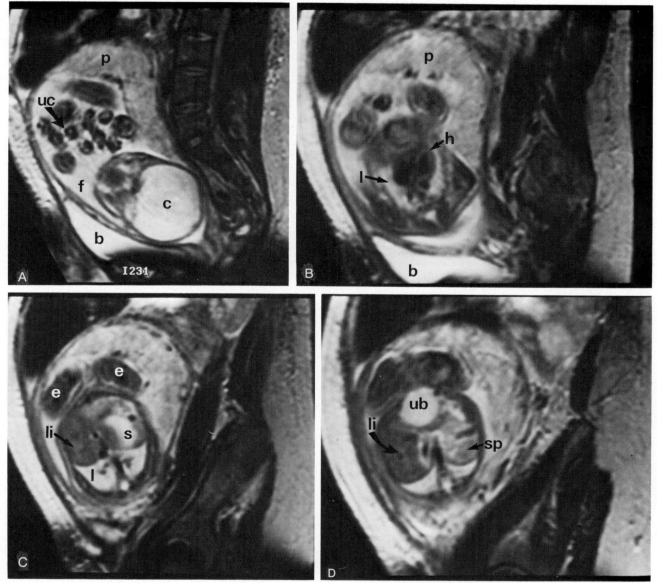

Figure 25–11. Serial fast spin-echo T2-weighted MR scans of a third-trimester pregnancy demonstrating normal maternal and fetal anatomy. *A.* Shown here are the placenta (p), fetal cranium (c), amniotic fluid (f), and umbilical cord (uc). Note that on this T2-weighted sequence, the amniotic fluid and urine in the maternal bladder (b) are of high signal intensity. The umbilical cord appears black owing to signal void from blood flow in the vessels. *B.* Image through the normal fetal thorax showing lungs (l) and heart (h). The lungs, because of their high fluid content, are of high signal intensity on this sequence. Flow void is seen within the cardiac chambers. p, placenta; b, maternal bladder. *C.* The fetal chest and abdomen are well seen. Noted are the liver (li), lungs (l), fluid-filled stomach (s), and lower extremities (e). *D.* The fetal spleen (sp) and urine-filled bladder (ub), as well as the liver (li), are well demonstrated.

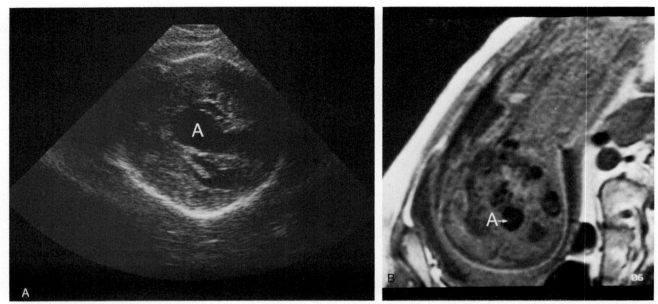

Figure 25–12. Vein of Galen aneurysm in a 39-week fetus. *A.* Sonogram of the fetal cranium demonstrates a large midline fluid-filled structure (A). *B.* Sagittal T1-weighted MR image. The aneurysm (A) demonstrates signal void due to blood flow.

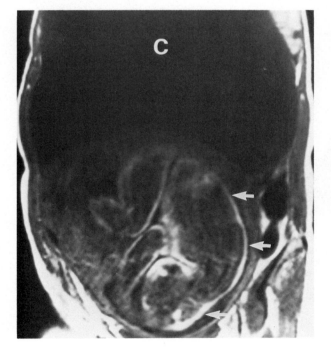

Figure 25–13. Coronal T1-weighted MR image of a normal fetus and coincidental maternal abdominal mass. The fetal subcutaneous fat (*arrows*) is bright and clearly distinguished from the dark amniotic fluid on this sequence. Also shown is a large maternal fluid-filled abdominal mass (C). This was a benign serous ovarian cystadenoma.

times and, therefore, less image degradation, and with fetally oriented imaging planes.[43–45] With such technical advances and additional clinical experience, MRI holds the potential to further supplement the diagnostic capabilities of ultrasonography in the evaluation of the pregnant patient.

References

1. Mole RH: Childhood cancer after prenatal exposure to diagnostic x-ray examination in Britain. Br J Cancer 62:152, 1990.
2. Bithell JF, Stiller CA: A new calculation of the carcinogenic risk of obstetric x-raying. Stat Med 7:857, 1988.
3. Ginsberg JS, Hirsh J, Rainbow AJ, et al: Risks to the fetus of radiologic procedures used in the diagnosis of maternal venous thromboembolic disease. Thromb Haemost 61:189, 1989.
4. Kopelman JN, Duff P, Karl RT, et al: Computed tomographic pelvimetry in the evaluation of breech presentation. Obstet Gynecol 68:455, 1986.
5. Federle MP, Cohen HA, Rosenwein MF, et al: Pelvimetry by digital radiography: A low-dose examination. Radiology 143:733, 1982.
6. Moore MM, Shearer DR: Fetal dose estimates for CT pelvimetry. Radiology 171:265, 1989.
7. Carlan SJ, Angel JL, Sawai SK, et al: Late diagnosis of nonconjoined monoamniotic twins using computed tomographic imaging: A case report. Obstet Gynecol 76:504, 1990.
8. Sargent SK, Young W, Crow P, et al: CT amniography: Value in detecting a monoamniotic pair in a triplet pregnancy. AJR 156:559, 1991.
9. Finberg HJ, Clewell WH: Definitive prenatal diagnosis of monoamniotic twins. J Ultrasound Med 10:513, 1991.
10. Budinger TF: Nuclear magnetic resonance (NMR) in vivo studies: Known thresholds for health effects. J Comput Assist Tomogr 5:800, 1981.
11. Wolff S, Crooks LE, Brown P, et al: Tests for DNA and chromosomal damage induced by nuclear magnetic resonance imaging. Radiology 136:707, 1980.
12. Thomas A, Morris PG: The effects of NMR exposure on living organisms: I. A microbial assay. Br J Radiol 54:615, 1981.
13. Cooke P, Morris PG: The effects of NMR exposure on living organisms. II. A genetic study of human lymphocytes. Br J Radiol 54:622, 1981.
14. Reid A, Smith FW, Hutchison JMS: Nuclear magnetic resonance imaging and its safety implications: Follow-up of 181 patients. Br J Radiol 55:784, 1982.
15. Schwartz JL, Crooks LE: NMR imaging produces no observable mutations or cytotoxicity in mammalian cells. AJR 139:583, 1982.
16. National Radiological Protection Board: Revised guidance on acceptable limits of exposure during nuclear magnetic resonance imaging. Br J Radiol 56:974, 1983.
17. Weinreb JC, Lowe T, Cohen JM, et al: Human fetal anatomy: MR imaging. Radiology 157:715, 1985.
18. McCarthy SM, Filly RA, Stark DD, et al: Obstetrical magnetic resonance imaging: Fetal anatomy. Radiology 154:427, 1985.
19. Lenke RR, Persutte WH, Nemes JM: Use of pancuronium bromide to inhibit fetal movement during magnetic resonance imaging: A case report. J Reprod Med 34:315, 1989.
20. Horvath L, Seeds JW: Temporary arrest of fetal movement with pancuronium bromide to enable antenatal magnetic resonance imaging of holoprosencephaly. Am J Perinatol 6:418, 1989.
21. Daffos F, Forestier F, MacAleese J, et al: Fetal curarization for prenatal magnetic resonance imaging. Prenat Diagn 8:311, 1988.
22. Stark DD, McCarthy SM, Filly RA, et al: Pelvimetry by magnetic resonance imaging. AJR 144:947, 1985.
23. McCarthy SM, Stark DD, Filly RA, et al: Obstetrical magnetic resonance imaging: Maternal anatomy. Radiology 154:421, 1985.
24. Johnson IR, Symonds EM, Kean DM, et al: Imaging the pregnant human uterus with nuclear magnetic resonance. Am J Obstet Gynecol 148:1136, 1984.
25. Yuh WTC, DeMarino GB, Ludwig WD, et al: MR imaging of pregnancy in bicornuate uterus. J Comput Assist Tomogr 12:162, 1988.
26. Hricak H, Chang YCF, Cann CE, et al: Cervical incompetence: Preliminary evaluation with MR imaging. Radiology 174:821, 1990.
27. Kier R, McCarthy SM, Scoutt LM, et al: Pelvic masses in pregnancy: MR imaging. Radiology 176:709, 1990.
28. Weinreb JC, Brown CE, Lowe TW, et al: Pelvic masses in pregnant patients: MR and US imaging. Radiology 159:717, 1986.
29. Powell MC, Buckley J, Price H, et al: Magnetic resonance imaging and placenta previa. Am J Obstet Gynecol 154:565, 1986.
30. Weinreb JC, Lowe T, Cohen JM, et al: Human fetal anatomy: MR imaging. Radiology 157:715, 1985.
31. Powell MC, Worthington BS, Buckley JM, et al: Magnetic resonance imaging in obstetrics: II. Fetal anatomy. Br J Obstet Gynecol 95:38, 1988.
32. McCarthy SM, Filly RA, Stark DD, et al: Magnetic resonance imaging of fetal anomalies in utero: Early experience. AJR 145:677, 1985.
33. Williamson RA, Weiner CP, Yuh WT, et al: Magnetic resonance imaging of anomalous fetuses. Obstet Gynecol 73:952, 1989.
34. Benson RC, Colletti PM, Platt LD, et al: MR imaging of fetal anomalies. AJR 156:1205, 1991.
35. Lowe TW, Weinreb J, Santos-Ramos R, et al: Magnetic resonance imaging in human pregnancy. Obstet Gynecol 66:629, 1985.
36. Weinreb JC, Lowe TW, Santos-Ramos R: Magnetic resonance imaging in obstetric diagnosis. Radiology 154:157, 1985.
37. Angtuaco TL, Shah HR, Mattison DR, et al: MR imaging in high-risk obstetric patients: A valuable complement to US. Radiographics 12:91, 1992.
38. Dinh DH, Wright RM, Hanigan WC: The use of magnetic resonance imaging for the diagnosis of fetal intracranial anomalies. Childs Nerv Syst 5:212, 1990.
39. Deans HE, Smith FW, Lloyd DJ, et al: Fetal fat measurement by magnetic resonance imaging. Br J Radiol 52:603, 1989.
40. Stark DD, McCarthy SM, Filly RA, et al: Intrauterine growth retardation: Evaluation by magnetic resonance. Radiology 155:425, 1985.
41. Brown CE, Weinreb JC: Magnetic resonance imaging appearance of growth retardation in a twin pregnancy. Obstet Gynecol 71:987, 1988.
42. Borcard B, Hiltbrand E, Magnin P, et al: Estimating meconium concentration in human amniotic fluid by nuclear magnetic resonance. Physiol Chem Phys 14:189, 1982.
43. Garden AS, Griffiths RD, Weindling M, et al: Fast-scan magnetic resonance imaging in fetal visualization. Am J Obstet Gynecol 164:1190, 1991.
44. Smith FW, Sutherland HW: Magnetic resonance imaging: The use of the inversion recovery sequence to display fetal morphology. Br J Radiol 61:338, 1988.
45. Johnson IR, Stehling MK, Blamire AM, et al: Study of internal structures of the human fetus in utero by echo planar magnetic resonance imaging. Am J Obstet Gynecol 163:601, 1990.

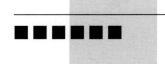

CHAPTER 26

Prenatal Management of the Fetus With a Correctable Defect

MICHAEL R. HARRISON, M.D.
N. SCOTT ADZICK, M.D.
ALAN W. FLAKE, M.D.

The diagnosis and treatment of human fetal defects have evolved rapidly over the past 2 decades owing to improved fetal imaging techniques and better understanding of fetal pathophysiology derived from animal models and increasing clinical experience.[1] Although some fetal malformations with a known pattern of inheritance may be specifically sought, many are identified serendipitously during obstetric ultrasonography. Until recently, the only question raised by the prenatal diagnosis of a fetal malformation was whether the fetus should be aborted, but other therapeutic alternatives are now available. The detection of a fetal abnormality may now lead to a change in the timing of delivery, a change in the mode of delivery, and, in selected cases, prenatal treatment.

Since most diagnostic and therapeutic maneuvers involve some risk to the fetus and mother, there must be a reasonable expectation that a procedure is feasible, safe, and effective before it can be attempted in humans.[2] This requires reliable information about the pathophysiology and natural history of the disease process, the efficacy of intervention in ameliorating the disease, and the feasibility and safety of the proposed intervention. We have tentatively outlined the diagnostic and therapeutic alternatives for the management of specific fetal malformations that can be recognized in utero.[3, 4]

MALFORMATIONS BEST TREATED AFTER TERM DELIVERY

Most correctable malformations that can be diagnosed in utero are best managed by appropriate medical and surgical therapy after delivery at term. The term infant is a better anesthetic and surgical risk than the preterm infant. Examples of such malformations that have been diagnosed in utero are given in Table 26–1. Although this list is not exhaustive, most neonatal surgical disorders fall into this category. Knowledge that a fetus has one of these anomalies may improve perinatal management by allowing preparation for appropriate postnatal care.

Therapy for polyhydramnios and premature labor may be desirable to allow the fetus to remain in utero as long as possible. The delivery can be planned so that appropriate personnel (neonatologist, anesthesiologist, pediatric surgeon) are available. When the neonate will require highly specialized services, transporting the fetus in situ (maternal transport) may be preferable to postnatal transport of the fragile neonate.

MALFORMATIONS USUALLY MANAGED BY SELECTIVE ABORTION

When serious malformations incompatible with normal postnatal life are diagnosed early enough, the mother has the option of terminating the pregnancy. When these malformations are recognized too late for safe termination, the mother can be counseled and appropriate postnatal management arranged. Table 26–2 lists examples of severe anatomic malformations that are considered indications for selective termination. These anatomic abnormalities join a long list of inherited chromosomal and metabolic disorders that can be diagnosed in utero and may lead to selective termination of pregnancy.

PRENATAL DIAGNOSIS LEADING TO EARLY DELIVERY

Early delivery may be indicated for certain fetal anomalies that require correction as soon as possible after diagnosis (Table 26–3). In each of these cases, the risk of premature delivery must be weighed against the risk of continued gestation. This approach has already proven beneficial in managing the fetus with hydrops fetalis and intrauterine growth retardation. Advances in stimulating fetal surfactant production with corticosteroids, exogenous surfactant administra-

---

Table 26–1. MALFORMATIONS DETECTABLE IN UTERO BUT BEST CORRECTED AFTER DELIVERY AT TERM

Esophageal, duodenal, jejunoileal, and anorectal atresias
Meconium ileus (cystic fibrosis)
Enteric cysts and duplications
Small intact omphalocele
Small intact meningocele, myelomeningocele, and spina bifida
Unilateral multicystic dysplastic kidney
Craniofacial, extremity, and chest wall deformities
Cystic hygroma
Small sacrococcygeal teratoma
Ovarian cysts

Table 26–2. MALFORMATIONS USUALLY MANAGED BY SELECTIVE ABORTION

Anencephaly, porencephaly, encephalocele, and giant
  hydrocephalus
Severe anomalies associated with chromosomal abnormalities
  (trisomy 13, trisomy 18, and similar conditions)
Bilateral renal agenesis or bilateral infantile polycystic kidney
  disease
Inherited chromosomal, metabolic, and hematologic abnormalities
  (hemoglobinopathies, Tay-Sachs disease, and similar conditions)

tion, and ventilation of small infants have greatly improved the outcome for premature infants with respiratory distress syndrome.

The rationale for early correction is unique to each anomaly, but the principle remains the same: continued gestation would have a progressive ill effect on the fetus. In some cases, the function of a specific organ system is compromised by the lesion and will continue to deteriorate until it is corrected. In congenital hydronephrosis, unrelieved urinary tract obstruction results in progressive deterioration of renal function. Preterm delivery for early decompression of the urinary tract should reverse the renal maldevelopment at the earliest possible time, maximizing subsequent renal growth and development.[5] In obstructive hydrocephalus, high intraventricular pressure compresses the developing brain. Early delivery for ventricular decompression should maximize the opportunity for subsequent brain development and may avoid the difficult obstetric problem of delivering the neonate with an abnormally large head.

Anomalies associated with progressive organ ischemia should be corrected as soon as possible. Volvulus associated with intestinal malrotation or meconium ileus may lead to intestinal gangrene, perforation, and meconium peritonitis. Early delivery for correction of this type of bowel lesion would be aimed at minimizing the amount of bowel lost to the ischemic process. In some malformations, the progressive ill effects on the fetus result directly from being in utero. In the amniotic band complex, a fetal part is compressed or strangulated by herniation through a defect in the fetal membranes, resulting in amputation or deformity. This simple mechanical restriction to growth and development should be relived at the earliest possible time to prevent further deformity.

Table 26–3. MALFORMATIONS THAT MAY REQUIRE INDUCED PRETERM DELIVERY FOR EARLY CORRECTION EX UTERO

Obstructive hydronephrosis
Obstructive hydrocephalus
Gastroschisis or ruptured omphalocele
Intestinal ischemia/necrosis secondary to volvulus, meconium ileus,
  and similar conditions
Hydrops fetalis
Intrauterine growth retardation

Abdominal Wall Defects

Optimal perinatal management of abdominal wall defects depends on distinguishing before birth those lesions with a good prognosis (gastrochisis, hernia of the cord, small omphalocele) from those lesions with a high associated perinatal morbidity and mortality (giant omphalocele with associated anomalies or syndrome related omphalocele). Clinical experience and laboratory data support the following approach to diagnosis and management (Fig. 26–1).[6] All abdominal wall defects should undergo detailed sonographic evaluation to determine the type of defect. Important features are the size of the defect, presence of a sac, relationship of the umbilical cord to the defect, and presence or absence of extruded liver. Next, particularly in the case of omphalocele, associated anomalies should be sought. Karyotype analysis and careful sonographic assessment for other structural anomalies should be done. Common associations include pentalogy of Cantrell (omphalocele, ectopia cordis, Morgagni diaphragmatic hernia, sternal/pericardial defects), trisomy syndromes, Beckwith-Wiedeman syndrome, and the amniotic band syndrome, which may be associated with gastroschisis. Elective termination may be advisable for fetuses with lethal associated anomalies or chromosomal abnormalities.

Appropriate timing and mode of delivery remain controversial. Gastroschisis and omphalocele can be followed to term in most cases. However, experimental observations suggest that both amniotic fluid contact and bowel constriction are important in the etiology of bowel damage in gastroschisis, and both experimental and clinical data suggest that the most severe bowel damage (ischemic injury, atresia) in gastroschisis is related to bowel constriction by the umbilical ring late in gestation.[7, 8] The authors therefore recommend frequent sonography after 28 weeks' gestation. The evolution of small bowel distention or bowel wall thickening suggests ischemia and may be an indication for early delivery and repair ex utero. Despite some theoretical advantages (sterility and avoiding visceral injury), cesarean delivery has little if any advantage over vaginal delivery in management of most abdominal wall defects.

PRENATAL DIAGNOSIS LEADING TO CESAREAN DELIVERY

Elective cesarean delivery rather than a trial at vaginal delivery may be indicated for the fetal malformations listed in Table 26–4. In most cases, this is because the malformation would cause dystocia. Another indication for elective cesarean delivery is a malformation requiring immediate surgical correction best performed in a sterile environment. A good example is an uncovered meningomyelocele. In this circumstance, the neonate can be resuscitated in an adjacent sterile operating room and undergo immediate surgical correction. Finally, a cesarean delivery may be required if preterm delivery of an affected

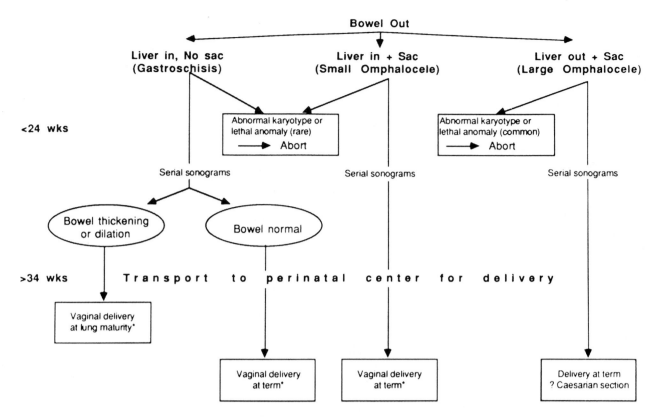

Figure 26–1. Management scheme for the fetus with an abdominal wall defect. (From Langer JC, Harrison MR, Adzick NS, et al: Perinatal management of the fetus with an abdominal wall defect. Fetal Ther 2:216, 1987; with permission of S. Karger AG, Basel.)

fetus is elected but labor is inadequate or if the fetus does not tolerate labor as determined by fetal monitoring.

PRENATAL DIAGNOSIS LEADING TO INTERVENTION BEFORE BIRTH

Fetal Deficiencies

Some fetal deficiency states may be alleviated by treatment before birth (Table 26–5). In respiratory distress syndrome, glucocorticoids given to the mother increase deficient fetal pulmonary surfactant and alleviate the disease. Fetal anemia secondary to isoimmunization-induced hemolysis can be treated by transfusing red blood cells into the fetus. A fetus with vitamin B_{12}–responsive methylmalonic acidemia has been treated in utero by giving massive doses of vitamin B_{12} to the mother. A fetus with biotin-dependent multiple carboxylase deficiency has been treated by giving the mother pharmacologic doses of biotin during the last half of pregnancy.

Medications and nutrients injected into the amniotic

Table 26–4. MALFORMATIONS THAT MAY REQUIRE CESAREAN DELIVERY

Conjoined twins
Giant omphalocele
Large hydrocephalus
Large sacrococcygeal teratoma
Large cystic hygroma
Large or ruptured meningomyelocele
Malformations requiring preterm delivery in the presence of inadequate labor or fetal distress

Table 26–5. FETAL CONDITIONS THAT MAY REQUIRE MEDICAL TREATMENT BEFORE BIRTH

Disorder	Treatment
Erythroblastosis fetalis (red blood cell deficiency)	Red blood cells—intraperitoneal or intravenous
Pulmonary immaturity (surfactant deficiency)	Glucocorticoids—transplacental
Metabolic block (e.g., methylmalonic acidemia, multiple carboxylase deficiency)	Vitamin B_{12}—transplacental Biotin—transplacental
Cardiac arrhythmia (e.g., supraventricular tachycardia)	Digitalis, propranolol, procainamide—transplacental
Endocrine deficiency (e.g., hypothyroidism, adrenal hyperplasia)	Thyroid—transamniotic Corticosteroids—transplacental
Nutritional deficiency (e.g., intrauterine growth retardation)	? Protein-calories—transamniotic or intravenous
Cellular deficiency (e.g., severe combined immunodeficiency)	? Stem cell reconstitution

fluid are swallowed and absorbed by the fetus. Intra-amniotic thyroid hormone can be used to treat congenital hypothyroidism and goiter and to help mature the fetal lung. The intrauterine growth retarded fetus might be fed orally by instilling nutrients into the amniotic fluid.[9] In the future, it is possible that deficiencies in cellular function will be corrected by providing the appropriate stem cell graft.[10]

Anatomic Malformations

Correcting an anatomic malformation in utero is more difficult than providing a missing substrate, hormone, or medication to the fetus. The only anatomic malformations that warrant consideration are those that interfere with fetal organ development and that, if alleviated, would allow normal fetal development to proceed. At present, only four anatomic malformations deserve consideration (Table 26–6).

Congenital Hydronephrosis. Congenital hydronephrosis secondary to urethral obstruction is an excellent example of an anatomically simple lesion having devastating consequences on the developing fetus that may be prevented by correction before birth. Fetal hydronephrosis is being recognized with increasing frequency because fluid-filled masses are particularly easy to detect by sonography and because associated oligohydramnios is a common obstetric indication for sonography. We have managed more than 200 fetuses with urinary tract malformations and have developed an approach based on the predictable pathophysiologic consequences of obstruction on renal and pulmonary

Table 26–6. ANATOMIC DEFECTS THAT INTERFERE WITH DEVELOPMENT AND MAY REQUIRE EARLY SURGICAL RELIEF

Malformation	Effect on Development
Urethral obstruction	Hydronephrosis/lung hypoplasia
	Renal/respiratory failure
Diaphragmatic hernia	Lung hypoplasia
	Respiratory failure
Aqueductal stenosis	Hydrocephalus
	Brain damage

development.[5, 11, 12] The algorithm is presented in Figure 26–2.

The fetus with unilateral hydronephrosis or mild bilateral hydronephrosis with evidence of continuing good renal function does not require prenatal intervention but will benefit from early recognition and prompt postnatal treatment. Conversely, the fetus with severe irreversible renal damage, as evidenced by oligohydramnios or severe renal dysplasia before 20 weeks, probably cannot be salvaged.[12]

The fetus with bilateral hydronephrosis secondary to urethral obstruction who develops oligohydramnios after 20 weeks may benefit from early decompression to halt the ongoing damage to the developing kidneys and lungs. The fetus older than 32 weeks can be delivered early and decompressed ex utero. For the younger fetus, decompression in utero may be necessary.

Selecting appropriate management for the fetus with obstructive uropathy depends on the ability to accu-

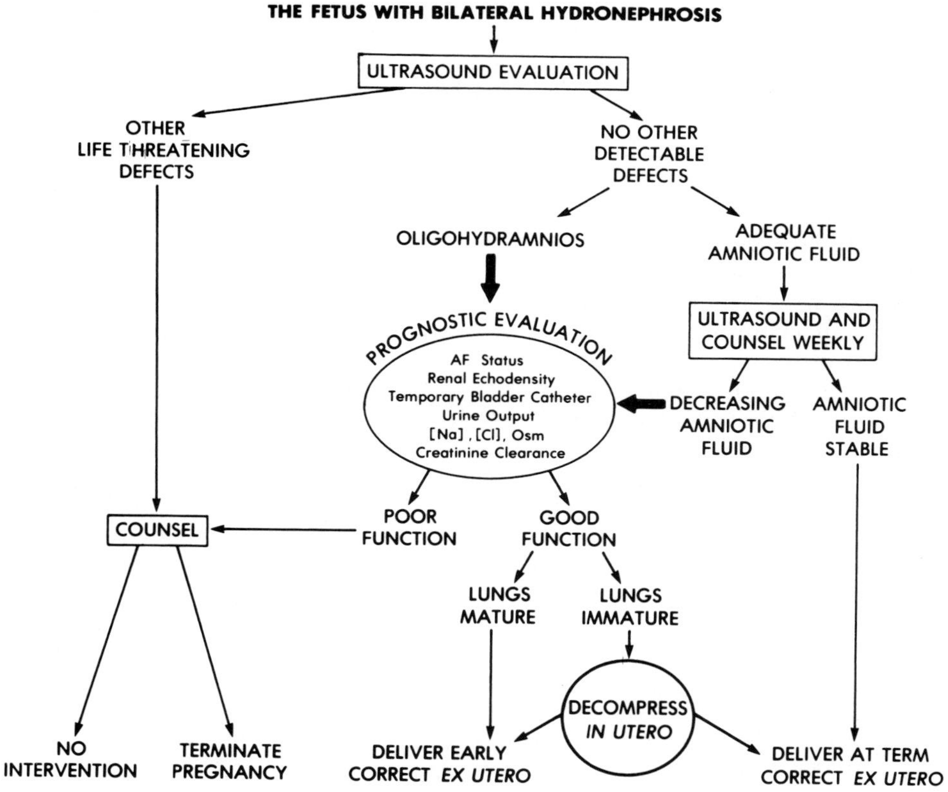

Figure 26–2. Management scheme for the fetus with bilateral hydronephrosis. (From Adzick NS, Flake AW, Harrison MR: Recent advances in prenatal diagnosis and treatment. Pediatr Clin North Am 32:1103, 1985.)

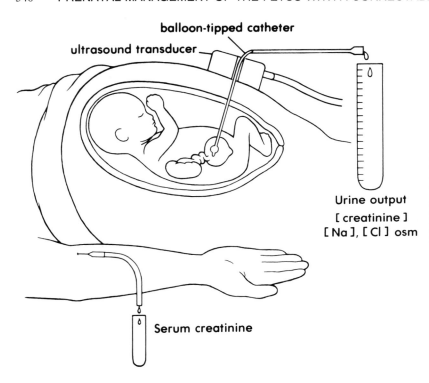

ultrasound transducer
balloon-tipped catheter

Urine output
[creatinine]
[Na], [Cl] osm

Serum creatinine

Figure 26–3. Current clinical technique for diagnostic urinary catheterization. A No. 4 French balloon-tipped catheter is placed into the distended fetal bladder. Fetal urine output, urinary electrolytes, and creatinine clearance can be determined with this method. (From Adzick NS, Flake AW, Harrison MR: Recent advances in prenatal diagnosis and treatment. Pediatr Clin North Am 32:1103, 1985.)

rately assess the severity of existing renal damage and to predict the potential for recovery of renal function if the obstruction is relieved. Clinical assessment of the functional potential of the obstructed fetal urinary tract has proven to be difficult. Evaluative tests using either urine reaccumulation after bladder aspiration[13] or furosemide (Lasix) stimulation of urine output[14] are unreliable. Amniotic fluid status is predictive only in the extremes (i.e., normal volume late in gestation suggests adequate function whereas severe oligohydramnios early in gestation suggests poor function.[12] Similarly, the sonographic appearance of the fetal kidneys lacks the sensitivity and specificity to be used as the sole predictor of function.[15] Clinical use of diagnostic fetal bladder catheterization to assess urine sodium and chloride concentration and hourly urine output has proven to be extremely helpful (Figs. 26–3 and 26–4). Normal fetal urine is hypotonic,[16] whereas our clinical work has demonstrated that human fetuses with obstructive uropathy and renal dysplasia produce minimal amounts of nearly isotonic urine.[11] Specific criteria for "good" or "poor" fetal renal function have been generated. Although these criteria are based on retrospective analysis, the utility of these parameters has been confirmed in recent prospective and retrospective studies as well as by our own clinical experience.[17, 18] Finally, laboratory studies suggest that fetal creatinine clearance will allow a simple, quantitative estimate of fetal renal function.[19] Since maternal and fetal serum creatinine levels are equal,[20–22] fetal creatinine clearance can be determined by fetal urine collection and maternal blood sampling alone, obviating the need for simultaneous fetal blood sampling.

Experimentally, prenatal decompression arrests the adverse effects on renal development and reverses

otherwise lethal pulmonary hypoplasia.[23–26] Prenatal intervention is safe and feasible in a rigorous primate model.[27–29] We have developed techniques for sonographically guided percutaneous placement of fetal shunt catheters (Fig. 26–5) and for surgical exteriorization of the fetal urinary tract and have begun to apply these techniques in highly selected cases.[11, 12, 30] Although percutaneous drainage has been successful, all catheters are prone to obstruction and migration, necessitating close observation and frequent catheter replacement. We favor surgical decompression by bladder marsupialization for the singleton fetus with posterior urethral valves who has evidence of compromised renal function and is too immature to be delivered for postnatal decompression.[11]

Congenital Diaphragmatic Hernia. Congenital diaphragmatic hernia (CDH) is an anatomically simple defect that is easily correctable after birth by removing the herniated viscera from the chest and closing the diaphragm. However, 50% to 80% of all infants with CDH die of pulmonary insufficiency despite optimal postnatal care because their lungs are too hypoplastic to support extrauterine life even at term.[31, 32] Since the pulmonary hypoplasia appears to be a developmental consequence of compression by the herniated viscera, removal of this space-occupying lesion in utero should allow pulmonary development to proceed so that pulmonary function will be adequate to support life at birth.

We have demonstrated in fetal lambs that compression of the lung during the last trimester results in fatal pulmonary hypoplasia and that removal of the compressing lesion allows the lung to grow and develop sufficiently to reverse the fatal pulmonary hypoplasia and allow survival at birth.[33–36] The hidden mortality

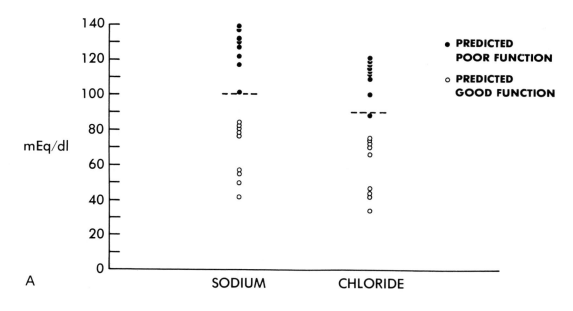

URINARY ELECTROLYTES IN THE HUMAN FETUS WITH BILATERAL OBSTRUCTIVE UROPATHY

Predicted Function	Amniotic Fluid Status At the Time of Initial Presentation	Sonographic Appearance of Kidneys	Fetal Urine			
			Sodium (mEq/mL)	Chloride (mEq/mL)	Osmolarity (mosm)	Output (mL/H)
Poor	Moderate to severely decreased	Echogenic to cystic	> 100	> 90	> 210	< 2
Good	Normal to moderately decreased	Normal to echogenic	< 100	< 90	< 210	> 2

Figure 26–4. *A.* Graph of fetal urinary sodium and chloride concentrations in fetuses with good and poor function. Fetuses with poor renal function have "salt wasting" and urinary sodium levels greater than 100 mEq/dL. *B.* Prognostic criteria for the fetus with bilateral obstructive uropathy. (From Glick PL, Harrison MR, Golbus MS, et al: Management of the fetus with congenital hydronephrosis: II. Prognostic criteria and selection for treatment. J Pediatr Surg 20:376, 1985.)

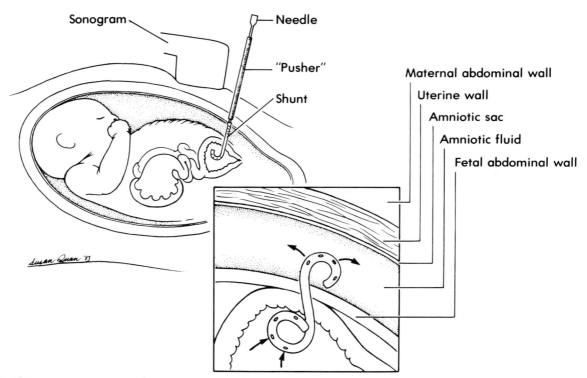

Figure 26–5. Placement of a fetal bladder shunt depicted schematically. The double pigtail catheter is pushed off the needle so that one end is in the bladder and the other end is in the amniotic space. (From Adzick NS, Flake AW, Harrison MR: Recent advances in prenatal diagnosis and treatment. Pediatr Clin North Am 32:1103, 1985.)

of CDH has been well documented, resulting in a selection bias for good outcome in all postnatal series of CDH.[37] The true natural history of CDH can only be defined by examination of outcome of fetuses prenatally diagnosed with CDH. A number of large series of prenatally diagnosed CDH have now been published.[38–41] The overall mortality of isolated, prenatally diagnosed CDH has varied between 62% and 80%, in spite of the availability of optimal postnatal care and, in some series, extracorporeal membrane oxygenation. Defining prognostic criteria in individual cases of prenatally diagnosed CDH has been more difficult. Clearly there are prenatally diagnosed cases that will do well with conventional therapy and are therefore "too good" for consideration of fetal surgery, whereas others are "too bad" or beyond salvage by fetal surgery. In our experience, the early appearance (<24 weeks' gestation) of a large volume of visceral herniation, as suggested by the presence of a herniated stomach and left lobe of the liver in the fetal chest and quantified by a decreased lung to thorax ratio at the level of a four-chamber view of the heart, is associated with a poor prognosis.

After a decade of experimental work in animal models, techniques have now been developed to successfully repair CDH in utero.[42, 43] Our current recommendations are that all fetuses with CDH diagnosed before 28 weeks' gestation undergo a detailed ultrasound evaluation, amniocentesis, or percutaneous umbilical blood sampling for karyotype determination and a fetal echocardiogram to exclude other anomalies (Fig. 26–6). If a lethal associated anomaly is found,

the parents are counseled and the fetus is managed expectantly or by elective termination. If an isolated CDH is present, detailed prognostic evaluation should be performed. The presence of early gestation (<24 weeks), of stomach and/or liver in the chest, of a low lung to thorax ratio, and of the early appearance of polyhydramnios places the fetus in an early/severe category with a dismal prognosis. In these cases, fetal surgical repair is recommended in the context of a clinical trial. Honest evaluation of the efficacy of fetal surgery for CDH can only be done through conductance of a prospective randomized trial that we are now pursuing.

The repair of human fetal CDH remains a formidable challenge that should not be attempted under any but the most rigorous conditions. Diaphragmatic hernia remains the best studied and most compelling example of a defect requiring correction before birth.

Congenital Cystic Adenomatoid Malformation. Congenital cystic adenomatoid malformation (CCAM) represents a spectrum of disease characterized by cystic lesions of the lung. In the majority of cases, CCAM becomes manifest after birth and is easily treated ex utero. As with CDH, however, prenatal experience has uncovered a "hidden" mortality for CCAM. We previously reported our experience with 12 cases of prenatally diagnosed CCAM and proposed a classification based on prenatal sonographic appearance, gross anatomy, and prognosis.[44] CCAM can be divided into macrocystic and microcystic types depending on the presence or absence of cysts greater than 5 mm in diameter, respectively. The macrocystic lesion was

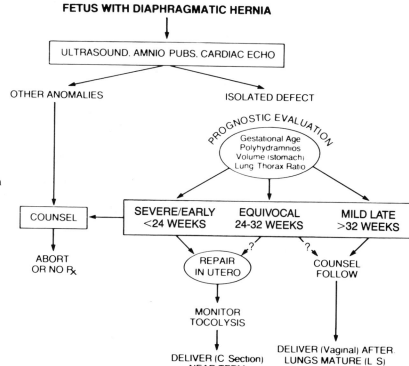

FETUS WITH DIAPHRAGMATIC HERNIA

Figure 26–6. Management scheme for the fetus with congenital diaphragmatic hernia.

associated with a relatively favorable prognosis. The microcystic or solid lesion, however, frequently induces fetal hydrops, which uniformly results in rapid fetal death.

The fatal outcome seen with large CCAMs is related to several factors including development of hydrops, hypoplasia of the lung secondary to prolonged compression in utero, and, in some cases, lack of immediate diagnosis and postnatal surgery. The etiology of hydrops remains speculative but most likely results from vena caval obstruction or cardiac compression from extreme mediastinal shift associated with these lesions. Subsequent experience with over 30 cases of prenatally diagnosed CCAM has confirmed the overriding importance of the presence or absence of hydrops as a harbinger of fetal death. We therefore postulated that prenatal resection of the pulmonary mass might reverse the hydrops and allow sufficient lung growth to permit survival in these selected severe cases. Experimental work in the lamb model confirmed the feasibility of pulmonary resection and demonstrated compensatory growth of the opposite lung.[45] Subsequent clinical experience with the prenatal resection of CCAM in cases of fetal hydrops has confirmed the efficacy of resection in reversing fetal hydrops and allowing survival of an otherwise doomed fetus.[46, 47]

We currently give the following recommendations for management of a fetus with prenatally diagnosed CCAM (Fig. 26–7). All fetuses should undergo detailed sonography to confirm the diagnosis, evaluate for hydrops, determine the appearance of the lesion, and rule out other life-threatening anomalies. The majority of these fetuses will have isolated, small CCAM without hydrops and will best be treated by surgical resection after term delivery. When a large CCAM (particularly microcystic) is diagnosed early in gestation, there is a much higher probability of development of hydrops and these cases should be followed by frequent serial sonography. Recommendations for management depend on the presence or absence of associated hydrops and gestational age. The immature fetus (<28 weeks' gestation) with a large CCAM and evolution of hydrops should be immediately considered for in utero resection of the tumor. If pulmonary maturity is established and hydrops evolves, the fetus should be emergently delivered and undergo resection ex utero. Fetuses that are between 28 weeks' gestation and lung maturity with evolving hydrops should undergo an attempt at steroid-induced lung maturation and early delivery, with surfactant administration and tumor resection immediately after birth.

Fetal Sacrococcygeal Teratoma. Sacrococcygeal teratoma (SCT) is the most common tumor of the neonate.[48] The majority of cases remain asymptomatic in utero and are diagnosed after birth. To define the natural history of SCT, we reviewed our own experience with prenatally diagnosed SCT and that of the literature.[49] Once again, a significant hidden mortality of SCT became apparent. The majority of fetuses in this series died of their SCT, but not by the mechanism usually responsible for death in postnatal series (i.e., malignancy). Instead, death appeared to result from secondary effects of the SCT. Tumor mass and associated polyhydramnios frequently caused preterm labor and delivery with fetal survival depending on lung maturity. Massive hemorrhage into the tumor with secondary fetal exsanguination may occur spontaneously in utero or be precipitated by labor and

FETUS WITH CYSTIC ADENOMATOID MALFORMATION

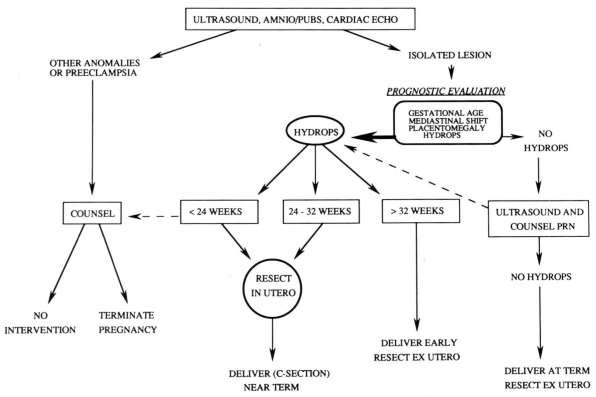

Figure 26–7. Management scheme for the fetus with cystic adenomatoid malformation of the lung.

delivery. Dystocia, secondary to tumor bulk or tumor rupture, may occur complicating delivery. Finally, in a few cases, placentomegaly and/or hydrops evolves, precipitating rapid fetal death.

These observations were confirmed in more recent reviews of our experience combined with survey data. In total, 22 of 42 fetuses prenatally diagnosed with SCT died. When placentomegaly or hydrops was present, death occurred precipitously in 15 of 15 fetuses. A postulated mechanism for hydrops was high output failure secondary to tumor steal.[50] This mechanism was confirmed in one case[51] using duplex Doppler sonography by documenting augmented descending aortic flow in combination with decreased umbilical arterial blood flow and increased vena caval diameter. This constellation of findings was only consistent with diversion of blood from the placenta and toward the tumor, confirming the hypothesis of a vascular steal phenomenon. The uniform association of precipitous death in utero after the appearance of placentomegaly/hydrops and confirmation of a vascular steal etiology of hydrops suggested our current belief that prenatal tumor resection might reverse hydrops and result in fetal salvage.

Our recommendation (Fig. 26–8) is that all fetuses diagnosed with SCT undergo detailed sonographic evaluation to confirm the diagnosis, rule out associated anomalies (rare), and assess placental size, type of SCT, and the presence or absence of hydrops. If diagnosis is serendipitous and the tumor is small, an optimistic outlook can be given and the pregnancy

followed by infrequent sonography to term vaginal delivery. If the tumor is large a guarded prognosis should be given and the pregnancy followed by frequent sonography. If no placentomegaly or hydrops evolves, the fetus should be delivered by elective cesarean section to avoid dystocia or tumor rupture and hemorrhage. If placentomegaly/hydrops evolves after fetal pulmonary maturity is established, the fetus should be delivered by emergent cesarean section and treated ex utero. If placentomegaly/hydrops evolves before 28 weeks' gestation and the tumor is anatomically amenable to easy resection (APSA type I), in utero resection should be considered (Fig. 26–9).

THE FUTURE OF FETAL TREATMENT

Prenatal diagnosis offers new hope for improved management of the fetus with a congenital defect, but the more invasive diagnostic and therapeutic procedures involve significant risks for both fetus and mother, raising difficult ethical questions about risks versus benefits and about the rights of the fetus and mother. A great deal of clinical and laboratory experience will be required to establish which procedures are truly safe and feasible. In the meantime, it is important to maintain a healthy skepticism about fetal treatment. Because a procedure can be done does not mean that it should be done.

At this very early stage, fetal intervention should be

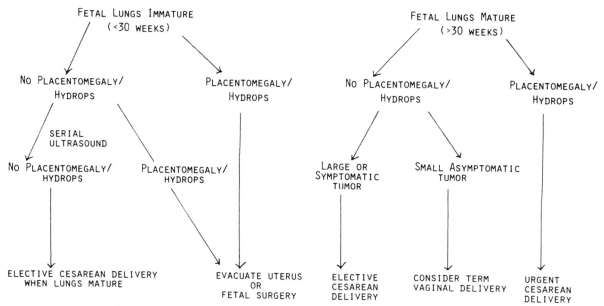

FETUS WITH
SACROCOCCYGEAL TERATOMA

FETAL LUNGS IMMATURE
(<30 WEEKS)

FETAL LUNGS MATURE
(>30 WEEKS)

NO PLACENTOMEGALY/
HYDROPS

PLACENTOMEGALY/
HYDROPS

NO PLACENTOMEGALY/
HYDROPS

PLACENTOMEGALY/
HYDROPS

SERIAL
ULTRASOUND

NO PLACENTOMEGALY/
HYDROPS

PLACENTOMEGALY/
HYDROPS

LARGE OR
SYMPTOMATIC
TUMOR

SMALL ASYMPTOMATIC
TUMOR

ELECTIVE CESAREAN DELIVERY
WHEN LUNGS MATURE

EVACUATE UTERUS
OR
FETAL SURGERY

ELECTIVE
CESAREAN
DELIVERY

CONSIDER TERM
VAGINAL DELIVERY

URGENT
CESAREAN
DELIVERY

Figure 26–8. Management scheme for the fetus with a sacrococcygeal teratoma.

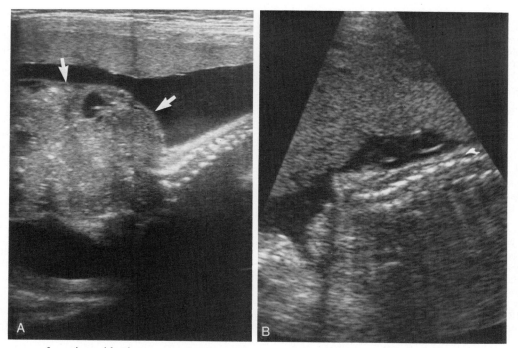

Figure 26–9. Sonogram of a patient with a large sacrococcygeal teratoma. *A.* Preoperative sonogram showing a large mass (*arrows*) emanating from the lower fetal spine. *B.* Postoperative sonogram demonstrates small residual tissue at the resection site.

pursued only in centers committed to research and development as well as (and before) responsible clinical application. The minimum requirments for fetal intervention include the cooperative efforts of an obstetrician experienced in prenatal intervention, a sonologist experienced and skilled in fetal diagnosis, a surgeon experienced in operating on tiny preterm neonates and in performing fetal procedures in the laboratory, a perinatologist working in a high-risk obstetric unit associated with a tertiary intensive care nursery, a reasonable and compassionate bioethicist, and uninvolved professional colleagues who will monitor such innovative therapy (i.e., a committee on human research). Since there is considerable potential for doing harm, a fetal abnormality of any type should never be treated simply "because it is there" and never by someone unprepared for this fearsome responsibility. The responsibility of those undertaking fetal therapy includes an obligation to report to the medical profession all results, good or bad, so that the merits and liabilities of fetal treatment can be established as soon as possible.

The ability to diagnose fetal birth defects has achieved considerable sophistication. Treatment of several fetal disorders has proved feasible, and treatment of more complicated lesions will undoubtedly expand as techniques for fetal intervention improve.

References

1. Harrison MR, Golbus MS, Filly RA (eds): The Unborn Patient, 2nd ed. Philadelphia, WB Saunders, 1990.
2. Harrison MR, Golbus MS, Filly RA, et al: Fetal treatment 1982. N Engl J Med 307:1651, 1982.
3. Harrison MR, Golbus MS, Filly RA: Management of the fetus with a correctable congenital defect. JAMA 246:774, 1981.
4. Harrison MR, Adzick NS: The fetus as a patient: Surgical considerations. Ann Surg 213:279, 1991.
5. Harrison MR, Filly RA, Parer JT: Management of the fetus with a urinary tract malformation. JAMA 246:635, 1981.
6. Langer JC, Harrison MR, Adzick NS, et al: Perinatal management of the fetus with an abdominal wall defect. Fetal Ther 2:216, 1987.
7. Langer JC, Longaker MT, Crombleholme TM, et al: Etiology of intestinal damage in gastroschisis: I. Effects of amniotic fluid exposure and bowel constriction in a fetal lamb model. J Pediatr Surg 24:992, 1989.
8. Langer JC, Bell JG, Castillo RO, et al: Etiology of intestinal damage in gastroschisis: II. Timing and reversibility of histologic changes, mucosal function, and contractility. J Pediatr Surg 25:1122, 1990.
9. Flake AW, Laberge JM, Adzick NS, et al: Trans-amniotic fetal feeding: III. The effect of nutrient infusion on intrauterine growth retardation. J Pediatr Surg 21:481, 1986.
10. Flake AW, Harrison MR, Adzick NS, et al: Transplantation of fetal hematopoietic stem cells in utero: The creation of hematopoietic chimeras. Science 233:776, 1986.
11. Glick PL, Harrison MR, Golbus MS, et al: Management of the fetus with congenital hydronephrosis: II. Prognostic criteria and selection for treatment. J Pediatr Surg 20:376, 1985.
12. Harrison MR, Golbus MS, Filly RA, et al: Management of the fetus with congenital hydronephrosis. J Pediatr Surg 17:728, 1982.
13. Bellinger MF, Comstock C, Grosso D, et al: Fetal posterior urethral valves and renal dysplasia at 15 weeks' gestational age. J Urol 129:1238, 1983.
14. Wladimiroff JW: Effect of furosemide on fetal urine production. Br J Obstet Gynaecol 82:221, 1975.
15. Mahony BS, Filly RA, Callen PW, et al: Sonographic evaluation of fetal renal dysplasia. Radiology 152:143, 1984.
16. McGrory WW: Development of renal function in utero. In Developmental Nephrology, pp 51–78. Cambridge, MA, Harvard University Press, 1972.
17. Crombleholme TM, Harrison MR, Golbus MS, et al: Fetal intervention in obstructive uropathy: Prognostic indicators and efficacy of intervention. Am J Obstet Gynecol 162:1239, 1990.
18. Muller F, Dumez Y, Dommergues M, et al: Can fetal urinary biochemistry predict postnatal renal function. Fetal Ther, in press.
19. Adzick NS, Harrison MR, Flake AW, et al: Development of a fetal renal function test using endogenous creatinine clearance. J Pediatr Surg 20:602, 1985.
20. Hodari AA, Mariona FG, Houlihan RT, et al: Creatinine transport in the maternal-fetal complex. Obstet Gynecol 41:55, 1973.
21. Hutchinson DL, Bashore RA, Will DW: Creatinine equilibrium between mother and nephrectomized primate fetus. Proc Soc Exp Biol Med 110:395, 1962.
22. McGaughey HS, Corey EL, Scoggin WA, et al: Creatinine transport between baby and mother at term. Am J Obstet Gynecol 80:108, 1960.
23. Glick PL, Harrison MR, Noall R, et al: Correction of congenital hydronephrosis in utero: III. Early mid-trimester ureteral obstruction produces renal dysplasia. J Pediatr Surg 18:681, 1983.
24. Glick PL, Harrison MR, Adzick NS, et al: Correction of congenital hydronephrosis in utero: IV. In utero decompression prevents renal dysplasia. J Pediatr Surg 19:649, 1984.
25. Harrison MR, Ross N, Noall R, et al: Correction of congenital hydronephrosis in utero: I. The model: Fetal urethral obstruction produces hydronephrosis and pulmonary hypoplasia in fetal lambs. J Pediatr Surg 18:247, 1983.
26. Harrison MR, Nakayama DK, Noall R, et al: Correction of congenital hydronephrosis in utero: II. Decompression reverses the effects of obstruction on the fetal lung and urinary tract. J Pediatr Surg 17:965, 1982.
27. Adzick NS, Harrison MR, et al: Fetal surgery in the primate: III. Maternal outcome after fetal surgery. J Pediatr Surg 21:477, 1986.
28. Harrison MR, Anderson J, Rosen MA, et al: Fetal surgery in the primate: I. Anesthetic, surgical, and tocolytic management to maximize fetal-neonatal survival. J Pediatr Surg 17:115, 1982.
29. Nakayama DK, Harrison MR, Seron-Ferre M, Villa RL: Fetal surgery in the primate: II. Uterine electromyographic response to operative procedures and pharmacologic agents. J Pediatr Surg 19:333, 1984.
30. Harrison MR, Golbus MS, Filly RA, et al: Fetal surgery for congenital hydronephrosis. N Engl J Med 306:591, 1982.
31. Harrison MR, Bjordal RI, Landmark F, et al: Congenital diaphragmatic hernia: The hidden mortality. J Pediatr Surg 13:227, 1979.
32. Harrison MR, deLorimier AA: Congenital diaphragmatic hernia. Surg Clin North Am 61:1023, 1981.
33. Adzick NS, Outwater KM, Harrison MR, et al: Correction of congenital diaphragmatic hernia in utero: IV. An early gestational model for pulmonary vascular morphometric analysis. J Pediatr Surg 20:673, 1985.
34. Harrison MR, Jester JA, Ross NA: Correction of congenital diaphragmatic hernia in utero: I. The model: Intrathoracic balloon produced fetal pulmonary hypoplasia. Surgery 88:174, 1980.
35. Harrison MR, Bressack MA, Churg AM: Correction of congenital diaphragmatic hernia in utero: II. Simulated correction permits fetal lung growth with survival at birth. Surgery 88:260, 1980.
36. Harrison MR, Ross NA, deLorimier AA: Correction of congenital diaphragmatic hernia in utero: III. Development of a successful surgical technique using abdominoplasty to avoid compromise of umbilical blood flow. J Pediatr Surg 16:934, 1981.
37. Harrison MR, Bjordal RI, Landmark F: Congenital diaphragmatic hernia: The hidden mortality. J Pediatr Surg 13:227, 1978.
38. Adzick NS, Harrison MR, et al: Diaphragmatic hernia in the fetus: Prenatal diagnosis and outcome in 94 cases. J Pediatr Surg 20:357, 1985.

39. Benacerraf B, Adzick NS: Fetal diaphragmatic hernia: Ultrasound diagnosis and clinical outcome in 19 cases. Am J Obstet Gynecol 156:573, 1987.
40. Nakayama DK, Harrison MR, Chinn DH, et al: Prenatal diagnosis and natural history of the fetus with a congenital diaphragmatic hernia: Initial clinical experience. J Pediatr Surg 20:118, 1985.
41. Sharland G, Lockhart SM, Heward AJ, et al: Prognosis in fetal diaphragmatic hernia. Am J Obstet Gynecol 166:9, 1992.
42. Harrison MR, Adzick NS, Longaker MT, et al: Successful repair in utero of a fetal diaphragmatic hernia after removal of herniated viscera from the left thorax. N Engl J Med 322:1582, 1990.
43. Harrison MR, Langer JC, Adzick NS, et al: Correction of congenital diaphragmatic hernia in utero: V. Initial clinical experience. J Pediatr Surg 25:47, 1990.
44. Adzick NS, Harrison MR, Glick PL, et al: Fetal cystic adenomatoid malformation: Prenatal diagnosis and natural history. J Pediatr Surg 20:483, 1985.
45. Adzick NS, Harrison MR, Hu LM, et al: Compensatory lung growth after pneumonectomy in fetal lambs: A morphometric study. Surg Forum 37:648, 1986.
46. Adzick NS, Harrison MR, Flake AW, et al: Open fetal surgery for congenital cystic adenomatoid malformation. J Pediatr Surg 28:806, 1993.
47. Harrison MR, Adzick NS, Jennings RW, et al: Antenatal intervention for congenital cystic adenomatoid malformation. Lancet 336:965, 1990.
48. Pantoja E, Llobet R, Gonzalez-Flores B: Retroperitoneal teratoma: Historical review. J Urol 115:520, 1976.
49. Flake AW, Harrison MR, Adzick NS, et al: Fetal sacrococcygeal teratoma. J Pediatr Surg 21:563, 1986.
50. Bond SJ, Schmidt KG, Silverman NH, et al: Death due to high output cardiac failure in fetal sacrococcygeal teratoma. J Pediatr Surg 25:1287, 1990.
51. Langer JC, Harrison MR, Schmidt KG, et al: Fetal hydrops and demise from sacrococcygeal teratoma: Rationale for fetal surgery. Am J Obstet Gynecol 160:1145, 1989.

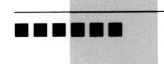

CHAPTER 27

Normal Anatomy of the Female Pelvis

SUSAN C. HOLT, M.D.
CLIFFORD S. LEVI, M.D.
EDWARD A. LYONS, M.D.
DANIEL J. LINDSAY, M.D.
GERALDINE BALLARD, R.D.M.S.
SIDNEY M. DASHEFSKY, M.D.

The advent of endovaginal scanning (EVS) has vastly increased the amount of information attainable in assessing the female pelvis. Cyclical changes related to hormonal stimulation and age-related changes are now seen in greater detail than ever before. Color Doppler imaging has added a new dimension to the study of pelvic hemodynamics, further detailing normal from pathologic blood flow. EVS is now being used frequently to augment the traditional method of pelvic scanning through the distended urinary bladder known as transabdominal sonography (TAS).[1] In fact, in our practice, EVS is performed on all patients with no contraindication who present for gynecologic or first-trimester ultrasound examination.

The anatomy pertinent to obstetric and gynecologic ultrasonography is discussed in this chapter. The chapters dealing with ultrasound evaluation of the uterus and ultrasound evaluation of the ovary include a discussion of physiologic changes and pathology of these organs.

The pelvis is arbitrarily divided into two structurally continuous compartments: the true and false pelves. The division is defined by the sacral promontory and the lineae terminales. The lineae terminales are the arcuate line of the ilium, the iliopectineal line, and the crest of the pubis. The false pelvis is bounded by the flanged portions of the iliac bones, the base of the sacrum posteriorly, and the abdominal wall anteriorly and laterally. The true pelvis is bounded anteriorly by the pubis and pubic rami, posteriorly by the sacrum and coccyx, and laterally by the fused ilium and ischium. With the muscles of the pelvic floor in place, the true pelvis forms a basin.

On TAS a full bladder is required to displace small bowel out of the true pelvis into the false pelvis and to provide a "sonic window" to view the pelvic contents (Fig. 27–1). Thus, visualization of the pelvic organs is limited by body habitus owing to sonic attenuation of the intervening anterior abdominal wall, subcutaneous and properitoneal fat, and fat in the mesentery and omentum. As a result of this attenuation and the distance of the area of interest from the anterior abdominal wall, it is often not possible to use high-frequency transducers and benefit from their inherent enhanced axial and lateral resolution. In our practice, although a 5.0-MHz transducer is used whenever possible, most transvesical examinations are performed with a 3.5-MHz transducer.

Endovaginal scanning has numerous advantages over traditional transvesical scanning. Because of the proximity of the vaginal fornices to the uterus and adnexa, the problem of sonic attenuation is much less significant with EVS in the evaluation of the viscera of the true pelvis. As a result, higher frequency transducers can be used in EVS. The endovaginal scans shown in this chapter were performed with transducers of various frequencies, ranging from 5.0 to 7.5 MHz. The normal and pathologic anatomy of the uterus, ovaries, and uterine tubes, if within the field of view of the transducer, is demonstrated to better advantage using the endovaginal rather than the transvesical approach (Fig. 27–2). In our experience, patient acceptance of EVS is actually better than for the transvesical approach because EVS obviates the need for a full bladder.

The disadvantages of EVS when compared with TAS include a limited field of view and an inability to examine the false pelvis adequately. The full urinary bladder in TAS provides a window to examine the true pelvis by displacement of bowel but may also inadvertently displace pathologic structures into the false pelvis.[3, 4] A quick scan of the true and false pelves at the end of the study after the patient has voided is part of a routine examination. It will allow one to detect large masses that have been displaced by the full bladder and masses that mimic a full bladder (Fig. 27–3). On the postvoid examination, it is often necessary to use compression to displace gas in loops of small bowel and colon, especially when searching for a small mass in the false pelvis.

When EVS is used, free fluid is often demonstrated in the posterior cul-de-sac in normal patients (Figs. 27–4 and 27–5). The presence of fluid in the anterior cul-de-sac or lateral pelvic recesses or a large amount of fluid in the posterior cul-de-sac suggests the presence

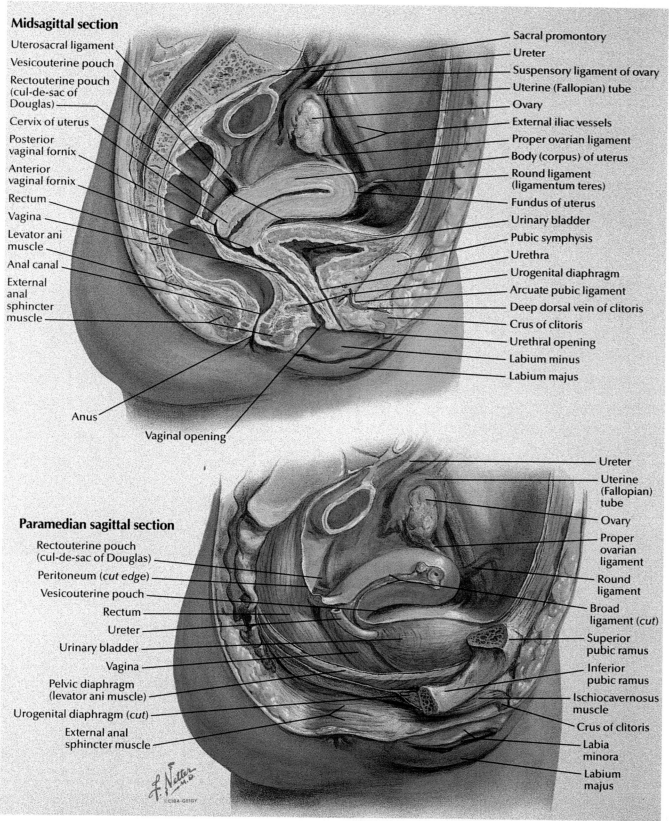

Midsagittal section

Uterosacral ligament
Vesicouterine pouch
Rectouterine pouch (cul-de-sac of Douglas)
Cervix of uterus
Posterior vaginal fornix
Anterior vaginal fornix
Rectum
Vagina
Levator ani muscle
Anal canal
External anal sphincter muscle
Anus
Vaginal opening

Sacral promontory
Ureter
Suspensory ligament of ovary
Uterine (Fallopian) tube
Ovary
External iliac vessels
Proper ovarian ligament
Body (corpus) of uterus
Round ligament (ligamentum teres)
Fundus of uterus
Urinary bladder
Pubic symphysis
Urethra
Urogenital diaphragm
Arcuate pubic ligament
Deep dorsal vein of clitoris
Crus of clitoris
Urethral opening
Labium minus
Labium majus

Paramedian sagittal section

Rectouterine pouch (cul-de-sac of Douglas)
Peritoneum (cut edge)
Vesicouterine pouch
Rectum
Ureter
Urinary bladder
Vagina
Pelvic diaphragm (levator ani muscle)
Urogenital diaphragm (cut)
External anal sphincter muscle

Ureter
Uterine (Fallopian) tube
Ovary
Proper ovarian ligament
Round ligament
Broad ligament (cut)
Superior pubic ramus
Inferior pubic ramus
Ischiocavernosus muscle
Crus of clitoris
Labia minora
Labium majus

Figure 27–1. *A.* Midsagittal section diagram of the female pelvis demonstrating the relationship of the uterus, urinary bladder, rectum, and adnexal structures. (*A* from Netter FH: Atlas of Human Anatomy, plate 341. West Caldwell, NJ, CIBA-Geigy Co, 1989.)

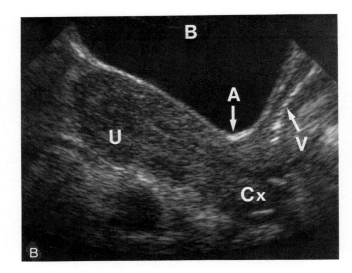

Figure 27–1. *Continued B.* Midline sagittal transabdominal sonogram through the distended urinary bladder (B). The cervix lies posterior to the angle (A) of the bladder. U, uterus; V, vagina; Cx, cervix.

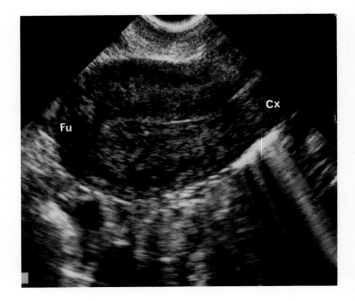

Figure 27–2. Endovaginal sagittal sonogram through the uterine fundus (Fu) and proximal portion of the cervix (Cx).

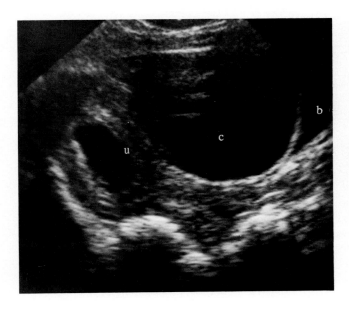

Figure 27–3. Transabdominal midline longitudinal sonogram of a large serous cystadenoma (c) anterior to the uterus, mimicking a full bladder (b). u, uterus.

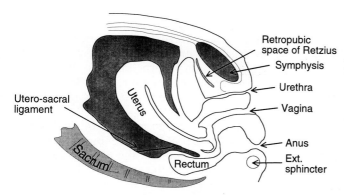

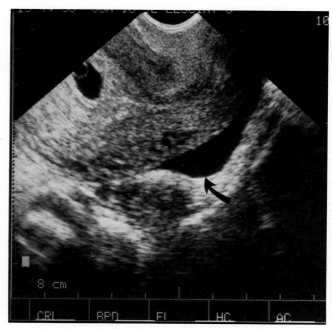

Figure 27–4. Diagram of a midline sagittal section through the pelvis showing the peritoneal reflections including the anterior cul-de-sac (vesicouterine recess) and the posterior cul-de-sac (rectouterine recess). The posterior cul-de-sac is closely related to the posterior fornix of the vagina.

of a large intraperitoneal fluid collection (Fig. 27–6). The volume of fluid may be estimated by examining the hepatorenal space (Morrison's pouch).

THE PELVIC MUSCULATURE AND FASCIAL PLANES

The superficial or subcutaneous fascia is areolar in texture and contains varying amounts of fat. The subcutaneous fascia is continuous with the superficial fascia of the thigh, labia majora, and perineum. The anterior and lateral walls of the false pelvis are the anterior and lateral muscles of the abdominal wall. Laterally, these muscles include the external and internal obliques and the transversus abdominis, which is the inner muscle layer (Fig. 27–7).[5, 6] The rectus

Figure 27–5. Free fluid *(curved arrow)* posterior to the cervix on a endovaginal longitudinal sonogram in a pregnant patient.

abdominis muscles are paired paramedian muscles oriented longitudinally on either side of the linea alba (see Figs. 27–7 and 27–8). The pelvic attachment of the rectus abdominis muscles is the crest of the pubis. The aponeuroses of the external and internal obliques and transversus muscles fuse with the anterior rectus abdominis fascia to form the linea alba in the midline. It should be noted that the anatomy of the rectus sheath is different above and below the arcuate line.[5] Below the arcuate line, a rectus sheath hematoma may

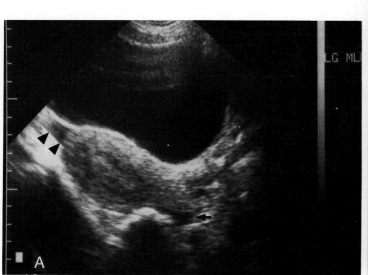

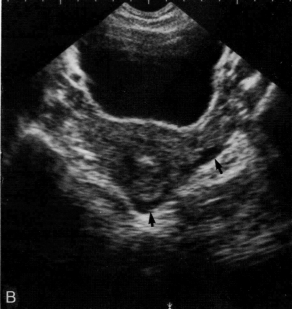

Figure 27–6. Transabdominal midline longitudinal *(A)* and transverse *(B)* sonograms with free intraperitoneal fluid in the posterior cul-de-sac *(arrows)* and anterior cul-de-sac *(arrowheads)*.

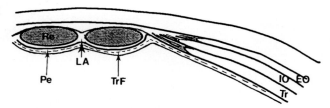

Figure 27–7. Diagram of a transverse section through the anterior abdominal wall, inferior to the arcuate line. Re, rectus abdominis; EO, external oblique; IO, internal oblique; Tr, transversus abdominis; Pe, peritoneum; LA, linea alba; TrF, transversalis fascia.

extend across the midline and displace the bladder posteriorly.[7] Above the arcuate line, however, a hematoma will be confined and not cross the midline. Without careful evaluation of the abdominal wall and the epicenter of the mass, a hematoma of the rectus sheath may be mistaken for a mass of pelvic origin.

Masses in the space of Retzius (also known as the prevesical or retropubic space) may also be confused with masses arising from the pelvic viscera. The space of Retzius is situated between the transversalis fascia and the extraperitoneal fascia (see Figs. 27–4 and 27–7).[5, 6] The transversalis fascia is a thin layer of connective tissue separating the transversus abdominis from the extraperitoneal fascia (see Fig. 27–7). Below the umbilicus, the extraperitoneal fascia presents two well-defined layers. The umbilical vesical fascia is the deeper of the two and is continuous with the vesical fascia. The umbilical prevesical fascia lies between the transversalis and umbilical vesical fasciae and is fused to the latter. It is also fused to the transversalis fascia along the medial umbilical ligaments and at the umbilicus. The resultant space between the transversalis fascia and the umbilical prevesical fascia is the space of Retzius. Sonographically, masses in the space of Retzius (usually hematomas or abscesses) displace the bladder posteriorly and can be differentiated from pelvic or abdominal masses that displace the bladder inferiorly or anteriorly.[8]

Muscles of the pelvis include those of the lower limb (psoas major, iliacus, piriformis, obturator internus) and the pelvic diaphragm (levator ani, coccygeus).[6, 9] The psoas major is a large triangular muscle that arises

from the lumbar transverse processes and the vertebral bodies and the disks of T12 to L2. It descends through the false pelvis on the pelvic sidewall anteriorly and exits posterior to the inguinal ligament (Fig. 27–9). It converges with the iliacus to form a tendon that inserts on the lesser trochanter of the femur. The iliacus arises from the concavity of the upper two thirds of the iliac fossa.

Sonographically, the psoas is seen in the lower abdomen in a paravertebral position. In a transverse sonogram of the lower abdomen, the psoas is rounded and hypoechoic. As the transducer is angled inferiorly, the psoas muscles diverge laterally and, in the false pelvis, assume a position medial and slightly anterior to the iliacus muscle (see Figs. 27–9 and 27–10). In the false pelvis, the iliac wings are identified as brightly echogenic linear structures with loss of distal sonic information (see Fig. 27–10). More inferiorly, within the true pelvis the iliacus/psoas muscle is seen as a hypoechoic, discretely marginated muscle with its two component muscles separated by a brightly echogenic line, which represents interposed fascia continuous with the psoas tendon (Fig. 27–11). The psoas may be demonstrated in its long axis by scanning in a longitudinal oblique plane (Fig. 27–12). In thin patients, the fasciculi of the psoas muscle may be identified (see Fig. 27–12). Movement of the normal psoas muscle may be seen with flexion of the hip.

The piriformis muscle arises from the sacrum between the pelvic sacral foramina and from the gluteal surface of the ilium (Fig. 27–13).[6, 9] On pelvic sonography, the piriformis can be identified posteriorly within the pelvis until it passes through the greater sciatic notch (Fig. 27–14) to insert onto the greater trochanter of the femur. The obturator internus muscle arises from the anterolateral pelvic wall surrounding the obturator foramen and passes through the lesser sciatic foramen to insert on the greater trochanter of the femur (Fig. 27–15).

The pelvic diaphragm is formed by the levator ani and coccygeus muscles. This is the most caudal structure of the pelvic cavity and can be routinely identified on TAS when the transducer is angled inferiorly (Fig. 27–16).

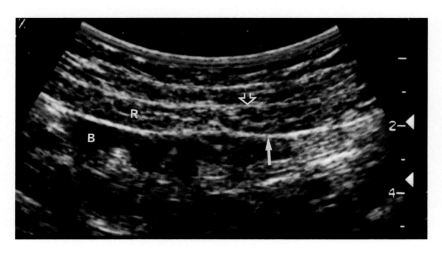

Figure 27–8. Transverse sonogram of anterior abdominal wall showing the anterior *(open arrow)* and posterior *(solid arrow)* rectus sheath. R, rectus abdominis muscle; B, bowel loops in the peritoneal cavity.

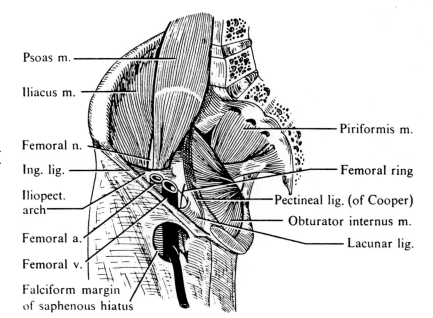

Figure 27–9. Diagram of the pelvic musculature. (From Pansky B: Review of Gross Anatomy, 5th ed. New York, Macmillan, 1987.)

Psoas m.

Iliacus m.

Femoral n.

Ing. lig.

Iliopect. arch

Femoral a.

Femoral v.

Falciform margin of saphenous hiatus

Piriformis m.

Femoral ring

Pectineal lig. (of Cooper)

Obturator internus m.

Lacunar lig.

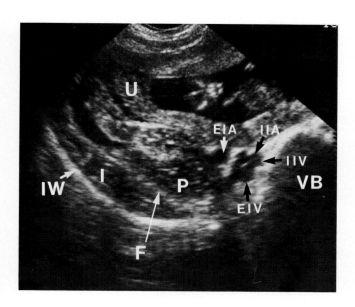

Figure 27–10. Transverse sonogram through the right iliac fossa, using the gravid uterus (U) as a sonic window, showing the relative positions of the iliacus (I) and psoas major (P) muscles separated by a fascial plane (F) in the false pelvis. The iliac vessels are medial to the psoas. EIA, external iliac artery; IIA, internal iliac artery; EIV, external iliac vein; IIV, internal iliac vein; VB, vertebral body; IW, iliac wing.

Figure 27–11. Transverse sonogram through the pelvic side wall, angled to the right to visualize the psoas major (P), the iliacus muscle (I), and the psoas tendon (Pt). The external iliac artery (EIA) and vein (V) are anterior to the iliopsoas muscle bundle.

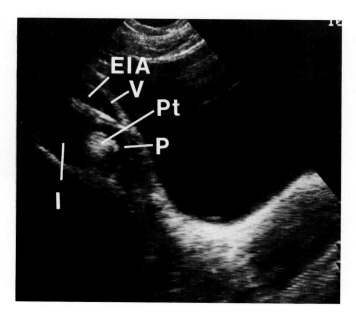

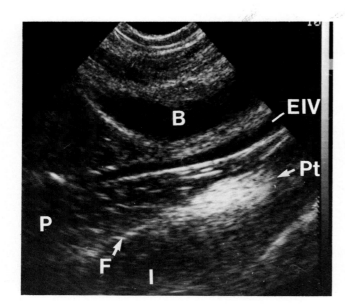

Figure 27–12. Coronal sonogram through the distended urinary bladder (B), with the transducer situated medially and angled laterally to visualize the psoas major (P) and the iliacus muscles (I) in their long axes. F, iliopsoas fascial plane; Pt, psoas tendon; EIV, external iliac vein.

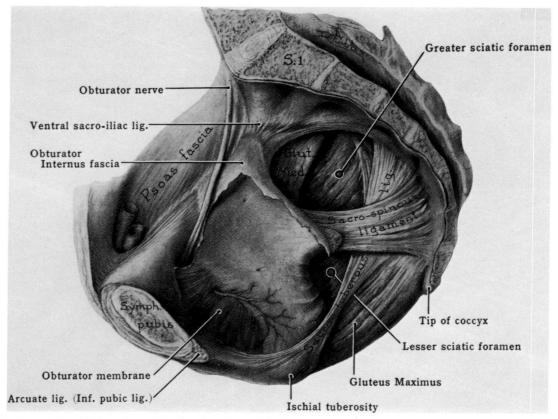

Figure 27–13. The muscles and ligaments of the lateral pelvic wall as viewed from the pelvis. (From Grant JCB: Grant's Atlas of Anatomy, 5th ed, p 217. Baltimore, Williams & Wilkins, 1962. Copyright 1962, the Williams & Wilkins Company.)

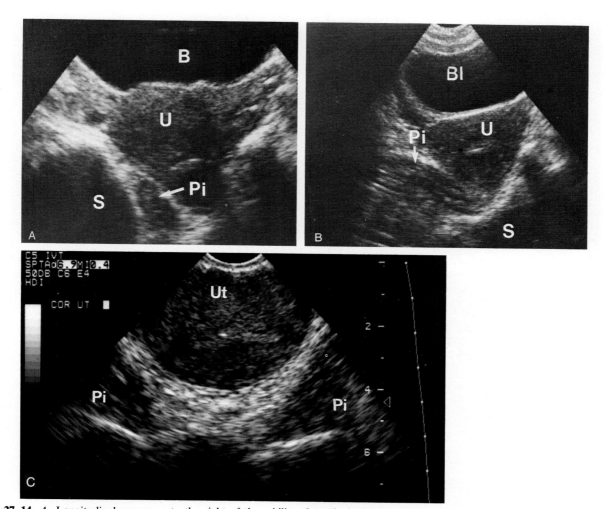

Figure 27–14. *A.* Longitudinal sonogram to the right of the midline through the bladder (B), showing the right piriformis muscle (Pi) in cross section. *B.* Transverse sonogram through the bladder (Bl), angled to the right, showing the right piriformis muscle (Pi) in its length. U, uterus; S, sacrum. *C.* Endovaginal coronal sonogram of the uterus anterior to the paired piriformis muscles.

Figure 27–15. Transverse sonogram through the bladder (B), at the level of the vagina (V), showing the obturator internus muscles (OI) bilaterally.

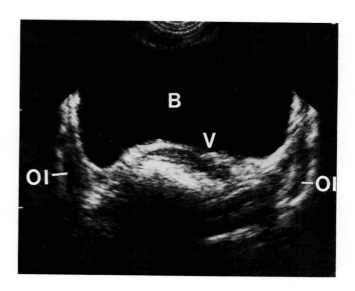

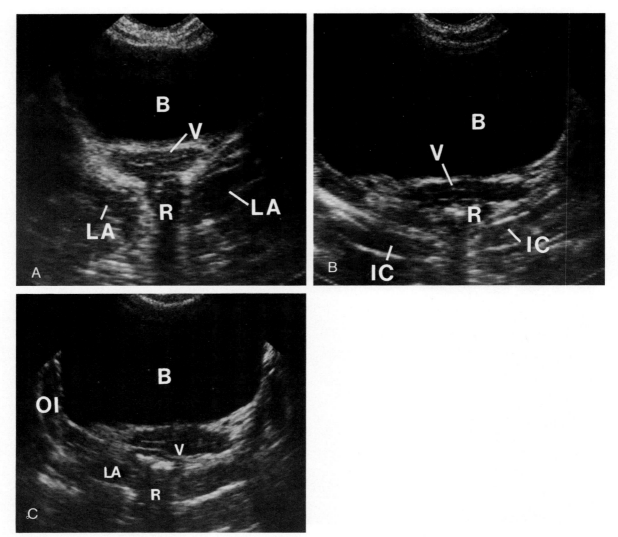

Figure 27–16. *A* and *B.* Transverse sonogram through the bladder (B), angled caudally, showing the levator ani (LA) and iliococcygeus (IC) muscles. *C.* Transverse sonogram with slightly less caudal angulation than in *A* or *B,* showing the obturator internus (OI) and levator ani (LA) muscles. R, anal canal; V, vagina.

VASCULAR ANATOMY

The common iliac arteries course anteriorly and medially to the psoas muscles (Fig. 27–17).[6, 10, 11] The right common iliac vein ascends posteriorly and then laterally to the right common iliac artery. The left common iliac vein ascends medially and then posteriorly to the left common iliac artery. The common iliac arteries bifurcate to form the external and internal iliac arteries. The external iliac arteries supply most of the lower limbs. The internal iliac arteries supply the pelvic viscera, walls of the pelvis, perineum, and gluteal regions (Fig. 27–18).

The external iliac arteries course through the false pelvis without entering the true pelvis. In the nongravid state, the caliber of the external iliac arteries is greater than that of the internal iliac arteries. The external iliac arteries assume a course adjacent to the medial psoas border and exit the pelvis through the femoral canals at the level of the inguinal ligaments (see Figs. 27–9, 27–10, and 27–17). The right external iliac vein ascends medially and then posteriorly to the right external iliac artery. The left external iliac vein is medial to the left external iliac artery.[6, 10, 11] The internal iliac arteries arise at the bifurcation of the common iliac arteries at the level of the L5/S1 disk immediately anterior to the sacroiliac joints. They course approximately 4 cm posteriorly to the superior margin of the greater sciatic foramen. The internal iliac arteries divide into anterior and posterior trunks, which pass posteriorly into the greater sciatic foramina. The anterior division divides into seven branches: (1) umbilical and superior vesicle; (2) uterine; (3) vaginal; (4) middle rectal; (5) obturator; (6) internal pudendal; and (7) inferior gluteal. The posterior division divides into the iliolumbar, lateral sacral, and superior gluteal (see Fig. 27–18). High-velocity, high-impedance flow is the characteristic Doppler signal of the internal and external iliac arteries (Fig. 27–19).[12] Anterior to the internal iliac arteries are the ureters, ovaries, and fimbriated ends of the uterine tubes (see Fig. 27–17). The internal iliac veins are posterior to their respective arteries.

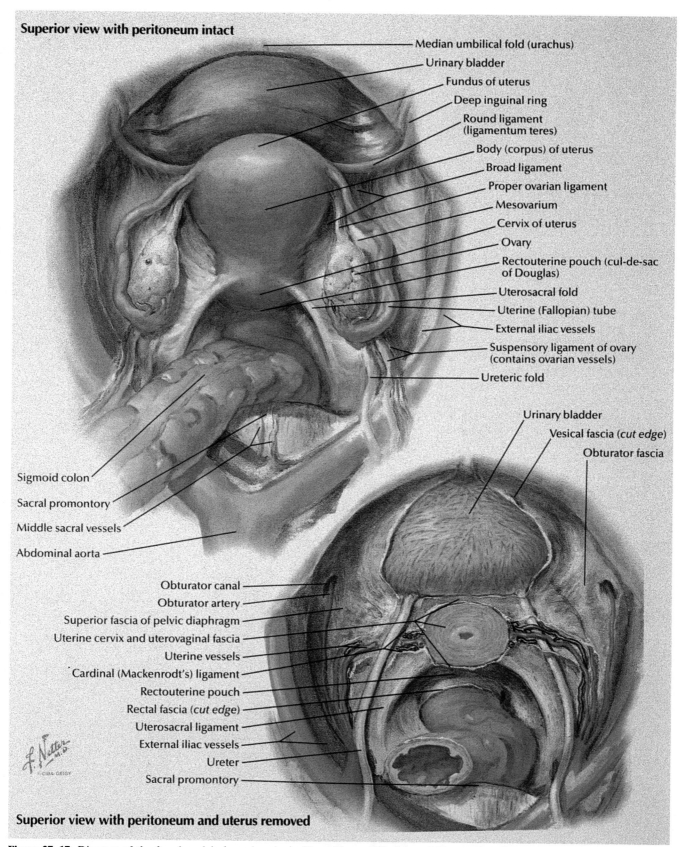

Superior view with peritoneum intact

Median umbilical fold (urachus)
Urinary bladder
Fundus of uterus
Deep inguinal ring
Round ligament (ligamentum teres)
Body (corpus) of uterus
Broad ligament
Proper ovarian ligament
Mesovarium
Cervix of uterus
Ovary
Rectouterine pouch (cul-de-sac of Douglas)
Uterosacral fold
Uterine (Fallopian) tube
External iliac vessels
Suspensory ligament of ovary (contains ovarian vessels)
Ureteric fold

Sigmoid colon
Sacral promontory
Middle sacral vessels
Abdominal aorta

Urinary bladder
Vesical fascia (cut edge)
Obturator fascia

Obturator canal
Obturator artery
Superior fascia of pelvic diaphragm
Uterine cervix and uterovaginal fascia
Uterine vessels
Cardinal (Mackenrodt's) ligament
Rectouterine pouch
Rectal fascia (cut edge)
Uterosacral ligament
External iliac vessels
Ureter
Sacral promontory

Superior view with peritoneum and uterus removed

Figure 27–17. Diagram of the female pelvis (superior view). (From Netter FH: Atlas of Human Anatomy, plate 348. West Caldwell, NJ, CIBA-Geigy Co, 1989.)

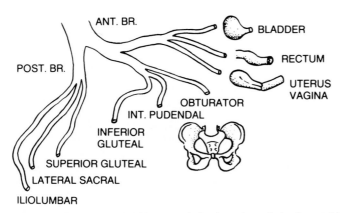

ANT. BR.
BLADDER
POST. BR.
RECTUM
UTERUS
VAGINA
OBTURATOR
INT. PUDENDAL
INFERIOR GLUTEAL
SUPERIOR GLUTEAL
LATERAL SACRAL
ILIOLUMBAR

Figure 27–18. Schematic diagram of the branches of the internal iliac arteries and the pelvic viscera that they supply.

Occasionally, the division of the internal iliac artery into the anterior and posterior branches can be seen on EVS (Fig. 27–20).

The uterine artery, an important branch of the anterior trunk, runs medially on the levator ani to the cervix. Approximately 2 cm from the cervix, it crosses superiorly and anteriorly to the ureter (Fig. 27–21). The uterine artery ascends lateral to the uterus in the broad ligament to the junction of the fallopian tubes and the uterus (Fig. 27–22). From the cornua of the uterus, the uterine artery courses laterally to reach the hilum of the ovary, and it ends by joining with the ovarian artery. The uterine arteries anastomose extensively with each other across the midline through anterior and posterior arcuate arteries.[6, 11, 13] The arcuate arteries run within the broad ligament and then enter the myometrium (see Figs. 27–17 and 27–21).

Doppler waveforms of uterine artery flow are typically a high-velocity, high-resistance pattern.[14]

The uterine plexus of veins accompanies the arcuate arteries, passing circumferentially within the myometrium. The venous plexus is larger than the associated arterial channels and is frequently identified sonographically by both the transabdominal and endovaginal approaches (Figs. 27–23 and 27–24).

The ovarian arteries arise from the lateral margin of the aorta at a level slightly inferior to the renal arteries. At the pelvic brim, they cross the external iliac artery and vein and course medially within the suspensory (infundibulopelvic) ligament of the ovary (see Figs. 27–21 and 27–25). The ovarian artery passes posteriorly in the mesovarium and breaks up into branches (see Fig. 27–25).[10]

The right ovarian vein empties into the inferior vena cava just below the renal vein. The left ovarian vein empties into the left renal vein. Physiologic variations of the Doppler waveforms of the ovarian artery are seen with cyclical changes. The phase just preceding ovulation and the secretory phase typically demonstrate high systolic and high diastolic flow.[14] Low-velocity, high-resistance flow is seen in the dormant ovary (Fig. 27–26).[12, 15]

The lymph nodes and lymphatic channels are not normally visualized by sonography. However, knowledge of the location of the major lymph node groups is important to recognize them when they are pathologically enlarged. The main groups are (1) the common iliac lymph nodes that accompany the common iliac artery; (2) the external iliac lymph nodes that are situated in the false pelvis and pelvic side wall lateral to the bladder and are associated with the external

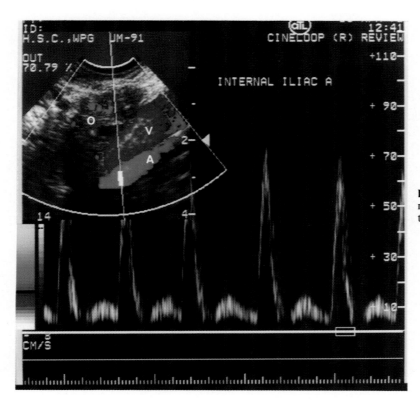

Figure 27–19. Color and pulsed-wave Doppler examination of the internal iliac artery demonstrating characteristic high-velocity, high-impedence flow.

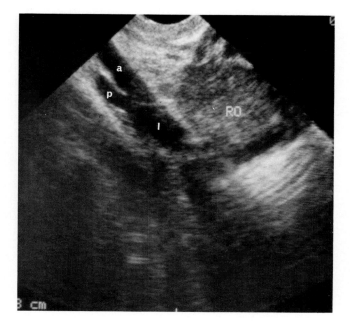

Figure 27–20. Endovaginal sonogram through the right pelvis showing the internal iliac artery (I) and the posterior (p) and anterior (a) divisions. RO, right ovary.

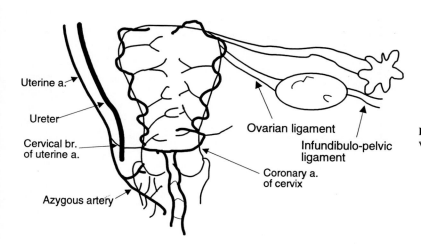

Figure 27–21. Diagram of the ovarian, uterine, and vaginal arteries and the ipsilateral ureter.

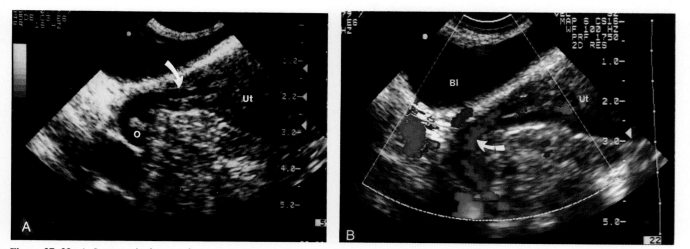

Figure 27–22. *A.* Endovaginal coronal sonogram through the right adnexal region showing vessels *(curved arrow)* as they enter the uterus at the junction of the uterus (U) and right fallopian tube. o, ovary. *B.* Similar view with color Doppler study showing precisely the location of the arteries and veins. Bl, bladder.

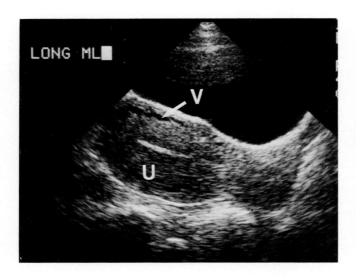

Figure 27–23. Longitudinal midline sonogram of the uterus (U) through the bladder, demonstrating the uterine plexus of veins (V) within the myometrium, between the middle and outer layers.

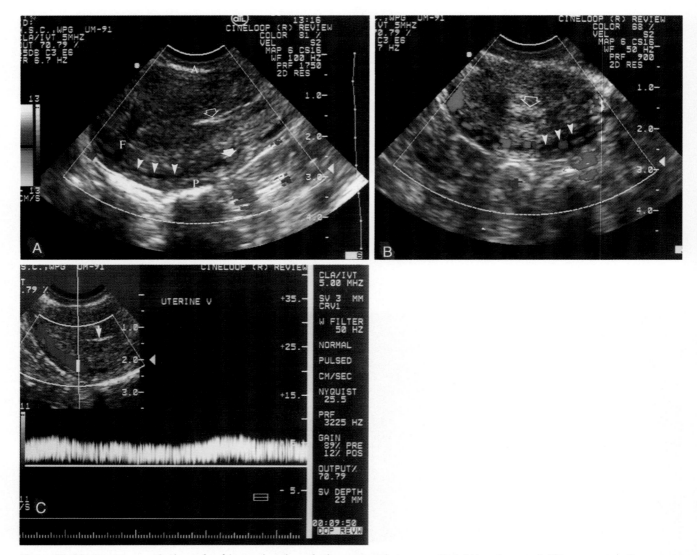

Figure 27–24. Arcuate vessels *(arrowheads)* coursing through the myometrium on sagittal *(A)* and coronal *(B)* sonograms. Open arrow indicates endometrium. F, uterine fundus; A, anterior; P, posterior. *C.* Endovaginal coronal sonogram with color Doppler and pulsed Doppler waveform of the arcuate veins *(cursor)* in the myometrium. Arrow points to endometrium.

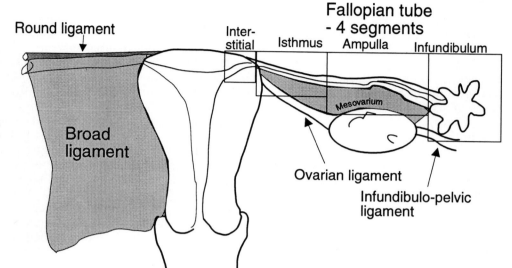

Figure 27–25. Diagram of the ovary, uterus, and adjacent peritoneal reflection and ligaments.

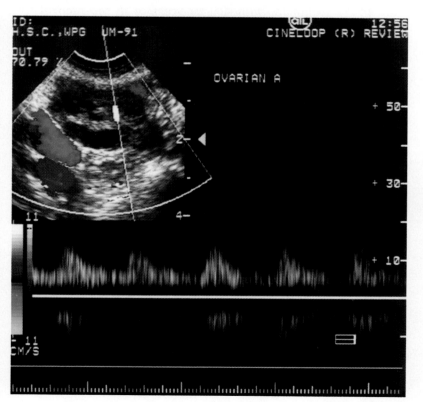

Figure 27–26. Pulsed Doppler scan through a terminal branch of the ovarian artery *(cursor)* showing low-velocity, low-resistance flow.

iliac artery and vein; and (3) the internal iliac lymph nodes that surround the internal iliac vessels. Outlying groups include the sacral and obturator nodes.

The lymphatic drainage of the pelvic viscera is variable. The following is a general guideline to drainage of specific viscera, which is important in assessing nodal spread in neoplasia:

1. *Ovaries*: The lymphatic channels ascend along the ovarian arteries to the lateral aortic and periaortic nodes at the level of the renal hila.

2. *Cervix*: The lymphatic channels course lateral in the parametrium to the external iliac nodes, posterolateral to the internal iliac nodes, and posterior to the rectal or sacral nodes.

3. *Uterus, lower corpus*: The lymphatics course lateral to the external iliacs through the parametrium.

4. *Uterus, lower corpus, fundus, and tube*: The lymphatics accompany the ovarian channels.

5. *Vagina*: The lymphatics of the upper vagina accompany the uterine artery to the internal and external iliac lymph nodes, whereas those of the midvagina accompany the vaginal artery to the internal iliac lymph nodes. The vagina external to the hymen drains to the superficial inguinal nodes.[16] This reflects the embryologic origin of the vagina, in which the fibromuscular wall of the upper two thirds of the vagina arises from the paramesonephric (müllerian) duct, which also gives rise to the uterus and fallopian tubes. The lower one third of the vagina arises from the urogenital sinus and therefore shares the lymphatic drainage with the external genitalia.

THE OVARIES

The ovaries are ellipsoid, with the long axis usually oriented vertically when the bladder is empty. Ovarian location is variable, especially in women who have been pregnant. In the nulliparous female, the ovaries are situated in the ovarian fossa (also known as the fossa of Waldeyer (Fig. 27–27).[6, 17, 18] The ovarian fossa is situated on the lateral pelvic wall and is bounded by the obliterated umbilical artery anteriorly, the ureter and internal iliac artery posteriorly, and the external iliac vein superiorly. On the superior surface of the ovary are attached the ovarian fimbria of the uterine tube and suspensory ligament of the ovary (see Fig. 27–25). The suspensory ligament of the ovary is a fold of peritoneum that arises from the pelvic sidewall and contains the ovarian vessels and nerves. The ovarian ligament extends between the medial pole of the ovary and the ipsilateral uterine cornua. Ovarian size varies depending on age, menstrual status, pregnancy status, body habitus, and phase of the menstrual cycle.[19] Cohen and colleagues[20] measured ovarian volumes in premenarchal, menstruating, and postmenopausal subjects. In menstruating subjects the mean ovarian volume was 9.8 cm³ with 5% and 95% confidence intervals of 2.5 and 21.9 cm³. For premenarchal girls the mean was 3.0 cm³ with 5% and 95% confidence intervals of 0.2 and 9.1 cm³, and for postmenopausal patients the mean was 5.8 cm³ with confidence intervals of 1.2 and 14.9 cm³. Minor cyclical changes in volume were also identified, with highest volumes in the preovulatory phase and lowest volumes in the luteal phase.

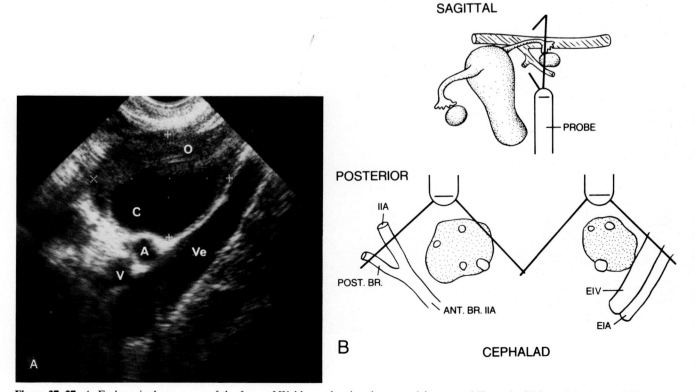

Figure 27–27. *A*. Endovaginal sonogram of the fossa of Waldeyer showing the ovary (o), external iliac vein (Ve), and the internal iliac artery (A) and vein (V). c, ovarian cyst. *B*. A schematic diagram of the scan plane of *A*. The transducer was initially in the sagittal plane and angled to the right to obtain the image of the fossa of Waldeyer and the surrounding vessels.

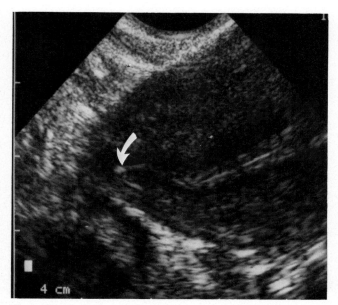

Figure 27–28. Endovaginal coronal sonogram angled to the right showing the uterus and interstitial portion of the fallopian tube *(curved arrow).*

THE FALLOPIAN (UTERINE) TUBE

The fallopian tube is approximately 10 cm in length and lies in the superior part of the broad ligament. The fimbriated end is open to the peritoneal cavity and has an ostium measuring approximately 3 mm in diameter. The medial third is referred to as the isthmus, which is round and cordlike (see Fig. 27–25). The intramural or interstitial portion of the fallopian tube is approximately 1 cm in length[17, 21] and is well seen with EVS (Fig. 27–28). The isthmus and ampullary

portions of the tube are usually visualized only when diseased (i.e., filled with fluid or when surrounded by fluid).

THE UTERUS AND VAGINA

The uterus is located in the true pelvis, between the urinary bladder anteriorly and the rectosigmoid posteriorly. Uterine position is highly variable and changes with varying degrees of bladder and rectal distention. The cervix projects through the anterior vaginal wall, separating the vagina into the anterior, posterior, and two lateral fornices. The cervix can be identified sonographically in the sagittal plane as that portion of the uterus immediately posterior to the angle of the bladder (see Fig. 27–1). The cervix is anchored at the angle of the bladder by the parametrium and is less freely movable than the corpus and fundus. The cervix and the vagina form a 90° angle, a condition referred to as anteversion. The more movable corpus is usually flexed anteriorly on the cervix (anteflexed). Filling of the bladder usually straightens out the uterus so that on TAS the uterus does not appear anteflexed and the angle between the cervix and vagina is greater than 90°. Retroversion of the uterus and tilting of the uterus to the right or the left are considered to be normal variants in position.[17] Retroversion of the uterus can result in poor visualization of the endometrial canal on TAS and widening of the adnexa due to visualization of the broad ligaments. In addition, because of attenuation of sound by the uterus, the fundus of a retroverted uterus may be "echo poor" in appearance (Fig. 27–29A). This "dropout" phenomenon may simulate the appearance of a fundal fibroid. The differentiation between the fundal fibroid and dropout of sound may

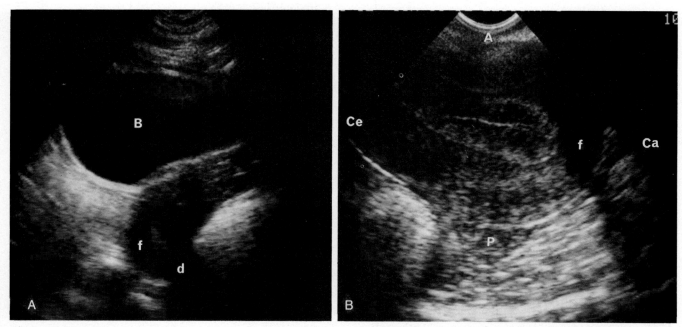

Figure 27–29. *A.* Longitudinal transvesical sonogram of a retroverted uterus demonstrating "dropout" (d) artifact in the uterine fundus (f). B, bladder. *B.* Endovaginal sonogram in the sagittal plane of a retroverted uterus. The fundus (f) is directed caudally and displayed on the right of the image. A, anterior; P, posterior; Ce, cephalad; Ca, caudad.

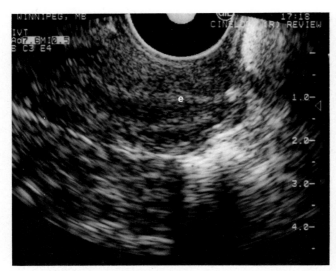

Figure 27–30. Endovaginal sonogram through the cervix showing the endocervical stripe (e), a continuation of the endometrium from the fundus and body of the uterus.

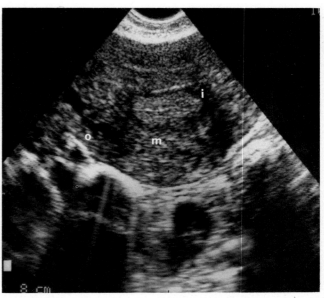

Figure 27–32. The three zones of the myometrium: hypoechoic inner layer (i), middle zone (m), and outer layer (o).

be made by the lack of displacement of the endometrial canal and the lack of a contour abnormality of the latter. Alternatively, dropout in the fundus of a retroverted uterus is usually not a problem in EVS (Fig. 27–29B). The endovaginal approach may be used to assess the presence or absence of a fibroid when the fundus of a retroverted uterus is echo poor on TAS.

The cervix is best visualized endovaginally with the tip of the probe about 2 to 3 cm from it. The endocervical canal is a continuation of the endometrial canal, appearing as a thin echogenic stripe (Fig. 27–30). Fluid is sometimes seen in the endocervical canal, particularly in the preovulatory period. Occasionally, air can be seen in the vaginal fornices surrounding the cervix (Fig. 27–31).

The three zones of the myometrium consist of a hypoechoic inner layer, the thicker more echogenic middle zone, and the outer layer, which is separated from the middle zone by the arcuate plexus of arteries and veins (Fig. 27–32).

The endometrium varies in thickness and echogenicity depending on the menstrual phase, age, parity, and estrogen replacement therapy.[22] Total endometrial thickness should not exceed 14 to 16 mm premenopausally and 0.8 mm in the postmenopausal patient.[23, 24] The sonographic appearance of the endometrium changes cyclically with the menstrual cycle. In the early proliferative phase (days 5 to 9), the endometrium is seen as a thin echogenic line (see Fig. 27–24C). In the late proliferative phase (days 10 to 14), the functional zone of the endometrium increases in thickness under the influence of estrogen and is hypoechoic compared with the echogenic basal layer (Fig. 27–33). During the secretory phase (days 15 to 28), the functional layer of the endometrium becomes thickened, soft, and edematous under the influence of progesterone. The glandular epithelium secretes a glycogen-rich fluid, and the spiral arteries become tortuous. The combination of these factors results in increased echogenicity of the functional layer, which becomes isoechoic with the basal layer (see Fig. 27–32).

The anterior surface of the uterus is covered with peritoneum to the level of the junction between the uterine corpus and cervix.[17] The peritoneal space anterior to the uterus is the vesicouterine pouch or anterior cul-de-sac (see Fig. 27–4). This space is usually empty but may contain loops of small bowel. Posteriorly, the peritoneal reflection extends to the posterior fornix of the vagina, forming the posterior cul-de-sac. Laterally, the peritoneal reflection forms the broad ligaments.

The vagina is seen as a hypoechoic tubular structure with an echogenic lumen that curves inferiorly over

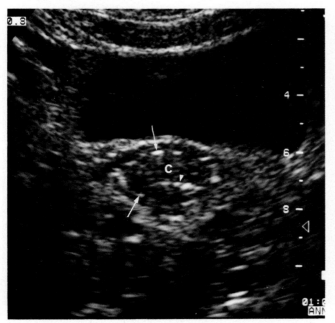

Figure 27–31. Air in the vaginal fornices surrounding the cervix (c, *arrows*). Cervical os is indicated by arrowhead.

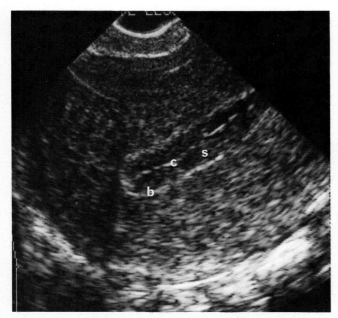

Figure 27–33. Endovaginal sonogram demonstrating the three layers of the endometrium: compact inner layer (c), deeper spongy layer (s), and basal layer (b).

the muscular perineal body at the introitus (Fig. 27–34). The bladder, trigone, and urethra are anterior to the vagina, and the rectum is posterior. The distal ureters are lateral to the upper vagina and pass anteriorly to enter the bladder.[17, 25] The posterior fornix of the vagina is closely related to the rectouterine recess of the peritoneal cavity (posterior cul-de-sac)[17] and is separated by the thickness of the vaginal wall and peritoneal membrane (see Figs. 27–4 and 27–6).

THE URETERS

The ureters are muscular tubes that measure 25 to 30 cm in length in the adult. In the pelvis, the ureters course within the extraperitoneal areolar tissue. In the true pelvis the ureter begins anterior to the internal iliac artery and posterior to the ovary (Fig. 27–35). From there it courses anteriorly and medially to lie within the inferior medial portion of the broad ligament, where it is in close proximity to the uterine artery. The ureter then runs anterior, situated in front of the lateral fornices of the vagina, about 2 cm lateral to the supravaginal cervix, and then passes medially to enter the trigone of the bladder anterior to the vagina (Fig. 27–36).[25] The relationships of the ureter to the ovary, cervix, uterine artery, and vagina are of clinical importance because pelvic pathology may result in secondary hydronephrosis due to ureteric obstruction (Fig. 27–37). As a result, we routinely evaluate the kidneys after the postvoid examination during gynecologic sonography. This is done to confirm the presence of two kidneys, to assess their position, and to identify any degree of obstructive uropathy.

THE URINARY BLADDER

The bladder is a distensible reservoir for urine. Its shape depends on the degree of distention of itself and neighboring viscera. The bladder is fixed inferiorly at the urethral orifice, base, and angle; and as it fills, the remainder of the walls displace moveable viscera and conform to the space available within the confines of the true pelvis.[25] A transverse scan through the bladder superiorly gives it a rounded appearance. More inferiorly, the pelvic musculature and bones cause the bladder to appear square in the transverse plane (Fig. 27–38). The bladder wall is echogenic and should be of uniform thickness.

Endovaginal scanning enables better visualization of the trigone, posterior wall, and urethra. The ureteric

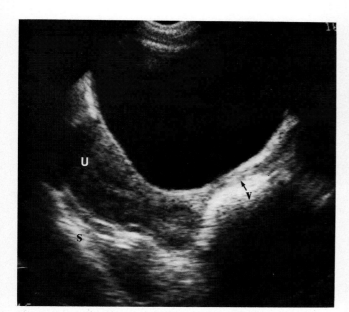

Figure 27–34. Midline longitudinal transabdominal sonogram of the uterus (u) and vagina (v). The vagina curves inferiorly over the perineal body. s, sacrum.

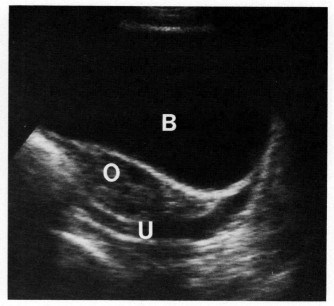

Figure 27–35. Longitudinal transabdominal sonogram of the right ovary (O) with a dilated ureter (U) demonstrated immediately posterior. B, bladder.

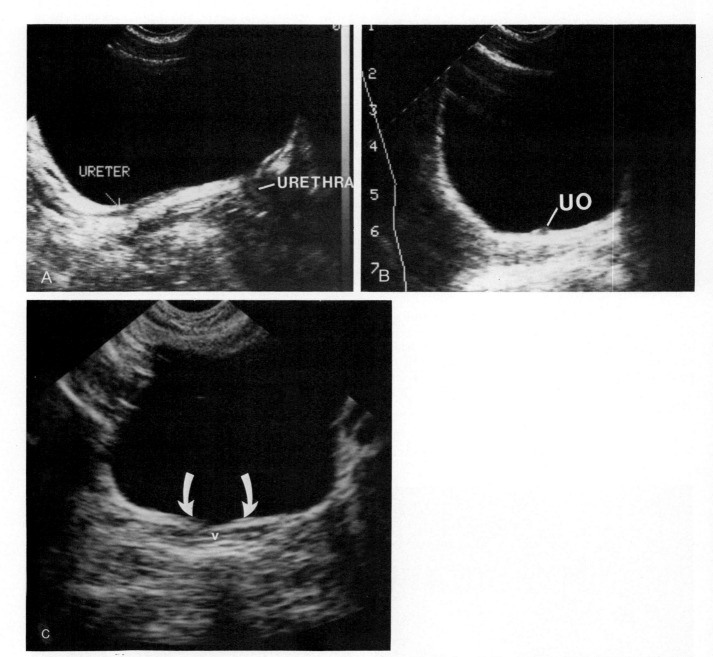

Figure 27–36. *A.* Longitudinal transabdominal sonogram of the right ureter and the urethra. *B.* Longitudinal transabdominal sonogram of the right ureteric orifice (uo). *C.* Transverse transabdominal sonogram of both ureteric orifices *(curved arrows).* V, vagina.

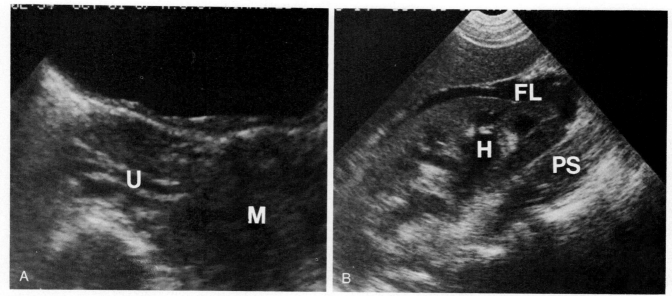

Figure 27–37. *A.* Longitudinal transvesical sonogram of the distal right ureter (U). A mass (M) is noted encasing and obstructing the distal ureter in this patient with carcinoma of the cervix with direct local extension. *B.* Coronal sonogram of the right kidney. There is hydronephrosis (H) secondary to the distal ureteric obstruction. A urinoma (FL) is present within the perirenal space. Ps, psoas major.

and urethral orifices are visualized at the base and neck of the bladder, respectively. The urethra can be seen throughout its length by translabial scanning. The probe is placed at the introitus or just partially inserted into the vagina.

THE LIGAMENTS

The broad ligaments extend from the lateral aspect of the uterus to the lateral pelvic sidewalls (see Fig.

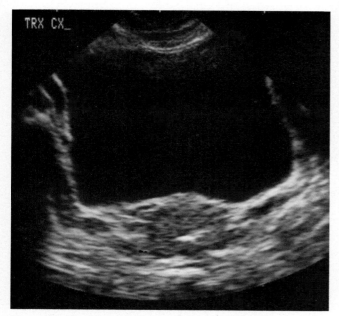

Figure 27–38. "Square" shape of the bladder on a transverse sonogram through the inferior portion of the pelvis.

27–25). The free border of the broad ligament contains the uterine (fallopian) tube.

The broad ligaments may be identified sonographically when they are outlined by free intraperitoneal fluid (Fig. 27–39) or when the uterus is retroverted. The portion of the broad ligament between the fallopian tube and the ligament of the ovary and mesovarium is the mesosalpinx. The ovary is attached to the posterior layer of the broad ligament by the mesovarium.[6, 17]

The portion of the ligament that extends from the infundibulum of the tube and upper pole of the ovary to the pelvic sidewall is referred to as the suspensory ligament of the ovary. In it course the ovarian vessels and nerves. The round ligaments arise in the uterine cornua, anterior to the fallopian tubes in the broad ligaments, and extend anterolaterally to run beneath the inguinal ligament and insert into the fascia of the labia majora. The mesovarium, mesosalpinx, and round ligaments are not identified sonographically. The suspensory ligament of the ovary is usually not seen; however, the ovarian artery within the ligament may be identified occasionally with TAS or EVS.

THE RECTOSIGMOID COLON

The sigmoid colon begins at the inlet of the true pelvis and is extremely variable in length. It has a mesentery, and its course is variable, looping either to the left or right before ascending on the left to join the descending colon. The rectum begins at the third sacral vertebra and is fixed in position.[6]

The rectosigmoid colon usually contains gas and fecal material that cast an acoustic shadow and may make

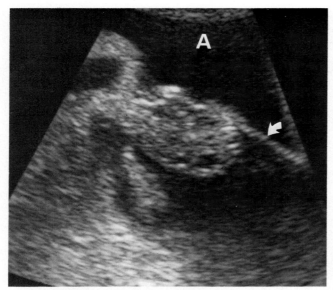

Figure 27–39. Transverse sonogram in a patient with gross ascites *(A)*. The broad ligament *(arrow)* is well visualized.

identification or differentiation from pelvic masses difficult. Often the differentiation between a pelvic mass and the rectosigmoid colon can be made by real-time imaging if peristalsis can be visualized. Differentiation between bowel contents and a mass is not usually a problem if the endovaginal approach is used (Fig. 27–40).

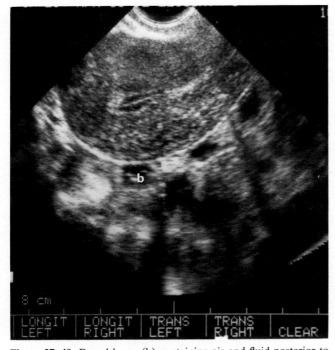

Figure 27–40. Bowel loops (b) containing air and fluid posterior to uterus on an endovaginal sagittal sonogram.

References

1. Kurtz AB, Rifkin MD: Normal anatomy of the female pelvis. In Callen PW (ed): Ultrasonography in Obstetrics and Gynecology, pp 193–208. Philadelphia, WB Saunders, 1983.
2. Osteology: Skeleton of lower limb. In Williams PM, Warwick R (eds): Gray's Anatomy, 36th ed, pp 378–390. Edinburgh, Churchill Livingstone, 1980.
3. Fiske CE, Callen PW: Fluid collections ultrasonically simulating urinary bladder. J Can Assoc Radiol 31:254, 1980.
4. Levi CS, Lyons EA, Schollenberg J, Bristowe JRB: The value of post void scans in the diagnosis of ruptured ectopic pregnancy. J Ultrasound Med 1:253, 1982.
5. Myology: Fasciae and muscles of the trunk. In Williams PM, Warwick R (eds): Gray's Anatomy, 36th ed, pp 551–564. Edinburgh, Churchill Livingstone, 1980.
6. Gardner E, Gray DJ, O'Rhahilly R: The pelvis. In: Anatomy: A Regional Study of Human Structure, 5th ed, pp 445–512. Philadelphia, WB Saunders, 1986.
7. Benson M: Rectus sheath haematomas simulating pelvic pathology: The ultrasound appearances. Clin Radiol 33:651, 1982.
8. Spring DB, Deshon GE Jr, Babu S: The sonographic appearance of fluid in the prevesical space. Radiology 147:205, 1983.
9. Myology: Fasciae and muscles of the lower limb. In Williams PM, Warwick R (eds): Gray's Anatomy, 36 ed, pp 593–595. Edinburgh, Churchill Livingstone, 1980.
10. Angiology: Iliac arterial system. In Williams PM, Warwick R (eds): Gray's Anatomy, 36th ed, pp 719–724. Edinburgh, Churchill Livingstone, 1980.
11. Angiology: Veins of the abdomen and pelvis. In Williams PM, Warwick R (eds): Gray's Anatomy, 36th ed, pp 759–765. Edinburgh, Churchill Livingstone, 1980.
12. Thaler I, Manor D, Rottem S, et al: Hemodynamic evaluation of the female pelvic vessels using a high-frequency transvaginal image-directed Doppler system. J Clin Ultrasound 18:364, 1990.
13. DuBose TJ, Hill LW, Hennigan HW Jr, et al: Sonography of arcuate uterine blood vessels. J Ultrasound Med 4:299, 1985.
14. Kurjak A, Zaker D, Kupesic-Urek S: Normal pelvic blood flow. In Kurjak A (ed): Transvaginal Color Doppler. Park Ridge, NJ, Parthenon Publishing Group, 1991.
15. Taylor KJW, Burns PN, Wells RJT, et al: Ultrasound Doppler flow studies of the ovarian and uterine arteries. Br J Obstet Gynecol 92:249, 1985.
16. Angiology: The lymphatic drainage of the abdomen and pelvis. In Williams PM, Warwick R (eds): Gray's Anatomy, 36th ed, pp 793–798. Edinburgh, Churchill Livingstone, 1980.
17. Splanchnology: Reproductive organs of the female. In Williams PM, Warwick R (eds): Gray's Anatomy, 36th ed, pp 1423–1433. Edinburgh, Churchill Livingstone, 1980.
18. Hall DH: Sonographic appearance of the normal ovary, of polycystic ovary disease, and of functional ovarian cysts. Semin Ultrasound 4:149, 1983.
19. Fleischer AC, McKee MS, Gordon AN, et al: Transvaginal sonography of post-menopausal ovaries with pathologic correlation. J Ultrasound Med 9:637, 1990.
20. Cohen H, Tice H, Mandel F: Ovarian volumes measured by ultrasound: Bigger than we think. Radiology 177:189, 1990.
21. Timor-Tritsch IE, Rottem S: Transvaginal ultrasonographic study of the fallopian tube. Obstet Gynecol 70:424, 1987.
22. Mendelson EB, Bohm-Velez M, Neiman HL, et al: Transvaginal sonography in gynecological imaging. Semin Ultrasound CT MR 9:102, 1988.
23. Mendelson EB, Bohm-Velez M, Joseph N, et al: Endometrial abnormalities: Evaluation with transvaginal sonography. AJR 150:139, 1988.
24. Lin MC, Gosink BB, Wolf SI, et al: Endometrial thickness after menopause: Effect of hormone replacement. Radiology 180:427, 1991.
25. Splanchnology: The urinary organs. In Williams PM, Warwick R (eds): Gray's Anatomy, 36th ed, pp 1387–1423. Edinburgh, Churchill Livingstone, 1980.

CHAPTER 28

Ultrasound Evaluation of Normal and Induced Ovulation

WILLIAM G. M. RITCHIE, M.D.

Before the advent of ultrasonography, only presumptive evidence of follicular development and ovulation was readily available. The widespread use of ultrasound evaluation and a growing interest in female infertility have dramatically increased our understanding of the ovulatory cycle. In this chapter we provide an overview of the sonographic findings in normal and induced ovulatory functions. A thorough understanding of these features is essential for correct interpretation of routine female pelvic sonograms and follicular development studies performed for the management and treatment of infertility.

The periodic release of oocytes is the primary function of the ovary, and this process is associated with the cyclic release of the steroid hormones, estrogen and progesterone. At birth, the ovaries contain at least 150,000 eggs, each consisting of an oocyte that has already entered the maturation cycle and is arrested in the prophase of the first maturation division. No further formation of eggs occurs after birth, and some of these eggs must lie dormant in the ovary for more than 40 years before they either complete their maturation and ovulate or degenerate.[1] The primary oocyte is surrounded by a single layer of granulosa cells to form a primordial follicle (Fig. 28–1). The initiation of early

follicular growth to the next stage of maturation, with formation of a preantral follicle, is a continous process independent of neuroendocrine control. This process starts before birth so that even by menarche there has been a significant depletion of the initial pool of primordial follicles. This process continues throughout the reproductive life, remaining uninterrupted even during pregnancy, until the supply of primordial follicles is depleted. Of the initial large number of primordial follicles, only about 400 undergo the full maturation process to develop into antral or graafian follicles capable of ovulating during the reproductive life of the woman; the remainder undergo limited or incomplete maturation and subsequently become atretic and degenerate.[1]

Puberty is heralded by the onset of the pulsatile release of gonadotropin releasing hormone (GnRH) from the hypothalamus. With activation of the hypothalamic-pituitary-ovarian endocrine axis, repetitive cyclic follicular development, beyond the preantral phase, occurs with follicular maturation and ovulation, corpus luteum formation, and regression (Fig. 28–2). This pattern continues throughout the reproductive lifetime, being interrupted normally only by pregnancy. The rate at which inactive primordial follicles begin to

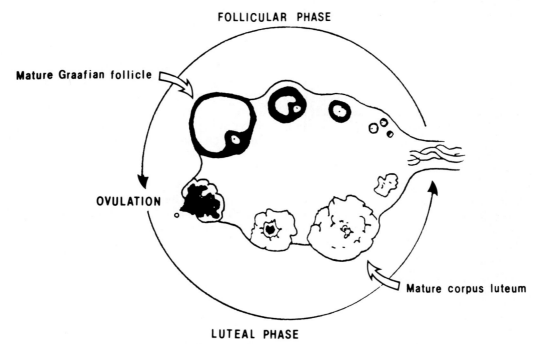

Figure 28–1. Diagrammatic representation of the ovulatory cycle demonstrating follicular maturation and ovulation with subsequent corpus luteum formation. (From Ritchie WGM: Sonographic evaluation of normal and induced ovulation. Radiology 161:1, 1986.)

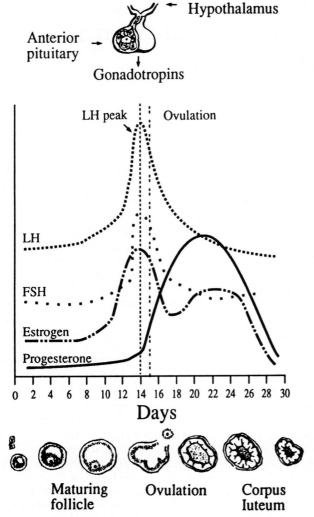

Figure 28–2. The temporal relationship of gonadotropin (follicle-stimulating hormone [FSH] and luteinizing hormone [LH]) and ovarian steroid (estrogen and progesterone) secretion in the normal menstrual cycle.

Under the influence of FSH there is proliferation of the granulosa cells of the follicle with production of estrogen, accumulation of antral fluid, and induction of LH receptors. All of these events lead to the formation of a mature antral graafian follicle that secretes large amounts of estrogen into the circulation. The increase of circulating estrogen triggers the release of LH, which induces luteinization of the granulosa cells and initiates progesterone production, rupture of the follicle with expulsion of the egg, and subsequent formation of a corpus luteum with continued progesterone production. As the effect of LH on the corpus luteum regresses, production of estrogen and progesterone declines and endometrial shedding (menstruation) occurs.[2]

SONOGRAPHIC FEATURES OF THE NORMAL CYCLE

With activation of the hypothalamic-pituitary-ovarian endocrine axis at puberty, the ovaries and uterus rapidly enlarge to their adult configuration and size. Ovarian growth and the appearance of cysts may be noted several years before puberty. The change in uterine size is much more abrupt. The ovaries are the only organ in the peritoneal cavity not invested in the peritoneum.[1] They are covered by a single layer of germinal epithelium in continuity with the squamous epithelium of the peritoneum. Beneath the germinal layer is the fibrous capsule of the ovary, the tunica albuginea. The remaining ovarian stroma is divided into an inner medullary layer and an outer cortical layer, where the developing follicles are found. The ovaries are attached to the uterus and pelvic sidewalls by pliable adnexal structures, the utero-ovarian and infundibulo-ovarian ligaments, respectively. The broad ligaments, extending from the uterus to the pelvic sidewall, enfold the fallopian tubes, which are draped over the ovaries. An extension of the broad ligament, the mesosalpinx, maintains close approximation of the ovary to the fallopian tube.

The ovaries may be visualized transabdominally, through the distended bladder,[3, 4] but endovaginal imaging affords better visualization of ovarian morphology.[5, 6] By using the distended bladder technique, one can image the ovaries in variable cephalo-caudad locations, lateral to the uterus lying in the shallow fossa of Waldeyer between the external iliac vessels and the ureter, often in front of the internal iliac vessels. The ovarian artery and vein are sometimes identified entering the upper or tubal pole of the ovary through the infundibulopelvic ligament. The normal ovaries are relatively mobile in the pelvis and tend to lie more cephalad when the bladder is distended. With an empty bladder and endovaginal imaging, the ovaries are detected lying lateral to the body of the uterus overlying the internal iliac vessels. This approach allows more frequent detection and better visualization of the ovaries and has a high acceptance rate by the majority of women.[5, 6]

The adult ovary measures 2.5 to 5.0 cm long, 1.5 to

grow appears directly proportional to the number of follicles remaining in the ovaries and decreases with advancing age until the supply of follicles is depleted. At the onset of menopause, follicular maturation and ovulation become less frequent, eventually stopping completely.

In the process of oogenesis, the ovary secretes the steroid hormones estrogen and progesterone. The control of follicular development and steroid hormone production require the cyclic influence of the pituitary gonadotropins follicle-stimulating hormone (FSH) and luteinizing hormone (LH). Mature hypothalamic function is characterized by hourly (60 to 120 minutes) pulses of GnRH that are essential stimuli to the pituitary gland for the synthesis of FSH and LH. Neither the hypothalamus nor the pituitary has innate cyclicity. It is ovarian estrogen production that determines the cyclic pattern of FSH and LH in the normal menstrual cycle by a negative feedback mechanism. Under the influence of pulsatile GnRH release, FSH and LH production incites follicular growth and maturation.

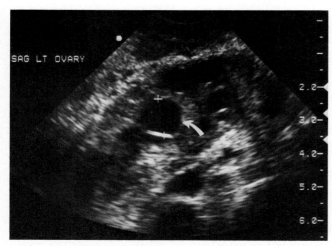

Figure 28–3. Sagittal sonogram of a normal ovary in the follicular phase (day 9) demonstrates an early dominant follicle that measures 11 mm *(curved arrow)* and other smaller subordinate follicles.

3.0 cm wide, and 0.6 to 1.5 cm thick with volumes ranging from 1.2 to 11.8 mL.[7] The normal range of size may be even greater, and an average volume of 9.8 mL with a 95% confidence interval of 2.7 to 23.3 mL has been suggested.[8] The ovarian size peaks in the third decade and declines slowly through menopause. The ovarian volumes may be adequately determined by the simplified formula for a prolate ellipse ($\frac{1}{2}$ × length × width × thickness). There does not appear to be any correlation of ovarian size with body weight or size. A varying number of maturing follicles will be visible as small cystic structures within the ovaries. The number of follicles visible is usually about 5 but may be up to 11 in each ovary,[9] and these multiple small cysts give the ovary its typical appearance (Fig. 28–3). At menopause, with the depletion of follicles and cessation of ovulation and menstruation, the ovaries diminish in size and become more difficult to visualize but may often be seen for the first 2 decades of the menopause.

The development and fate of ovarian follicles have been documented by sequential scanning throughout the normal menstrual cycle.[10–12] The recruitment of several follicles, with the subsequent selection of a dominant follicle, maturation of the dominant follicle, ovulation, and the subsequent development of a corpus luteum may be observed and related to the complex hormonal events that control ovulation.[13] Under the influence of pituitary gonadotropins, the ovary goes through three phases during each menstrual cycle: (1) the follicular phase, (2) ovulation, and (3) the luteal phase.

FOLLICULAR PHASE

The follicular phase begins on the first day of menses and continues until the follicle matures and ovulation occurs, which is usually day 14 of a 28-day cycle. The ovarian follicle destined to ovulate is derived from a cohort of developing follicles.[14] In the follicular phase

under the influence of FSH, secreted in response to the pulsatile release of GnRH, a variable number of preantral follicles undergo further development with initiation of estrogen production by the granulosa cells. The rising estrogen level acts synergistically with FSH to bring about the accumulation of follicular fluid in the intercellular spaces of the granulosa with the formation of antral follicles. By way of a negative feedback mechanism, the increasing estrogen production effects a decline in the FSH, and this may be important in inducing atresia in all but one of the follicles, which becomes the dominant follicle. At the same time, this mid-follicular phase rise in estrogen exerts a positive influence on the LH. The resulting mid-cycle LH surge from the pituitary gland completes follicular maturation with reduction division in the oocyte and luteinization of the granulosa cells with synthesis of progesterone. The mid-cycle LH surge is accompanied by simultaneous release of FSH that causes cumulus expansion, allowing the cumulus-oocyte cell mass attached to the follicular wall to loosen and become free floating in the antral fluid, just before follicular rupture.[1]

The primordial and preantral follicles are too small to be defined sonographically. In optimal conditions, cystic structures as small as 2 to 4 mm in diameter may be imaged within the ovaries, and as the antral follicles develop they become large enough to be detected. Early in the menstrual cycle, a varying number of follicles, typically five to eight, will have been recruited and by cycle days 5 to 7 will be readily visible as tense, circular or oval echo-free cysts sharply demarcated from the surrounding ovarian tissue. The selection of the dominant follicle occurs normally by cycle days 5 to 7,[15, 16] and this may be detected by endovaginal sonography at about day 8, between 9 and 6 days before the LH surge. The dominant follicle will measure about 10mm (9.9 ± 3.0 mm) at this time and may be recognized because its size begins to exceed that of its fellow subordinate antral follicles that will subsequently undergo atresia (see Fig. 28–3). Growth of nondominant follicles occurs in both the dominant and nondominant ovary until the time of selection. During the late follicular and luteal phases, a decrease in mean size of the nondominant follicles may be observed in the dominant ovary only with limited follicular growth continuing in the nondominant ovary (Fig. 28–4). This suggests that there is active suppression of growth of the nondominant ipsilateral follicles by some intraovarian paracrine mechanism. The nondominant follicles rarely exceed 11 mm in diameter. A follicle that is much greater than 11 mm in diameter is a dominant follicle and is destined to ovulate.[16] The dominant and lesser order follicles are distributed randomly in both ovaries during single and sequential cycles. In 5% to 11%, two dominant follicles may develop but invariably in opposite ovaries.[17] Each dominant follicle usually contains a cumulus mass with a single oocyte. Rarely, two or more oocytes may coexist in a single follicle. The incidence of this phenomenon is higher in early life and becomes sporadic in adults but probably occurs in about 5% of reproductive aged women.[18] It is

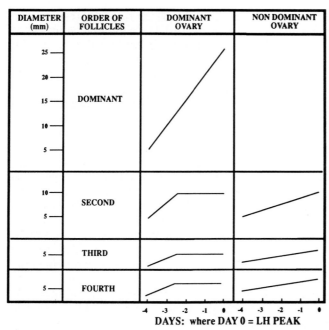

DIAMETER (mm)	ORDER OF FOLLICLES	DOMINANT OVARY	NON DOMINANT OVARY
25 20 15 10 5	DOMINANT		
10 5	SECOND		
5	THIRD		
5	FOURTH		

DAYS: where DAY 0 = LH PEAK

Figure 28–4. Follicular growth of the dominant and subordinate follicles. The growth rate of the dominant follicle exceeds the others and exerts a local suppressive effect on the development of the subordinate follicles in the dominant ovary but not in the contralateral nondominant ovary.

probable that only one of these oocytes is mature and able to be fertilized.

Once the dominant follicle is recognized, its size may be followed to the immediate preovulatory period. During this time the follicle grows rapidly in a linear manner, by 2 to 3 mm a day, and reaches a mean diameter of about 20 to 24 mm by the time of ovulation.[17, 19] The maximum preovulatory diameters, however, may vary widely from 15 to 30 mm, and this limits the value of follicular diameter alone as an absolute predictor of the time of ovulation.

The relative accuracy of sonographic measurements of preovulatory follicular size has been confirmed by laparoscopic studies, at which time the follicles were aspirated and the follicular diameters were directly measured or estimated from the volume of aspirated fluid.[20] As might be expected, both interobserver and intraobserver measurement errors have also been documented.[21, 22] Repeated measurements by a single observer appear to be less variable than observations by multiple observers. In one well-controlled study, the 95% confidence interval for a follicle measured at 15 mm by a single observer was 13 to 17 mm, whereas for multiple observers the 95% confidence interval was 12 to 18 mm. Errors were also noted to be greater for larger diameter follicles.[22] These errors may account, at least in part, for the inability of follicular size measurements alone to predict ovulation.[23]

Endocrine events correlate well with sonographic documentation of follicular growth in spontaneous cycles. There is a linear correlation between dominant follicular diameter and plasma estradiol level.[10, 17, 24] A higher concentration of estradiol has also been observed in venous plasma draining the ovary containing

at least one large follicle greater than 10 mm in size. Intrafollicular androgen/estrogen ratios are regulated by the granulosa cell enzyme aromatase, and it has been noted that aromatase activity is restricted in follicles up to 10 mm in diameter, whereas in larger follicles this activity is greatly enhanced, resulting in high estradiol levels in the follicular fluid. This information supports the role of the dominant follicle as the major preovulatory estrogen source in spontaneous cycles.[16] The hormonal contribution of the accompanying nondominant follicles is minimal despite the parallel growth changes noted.

Certain sonographic features that may be observed in the immediate preovulatory period may be helpful in predicting impending ovulation. These changes reflect the hormonally induced morphologic changes occurring in the preovulatory follicle following the onset of the LH surge. With the LH surge, the thecal tissue becomes hypervascular and edematous, and the granulosa cell layer begins to separate from the thecal cell layer. These features may be appreciated sonographically and may be detected by the appearance of a line of decreased reflectivity around the follicle. This feature is seen within 24 hours of ovulation and is associated with increasing plasma progesterone levels. Advanced folding and separation of the granulosa cell layer may produce a crenated pattern to the lining of the follicle (Fig. 28–5). This latter sign is less consistently seen but occurs when ovulation is imminent.[25, 26]

Another sign of follicular maturity is the detection of a small crescent-shaped echogenic rim or mound with an internal hypoechoic area measuring from 3 to 4 mm. This represents the cumulus oophorus and its surrounding complement of granulosa cells (Fig. 28–6).[27, 28] This may be visualized in more than 80% of follicles greater than 17 mm in diameter.[12] Identification of the cumulus oophorus confirms that a cystic structure is indeed an oocyte-containing follicle and that ovulation will occur within 36 hours. The occasional presence of a free-floating cumulus mass has also been observed in the immediate preovulatory period. Other authors have questioned the ability to define the cumulus oophorus,[23] suggesting that the structure represents artifactual echoes, either side-lobe

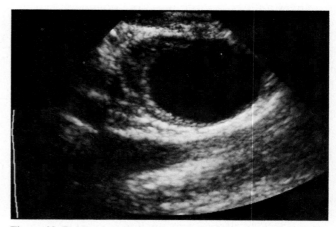

Figure 28–5. Mature follicle. There is a follicle measuring 21 mm average diameter with a slightly crenated echogenic rim.

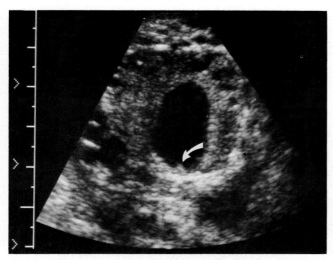

Figure 28–6. Mature follicle. There is a mature follicle measuring 19 mm average diameter with a small echogenic focus on the wall *(curved arrow)* representing a cumulus oophorus.

or slice-thickness artifact, projecting into the anechoic follicle or adjacent small follicles misinterpreted as intrafollicular because of slice-thickness artifact.

OVULATION

The changes associated with ovulation have been documented, and actual follicular rupture has been observed sonographically.[19, 28, 29] When the follicle ruptures with presumed release of the ovum, there is a sudden decrease in follicular size and an escape of fluid into the periovulatory area or cul-de-sac. In about 90% of cases, the follicle disappears immediately after ovulation.[19, 23] In the remainder, the follicle decreases in size and develops a crenated wall.

With daily scanning, ovulation may be detected in more than 90% of cases (Fig. 28–7). Sonographically detected ovulation usually occurs within 24 to 36 hours after onset of the LH surge.[29–31] Laparoscopic examination of the ovary immediately following ovulation will demonstrate a crater or hole, often with a surrounding vascularized collar, in the wall of the corpus luteum. This stigma closes and reepithelializes within 2 to 5 days of ovulation. Progesterone and estrogen levels in the peritoneal fluid reflect closure of the corpus luteum with very high hormone concentrations in the immediate postovulatory period and a very sharp decline as early as the second and third day after ovulation.[32]

The occurrence of sonographically detectable fluid in the cul-de-sac is seen following ovulation in the majority of patients. Although small amounts of fluid may be detected before ovulation, the volume increases progressively during the follicular phase, with an abrupt increase following ovulation and peak volumes detected in the early luteal phase (see Fig. 28–7).[29] This has been measured by laparoscopic aspiration to be about 15 to 25 mL, which greatly exceeds the amount (4 to 6 mL) released by follicular rupture. It has been inferred that the peritoneal fluid is predomi-

nantly formed by exudation from the active ovary, and this is strongly supported by the higher concentrations of ovarian steroid hormones found in the peritoneal fluid than in the plasma. This mid-cycle fluid is not observed when ovarian function is suppressed, as with oral contraceptives.

The occurrence of mittelschmertz ("middle pain") is also closely associated with the process of follicular rupture and was initially believed to be caused by peritoneal irritation from blood and follicular contents following ovulation. Mid-cycle sonographic surveillance of the ovaries has shown that in the majority of cases the symptoms precede ovulation and are present on the side with the dominant follicle, suggesting local effects of the enlarging follicle.[10] It has also been shown that 77% of women with mittleschmertz experienced the symptoms on the same day as the peak plasma LH, and, in 97%, the pain preceded follicular rupture.[30]

A significant rise in the basal body temperature (BBT) does not occur until 2 days after the LH peak, coinciding with increasing amounts of plasma progesterone. Sonographic correlation with BBT has demonstrated that ovulation precedes the initial rise in temperature in most individuals, confirming the limited value of the rise of the BBT as a predictor of impending ovulation and thus as a reliable method of contraception.[10]

LUTEAL PHASE

After ovulation the wall of the follicle becomes convoluted and the antrum fills with blood and lymph to form a corpus hemorrhagicum. The remaining granulosa cells enlarge and accumulate lipid and a yellow pigment, called lutein, and vascularization of the granulosa occurs to form a corpus luteum. The corpus luteum produces progesterone, which is necessary for the maintenance of the secretory phase of the endometrial lining to ensure successful implantation should a pregnancy supervene.

Although the length of the follicular phase is variable, the life span of the corpus luteum is a constant 14 days, and it will rapidly degenerate after this time without an intervening pregnancy. Human chorionic gonadotropin (hCG) from a fertilized ovum prevents corpus luteum regression, and, under the stimulation of hCG, steroidogenesis continues in the corpus luteum until placental production is established, usually by the 10th week of gestation.

Following ovulation the process may vary with sonographic evidence of replacement of the echo-free follicle by an echogenic structure representing invasion of the follicle by blood clot and fibroblasts with or without the reappearance of a cystic corpus luteum.[12, 33] A mature corpus luteum is seen sonographically in only about 50% of persons. The most frequent pattern is the detection of a small irregular cyst with echogenic crenated walls, the corpus hemorrhagicum, containing numerous echoes that probably originate from blood (Fig. 28–8). Once found, the echogenic corpus luteum

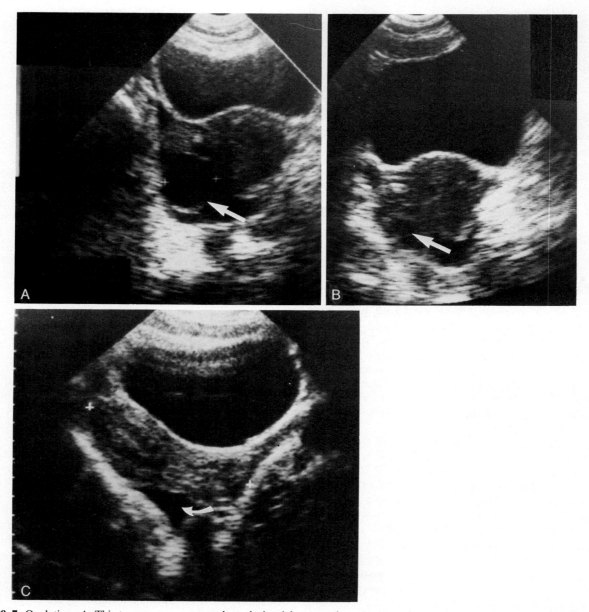

Figure 28–7. Ovulation. *A.* This transverse sonogram through the right ovary demonstrates a large preovulatory follicle with echogenic rim *(arrow).* *B.* A comparable sonogram 2 days later demonstrates a much smaller irregular cyst containing internal echoes representing the collapsed follicle with development of a corpus hemorrhagicum *(arrow).* *C.* A longitudinal sonogram through the uterus demonstrates a sudden and significant increase in the amount of fluid in the cul-de-sac *(curved arrow).* (From Ritchie WGM: Sonographic evaluation of normal and induced ovulation. Radiology 161:1, 1986.)

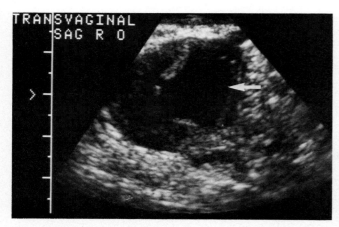

Figure 28–8. A corpus luteum was demonstrated as a partially collapsed cyst with a 15-mm diameter, a thick echogenic rim, and internal debris *(arrow)*.

remains almost unchanged throughout the luteal phase. In a significant number of patients, the follicle will disappear and no corpus luteum may be identified. In this situation, the presence of a functioning corpus luteum can often be detected by the recognition of the typical "ring" color flow Doppler pattern around the wall of an isoechoic corpus luteum. In a few patients a well-defined cyst will develop and grow slowly and may reach 25 to 40 mm in diameter. It remains unclear how these structural differences relate to the adequacy of ovulation and corpus luteum function. Corpora lutea disappear shortly before or with the onset of menstruation and should not be visible beyond 72 hours of the subsequent cycle.

This pattern of follicular development continues throughout the reproductive life of the woman. As the stock of primordial follicles is depleted, there are fewer preantral follicles available to undergo maturation, ovulatory cycles become less frequent and eventually stop completely. In the absence of estrogen production by developing follicles, there is no negative feedback mechanism to suppress gonadotropin release from the pituitary and the menopause is characterized by extremely high levels of circulating and urinary FSH and LH. The size of the ovary after menopause diminishes but is still visible in about 50% and 25% of women in the sixth and seventh decades of life, respectively, using endovaginal sonography. The volume of the postmenopausal ovary is about 6 mL.[8] The multiple, small antral follicles visible in the reproductive life are not apparent, and the ovaries have a more uniform texture. The presence of nonactive cysts, however, is not uncommon and may be seen in as many as 17% of asymptomatic postmenopausal women; about 50% of these cysts will resolve spontaneously.[34]

UTERINE CHANGES

The normal postpubertal nulliparous uterus measures 5.0 to 8.0 cm long and 1.6 to 3.0 cm in the anteroposterior diameter.[4] The endometrial canal may be easily identified lying centrally within the uterine body, and the vagina may be visualized in continuity with the cervix. The position of the uterus varies with the uterine fundus lying on either size of the pelvis. The body of the uterus is normally anteverted in relation to the vagina but may be retroverted or retroflexed, and, in these positions, the endometrial canal may be more difficult to image.

ENDOMETRIAL CHANGES

The sonographic appearances of the endometrium during the menstrual cycle may be correlated with changes in its histologic anatomy.[30, 35, 36] There are two main layers of the endometrium: (1) the functionalis layer consisting of a compactum and spongiosum stratum that thickens and is shed with each menses and (2) the basalis layer remains intact throughout the cycle and contains the nutrient vessels that elongate to supply the endometrium when it thickens. The endometrial changes may be divided into three phases: proliferative, secretory, and menstrual. The first two phases coincide with the mid- to late follicular and luteal phases of the ovulatory cycle.

There is progressive thickening of the endometrium during the cycle. Endometrial thickness is usually measured from the echogenic interface of the junction of endometrium and myometrium and represents two layers of endometrium. This double endometrial thickness measurement represents the spongiosum and compactum layers. The thin hypoechoic halo is not included in the measurement because this represents the basalis layer and inner layer of the compactum.[36] The endometrium measures 4 to 5 mm by day 7 or 8 of the cycle and increases in thickness during the follicular phase to 8 to 12 mm, plateauing in the luteal phase.[36, 37] This increase in thickness is accompanied by changes in endometrial reflectivity. During the early proliferative or follicular phase a hypoechoic area develops around a prominent midline echo (Fig. 28–9A). By the late proliferative phase, the endometrium has thickened and becomes isoechoic with the endometrium. In the luteal phase, the endometrium becomes hyperechoic, often blurring the midline echo (see Fig. 28–9B). These changes reflect the histologic and morphologic changes during the menstrual cycle, and the increasing reflectivity seems to be related to increasing length and tortuosity of endometrial glands with mucin and glycogen storage within the functionalis layer. The thickened echogenic endometrium persists until the onset of the menses. In the menstrual phase, as the functionalis layer of the endometrium is shed, the endometrium appears sonographically as a thin, slightly irregular echogenic interface (see Fig. 28–9C).

It has long been recognized that the uterus has inherent contractility. Two types of contraction have been observed. Random contractions of the entire myometrium occur, and these become markedly diminished in the periovulatory period. More recently, subtle wavelike subendometrial contractions have been observed sonographically.[38, 39] Appreciation of these progressive contractions of the inner third of the myo-

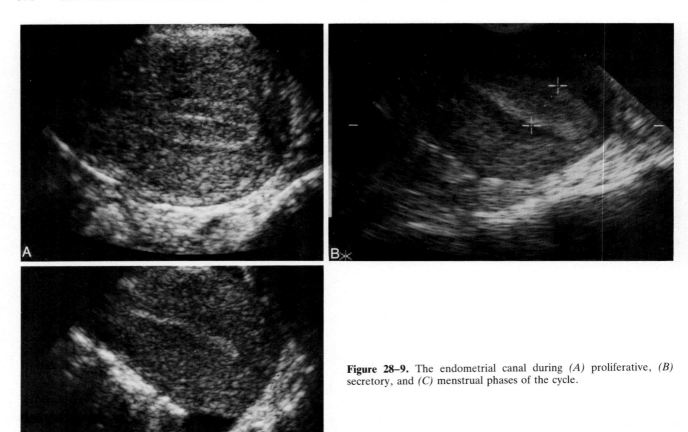

Figure 28–9. The endometrial canal during *(A)* proliferative, *(B)* secretory, and *(C)* menstrual phases of the cycle.

metrium is enhanced by reviewing taped real-time images at five times regular speed. Retrograde contractions spreading from the cervix increase in frequency, amplitude, and percentage toward the fundus throughout the follicular and periovulatory phases. These waves occur with a frequency of about 3 cycles per minute in the periovulatory period. The pattern is essentially reversed in the luteal phase. Unlike the contractions described with dysmenorrhea or during pregnancy (Braxton-Hicks contractions), women are unaware of these subendometrial contractions. The role that these contractions play in sperm transport is conjectural. The physiologic mechanism that controls these contractions is unknown, but the pattern of follicular rise and luteal fall in activity is suggestive of a stimulatory effect of estrogen at mid cycle and an inhibitory effect of estrogen plus progesterone. This hypothesis is supported by the observations that the subendometrial contractions are less prominent in women taking oral contraceptives.

OVARIAN AND UTERINE DOPPLER

A pattern of pulsed and color flow Doppler observations in the ovary and uterus is evolving, but clinical application of these qualitative observations and quantitative measurements must await expansion and con-

firmation of these findings. Nevertheless, important and consistent observations have been made.[40–47]

The ovary has a dual blood supply: (1) one derived from the adnexal branch of the uterine artery and (2) one as a dedicated ovarian branch arising directly from the abdominal aorta passing to the ovary in the infundibulopelvic ligament.[1] Recognition of these vessels is assisted with endovaginal color flow Doppler imaging with subsequent evaluation of ovarian flow by pulsed Doppler study. The best quantitative information may be obtained from interrogation of the true ovarian artery in the infundibulopelvic ligament or from recordings obtained from intraovarian vessels. Resistive and pulsatility indices are used to quantitate blood flow in the ovary as they are angle independent and unitless. The resistive index is defined as the systolic peak minus the diastolic peak divided by the systolic peak and ranges from 1.0 to 0, with 1.0 representing the highest resistance to forward flow and 0 reflecting the absence of end-diastolic forward flow. The pulsatility index, however, is probably a better physiologic measurement taking into account more of the frequencies in the waveform by measuring the envelope of all of the recorded frequencies during a complete cardiac cycle to define a mean flow velocity. The pulsatility index is defined as the systolic peak minus the diastolic peak divided by the mean. Since the frequency envelope is usually measured manually, the pulsatility index is more prone to interobserver and intraobserver error.

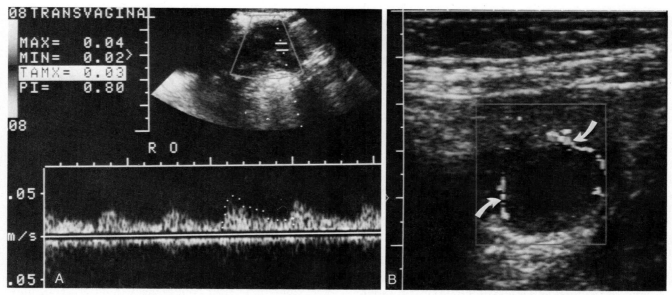

Figure 28–10. *A.* Pulsed Doppler interrogation of the wall of a corpus luteum demonstrating low resistance (PI = .80) flow. *B.* A color flow Doppler "ring" pattern *(curved arrows)* around a cystic corpus luteum reflecting neovascularity in the wall of the cyst.

Pulsed Doppler studies of ovarian artery flow demonstrate a high impedance waveform with low amplitude and little or no diastolic flow in the early follicular phase of the cycle (days 1 to 10). The ovary developing the dominant follicle begins to show diastolic flow and an increased amplitude waveform, which increases rapidly about 2 days before ovulation, reflecting increased flow and diminished vascular resistance.[39–41] This coincides with the LH surge and reflects neovascularization and luteinization of the granulosa cells of the maturing follicle. This increased amplitude, low resistance flow increases through the periovulatory period, remaining at this level for 4 to 5 days into the functioning period of the corpus luteum (Fig. 28–10). It then gradually returns to a higher resistance pattern with lower amplitude flow and less diastolic flow, finally reverting to the inactive high resistance pattern during the menstrual period. The contralateral ovary maintains the same high impedance pattern throughout the cycle (Fig. 28–11).[42–44]

The normal ranges for both ovarian Doppler resistive and pulsatility indices are fairly wide and, as isolated measurements, are of little predictive value in defining the active ovary. Comparison of indices from both ovarian arteries, however, will readily document lower resistance flow in the ovary harboring the dominant follicle or functioning corpus luteum.

Doppler interrogation of the uterine artery does not always reflect the changes occurring in the ipsilateral ovary and may reflect more the direct effect of increasing estrogen levels on the uterine arteries.[45] It has also been suggested that there is persistence of a vasodilative effect from previous pregnancies and lower resistance flow is found in parous subjects.[46, 47] This hypothesis is supported by the frequent observation of many uterine and adnexal vessels in parous women, a finding that is extremely uncommon in nulliparous patients.

ABNORMAL CYCLES

With such a complicated process involved in ovulation, it is not surprising that both random and persistent defects in ovulation are encountered. Some of these syndromes may be suspected and confirmed clinically by appropriate hormonal assays. The addition of sonography has correlated many of the morphologic and hormonal findings and often affords a simple noninvasive method to detect abnormal ovulatory cycles.

Although there is considerable debate about the frequency and significance of spontaneously occurring abnormal cycles, there appear to be at least three types

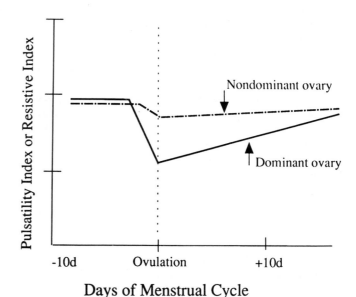

Figure 28–11. A diagrammatic representation of the ovarian flow profile (pulsatility index or resistive index) in the dominant and nondominant ovary during the ovarian cycle.

of sonographically detectable abnormal cycles: (1) anovulatory cycles with follicular atresia, (2) empty follicle syndrome, and (3) luteinized unruptured follicles. These abnormal cycles may be suspected by careful sonographic examination in the periovulatory period. There are also three types of chronic or persistent anovulatory syndromes.

Randomly occurring anovulatory cycles occur in about 7% of cycles, but sonographic studies of apparently normal cycles with biphasic BBT curves and normal cycle length suggest that abnormal cycles may be significantly more frequent.[48] In such cycles there is asynchrony between the E_2 peak and the LH surge and the growth and disappearance of ovarian follicles. These cycles may be recognized during serial sonographic observations of follicular development, when the poor follicular size or premature disappearance of the follicle in relation to the hormonal changes will be detected. In this situation, the follicle rarely reaches 14 mm and either collapses prematurely or rapidly becomes atretic.[48] A similar pattern or aborted follicular development may be seen in women taking oral contraceptives.

Another type of anovulatory cycle has also been described—the empty follicle syndrome.[49–52] It was first described in stimulated cycles following the observation that some follicular aspirates contain no ova.[49, 50] Sonographic recognition of this syndrome has depended on the inability to demonstrate a cumulus oophorus in a mature follicle. Since detection of the cumulus is, at best, very time consuming and technologically demanding, the validity of this finding must be questioned until correlation with follicular aspiration studies is available. The sonographic incidence of this phenomenon in a normal population of women is unknown but has been reported to be about 36% in an infertile population.[51, 52]

In a small number of women following an appropriate LH surge, the luteinized follicle fails to rupture and release the oocyte—luteinized unruptured follicle (LUF) syndrome.[53–56] In the past, this diagnosis depended on the failure of laparoscopic demonstration of an ovulation stigma in the early luteal phase in a patient with apparent normal ovulatory cycles. This was further supported by recovery of an oocyte from the unruptured follicle. The concept was also supported by the observation that the amount of peritoneal fluid and concentration of progesterone and estrogen were significantly lower in those cases in which the luteinized follicle failed to rupture when these cycles were compared with normal ovulatory cycles.[29] The presence of LUF may now be demonstrated sonographically by sequential scanning beyond the LH peak.[53–56] The persistence of a dominant follicle with an echo-free cystic appearance beyond 48 hours after the LH peak, with no sign of collapse, is abnormal and may be taken as evidence of failure of ovulation. In most of these unruptured follicles, the normally sharp definition between the follicle wall and follicular fluid becomes an ill-defined gray zone caused by an echogenic interface of low-density echoes. This appearance is similar to that seen in the immediate preovulatory follicle but becomes more marked in the LUF syndrome, where the sonographic gray zone may be 4 to 7 mm thick and probably reflects imaging of the hypertrophied and luteinized granulosa cells. The patterns of LH, estrogen, and progesterone secretion do not differ from those in subjects ovulating normally and suggest that the LUF behaves steroidogenically as a corpus luteum with a luteal phase of normal length. The frequency of this syndrome is uncertain but has been reported in approximately 11% of cycles in normal women.[54, 57] Although sonography may provide serial observations of follicle activity, it may not be as accurate as laparoscopy. False-positive predictions of LUF in 14% of patients undergoing both procedures have been reported, and the incidence of LUF is higher when diagnosed by laparoscopy. It appears to be much more common in patients with unexplained infertility, occurring in more than 50% of cycles,[55] and may be associated with the empty follicle syndrome.[51] This syndrome may occur continuously in all cycles or may be intermittent and may account for some cases of otherwise unexplained infertility.

As well as randomly occurring anovulatory cycles, three chronic anovulatory syndromes occur. They are related to failure in the hypothalamic-pituitary-ovarian axis control system. Three categories of women fail to ovulate: (1) those with hypergonadotropism, (2) those with hypogonadotropism, and (3) those with chronic anovulatory syndrome or polycystic ovarian disease.

The first two conditions are characterized by anestrogenic amenorrhea. Since there is no estrogen production, no withdrawal bleeding occurs following a suitable progestational stimulus. If the LH and FSH levels are elevated in this group (hypergonadotropism), the patient has primary ovarian failure, major causes of which are premature menopause, autoimmune ovarian insensitivity, and sex chromosmal mosaicism. In this situation small, postmenopausal sized ovaries with extremely few, small, or no developing follicles will be imaged. With the possible exception of cases of autoimmune ovarian insensitivity that respond to steroids or immunosuppressive therapy, it is not possible to induce ovulation in this group since there are no follicles remaining in the ovaries.

In the second group the LH and FSH levels are very depressed (hypogonadotropism), and these patients must be evaluated for pituitary and parasellar tumors or other hypothalamic abnormalities interfering with GnRH or FSH and LH release. Surgical removal of pituitary microadenomas or other tumors may be accompanied by return of normal ovulatory cycles.

Most infertile patients who require ovulation induction have polycystic ovary disease (PCOD). These patients have amenorrhea or oligomenorrhea and will have withdrawal bleeding after progestin treatment. They release gonadotropins and their ovaries respond, but the pituitary-ovarian axis is acyclic. The ovaries secrete predominantly the male hormone androstenedione, and most of the estrogen is formed in extraglandular sites, such as fat tissue. Thus, even though there is no potent follicular estradiol secretion, the patients are estrogenized and their menstrual episodes typically represent estrogen breakthrough bleeding. These patients usually exhibit elevated LH levels and depressed FSH levels with an elevated LH/FSH ratio; the minimal FSH release is probably not enough to initiate follicular growth and maturation, and the patients are anovulatory.

The sonographic features of PCOD reflect the morphologic changes occurring in the ovary with multiple, poorly developed atretic follicles in an enlarged ovary demonstrating stromal hypertrophy.[57, 58] The ovarian enlargement becomes more apparent with increased duration of disease, and about 33% of patients will still have normal-sized ovaries. In the remainder, the ovaries are obviously enlarged (>6 cm³) and are usually twice normal size. As the ovaries become enlarged they become more spheroidal and the ovarian diameter often exceeds the anteroposterior diameter of the fundus of the uterus.[58] Using transabdominal sonography, the number of follicles necessary to establish the diagnosis of PCOD has been reported to vary from about 5 to at least 15. In a more recent endovaginal study,[9] the maximum number of developing follicles found in control subjects was 11. Although the majority of patients with PCOD had more than 11 follicles, a significant number had less than 11 follicles, reducing the sensitivity of follicular numbers alone as a predictor of PCOD. The follicles, however, are smaller without evidence of a dominant follicle, and the ovarian volume and stromal echogenicity are greater (Fig. 28–12). Median values of the mean size and number of follicles, ovarian volume, and percentage with moderate or markedly increased stromal echogenicity were, respectively, 5.1 mm, 5.0, 5.9 mL, and 10% in control subjects and 3.8 mm, 9.8, 9.8 mL, and 94% in patients with PCOD.[9] The presence of multiple small follicles in an enlarged ovary especially when associated with increased stromal echogenicity should raise the possibility of PCOD. When such polycystic ovaries are encountered incidentally in women referred for gyne-

cologic ultrasound evaluation, about 50% of the patients will have the classic signs and symptoms associated with PCOD. Twenty-five percent will have a variant of the syndrome, and in another 25% no clinical abnormality will be evident at the time of the examination.[58] Polycystic ovaries may also be associated with other clinical situations, such as Cushing syndrome, basophilic pituitary adenoma, and other unexplained causes of infertility, including endometriosis.

The important drugs used in ovulation induction are clomiphene citrate, hMG, and the gonadotropin-releasing hormone agonist leuprolide acetate.[59, 60]

Clomiphene requires an intact hypothalamic-pituitary-ovarian axis. It is indicated when there is evidence of follicular function with adequate endogenous estrogen production but no cyclic stimulation by pituitary gonadotropin. It is the drug of choice in the treatment of anovulation because of PCOD, oligo-ovulation, post-pill amenorrhea, and some cases of amenorrhea-galactorrhea. Starting on day 5, following progesterone-induced endometrial bleeding, 50 to 150 mg of clomiphene is given daily for 5 days. Clomiphene is considered an estrogen antagonist and exerts its effect by binding estrogen receptors in the pituitary and hypothalamus. This effect leads to increased FSH secretion by the pituitary with recruitment of several follicles overcoming the process of selection and dominance of a single follicle. This process results in the development of multiple relatively synchronous follicles. Although a preovulatory estrogen-LH feedback may be intact in the clomiphene-treated patient with an intact hypothalamus, most patients are given hCG to induce final follicular post-pill amenorrhea, and virilizing ovarian or adrenal tumors.

INDUCED OVULATION

Disorders of ovulation are present in 15% to 25% of infertile women. Depending on the cause, appropriate therapy may be used to induce ovulation and allow conception. In the absence of premature menopause and hyperprolactinemia, most ovulatory disorders are treated with clomiphene citrate and human menopausal gonadotropin (hMG) therapy or more recently with gonadotropin releasing factor and its synthetic analogues. The aim of therapy is to induce satisfactory ovulation of one or more follicles and to avoid multiple follicular development, hyperstimulation, and multiple pregnancies.[59, 60]

In the past decade, the development of assisted reproductive technologies such as in vitro fertilization with embryo transfer (IVF-ET) and gamete and zygote intrafallopian transfer (GIFT and ZIFT) have expanded the use of superovulation programs to include women with normal ovulatory cycles and other mechanical forms of infertility. Over 24,000 ovarian stimulation cycles were reported by the United States Registry of IVF-ET and related practices in 1989.[61] In these women, the aim is to produce multiple follicles to allow oocyte harvesting, gamete replacement, or IVF-ET to improve the pregnancy rate. Despite the

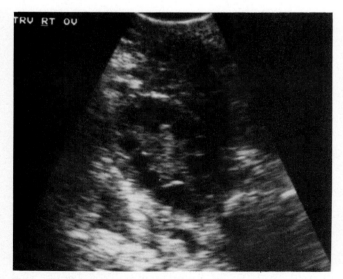

Figure 28–12. Polycystic ovarian disease. This sonogram through an enlarged ovary demonstrates multiple small peripherally placed poorly developed follicles.

implantation of multiple embryos, the overall success rate per IVF cycle is 13% to 20% or about 50% of the conception rate per menstrual cycle for a normal couple of reproductive age having unprotected intercourse.[62] Although the pregnancy rate increases as a function of the number of oocytes fertilized and embryos transferred, it is simplistic to think that superovulation per se accounts for all of the improvement in pregnancy rate. It has long been appreciated that treatment-associated pregnancies occurred in patients whose oocyte retrievals were cancelled and insemination occurred spontaneously (coital) or after intrauterine or cervical insemination of the already donated semen. Pregnancy rates in some of these groups approached the rate achieved by IVF or GIFT programs, supporting the contention that superovulation may be successful in achieving pregnancy because there is associated improved ovarian follicular and corpus luteal function, improved cervical mucus production, and control of ovulation that may allow improved timing of insemination. Thus, superovulation programs, as well as overcoming a variety of ovulation defects, may improve tubal and uterine motility, endometrial preparedness and luteal phase deficiency, cervical hospitality to sperm, even in the face of oligoasthenospermia, and oocyte maturation.

Pergonal (hMG) is a preparation of gonadotropins, FSH, and LH obtained from postmenopausal urine. It is a potent direct stimulator of ovarian folliculogenesis and does not require an intact hypothalamic-pituitary-ovarian axis.[63] The process of selection is overriden, and many follicles may develop. Two patterns of response may be identified. In amenorrheic women with no exogenous estrogenic activity, the dormant ovaries are induced to produce a small cohort of relatively synchronously developing follicles. The growth rate and E_2 secretion are linear, and good pregnancy rates are achieved. In contrast, women with estrogenic activity who harbor antral follicles at various stages of development, typically patients with PCOD, tend to be very sensitive to hMG stimulation. Stimulation of these patients results in the recruitment of many follicles with different growth rates and varying degrees of estrogen secretory capacity with estradiol levels correlating best with the diameter of the leading follicle.[64] A spontaneous LH surge is less frequent when stimulating with hMG, and hCG is usually given to induce final follicular maturation.

With the elucidation of the structure of GnRH and the importance of the pulsatile nature of its secretion, pulsatile administration of GnRH has been successfully used to induce ovulation in hypothalamic amenorrhea.[65] Subsequent use in patients with PCOD has been less successful. Soon after the structure of GnRH was described, analogues with prolonged action were developed. These analogues had a paradoxic effect; however, their prolonged binding to pituitary GnRH receptors initially resulted in stimulation of FSH and LH release and ultimately led to down-regulation and decreased gonadotropin and ovarian secretion. This phenomenon allows the induction of hypothalamic amenorrhoea or a reversible "medical menopause."

This drug has proved useful especially in PCOD; without any gonadotropin stimulation follicular development is suppressed, and this can be followed by induction of ovulation using hMG. This regimen is very successful in attaining multiple synchronous follicular development, but there is a high incidence of hyperstimulation and multiple pregnancies and, thus, this regimen is better suited to IVF programs.

The number of follicles developing in any cycle depends, to a certain extent, on the dose of each drug, but it is usual to see fewer follicles developing with clomiphene cycles than with hMG cycles. Although two follicles develop in 5% to 11% of spontaneous cycles, multiple follicular development is seen in 35% to 60% of clomiphene cycles and in up to 80% of gonadotropin cycles.[66] Not only the frequency with which multiple follicular development occurs but also the numbers of follicles developing in these cycles tend to be greater with gonadotropins than with clomiphene, usually averaging about four to six follicles in well-controlled cycles. In IVF, in which the aim is for controlled superovulation with oocyte retrieval, the number of follicles tends to be even greater. Although the rate and patterns of follicular development differ somewhat with the different therapeutic regimens, the principles of sonographic surveillance in all induced cycles is similar and is tailored to demonstrate the number of recruited follicles and to follow their development to maturity and to assist in timing of hCG administration to precipitate ovulation (Fig. 28–13). Evaluation of the endometrial canal thickness has a role in predicting the outcome of the cycle.

A baseline study may be performed. The follicular surveillance studies are best performed using an endovaginal probe, but there is some utility in including a transabdominal study in the baseline examination to allow a larger global view of pelvic structures, especially if abnormalities in the uterus or adnexal structures are suspected. A baseline study should also be performed if there have been recent induced cycles to exclude the presence of residual cysts. The presence of baseline ovarian cysts has been a frequent cause for cancellation of a cycle on account of the concern that the cyst may grow further, undergo torsion, rupture, or compromise the potential for follicular development. Poorer outcomes for induced cycles with baseline cysts have been noted, and although this has not been substantiated by others, several programs now perform endovaginal aspiration of these cysts before ovulation induction rather than cancelling or postponing the cycle.[67]

Following a baseline study early in the cycle, serial monitoring is usually started on cycle days 8 to 10. At this time the recruited follicles should be readily visible, approaching 8 to 10 mm in diameter, giving an early idea of the response to therapy. Daily or alternate-day scanning is then performed until the lead follicle or follicles approach mature size. When many follicles develop in an ovary, they may be distorted and compressed by adjacent follicles, and these factors can make accurate measurement difficult. Careful assessment of the lead follicle size is very important. Allow-

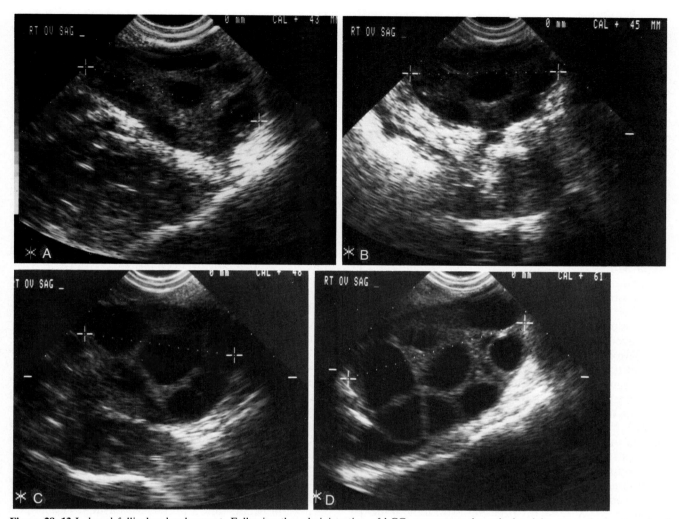

Figure 28–13. Induced follicular development. Following the administration of hCG, sonograms through the right ovary obtained on day 8 *(A)*, day 10 *(B)*, day 12 *(C)*, and day 14 *(D)* show the development of multiple follicles to a mature size.

ing a follicle to grow beyond predicted mature size while waiting for other follicles to mature is risking the possibility of spontaneous ovulation or luteinization of an unruptured follicle and thus sacrificing that cycle. Sonographic observation of any of the periovulatory phenomena seen in normal spontaneous cycles (sonolucent perifollicular halo with marginal crenation or observation of a cumulus oophorus) suggests that a spontaneous LH surge has occurred. This may be confirmed by measurement of LH or progesterone. Likewise, the observation of a sudden increase in the amount of fluid in the cul-de-sac or collapse of follicle is highly suspicious for spontaneous ovulation. It is easy, however, to overlook the collapse of a follicle in the presence of multiple follicular development, and a moderate amount of fluid is occasionally seen in stimulated women without ovulation having occurred. Suspected spontaneous ovulation should be confirmed biochemically rather than sacrifice a cycle. In induced cycles with normal fertilization it is usual to administer hCG when the follicles approach an average diameter of 18 mm. Using follicle diameter as a guide to hCG administration assumes that maturation of the oocyte can be equated with follicular size. However, oocyte retrieval in IVF programs has shown a poor correlation, and mature oocytes may be retrieved from follicles ranging from 10 to more than 20 mm in diameter. Within this range there is no significant difference in the percentage of mature oocytes retrieved or in the fertilization rates. The embryo quality does appear to improve with follicular size, although the difference is not marked enough to recommend nonaspiration of small follicles.[68] For this reason many IVF-ET groups will administer hCG when follicles reach 15 mm in diameter rather than risk spontaneous ovulation with loss of the cycle. Apparent maturity of follicles as small as 15 mm, however, may also reflect interobserver or intraobserver errors, as discussed earlier, and ideally a single skilled observer should perform all of the studies in any cycle.[22] Following hCG administration, a follicle will usually grow by 2 to 4 mm before ovulation occurs. If the patient is scanned following hCG administration the previously described periovulatory phenomena can be observed, allowing more accurate prediction of the number of follicles that are likely to ovulate. Cumuli are seen most frequently in follicles more than 18 mm in diameter and can be seen in about 50% of follicles immediately before retrieval in IVF-ET programs.[69]

Simultaneous biochemical and morphologic assessments of oocyte maturation are required for optimal results in most situations. The most frequently used variable is the estradiol level, and levels of 400 pg/mL per preovulatory follicle are suggestive of maturity.[70] A wide range of estradiol responses is encountered, and, in this situation, ultrasonography is able to differentiate whether an elevated estradiol level is due to multiple small follicles or a single mature follicle. It is, therefore, generally accepted that ultrasonography and estradiol levels are complementary in their ability to monitor ovulation induction therapy by allowing correct timing of hCG administration and to help avoid hyperstimulation and multiple gestations by indicating when hCG may be safely given.

Considerable interest has been shown in observation of the endometrium to assess follicular maturity and preparedness of the endometrium for implantation of the fertilized oocyte.[37, 64] In hMG-stimulated cycles the endometrial thickness in the proliferative phase tends to be greater than in normal cycles and uterine size and endometrial thickness increase to a maximum value around the time of ovulation and show a positive correlation with estradiol levels.[64] A significant difference in the degree of endometrial thickness measured at the time of hCG administration in conception and nonconception cycles has been observed, with no conceptions occurring when the endometrium is less than 7 mm.[37, 64] The underdeveloped endometrium probably reflects endometrial inability to respond to estrogen since estradiol levels are not significantly different in the groups with and without satisfactory endometrial development. Poor endometrial development is found more frequently in clomiphene-stimulated cycles, and this is probably related to the antiestrogenic effect of clomiphene.

Sonographic observation of the cervical canal in the immediate preovulatory period will often show changes in response to elevated estradiol levels coinciding with the clinically apparent preovulatory production of copious thin cervical mucus. These changes, however, are not consistent. Hypertrophy of the cervical mucous glands may have several appearances. The earliest noticeable change is a zone of increased echogenicity around the cervical canal. When the secretions become copious, fluid may be seen in the canal. Occasionally, discrete fluid-filled glands may be seen in the wall of the cervical canal. These have an appearance similar to that of nabothian cysts but disappear rapidly after ovulation.

The success rate for conception in induced cycles, both in vivo and in vitro, falls short of the rate of conception in normal cycles with comparable optimal timing of fertilization.[62] Although not all failures are attributable to failure of folliculogenesis, sonographic observations have assisted in the recognition of several patterns of abnormality. These unsuccessful cycles fall into three categories. Both follicular atresia and LUF as seen in normal cycles occur, but ovarian hyperstimulation syndrome (OHSS) is unique to stimulated cycles.

In the first group, poor follicular development with slow or irregular growth of follicles may be observed. This phenomenon is usually associated with low or fluctuating estradiol levels and is most often seen with inadequate gonadotropin administration. These follicles will become atretic before ovulation unless the dose of gonadotropin is increased.

In the second group, following hCG administration, the LUF syndrome may occur.[55, 71] This may be an expression of oocyte overexposure in hMG and may coincide with the aspiration of postmature oocytes in IVF programs. This phenomenon is also, but less frequently, seen in clomiphene-induced cycles. There are no sonographic features to allow identification of these follicles before hCG administration. Following the administration of hCG, changes similar to those occurring in spontaneous cycles may be seen, with absence of follicular collapse and the development of a thick gray zone around the follicle and the low level internal echoes. In the presence of multiple follicles, this feature may not always be appreciated, and satisfactory ovulation may still occur from other mature follicles.

In the third group, OHSS may occur.[72] Hyperstimulation is the most serious complication of ovulation induction with clomiphene and gonadotropins but has also been reported with gonadotropin-releasing factor therapy. OHSS is unlikely in women whose ovaries contain several large follicles (>15 mm) but tends to occur when there are multiple small or intermediate follicles. With OHSS, multiple follicles are induced with the development of multiple corpus luteum cysts after ovulation. Although the ovaries may become extremely large and the estrogen levels may be very high, the full clinical syndrome of OHSS rarely occurs unless hCG has been administered or spontaneous ovulation occurs and a pregnancy ensues. The clinical symptoms usually appear 5 to 7 days after ovulation. Three degrees of OHSS are distinguished clinically: (1) mild, (2) moderate, and (3) severe. Mild hyperstimulation is associated with lower abdominal discomfort but with no significant weight gain. The ovaries are enlarged but are less than 5 cm in average diameter (Fig. 28–14A). With severe hyperstimulation, the ovaries are markedly enlarged (> 10 cm in diameter) and at risk of rupture or torsion. The development of large amounts of ascites and pleural effusions leads to hemoconcentration, with hypotension, oliguria, and electrolyte imbalance. In these cases, hospitalization may be required. Intra-abdominal hemorrhage caused by ovarian rupture or ruptured ectopic pregnancy must also be considered in the differential diagnosis. The sonographic appearance of the ovaries is distinctive. The ovarian enlargement is mainly caused by the presence of numerous large thin-walled cysts that are usually peripherally placed and may replace most of the ovary. The fluid exuded from the enlarged ovaries is easily detected in the pelvis and abdomen (see Fig. 28–14B). If the patient does not become pregnant, the syndrome resolves in 3 to 7 days or at the onset of the next menstrual cycle. It is probable that OHSS is seen more commonly when a pregnancy occurs; and, in this situation, ovarian enlargement and symptoms may persist with slow improvement occurring over a time frame of 6 to 8 weeks.

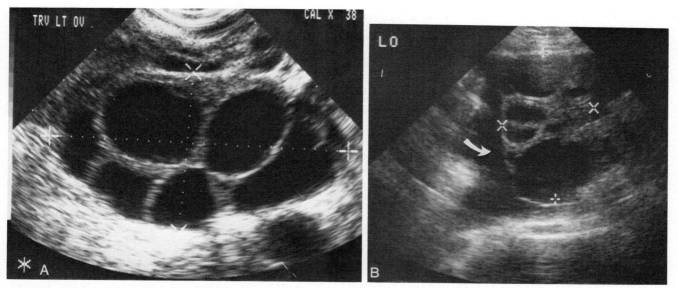

Figure 28–14. Ovarian hyperstimulation syndrome. *A.* There is mild disease with an enlarged ovary (6.8 × 3.8 × 6.2 cm) with multiple large theca lutein cysts. *B.* In this example of more severe disease there is an enlarged ovary (5.6 × 8.8 × 8.0 cm) and a moderate amount of ascites *(arrows).*

Sonographically, the potential for the development of OHSS should be suspected when multiple (more than eight) follicles develop; however, this is not as accurate as plasma estradiol levels in predicting OHSS. Although mild or moderate hyperstimulation may be encountered with estradiol levels in the 1000 to 4000 pg/mL range, the risk of severe hyperstimulation becomes very significant with estradiol levels greater than 4000 pg/mL at the time of hCG administration.[73] At these levels, OHSS is particularly likely if pregnancy occurs. Despite superovulation induction, OHSS is less often seen in IVF programs, probably because the follicles are damaged at the time of oocyte aspiration and there is consequently poor corpus luteum development, although this is rarely clinically apparent.

ULTRASOUND-GUIDED OOCYTE RETRIEVAL AND EMBRYO/GAMETE TRANSFER

Endovaginal oocyte retrieval has replaced laparoscopic retrieval in the majority of infertility programs. The major advantages include decreased exposure to general anesthesia, lower chances of procedural complications, and the ability to perform the procedure in an outpatient setting. The endovaginal sonographic approach has significant advantages over transabdominal[74] and periurethral sonographic approaches,[75] although these techniques may have a role in abnormally positioned ovaries that are not accessible endovaginally. Endovaginal sonographic retrieval is performed after appropriate premedication and placement of a paracervical block. A relatively large-gauge needle, greater than 18F, with a large internal bore, a beveled tip, and occluding stylet is recommended because of the size of the expanded preovulatory cumulus mass that is just visible to the naked eye. Teflon coating of

the needle tip may assist in sonographic recognition and ease of passage through pelvic tissues especially in the presence of adhesions. With the use of a needle guide on the transducer, the needle is introduced sequentially into follicles. After initial aspiration, the follicle is filled with buffered medium and flushed so that the chances for retrieving a mature oocyte are maximized. The needle is not withdrawn between punctures unless an endometrioma is encountered, which requires removal of the needle and flushing of the system. This technique is associated with a low complication rate, but the inadvertent introduction of the needle into a vessel, usually the iliac vein, may occur. This probably could be avoided by examination of all apparently round structures in both the long and short axis or by the use of color flow Doppler imaging. The success rate, as determined by the number of fertilizable oocytes retrieved and pregnancies produced, is comparable with that of the laparoscopic technique.[61]

Endovaginal sonography is also used for cannulization of the uterine and tubal lumen allowing placement of a catheter into the fallopian tube for GIFT. Embryo or ZIFT may also be performed. A catheter is placed transcervically and manipulated into the area of the uterine cornu. Under sonographic guidance, the catheter is then advanced into the distal tube where the sperm and ova (GIFT) or zygote (ZIFT) are deposited.[61]

References

1. Davies J, Hafez ESE, Ludwig H: Microscopic anatomy of the female reproductive tract and pituitary. In Danforth DN, Scott JR (eds): Obstetrics and Gynecology, 5th ed, p 78. Philadelphia, JB Lippincott, 1986.
2. Coulam CB: Cyclic ovarian function and its neuroendocrine control. In Danforth DN, Scott JR (eds): Obstetrics and Gynecology, 5th ed, p 120. Philadelphia, JB Lippincott, 1986.

3. Sample WF, Lippe BM, Gyepes MT: Gray-scale ultrasonography of the normal female pelvis. Radiology 125:477, 1977.

4. Hall DA, Hann LE, Ferrucci JT, et al: Sonographic morphology of the normal menstrual cycle. Radiology 133:185, 1979.

5. Fleischer AC, Herbert CM, Hill GA, Kepple DM: Transvaginal sonography: Applications in infertility. Semin Ultrasound CT MR 11:71, 1990.

6. Meldrum DR, Chetkowski RJ, Steingold KA, Randle D: Transvaginal ultrasound scanning of ovarian follicles. Fertil Steril 42:803, 1984.

7. Hall DA: Sonographic appearance of normal ovary, of polycystic disease, and of functional ovarian cysts. Semin Ultrasound 4:149, 1983.

8. Cohen HL, Tice HM, Mandel FS: Ovarian volumes measured by US: Bigger than we think. Radiology 177:189, 1990.

9. Pache TD, Wladimiroff JW, Hop WCJ, Fauser BCJM: How to discriminate between normal and polycystic ovaries: Transvaginal US study. Radiology 183:421, 1992.

10. Hackeloer BJ, Fleming R, Robinson HP, et al: Correlation of ultrasonic and endocrinologic assessment of human follicular development. Am J Obstet Gynecol 135:122, 1979.

11. Fleischer AC, Darnell J, Rodier J, et al: Sonographic monitoring of ovarian follicular development. J Clin Ultrasound 9:275, 1981.

12. Lenz S: Ultrasonic study of follicular maturation, ovulation and development of corpus luteum during normal menstrual cycles. Acta Obstet Gynecol Scand 64:15, 1985.

13. Hackeloer BJ: Ultrasound scanning of the ovarian cycle. J In Vitro Fertil Embryo Transfer 1:217, 1984.

14. Hodgen GD: The dominant ovarian follicle. Fertil Steril 38:281, 1982.

15. Fritz MA, Speroff L: The endocrinology of the menstrual cycle: The interaction of folliculogenesis and neuroendocrine mechanisms. Fertil Steril 38:509, 1982.

16. Pache TD, Wladimiroff JW, deJong FH, et al: Growth patterns of nondominant ovarian follicles during the normal menstrual cycle. Fertil Steril 54:638, 1990.

17. Kerin JF, Edmonds DK, Warnes GM, et al: Morphological and functional relations of graafian follicle growth to ovulation in women using ultrasonic, laparoscopic and biochemical measurements. Br J Obstet Gynaecol 88:81, 1981.

18. Ron-El R, Nachum H, Golan A, et al: Binovular human ovarian follicles associated with in vitro fertilization: Incidence and outcome. Fertil Steril 54:869, 1990.

19. Queenan JT, O'Brien GD, Bains LM, et al: Ultrasound scanning of ovaries to detect ovulation in women. Fertil Steril 34:99, 1980.

20. O'Herlihy C, deCrespigny LJ, Lopata A, et al: Preovulatory follicular size: A comparison of ultrasound and laparoscopic measurements. Fertil Steril 34:24, 1980.

21. Eissa MF, Hudson K, Docker MF, et al: Ultrasound follicle diameter measurement: An assessment of interobserver and intraobserver variation. Fertil Steril 44:751, 1985.

22. Forman RG, Robinson J, Yudkin P, et al: What is the true follicular diameter: An assessment of reproducibility of transvaginal ultrasound monitoring in stimulated cycles. Fertil Steril 56:989, 1991.

23. Zandt-Stastny D, Thorsen MK, Middleton WD, et al: Inability of sonography to detect imminent ovulation. AJR 152:91, 1989.

24. O'Herlihy C, deCrespigny LJ: Monitoring ovarian follicular development with real-time ultrasound. Br J Obstet Gynaecol 87:613, 1980.

25. Schwimer SR, Lebovic J: Transvaginal pelvic ultrasonography: Accuracy in follicle and cyst size determination. J Ultrasound Med 4:61, 1985.

26. Picker RH, Smith DH, Tucker MH, Saunders DM: Ultrasonic signs of imminent ovulation. J Clin Ultrasound 11:1, 1983.

27. Marinho AO, Sallam HN, Goessens LKV, et al: Real-time pelvic ultrasonography during the periovulatory period of patients attending an artificial insemination clinic. Fertil Steril 37:633, 1982.

28. Nitschke-Dabelstein S, Hackeloer BJ, Sturm G: Ovulation and corpus luteum formation observed by ultrasonography. Ultrasound Med Biol 7:33, 1980.

29. Koninckx PR, Renaer M, Brosens IA: Origin of peritoneal fluid in women: An ovarian exudation product. Br J Obstet Gynaecol 87:177, 1980.

30. O'Herlihy C, Robinson HP, deCrespigny LJ: Mittelschmerz is a preovulatory symptom. Br Med J 280:986, 1980.

31. Wetzels LCG, Hoogland HJ: Relation between ultrasonographic evidence of ovulation and hormonal parameters: Luteinizing hormone surge and initial progesterone rise. Fertil Steril 37:336, 1982.

32. Scheenjes E, te Velde ER, Kremer J: Inspection of the ovaries and steroids in serum and peritoneal fluid at various time intervals after ovulation in fertile women: Luteinized unruptured follicle syndrome. Fertil Steril 54:38, 1990.

33. deCrespigny LJ, O'Herlihy C, Robinson HP: Ultrasonic observations of the mechanisms of human ovulation. Am J Obstet Gynecol 1939:636, 1981.

34. Levine D, Gosink BB, Wolf SI, et al: Simple adnexal cysts: The natural history in post menopausal women. Radiology 184:653, 1992.

35. Fleischer AC, Kalemeris GC, Entman SS: Sonographic depiction of the endometrium during normal cycles. Ultrasound Med Biol 12:271, 1986.

36. Fleischer AC, Kalemeris CG, Machin JE, et al: Sonographic depiction of normal and abnormal endometrium with histopathologic correlation. J Ultrasound Med 8:445, 1986.

37. Randall JM, Fisk NM, McTavish A, Templeton AA: Transvaginal ultrasonic assessment of endometrial growth in spontaneous and hyperstimulated menstrual cycles. Br J Obstet Gynaecol 96:954, 1989.

38. Lyons EA, Taylor PJ, Zheng HX, et al: Characterization of subendometrial myometrial contractions throughout the menstrual cycle in normal fertile women. Fertil Steril 55:771, 1991.

39. Abramowicz JS, Archer DF: Uterine endometrial peristalsis—a transvaginal ultrasound study. Fertil Steril 54:451, 1990.

40. Farquhar CM, Rae T, Thomas DC, et al: Doppler ultrasound in the nonpregnant pelvis. J Ultrasound Med 8:451, 1989.

41. Taylor JW, Burns PN, Woodcock JP, Wells PNT: Blood flow in deep abdominal and pelvic vessels: Ultrasonic pulsed Doppler analysis. Radiology 154:487, 1985.

42. Dillon EH, Taylor KJW: Doppler ultrasound in the female pelvis in first trimester of pregnancy. Clin Diag Ultrasound 26:93, 1990.

43. Kurjak A, Kupesic-Urek S, Schulman H, Zalud I: Transvaginal color flow Doppler in the assessment of ovarian and uterine flow in infertile women. Fertil Steril 56:870, 1991.

44. Scholtes MCW, Wladimiroff JW, van Rigen HJM, Hop WCJ: Uterine and ovarian flow velocity waveforms in the normal menstrual cycle: A transvaginal Doppler study. Fertil Steril 52:981, 1989.

45. deZiegler D, Bessis R, Frydman R: Vascular resistance of uterine arteries: Physiological effect of estradiol and progesterone. Fertil Steril 55:775, 1991.

46. Goswamy RK, Steptoe PC: Doppler ultrasound studies of the uterine artery in spontaneous ovarian cycles. Human Reprod 3:721, 1988.

47. Thaler I, Manor D, Rotten S, et al: Hemodynamic evaluation of the female pelvic vessels using high-frequency transvaginal image-directed Doppler system. J Clin Ultrasound 18:364, 1990.

48. Polan ML, Totora M, Caldwell BV, et al: Abnormal ovarian cycles as diagnosed by ultrasound and serum estradiol levels. Fertil Steril 37:342, 1982.

49. Coulman CB, Bustillo M, Schulman JD: Empty follicle syndrome. Fertil Steril 46:1153, 1986.

50. Ben-Shlomo I, Schiff E, Levran D, et al: Failure of oocyte retrieval during in vitro fertilization: A sporadic event rather than a syndrome. Fertil Steril 55:324, 1991.

51. Hilgers TA, Kimball CR, Keck SJ, et al: Assessment of the empty follicle syndrome by transvaginal sonography. J Ultrasound Med 11:313, 1992.

52. Hilgers TW, Dvorak AD, Tamisiea DF, et al: Sonographic definition of the empty follicle syndrome. J Ultrasound Med 8:411, 1989.

53. Coulam CB, Hill LM, Breckle R: Ultrasonic evidence for luteinization of unruptured preovulatory follicles. Fertil Steril 37:524, 1982.

54. Kerin JF, Kirby C, Morris D, et al: Incidence of luteinized unruptured follicle phenomenon in cycling women. Fertil Steril 40:620, 1983.

55. Liukkonen S, Koskimies AI, Tenhunen A, Ylostalo P: Diagnosis

of luteinized unruptured follicle (LUF) syndrome by ultrasound. Fertil Steril 41:26, 1984.

56. Killick S, Elstein M: Pharmacologic production of luteinized unruptured follicles by prostaglandin synthetase inhibitors. Fertil Steril 5:773, 1987.

57. Parisi L, Tramonti M, Derchi LE, et al: Polycystic ovarian disease: Ultrasonic evaluation and correlations with clinical and hormonal data. J Clin Ultrasound 12:21, 1984.

58. Swanson M, Sauerbrei EE, Cooperberg PL: Medical implications of ultrasonically detected polycystic ovaries. J Clin Ultrasound 9:219, 1981.

59. Worley R: Ovulation induction. In Garcia CR, Mastroianni L, Amelar RD, Dublin L (eds): Current Therapy in Infertility 3, pp 106–110. Toronto, BC Decker, 1988.

60. Thanki KH, Schmidt CL: Follicular development and oocyte maturation after stimulation with gonadotropins versus leuprolide acetate/gonadotropins during in vitro fertilizations. Fertil Steril 54:656, 1990.

61. Medical Research International. In vitro fertilization–embryo transfer (IVF-ET) in the United States: 1990 results from the IVF-ET Registry. Fertil Steril 57:15, 1992.

62. Soules MR: The in vitro fertilization pregnancy rate: Let's be honest with one another. Fertil Steril 43:511, 1985.

63. Corson GH, Kemmann E: The role of superovulation with menotropins in ovulatory infertility: A review. Fertil Steril 55:468, 1991.

64. Shoham Z, DiCarlo C, Patel A, et al: Is it possible to run a successful ovulation induction program based solely on ultrasound monitoring? The importance of endometrial measurements. Fertil Steril 56:836, 1991.

65. Zacur HA: Ovulation with gonadotropin-releasing hormone. Fertil Steril 44:435, 1986.

66. Ritchie WGM: Sonographic evaluation of normal and induced ovulation. Radiology 161:1, 1986.

67. Goldberg JM, Miller FA, Friedman CI, et al: Effect of baseline ovarian cysts on in vitro fertilization and gamete intrafallopian transfer cycles. Fertil Steril 55:319, 1991.

68. Haines CJ, Emes A: The relationship between follicle diameter, fertilization rate, and microscopic embryo quality. Fertil Steril 55:205, 1991.

69. Cacciatore B, Liukkonen S, Koskimies AI, Ylostalo P: Ultrasonic detection of cumulus oophorus in patients undergoing in vitro fertilization. J In Vitro Fertil Embryo Transfer 2:224, 1985.

70. Marrs RP, Vargyas JM, March CM: Correlation of ultrasonic and endocrinologic measurements in human menopausal gonadotropin therapy. Am J Obstet Gynecol 145:417, 1983.

71. Bateman BG, Kolp LA, Nunley WC, et al: Oocyte retention after follicle luteinization. Fertil Steril 54:793, 1990.

72. McArdle C, Seibel M, Hann LE, et al: The diagnosis of ovarian hyperstimulation (OHS): The impact of ultrasound. Fertil Steril 39:464, 1983.

73. Haning RV, Austin CW, Carlson IM, et al: Plasma estradiol is superior to ultrasound and urinary estriol glucuronide as a predictor of ovarian hyperstimulation during induction of ovulation with menotropins. Fertil Steril 40:31, 1983.

74. Lenz S: Ultrasonic-guided follicle puncture under local anesthesia. J In Vitro Fertil Embryo Transfer 1:239, 1984.

75. Parsons J, Riddle A, Booker M, et al: Oocyte retrieval for in vitro fertilization by ultrasonically guided needle aspiration via the urethra. Lancet 1:1076, 1985.

CHAPTER 29

Ultrasound Evaluation of the Uterus

DEBORAH A. HALL, M.D.
ISABEL C. YODER, M.D.

The uterus is one of the most dynamic organs in the human body. It grows in size and changes in configuration with the hormonal influence of puberty and then atrophies again with menopause. During the reproductive years the endometrium is continuously undergoing cyclic renewals. During pregnancy the uterus must remarkably grow and change to protect, support, and finally deliver the developing fetus. In addition to these obvious transformations, it has been demonstrated that the uterus has a complex system of internal contractions.[1] Submyometrial contractions occur with a wave from the cervix to the fundus, and they occur with increasing frequency and amplitude during the periovulatory period, as studied with endovaginal ultrasonography and videotape. Perhaps this activity assists in the complex mechanism of sperm transportation and subsequent fertilization. With recent advances in color and Doppler ultrasonography, vascular alterations during the uterine cycle are now obvious and our understanding of these events might be helpful diagnostically and therapeutically.

Since the arrival of clinical ultrasonography in the late 1970s, it has been the major focus and "gold standard" of uterine imaging. The advent of endovaginal sonography in the 1980s solidified this position by providing a closer and more accurate ultrasound appraisal of the uterus. Now in the 1990s with improvements in computed tomography (CT), hysterosalpingography, and the rapidly developing magnetic resonance imaging (MRI) technology, these other modalities can complement the traditional sonographic evaluation. The focus in this chapter is on the transabdominal and endovaginal sonographic study of the uterus. There will be incorporation of other modalities for specific indications and illustrative purposes. The anatomy, embryology, and physiology of the uterus as well as benign and malignant conditions will be reviewed. Issues related to fertility are included, but all aspects of pregnancy are discussed elsewhere in this book.

SCANNING TECHNIQUES

Any discussion of uterine sonography must include both transabdominally and endovaginally performed examinations. It should be an unusual occurrence in most ultrasound departments to perform only one of these examinations as a diagnostic study. Obviously, endovaginal scanning is inappropriate in prepubertal children and some adolescent patients. Endovaginal

scanning may be also difficult or impossible for some premenopausal or postmenopausal women as well. Recent endometrial, cervical, or vaginal instrumentation is a relative contraindication to endovaginal scanning. Most fertility patients undergoing ovulation induction with frequent sonographic examinations for follicular assessment need only have an endovaginal scan. For other indications such as pelvic pain, pelvic mass, or bleeding the majority of patients should have both a transabdominal and an endovaginal study as part of the primary workup.

Patients should be encouraged to arrive in the ultrasound department with a full urinary bladder. This displaces small and large bowel away from the central pelvis and allows the use of the bladder as an acoustical window to the uterus and ovaries. Uterine and ovarian sizes can be measured and abnormal morphologic structures detected. Masses can be identified as to origin and then characterized. Associated findings such as cul-de-sac fluid, abdominal fluid, abdominal masses, or hydronephrosis should be noted. Since the gynecologist may be the primary physician for many women, all pelvic masses may not be gynecologic in origin and bowel, nodal, vascular, and other etiologies should be considered by the sonographer.

The uterus can be sonographically identified by its usual central location, by its continuity with the vagina, and by the endometrial stripe or echo. The sonographic appearance of the uterine cavity was described in the early ultrasound literature.[2] It represents the echoes reflecting from the apposed endometrial surfaces, and the cyclic variations during the normal and induced menstrual cycle.[3–5] The uterus is scanned in longitudinal and transverse planes transabdominally and in sagittal and coronal planes endovaginally (Fig. 29–1). Obliquing or angling the transducers both transabdominally and endovaginally is often necessary since the uterus may not be oriented directly in the midline. The highest-frequency transducer possible provides a more detailed image of the uterine structure. This is usually a 3.5- or 5-MHz transabdominal scanner. Endovaginal probes usually range from 5 to 8 MHz.

Emptying the full urinary bladder is necessary for endovaginal scanning to bring the uterus into the short focal zone of the endovaginal transducer. With large masses, an empty or partially full urinary bladder may also help with transabdominal scanning. For example, a small anterior uterus may be compressed against the full urinary bladder and not separately resolved from a large ovarian or other adnexal mass. Using a higher-

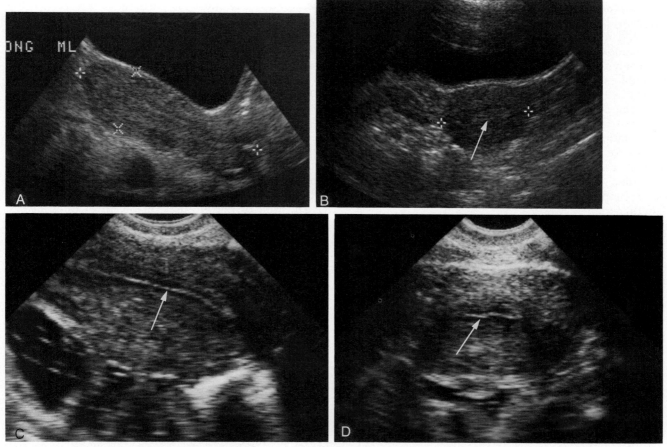

Figure 29–1. The normal uterus. Sagittal (*A*) and transverse (*B*) transabdominal sonograms of an adult uterus using the full urinary bladder as an acoustical window and a 3.5-MHz transducer. Sagittal (*C*) and coronal (*D*) endovaginal sonograms after voiding and the insertion of a 6.5-MHz probe. Arrow indicates endometrial canal.

frequency transducer and/or emptying the bladder may help to visualize the uterus separate from the mass.

Endovaginal scanning is performed with a protective covering, usually a condom over the transducer. Acoustical gel can be used both within the condom and as a lubricant over the condom. However, in infertility patients, this gel may be spermatocidal or may change the cervical mucus characteristics and only water should be used as a lubricant for insertion. Endovaginal scanning of the uterus can be performed with the patient in stirrups on a gynecologic table or with the patient's hips elevated on a pillow on a flat table. This allows manueverability of the transducer handle to visualize the severely anteverted uterus. The retropositioned uterus is easier to visualize and best seen endovaginally.

As with any ultrasound examination, the uterus should be examined with real-time imaging to avoid confusion with bowel loops or other pelvic structures. Static images are obtained to document the anatomy and any findings. Water enemas are rarely necessary anymore but occasionally may help in clarifying the retrouterine space.[6]

ANATOMY

As in all aspects of imaging, it is critical to understand normal anatomy and how it is reflected in the normal radiographic or sonographic images. Before abnormal morphology can be recognized or explained, all aspects of normal and normal variants need to be understood. The adult uterus is a thick-walled muscular structure that is usually anteverted, forming nearly a right angle with the vagina. It is situated between the bladder anteriorly and inferiorly and the sigmoid colon and rectum posteriorly. In *Gray's Anatomy* the uterus is described as 7.5 cm in length, 5 cm in width, and 2.5 cm thick and as weighing 30 to 40 grams.[7]

Many sonographic studies have tried to refine these values by correlating age, parity, and menstrual status.[8] In general, the pediatric uterus (under 7 years of age) measures less than or equal to 3.5 cm in length on sagittal ultrasound images. The cervix is more prominent in the prepubertal uterus and the ratio of cervix to fundus anteroposterior diameters is 2:1.[9] Under the influence of pubertal gonadotropins the uterus begins to increase in size around 8 years and measures 6 cm in length by approximately age 13. The cervix to fundus ratio remains 2:1. Transversely the uterus may measure 3 cm at this point. With the onset of true puberty and adulthood the normal uterus will measure less than or equal to 10 cm in length, less than or equal to 5 cm in width, and less than or equal to 4 cm in height. Parity may increase the overall uterine size and weight or volume. Under the influence of pubertal hormones the cervix to fundus ratio becomes 1:2 with development of the uterine fundus (Fig. 29–2). In menopause the uterus will undergo progressive atrophy with increasing age and all measurements should be less than seen premenopausally. The cervix to fundus ratio will theoretically return to a 2:1 situation. However, given an isolated examination on a postmenopausal uterus it is difficult to know if that uterus is enlarged relative to its premenopausal status. Fibroids, parity, and surgery can cause such distortion and variability that clinical examinations and sequential sonograms are more accurate for assessing the significance of uterine size. The average postmenopausal uterus should measure less than 9 cm in length and by 15 or 20 years postmenopausally may only measure 5 to 6 cm in length.

The uterus is divided into the fundus, body, and cervical regions. The sonographic sagittal appearance is a dumbbell-shaped organ with a more bulbous fundus and cervix and a narrower middle body. The part of the uterus above the insertion of the fallopian tubes is termed the *fundus*. The lateral funnel-shaped horns of the uterus where the fallopian tubes insert are called the *cornua*. The uterus is partially covered anteriorly by peritoneum reflecting off the posterior bladder and forming the vesicouterine pouch and then covering the body and fundus. The peritoneum continues posteriorly to create the deeper posterior uterorectal pouch of Douglas or cul-de-sac. Thus all but the anterior low body and cervix of the uterus are covered by peritoneum. This anatomic situation allows cesarean sections to be performed extraperitoneally when a low transverse uterine incision is used. The cervix is less mobile than the body of the uterus. Its inferior aspect protrudes into the vagina. The cervical canal connects the uterine cavity to the vagina through the internal and external os.

The wall of the uterus is made up of three layers. The overall covering of the peritoneum is the serosal or external surface. The second or muscular layer of the myometrium accounts for the bulk of the uterine wall. Nonstriated muscle fibers are woven with loose connective tissue, blood vessels, lymph channels, and nerves. With pregnancy the myometrium hypertrophies and three layers of the myometrium become more

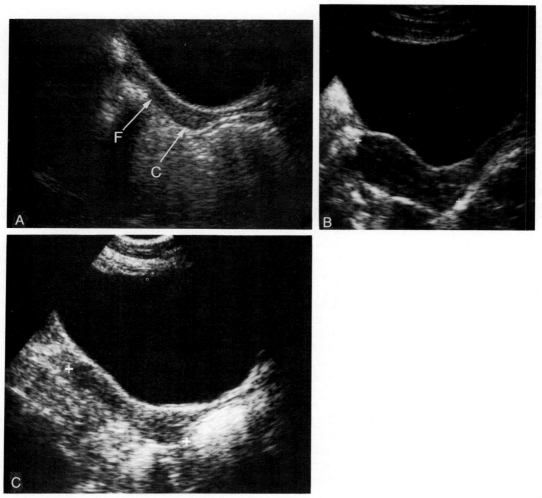

Figure 29–2. Uterine morphology. *A.* The prepubertal uterus has a bulbous cervix (C) in comparison to the rudimentary fundus (F). This sagittal sonogram of a 7-year-old child demonstrates a normal cervical/fundal anteroposterior ratio of 2:1. *B.* With puberty the fundus develops and the uterus assumes a more "hourglass" shape with a C/F ratio of 1:2. *C.* After menopause the uterus will atrophy and its configuration may return to a prepubertal C/F ratio of 2:1. This image of a postmenopausal uterus demonstrates that the cervix is slightly more prominent than the fundus.

distinct. The outer or external layer is composed of mostly longitudinally oriented fibers. The intermediate layer is the widest with longitudinal, transverse, and oblique fibers and contains the larger blood vessels, for which it is named the stratum vasculare. The internal or inner layer has longitudinal and circular fibers and contains the deepest part of the tortuous endometrial uterine glands. The muscle layers of the cervix contain more elastin and collagen than do the muscle layers of the myometrium.

The third or inner layer of the uterus is the highly specialized mucosa or endometrium. It contains connective tissue and tubular glands that undergo cyclic response to ovarian hormones. The endometrium is continuous with the vaginal mucosa through the cervical canal and with the peritoneum through the tubal lining. The upper two thirds of the endocervical epithelium is made of mucin-secreting columnar cells. The lower cervical epithelium is stratified squamous epithelium continuous with the vaginal lining. The transitional zone of cervical epithelium undergoes constant change, and it is in this junctional area that squamous carcinoma of the cervix is likely to develop.

The uterus is supported and suspended in the pelvis by a combination of true fibrous ligaments and filamentous folds of the peritoneum that offer little support. The uterosacral ligaments are composed of fibrous tissue and nonstriated muscle that extend from the cervix posteriorly on either side of the rectum to attach to the sacrum. The round ligaments also contain nonstriated muscle, especially near their origin along the lateral uterine body below the cornu. These bands travel anteriorly and laterally along the pelvic side wall to enter the inguinal canal (Fig. 29–3). The cardinal ligaments or ligaments of Mackenrodt are also supportive and extend from the cervix to the vaginal vault. Thus the uterus has some fixation to the sacrum posteriorly, the inguinal canal region anteriorly, and caudally to the vagina. The broad ligament is the folded peritoneum covering the fundus and extending laterally to the pelvic wall and to the pelvic floor inferiorly. It is simply connective tissue and not truly supporting. It is continuous with the mesosalpinx and the mesometrium, which are leaves of mesentery suspending the ovary from the tube and from the ovarian ligament that extends laterally from the uterus. The lateral

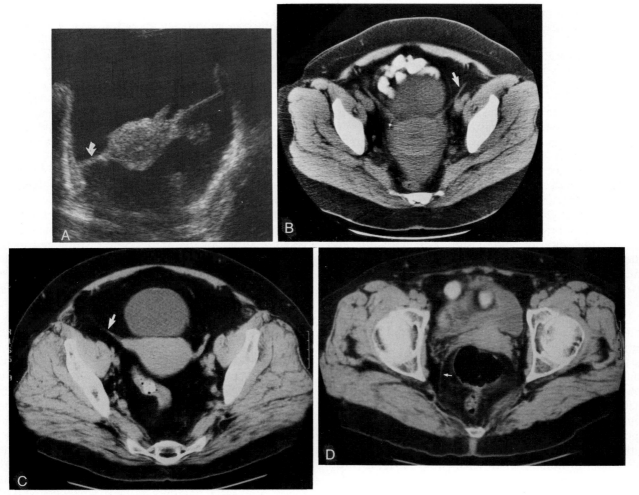

Figure 29–3. Uterine ligaments. *A*. Transverse sonogram of the pelvis in a patient with a large amount of ascites secondary to liver disease demonstrates a small uterus suspended in the fluid by the broad ligaments and infundibular pelvic ligaments (*arrows*). *B* and *C*. Two CT scans demonstrating the round ligaments of the uterus, which extend anterior and laterally from the uterine body to the inguinal canal (*arrows*). *D*. Transverse CT scan lower in the pelvis of another patient demonstrates the uterosacral ligaments extending posteriorly from the cervix around the rectum to attach to the sacrum (*arrow*).

aspect of the broad ligament forms a more prominent fold called the infundibular pelvic ligament or the suspensory ligament of the ovary and contains the ovarian vessels and nerves extending laterally to the external iliac vessels. This flexible arrangement of support allows uterine mobility with a variety of possible positions. The cervical axis is relatively fixed in the midline but the axis of the uterine body may join the cervix from any obliquity. The status of the other pelvic organs and any abnormal masses may change the uterine position and orientation. The full urinary bladder also changes the uterine relationships during transabdominal ultrasound scanning.

The uterus usually assumes a position that is both anteverted and anteflexed (Fig. 29–4). Version refers to the axis of the cervix in relationship to the vagina. When the bladder is empty, the axis of the cervix to the vagina is about 90° or in anteversion. Retroversion occurs when the angle of the cervix with the vagina is greater than 90°. Flexion refers to the axis of the body of the uterus in relationship to the cervix. The uterus is usually anteflexed with an approximately 20° angle between the body and cervix. Similarly, the body can be retroflexed posteriorly in relationship to the cervix. With the full urinary bladder necessary for transabdominal examinations the uterus assumes a more repositioned orientation than it does naturally (see Fig. 29–4).

The main arterial blood supply to the uterus is the uterine artery from the internal iliac artery, which is the major arterial source for the pelvis through its many branches. The uterine artery branch travels in the cardinal ligament to the lower body of the uterus. Cervical and vaginal arteries branch from it, and then the uterine artery courses toward the fundus lateral to the uterine wall in the broad ligament. It anastomoses with the ovarian artery, which arises from the aorta and has reached the ovary by way of the infundibular pelvic ligament to create a vascular plexus supplying the ovary, tube, and round ligament. The uterine arteries send branches into the uterine wall, which become the anterior and posterior arcuate arteries. These arteries course transversely in the myometrium and anastomose across the midline. These arcuate arteries send radial branches centrally through the myometrium to reach the endometrium.

The arcuate arteries were first described with transabdominal sonography in 1985 as hypoechoic areas in the outer myometrium at regular intervals.[10] These vascular channels are now well recognized in routine scanning with the endovaginal probe and the use of color flow Doppler scanning. Calcifications in the arcuate arteries in the older or diabetic uterus are also commonly seen.[11] These typical calcifications are peripheral, regularly spaced, and linear echogenic areas with shadowing. This description aids in differentiating this common finding from calcified leiomyomas. The uterine veins parallel the arterial arrangement but are generally larger. This vascular anatomy can be elegantly displayed with ultrasonography, Doppler ultrasonography, and color flow Doppler imaging (Fig. 29–5).[12]

The lymphatic drainage of the uterus can follow a number of routes. A major pathway is along the uterine vessels to the internal iliac nodes. There may be direct connections to the external iliac or obturator nodes. Minor pathways travel along the ovarian vessels to the para-aortic nodes, along the round ligament to the inguinal nodes, and along the uterosacral ligament to the presacral nodes. These nodes are not normally seen on ultrasound evaluation but may be seen if they are enlarged. CT and MRI are better imaging modalities to visualize the lymph node chains.

Directly correlating the gross anatomy of the uterus with the ultrasound appearance is difficult. The apposed endometrial surfaces of the endometrial cavity create the hyperechoic central uterine echo. The cyclic ultrasound appearance of the endometrium has been extensively studied and will be discussed subsequently in the next section. Surrounding the endometrial complex is a hypoechoic area or ring. This may represent the inner myometrium with more compacted myometrial cells and less connective tissue. However, this has no real histologic counterpart.[3–5] The outer layer of myometrium is thicker and has a more homogeneous appearance with moderate echogenicity (Fig. 29–6).

All the advantages of ultrasonography, including nonionizing radiation, ability to scan in multiple planes, ease of examination, relatively low cost, and noninvasiveness, make it ideally suited to image the uterus. CT, which is generally limited to the transverse axial projection, involves ionizing radiation, often employs intravenous contrast agents, and offers a less sensitive and less specific uterine image since the attenuation values of normal uterus and uterine abnormalities are so similar. CT, however, is critical in staging disease and detecting other abdominal and pelvic abnormalities.

Magnetic resonance imaging uniquely combines features that add specificity to abnormalities detected on ultrasound evaluation. MRI does not use ionizing radiation, and images can be obtained in multiple planes. In particular, T2-weighted images delineate a zonal anatomy of the uterus. On T1-weighted images the uterine signal is homogeneous and low to intermediate. With T2-weighted sequences, three separate zones are apparent in the uterus. A high or bright signal is believed to represent the endometrium. Surrounding the endometrium is a junctional zone of low signal intensity. The outer layer has an intermediate signal (Fig. 29–7). It is unclear what these layers or zones represent histologically and anatomically. Studies have shown that the low junctional zone signal may be secondary to its lower water content.[13] Other studies show no correlation between the described sonographic layers and the zonal layers of MRI.[14] These layers both on ultrasonography and MRI vary with the phases of the menstrual cycle. Surprisingly, even after a dilatation and curettage there is no MRI change in the width of the endometrial signal.[15] In addition, ultrasonography and MRI anatomy do not correlate with the histologic differences in the myometrium. However, despite the unexplained etiology of "zonal anatomy," MRI does afford a more detailed evaluation of the

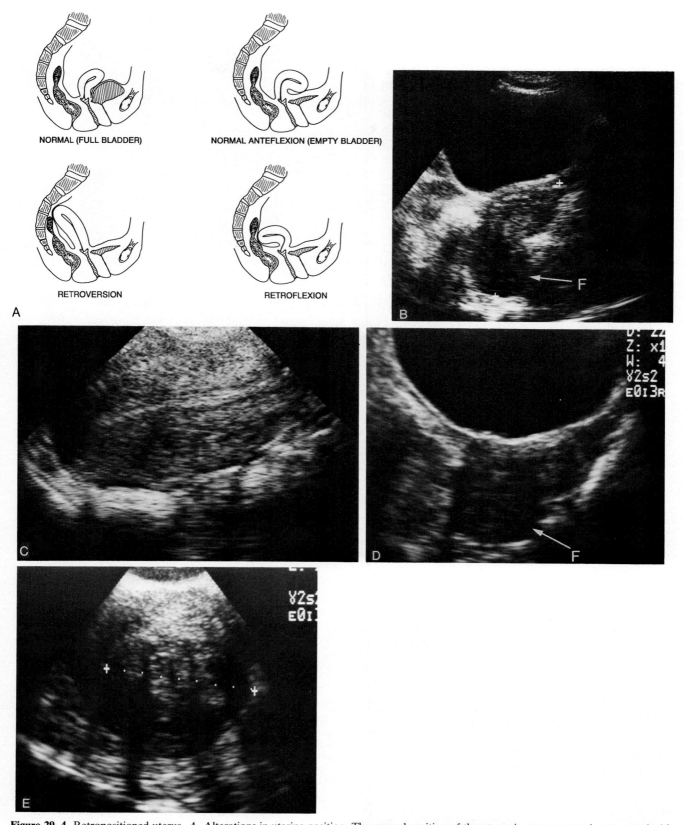

Figure 29–4. Retropositioned uterus. *A.* Alterations in uterine position. The normal position of the uterus in most women is anteverted with a mild degree of anteflexion. In retroversion, the long axis of the uterus and cervix points more posteriorly than the long axis of the vagina. In retroflexion, the body of the uterus is angled posteriorly relative to the cervix. *B.* The uterus in this sagittal transabdominal sonogram has assumed a severely retroverted and retroflexed position. The uterine fundus is hypoechoic and the distinction from a fundal fibroid is difficult. With retroflexion and a full urinary bladder the fundus is often displaced beyond the focal zone of the ultrasound beam and the beam is attenuated. *C.* A sagittal endovaginal sonogram of the same patient as *B* demonstrates a remarkably normal-appearing uterine fundus. *D.* In this less severely retropositioned uterus the fundus on this sagittal sonogram is also relatively hypoechoic. *E.* Endovaginal sonogram in the sagittal plane confirms the presence of a fundal fibroid (*cursors*) in this patient.

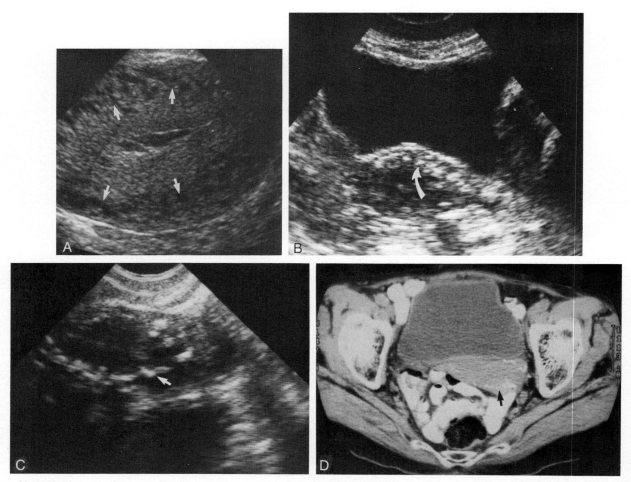

Figure 29–5. Uterine vasculature. *A.* Very prominent arcuate vessels that are most likely veins are seen in this coronal endovaginal sonogram (*arrows*). *B.* Transverse transabdominal sonogram in a postmenopausal woman demonstrates hyperechoic foci in a peripheral distribution in the uterus (*arrow*). *C.* Endovaginal coronal sonogram through the same uterus demonstrates again the peripheral circumferential nature of these calcified foci (*arrow*). *D.* A CT scan in the same patient elegantly confirms the calcified arcuate arteries (*arrow*).

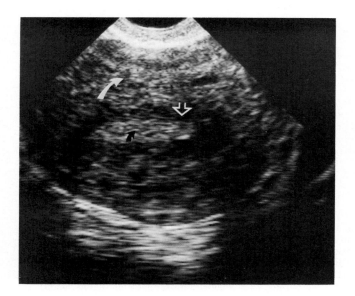

Figure 29–6. Uterine echotexture. This endovaginal coronal sonogram displays the normal sonographic appearance of the uterine wall. The central echogenic endometrium (*black arrow*) is surrounded by a hypoechoic layer, which may be the inner myometrium (*open arrow*). The outer myometrium is more echogenic and contains the vascular channels (*white arrow*).

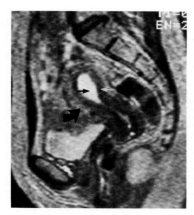

Figure 29-7. Magnetic resonance image of the uterus. T2-weighted midline sagittal image of the normal adult uterus reveals three zones or layers of the uterine wall: the high-signal or white endometrium (*small black arrow*), the low-signal junctional zone (*small white arrow*), and the outer moderate signal myometrium (*larger black arrow*).

uterine wall for specific indications, such as location of a leiomyoma and depth of invasion of endometrial carcinoma.

EMBRYOLOGY AND ANOMALIES

Embryology

It is no longer acceptable to classify a uterine duplication anomaly vaguely as a "double uterus." Accurate delineation of the uterus with endovaginal sonography, coupled with knowledge of the basic embryologic development of the uterus, allows a more specific diagnosis of the exact anomaly involved (Fig. 29–8). The uterus originates from paired müllerian ducts, and most uterine malformations stem from partial failure of fusion or from failure of septum resorption of these ducts. The müllerian or paramesonephric ducts appear on the posterior abdominal wall of the 6-week embryo.[16] The cranial portion of the müllerian ducts develops lateral and parallel to the mesonephric ducts, but on reaching the pelvic region the müllerian ducts cross the mesonephric ducts ventrally and fuse as they approach each other in the midline. Canalization of the müllerian ducts occurs during their downward growth. The fallopian tubes are derived from the cranial unfused portions while the uterus is derived from the fusion of the caudal part of the hollow müllerian ducts. At first a septum exists between the ducts, and its subsequent resorption results in a single uterine cavity.

Complete failure of fusion of the müllerian ducts gives rise to the uterus didelphys, a rare complete duplication of the uterus, often associated with a sagittal vaginal septum. More commonly only the fundus fails to fuse while the cervix fuses normally giving rise to the bicornuate uterus. The mildest fusion anomaly is the uterus arcuatus, which results from minor lack of fusion of the fundus and is considered a normal variant. If fusion occurs but the median septum fails

to resorb totally or partially, the uterus is classified as septus or subseptus. Rarely a combination anomaly is seen in which the fundus is bicornuate and the cervix is septate; this is known as a uterus bicornis bicollis.

The unicornuate uterus results from development of only one müllerian duct and varying degrees of atresia of the contralateral system. Aplasia of both müllerian ducts is very rare and results in congenital absence of the uterus, often associated with absence or shortening of the vagina. Uterine malformations are frequently associated with urinary tract abnormalities. Approximately one third of women with abnormal genital tracts will have unilateral renal agenesis or renal ectopia.[17] Ultrasonography provides the ideal diagnostic tool for simultaneous evaluation of the genital and urinary tracts.

Ultrasonography

Ultrasonography can detect most uterine anomalies because it demonstrates the external outline of the uterus and the presence of two endometrial echo complexes.[18] When there is lack of fusion of the fundus, as seen in the didelphys and the bicornuate uterus, the sonogram shows a deep fundal notch. In a septate uterus the fundal notch is shallow and much less evident. In addition, the endometrial cavities of the didelphys and bicornuate uterus are widely separated by a full complement of myometrium while the endometrial cavities in septate and subseptate uterus are closer together and separated only by a thin echogenic fibrous septum (see Fig. 29–8). Combining the sonographic findings with hysterosalpingography provides a 90% accuracy in distinguishing a septate from a bicornuate abnormality.[19] This differentiation is important because the septate uterus, often associated with multiple second-trimester miscarriages, can easily be treated by hysteroscopic resection of the septum. To achieve unification of the bicornuate uterus, on the other hand, requires abdominal surgery.

More complex uterine anomalies such as uterus didelphys associated with a unilateral hematocolpos are well demonstrated by ultrasound imaging.[20] The hematocolpos presents as a large vaginal echogenic cystic mass, often producing hematometros and hematosalpinx on the affected side, and is associated with a relatively normal contralateral uterine horn. The differential diagnosis includes a large Gartner's duct cyst, not usually associated with a uterine duplication anomaly. Agenesis of the kidney on the same side as the vaginal obstruction almost always accompanies unilateral hematocolpos.

The unicornuate uterus is difficult to recognize sonographically. The opposite dilated rudimentary horn may be erroneously diagnosed as a uterine or adnexal mass. Complete evaluation of these cases requires hysterosalpingography or MRI, which provides more accurate delineation of uterine anomalies. The relatively high cost of MRI reserves its use for preoperative evaluation of the more confusing or complicated genital anomalies.

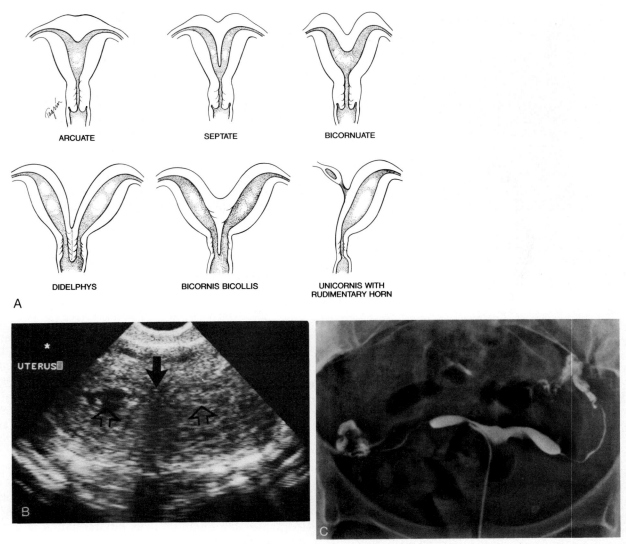

Figure 29–8. Uterine anomalies. *A.* Diagram of uterine anomalies. *B.* Coronal endovaginal sonogram through the fundus of a bicornuate uterus demonstrates the two endometrial cavities (*open arrows*) separated by the uterine musculature (*arrow*). *C.* Two separate cavities with patent tubes are seen on the hysterosalpingogram.

In utero exposure to diethylstilbestrol causes uterine abnormalities that are not fusion defects. Diethylstilbestrol given during the first trimester crosses the placenta and exerts a direct effect on the müllerian system of the fetus. The uterus in these patients is small, and the uterine cavity is irregular and T shaped. Ultrasonography may demonstrate a diffuse decrease in the size of the uterus.[21]

UTERINE PHYSIOLOGY

The endometrium is under direct influence of the ovarian hormones estrogen and progesterone and responds in a cyclic manner that is easily recognized sonographically. Early transabdominal studies of the endometrium were done of both normal and stimulated cycles.[3, 4] Recently, similar studies have been performed using endovaginal sonography with elegant histologic correlation.[15, 22] The endometrium or mucosal surface of the uterus is composed of columnar epithelial cells, deep endometrial glands, and the lamina propria or stroma. It can be roughly divided into a superficial or functional layer and a thin deeper basal layer. The uterine cycle consists of the proliferative, secretory, and menstrual phases. Under the influence of rising estrogens from folliculogenesis in the ovary, the endometrial cells proliferate and increase in size. The spiral arteriolar capillary bed of the functional layer also enlarges. Endovaginal ultrasound scanning during this proliferative phase demonstrates a "triple lined appearance" to the endometrium (Fig. 29–9). The hypoechoic appearance of the functional layer may be related to the orderly arrangement of glands and lack of secretions. Measuring the normal proliferative endometrium in the sagittal projection from basalis to the basalis gives a range of 4 to 8 mm.[5]

With ovulation and the production of progesterone from the corpus luteum, the secretory phase of the endometrium begins with glandular elongation and tortuosity and with the production of secretory vacuoles. The glandular lumina contain secretions and the

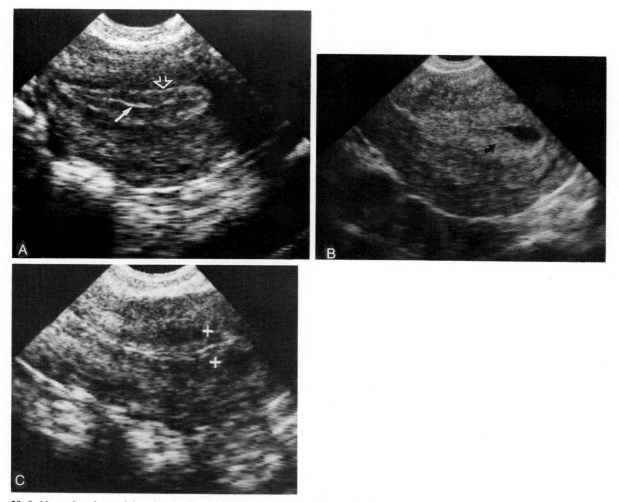

Figure 29–9. Normal endometrial cycle. *A.* The "triple-line" appearance of proliferative endometrium during the first half of the menstrual cycle is demonstrated in this sagittal endovaginal sonogram. The apposed endometrial surfaces comprise the central echogenic line (*arrow*), which is surrounded by the hypoechoic developing functional layer. The outer echogenic layer (*open arrow*) is the basal layer. *B.* After ovulation, maturation of the glands and the increasing tortuousity of the spiral arteries results in the echogenic or bright appearance of the functional layer (*arrow*). In this endovaginal sagittal sonogram there is a small amount of black fluid in the endometrial cavity. *C.* The sonographic appearance of the endometrium during menses is variable. In this sagittal endovaginal sonogram the patient's endometrium (*cursors*) is thin and slightly echogenic.

arteriolar bed becomes more tortuous. The stroma becomes edematous. These changes are reflected ultrasonographically by increasing echogenicity of the functional layer, perhaps because of the increasing number of acoustical interfaces of glands, secretions, and arteries (see Fig. 29–9). Normal measurements of the secretory phase are 7 to 14 mm. The corpus luteum begins to regress after 12 days and is totally nonfunctional by day 14 after ovulation. With the decreasing levels of progesterone (and without human chorionic gonadotropin from a developing pregnancy) the endometrium loses its support and undergoes anoxic periods with loss of blood supply and subsequent necrosis and sloughing—the menstrual phase.

During menstruation the functional layer is lost and only the thin basal layer remains with the glandular remnants from which to regenerate a new endometrium during the next cycle. The endovaginal appearance of the menstrual endometrium is variable in both echogenicity and measurements. The amount of blood or

clot present affects the appearance and the echotexture (see Fig. 29–9).

Measuring the pulsatility index of a vessel is an indication of blood flow impedance. Ultrasound studies of the uterine artery during the menstrual cycle suggest a lower pulsatility index value during the secretory phase with higher impedance during the menstrual phase.[23, 24] Knowledge of normal waveforms during the cycle may one day help in assessing the readiness of the endometrium for implantation.

Postmenopausally, without hormonal fluctuations, the endometrium is atrophic and is seen sonographically as a thin echogenic line measuring 4 to 8 mm (Fig. 29–10). Any variation in the size or appearance of the postmenopausal endometrial stripe needs to be fully investigated by endovaginal scanning and, when indicated, by endometrial sampling. Many postmenopausal women are on hormonal replacement regimens for relief of menstrual symptoms and prevention of further osteoporosis. Early guidelines suggest unop-

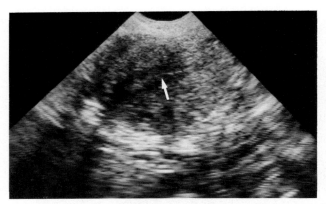

Figure 29–10. Postmenopausal endometrium. In the postmenopausal patient, the endometrium should atrophy. This sagittal endovaginal sonogram demonstrates the normal thin echogenic line that represents the postmenopausal endometrium. It should measure between 4 and 8 mm (*arrow*).

posed estrogen or continuous combined estrogen and progesterone therapy; these can increase the thickness of the normal postmenopausal endometrial stripe.[25] However, patients receiving sequential replacement with estrogen and progesterone should have an endometrial appearance similar to the normal cyclical premenopausal endometrium. Perhaps these patients should be evaluated sonographically after finishing the progesterone phase of their therapy. Specific normal values for endometrial measurements of asymptomatic postmenopausal patients on hormonal replacement therapy have not evolved yet. Perhaps the measurement of 1 cm will emerge as the norm for such women. Above this width of endometrium even asymptomatic postmenopausal patients who are on hormonal replacement therapy may need to undergo endometrial biopsy or have follow-up observation.

Similar to the effect of hormonal replacement is the occasional effect of tamoxifen therapy on the postmenopausal uterus. Tamoxifen is a widely used non-steroidal antiestrogen used as a chemotherapeutic agent in women with estrogen receptor-positive breast carcinoma. Although its primary action is competitive binding to estrogen receptors, it has a stimulatory or positive effect on the endometrium in some patients.[26] Endometrial polyps, endometrial hyperplasia, and endometrial carcinoma are reported complications of tamoxifen therapy.[27–29] As with hormonal replacement therapy no guidelines are available yet for the upper limit of normal endometrial measurement in asymptomatic patients on tamoxifen (Fig. 29–11).

The guidelines for endometrial width by sonography are more established for symptomatic patients with postmenopausal bleeding. In studies assessing the endometrial appearance and size in patients undergoing endometrial sampling for bleeding, an endometrium that measures less than or equal to 5 mm was never associated with significant morphology. Atrophic endometrium, cellular debris, and insufficient tissue were reported in these patients. These studies included a mixed population of women both with and without hormonal replacement therapy.[30, 31] This suggested limit is also supported by a retrospective comparison study of patients with endometrial hyperplasia. No patient with endometrial hyperplasia had an endometrial measurement of less than 8 mm.[32] Therefore, in the postmenopausal patient with bleeding an endometrial measurement of less than or equal to 5 mm suggests no significant abnormality is present and perhaps a biopsy or dilatation and curettage can be avoided.

All endometrial causes of abnormal postmenopausal bleeding such as endometrial hyperplasia, endometrial polyps, tamoxifen effect, and endometrial carcinoma can have similar sonographic appearances. Endometrial polyps and endometrial carcinoma may be more masslike or eccentric to the endometrial stripe (Fig. 29–12). Any such appearance regardless of the endometrial measurement should be investigated by endometrial sampling.

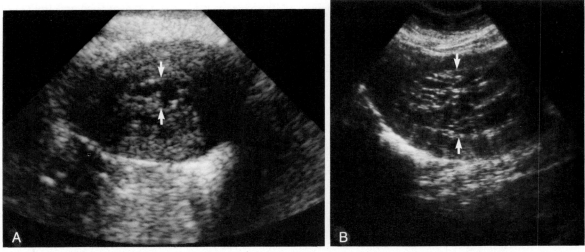

Figure 29–11. The tamoxifen effect. *A.* A coronal endovaginal sonogram of a postmenopausal patient with breast cancer on tamoxifen. The area between the arrows represents the endometrial cavity, which is filled by an endometrial polyp. *B.* Both endometrial hyperplasia and endometrial polyps were found in this postmenopausal patient on tamoxifen when she had vaginal bleeding. This coronal endovaginal examination demonstrates a mixed echogenic and hypoechoic appearance to the endometrium (*arrows*).

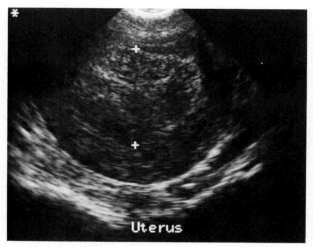

Figure 29–12. Endometrial carcinoma. A coronal endovaginal sonogram of a postmenopausal patient with bleeding and proven endometrial carcinoma. The endometrial carcinoma (*cursors*) has a mass-like effect in the central uterus.

BENIGN CERVICAL CONDITIONS

The cervix is somewhat difficult to examine sonographically. The usual position of the cervix deep to the bladder and low in the pelvis places it outside the usual focal zone of the ultrasound beam and resolution is diminished. Cervical visualization is generally improved with endovaginal scanning. However, depending on body habitus, cervical and uterine position, patient tolerance, and probe placement the cervical region of the uterus may still not be fully visualized. Fortunately, few conditions occur in the cervix for which sonographic imaging can be diagnostic or helpful.

Some degree of cervicitis and chronic inflammation is normal in most women. The cervix is exposed to the mixed bacterial flora of the vagina as well as to the sexually transmitted organisms and viruses. When severe infections occur, diagnosis is by history, symptoms, and cultures.

Nabothian cysts are common sonographic findings, especially on endovaginal examinations (Fig. 29–13). The nabothian cyst is simply an obstructed and dilated endocervical gland, and it is also called an epithelial inclusion cyst. They are most common in adult premenopausal women and may often be multiple or occur in clusters. They are asymptomatic and have no clinical or pathologic significance.

One of the frequent causes of intermenstrual bleeding or spotting is cervical polyps. Like cervicitis, cervical polyps is not an ultrasound diagnosis. Cervical polyps arise from the hyperplastic protrusion of the epithelium of the endocervix or ectocervix. Chronic inflammation is probably the etiologic factor. These polyps may be broad based or pedunculated. They occur at any time but usually in the fifth or sixth decade and are usually seen in patients who are multigravidas. They are benign and have no relationship to cervical carcinoma.

Cervical stenosis is a condition with several causes. Sonography can readily diagnose cervical stenosis but not necessarily its etiologic factor. It is an acquired condition with obstruction of the cervical canal at the internal or external os. Cervical stenosis may be caused by iatrogenic manipulations such as conizations, cryotherapy, obstetric trauma, and radiation, or the cervix may simply atrophy after menopause. Rarely, a cervical or uterine fibroid or polyp may obstruct the canal. The most serious cause to be excluded is cervical carcinoma or, less likely, endometrial carcinoma. Premenopausal patients may experience oligomenorrhea or amenorrhea with cramping or dysmenorrhea. Symptoms are less frequent in postmenopausal patients in whom the uterus slowly enlarges with the accumulation of blood and secretions. In either case, cervical stenosis should be rapidly treated since the obstructed uterine contents are ripe for infection and pyometria and also because malignancy needs to be excluded.

Either transabdominal or endovaginal sonography will show fluid or debris or a fluid-debris level in the endometrial cavity (Fig. 29–14). A lobulated or distorted cervix may suggest carcinoma or fibroids as the cause. Clinically, the obstructed cervical os may be difficult to find, especially in postmenopausal patients or patients after pelvic irradiation. Transabdominal ultrasound guidance may help by directing the probe or sound during gynecologic procedures to drain the uterus.

Eight percent of all leiomyomas are cervical in origin. They are usually small and asymptomatic but may enlarge and cause bladder or bowel symptoms or pain and bleeding. They may be pedunculated and prolapse through the cervical canal into the vagina. Ultrasonography and CT scanning are usually nonspecific, demonstrating a bulbous or heterogeneous cervical stroma. Endovaginal scanning may demonstrate an eccentric cervical canal. If surgical intervention is necessary, MRI may help by defining the extent and location of the fibroid more clearly.

CERVICAL MALIGNANCIES

The vast majority of malignancies of the cervix, more than 90%, are squamous cell carcinomas that arise from the squamous epithelium of the exocervix. Adenocarcinoma of the cervix makes up the remaining 10% of cervical malignancies. It usually arises from the columnar epithelium of the endocervical canal and may grow within the cervix and not be obvious on external inspection. As with the usual adenocarcinoma, these tumors may vary from well to poorly differentiated. The primarily endocervical location of this tumor may lead to later detection and poorer prognosis because of larger size at diagnosis. Clear cell carcinoma of the cervix is a type of adenocarcinoma associated with exposure to diethylstilbestrol in utero. Occasionally cervical tumors contain both glandular and squamous cells. These tumors have a similar survival to pure squamous and adenocarcinomas and are called

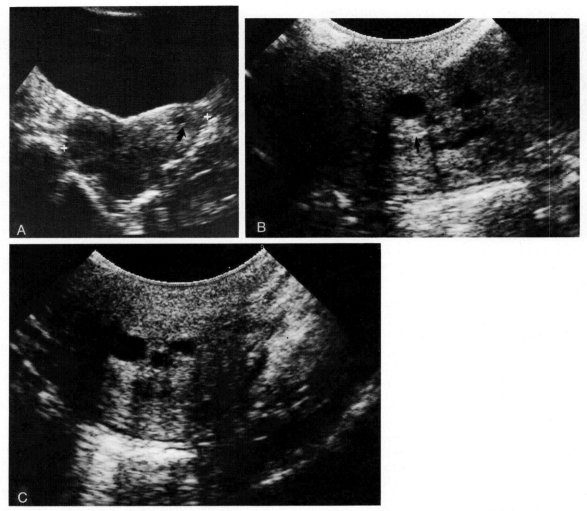

Figure 29–13. Nabothian cyst. *A.* On this sagittal transabdominal sonogram, a single nabothian cyst (*arrow*) is present in the cervix in this patient with a fibroid uterus. *B.* It is seen endovaginally as well. Note the echogenic line (*arrow*), which represents the endocervical canal. *C.* In another patient a cluster of nabothian cysts is seen surrounding the endocervical canal on this endovaginal sonogram.

adenosquamous or adenoepidermoid carcinomas. Even rarer cancers arising in the cervix include sarcomas, adenoid cystic melanomas, as well as lymphoma and metastatic disease.

Because of the effectiveness of the Papanicolaou smear screening test and improved treatment techniques the mortality from cervical cancer has decreased over the past 50 years. However, there are still approximately 15,000 new cases of invasive carcinoma of the cervix diagnosed in the United States every year.[33, 34] The mean age of presentation is 45 years. However, the peak age of carcinoma in situ is now 35 years and the trend is for increasingly younger women to develop dysplasia progressing to carcinoma in situ and ultimately invasive carcinoma. Carcinoma in situ is a curable disease and fortunately the diagnosis of carcinoma in situ is increasing as the incidence of invasive carcinoma of the cervix is decreasing.

Cervical carcinoma is a sexually transmitted disease with a high association with the human papillomavirus and the herpes simplex 2 virus, which may act as carcinogens. The preclinical stages of cervical intraepithelial neoplasia may take 10 years to evolve from dysplasia, to carcinoma in situ, to invasive carcinoma.

Interrelated risk factors include early sexual activity and child bearing, multiple sexual partners, and low socioeconomic status as well as smoking and immunosuppression.

Diagnosis is primarily made by inspection and the Papanicolaou smear. CT scanning and MRI and to a lesser extent ultrasonography also have a role in surveillance for recurrent disease and following the complications of therapy. Staging cervical cancer is performed primarily clinically with CT scanning and MRI as useful adjuncts. Squamous cell carcinoma spreads by direct local invasion or by the lymphatic system. Locally, carcinoma of the cervix extends into the endometrial cavity, into the vagina, or through the cervix into the paracervical or parametrial structures. The lymphatic route is through the paracervical channel to the obturator, external, and internal iliac chain and then to the common iliac and para-aortic node groups. Treatment is with a combination of surgical, radiation, and chemotherapeutic methods depending on the stage of the disease. Complications of primary or recurrent disease or therapy that often involve the radiologists include fistula formation, colostomies, and urinary diversion techniques, including percutaneous

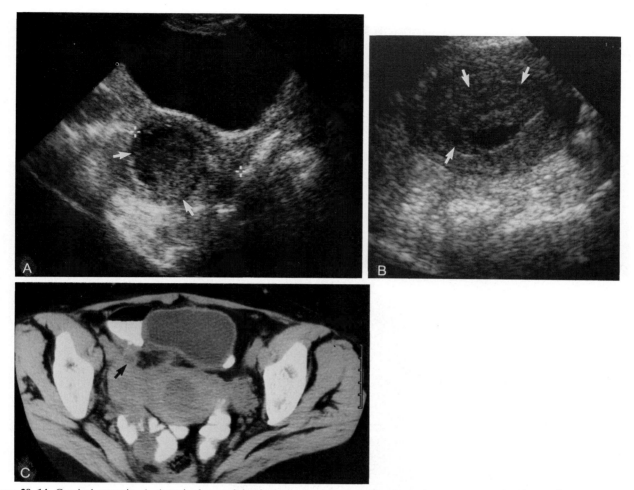

Figure 29–14. Cervical stenosis. *A.* A sagittal transabdominal sonogram through the uterus demonstrates a mass (*arrows*) in the mid uterus. *B.* Endovaginal sonogram shows this mass to represent fluid and debris (*arrows*) within a distended endometrial cavity. *C.* The CT scan in this patient confirms the pyometria in this patient with fever and pain and elevated white blood cell count. The cause of the pelvic inflammation (both adnexal and uterine) was found to be a ruptured appendix. Note the distended appendix on the CT scan (*arrow*).

nephrostomies. When invasive carcinoma of the cervix recurs it is usually at distant sites or centrally in the pelvis. Death is usually from extensive local disease and renal failure.

Computed tomography is not particularly helpful in defining the tumor and local spread. Since soft tissue contrast resolution is poor, CT cannot distinguish tumor from normal cervical stroma or always detect early parametrial involvement. Large bulky tumors can be visualized by their morphologic changes. CT is excellent for spread of disease to local lymph nodes and distant metastases (Fig. 29–15). MRI detects tumor by differences in signal intensity of the tumor. Many studies suggest MRI is significantly more accurate than CT in predicting the depth of tumor in the cervix and parametrial spread. In some instances, MRI is also more accurate than the clinical staging.[35–37] New MRI protocols and directed use of contrast agents may improve MRI's accuracy further in local staging of cervical carcinoma.[38, 39]

BENIGN UTERINE CONDITIONS

The correct position of the intrauterine contraceptive device (IUD) is within the endometrial cavity, where it prevents pregnancy by the mechanical prevention of the implantation or the minute presence of metal such as copper. The IUDs have a variety of shapes and configurations, but all should be detected by sonography. A highly reflective echo with an acoustical shadow is present. There are characteristic appearances of some IUDs such as the Lippes loop (Fig. 29–16). Endovaginal sonography can generally be diagnostic when the distinction between an endometrial stripe and an IUD cannot be made by transabdominal techniques. Myometrial penetration of the IUD may be seen as well. A kidney-ureter-bladder film will demonstrate the IUD and may show an IUD when none is seen on the sonogram, which indicates total perforation of the uterine wall (Fig. 29–17).

Endometritis may occur with pelvic inflammatory disease, in the puerperium, or post instrumentation such as after dilatation and curettage. In pelvic inflammatory disease whether of venereal or polymicrobial etiology, the uterus may be one route of ascending infection of the tubes and adnexa. Post partum 3% to 4% of patients develop endometritis, usually associated with prolonged labor, vaginitis, premature rupture of the membranes, or retained products of conception.[40] Sonograms of the uterus may demonstrate a prominent or irregular endometrium. Endometrial fluid, debris,

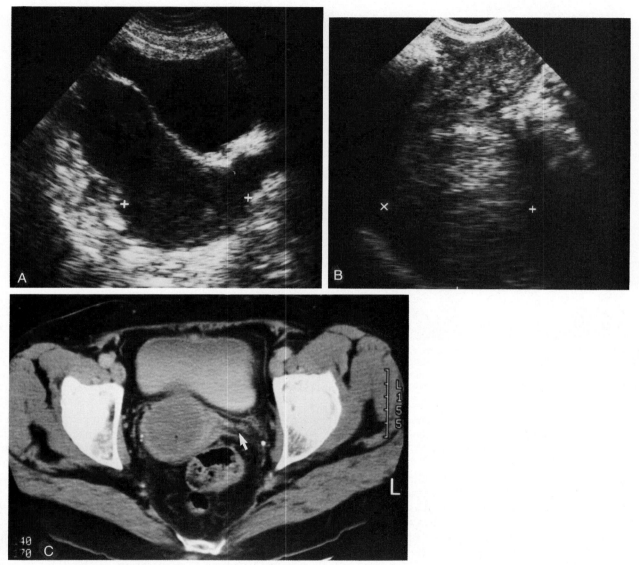

Figure 29–15. Cervical carcinoma. *A.* A sagittal transabdominal sonogram through the midline of the uterus demonstrates a bulky heterogeneous-appearing cervix (*cursors*). *B.* Endovaginal sonography in this patient is not particularly helpful but does demonstrate a masslike structure in the region of the cervix. *C.* The CT scan illustrates parametrial spread of the cervical carcinoma on the left (*arrow*). There is soft tissue infiltration of the parametrial fat. The CT scan was done before any surgical procedure or irradiation, both of which could account for stranding in the parametrial fat. Low attenuation fluid or debris is seen in the fundus of the endometrium on this CT scan.

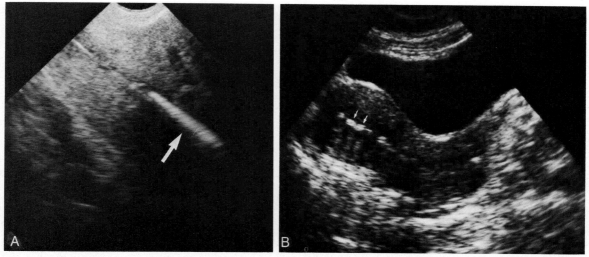

Figure 29–16. Intrauterine device. *A.* An endovaginal sonogram of a uterus that contains a Copper-7 intrauterine device (*arrow*). *B.* A transabdominal sagittal sonogram through the uterus in this patient with a Lippes loop demonstrates the typical appearance of interrupted echogenic foci in the uterine cavity with distal acoustical shadowing (*arrows*).

or gas may be present as demonstrated sonographically or by CT. Clinically, endometritis may be exquisitely painful even with minimal ultrasound findings.

Uterine polyps are pedunculated or sessile excrescences of endometrial tissue. They contain the glands, fibrous stroma, and vessels of the endometrium. The polyps may be single or multiple, small, or so large that they protrude through the cervical os. Polyps may be found in 10% of women.[41] Bleeding is the usual symptom, although many polyps are asymptomatic. Endometrial polyps rarely undergo malignant change, and only in the postmenopausal patient may there be

an ongoing surveillance after polyp removal. Since endometrial polyps may arise in an area of endometrial hyperplasia, endometrial carcinoma must be excluded. Ultrasound findings include nonspecific thickened endometrium, a focal echogenic area in the endometrium, or occasionally an endocavitary mass surrounded by fluid (Fig. 29–18).

Endometrial hyperplasia results from estrogen stimulation to the endometrium without the influence of progestin and is a frequent cause of bleeding. In the premenopausal patient, polycystic ovary disease and obesity may be causative with their elevated endogenous estrogen levels. Premenopausally and perimenopausally, anovulatory cycles and the use of exogenous estrogen are the primary causes. In any age group, estrogen-producing tumors such as granulosa theca cell tumors may cause endometrial hyperplasia. Endome-

Figure 29–17. This kidney-ureter-bladder view of the abdomen demonstrates a Lippes loop that has perforated through the uterus and is in the peritoneal cavity in the left upper quadrant (*arrow*).

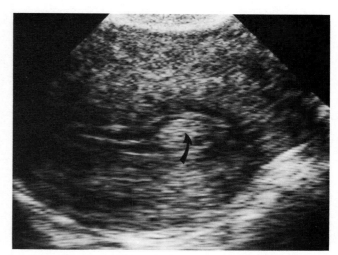

Figure 29–18. Endometrial polyp. This sagittal endovaginal sonogram demonstrates proliferative endometrium in this patient with intermenstrual bleeding. The central line of the opposed endometrium is splayed by an echogenic "mass"—the endometrial polyp (*arrow*).

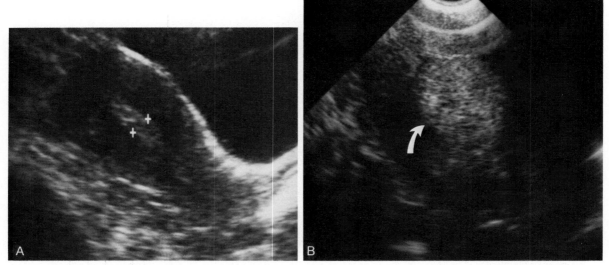

Figure 29–19. Endometrial hyperplasia. *A.* A transabdominal sagittal sonogram of a postmenopausal patient with bleeding demonstrates an abnormally thickened echogenic endometrium that proved on dilatation and curettage to be endometrial hyperplasia in this patient. *B.* Similar-appearing echogenic thickened endometrium in this endovaginal scan in another patient was also endometrial hyperplasia (*arrow*).

trial sampling, especially in the postmenopausal patient, is necessary to exclude endometrial carcinoma.

Histologically, endometrial hyperplasia can be categorized in three groups: cystic, adenomatous, or atypical adenomatous.[41] Cystic endometrial hyperplasia has large dilated glands. Adenomatous hyperplasia demonstrates glandular crowding with some branching glands but also maintains a single layer of columnar epithelium in these glands. Atypical adenomatous hyperplasia or dysplasia is a more complex histologic diagnosis with more crowding and abnormal glandular lining. When cytologic atypia is present, the risk of progression to endometrial carcinoma is significant. Medical therapy with cyclic progestins can suffice for cystic and adenomatous hyperplasia. Atypical adenomatous hyperplasia should probably be treated with hysterectomy if there are no contraindications to surgery. Unfortunately, the sonographic findings are again nonspecific (Fig. 29–19). A thickened postmenopausal endometrial stripe is abnormal, however.

Many references suggest normal measurements for the postmenopausal stripe. In the presence of bleeding, an endometrial stripe of less than or equal to 5 mm is unlikely to represent any significant abnormality. In these patients a dilatation and curettage may be able to be avoided.[30, 31] Postmenopausal hormonal replacement therapy may increase the threshold of these limits, as previously discussed.

ADENOMYOSIS

Adenomyosis is the ectopic occurrence of endometrial tissue within the myometrium. Although the pathology is similar to endometriosis, its etiology and presentation are very different. Endometriosis and adenomyosis occur together in only 20% of patients, and adenomyosis should not be thought of as "internal endometriosis."[41] Endometrial glands and stroma are scattered through the myometrium in one of two types. There is usually a tenuous connection to the endometrial cavity. Usually adenomyosis is diffuse with global infiltration of the endometrium. Less often, adenomyosis may be more focal with discrete masses or adenomyomas in the wall of the uterus.

Etiologic mechanisms for this seeding of the myometrium with endometrial tissue include multiple pregnancies and deliveries with subsequent uterine shrinking. Aggressive curettages and elevated estrogen levels may also promote the growth of myometrial islands of endometrial tissue. However, unlike endometriosis and normal endometrial tissue, the glands of adenomyosis are atrophic or underdeveloped and do not easily respond to hormonal control.

As might be predicted from the pathology, the clinical presentation of adenomyosis is dysmenorrhea, an enlarging uterus, and menorrhagia. This symptom complex and disease most often occur in multiparous women in their 40s or 50s. Treatment may be local excision of adenomyomas when possible or hysterectomy, depending on the patient's age and severity of symptoms.

The diagnosis is usually made clinically with radiology and ultrasonography offering little definitive or specific information. In the late 1980s there were several attempts to describe the ultrasound appearance of adenomyosis but the ultrasound findings are too nonspecific.[42, 43] The uterus may be enlarged, and there may be textural changes diffusely or focally. The specific differentiation from the more common fibroid uterus cannot be made. MRI may be helpful, since leiomyomas, despite varying degrees of degeneration, tend to be round, well defined, encapsulated masses with varying signal intensities depending on the degree of degeneration. Adenomyosis is a poorly demarcated or diffuse area without distinct margins or shape (Fig. 29–20). High-signal areas may represent foci of endometrial hemorrhage within the myometrium.[44]

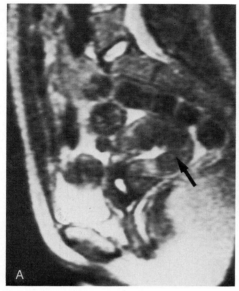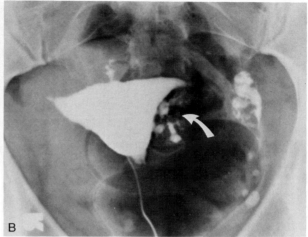

Figure 29–20. Adenomyosis. *A.* Sagittal midline MR image of a uterus that is diffusely involved with adenomyosis. Note the ill-defined low-signal areas obliterating the junctional zone (*arrow*). *B.* The hysterosalpingogram of the same patient demonstrates contrast agent filling the intramural glands of adenomyosis.

LEIOMYOMAS

Fibroids or uterine myomas occur in 20% to 50% of women and represent the most frequent gynecologic tumor.[41, 45] They may be single but are more commonly multiple. Depending on their location and size they may or may not be symptomatic. Myomas occur in all women but more frequently and at a younger age in the black population.

The fibroid is more correctly termed a *leiomyoma* since it arises from the smooth muscle of the uterine wall. Leiomyomas may occur in extrauterine sites such as the tube, cervix, vagina, or ligaments of the pelvis. They are most common in the uterus. The leiomyoma is actually a mass of smooth muscle proliferations in a whorled spherical configuration. They are encapsulated with a pseudocapsule and separate easily from the surrounding myometrium. With atrophy and vascular compromise, fibrotic changes and degeneration of the myomas occur. Liquefaction, necrosis, hemorrhage, and ultimate calcification may take place (Fig. 29–21).

Leiomyomas occurring in the uterine wall are either submucosal or adjacent to the endometrium, intramural, or subserosal. The symptoms and signs of leiomyomas depend on their size and location. Submucosal myomas may erode into the endometrial cavity and cause irregular or heavy bleeding, which may lead to anemia. Fertility may be affected by submucosal or intramural fibroids, which by their location may inhibit sperm transport down the tube, prevent adequate implantation, or cause recurrent miscarriages. Large cervical fibroids can prevent normal vaginal deliveries.

Intramural and subserosal fibroids do not usually cause the bleeding problems associated with submucosal fibroids. Intramural and subserosal myomas may enlarge and cause symptoms by pressure effect on adjacent organs such as the bladder, bowel, and ligaments of the pelvis. Thus leiomyomas may cause dysmenorrhea, dysuria, and constipation. Low back pain may be secondary to pressure on the pelvic ligaments or the lumbar plexus. Acute pelvic pain may be caused by torsion or necrosis of a previously asymptomatic myoma. Leiomyomas may be pedunculated and present as a separate pelvic mass. As cervical fibroids grow they often pedunculate into the endocervical canal, where ulceration and hemorrhage are common.

There is much evidence that leiomyomas are hormonally responsive. Estrogen and progestin receptors have been found in leiomyomas.[46] Myomas may rapidly enlarge under the influence of estrogen during pregnancy. At menopause, gradual shrinkage occurs with cessation of the estrogen stimulus. With hormonal replacement therapy some regrowth may occur. Administration of gonadotropin releasing hormone agonist to turn off the hypothalamic-pituitary-gonadal axis markedly decreases myoma size before surgery or can be used for the treatment of severe anemia without surgery. Because of other hypoestrogenic effects such as bone density loss and menopausal symptoms, long-term therapy is not practical with such agents.[47, 48] Even tamoxifen, the increasingly common adjuvant therapy for breast carcinoma, has been reported to cause growth in leiomyomas. Tamoxifen has both estrogen agonist and antagonist activity and presumably may stimulate leiomyoma growth.[49]

The frequency of myomas and the variability of their size and location and pathologic state hinder their ultrasound diagnosis. An enlarged uterus may be caused by diffuse small myomas and present sonographically as a diffusely heterogeneous and globular uterus. Myomas may be seen as discrete masses in the uterine wall, and endovaginal ultrasound scanning has certainly helped in the assessment of their relationship

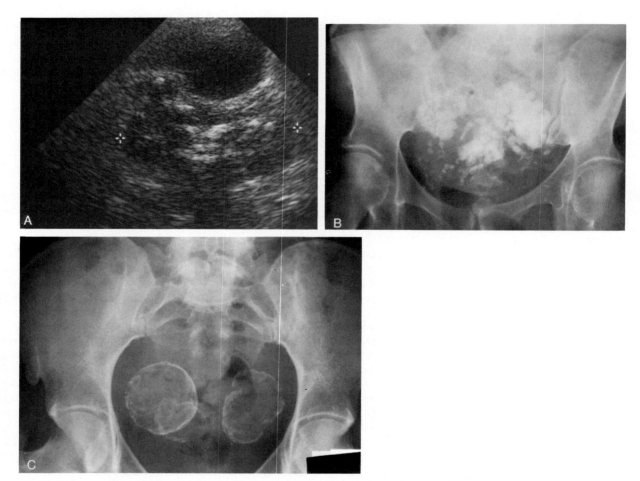

Figure 29–21. Leiomyomatous calcification. *A.* In this transverse transabdominal sonogram multiple high-amplitude echoes are seen within the uterus representing calcifications. *B.* A radiograph of this patient demonstrates the typical "popcornlike" calcifications typical of calcified uterine fibroids. *C.* In another patient, a rim or peripheral calcification is demonstrated.

to the endometrial cavity. The sonographic texture of leiomyomas may be homogeneous or heterogeneous and hypoechoic or hyperechoic. Dense fibrotic changes and/or calcification may cause attenuation of the sound transmission and make estimation of the size or position of myomas impossible (Fig. 29–22).

Computed tomography of leiomyomas is limited by the attenuation characteristics of leiomyomas, which are similar to the normal uterine musculature. Obviously, calcification is easily demonstrated by CT, but distinguishing between normal and abnormal uterine muscle is not possible (Fig. 29–23). The CT diagnosis of fibroids is usually based on the uterine contour or its lobulated abnormal shape. MRI offers the most sensitive imaging of leiomyomas. The signal intensity of leiomyomas distinguishes them from the normal uterine musculature when T1- and T2-weighted sequences are employed.[50] Exact size and location can be assessed (Fig. 29–24).

Treatment for myomas depends primarily on the clinical symptoms. Heavy bleeding necessitates therapy. Sudden growth in a dormant myoma is alarming, and malignancy may need to be excluded. Myomectomy may help in some cases of infertility. Myomectomies may be performed by the traditional transabdominal incision and, when appropriate, laparoscopically or hysteroscopically. Large myomas may be treated preoperatively with gonadotropin-releasing hormone agonist to shrink them before ultimate operative therapy. This may result in an easier and less destructive surgical procedure.[47, 48]

There are four unusual leiomyoma-type tumors. A rare type of leiomyoma contains varying amounts of fatty tissue. A pure lipoma of the uterus is a very rare

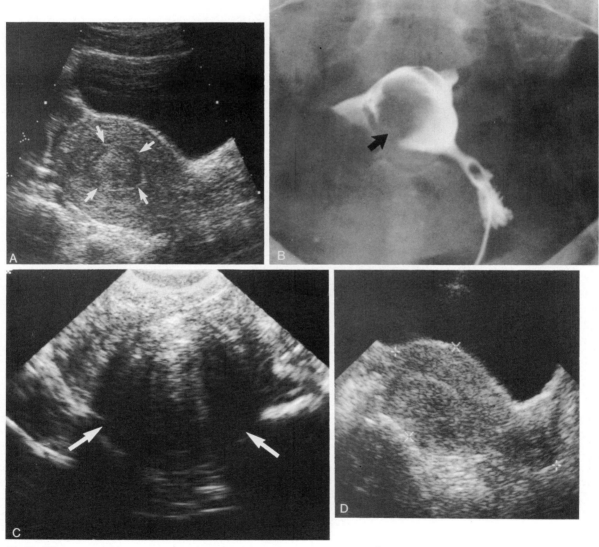

Figure 29–22. Ultrasonographic appearance of uterine leiomyomas. *A.* A transabdominal image demonstrates a poorly echogenic mass (*arrows*) apparently within the endometrial cavity in this young patient with heavy menstrual periods. Hysteroscopy confirmed the presence of a submucus fibroid. *B.* In another patient, a submucus fibroid is demonstrated by hysterosalpingography (*arrow*). *C.* This endovaginal coronal sonogram demonstrates the marked attenuation of the sound beam by a uterine leiomyoma (*arrows*). *D.* Longitudinal sonogram in a patient with pelvic pain. The uterus is enlarged and lobular with numerous myomas. This is a typical appearance for the fibroid uterus.

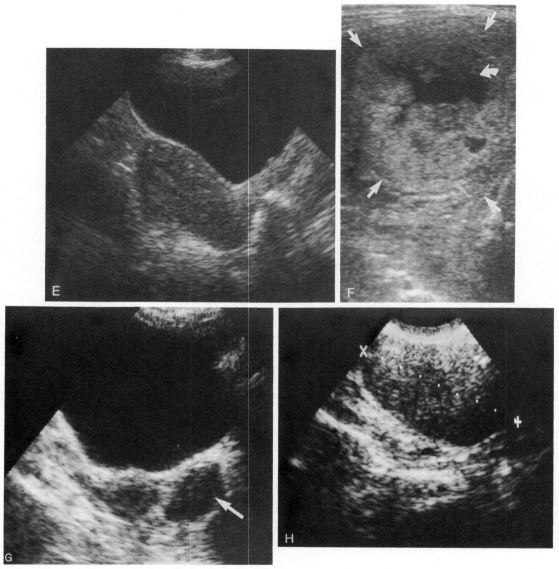

Figure 29–22 *Continued E.* Longitudinal sonogram in a postmenopausal patient. The uterus is somewhat heterogeneous and enlarged. Although no discrete myomas are seen, the uniform enlargement is most typical for a fibroid uterus. *F.* Longitudinal transabdominal sonogram in a patient with a painful pelvic mass. A large mass (*arrows*) is identified adjacent to the anterior abdominal wall. The uterine fibroid has outgrown its blood supply and become centrally necrotic (*curved arrow*). *G.* Transabdominal sonography in this patient with a left adnexal mass demonstrated a solid-appearing left adnexal mass (*arrow*). *H.* Endovaginal sonography demonstrated the homogeneous solid appearance of this mass. The differential diagnosis would include pedunculated subserosal leiomyoma as well as solid ovarian tumors. Laparoscopic diagnosis was a pedunculated leiomyoma.

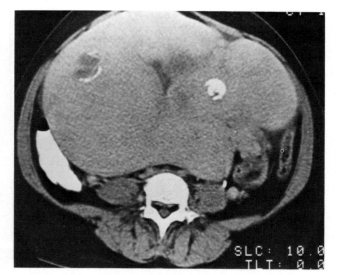

Figure 29–23. This patient presented with a very large abdominal mass on physical examination. The CT scan demonstrated a large solid mass of mixed attenuation with foci of calcification arising from the pelvis and extending into the abdomen. A large fibroid uterus with areas of necrosis and calcification was removed at surgery.

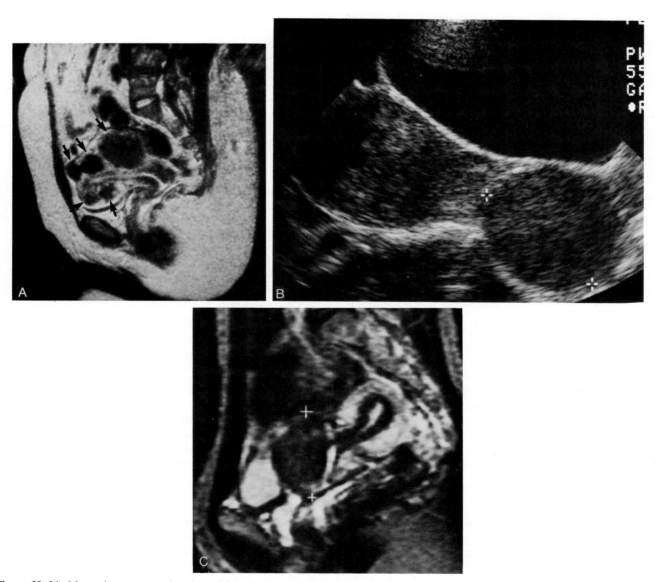

Figure 29–24. Magnetic resonance imaging of leiomyomas. *A.* This T2-weighted scan through the midline of the uterus demonstrates beautifully the zonal anatomy of the uterus. The low-signal leiomyomas (*arrows*) are well delineated. *B.* This transabdominal sagittal sonogram through the uterus of another patient demonstrates a large solid mass involving the cervix. *C.* The sagittal T2-weighted MR image demonstrates the low-signal cervical fibroid in the anterior aspect of the cervix.

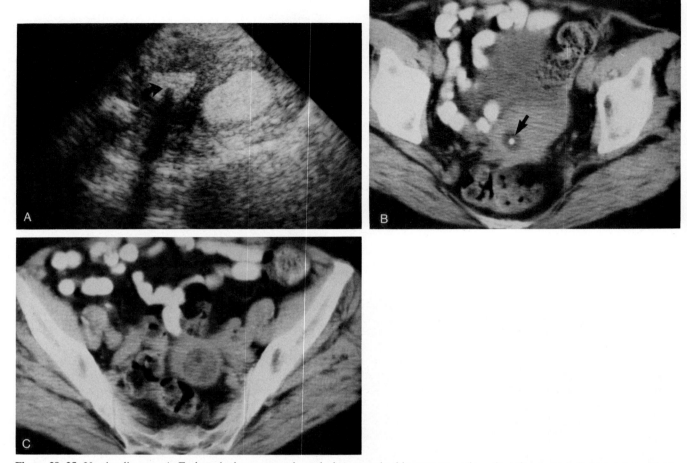

Figure 29–25. Uterine lipoma. *A.* Endovaginal sonogram through the uterus in this asymptomatic patient demonstrated at least three highly echogenic well-defined masses. One of the masses contained an echogenic area with marked beam attenuation (*arrow*). *B* and *C.* Two CT scans through the uterus in this patient demonstrate the low attenuation masses in the uterus consistent with uterine lipomas. Note the foci of calcification in one of the lipomas that accounted for the shadowing focus on the sonogram (*arrow on B*).

tumor occurring primarily in postmenopausal patients.[51] Its CT, MRI, and ultrasound appearance can be diagnostic (Fig. 29–25). Intravenous leiomyomatosis, leiomyomatosis peritonealis disseminata, and benign metastasizing leiomyoma are three unusual conditions in which nodules of histologically typically appearing leiomyoma are found in the blood vessels, the peritoneal cavity, the lungs, and other locations. Etiologies include spread of disease hematologically, intravenously, or lymphatically. The tumors are benign and can be surgically removed. They seem also to respond to estrogren deprivation or antiestrogen therapy.[41, 45, 52]

UTERINE MALIGNANCIES

Malignancies of the uterus other than the endometrium are rare and include sarcomas and, even more rarely, lymphomas. Sarcomas may arise primarily in the mesodermal tissues of the uterus or arise from malignant degeneration of an underlying myoma. The true incidence of each etiology is difficult to ascertain since leiomyomas are so common and sarcomas are relatively rare. Both incidences are probably 1% or less.[52, 53] Clinical symptoms include a sudden increase in uterine size, bleeding, weight loss, and other nonspecific symptoms. Treatment and survival depend on the stage of disease and the cytologic characteristics.

ENDOMETRIAL CARCINOMA

Adenocarcinoma of the endometrium is the most common occurring gynecologic cancer in the United States today. Over the past 50 years the incidence of endometrial carcinoma has been rising while the incidence of cervical carcinoma has been declining. The reasons for this increasing incidence in endometrial carcinoma are closely linked to the etiologic mechanisms and risk factors for development of endometrial carcinoma.

Endometrial carcinoma is primarily a disease of postmenopausal women, and the age of the population has been gradually increasing. There is a high occurrence of endometrial carcinoma in obese patients. Diabetes and hypertension have also been associated with endometrial carcinoma. A high-caloric and high-fat diet is associated with endometrial carcinoma as well.

The estrogen milieu is a major factor in endometrial carcinoma. Endometrial carcinoma occurs primarily in postmenopausal or theoretically relatively hypoestrogenic patients. However, estrogen is present even in the postmenopausal women. Estrogen is converted from adrenal and ovarian androgens in adipose tissue and is constantly circulating. When endometrial carcinoma occurs in premenopausal patients, as it does in approximately 10% of the time, there is a high incidence of anovulatory disorders, especially polycystic ovary disease in those patients. Chronic estrogen stimulation of the endometrium without the shedding caused by progesterone is causative. Patients with estrogen-producing tumors of the ovaries, such as granulosa cell tumors, also have an increase of endometrial carcinoma. Finally, data from patients on the early hormonal replacement therapy protocols indicate that estrogen replacement without progesterone is a definite risk factor.[34, 54] Thus the current regimen of hormonal replacement therapy includes both estrogen and progesterone.

Tamoxifen, which is primarily an antiestrogen used for adjuvant chemotherapy and estrogen receptor positive breast carcinoma, also has estrogen agonist effects on the endometrium. There is a definite association of tamoxifen therapy and risk of endometrial carcinoma and endometrial hyperplasia.[27, 29] Thus endometrial hyperplasia from whatever cause is the precursor for endometrial carcinoma.

Adenocarcinoma of the endometrium is usually a well-differentiated tumor, with the majority of the patients diagnosed with grade I or II disease. Poorly differentiated lesions and the depth of myometrial invasion are the most significant data for prognosis.

Endometrial carcinoma extends locally and then hematogenously and lymphatically.

Treatment is usually surgical with or without radiation therapy. Hormonal therapy with a progestin agent is occasionally successful in treating metastatic disease especially in the lung.

The diagnosis of endometrial carcinoma is usually made clinically since the majority of patients present with postmenopausal bleeding and have a dilatation or curettage or endometrial sampling procedure performed. Approximately one third of patients with postmenopausal bleeding will ultimately have endometrial carcinoma.

Since the diagnosis is usually made clinically and promptly when postmenopausal bleeding occurs, ultrasonography does not have a major role in detection at this time. The ultrasound appearance of endometrial carcinoma is usually normal or nonspecific endometrial thickening. The thickening of the endometrial stripe may be both echogenic or of mixed echogenicity (Fig. 29–26). Although less than or equal to 8 mm is considered normal for postmenopausal women, the diameters for the endometrium in patients on hormonal replacement therapy and other drugs such as tamoxifen are being studied. Studies using both transabdominal and endovaginal scanning to determine depth of invasion of endometrial carcinoma have been performed.[55, 56] Results demonstrate that sonography can reasonably predict the depth of myometrial invasion but not necessarily cervical extension. Endovaginal ultrasound scanning may ultimately be useful as a screening tool for endometrial carcinoma and especially in high-risk patients, such as patients with known endometrial hyperplasia, those on tamoxifen therapy,

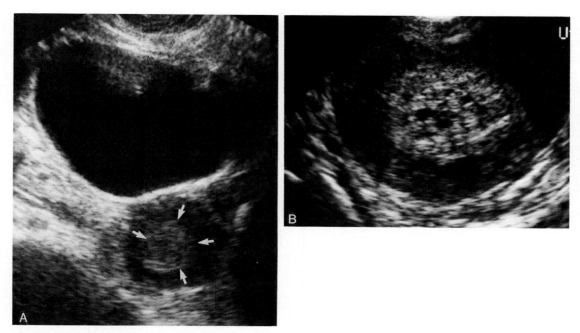

Figure 29–26. Endometrial carcinoma. *A.* This transabdominal sonogram of a postmenopausal patient with bleeding demonstrates a retropositioned uterus in the sagittal projection. There is an echogenic mass (*arrows*) within the uterine fundus. *B.* Endovaginal sonography demonstrates that the echogenic mass represents expansion of the endometrial cavity with a mass of mixed echogenic and cystic areas. This was grade I endometrial adenocarcinoma at surgery.

or those with a family history of disease or in patients with known breast or ovarian malignancies. Early reports suggest color flow imaging may be helpful in distinguishing the altered vascularity and low pulsatility index of vessels in a uterus in which there is endometrial carcinoma.[57]

Computed tomography contributes to endometrial carcinoma staging by the detection of lymph node enlargement and other signs of distant disease usually stage 3 or 4 disease. Recurrence in distant sites is also detected by CT. MRI can be useful in depicting the depth of myometrial invasion, especially in a uterus involved with leiomyomas. Cervical extension of the endometrial carcinoma can also be visualized with MRI. By accurately predicting these factors.[58, 59] MR images of a patient with endometrial carcinoma may affect treatment and thus prognosis.

FERTILITY AND THE FUTURE

The advances in radiologic imaging of the uterus have allowed ultrasonography, CT, and MRI to play a significant role not only in evaluation but also in the treatment of infertility patients. During ovulation induction therapy endovaginal ultrasound assessment of the endometrium is performed as well as follicular evaluation. Insufficient endometrial response to hormonal therapy may affect the dosage of the fertility agent or the time of ovulation or insemination. Certainly oocyte retrieval with endovaginal ultrasound guidance is much less invasive and stressful than previous laparoscopic, transvesicle, or transurethral techniques. Submucosal leiomyomas may interfere with implantation and cause habitual abortions. By clearly identifying the location of such leiomyomas, endovaginal ultrasound scanning and more accurately MRI can guide their hysteroscopic removal.

Hysterosalpingography has been the imaging standard for tubal evaluation. Recent more precise techniques now allow for better definition of the actual endometrial cavity. Anomalies of development, polyps, submucosal fibroids, and synechiae are detected. Intrauterine synechiae or adhesions, termed *Asherman syndrome,* is a condition in which the normal endometrial lining is ablated by adhesions. The adhesions may be partial or total. The etiology is usually secondary to deep curettage following miscarriage or delivery. The endometrium subsequently heals with fibrous bands traversing the endometrial cavity. Rarely such adhesions may be secondary to infectious causes such as tuberculosis or schistosomiasis. Symptoms include hypomenorrhea and dysmenorrhea. Infertility is a result, as are complicated pregnancies when implantation does occur. The ultrasound image of Asherman syndrome is usually unremarkable (Fig. 29–27). The endometrial stripe may be extremely thin when the cavity is completely ablated. After lysis of adhesions and hormonal stimulation, endovaginal sonography may be helpful in assessing restoration of the endometrium.

There are many avenues for further development of uterine sonography. Will endovaginal scanning be a useful adjuvant or screening tool for patients at high risk for endometrial carcinoma? Will endovaginal color flow Doppler examinations add to our knowledge of normal uterine physiology and other disorders? A recent report questions whether prominent periuterine venous plexi may be a cause of pelvic pain and other symptoms.[60] Finally, endoluminal ultrasound probes have been developed primarily for vascular and gastrointestinal lumen diagnosis. A specifically adapted ultrasound endoluminal probe has been developed for direct study of the endometrium and adjacent myometrium.[61] How this technology and other developing technologies will supplement the current endovaginal and transabdominal ultrasound techniques remains to be seen.

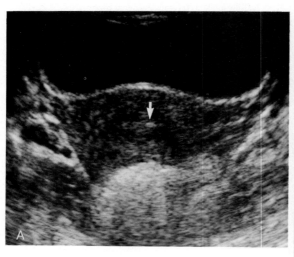 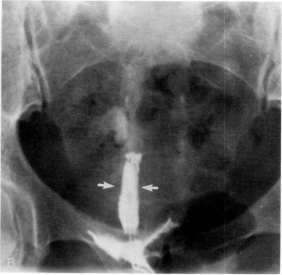

Figure 29–27. Asherman syndrome. *A.* Transverse transabdominal sonogram demonstrates a nonspecific appearance of the uterus. The endometrial stripe is thin and unremarkable (*arrow*). *B.* A radiograph from the hysterosalpingogram on this patient. Arrows outline the very abnormal adhesed and scarred endometrial cavity.

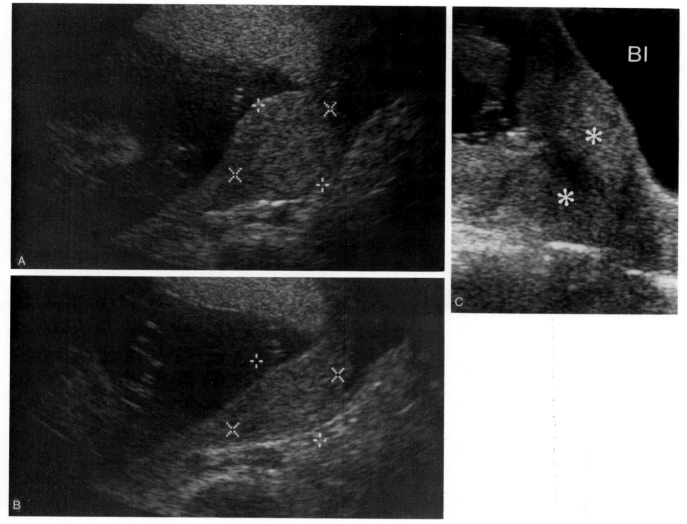

Figure 29–28. Myometrial contractions. *A.* A focal rounded mass is seen in the posterior myometrium in this patient (*cursors*). *B.* After 10 minutes of scanning this myometrial contraction has significantly reduced its size. *C.* In another patient contractions of the anterior and posterior lower uterine segment ("kissing contractions") (*asterisks*) simulate the anterior and posterior aspect of the cervix. This misinterpretation may make one wrongly conclude that this is the endocervical canal. Bl, bladder.

THE GRAVID UTERUS

There are several uterine conditions for which sonography is performed during pregnancy: abnormalities of structure or function of the cervix, status of uterine myomas during gestation, and the rare situation of incarcerated uterus or ruptured uterus. Uterine contractions can occur throughout pregnancy and early in pregnancy are not necessarily clinically apparent. Later in pregnancy when the patient can feel the contractions they are called Braxton Hicks contractions. A contraction will be seen sonographically as a focal thickening of the uterine wall and may last up to 45 minutes (Fig. 29–28). In contrast, labor contractions progress rhythmically from the fundus to the cervix. The sonographer must be aware of these silent contractions of the uterus since these contractions may mimic myomas during sonography. The contractions may also alter the apparent relationships of structures, especially the cervix and placenta (see Fig. 29–28).

Cervical incompetence is a functional condition whose hallmark is a history of recurrent, usually painless second-trimester spontaneous abortions. The etiologic factors are multifactorial and include congenital, traumatic, and hormonal causes. Patients exposed to diethylstilbestrol have an increased incidence of preterm labor and delivery and cervical incompetence. This may be in part secondary to structural changes such as the collars, hoods, septa, cockscombs, abnormal mucus, as well as functional abnormalities.[62] Cervical trauma from gynecologic or obstetric procedures or secondary to a previous precipitous delivery is another cause of cervical incompetence. The documentation of cervical effacement, dilatation, or shortening without labor developing in the early second trimester makes the clinical diagnosis of cervical incompetence. The ultrasound findings of a cervix of less than 3 cm, a gaping internal os, and funneling or tunneling of the patient's membranes into the endocervical canal are associated with preterm delivery (Fig. 29–29). There

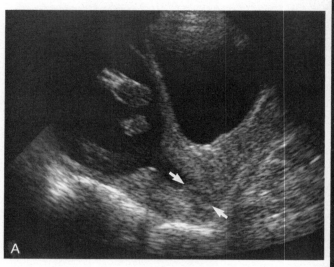
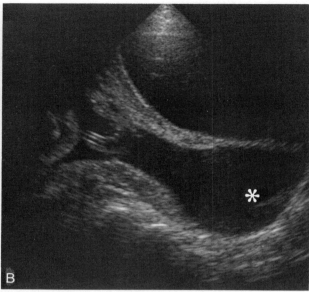

Figure 29–29. Cervical incompetence. *A.* A longitudinal sonogram in this patient with a 28-week gestation reveals a shortened cervix (*arrows*). The patient was asymptomatic and was being scanned for estimation of gestational age. *B.* A longitudinal sonogram in this patient reveals an incompetent cervix with ballooning of the membranes (*asterisk*).

are pitfalls in the transabdominal ultrasound diagnosis of cervical incompetence. A full urinary bladder will compress the lower uterine segment and may obliterate the ultrasound findings of the open internal os and bulging membranes. Also, as previously mentioned, contractions of the lower uterine segment may temporarily change the relationship of the cervix and lower uterus.[63] Scanning through the cervix should be done after voiding and performed several times during the general examination. When the presenting fetal part obscures the cervical detail endovaginal scanning or translabial scanning may be helpful.[64, 65]

Cervical cerclage is the treatment of choice for cervical incompetence (Fig. 29–30). Early second-trimester placement of elective cerclage is preferred. Fetal life and anatomy can be confirmed by ultrasound evaluation before the procedure. The elective cerclage has a better success rate than those procedures done after significant effacement and dilatation have occurred.[66]

Uterine myomas are so common that they will often be noted during obstetric examinations. Single or multiple myomas have been implicated in early spontaneous abortions secondary to poor implantation, in premature delivery, bleeding, premature rupture of the membranes, fetal malpresentations, as well as placental abruption. Myomas may initially grow during pregnancy with estrogen stimulation, but usually increasing progesterone will cause the myomas to decrease later during pregnancy. Half of all myomas may not change during pregnancy at all.[67] Myomas located in the lower uterine segment or cervix may inhibit or obstruct vaginal delivery (Fig. 29–31).

Uterine rupture may present with pain, bleeding, and shock. It is usually a life-threatening situation. Clinical signs and symptoms, however, may be silent or elusive. Rupture may occur at the site of former cesarean section scar, after therapeutic abortion and perforation, after rupture of a cornual pregnancy, or after the onset of labor when cerclage sutures are still

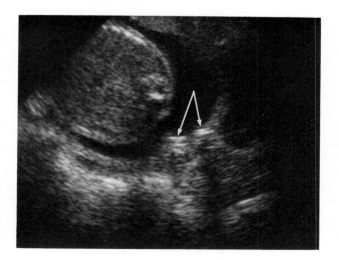

Figure 29–30. Cervical cerclage. A cerclage was placed in this patient owing to cervical incompetence. The highly reflective echoes (*arrows*) from the cerclage can be identified.

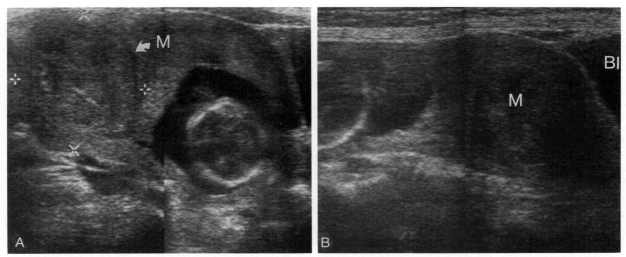

Figure 29–31. Uterine myomas. *A.* In this patient, a large fundal myoma (M) is identified. This patient was thought to be large for dates owing to the increased size of the uterus. *B.* A longitudinal sonogram through the gravid uterus reveals a large myoma (M) in the region of the lower uterine segment and cervix. This myoma obstructed the cervix and prevented the patient from having vaginal delivery. Bl, bladder.

in place. Sonographic examination may demonstrate free blood or hematoma in the cul-de-sac or peritoneal gutters, hemorrhage in the amniotic cavity, or retroplacental hemorrhage.[68] The gestational sac or fetal parts may be extruding from the uterus.

One other cause of uterine rupture is uterine incarceration in the pelvis when there is a persistently retropositioned uterus. Usually a retropositioned uterus will spontaneously reduce and rise out of the pelvis by the third month of gestation. If adhesions or other anatomic causes prohibit this reduction, the growing fetus becomes abnormally lodged deep in the pelvis. Thus the growing uterus may compress the bladder and bowel and cause extensive urinary and bowel symptoms. Vaginal delivery becomes nearly impossible and there is the potential for uterine rupture as well. The ultrasound examination will demonstrate the contained gestation abnormally located deep in the pelvis behind the bladder. Uterine tissue can usually be identified between the anterior bladder and the posterior growing gestation.[69] Occasionally, when this is recognized the uterus may be manually manipulated and reduced.

References

1. Lyons EA, Ballard G, Taylor PJ, et al: Characterization of subendometrial myometrial contractions throughout the menstrual cycle in normal fertile women. Fertil Steril 55:771, 1991.
2. Callen PW, DeMartini WJ, Filly RA: The central uterine cavity echo: A useful anatomic sign in the ultrasonographic evaluation of the female pelvis. Radiology 131:187, 1979.
3. Fleischer AC, Kalemeris GC, Entman SS: Sonographic depiction of the endometrium during normal cycles. Ultrasound Med Biol 12:271, 1986.
4. Fleischer AC, Pittaway DE, Beard LA, et al: Sonographic depiction of endometrial changes occurring with ovulation induction. J Ultrasound Med 3:341, 1984.
5. Fleischer AC, Gordon AN, Entman SS, et al: Transvaginal sonography (TVS) of the endometrium: Current and potential applications. Crit Rev Diagn Imag 30(2):85, 1990.
6. Rubin C, Kurtz AB, Goldberg BB: Water enema: A new ultrasound technique in defining pelvic anatomy. J Clin Ultrasound 6:28, 1978.
7. Williams PL, Warwick R, Dyson M, et al (eds): Gray's Anatomy, 37th ed. London, Churchill Livingstone, 1989.
8. Baltarowich OH: Female pelvic organ measurements. In Goldberg BB, Kurtz AB (eds): Atlas of Ultrasound Measurements. Chicago, Year Book Medical Publishers, 1990.
9. Orsini LF, Salardi S, Pilu G, et al: Pelvic organs in premenarchal girls: Real-time ultrasonography. Radiology 153:113, 1984.
10. DuBose TJ, Hill LW, Hennigan HW, et al: Sonography of arcuate uterine blood vessels. J Ultrasound Med 4:229, 1985.
11. Atri M, deStempel J, Senterman MK, et al: Diffuse peripheral uterine calcification (manifestation of Monckeberg's arteriosclerosis) detected by ultrasonography. J Clin Ultrasound 20:211, 1992.
12. Fleischer AC, Rao BK, Kepple DM: Transvaginal color Doppler sonography. In Fleischer AC, Kepple DM (eds): Transvaginal Sonography: A Clinical Atlas. Philadelphia, JB Lippincott, 1992.
13. McCarthy S, Scott G, Majumdar S, et al: Uterine junctional zone: MR study of water content and relaxation properties. Radiology 171:241, 1989.
14. Mitchell DG, Schonholz L, Hilpert PL, et al: Zones of the uterus: Discrepancy between US and MR images. Radiology 174:827, 1990.
15. Ascher SM, Scoutt LM, McCarthy SM, et al: Uterine changes after dilation and curettage: MR imaging findings. Radiology 180:433, 1991.
16. Snell RS: Clinical Embryology for Medical Students, 3rd ed. Boston, Little, Brown & Co 1983.
17. Fried AM, Oliff M, Wilson EA, et al: Uterine anomalies associated with renal agenesis: Role of gray scale ultrasonography. AJR 131:973, 1978.
18. Nicolini U, Bellotti M, Bonazzi B, et al: Can ultrasound be used to screen uterine malformations? Fertil Steril 47: 89, 1987.
19. Reuter KL, Daly DC, Cohen SM: Septate versus bicornuate uteri: Errors in imaging diagnosis. Radiology 172:749, 1989.
20. Rosenberg HK, et al: Duplication of the uterus and vagina, unilateral hydrometrocolpos, and ipsilateral renal agenesis: Sonographic aid to diagnosis. J Ultrasound Med 1:289, 1982.
21. Viscomi GN, Gonzalez R, Taylor KJW: Ultrasound detection of uterine abnormalities after diethylstilbestrol (DES) exposure. Radiology 136:733, 1980.
22. Grunfeld L, Walker B, Bergh PA, et al: High-resolution endovaginal ultrasonography of the endometrium: A noninvasive test for endometrial adequacy. Obstet Gynecol 78:200, 1991.
23. Fleischer AC: Ultrasound imaging-2000: Assessment of uteroovarian blood flow with transvaginal color Doppler sonography:

Potential clinical applications in infertility. Fertil Steril 55:684, 1991.

24. Steer CV, Campbell S, Pampiglione JS, et al: Transvaginal colour flow imaging of the uterine arteries during the ovarian and menstrual cycles. Hum Reprod 5:391, 1990.

25. Lin MC, Gosink BB, Wolf SI, et al: Endometrial thickness after menopause: Effect of hormone replacement. Radiology 180:427, 1991.

26. Jordan VC: Long-term adjuvant tamoxifen therapy for breast cancer. Breast Cancer Res Treat 15:125, 1990.

27. Cross SS, Ismail SM: Endometrial hyperplasia in an oophorectomized woman receiving tamoxifen therapy: Case report. Br J Obstet Gynaecol 97:190, 1990.

28. Corley D, Rowe J, Curtis MT, et al: Postmenopausal bleeding from unusual endometrial polyps in women on chronic tamoxifen therapy. Obstet Gynecol 79:111, 1992.

29. Malfetano JH: Tamoxifen-associated endometrial carcinoma in postmenopausal breast cancer patients. Gynecol Oncol 39:82, 1990.

30. Goldstein SR, Nachtigall M, Snyder JR, et al: Endometrial assessment by vaginal ultrasonography before endometrial sampling in patients with postmenopausal bleeding. Am J Obstet Gynecol 163:119, 1990.

31. Granberg S, Wikland M, Karlsson B, et al: Endometrial thickness as measured by endovaginal ultrasonography for identifying endometrial abnormality. Am J Obstet Gynecol 164:47, 1991.

32. Malpani A, Singer J, Wolverson MK, et al: Endometrial hyperplasia: Value of endometrial thickness in ultrasonographic diagnosis and clinical significance. J Clin Ultrasound 18:173, 1990.

33. Cervical cancer. In Clarke-Pearson DL, Dawood MY (eds): Green's Gynecology: Essentials of Clinical Practice. Boston, Little, Brown & Co, 1990.

34. Gusberg SB, Runowicz CD: Gynecologic cancers. In Holleb AI, Fink DJ, Murphy GP (eds): American Cancer Society Textbook of Clinical Oncology. Atlanta, American College of Radiology, 1991.

35. Sironi S, Belloni C, Taccagni GL, et al: Carcinoma of the cervix: Value of MR imaging in detecting parametrial involvement. AJR 156:753, 1991.

36. Kim SH, Choi BI, Lee HP, et al: Uterine cervical carcinoma: Comparison of CT and MR findings. Radiology 175:45, 1990.

37. Togashi K, Nishimura K, Sagoh T, et al: Carcinoma of the cervix: Staging with MR imaging. Radiology 171:245, 1989.

38. Yamashita Y, Takahashi M, Sawada T, et al: Carcinoma of the cervix: Dynamic MR imaging. Radiology 182:643, 1992.

39. Hricak H, Hamm B, Semelka RC, et al: Carcinoma of the uterus: Use of gadopentetate dimeglumine in MR imaging. Radiology 181:95, 1991.

40. Radecki PD, Lev-Toaff AS, Hilpert PL, et al: Inflammatory diseases. In Friedman AC, Radecki PD, Lev-Toaff AS, et al (eds): Clinical Pelvic Imaging: CT, Ultrasound and MRI. St. Louis, CV Mosby, 1990.

41. Benign diseases of the uterus: Leiomyomas, adenomyosis, hyperplasia, and polyps. In Clarke-Pearson DL, Dawood MY (eds): Green's Gynecology Essentials of Clinical Practice. Boston, Little, Brown & Co, 1990.

42. Bohlman ME, Ensor RE, Sanders RC: Sonographic findings in adenomyosis of the uterus. AJR 148:765, 1987.

43. Siedler D, Laing FC, Jeffrey RB, et al: Uterine adenomyosis: A difficult sonographic diagnosis. J Ultrasound Med 6:345, 1987.

44. Togashi K, Ozasa H, Konishi I, et al: Enlarged uterus: Differentiation between adenomyosis and leiomyoma with MR imaging. Radiology 171:531, 1989.

45. Entman SS: Uterine leiomyoma and adenomyosis. In Jones HW, Wentz AC, Burnett LS (eds): Novak's Textbook of Gynecology, 11th ed, p 443, Baltimore, Williams & Wilkins, 1988.

46. Pollow K, Geilfuss J, Boquoi E, et al: Estrogen and progesterone binding proteins in normal human myometrium and leiomyoma tissue. J Clin Chem Clin Biochem 16:503, 1978.

47. Filicori M, Hall DA, Loughlin JS, et al: A conservative approach to the management of uterine leiomyoma: Pituitary desensitization by an LHRH analogue. Am J Obstet Gynecol 147:726, 1983.

48. Friedman AJ, Lobel SM, Rein MS, et al: Efficacy and safety considerations in women with uterine leiomyomas treated with gonadotropin-releasing hormone agonists: The estrogen threshold hypothesis. Am J Obstet Gynecol 163:1114, 1990.

49. Dilts PV, Hopkins MP, Chang AE, et al: Rapid growth of leiomyoma in patient receiving tamoxifen. Am J Obstet Gynecol 166:167, 1992.

50. Olson MC, Posniak HV, Tempany CM, et al: MR imaging of the female pelvic region. Radiographics 12:445, 1992.

51. Jacobs JE, Markowitz SK: CT diagnosis of uterine lipoma. AJR 150:1335, 1988.

52. Jones HW: Sarcoma of the uterus. In Jones HW, Wentz AC, Burnett LS (eds): Novak's Textbook of Gynecology, 11th ed. Baltimore, Williams & Wilkins, 1988.

53. Leibsohn S, d'Ablaing G, Mishell DR, et al: Leiomyosarcoma in a series of hysterectomies performed for presumed uterine leiomyomas. Am J Obstet Gynecol 162:968, 1990.

54. Jones HW: Endometrial carcinoma. In Jones HW, Wentz AC, Burnett LS (eds): Novak's Textbook of Gynecology, 11th ed. Baltimore, Williams & Wilkins, 1988.

55. Fleischer AC, Dudley BS, Entman SS, et al: Myometrial invasion by endometrial carcinoma: Sonographic assessment. Radiology 162:307, 1987.

56. Gordon AN, Fleischer AC, Reed GW: Depth of myometrial invasion in endometrial cancer: Preoperative assessment by transvaginal ultrasonography. Gynecol Oncol 39:321, 1990.

57. Bourne TH, Campbell S, Steer CV, et al: Detection of endometrial cancer by transvaginal ultrasonography with color flow imaging and blood flow analysis: A preliminary report. Gynecol Oncol 40:253, 1991.

58. Posniak HV, Olson MC, Dudiak CM, et al: MR imaging of uterine carcinoma: Correlation with clinical and pathologic findings. Radiographics 10:15, 1990.

59. Hricak H, Stern JL, Fisher MR, et al: Endometrial carcinoma staging by MR imaging. Radiology 162:297, 1987.

60. Birnholz JC: Ultrasound links venous pathophysiology to pain. Diagn Imag 13:83, 1991.

61. Goldberg BB, Liu JB, Kuhlman K, et al: Endoluminal gynecologic ultrasound: Preliminary results. J Ultrasound Med 10:583, 1991.

62. Stillman RJ: In utero exposure to diethylstilbesterol: Adverse effects on the reproductive tract and reproductive performance in male and female offspring. Am J Obstet Gynecol 142:905, 1982.

63. Karis JP, Hertzberg BS, Bowie JD: Sonographic diagnosis of premature cervical dilatation: Potential pitfall due to lower uterine segment contractions. J Ultrasound Med 10:83, 1991.

64. Anderson HF: Transvaginal and transabdominal ultrasonography of the uterine cervix during pregnancy. J Clin Ultrasound 19:77, 1991.

65. Mahony BS, Nyberg DA, Luthy DA, et al: Translabial ultrasound of the third-trimester uterine cervix: Correlation with digital examination. J Ultrasound Med 9:717, 1990.

66. Parisi VM: Cervical incompetence and preterm labor. Clin Obstet Gynecol 31:585, 1988.

67. Lev-Toaff AS, Coleman BG, Arger PH, et al: Leiomyomas in pregnancy: Sonographic study. Radiology 164:375, 1987.

68. Gale JT, Mahoney BS, Bowie JD: Sonographic features of rupture of the pregnant uterus. J Ultrasound Med 5:713, 1986.

69. Laing FC: Sonography of a persistently retroverted gravid uterus. AJR 136:413, 1981.

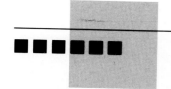

CHAPTER **30**

Ultrasound Evaluation of Gestational Trophoblastic Neoplasia

PETER W. CALLEN, M.D.

Although gestational trophoblastic neoplasia is one of the more potentially confusing diseases, it is also, fortunately, one of the gynecologic diseases with the most favorable cure rate. The confusion is due to the varied terminology used to describe this disease and also to the existence of a number of conditions that mimic gestational trophoblastic neoplasia. The favorable nature of this neoplasm is based on the fact that even in patients with high-risk metastatic disease, cure rates of 80% to 90% have been achieved.[1, 2]

TERMINOLOGY

Most practitioners are aware of the entity hydatidiform mole, but this is just one of the manifestations of gestational trophoblastic neoplasia. Gestational trophoblastic neoplasia is a proliferative disease of the trophoblast that may present as a relatively benign form, hydatidiform mole, or, in contrast, as the more malignant forms, invasive mole or choriocarcinoma. Although in one sense the division of this disease entity into these categories is useful for understanding the various manifestations and progression of the disease, it should be recognized that since the advent of an accurate immunologic biologic marker for this disease, specifically the β-subunit of human chorionic gonadotropin (β-hCG), this division has less clinical utility.

HYDATIDIFORM MOLE

Epidemiology

Hydatidiform mole is the most benign and most common form of trophoblastic disease. Its incidence varies geographically. In the United States, the incidence is approximately 1 in 1200 to 2000 pregnancies; in France, the incidence has been reported to be 1 in 500 pregnancies; and the greatest frequency is in the Far East, with a reported incidence of more than 1 in 100 pregnancies in some Indonesian hospitals.[3, 4] Age also appears to influence the risk of development of a hydatidiform mole. Those women who are at the end of their reproductive years have an increased incidence of trophoblastic disease, despite race or geography.[5, 6] Women who have had a previous hydatidiform mole have an increased risk of having another,[5, 6–8] ranging from 20 to 40 times that for the general population.[5, 6, 9] This risk may be less if these women have had one

or more normal pregnancies since the first hydatidiform mole.[5]

GENETICS

There are at least two different genetic types of hydatidiform mole, each with a different etiology.[5, 10–12] A complete or "classic" mole usually has a chromosomal makeup of 46,XX, which is derived entirely from the father.[5] This event likely results from an egg with an absent or inactivated nucleus in which there is fertilization by a haploid sperm that then duplicates to the normal diploid number.[5] The other genetic type of hydatidiform mole is one in which there is a 46,XY chromosomal complement. This is believed to result from fertilization of an egg with an absent nucleus by two different haploid sperm.[5, 13, 14] This likely occurs in only a small percentage of cases. In either case, the genetic origin of the nuclear DNA is paternal.

Pathophysiology

The standard explanation for the pathophysiology of a hydatidiform mole is that the chorionic villi of a blighted ovum in a missed abortion persist and continue to undergo hydatid swelling. This accounts for the characteristic vesicular appearance of the swollen chorionic villi but not for the primary pathologic feature of this disease—trophoblastic proliferation. Thus, some investigators have postulated that the primary event may well be abnormal proliferation of the trophoblast, with the hydropic change being a secondary phenomenon.

Pathology

The pathologic characteristics of hydatidiform mole are (1) marked edema and enlargement of the chorionic villi, (2) disappearance of the villus blood vessels, (3) proliferation of the lining trophoblast of the chorionic villi, and (4) absence of fetal tissue. As stated earlier, perhaps the most important characteristic that separates hydatidiform mole from other nontrophoblastic diseases is the proliferation of the lining trophoblast of the chorionic villi. Small islands of chorionic villus can be seen in the normal placenta with the trophoblastic elements forming a thin "limiting bor-

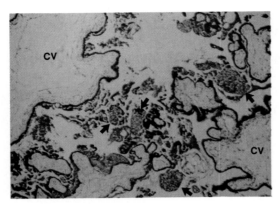

Figure 30–1. Photomicrograph from a patient with a hydatidiform mole. Abnormal nests of trophoblastic cells (*arrows*) are seen scattered among markedly swollen chorionic villi (CV). The degree of hydropic change of the chorionic villus, in addition to the presence of trophoblastic proliferation, distinguishes this from hydropic degeneration occurring in otherwise normal pregnancies.

der." In hydatidiform mole, the chorionic villus becomes markedly swollen with proliferating nests of trophoblastic cells scattered throughout (Fig. 30–1).

Sonographic Appearance

Characteristically, a hydatidiform mole appears as a large, moderately echogenic, soft tissue mass filling the uterine cavity. Numerous small, cystic, fluid-containing spaces are scattered throughout (Fig. 30–2A). When the tumor volume is small, the myometrium may be perceived as less echogenic soft tissue surrounding the more echogenic mass filling the uterine cavity (Fig. 30–2B).

Although these features have come to be recognized as typical of a hydatidiform mole, this appearance is only specific for a second-trimester mole.[15] Cases of first-trimester molar pregnancies have been widely reported in the literature and have a variable appearance. First-trimester moles, in some cases, may have an appearance simulating a blighted ovum or a threatened abortion; others may show a small echogenic

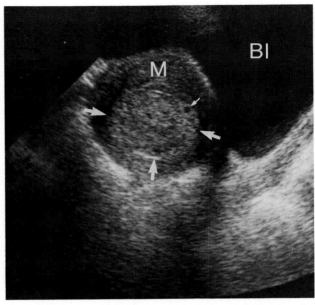

Figure 30–3. Longitudinal sonogram from a patient with a first-trimester hydatidiform mole. In this case, an echogenic mass (*arrows*) is seen filling the uterine cavity. Except for one small cyst (*small arrow*) there are virtually none of the cystic spaces that are characteristically seen in more advanced molar pregnancies. M, myometrium; Bl, bladder.

mass filling the uterine cavity without the characteristic vesicular appearance (Fig. 30–3).[16] In these cases, only a high index of suspicion in addition to correlation with the level of hCG will allow the sonographer to suggest the correct diagnosis.

In recent years, the addition of Doppler ultrasound technology has allowed the sonographer to evaluate blood flow and perfusion. Doppler evaluation of trophoblastic tissue reveals a low-impedance, high-flow state with high systolic and diastolic frequencies.[17, 18] This is different than the low-flow, higher-impedance states seen in patients with nonviable gestations or degenerating fibroids. When a patient presents with an echogenic mass within the uterus, Doppler interrogation of the mass, in addition to hCG evaluation, may help differentiate trophoblastic from nontrophoblastic disease.

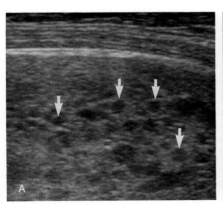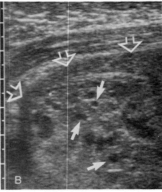

Figure 30–2. *A.* Longitudinal sonogram from a patient with a second-trimester hydatidiform mole. A large, moderately echogenic mass with numerous small cystic spaces (*arrows*) is seen filling the central uterine cavity. The cystic spaces undoubtedly represent the markedly hydropic chorionic villi. *B.* Sonogram from a patient with an early second-trimester hydatidiform mole. Numerous vesicles (*arrows*) and echogenic tissue are seen filling the uterine cavity. The adjacent, less echogenic myometrium is well seen (*open arrows*).

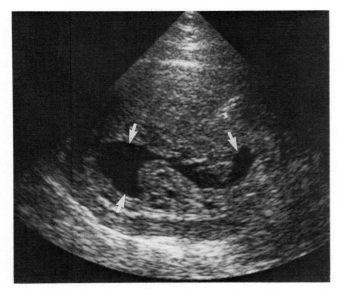

Figure 30–4. Transverse sonogram from a patient with a second-trimester hydatidiform mole. An irregularly shaped fluid collection (*arrows*) is seen that represents a large area of hemorrhage. This was initially thought to represent the amniotic fluid in a nonviable gestation.

COMPLICATIONS OF TROPHOBLASTIC DISEASE

Hemorrhage

Perhaps one of the most common complications of trophoblastic disease, which can be readily identified on the sonogram, is hemorrhage within this lesion or within adjacent tissues. The areas of hemorrhage usually appear as crescentic anechoic regions surrounding the tumor (Fig. 30–4).

Theca Lutein Cysts

The other feature frequently associated with hydatidiform mole and trophoblastic disease is theca lutein cysts. The incidence of theca lutein cysts in patients with trophoblastic disease is 20% to 50%. The number detected using ultrasonography is usually higher than that with clinical examination. This difference is probably because with excessive uterine enlargement the ovaries may be difficult to palpate, since they are displaced in a cephalic direction out of the true pelvis.

Theca lutein cysts are believed to be secondary to a markedly elevated circulating level of hCG. Analysis of the cysts shows them to be multilocular and to contain amber-colored or serosanguineous fluid.[19] The sonogram accurately depicts this pathologic description: multiseptated cysts are the most common presentation (Fig. 30–5). The sonographer should remember that it may take 2 to 4 months for these cysts to regress after molar evacuation; thus, they cannot be used as evidence of persistent or recurrent disease.[20]

DISEASES SIMULATING HYDATIDIFORM MOLE

The older literature about trophoblastic disease tended to be confusing since several diseases that were not truly hydatidiform moles, such as hydropic degeneration or partial moles, were included in this classification. If one adheres strictly to the pathologic criterion stated earlier for hydatidiform mole, one will be less prone to overestimate the prevalence of this disease. One entity that has been frequently included with hydatidiform mole and should remain separate is *hydropic degeneration of the placenta.*

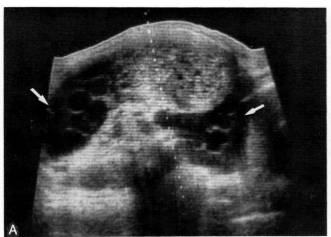
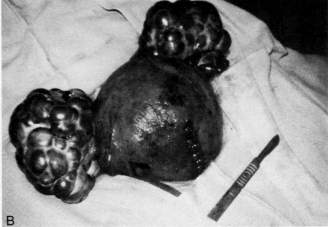

Figure 30–5. *A.* Transverse sonogram in a patient with a hydatidiform mole and theca lutein cysts. The characteristic multiseptated appearance (*arrows*) is seen. *B.* Intraoperative photograph of the postgravid uterus and ovaries in a patient with coexistent mole and live pregnancy. Bilateral theca lutein cysts are identified. The characteristic multilocular appearance is seen. (*B* from Yee B, Tu B, Platt LD: Coexisting hydatidiform mole with a live fetus presenting as a placenta previa on ultrasound. Am J Obstet Gynecol 144:726, 1982.)

Hydropic changes of the placenta may occur in 1% to 3% of pregnancies.[21] Although the chorionic villi may be engorged, a specific feature of trophoblastic disease, proliferation of the lining trophoblast of the chorionic villi, is not seen. The sonographer may find it extremely difficult to distinguish between a missed abortion, in which there is hydropic degeneration, and a molar pregnancy (Fig. 30–6). In these cases, determination of the levels of serum hCG as well as pathologic evaluation of the specimen will be needed to make this distinction.[22]

Although leiomyomas involving the uterus do not usually present a diagnostic dilemma, occasionally a leiomyoma with cystic degeneration may simulate the appearance of a hydatidiform mole (Fig. 30–7). In these cases, careful evaluation of the highly attenuating nature of myomatous disease may help distinguish it from trophoblastic disease.

FOLLOW-UP EVALUATION AND TREATMENT

The treatment and follow-up of trophoblastic disease are beyond the scope of this discussion, but some general points will be mentioned. Once hydatidiform mole has been diagnosed, suction evacuation of the uterus is usually performed, followed by curettage of

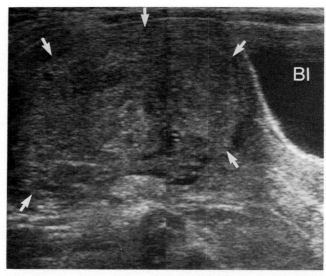

Figure 30–7. Longitudinal sonogram from a patient with vaginal bleeding and a large pelvic mass. Several poorly echogenic areas are seen within this mass that simulate a second-trimester hydatidiform mole. The serum β-hCG test was negative and may be useful in making the distinction between this leiomyoma (*arrows*) with cystic degeneration and a molar pregnancy. Bl, bladder.

the endometrium to determine if there is myometrial invasion. A baseline chest radiograph and computed tomogram of the chest are used to examine for evidence of metastatic disease. Declining serum levels of β-hCG may then be followed until the level is normal. Normally, the serum β-hCG level falls toward zero 10 to 12 weeks after evacuation of the molar pregnancy (Fig. 30–8).[20]

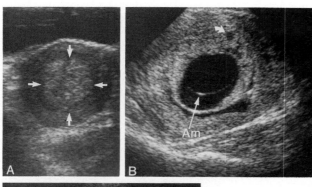

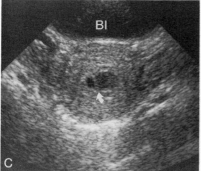

Figure 30–6. Three patients presented with vaginal bleeding and positive pregnancy tests. *A.* This patient has an echogenic mass (*arrows*) filling the uterine cavity. The appearance is quite similar to that of a first-trimester hydatidiform mole (compare with Fig. 30–3). This was a nonviable pregnancy ("missed abortion"). *B.* Sonogram in a patient with early pregnancy and vaginal bleeding. This pregnancy was nonviable. A small cystic area, probably representing hydropic change (*arrow*) is seen. Am, amnion. *C.* In this patient an irregular fluid collection (*arrows*) was seen in the uterine cavity. This has the appearance of a nonviable gestation. At pathologic evaluation there was evidence of trophoblastic proliferation consistent with a first-trimester hydatidiform mole. Bl, bladder.

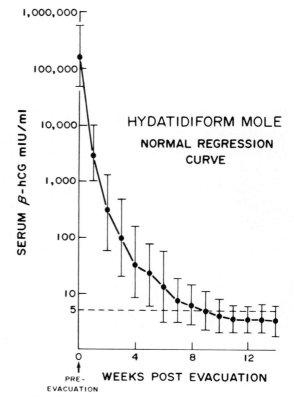

Figure 30–8. Normal regression curve after evacuation for patients with a hydatidiform mole. By 12 weeks after evacuation, the β-hCG level should have returned to near zero.

VARIATIONS OF MOLAR PREGNANCY

Coexistent Mole and Fetus

Several reports in the literature have noted that a living fetus was associated with a molar pregnancy.[23-25] Unfortunately, many patients were included in this category in whom there was hydropic degeneration or an incomplete mole rather than a true hydatidiform mole. Nevertheless, several well-documented cases of coexistent fetus and mole have been seen. Because absence of fetal structure is one of the pathologic requirements for a true hydatidiform mole, the presumed mechanism for coexistence of a true mole and normal fetus is molar transformation of one binovular twin placenta (Fig. 30–9). Although the diagnosis may be suggested and made with a high degree of certainty on the sonogram, it should be confirmed pathologically, since these lesions must be considered as having the same malignant potential as a more classically appearing molar pregnancy.

Incomplete or Partial Mole (Triploidy)

Several entities, including hydropic degeneration, have been placed in this category. The following pathologic findings for incomplete or partial moles are well presented in a review by Szulman and Surti:[26] (1) identifiable fetal tissues, (2) edematous chorionic villi with little or no trophoblastic proliferation, and (3) multiple congenital anomalies in which a chromosomal analysis usually reveals a triploid chromosomal complement usually resulting from fertilization of an apparently normal ovum by two sperm.

For the sonographer, the goal is to differentiate a partial or incomplete molar pregnancy from a true hydatidiform mole or a normal pregnancy with avillous areas within the placenta. Patients with a partial mole demonstrate a pregnancy with a "formed" placenta in which there are numerous cystic spaces (Fig. 30–10). This is quite different from a hydatidiform mole in which a globular echogenic mass, rather than a formed placenta, is seen within the uterus. In addition, in nearly all cases of partial mole, the fetus is growth retarded and/or dysmorphic.[27] If necessary, amniocentesis is helpful in demonstrating a triploid chromosomal complement.

In addition to identifying an abnormal fetus in these pregnancies, it is important to make the diagnosis for further follow-up. There have been cases of partial hydatidiform mole (2% to 4%) in which persistent trophoblastic disease requiring chemotherapy has developed after evacuation.[8, 27, 28]

Invasive Mole

In 80% of patients initially diagnosed as having hydatidiform mole, the disease will follow a benign course, with resolution after evacuation (Fig. 30–11). However, in 12% to 15% of patients, invasive mole develops, and in 5% to 8%, metastatic choriocarcinoma develops. The pathologic features of invasive mole are (1) extensive local invasion, (2) excessive trophoblastic proliferation, and (3) preservation of the villous pattern. The differentiating feature between invasive mole and choriocarcinoma is preservation of the villous pattern in invasive molar disease. Examination of a specimen from a patient with an invasive mole reveals that the characteristic elements seen with hydatidiform mole (nests of trophoblastic cells as well as swollen chorionic villi), rather than being within the central cavity of the uterus, are found within the myometrium.

Invasive mole is infrequently diagnosed without hys-

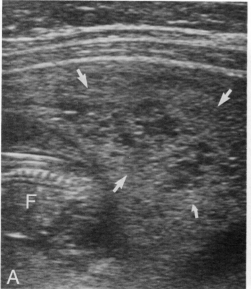
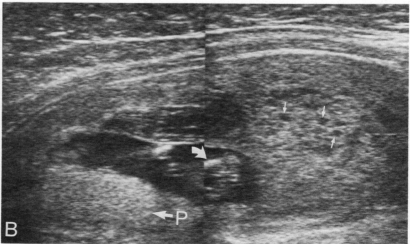

Figure 30–9. Sonogram in a patient with a coexistent pregnancy and true hydatidiform mole. *A.* In this plane of section the tissue characteristic of a true hydatidiform mole is seen (*arrows*). F, fetus. *B.* In this dual image scan the right side of the image demonstrates the hydatidiform mole with vesicles (*arrows*) clearly seen. On the left is the fetus (*curved arrow*) along with its more normal-appearing placenta (P).

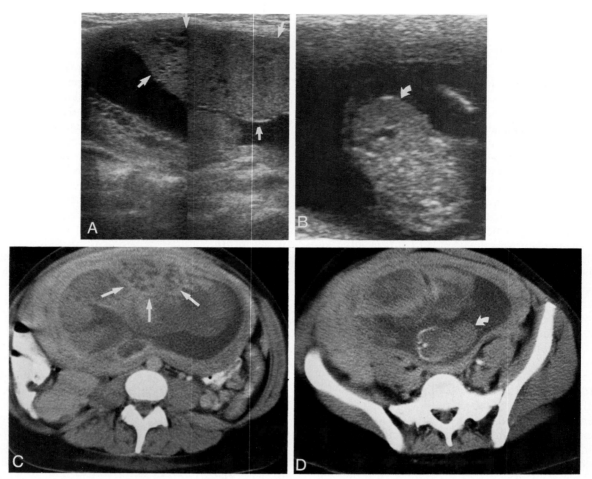

Figure 30–10. Partial hydatidiform mole. *A.* In this patient the placenta is enlarged (*arrows*) and contains numerous vesicles; however, it retains its normal overall shape. *B.* The fetus in this case was noted to be dysmorphic. A large abdominal wall defect was seen representing an omphalocele (*arrow*). *C.* A computed tomographic scan was performed because of a previous history of trophoblastic disease. The placenta, containing numerous cystic spaces, is evident (*arrows*). *D.* The abdominal wall defect (*arrow*) was also identified. The subsequent chromosomal analysis of the abortus was triploid.

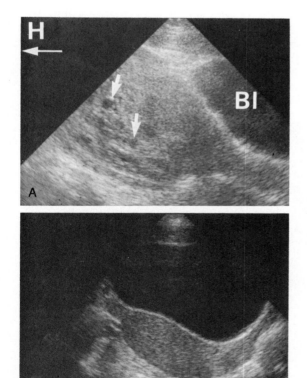

Figure 30–11. *A.* Uterine enlargement due to a hydatidiform mole. Cystic spaces are readily seen (*arrows*). Bl, bladder; H, head. *B.* Six weeks after molar evacuation the uterus has returned to normal size.

terectomy, since it is uncommon to obtain myometrium during curettage. Also, because hysterectomies are not commonly performed for any form of trophoblastic disease, the diagnosis may not be suspected by the clinician. The morbidity and mortality caused by invasive mole result from the penetration of the tumor through the myometrium and pelvic vessels, producing hemorrhage.[19–22] Although the sonographer may have a difficult time diagnosing this more aggressive form of the disease, hemorrhagic necrosis involving the myometrium and extending into the parametrial areas should make one suspect this entity (Fig. 30–12).

Choriocarcinoma

Choriocarcinoma is the most malignant form of trophoblastic disease, with an incidence of approximately 1 in 40,000 pregnancies in the United States. Approximately 50% of the cases of choriocarcinoma are preceded by a molar pregnancy; however, only 3% to 5% of all molar pregnancies result in choriocarcinoma. Approximately one half of cases of choriocarcinoma occur in association with a molar pregnancy, 25% occur after an abortion, 22% occur after normal pregnancy, and approximately 3% may occur after an ectopic pregnancy (Fig. 30–13).

Gross examination of the uterus in a patient with choriocarcinoma will reveal a dark hemorrhagic mass on the uterine wall, cervix, or vagina, which may show extensive ulceration and penetration of the tumor into the musculature (Fig. 30–14). Microscopically, the villous pattern is completely blotted out by the proliferating trophoblast (Fig. 30–15). This feature separates this disease entity from the less benign forms of trophoblastic disease.[19, 29] Choriocarcinoma is known to metastasize to the lung, brain, liver, bone, gastrointestinal tract, and skin. As such, the sonographer may help in evaluating the extent of the disease, particularly in the liver.

Placental Site Trophoblastic Tumor

Placental site trophoblastic tumor is a rare neoplasm that is considered by some to be a variant of choriocarcinoma. It arises within the trophoblastic tissue of the placental bed from the intermediate trophoblast cell.[30] The clinical course is benign for most persons; however, when disseminated, it is often fatal.

This neoplasm is distinguished from other forms of gestational trophoblastic neoplasia by the low level of hCG due to a paucity of syncytiotrophoblast. The major protein secreted by the predominant cell type in this disease is human placental lactogen.

Placental site trophoblastic tumor is distinguished from hydatidiform mole by the lack of chorionic villi and from choriocarcinoma by the lack of necrosis and hemorrhage. The sonographic appearance may be indistinguishable from that of an invasive mole.[31]

PROGRESSION OF DISEASE

As stated earlier, most patients originally diagnosed as having trophoblastic disease (i.e., hydatidiform mole) have resolution of their disease after evacuation of the molar pregnancy (approximately 80%). There are those patients, however, who may present initially with choriocarcinoma or develop persistent disease after a preceding pregnancy.

During the past 30 years, it has been recognized that trophoblastic disease is uniquely sensitive to systemic chemotherapy and thus potentially curable. Patients with persistent gestational trophoblastic neoplasia who are managed successfully with chemotherapy can expect normal reproduction in the future.[30–33] As with other malignancies, it has become important to define subgroups of these patients to determine adequate treatment regimens (Table 30–1). Thus, patients are divided into those groups with nonmetastatic and metastatic trophoblastic disease. The group with metastatic

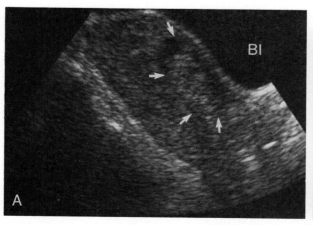
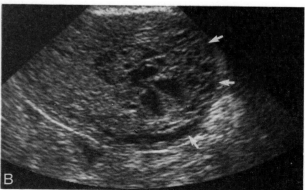

Figure 30–12. *A* and *B*. Extension of an invasive mole (*arrows*) into the myometrium in two patients with markedly elevated hCG levels. Bl, bladder.

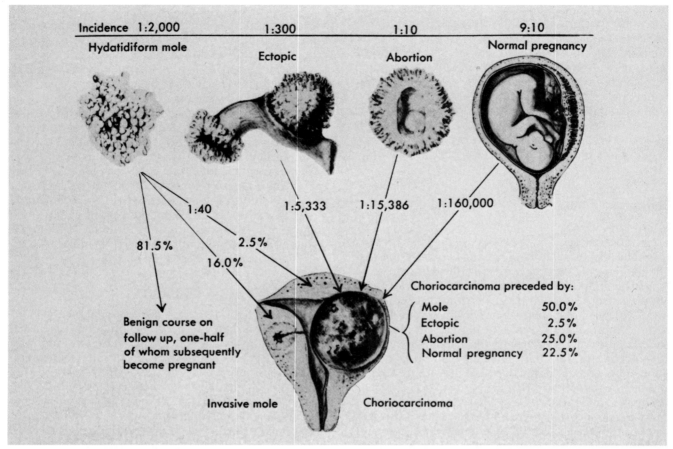

Figure 30–13. Origin and incidence of choriocarcinoma. (From Rosai J: Female reproductive system/placenta. In Ackerman's Surgical Pathology, 6th ed, p 1079, St. Louis, CV Mosby 1981.)

disease is subdivided into low-, intermediate-, and high-risk groups (Table 30–2).[34–37]

Role of the Sonologist in Persistent Gestational Trophoblastic Neoplasia

The sonographer or radiologist has two major goals in evaluating the patient suspected of having persistent trophoblastic disease: (1) to determine if the rise of hCG is due to a normal pregnancy rather than persistent disease and (2) to determine the sites of metastatic disease.

The major pathologic feature of trophoblastic disease is abnormal proliferation of trophoblastic tissue after a gestational event. Although pathologic confir-

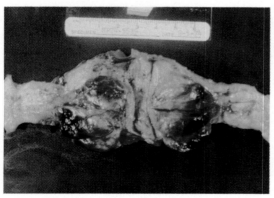

Figure 30–14. Pathologic specimen from a patient with choriocarcinoma. The bivalved uterus demonstrates a large, hemorrhagic necrotic mass involving the body of the uterus.

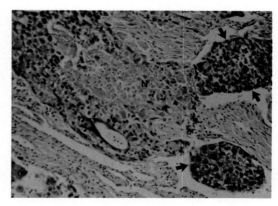

Figure 30–15. Photomicrograph from a patient with choriocarcinoma. Multiple cords (*arrows*) of malignant trophoblastic tissue infiltrate the uterine stroma. The absence of villi and the necrosis (N) of the tumor differentiate this process from invasive trophoblastic disease and a hydatidiform mole.

Table 30–1. INTERNATIONAL FEDERATION OF GYNECOLOGY AND OBSTETRICS STAGING FOR TROPHOBLASTIC TUMORS (GTT)

Stage	Description
I	Disease confined to the uterus
I A	Disease confined to the uterus with no risk factors
I B	Disease confined to the uterus with one risk factor
I C	Disease confined to the uterus with two risk factors
II	GTT extends outside of the uterus but is limited to the genital structures (adnexa, vagina, broad ligament)
II A	GTT involving genital structures without risk factors
II B	GTT extends outside of the uterus but limited to genital structures with one risk factor
II C	GTT extends outside of the uterus but limited to the genital structures with two risk factors
III	GTT extends to the lungs with or without known genital tract involvement
III A	GTT extends to the lungs with or without genital tract involvement and with no risk factors
III B	GTT extends to the lungs with or without genital tract involvement and with one risk factor
III C	GTT extends to the lungs with or without genital tract involvement and has two risk factors
IV	All other metastatic sites
IV A	All other metastatic sites without risk factors
IV B	All other metastatic sites with one risk factor
IV C	All other metastatic sites with two risk factors

The following factors should be considered and noted in reporting: (1) prior chemotherapy; (2) placental site tumors should be reported separately; and (3) histologic verification of disease is not required.

Risk factors affecting staging include the following: (1) HCG > 100,000 mIU/mL and (2) duration of disease > 6 months from termination of the antecedent pregnancy.

From Gynecology Oncology Committee of the International Federation of Gynecology and Obstetrics, Singapore, September 1991.

mation of choriocarcinoma is difficult because hysterectomies are now infrequently performed for this disease, correlation of the appearance of the uterus with an evaluation of known metastatic surveys as well as the level of serum β-hCG has proved interesting in assessing local involvement.[15] Patients with persistent

Table 30–2. MODIFIED NATIONAL INSTITUTES OF HEALTH CLASSIFICATION OF GESTATIONAL TROPHOBLASTIC DISEASE

Nonmetastatic Trophoblastic Disease
Hydatidiform mole
Undelivered
Delivered (>8 wk)
Persistent mole (>8 wk)
Invasive mole or choriocarcinoma confined to the uterus
Metastatic Trophoblastic Disease
Low risk
    Short duration (<4 mo)
    Low hCG titer (<100,000 mIU/24 h)
    Lung or vaginal metastasis
Intermediate risk
    Long duration (>4 mo)
    High hCG titer (>100,000 mIU/24 h)
    Metastasis other than to central nervous system or liver
High risk
    Central nervous system
    Liver metastasis

From Hilgers RA: Improving the outcome of high-risk gestational trophoblastic neoplasia. Contemp Obstet Gynecol 73:92, 1987.

trophoblastic disease may have focal areas of increased echogenicity within the myometrium as the only imaged evidence of disease. I hypothesize that trophoblastic disease appears on the sonogram as highly echogenic tissue within the uterus in which visualization depends on the amount of tissue present as well as on secondary changes.

If molar pregnancy is detected early, in a first-trimester mole or in cases of early detection of persistent or locally invasive disease, the vesicles that give hydatidiform mole its characteristic and easily recognizable appearance either may not be present or may be too small to be seen. Therefore, first-trimester molar pregnancies may often be misdiagnosed as a missed abortion or persistent disease may not be readily apparent on the sonogram. As the molar pregnancy progresses into the second trimester, the pathognomonic vesicles and theca lutein cysts become evident. This progression is supported by studies of Szulman and Surti,[36] who have established a roughly linear relationship between gestational age of the molar pregnancy and the microscopic size of the swollen chorionic villi. For example, their earliest hydatidiform mole, with a gestational age of 8.5 gestational weeks, yielded vesicles with a maximum diameter of 2 mm. This result contrasts to their most advanced case of 18.5 gestational weeks, yielding vesicles with a maximum diameter of 10 mm. As stated previously, in cases of first-trimester molar pregnancy or in cases of persistent or locally invasive disease when recurrence is detected by serial determinations of hCG levels, the characteristic vesicles may be too small to be imaged by ultrasound.

In addition to evaluation of the uterus, ultrasonography can determine if there is evidence of parametrial extension of disease or hepatic metastases. During the past several years, the newer imaging modalities of computed tomography and magnetic resonance imaging have shown the ability to detect metastatic disease that was not seen by conventional imaging methods.[38–41]

Knowledge of the various manifestations of trophoblastic disease as well as the complications that can be seen on the sonogram will aid the clinician in managing the disease. Differentiation between trophoblastic disease and a normal intrauterine pregnancy, as well as following the extent of spread of disease or response to therapy in advanced cases, may be accomplished using ultrasonography.

References

1. Lurain IR, Brewer JI, Torak EE, et al: Gestational trophoblastic disease: Treatment results at the Brewer Trophoblastic Disease Center. Obstet Gynecol 60:354, 1982.
2. Hammond CB, Weed JC, Currie JC: The role of operation in the current therapy of gestational trophoblastic disease. Am J Obstet Gynecol 136:844, 1980.
3. Sand PK, Lurain JR, Brewer JI: Repeat gestational trophoblastic disease. Obstet Gynecol 63:140, 1984.
4. Poen HJT, Djojopranoto M: The possible etiologic factors of hydatidiform mole and choriocarcinoma. Am J Obstet Gynecol 92:510, 1965.

5. Grimes DA: Epidemiology of gestational trophoblastic disease. Am J Obstet Gynecol 150:309, 1984.
6. Yen S, MacMahan B: Epidemiologic features of trophoblastic disease. Am J Obstet Gynecol 101:126, 1968.
7. MacGregor C, Ontiveros E, Vargas E, Valenzuela S: Hydatidiform mole. Obstet Gynecol 33:343, 1969.
8. Berkowitz RS, Goldstein DP: Pathogenesis of gestational trophoblastic neoplasms. Pathobiol Annu 11:391, 1981.
9. Rolan PA, deLopez BH: Epidemiologic aspects of hydatidiform mole in the Republic of Paraguay (South America). Br J Obstet Gynaecol 84:862, 1977.
10. Vassilahos P, Protton G, Kaju T: Hydatidiform mole: Two entities. Am J Obstet Gynecol 127:167, 1977.
11. Kaju T, Ohama K: Androgenetic origin of hydatidiform mole. Nature 268:633, 1977.
12. Szulman AE, Surti U: The syndromes of hydatidiform mole. Am J Obstet Gynecol 131:665, 1978.
13. Surti U, Szulman AE, O'Brien S: Complete (classic) hydatidiform mole with 46 XY karyotype of paternal origin. Hum Genet 51:153, 1979.
14. Ohami K, Kaju T, Ohamoto K, et al: Dispermic origin of XY hydatidiform moles. Nature 292:551, 1981.
15. Munyer TP, Callen PW, Filly RA, et al: Further observations on the sonographic spectrum of gestational trophoblastic disease. J Clin Ultrasound 9:349, 1981.
16. Woodward RM, Filly RA, Callen PW: First trimester molar pregnancy: Nonspecific ultrasonographic appearance. Obstet Gynecol 55:315, 1980.
17. Taylor KJW, Schwartz PE, Kohorn EI: Gestational trophoblastic neoplasia: Diagnosis with Doppler US. Radiology 165:445, 1987.
18. Desai RK, Desberg AL: Diagnosis of gestational trophoblastic disease: Value of endovaginal color flow Doppler sonography. AJR 157:787, 1991.
19. Kraus FT: Female genitalia. In Anderson WAD, Kissane JR (eds): Pathology, 7th ed. St. Louis, CV Mosby, 1977.
20. Goldstein DP, Berkowitz RJ, Cohen SM: The current management of molar pregnancy. Curr Probl Obstet Gynecol 3:1, 1979.
21. Hertig AT: Human Trophoblast, pp 228–237. Springfield, IL, Charles C Thomas, 1968.
22. Romero R, Horgan JG, Kohorn EF, et al: New criteria for the diagnosis of gestational trophoblastic disease. Obstet Gynecol 66:553, 1985.
23. Bree RL, Silver TM, Wichs JD, et al: Trophoblastic disease with coexistent fetus: A sonographic and clinical spectrum. J Clin Ultrasound 6:310, 1978.
24. Fleisher AC, James AD, Krause DA, et al: Sonographic patterns in trophoblastic diseases. Radiology 126:215, 1978.
25. Sauerbrei EE, Salem S, Fayle B: Coexistent hydatidiform mole and live fetus in the second trimester. Radiology 135:415, 1980.
26. Szulman AE, Surti U: The syndromes of hydatidiform mole: I. Cytogenic and morphologic correlations. Am J Obstet Gynecol 13:655, 1978.
27. Crane JP, Beaver HA, Cheung SW: Antenatal ultrasound finding in fetal triploidy syndrome. J Ultrasound Med 4:519, 1985.
28. Szulman AE, Ma HK, Wong LC, Hsu C: Residual trophoblastic disease in association with partial hydatidiform mole. Obstet Gynecol 57:392, 1981.
29. Jones HW III: Gestational trophoblastic disease. In Jones H, Jones GS (eds): Novak's Textbook of Gynecology, 10th ed. Baltimore, Williams & Wilkins, 1981.
30. Goldstein DP: Gestational trophoblastic neoplasia in the 1990s. Yale J Bio Med 64:639, 1991.
31. Caspi B, Elchalal U, Dgani R, et al: Invasive mole and placental site trophoblastic tumor: Two entities of gestational trophoblastic disease with a common ultrasonographic appearance. J Ultrasound Med 10:517, 1991.
32. Walden PAM, Bagshawe KD: Reproductive performance of women successfully treated for gestational trophoblastic tumors. Am J Obstet Gynecol 125:1108, 1976.
33. Sung HC, Wu PC, Wang Y, et al: Pregnancy outcomes after cytotoxic chemotherapy for choriocarcinoma and invasive moles: Long-term follow-up. Am J Obstet Gynecol 158:538, 1988.
34. Hilgers RD: Improving the outcome of high-risk gestational trophoblastic neoplasia. Contemp Obstet Gynecol 73:92, 1987.
35. Hilgers RD, Lewis JL Jr: Gestational trophoblastic disease. In Danforth DN (ed): Obstetrics and Gynecology, 4th ed, pp 393–406. Hagerstown, MD, Harper & Row, 1982.
36. Bagshawe KD: Risk and prognostic factors in trophoblastic neoplasia. Cancer 38:1373, 1976.
37. World Health Organization Scientific Group: Gestational trophoblastic diseases. WHO technical report series 692. Geneva, World Health Organization, 1983.
38. Szulman AE, Surti U: The syndromes of hydatidiform mole: II. Morphologic evolution of the complete and partial mole. Am J Obstet Gynecol 132:20, 1978.
39. Sanders C, Rubin E: Malignant gestational trophoblastic disease: CT findings. AJR 148:165, 1987.
40. Mutch DG, Soper JT, Baker ME, et al: Role of computed axial tomography of the chest in staging patients with nonmetastatic gestational trophoblastic disease. Obstet Gynecol 68:348, 1986.
41. Hricak H, Demas BE, Braga CA, et al: Gestational trophoblastic neoplasm of the uterus: MR assessment. Radiology 161:11, 1986.

CHAPTER 31

■■■■■■

Ovarian Masses . . . What to Look for . . . What to Do

ROY A. FILLY, M.D.

Ultrasonography is used extensively by gynecologists and radiologists to detect or assess gynecologic disease. Because pathology of the ovary is the most difficult gynecologic disease to evaluate clinically, the bulk of requests for sonographic imaging made by gynecologists involve questions regarding adnexal pathology. Mattingly[1] sums up the problem quite nicely:

> *Of all gynecologic diseases, tumors of the adnexa pose the most difficult of all diagnostic problems and offer the least reward for the greatest therapeutic effort. Strangely, the ovarian tumors which appear most frequently are usually physiologic in origin, produce acute symptoms, and receive the most radical of all surgical treatments. In contrast, malignant tumors of the ovary are the most lethal of all gynecologic tumors and usually remain silent until untreatable.*

TECHNIQUE

Usually the ovaries are not difficult to detect sonographically. Sonologic practitioners may favor endovaginal sonography for ovarian visualization, a concept with which I agree. However, a cohort of these practitioners favor exclusive use of the endovaginal probe, a concept with which I disagree strongly.

The goal of the examination is complete evaluation of the pelvis, not simple visualization of the ovaries. As well, there may be ancillary features that are important to demonstrate when an ovarian mass is detected (hydronephrosis, ascites [Fig. 31–1], pleural effusion, liver metastases [Fig. 31–2], peritoneal metastases or omental "cake"). Manufacturers have not developed a broad array of transducers so that we may select one per patient. The transducers are designed to do different tasks. These include providing a large field of view in the far field, a large field of view in the near field, deeper penetration, high resolution in the near field, and the ability to be placed in a confined space.

The expert sonologist evaluates the imaging problem and then selects the transducer or transducers that accomplish the task most efficiently and with the maximum diagnostic information. It is a serious mistake to fail to purchase an adequate number of transducers to perform the sonographic imaging tasks that are required. However, it is an even greater error to own transducers and fail to use them because one is locked into the concept that endovaginal transducers alone are adequate to the task. In the scanning laboratory, at my institution, patients are first scanned transabdominally through a distended urinary bladder and then endovaginally when appropriate. This approach,

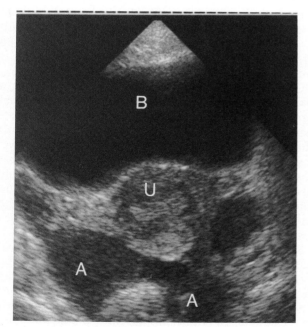

Figure 31–1. Transverse transabdominal sonogram of the pelvis demonstrating ascites in a patient with ovarian carcinoma. A, ascites; B, bladder; U, uterus.

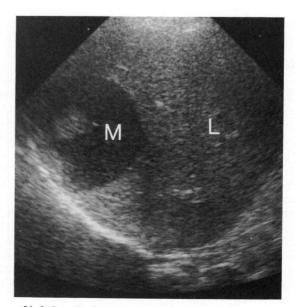

Figure 31–2. Longitudinal transabdominal sonogram of the liver (L) demonstrating an ovarian carcinoma metastasis (M).

while slightly more time consuming, has no imaging drawbacks and, when circumstances require it, can be modified toward a greater emphasis on transabdominal scanning or toward a greater emphasis on endovaginal scanning.

OVARIAN CANCER SCREENING

Sonography may ultimately impact on early detection of ovarian carcinoma with screening programs,[2–4] which are currently being evaluated in several centers. Ovarian cancer affects 20,000 American women per year, and approximately 12,000 per year die as a result of this disease process.[5, 6] At the present time, most cases (60% to 70%) are diagnosed in the more advanced stages of disease progression (stages III and IV). To alter this circumstance, screening programs are being developed that focus on serum CA-125 testing[7] and pelvic sonography [3, 4] or a combination of the two. Sonographic programs are analyzing both the morphology of the ovary on B-scan images as well as Doppler waveform analysis of arterial flow and color Doppler imaging.

All physicians would hope that these programs will be enormously successful. Although further testing and refinements of these techniques will continue, current results do not justify annual screening in all women. Prematurely adopted screening programs will not solve this problem.[8] Proposed screening protocols must be rigorously evaluated before implementation. The results of large-scale testing programs will need to be analyzed before routine screening is instituted.

Groups at higher risk than the general population, such as postmenopausal women (Fig. 31–3) and women with a relative afflicted with ovarian cancer, show more potential success in a screening setting.[5, 6] However, it remains unclear whether these groups are appropriate for annual screening. There is little dissension that women who have more than one relative with ovarian cancer have a high enough risk (50% over their lifetime) to warrant annual surveillance.[2, 6]

EVALUATION OF AN OVARIAN MASS

The purpose of this discussion is to analyze those sonographic features of ovarian masses that may help us to stay the surgeon's hand, as far as is safely possible, in patients who very likely have benign, self-limiting masses. The sonographic appearance of an adnexal mass is only one factor that may influence subsequent management. A key issue is symptomatology. For example, assume two lesions of identical size and morphology are found. However, one is found in a woman with severe acute symptomatology that likely is related to the mass while the other is detected in a reasonably asymptomatic woman. Even convincing sonographic features indicating benignancy may be overlooked in favor of surgical excision in the patient who is acutely symptomatic.

Similarly, the hormonal status of the patient may

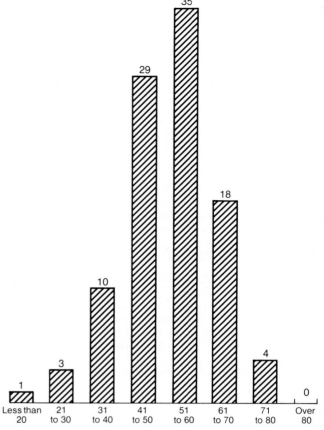

Figure 31–3. Primary ovarian carcinoma: frequency (percentage) as a function of years of age (665 cases). (From Zaloudek C: The ovary. In Gompel C, Silverberg SG (eds): Pathology in Gynecology and Obstetrics. Philadelphia, JB Lippincott, 1985).

influence management more than does the sonographic appearance. Identical appearing masses found in a premenopausal versus a postmenopausal woman will likely be greeted with a much different clinical reaction. Even premenopausal women who demonstrate an adnexal mass while on birth control pills will be viewed differently from normally ovulating women with a similar-appearing lesion.

Gynecologists may give patients hormones when a suspicious adnexal mass is detected. The hormonal suppression is given to stop formation of new cysts that may complicate clinical follow-up of the patient. The hormonal therapy is not given to "treat" the cyst that was discovered initially. Following such hormonal treatment, the originally identified cyst commonly takes 1 to 3 months to regress. Nonregressing cysts in patients who have undergone such treatment may be surgically excised even though sonographic features strongly suggest benignancy.

Sonography has its major benefits when clinical features have not already made the decision in the surgeon's mind. The sonologist should be aware of the clinical features that influence subsequent decisions regarding surgical excision versus monitored follow-up. A number of important questions should be asked of the patient before each gynecologic sonogram. The clinical history provided by the referring clinician may

PLEASE ANSWER THE FOLLOWING QUESTIONS ACCURATELY. THEY WILL HELP YOUR DOCTORS GET THE MOST INFORMATION FROM YOUR ULTRASOUND TEST. THANK YOU.

Name _____

My last menstrual period began on _____
month/day/year

If you have stopped having menstrual periods, check box ☐ and answer the following questions:

1.	My uterus was removed.	Yes _____	No _____
2.	I have been through menopause. (If you have been through menopause, do you take female hormone pills?)	Yes _____	No _____
		Yes _____	No _____

If you are still menstruating, answer the following:

I am currently using:
Birth control pills   Yes _____   No _____
An IUD   Yes _____   No _____

I am pregnant.   Yes _____   No _____   Maybe _____

My doctor did a pregnancy test on _____   Blood _____   Urine _____
month/day/year

The test was: Positive _____   Negative _____

All patients answer the following:

Symptoms:

I have or recently had vaginal bleeding.   Yes _____   No _____
I have pelvic pain _____.   Left side _____   Right side _____   Both _____
I have cramping.   Yes _____   No _____
Other symptoms: _____

Surgical History:

I have had an operation on my female organs.   Yes _____   No _____
My uterus was removed.   Yes _____   No _____
My ovary was removed.   Yes _____   No _____
   (Right ovary _____ Left Ovary _____ Both Ovaries _____)
I have been treated for cancer of my female organs.   Yes _____   No _____

Figure 31–4. Questionnaire for patients undergoing gynecologic sonography.

not include this important information. Therefore, I routinely have patients undergoing gynecologic sonography fill out a questionnaire (Fig. 31–4).

Physiologic Ovarian Cysts

During the course of a normal menstrual cycle, a woman develops a mature graafian follicle (occasionally more than one) and a number of smaller "support" follicles.[9] A mature graafian follicle would be seen at mid cycle and attains a size of approximately 20 mm, but not infrequently it achieves a size of 25 mm. Following ovulation, numerous capillaries from the theca interna spread between the granulosa cells. This

abundant vascularization may give rise to hemorrhage as the corpus luteum develops.[9] Granulosa cells continue their growth and become luteinized.

The corpus luteum itself usually attains a size of 1.5 cm, but after hemorrhage into the corpus luteum a corpus luteum cyst can develop. If it is a small cyst (up to 2.5 to 3.0 cm), this minor pathologic event is generally considered compatible with a normal cycle. Therefore, during normal menses, a woman may demonstrate a cyst of 2.5, or even 3.0 cm in either ovary, and often other smaller cysts. Thus, menstruating women who are not taking birth control pills should be considered *normal* when a unilocular cyst of 2.5 cm or less is seen in the ovary.

Table 31–1. CLASSIFICATION OF NONNEOPLASTIC CYSTS

Cyst Type	Hormone Activity	Hormone
Serous inclusion cyst	None	None
Follicular cyst	Possible	Estrogen
Corpus luteum cyst	Yes	Progesterone
Corpus albicans cyst	None	None
Theca lutein cyst	Yes	Estrogen

Nonneoplastic Ovarian Cysts

Nonneoplastic cysts are by far the most common pathologic masses to occur in the ovary.[10] They may be functional (i.e., associated with hormone production) or nonfunctional (Table 31–1). As a general rule, neoplastic masses of the ovary are removed even if one could be certain that the neoplasm was benign. Some gynecologists laparoscopically biopsy cystic masses and then fenestrate them if benign and aspirate the fluid, rather than surgically excising the mass or ovary.[11] Conversely, nearly all varieties of nonneoplastic cysts will resolve spontaneously and need not be removed unless torsion or rupture clinically forces a surgical exturpation.

Nonneoplastic cysts are seen frequently in menstruating women but may be seen in postmenopausal women as well. Most common nonneoplastic cysts are the result of "mishaps" during the normal menstrual cycle resulting in follicular or corpus luteum cysts. Follicular cysts are extremely common, unilocular cysts that are usually 5 cm or less, but occasionally larger (Fig. 31–5). These cysts have a smooth, thin wall lined with granulosa cells. When the cyst becomes large (i.e., clinically the most worrisome type) the pressure from the luminal cyst fluid may obliterate the lining cells. In this case the pathologist cannot recognize the

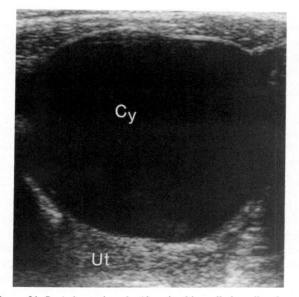

Figure 31–5. A large (nearly 10 cm), thin-walled, unilocular cyst (Cy) is seen depressing the uterus (Ut) posteriorly. This follicular cyst exceeded the usual size limit of these lesions.

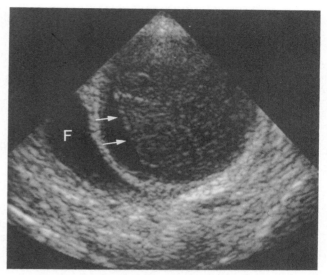

Figure 31–6. Adnexal mass with a mildly thickened wall. Numerous echoes are seen within the mass, but the mass demonstrates enhanced sound transmission. A small amount of free fluid (F) is seen adjacent to the mass. Note the flat margin (*arrows*) of the internal echoes that do not "obey the law of gravity." This is typical of layered, clotted blood. The lesion was never excised and disappeared within 6 weeks. It was presumed to be a corpus luteum cyst.

origin of the cyst and frequently calls these "simple cysts."

Corpora lutea are commonly complicated by hemorrhage, although hemorrhage is not necessary for the development of a corpus luteum cyst (Fig. 31–6). Progesterone production persists, resulting in delayed menstruation or persistent abnormal bleeding. Again, these cysts are unilocular and tend to be thin walled. However, they frequently demonstrate thrombus in the lumen. Ultimately, the luteal tissue regresses, but if the cyst cavity persists it is called a corpus albicans cyst.

Theca lutein cysts are not as common as the cysts described earlier. They occur when the ovary is hyperstimulated and are seen in clinically identifiable situations (twins, molar pregnancies, ovarian stimulating drugs, and pregnancies complicated by hydrops fetalis). Because these masses are not seen in clinical situations in which surgical excision is being contemplated they are not considered here.

The serous inclusion cyst, however, is a problem because these cysts are commonly found in postmenopausal women (although they may be encountered in the neonatal period and throughout life). These tend to be tiny but may be several centimeters in diameter. They typically are thin walled, are unilocular, and contain watery fluid. Occasionally, these cysts are hemorrhagic, particularly if torsion has occurred. Since they are functionless, they do not cause abnormal postmenopausal bleeding.

If one goes to the older gynecologic literature that predates sonographic imaging, it becomes obvious that on the basis of history and physical findings, clinicians cannot discriminate these benign nonneoplastic cysts from neoplasms (Table 31–2).[12] In an analysis of a large number of ovarian surgical specimens excised in

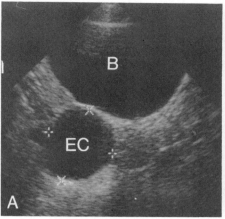
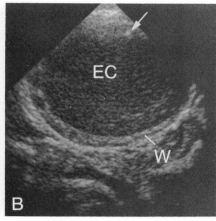

Figure 31–7. Endometriomas typically are filled with low-amplitude internal echoes. Transabdominal sonogram (A), generally obtained with lower-frequency transducers, does not show these echoes as well as an endovaginal sonogram (B) obtained with higher-frequency transducers. Arrow indicates bright reflector. B, bladder; EC, endometrial cyst; W, wall.

the late 1930s, nearly 80% were nonneoplastic cysts, only 6% were neoplasms, and less than 2% were malignancies. It is reasonable to assume that gynecologists of this era exercised reasonable caution before excising any palpable lesion. Therefore, one can assume that these nonneoplastic cysts were relatively large, symptomatic, or persistent. Even still, they constituted the vast preponderance of excised ovarian masses. Because large size, severe symptoms, and persistence are atypical of nonneoplastic cysts it is safe to say that their incidence is vastly greater than indicated in a surgical series. We should approach every identified ovarian mass in a premenopausal woman with the knowledge that the odds strongly favor that the mass is a nonneoplastic cyst even before we consider what the mass looks like on the sonogram.

Another ovarian mass that falls into the general category of nonneoplastic cyst is the endometrioma or endometrial cyst. The *oma* ending connotes neoplasm, which is clearly not the case, but the term *endometrioma* is now the most commonly used appellation to describe this lesion.

The ovary is involved in 80% of all cases of endometriosis. Eighteen percent of all laparotomies reveal microscopically proven endometriosis.[13] The prevalence increases to 33% if the laparotomy is performed for infertility. These masses may be large (15 to 20 cm) and are filled with old blood (the so-called chocolate cyst) (Figs. 31–7 and 31–8). However, clots may be present from recent bleeding (Fig. 31–9). They may be multiple and may have satellite cysts producing apparent "septations" (unlike other nonneoplastic cysts). Although the wall can be thin, it is often thick and may be very difficult to puncture. I have personally seen an endometrioma bend an 18-gauge needle and still not admit the needle tip. Bright reflectors are commonly seen in the wall (see Figs. 31–8 and 31–9).

Primary Ovarian Neoplasms

There is an extremely large variety of histologically identifiable types of ovarian neoplasms. Any good textbook of gynecologic pathology can acquaint you with the spectrum of lesions.[14–16] However, the vast

Table 31–2. SURGICALLY EXCISED OVARIAN MASSES BEFORE SONOGRAPHY

Lesion Type	%	
Follicular cyst	57	
"Simple" cyst	11	} 79%
Corpus luteum cyst	11	
Chronic "oophoritis"	10	
Hemorrhagic cyst	5	
Benign neoplasms	4.8	
Primary malignancy	0.6	
Secondary malignancy	0.6	

Modified from Carpenter CC: Considerations of physiology and pathology in gynecology: Analysis of 2933 surgical specimens. Trans Med Soc NC 83:236, 1936.

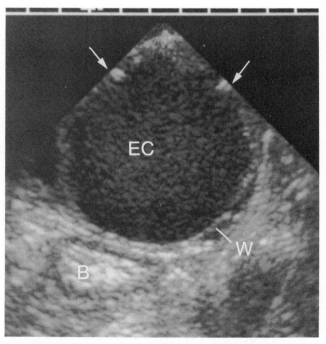

Figure 31–8. Endovaginal sonogram of a typical endometrial cyst (EC). In the absence of fresh thrombus, these lesions demonstrate diffuse low-amplitude internal echoes, enhanced sound transmission, and a visible wall (W), which is often thin (as seen here) but may be mildly thickened (see Fig. 31–7). As well, these lesions commonly demonstrate bright reflectors in the wall (*arrows*). B, bowel.

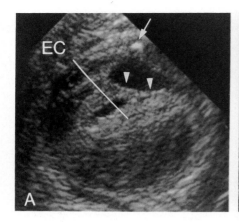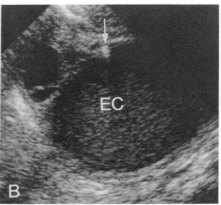

Figure 31–9. Endovaginal sonograms of an endometrial cyst (EC) obtained 6 months apart. The apparent change is likely secondary to acute hemorrhage (A) that has clotted. Note the concave margin (*arrowheads*) of the internal echoes. Later (B) the endometrial cyst has a more typical appearance. Arrow indicates bright wall reflector.

majority of benign ovarian neoplasms is encompassed by a small minority of histologic types.[17]

Everyone agrees on which types (e.g., epithelial, germ cell, stromal) are the most common, but interestingly there is considerable controversy about precisely which tumor is the most common. Various reports find either serous cystadenoma (Fig. 31–10) or cystic teratoma (dermoid) (Figs. 31–11 and 31–12) to be the winner.

By analyzing a review[17] that spans the 10 years that would encompass real-time sonography (without endovaginal capability) we can develop several concepts. These researchers evaluated 861 surgically confirmed ovarian neoplasms. In their series, cystic teratoma was the most prevalent neoplasm, accounting for 44% of all ovarian tumors and being 57% more frequent than serous tumors (Table 31–3). The risk of malignancy was not related statistically to the size of an ovarian

neoplasm in their series, although the average size of malignant lesions (12 cm) was greater than benign lesions (9 cm). By size, 28% of the neoplasms were less than 6 cm, 53% ranged from 6 to 11 cm, and 19% were larger than 11 cm. Seventy-five percent of masses were excised from premenopausal women, but 75% of malignancies were excised from postmenopausal women. In premenopausal women, only 13% were malignant. From the second decade to the sixth decade, the risk of malignancy in an ovarian neoplasm increased 12-fold. Of all the lesions excised, 75% were benign, 21% were malignant, and 4% were of low malignant potential. Recall that in Carpenter's 1936 series of excised ovarian neoplasms,[12] there was a similar breakdown: 80% benign and 20% malignant. The data of interest from the study of Koonings and colleagues[17] are summarized in Tables 31–3 through 31–5.

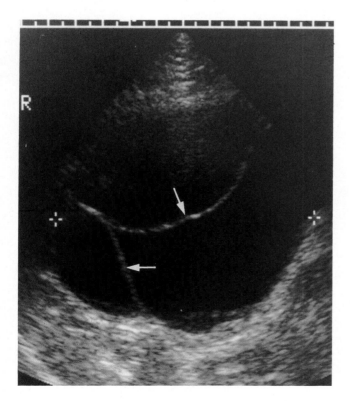

Figure 31–10. This relatively large mass (nearly 10 cm) demonstrates a thin wall and two thin septa (*arrows*). Although lesions of several histologic types could potentially demonstrate this appearance, the probability is high that regardless of histologic type the lesion would be benign although neoplastic. This lesion was a serous cystadenoma, the most common type to demonstrate this appearance.

Figure 31–11. *A* and *B*. Two sonograms of a cystic teratoma. In *A*, a thick wall (*arrow*) and numerous bright echoes are seen. In *B*, a highly echogenic "dermoid plug" (*curved arrow*), which casts an acoustic shadow (*arrowheads*), is seen. This appearance is highly characteristic of a cystic teratoma. Although cystic teratomas manifest multiple appearances, the features that are highly characteristic are bright echoes and shadowing. (See also Fig. 31–12.)

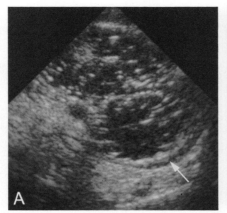 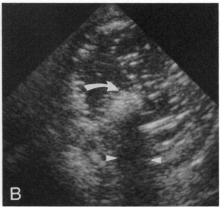

Table 31–3. OVARIAN NEOPLASM (861 CASES)

Type	Occurrence
Premenopausal	75% (13% malignant)
Postmenopausal	25% (45% malignant)
Benign	75%
Malignant	21%
Low malignancy potential	4%

Modified from Koonings PP, Campbell K, Mishell DR, Grimes DA: Relative frequency of primary ovarian neoplasms: A 10-year review. Reprinted with permission from The American College of Obstetricians and Gynecologists (Obstetrics and Gynecology, 1989, 74:921).

Table 31–4. BENIGN OVARIAN NEOPLASMS

Type	Occurrence
Cystic teratoma	58%
Serous cystadenoma	25%
Mucinous cystadenoma	12%
Benign stromal	4%
Brenner tumor	1%

Modified from Koonings PP, Campbell K, Mishell DR, Grimes DA: Relative frequency of primary ovarian neoplasms: A 10-year review. Reprinted with permission from The American College of Obstetricians and Gynecologists (Obstetrics and Gynecology, 1989, 74:921).

Table 31–5. MALIGNANT OVARIAN NEOPLASM

Type	Occurrence
Serous cystadenocarcinoma	43%
Undifferentiated carcinoma	14%
Endometrioid carcinoma	11%
Mucinous cystadenocarcinoma	9%
Germ cell carcinoma	7%
Sex cord carcinoma	7%

Modified from Koonings PP, Campbell K, Mishell DR, Grimes DA: Relative frequency of primary ovarian neoplasms: A 10-year review. Reprinted with permission from The American College of Obstetricians and Gynecologists (Obstetrics and Gynecology, 1989, 74:921).

As stated earlier, cystic teratoma was the most common neoplasm encountered by Koonings and colleagues (see Table 31–4).[17] One must consider the possibility that sonography impacted on this result. As will be discussed in detail later, but likely already familiar to the reader, is the concept that thin-walled, unilocular cysts smaller than 6 cm in diameter are virtually never malignant. Surgeons have a tendency to observe rather than excise such lesions. Serous cystadenomas commonly demonstrate such morphology, but cystic teratomas rarely do so. Therefore, it is unlikely that many cystic teratomas were observed (or more appropriately lost to follow-up). That outcome would be more likely for serous cystadenomas.

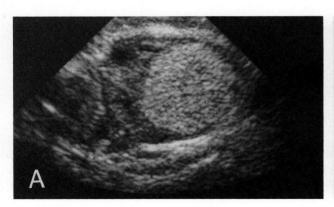 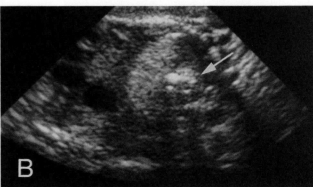

Figure 31–12. *A* and *B*. Two endovaginal sonograms of a cystic teratoma. This lesion is small and does not deform the outer contours of the ovary. Although it is quite different in appearance from Figure 31–11, it has the sonographic hallmarks of this lesion (bright echoes and shadowing echodensities [*arrow*]). A diagnosis can be made with confidence.

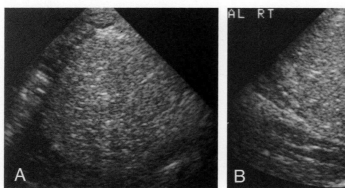

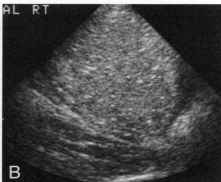

Figure 31–13. *A* and *B*. Two endovaginal sonograms of an ovarian mass interpreted as a solid mass with our usual differential diagnosis including ovarian carcinoma, Brenner tumor, ovarian fibroma, and thecoma. The mass was a cystic teratoma.

Figure 31–14. *A*. Small ovarian mass with a possible septation (*arrow*) versus resolving thrombus. The appearance overlaps that of a serous cystadenoma. However, it is practical and safe to observe such lesions for 4 to 6 weeks. *B*. Sonogram 6 weeks later demonstrates complete resolution of the mass. Bl, bladder; O, ovary.

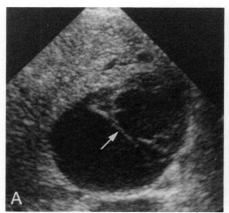

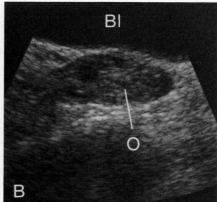

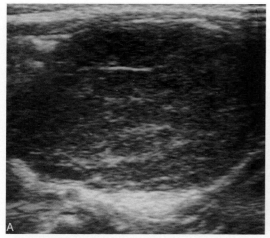

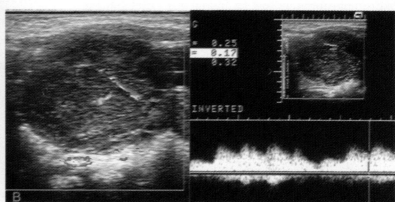

Figure 31–15. *A*. Solid ovarian mass seen in a young girl with precocious puberty. One can predict that the mass is likely to be a granulosa cell tumor producing estrogen. *B*. The lesion shows strong color Doppler signals and a resistive index of 0.32. These features erroneously predict malignancy in a lesion known to be almost universally benign.

Sonographic Appearance of Ovarian Masses

The sonographic literature is replete with articles dealing with the "spectrum" of sonographic findings in this or that gynecologic pathologic entity (Fig. 31–13). A further large compendium deals with the overlap in appearance of neoplastic and nonneoplastic diseases (Fig. 31–14). Still further, a large number of articles confirm that sonography cannot distinguish malignant and benign neoplasms with the accuracy necessary to avert surgery. One wonders why we do so much gynecologic sonography if the technique commonly fails to draw clinically useful conclusions. The answer, of course, is that sonography commonly provides useful information even when it cannot histologically categorize the abnormality. Indeed, a few straightforward observations can greatly assist the gynecologist in deciding whether surgery is indicated.

The first observation is whether the mass is solid or cystic. The object of this discussion is not to review the fundamentals of sonographic interpretation of "cyst versus solid" mass, but a few salient observations are important. A solid mass virtually ensures that an ovarian lesion is neoplastic (Figs. 31–15 through 31–17). However, solid ovarian masses are extremely uncommon. Of all solid pelvic masses in females, leiomyomas are vastly more common than solid ovarian tumors. However, sonographically one can nearly always be confident that myomas are intrauterine and not adnexal. However, I live by the rule that uncommon manifestations of common diseases account for more cases than all of the rare diseases combined. Therefore, an exophytic or pedunculated myoma is more likely to account for a solid adnexal mass than is a solid ovarian tumor. Features that assist in concluding that a solid adnexal mass is a myoma are as follows:

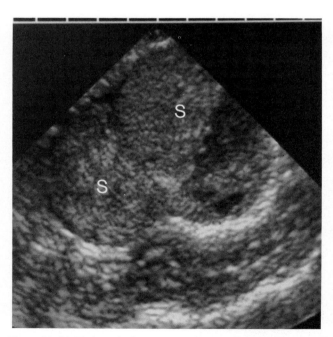

Figure 31–16. Endovaginal sonogram of an ovarian mass less than 6 cm but predominantly solid (S). A strong concern for malignancy exists in such a lesion. Ovarian carcinoma was proven.

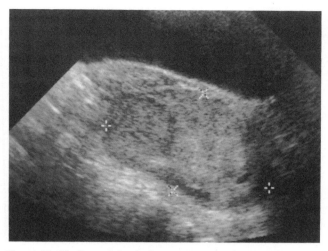

Figure 31–17. Transabdominal sonogram of a large, solid ovarian mass (*cursors*). This turned out to be metastatic disease from gastric carcinoma.

1. The normal ovary is seen as distinct from the mass (exophytic ovarian masses are extremely uncommon).
2. The mass has characteristics typical of a myoma (relatively hypoechoic and attenuating).
3. Other myomas are seen in the uterine corpus (guilt by association).

Further consideration can be given to computed tomography or magnetic resonance imaging to further assess solid adnexal masses regarding the probability that the lesion is an exophytic myoma. Finally, endovaginal or transabdominal fine-needle biopsy can be performed to cytologically evaluate the lesion, but this is rarely employed for this purpose.

If after careful evaluation the mass is possibly ovarian, laparoscopy and/or surgical excision is warranted owing to the relatively high risk of malignancy in solid ovarian neoplasms (see Figs. 31–15 through 31–17). Recall that a number of benign ovarian neoplasms are solid, including ovarian fibromas, adenofibromas, thecomas, and Brenner tumors among others that are even less common.

It is important to remember that echoes, even numerous echoes, within a mass do not sonographically confirm that the mass is solid (see Figs. 31–6 through 31–13). As noted earlier, the cystic teratoma is probably the single most common ovarian neoplasm and is universally benign. The masses are frequently characterized by numerous bright echoes (see Fig. 31–12). Such echoes do not indicate that this cystic mass is "solid," and an interpretation that the mass is "solid" is erroneous. Even though surgical excision is usually the preferred course of action when a cystic teratoma is identified, that does not excuse misinforming the gynecologist that a solid adnexal mass is present.

The most likely appearance of an ovarian mass will be to identify a thin-walled unilocular cyst (see Fig. 31–5). The identification of unilocularity has extremely important implications for subsequent management. A unilocular cyst is almost universally benign (see Figs. 31–5, 31–7, and 31–8; Table 31–6).

Table 31–6. UNILOCULAR CYSTS

Very Common
Follicular cyst
Corpus luteum cyst
Endometrial cyst
Less Common
Paraovarian cyst
Serous inclusion cyst
Serous cystadenoma
Uncommon
Cystic teratoma
Mucinous cystadenoma
Cystadenofibroma
Rare
Cystadenoma of low malignant potential
Cystadenocarcinoma

Compelling evidence to verify this concept comes from several recent publications.[18–21] The evidence for benignancy of unilocular cysts identified sonographically is all the more convincing when looked at in the postmenopausal woman. In 30 unilocular cysts followed prospectively[18] in postmenopausal women, no malignancies were identified and 12 spontaneously resolved in 7 months or less. Goldstein and colleagues[19] reporting on 42 postmenopausal women with a unilocular cyst of 5 cm or less found no malignancies.

Hurwitz and associates[21] reported on 52 unilocular cysts in women of all ages that persisted when the patient was placed on oral contraceptives. Again, there were no malignancies. Indeed it is quite difficult to find documentation of unilocularity with modern sonographic equipment in a malignant ovarian neoplasm. I am aware of only five cases in the literature of the past decade in which unilocular cystic masses were "malignant." Hermann and coworkers[22] reported on 58 "purely" cystic neoplasms examined sonographically.[22] Forty-eight lesions were 10 cm or less in size, and none was malignant. Of 10 masses greater than 10 cm in size, one was malignant, but this lesion was not depicted in the article to confirm their impression (Hermann and coworkers used scanners that are obsolete by modern standards). The second lesion was

reported by Hall and McCarthy.[20] This is an often-quoted identification of a 3.5-cm "simple" adnexal cyst that was malignant. What is not quoted but clearly stated in the article is that the lesion was not frankly malignant but of "borderline" or low malignant potential and was found in an 84-year-old woman. Although I agree that the lesion is relatively innocuous in appearance, it is also true that the image presented in the manuscript demonstrates irregular margins and a small mural nodule. All other "simple" cysts found in postmenopausal women reported from their institution were benign. The third lesion was reported by Moyle and coworkers.[23] They had one unilocular cystadenocarcinoma among 106 neoplasms of the ovary. However, the lesion was 10 cm in diameter and demonstrated a 2-cm irregular mural nodule. Finally, Luxman and colleagues[24] state that two "simple" cysts less than 5 cm among 102 postmenopausal women with ovarian neoplasms had ovarian cancer but do not illustrate the lesions, and they do not further comment on whether the gross pathology also showed a unilocular cyst. These investigators employed transabdominal transducers.

This brings us to another important sonographic observation. Unilocularity alone in a cystic mass is compelling evidence that the lesion is benign, but if in addition the mass has a thin wall (no diffuse or focal thickening—mural nodules), one can be virtually certain that the mass is benign (see Fig. 31–5).[20, 21] The presence of a mural nodule or septations is strong evidence that an ovarian mass is a neoplasm (Figs. 31–18 through 31–21) (although it is still quite possible that the mass is benign). Once one is convinced that an ovarian mass is a neoplasm, it is then difficult to be certain that a mass is unambiguously benign.[22]

Hermann and colleagues attempted to predict benignancy versus malignancy based on the sonographic appearance of a large number of ovarian neoplasms.[22] They considered a lesion malignant if it showed thick septa (see Fig. 31–5), irregular solid areas, poorly defined margins, ascites, or matted bowel loops. These are certainly reasonable criteria if specificity is one's goal, but such findings would not be highly sensitive

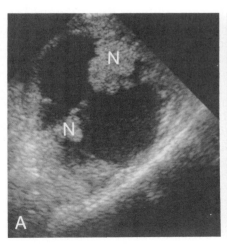

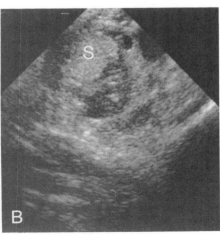

Figure 31–18. Endovaginal sonogram of the left (*A*) and right (*B*) ovaries in a postmenopausal women. A large cystic mass is seen in *A* that demonstrates mural nodules (N). Note that these nodules have convex borders. In the opposite ovary a small solid mass (S) is seen.

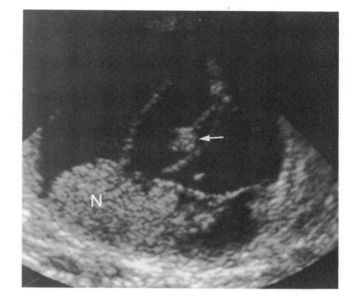

Figure 31–19. A 5-cm cystic mass is seen that has a large mural nodule (N) and a septal nodule (*arrow*). Although the mass is relatively small, it is highly suggestive of a malignant neoplasm.

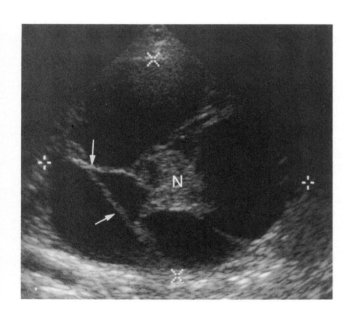

Figure 31–20. A cystic mass with septations (*arrows*) and a large septal nodule (N) is seen. Again, such lesions are highly suggestive of ovarian carcinoma.

Figure 31–21. A large cystic ovarian mass with thick, irregular septa. Ovarian carcinoma is the leading consideration.

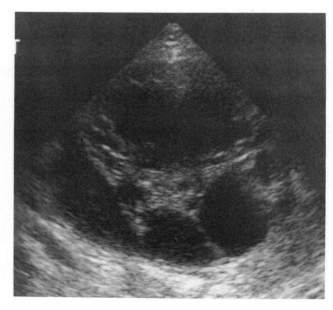

for malignancy. Indeed, when the authors concluded that a lesion was malignant, they were correct 73% of the time (positive predictive value = 73%). When they concluded it was benign they were correct 96% of the time (negative predictive value = 96%). Granberg and associates[25] used criteria that would be highly sensitive for segregating malignant from benign masses. These included a mass greater than 10 cm in diameter (excluding thin-walled, unilocular cysts), the presence of echogenic nodules in a cyst, and more than one thick septation. Using these criteria they achieved a 100% negative predictive value and a positive predictive value of 73%.

Overall, a few observations are pertinent from my experience. I have seen only two malignant unilocular cysts (both masses were large [>10 cm] and one had a small mural nodule). I have seen only one ovarian cancer that did not deform the ovary (I missed it). I agree that an attempt to correlate the sonographic appearance of the mass with the histologic diagnosis can be extremely frustrating (not infrequently a lesion judged to be a specific histologic type of ovarian neoplasm is not even a neoplasm at all and is not even a lesion of the ovary).

Special Observations

HEMORRHAGIC CYSTS

It is common to find evidence of hemorrhage in unilocular cysts.[26–29] The sonographic appearance generated by fibrin, clot, and fresh blood may undermine one's resolve that the lesion is benign and likely nonneoplastic. In fact, the opposite situation exists. Confident identification of hemorrhage into a unilocular cyst is excellent evidence of benignancy. Elements of new or old hemorrhage frequently have a characteristic appearance (Figs. 31–6 through 31–8, 31–22, and 31–23). These findings are important to recognize to avoid erroneous interpretations that a cystic mass is solid (because it has diffuse internal echoes) (see Figs. 31–3, 31–7, and 31–8), that it has a mural nodule (because of clot adherent to the wall), or that it is septate (because of fibrin strands within thrombus or crossing the lumen) (see Figs. 31–14, 31–22, and 31–23).

Once a hemorrhagic ovarian mass is seen, statistics strongly favor that the lesion is nonneoplastic. Obviously, corpus luteum cysts and endometrial cysts are extremely common and largely the result of pathologic bleeding events. This is not to say that ovarian neoplasms do not have hemorrhagic events, but when they do it is usually secondary to torsion with subsequent internal bleeding within the cyst cavity. Torsion is highly atypical of ovarian malignancies, which tend to rapidly penetrate the capsule and adhere to adjacent structures. This sequence of events makes torsion virtually impossible.

Thus, hemorrhage is excellent evidence that the mass is benign. Recent literature bears this out. Well over 100 hemorrhagic ovarian cysts have been reported in the sonographic literature.[27–29] Of these, greater than 98% were nonneoplastic and the remainder (three lesions) were benign ovarian neoplasms. No malignancies occurred in these reports. The history also may point toward a hemorrhagic cyst. In 90% of cases in one report[27] there was an abrupt onset of lower abdominal pain.

Although hemorrhage may make the sonographic appearance confusing, there are certain patterns that are typical of a hemorrhagic cyst or an endometrial cyst (endometrioma). One pattern is diffuse low-amplitude echoes in a mass that transmits sound with enhancement. This is a particularly prevalent appearance of endometrial cysts (see Figs. 31–7B, 31–8, and 31–9B). Another pattern is that of fibrin strands. Unlike septations, fibrin strands are weak reflectors and are thin rather than sheetlike (see Fig. 31–23). Finally, clot usually appears different from a mural nodule. Clot may have one or more convex borders indicating retraction (see Fig. 31–9A). Furthermore, fibrinous bands may pass through a clot. A clot may have a flat margin where a layer of blood in the dependent portion of the cyst congealed (see Fig. 31–6). Once congealed, this "fluid-fluid" level no longer obeys the law of gravity. Hemorrhagic cysts commonly have a mildly thickened wall. When sonographic findings suggest hemorrhage, benignancy should be pre-

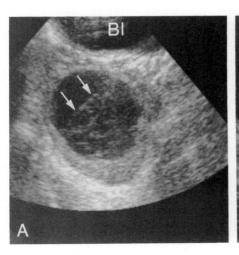

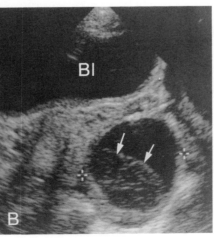

Figure 31–22. *A* and *B*. Transabdominal sonograms of a left ovarian mass taken 1 week apart. The mass was diagnosed as a hemorrhagic cyst containing thrombus. The attending gynecologist was concerned and requested a repeat examination in 1 week. The retracting thrombus seen in *A* (*arrows*) has further retracted during the week. Bl, bladder.

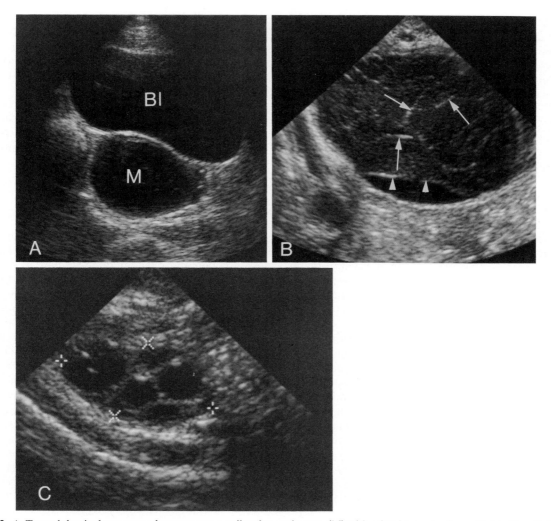

Figure 31–23. *A.* Transabdominal sonogram demonstrates a unilocular cystic mass (M) with a few internal echoes. Bl, bladder. *B.* Endovaginal sonography demonstrates typical internal thrombus including clot retraction (*arrowheads*) and fibrin strands (*arrows*) coursing through the thrombus. It is appropriate to examine such a mass with color Doppler scanning set for slow flow detection. The expectation is that no vessels will be seen in the interior of the mass (compare with Fig. 31–15*B*). *C.* Follow-up examination 6 weeks later shows complete resolution and a normal ovary.

sumed and the lesion followed for resolution by sonography (see Fig. 31–23).

CYSTIC TERATOMAS

Cystic teratomas are probably the most common ovarian neoplasm in patients younger than the age of 50 (see Table 31–4).[17] They have a broad spectrum of appearance.[30] Many have a highly characteristic appearance, but this appearance is not that of the usual "cyst" on sonography (see Figs. 31–11 and 31–12). Indeed, the common error is to diagnose these lesions as "solid masses" because they demonstrate numerous high-amplitude echoes and transmit sound poorly or not at all. The bulk of dermoid cysts can be recognized by this approach (see Figs. 31–11 and 31–12). When you observe one of these highly echogenic masses do not foolishly describe the lesion as solid and then conclude that it is a cyst.

Dermoid cysts may appear as a unilocular anechoic or hypoechoic cyst with a thin or somewhat thickened wall. They may be a hypoechoic or an anechoic unilocular cyst with a mural nodule (the so-called dermoid plug or Rokitansky protuberance). They may be a septated cyst. However, most commonly they demonstrate diffuse or focal areas of greatly increased echogenicity, often with shadowing. Fat (sebum) mixed with hair generates very high-amplitude echoes.[30] This is also true of fat in the dermoid plug (see Fig. 31–11*B*). Conversely, pure sebum tends to be anechoic or hypoechoic. When doubt exists, computed tomography has great ability to detect even small amounts of fat. Teeth (7%) or bone fragments (18%) may also be seen on computed tomography and may generate focal high-amplitude shadowing structures on sonography.[30]

Dermoid cysts are not culprits in mistaking malignant lesions for benign ones. These cysts are virtually all benign. Their sonographic appearance is, if anything, overread toward being worrisome for solid neoplasia. Dermoid cysts (other than very small ones) are virtually always removed once diagnosed to avoid the serious complications of rupture or torsion.

Table 31–7. OVARIAN TUMOR SIZE AND MALIGNANCY

Tumor Size	Total	Malignancies
<5 cm	32	1
5–10 cm	55	6
>10 cm	63	40

From Rulin MC, Preston AL: Adnexal masses in postmenopausal women. Reprinted with permission from The American College of Obstetricians and Gynecologists (Obstetrics and Gynecology, 1987, 70:578).

OVARIAN MALIGNANCY

The focus of this discussion has been to recognize those lesions that are typically benign and likely to disappear without surgical treatment. However, a few points regarding malignant ovarian lesions are appropriate. The chance of detecting an ovarian cancer during a routine pelvic examination in an asymptomatic woman is approximately 1 in 10,000. However, as stated earlier, age greatly alters this probability. Adnexal masses in postmenopausal women carry an unacceptably high risk of malignancy,[31] unless they are small, thin-walled, unilocular cysts; and even then they should be observed carefully for growth. One should not be surprised to see such a lesion[32] and, once seen, to demonstrate that it subsequently disappears.[18, 33] The postmenopausal ovary is a far more dynamic organ than previously thought. One should not be in an inordinate rush to excise small unilocular, thin-walled cysts simply because a patient is postmenopausal. These cysts may simply go away on their own.[33]

Tumor size is important. In 150 postmenopausal women with pathologic evaluation of their ovarian lesions, Rulin and Preston[31] found that the larger the size of the lesion, the higher the likelihood of malignancy (Table 31–7). Large size also indicates that the mass has persisted for some time.

It is also important to realize that the ovary is a relatively common site for metastatic disease (see Fig. 31–17).[34] The primary neoplasms that most commonly metastasize to the ovary are colon, breast, and gastric carcinomas. These lesions cannot be discriminated from primary cancers based on their gross pathologic appearance. Therefore, imaging studies cannot segregate primary from metastatic deposits.

DOPPLER EVALUATION OF OVARIAN MASSES

There is an increasing interest in the Doppler evaluation of ovarian masses to determine whether the lesion is benign or malignant.[35–39] Ovarian carcinomas, as a rule, are vascular.[40, 41] Tumor angiogenesis results in proliferation of sinusoidal type vessels that lack smooth muscle in the vessel wall.[40] This results in a low-resistance vascular network that can be analyzed with color Doppler imaging and Doppler waveform analysis.[35] Color Doppler imaging can detect flow patterns associated with tumor neovasculature.[36–38] Vessels can then be selected for duplex Doppler waveform analysis.

The Doppler waveform is analyzed for resistance by a variety of indicators, including systolic/diastolic ratio, resistive index, or pulsatility index. Typically, malignant lesions demonstrate pulsatility indices less than 1.0[36] and resistive indices less than 0.40.[37] By comparison, normal kidneys generally have low resistive indices ranging from 0.45 to 0.70. Thus, one can appre-

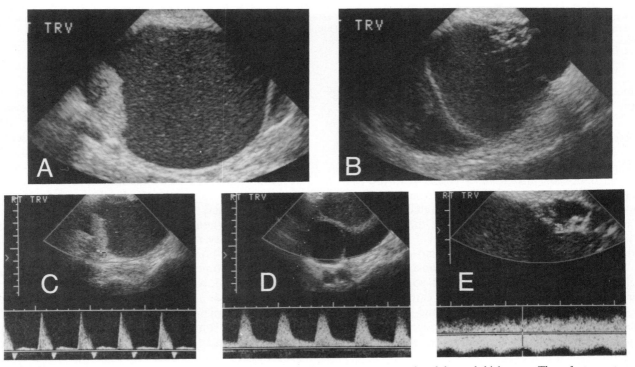

Figure 31–24. *A* and *B*. Endovaginal sonograms of an ovarian mass that demonstrates mural nodules and thick septa. These features strongly suggest malignancy. *C* through *E*. Doppler waveforms obtained from three differing vessels within the mass. The waveforms in *C* and *D* are clearly "benign" appearing, while the very low resistance pattern in *E* has a "malignant" appearance. Such variation can create confusion.

ciate that there is a remarkable amount of diastolic flow in malignant ovarian neoplasms.

Tumor vessels tend to be very tortuous. Therefore, angle-corrected velocity measurements are not possible. However, one can assume that peak velocities are recorded from vessels that are being insonated at a Doppler angle of 0°. Fortunately, since they are ratios of velocity, resistive and pulsatility indices are not dependent on the angle of Doppler insonation.

Problems arise because inflammatory masses and corpus luteum cysts also may demonstrate low resistance to flow as measured by Doppler waveform analysis.[35, 36] Furthermore, there is overlap between resistive indices of benign and malignant lesions.[37] Early evidence is encouraging, although some have reported an unacceptably high interobserver and intraobserver variation when obtaining ovarian Doppler resistance measurements (Fig. 31–24).[39] At the present time, it seems appropriate to be concerned about an adnexal mass that appears "benign" by morphologic criteria if the mass demonstrates low resistance on Doppler waveform measurements. However, I believe it would be imprudent to assume a lesion that appeared malignant by morphologic criteria was benign because it demonstrated a resistive index greater than 0.40.

Table 31–8. RECOMMENDATIONS FOR MANAGEMENT OF OVARIAN MASSES

Premenopausal	Recommendation
Unilocular cyst 2.5 cm or less ± hemorrhage	Normal; no follow-up unless on birth control pills
Unilocular cyst (thin wall, no hemorrhage) 2.5 to 6 cm	Clinical or sonographic follow-up in 1 to 2 months; consider addition of hormones to patient management
Unilocular cyst with hemorrhage 3 to 6 cm	Sonographic follow-up in 1 month ± addition of hormones to patient management
Unilocular cyst <6 cm (Doppler resistive index > 0.40)	Benign ovarian neoplasm is a strong consideration. Such patients usually undergo surgery but follow-up ± addition of hormones to patient management is done as clinically indicated.
Adnexal mass with one or more of the following features: Septation(s) Mural nodule(s) Irregular wall thickening Brightly echogenic (in toto or in part) Shadowing echodensity in wall Solid (without visualization of normal ipsilateral ovary)	Strongly consider ovarian neoplasm (malignancy difficult to exclude unless mass is a typical dermoid cyst). Color Doppler imaging and Doppler waveform analysis may be beneficial in this group.
Unilocular, thin-walled, smoothly contoured cyst < 5 cm	Consider serial follow-up (especially if on hormonal therapy and if the Doppler waveform analysis demonstrated high resistance)
Any other appearance	High probability of neoplasm. Malignancy cannot be excluded with certainty; especially worrisome if resistive index < 0.40 and pulsatility index < 1.0

Recommendations

Table 31–8 is a list of my recommendations for the management of asymptomatic or mildly symptomatic adnexal (ovarian) masses detected sonographically. These recommendations are heavily weighted toward conservative management. Nonetheless, as soon as one establishes morphologic criteria for management of ovarian masses there will be a malignant lesion that eventually fails to follow the rules. A balance must be drawn between our desire to sonographically identify every ovarian malignancy and our desire to avoid unnecessary surgery. The equation should be heavily weighted toward malignancy identification. However, we are obligated to make some decisions. The features described previously are reliable and may be trusted. They are not perfect.

References

1. Mattingly RF: Adnexal tumors. In Mattingly RF (ed): Te Linde's Operative Gynecology, pp 809–853. Philadelphia, JB Lippincott, 1977.
2. Goswamy RK, Campbell S, Whitehead MI: Screening for ovarian cancer. Clin Obstet Gynecol 10:621, 1983.
3. Campbell S, Bhan V, Royston P, et al: Transabdominal ultrasound screening for early ovarian cancer. Br Med J 299:1363, 1989.
4. Van Nagell JR, Higgins RV, Donaldson ES, et al: Transvaginal sonography as a screening method for ovarian cancer. Cancer 65:573, 1990.
5. Greene MH, Clark JW, Blayney DW: The epidemiology of ovarian cancer. Semin Oncol 11:209, 1984.
6. Schildkraut JM, Thompson WD: Familial ovarian cancer: A population-based case-control study. Am J Epidemiol 128:456, 1988.
7. Malkasian GD, Knapp RC, Laving PT, et al: Preoperative evaluation of serum CA 125 levels in premenopausal and postmenopausal patients with pelvic masses. Am J Obstet Gynecol 159:341, 1988.
8. Mant D, Fowler G: Mass screening: Theory and ethics. Br Med J 300:916, 1990.
9. Blaustein A: Anatomy and histology of the human ovary. In Blaustein A (ed): Pathology of the Female Genital Tract, p 365. New York, Springer-Verlag, 1977.
10. Blaustein A: Nonneoplastic cysts of the ovary. In Blaustein A (ed): Pathology of the Female Genital Tract, p 393, New York, Springer-Verlag, 1977.
11. Larsen JF, Pederson OD, Gregerson E: Ovarian cyst fenestration via a laparoscope: A laparoscopic method for treatment of non-neoplastic ovarian cysts. Acta Obstet Gynecol Scand 65:539, 1986.
12. Carpenter CC: Considerations of physiology and pathology in gynecology: Analysis of 2933 surgical specimens. Trans Med Soc NC 83:236, 1936.
13. Blaustein A: Pelvic endometriosis. In Blaustein A (ed): Pathology of the Female Genital Tract, p 404. New York, Springer-Verlag, 1977.
14. Czernobilzky B: Primary epithelial tumors of the ovary. In Blaustein A (ed): Pathology of the Female Genital Tract, p 453. New York, Springer-Verlag, 1977.
15. Scully RE: Sex cord-stromal tumors. In Blaustein A (ed): Pathology of the Female Genital Tract, p 505. New York, Springer-Verlag, 1977.
16. Talerman A: Germ cell tumors of the ovary. In Blaustein A (ed): Pathology of the Female Genital Tract, p 527. New York, Springer-Verlag, 1977.
17. Koonings PP, Campbell K, Mishell DR, Grimes DA: Relative frequency of primary ovarian neoplasms: A 10-year review. Obstet Gynecol 74:921, 1989.

18. Andolf E, Jorgensen C: Simple adnexal cysts diagnosed by ultrasound in postmenopausal women. J Clin Ultrasound 16:301, 1988.
19. Goldstein SR, Subramanyam B, Synder JR, et al: The postmenopausal cystic adnexal mass: The potential role of ultrasound in conservative management. Obstet Gynecol 73:8, 1989.
20. Hall DA, McCarthy KA: The significance of the postmenopausal simple adnexal cyst. J Ultrasound Med 5:503, 1986.
21. Hurwitz A, Yagel S, Zion I, et al: The management of persistent clear pelvic cysts diagnosed by ultrasonography. Obstet Gynecol 72:320, 1988.
22. Hermann UJ, Locher GW, Goldhirsch A: Sonographic patterns of ovarian tumors: Prediction of malignancy. Obstet Gynecol 69:777, 1987.
23. Moyle JW, Rochester D, Sider L, et al: Sonography of ovarian tumors: Predictability of tumor type. AJR 141:985, 1983.
24. Luxman D, Bergman A, Sagi J, David MP: The postmenopausal adnexal mass: Correlation between ultrasonic and pathologic findings. Obstet Gynecol 77:726, 1991.
25. Granberg S, Norstrom A, Wikland M: Comparison of endovaginal ultrasound and cytologic evaluation of cystic ovarian tumors. J Ultrasound Med 10:9, 1992.
26. Nishimura K, Togashi K, Itoh K, et al: Endometrial cyst of the ovary: MR imaging. Radiology 162:315, 1987.
27. Reynolds T, Hill MC, Glassman LM: Sonography of hemorrhagic ovarian cysts. J Clin Ultrasound 14:449, 1986.
28. Baltarowich OH, Kurtz AB, Pasto ME, et al: The spectrum of sonographic findings in hemorrhagic ovarian cysts. AJR 148:901, 1987.
29. Bass IS, Haller JO, Freidman AP, et al: The sonographic appearance of the hemorrhagic ovarian cyst in adolescents. J Ultrasound Med 3:509, 1984.
30. Sheth S, Fishman EK, Buck JL, et al: The variable sonographic appearance of ovarian teratomas: Correlation with CT. AJR 151:331, 1988.
31. Rulin MC, Preston AL: Adnexal masses in postmenopausal women. Obstet Gynecol 70:578, 1987.
32. Wolf SI, Gosnink BB, Feldesman MR, et al: Prevalence of simple adnexal cysts in postmenopausal women. Radiology 180:65, 1991.
33. Levine D, Gosink BB, Wolf SL, et al: Simple adnexal cysts: The natural history in postmenopausal women. Radiology 184:653, 1992.
34. Megibow AJ, Hulnick DH, Bosniak MA, Balthazar EJ: Ovarian metastases: Computed tomographic appearances. Radiology 156:161, 1985.
35. Taylor KJW, Ramos I, Carter D, et al: Correlation of Doppler US tumor signals with neovascular morphologic features. Radiology 166:57, 1988.
36. Fleischer AC, Rodgers WH, Rao BK, et al: Assessment of ovarian tumor vascularity with transvaginal color Doppler sonography. J Ultrasound Med 10:563, 1991.
37. Kurjak A, Jurkovic D, Alfirevic Z, Zalud I: Transvaginal color Doppler imaging. J Clin Ultrasound 18:227, 1990.
38. Bourne T, Campbell S, Steer C, et al: Transvaginal colour flow imaging: A possible new screening technique for ovarian cancer. Br Med J 299:1367, 1989.
39. Farquhar CM, Rae T, Wadsworth TJ, Beard RW: Doppler ultrasound in the nonpregnant pelvis. J Ultrasound Med 8:451, 1989.
40. Folkman J, Watson K, Ingber D, Hanahan D: Induction of angiogenesis during the transition from hyperplasia to neoplasia. Nature 339:58, 1989.
41. Ramos I, Fernandez IA, Morse SS, et al: Detection of neovascular morphologic features. Radiology 166:57, 1988.

CHAPTER 32

Ectopic Pregnancy

ROY A. FILLY, M.D.

The first documented autopsy performed in the United States, circa 1638 or 1639, identified an ectopic pregnancy as the cause of death.[1] This disease process has been a continuing problem since then and has probably never been more in the minds of practicing clinicians than it is today. During the 1970s, the number of hospitalizations for ectopic pregnancy more than doubled (Fig. 32–1) (by 1990 it had easily tripled) and ectopic pregnancy has emerged as a leading cause of maternal death.[2, 3] Fortunately, the risk of death has declined despite the increasing incidence of the disease.

Estimates of the death rate from ectopic pregnancy are approximately 1 in 1000 cases. However, lest this low death rate calm one's anxiety, it should be noted that ectopic pregnancy has a relative risk of death 10 times greater than that of childbirth and 50 times greater than that of a legal induced abortion.[2, 4] A most troublesome fact is that this disease can result in the death of young women of childbearing age who are, for all intents and purposes, otherwise free of disease and in whom eradication of the ectopic pregnancy ends their current risk.

Ectopic pregnancy has a well-recognized association with infertility. Among women who have had an ectopic pregnancy, the subsequent overall conception rate is approximately 60%. Of those who conceive, only 80% have intrauterine gestations while 20% have repeat ectopic gestations.[5–7] This association is probably due to the etiologic relationship of tubal scarring to both the implantation of ectopic pregnancies and infertility; 97% of ectopic pregnancies are tubal in location (Fig. 32–2).

Misdiagnosed ectopic pregnancies not uncommonly lead to medical malpractice litigation.[8, 9] The latter clearly affects the frequency with which tests are ordered to investigate the possible presence of an ectopic gestation. "Overordering" of tests decreases the prevalence of disease in the test population. Statistically, this will adversely affect the predictive accuracy for ectopic pregnancy by any test, including sonography.[10, 11]

The above observations discussed earlier document the importance of ectopic pregnancy as a medical entity. Numerous diagnostic strategies have been proposed for the evaluation of patients suspected of harboring an extrauterine gestation. The focus in the following discussion is on the usefulness of sonography in this difficult patient group.

WHO IS AT RISK?

The clinical diagnosis of ectopic pregnancy is not at all straightforward. The "classic" clinical triad of pain, abnormal bleeding, and palpable adnexal mass is not commonly present and, when present, may erroneously lead to a diagnosis of ectopic pregnancy. In a review of 154 patients with extrauterine gestation pain was present in 97% and abnormal bleeding was noted in 86%.[3] Only 61% of patients reported "missing" a menstrual period. A pelvic mass was palpated in 41% and was equivocally present in 23%. No mass was palpable in the remaining patients. The average duration from last menstrual period to surgery was approximately 7.5 weeks. One patient's ectopic pregnancy eluded diagnosis for more than 17 menstrual weeks. These clinical results are similar to those reported in 1970.[12] The emphasis that clinicians place on history and physical findings varies. However, when an ectopic pregnancy is suspected, the examining sonologist should consistently attempt to document a sequence of observations. Subsequently, the interpretation of findings should not be based on the strength or weakness of the clinical history.

Some women are at especially high risk for harboring an ectopic gestation (Table 32–1). The relatively high recurrence risk of ectopic pregnancy has already been noted.[5–7] Women with a documented history of pelvic inflammatory disease are at an increased risk of devel-

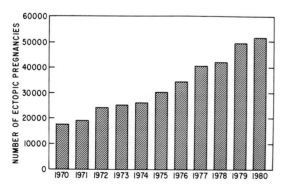

Figure 32–1. Number of hospitalizations for ectopic pregnancy from 1970 through 1980. (From Dorfman SF: Deaths from ectopic pregnancy, United States: 1979 to 1980. Obstet Gynecol 62:334, 1983.)

Table 32–1. PATIENT GROUPS AT INCREASED RISK FOR ECTOPIC PREGNANCY

Prior ectopic pregnancy
Pregnant with intrauterine device in place
History of pelvic inflammatory disease
Prior tubal reconstructive surgery
Pregnancy by in vitro fertilization
Pregnancy following laparoscopic tubal coagulation

SITES OF ECTOPIC PREGNANCY

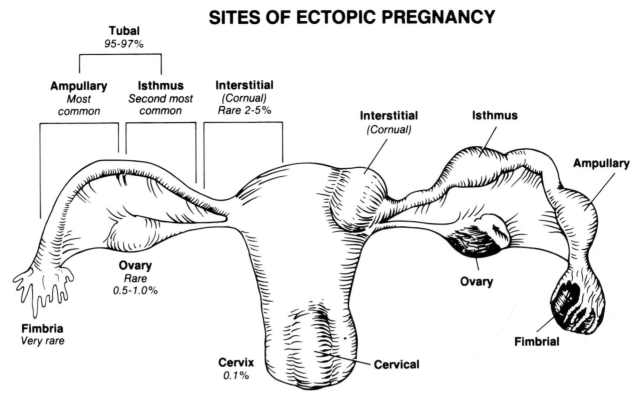

Figure 32–2. Diagram of the common locations of ectopic pregnancy. Note that 95% to 97% of ectopic pregnancies occur somewhere along the course of the fallopian tube. (Modified from Benson RC: Handbook of Obstetrics & Gynecology, 8th ed. Los Altos, Lange Medical Publications, 1983; and from Schoenbaum S, Rosendorf L, Kappelman N, Rowan T: Gray-scale ultrasound in tubal pregnancy. Radiology 127:757, 1978.)

oping an ectopic pregnancy. Thirty to 50% of women with ectopic pregnancies have a history of prior acute salpingitis, and chronic salpingitis is histologically documented in a substantial percentage of surgical specimens from ectopic pregnancies.[3, 12, 13]

Women who are pregnant and have an intrauterine contraceptive device in place are at an increased risk of ectopic pregnancy.[14] This is not to say that intrauterine devices cause ectopic pregnancy, although some investigators consider this plausible. However, most agree that an intrauterine device is far more effective at preventing implantation in the uterus than it is at preventing implantation in an ectopic location. Thus, a woman *who is pregnant* and has an intrauterine device in place has a substantially greater risk of harboring an extrauterine gestation than a pregnant woman without an intrauterine device in place.

Other groups of patients, although small, are also at high risk. Certain infertile women with known tubal disease who become pregnant after tubal microsurgery or by in vitro fertilization are at increased risk. One very small group is at exceptional risk.[15] These are women who become pregnant following a laparoscopic tubal coagulation. As expected, the incidence of pregnancy in this group is quite low, but among those unfortunate women who become pregnant after this attempted procedure to induce permanent sterility, more than one half have ectopic pregnancies. Despite the numerous groups at especially high risk of ectopic pregnancy, the only safe rule to remember is as follows:

all women of childbearing age are at risk of harboring an ectopic gestation. From a sonologic perspective, the following philosophy is highly recommended: the location of a gestation should be firmly established in the first trimester in any pregnant woman who presents for sonography. If the pregnancy cannot be documented as intrauterine, the patient should be considered at risk for an ectopic gestation and appropriate steps taken to determine the patient's status through subsequent testing.

PREGNANCY TESTING

The single most significant advancement in the management of patients suspected of harboring an ectopic gestation has been the appearance of highly sensitive radioimmunoassays to detect human chorionic gonadotropin (hCG). The antibodies employed in these hCG tests are specific for the β-subunit of the hormone. Indeed, as will be pointed out, the interpretation of the sonogram is predicated on the results of this test.

In the era when hemagglutination-inhibition tests were employed to chemically confirm pregnancy, a substantial number of patients who were pregnant but in whom the pregnancy was ectopically located failed to test positively. This was due to two important factors. First, ectopic pregnancies produce hCG at a slower rate than normally implanted pregnancies.[16] Second, pregnancy tests of the hemagglutination-inhibition variety were relatively insensitive to the detection of hCG. Thus, one can easily imagine the consternation of the clinician when previously dealing with a suspected case. Neither a positive nor a negative test was particularly helpful. If the pregnancy test was positive, the location of the pregnancy remained in doubt. If the pregnancy test was negative, the patient remained in the group at risk. The latter extraordinarily difficult patients (i.e., negative pregnancy test group) were frequently referred for sonograms, but this was of little help in managing these patients.[17]

Fortunately for all concerned, the newer radioimmunologic tests can detect extraordinarily small quantities of hCG. By comparison, radioimmunologic tests can detect 1 to 2 IU/L of hCG whereas hemagglutination-inhibition tests detect 1000 to 2000 IU/L. It is important that sonologists be aware that more than one standard exists for the measurement of hCG biologic activity.[18] The Second International Standard (2nd IS) was described in the 1960s. Later, a purer standard was defined and is termed the International Reference Preparation (IRP). Both standards are in use. A given numeric value of hCG in biologic units varies by an approximate factor of 2 between these standards (i.e., 100 IU/L [2nd IS] equals approximately 200 IU/L [IRP]). To add to the potential confusion, some laboratories report results in nanograms per milliliter.[19] Although this appears to be the preferable method, it is not the accepted standard. Conversion factors are available for changing nanograms per milliliter to international units per liter for both commonly used standards of biologic activity. As a rough guideline, 1 ng/mL = 5 to 6 IU/L (2nd IS) and 10 to 12 IU/L (IRP). Awareness of the standard employed by the referring clinician's laboratory is of major importance when quantitated levels of hCG are being compared with the sonographic results. These standards are also important for understanding the lower limit of sensitivity in qualitative testing.[20–27] Differences in standards do not affect the interpretation of serial quantitated levels performed on an individual patient when measured in the same laboratory. Remember, patients will likely be referred by clinicians who use different laboratories that may well employ different standards.

Romero and associates[25] found a 0.5% false-negative rate among patients with ectopic pregnancy when the hCG level was less than 10 IU/L (IRP). The false-negative rate increased, as one might suspect, as the lower limit was raised.[25] These results are similar to those of Olson and coworkers,[26] who found 100% sensitivity for ectopic pregnancy employing a test cutoff level of less than 3 IU/L. Longer incubation times are required[25] to achieve greater sensitivity for hCG. Speed may be clinically necessary in some cases suspected of ectopic pregnancy; however, only a few hours of incubation are required to achieve a sensitivity of 30 IU/L (IRP).

There is reasonably good evidence that the embryos in many ectopic pregnancies exhibiting very low hCG levels are already dead.[26] The natural history of ectopic pregnancy almost certainly includes those embryos that implant, die, and are reabsorbed without being clinically recognized.

SONOGRAPHY

Elevation of the hCG assists the gynecologist in confirming the pregnant state but, at least as an initial screening, does not permit distinction between intrauterine pregnancies (either normal or abnormal), recent spontaneous abortions, and extrauterine gestations. Numerous relatively invasive procedures short of laparotomy, such as culdocentesis, laparoscopy, and dilatation and curettage for microscopic evaluation of the endometrium, increase diagnostic accuracy but involve increased risk to the patient.[28] Laparoscopy, while not 100% accurate in very early ectopic pregnancies, is the single most accurate method of confirming the presence of an ectopic pregnancy before surgery. However, routine use of laparoscopy in suspected cases of ectopic pregnancy is impractical. This procedure is highly invasive. Furthermore, the prevalence of ectopic pregnancy in a clinically suspected group is relatively low, ranging from 10% to 16%.[29–31] Thus, most patients would needlessly undergo a laparoscopic examination. Finally, laparoscopy may lead to the iatrogenic compromise of a normal intrauterine pregnancy.[8]

One would like, if possible, to greatly increase the prevalence of ectopic pregnancy among the group being considered for laparoscopy. Accomplishing this end requires a level of testing interposed between the clinical suspicion of an ectopic pregnancy and the performance of a laparoscopic examination. Gynecologists, at this juncture of the diagnostic workup, will commonly choose, albeit not exclusively, between culdocentesis and sonography. Culdocentesis, although invasive, is substantially less so than laparoscopy. Aspiration of nonclotting blood from the cul-de-sac, especially if the hematocrit is greater than 15%, indicates a high probability that the patient harbors an extrauterine gestation.[28] Gynecologists commonly proceed directly to laparotomy if the culdocentesis is positive. Negative aspirations are unreliable for excluding an extrauterine gestation. This is unfortunate because most suspected pregnancies are not, in fact, extrauterine but instead are normal or abnormal intrauterine pregnancies. This larger patient group will have a negative culdocentesis result. Further testing is then required.

Previous reports emphasize different approaches in the sonographic evaluation of ectopic pregnancy. One group of investigators have attempted to recognize the presence of an ectopic pregnancy on the basis of the adnexal sonographic findings.[30–34] Other groups[23, 35–37] stress that sonography's primary utility is its ability to recognize intrauterine pregnancies. Both aspects are important, but not equally so.

The value of demonstrating an intrauterine pregnancy in a patient suspected of harboring an extrauterine gestation is based on the well-established clinical observation that the concomitant occurrence of an

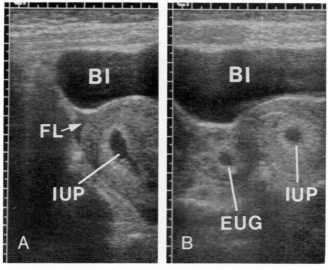

Figure 32–3. Longitudinal (*A*) and transverse (*B*) transabdominal sonograms of a patient with simultaneous intrauterine pregnancy (IUP) and extrauterine gestation (EUG). The intrauterine pregnancy demonstrated a living embryo. A simultaneous extrauterine gestation is extremely improbable but is becoming somewhat more common with the use of ovulation-induction agents. Fortunately, a typical-appearing "ringlike" adnexal mass and pelvic fluid (FL) led to the correct diagnosis. Bl, bladder.

intrauterine pregnancy and an extrauterine gestation (heterotopic pregnancy) is a rare event.[38-40] In patients who have no special risk factors, the expected rate of concomitancy is extremely low, originally quoted as 1 in 30,000 pregnancies.[38] More recent estimates suggest that the rate may be as low as 1 in 4000.[40] Furthermore, gynecologists are currently performing procedures that can alter this frequency.[41, 42] Patients undergoing ovulation induction produce multiple ova per cycle and thus are at greater risk. Such patients have been estimated as having an increased incidence of combined intrauterine pregnancy and extrauterine gestation.[41, 43]

Women undergoing in vitro fertilization may have a risk as high as 1 in 100.[44, 45]

There is no question that concomitant intrauterine pregnancy and extrauterine gestation occurs and that the incidence is increasing (Fig. 32–3).[38-45] However, it is impractical to manage every suspected case of ectopic pregnancy based on the possibility that a heterotopic pregnancy has occurred, even in patients undergoing in vitro fertilization. This is especially true since the alternative diagnostic pathway includes invasive procedures in virtually every case. Women who have a very high risk for ectopic pregnancy should have an early sonogram to establish the location of their pregnancy, whether or not they are symptomatic. If these women also are in a group in which heterotopic pregnancies occur at a much increased rate,[44, 45] they must be instructed of the warning signs and symptoms of ectopic pregnancy even though an intrauterine pregnancy has been demonstrated.

Sonographic Diagnosis of Intrauterine Pregnancies

Sonographic demonstration of an intrauterine pregnancy represents extremely valuable evidence against the possibility of an ectopic pregnancy. However, a variety of morphologic observations may be made by the interpreting sonologist when diagnosing an early intrauterine pregnancy (see Chapter 6). Some of these observations are more reliable than others for this purpose. Researchers who first described early intrauterine gestations considered their appearance to be typical. However, subsequent observations have disclosed that stimulation of the uterine lining with hormones produced by an ectopic pregnancy can, unfortunately, result in endometrial changes that are quite similar in appearance to those seen with an early intrauterine pregnancy.[35-37, 46-51] This stimulation is histologically recognizable in approximately half of patients with an ectopic pregnancy (decidual cast) (Fig. 32–4) but simulates the sonographic appearance of an early pregnancy (pseudogestational sac of ectopic pregnancy) in a much smaller percentage of cases (Table 32–2; Fig. 32–5).[46] This potential for confusion mandates that sonologists be extremely cautious when diagnosing an intrauterine pregnancy in a patient sus-

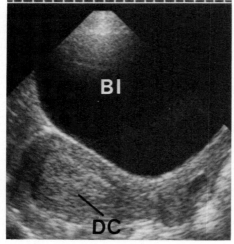

Figure 32–4. Longitudinal transabdominal sonogram of the uterus in a patient with an ectopic pregnancy. The sonogram shows a large decidual cast (DC) within the uterus. This would not likely be mistaken for an intrauterine pregnancy. Bl, bladder.

Table 32–2. APPEARANCE OF THE ENDOMETRIAL CAVITY ON TRANSABDOMINAL SONOGRAPHY IN 39 PATIENTS WITH PROVEN ECTOPIC PREGNANCY

Finding	No.
Normal	21 (54%)
Gestational sac like	8 (20%)
Prominent central echoes	5 (13%)
Other (including fluid collection not typical of gestational sac, a gestational sac–like appearance, and prominent central echoes)	5 (13%)

Modified from Marks WM, Filly RA, Callen PW, et al: The decidual cast of ectopic pregnancy: A confusing ultrasonographic appearance. Radiology 133:451, 1979.

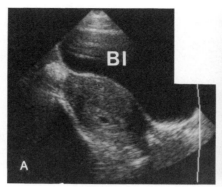
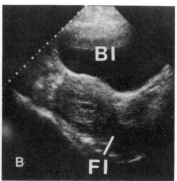

Figure 32–5. *A.* Longitudinal transabdominal sonogram of a patient suspected of harboring an extrauterine gestation. However, an intrauterine fluid collection surrounded by a double decidual sac is clearly identified, indicating a normal position of the pregnancy. *B.* Conversely, in a patient with a similar clinical history there is an intraendometrial fluid collection surrounded by a single rim of echoes. This is a pseudogestational sac of an ectopic pregnancy. Note that this patient also has fluid (Fl) in the cul-de-sac. Bl, bladder.

pected of harboring an extrauterine gestation. Specific morphologic criteria should be applied.

Endovaginal transducers greatly enhance visualization of very early pregnancies.[52–54] Such transducers result in a decrease in distance from the transducer face to the endometrial cavity. This enables the sonographer both to use higher-frequency transducers and to scan the endometrial cavity in a portion of the beam that is more easily focused by manufacturers. Both advantages result in superior resolution. The widespread use of endovaginal transducers has resulted in an ability to resolve pregnancies earlier (Fig. 32–6) and features that reliably distinguish true pregnancies from the pseudogestational sac of ectopic pregnancy (i.e., yolk sac identification, embryonic visualization) (Figs. 32–7 and 32–8).

Normal intrauterine pregnancies can first be detected with endovaginal sonography as an intraendometrial fluid collection surrounded by an echogenic margin at approximately 4.5 menstrual weeks (2.5 weeks after conception) (see Fig. 32–6).[19, 20] When the mean sac diameter of the gestation sac reaches approximately 10 mm, the yolk sac becomes consistently visible within the developing gestational sac, and when the gestation sac reaches approximately 16 mm an embryo can be consistently detected.[51, 55, 56] With modern equipment, the fetal heartbeat is consistently visible when the embryo reaches a crown-rump length of 5 mm.[56] Identification of embryonic components of the pregnancy (yolk sac, embryo, and especially a living embryo) are highly reliable indicators of a true intrauterine pregnancy (see Figs. 32–7 through 32–9). It is during the brief but important period (4.5 to 5.5 menstrual weeks) when the pregnancy first becomes visible and more definitive signs of an intrauterine pregnancy appear (yolk sac or embryo) that one must be cautious not to interpret a pseudogestational sac of ectopic pregnancy as a true intrauterine pregnancy (Figs. 32–10 and 32–11). However, the major source of confusion between pseudogestational sacs and intrauterine pregnancies is not the normal early intrauterine pregnancy but occurs when the gestation is abnormal and does not meet expected developmental landmarks (Fig. 32–12).

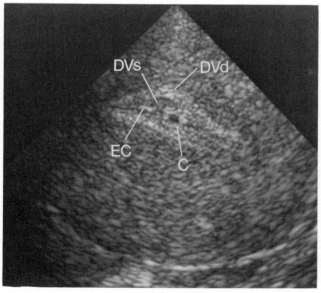

Figure 32–6. Endovaginal sonogram of a very early pregnancy. This sonogram demonstrates the origins of the so-called double decidual sac sign. The inner ring is formed by the margin of chorionic villi (C). The outer ring is the deeper layer of decidua vera (DVd). The separating lucent zone is the more superficial decidua vera (DVs). EC, endometrial cavity.

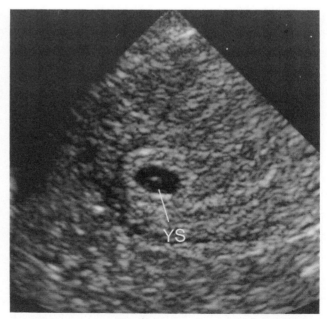

Figure 32–7. Endovaginal sonogram demonstrates the double decidual sac sign but also demonstrates the more reliable feature of a yolk sac (YS).

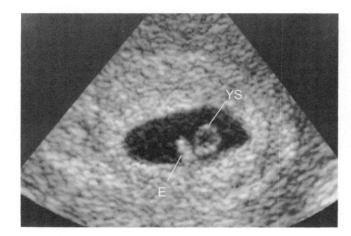

Figure 32–8. Endovaginal sonogram demonstrating an early embryo (E) (less than 5 mm crown-rump length). YS, yolk sac.

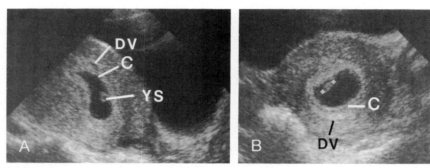

Figure 32–9. Longitudinal (*A*) and transverse (*B*) transabdominal sonograms of patient with a differential diagnosis of threatened abortion versus ectopic pregnancy. By this stage of development, all of the features seen in early pregnancy can be noted. These include the double decidual sac sign, consisting of the concentric rings of the deep decidua vera (DV) and chorionic villi (C). Additionally, the yolk sac (YS) and a living embryo (*cursors*) can be detected. When definitive features of an intrauterine pregnancy are seen on transabdominal sonography, further evaluation with endovaginal sonography is not required.

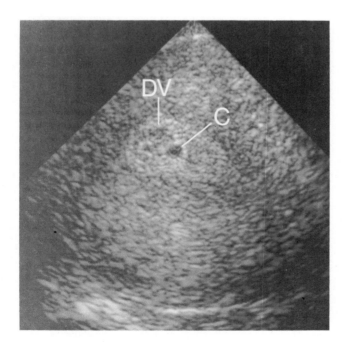

Figure 32–10. Early pregnancy demonstrating a double decidual sac sign but no yolk sac or embryo. A confident diagnosis of intrauterine pregnancy still can be made. C, chorionic villi; DV, deep decidua vera.

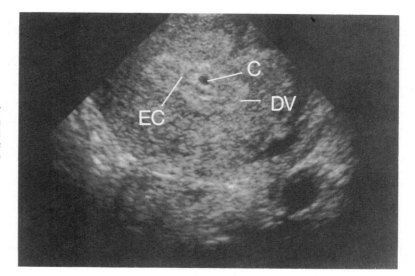

Figure 32–11. Another example of an early pregnancy in which the double decidual sac sign is easily seen when no yolk sac or embryo is visible. Note that the gestational sac is within the endometrium by observing the eccentric endometrial cavity (EC). C, chorionic villi; DV, deep decidua vera.

In my experience, endovaginal sonography has significantly enhanced our recognition of early pregnancies.[57] Indeed, in the area of ectopic pregnancy diagnosis, this has been a major area of improvement (if not the most significant improvement) in sonography's abilities to assist in the assessment of patients suspected of harboring an extrauterine gestation. Before the availability of endovaginal sonography our laboratory recognized an intrauterine pregnancy at first visit in only 58% of patients at risk for an extrauterine gestation.[29] After the introduction of endovaginal sonography the proportion increased to 72% (Fig. 32–13).[57] Furthermore, our laboratory now identifies 85% of intrauterine pregnancies at first examination and one institution has published a 95%[56] recognition of intrauterine pregnancies during the first clinical sonographic examination.

The "double decidual sac (DDS) sign" has been suggested as a finding that characterizes an early intrauterine pregnancy and reliably discriminates a true gestational sac from the pseudogestational sac of ectopic pregnancy[37, 50] before the ability to recognize either the yolk sac or embryo. The double sac, which consists of two concentric rings surrounding a portion of the gestational sac, originally was thought to represent the decidua parietalis (decidua vera) adjacent to the decidua capsularis (Fig. 32–14). Some authors differed in their judgments as to the origin of the double concentric rings.[29, 36, 59, 60] Observations with endovaginal sonography now suggest that the inner ring is composed of the chorionic villi proliferating around the developing gestation while the outer ring is the deeper and more echogenic layer of the decidua vera (see Figs. 32–6 and 32–10). When the decidua

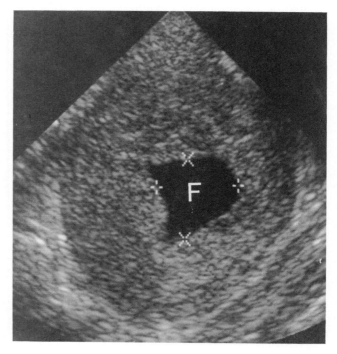

Figure 32–12. An irregular fluid (F) collection is seen in the uterus. No double decidual sac sign, yolk sac, or embryo is seen. The mean sac diameter is 17 mm. Therefore, an intrauterine pregnancy cannot be diagnosed. However, one can state that if this is an intrauterine pregnancy, it is not viable (see Chapter 6). Therefore, the uterus can be safely evacuated and the products examined for chorionic villi. If chorionic villi are found, an abnormal intrauterine pregnancy is established and the patient's risk for extrauterine gestation is eliminated.

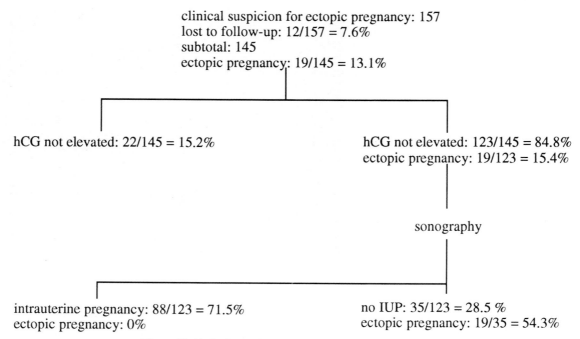

clinical suspicion for ectopic pregnancy: 157
lost to follow-up: 12/157 = 7.6%
subtotal: 145
ectopic pregnancy: 19/145 = 13.1%

hCG not elevated: 22/145 = 15.2%

hCG not elevated: 123/145 = 84.8%
ectopic pregnancy: 19/123 = 15.4%

sonography

intrauterine pregnancy: 88/123 = 71.5%
ectopic pregnancy: 0%

no IUP: 35/123 = 28.5 %
ectopic pregnancy: 19/35 = 54.3%

Figure 32–13. Patient cohort initial sonographic categorization.

vera is uniformly echogenic throughout its entire thickness a true DDS sign cannot be demonstrated (Fig. 32–15). Despite the erroneous name, this finding remains valuable to sonologists. In contradistinction to the DDS sign, the pseudogestational sac of ectopic pregnancy is composed of a single echogenic ring surrounding either an intraendometrial fluid collection or the more echogenic deeper layer of decidua "surrounding" the less echogenic superficial layer (see Figs. 32–5 and 32–16). Several investigations have been done to establish the validity of the DDS sign.[29, 36, 50, 59] The weight of evidence indicates that this sign is highly reliable in discriminating pseudogestational from true gestational sacs. However, *the DDS sign does not absolutely exclude a pseudogestational sac nor does its presence confirm that an intrauterine pregnancy is normal.*[50, 55, 60] Therefore, when employed in patients suspected of harboring an extrauterine gestation, follow-up examinations may be beneficial. With endovaginal sonography the number of instances in which a pseu-

dogestational is erroneously interpreted as a true gestational sac has decreased, as has our reliance on the DDS sign.[57]

Before the onset of our utilization of endovaginal sonography 37.5% of early intrauterine pregnancies were diagnosed in the laboratory at my institution based on the DDS sign.[29] However, since the advent of endovaginal sonography this proportion has been reduced to 10%.[57] The DDS sign may be observed in transabdominal scanning 5 weeks from commencement of the last menstrual period and the yolk sac may be seen from 7 weeks onward. Therefore, the most useful period for the application of the DDS sign previously

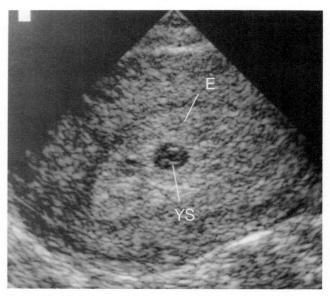

Figure 32–14. Longitudinal transabdominal sonogram of the uterus, demonstrating the double decidual sac sign before visualization of either the yolk sac or the embryo. The double decidual sac is composed of the deep decidual vera (DV) surrounding the chorionic villi (C). EC, endometrial cavity.

Figure 32–15. When the endometrium (E) is uniformly echogenic the double decidual sac sign cannot be demonstrated. However, in this case a yolk sac (YS) is detected.

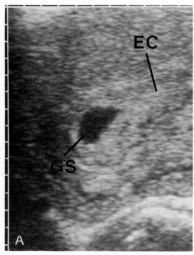
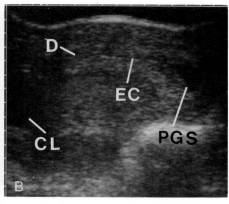

Figure 32–16. *A.* Transverse magnified high-resolution transabdominal sonogram of a patient with an early intrauterine pregnancy. Notice that the gestational sac (GS) is eccentrically positioned within the endometrial cavity (EC). This is a useful feature for discriminating early pregnancies from the pseudogestational sac of ectopic pregnancy, which commonly fills the entire uterine cavity symmetrically (see Fig. 32–5*B*). *B.* However, like all features designed to distinguish the pseudogestational sac from true intrauterine pregnancies, failures may be anticipated. The pseudogestational sac (PGS) in this transverse magnified high-resolution sonogram of a patient with an ectopic pregnancy is eccentrically positioned within the endometrial cavity (EC). D, decidualized endometrium; CL, corpus luteum cyst.

was between 5 and 7 weeks when transabdominal scanning dominated early pregnancy visualization. With the use of endovaginal sonography this time period is effectively reduced by 1 week owing to the earlier visualization of the yolk sac, which is a more reliable morphologic criterion for early pregnancy diagnosis. Therefore, endovaginal sonography has reduced but not eliminated reliance on the DDS sign to diagnose early intrauterine pregnancies (see Figs. 32–10 and 32–11).

Evaluation of the morphology of intrauterine contents, beyond exclusion of an intrauterine pregnancy does not improve diagnostic accuracy. A pseudogestational sac has been reported as a finding in 8%[61] to 33.3%[62] of cases with a proven ectopic pregnancy, and its potential confusion with a normal gestational sac emphasized. More recent experience indicates that only 5% of ectopic pregnancies have a pseudogestational sac, and currently this causes little difficulty in scan interpretation.[57] It is likely that improved visualization of the endometrial tissues and the contents of the endometrial cavity decreases the likelihood that pseudogestational sacs will cause false results.

Evaluation of the Patient At Risk

When either a transabdominal or endovaginal sonogram documents the presence of an intrauterine pregnancy, the extremely low occurrence rate of concomitant intrauterine pregnancy and extrauterine gestation (heterotopic pregnancies) effectively excludes the diagnosis of ectopic pregnancy (see Fig. 32–13). Sonographic visualization of an intrauterine pregnancy, by demonstration of a DDS sign, a yolk sac, or an embryo, therefore, is the most beneficial finding in the exclusion of ectopic pregnancy. When used as a screening test, sonographic documentation of an intrauterine pregnancy provides the only convincing evidence for the absence of an extrauterine gestation.[57, 58, 61–66]

Several studies document the utility and accuracy of the DDS sign in confirming the presence of an intrauterine pregnancy before a stage of development when

a yolk sac or embryo can be seen. Special care must be taken to unequivocally document the DDS sign. Erroneous interpretation of a pseudogestational sac as an intrauterine pregnancy could lead to a false diagnosis and a potentially catastrophic outcome. Subjects whose sonograms do not confirm an intrauterine pregnancy immediately enter a high-risk category. The risk is substantially higher if no intrauterine pregnancy is seen with endovaginal transducers (54%) than transabdominal transducers (43%) although both are quite high.[57] This is due to the greater number of intrauterine pregnancies recognized by endovaginal transducers (see Fig. 32–13). Thus, the risk of extrauterine gestation increases among the residual patients.

Characterization of the adnexal findings in the group without a demonstrable intrauterine pregnancy improves the ability of sonography to predict the presence of an ectopic gestation using either technique (Fig. 32–17; Table 32–3). Patients with no visible intrauterine pregnancy who in addition demonstrate either an adnexal mass (Figs. 32–18 through 32–21) or cul-de-sac fluid (Figs. 32–22 and 32–23) move into a category of even greater risk (approximately 70% with either finding) (see Fig. 32–17 and Table 32–3). Combining adnexal findings further improves specificity and posi-

Table 32–3. SONOGRAPHIC FINDINGS VERSUS RISK OF ECTOPIC PREGNANCY

	% Risk of Ectopic Pregnancy	
Finding	**Transabdominal Study***	**Endovaginal Study†**
Adnexal embryo	100	100
Mass and large to moderate amounts of fluid	100	100
Mass and fluid	85	78
Any fluid	71	75
Any mass	71	69
No mass or fluid	20	33

*Data from Mahony BS, Filly RA, Nyberg DA, et al: Sonographic evaluation of ectopic pregnancy. J Ultrasound Med 4:221, 1985.

†Data from Cadkin AV, McAlpin J: Detection of fetal cardiac activity between 41 and 43 days' gestation. J Ultrasound Med 3:499, 1984.

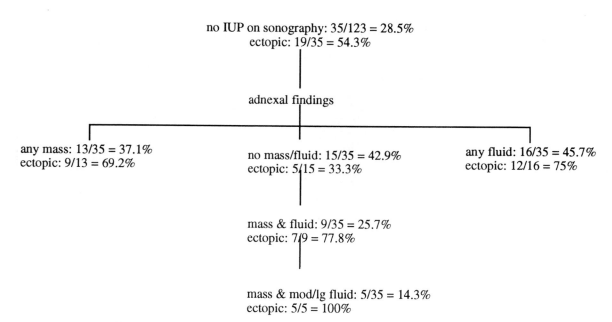

no IUP on sonography: 35/123 = 28.5%
ectopic: 19/35 = 54.3%

adnexal findings

any mass: 13/35 = 37.1%
ectopic: 9/13 = 69.2%

no mass/fluid: 15/35 = 42.9%
ectopic: 5/15 = 33.3%

any fluid: 16/35 = 45.7%
ectopic: 12/16 = 75%

mass & fluid: 9/35 = 25.7%
ectopic: 7/9 = 77.8%

mass & mod/lg fluid: 5/35 = 14.3%
ectopic: 5/5 = 100%

Figure 32–17. Further sonographic segregation of the group at special risk for ectopic pregnancy.

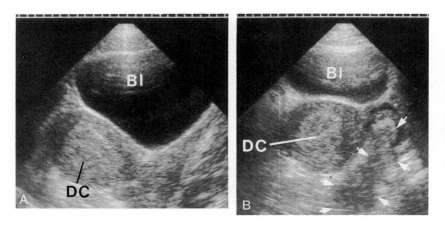

Figure 32–18. Longitudinal (A) and transverse (B) transabdominal sonograms of a patient with an ectopic pregnancy. There is a large decidual cast (DC) and a vague elliptical echogenic mass in the left adnexa, extending into the cul-de-sac (arrows). A patient who fails to demonstrate an intrauterine pregnancy and also demonstrates an echogenic mass has approximately an 85% risk of having an ectopic pregnancy. Masses of this type generally represent a hematosalpinx. Bl, bladder.

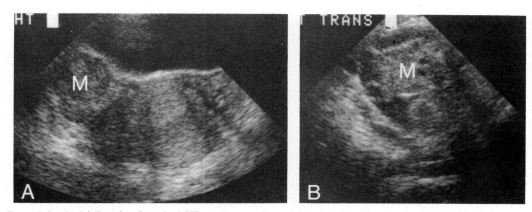

Figure 32–19. Transabdominal (A) and endovaginal (B) sonograms of an echogenic right adnexal mass (M) in a patient suspected of harboring an ectopic pregnancy and in whom no intrauterine pregnancy was demonstrated. This mass was a hemorrhagic corpus luteum cyst.

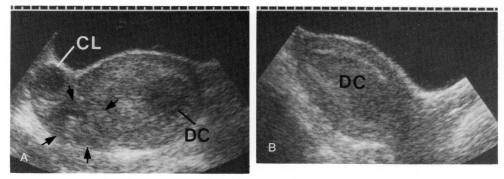

Figure 32–20. Transverse (*A*) and longitudinal (*B*) transabdominal sonograms of a patient with an ectopic pregnancy. A large and somewhat eccentric decidual cast (DC) is seen within the uterus. Decidual casts of this appearance probably "mature" into pseudogestational sacs. No fluid is seen in the cul-de-sac. A relatively typical corpus luteum (CL) is seen in the right ovary. Additionally, an echogenic mass (*arrows*) is wedged between the right ovary and the uterus. This is a relatively typical location and appearance for an ectopic gestation.

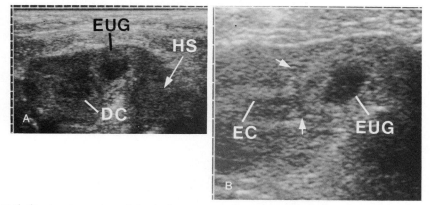

Figure 32–21. *A*. High-resolution transverse transabdominal sonogram of a patient with an ectopic gestation (EUG) in the cornual portion of the tube. A decidual cast (DC) is clearly identified and marks the endometrial cavity. Distal to the ectopic gestation, an enlarged tube caused by a hematosalpinx (HS) is identified. *B*. Magnified view of *A* demonstrates effacement of the decidualized endometrium (*arrows*) by the cornual ectopic gestation (EUG). This type of ectopic gestation is particularly hazardous because of the extensive vasculature generally associated with pregnancies contained in this portion of the tube. EC, endometrial cavity.

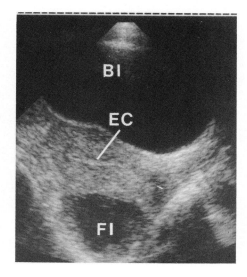

Figure 32–22. Longitudinal transabdominal sonogram of a patient suspected of harboring an ectopic pregnancy. There is no evidence of an intrauterine pregnancy within the endometrial cavity (EC). A moderate amount of echogenic fluid (Fl) is seen in the cul-de-sac. The absence of an intrauterine pregnancy in the presence of a moderate amount of cul-de-sac fluid places this patient at high risk for an ectopic pregnancy. Bl, bladder.

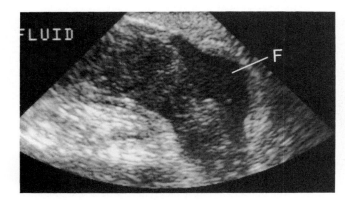

Figure 32–23. Endovaginal sonogram demonstrating a small amount of echogenic fluid (F). Any fluid seen in a patient without a demonstrable intrauterine pregnancy is worrisome for extrauterine gestation. However, echogenic fluid is even more suggestive.

Figure 32–24. Transverse (*A*) and left longitudinal (*B*) transabdominal sonograms of a patient suspected of harboring an ectopic pregnancy. No pregnancy is seen within the endometrial cavity (EC). Additionally, a moderate amount of fluid (Fl) is noted in the cul-de-sac, extending into the left adnexa, where a moderately echogenic (*arrows*) ringlike mass (M) is identified. The combination of moderate fluid, a ringlike mass, and the absence of an intrauterine pregnancy virtually confirms the presence of an ectopic pregnancy. Bl, bladder.

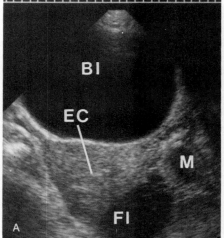
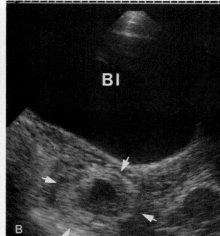

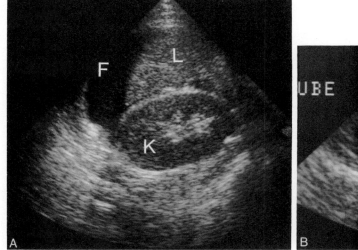
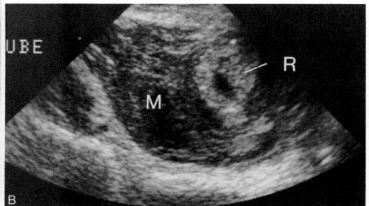

Figure 32–25. *A.* Endovaginal sonogram demonstrating an adnexal mass (M) with an echogenic ringlike component (R). *B.* Transabdominal sonogram demonstrating a large amount of echogenic fluid (F) in the upper abdomen. Such features are virtually diagnostic of ectopic pregnancy and further indicate that laparotomy, rather than laparoscopic surgery or cytotoxic therapy, is indicated. L, liver; K, kidney.

Figure 32–26. Transverse (A) and right longitudinal (B) transabdominal sonograms of a patient with moderately severe abdominal pain and a positive pregnancy test. The uterus (U) is partially obscured by contiguous echogenic hemorrhagic fluid (H) and an extrauterine echogenic ringlike mass representing the extrauterine gestation (EUG). These features alone virtually confirm an ectopic pregnancy, but the identification of the living adnexal embryo (E) conclusively documents that the patient has an ectopic pregnancy, which is leaking blood. Bl, bladder.

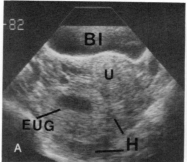
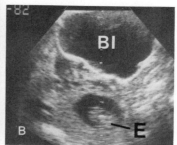

tive predictive accuracy (see Figs. 32–17, 32–24, and 32–25). However, each refinement concomitantly reduces sensitivity and the accuracy of a negative prediction. For example, demonstration of a living adnexal embryo is 100% specific for an extrauterine gestation (Figs. 32–26 through 32–28). Unfortunately, sensitivity drops to approximately 15% with transabdominal sonography.[63] Endovaginal sonography can detect living embryos in approximately 30% of ectopic pregnancies.[61–67] Furthermore, improved resolution has enabled confirmation of an adnexal gestation by visualization of a yolk sac independent of embryo visualization (Figs. 32–29 and 32–30).

Although sonographic documentation of an adnexal mass or pelvic intraperitoneal fluid in a woman with measurable circulating hCG and no evidence of an intrauterine pregnancy substantially increases her risk of harboring an extrauterine gestation, the absence of these findings does not exclude an ectopic pregnancy (Fig. 32–31).[61–66] Up to one third of women with a confirmed extrauterine gestation had no sonographic evidence of either an adnexal mass or cul-de-sac fluid

even employing endovaginal sonography on initial examination.[57] The only sonographic feature that reliably excludes a patient from the group at risk for extrauterine gestation is demonstration of an intrauterine pregnancy. If no intrauterine pregnancy is demonstrated, a variety of adnexal findings may effectively increase a patient's risk, but the absence of sonographic abnormalities in the adnexal region cannot decrease the patient's risk to an acceptably low level. The life-threatening nature of this entity necessitates further investigation in these cases. At the present time, the appropriate course of action is to consider patients with measurable levels of hCG and absent adnexal findings still to be at risk for an extrauterine gestation when no intrauterine pregnancy can be demonstrated.

Direct visualization of the ectopic embryo has been documented in 16%[57] to 32.5%[67] of cases on endovaginal scanning. In the absence of detection of the embryo in an adnexal location, an adnexal "ringlike" structure has been found by many studies[29, 58, 61, 68, 69] to be both a frequent (14%[58] to 69%[66]) and specific observation for ectopic pregnancy. However, my col-

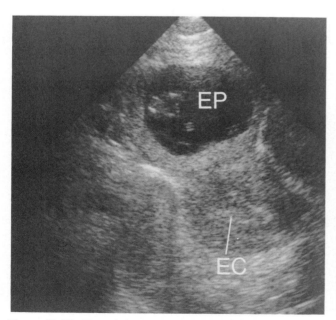

Figure 32–27. Transabdominal sonogram demonstrating a large ectopic pregnancy (EP) that is difficult to separate from the uterus. However, the empty endometrial cavity (EC) is seen.

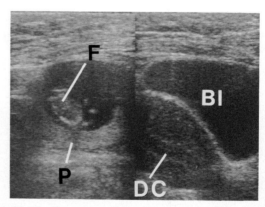

Figure 32–28. Composite, linear-array real-time transabdominal sonogram of a patient suspected of harboring an ectopic pregnancy. Indeed, an extremely large ectopic gestation is seen superior to the fundus of the uterus. A fetus (F), whose biparietal diameter was easily measured, can be identified. Additionally, there is a well-developed placenta (P). Only a decidual cast (DC) is seen within the uterus. Although large and easily seen, such ectopic pregnancies may be misdiagnosed as intrauterine if the sonologist fails to observe a line of demarcation between the ectopic gestation and the uterine fundus. When this separation is not noted, the ectopic gestation is mistakenly incorporated into the uterine fundus. This error can be devastating to the patient. Bl, bladder.

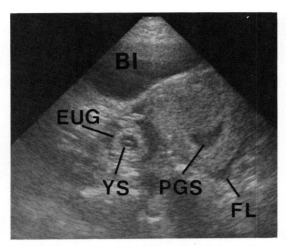

Figure 32–29. Transverse transabdominal sonogram of a patient suspected of harboring an ectopic pregnancy. A pseudogestational sac (PGS) is seen within the uterus. There is fluid in the cul-de-sac (FL), extending to the right adnexa, where an adnexal ring containing a yolk sac (YS) confirms this mass as an extrauterine gestation (EUG). Just as a yolk sac within an intraendometrial fluid collection confirms an intrauterine pregnancy, a yolk sac within an adnexal mass confirms an extrauterine pregnancy. Bl, bladder.

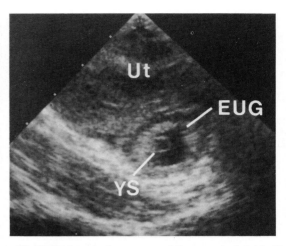

Figure 32–30. Endovaginal sonogram of the mass depicted in Figure 32–32. As viewed with this newer technology, the thick-walled adnexal cyst demonstrates an unequivocal yolk sac (YS), discriminating this adnexal ring from a corpus luteum cyst and confirming it as an extrauterine gestation (EUG). The uterus (Ut) represents the tissue lying in front of the unruptured ectopic pregnancy.

leagues and I have not observed this feature as commonly as other investigators.[57] This may be a reflection of the proportion of ectopic pregnancies that have ruptured. Those researchers who found the highest incidence of the "ringlike" adnexal structures reported the lowest proportion of ruptured ectopic pregnancies.[66, 67, 70] This controversy does not alter the predictive value of an adnexal "ring" when present but does call into question the ease of making this observation in at-risk patients (see Figs. 32–3B, 32–21, 32–24, 32–25A, and 32–32). Other than visualization of an ectopic embryo or "adnexal ring," the combination of a pelvic mass and free pelvic fluid carries the highest risk (77.8%) for an ectopic pregnancy, which is increased still further to 100% if the volume of free fluid is judged subjectively to be moderate to large (see Table 32–3).[57] These findings do not differ substantially from those reported from this laboratory before the introduction of endovaginal probes.[29]

Doppler Sonography in Extrauterine Gestation

Both color and gated Doppler sonography have been employed to enhance the examination of patients at increased risk for an ectopic pregnancy (i.e., those who do not demonstrate an intrauterine pregnancy).[71, 72] Such patients who additionally demonstrate an adnexal embryo or yolk sac, an "adnexal ring," or a mass and a moderate to large amount of fluid may be confidently diagnosed as having an ectopic pregnancy. However, those patients with a nondescript mass (Figs. 32–33 and 32–34), a small to moderate amount of pelvic fluid, or no findings at all in the adnexa or cul-de-sac constitute a difficult diagnostic

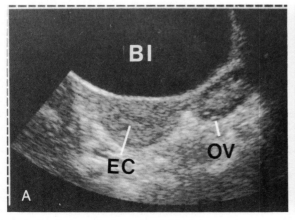

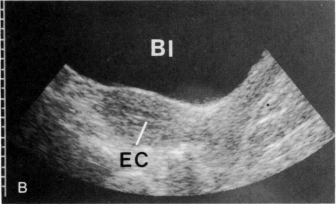

Figure 32–31. Transverse (*A*) and longitudinal (*B*) high-resolution transabdominal sonograms of a patient suspected of harboring an ectopic pregnancy. No intrauterine pregnancy is identified within the endometrial cavity (EC). The adnexa are unremarkable. The left ovary (OV) is clearly identified. There is no fluid in the cul-de-sac. Despite the essentially normal appearance of this pelvis, there is an ectopic pregnancy. It is extremely important to remember that a normal pelvic sonogram does not exclude an ectopic pregnancy. Bl, bladder.

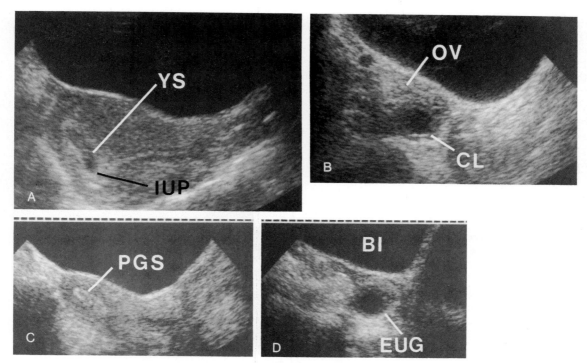

Figure 32–32. Two patients presented with intrauterine "sacs" and adnexal "masses." *A.* Longitudinal transabdominal sonogram of the uterus in a patient suspected of harboring an ectopic pregnancy. An intrauterine pregnancy (IUP) is confirmed by demonstration of a yolk sac (YS). *B.* In the left adnexa, this patient demonstrates a thick-walled adnexal cystic ringlike mass. This may be safely presumed to represent a corpus luteum (CL) in the ovary (OV). *C.* By contrast, a longitudinal sonogram of the uterus in another patient demonstrates a small intrauterine fluid collection without the definitive morphologic criteria for an intrauterine pregnancy. Indeed, this proved to be a pseudogestational sac (PGS) of an ectopic pregnancy. *D.* In the right adnexa, a thick-walled adnexal ringlike cystic mass, quite similar in appearance to that in *B,* was identified. This mass, however, turned out to be an ectopic gestation (EUG) (see Fig. 32–30). On the basis of the adnexal findings, one could not reasonably discriminate the masses in *B* and *D*. It is the identification of the intrauterine pregnancy in *A* that effectively excludes this patient from the group at risk for ectopic pregnancy. Bl, bladder.

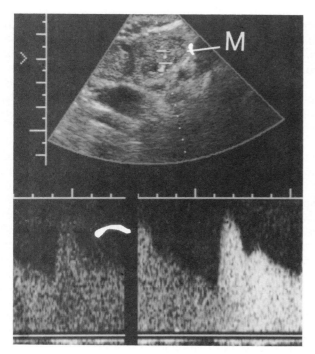

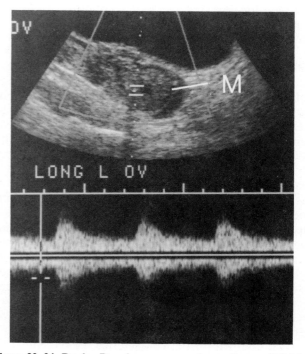

Figure 32–33. Duplex Doppler sonogram of a small adnexal mass (M) seen in a patient suspected of harboring an EUG. The low-resistance arterial signal adds further confirmation that this mass represents the ectopic pregnancy.

Figure 32–34. Duplex Doppler sonogram of a small mass (M) lying adjacent to or within the left ovary. The Doppler profile does not show very high diastolic flow. In this situation Doppler scanning may only add to the confusion about the findings. This mass was an ectopic pregnancy.

problem. The addition of Doppler sonography may quickly point toward the correct diagnostic conclusion.

Although color and pulsed Doppler sonography can be performed either transabdominally or endovaginally, they are best performed by the latter technique.[71, 72] Both modalities can assist in the confirmation that a small intrauterine fluid collection is indeed a gestational sac even though it fails to fulfill acceptable morphologic criteria (DDS sign or visualization of a yolk sac).[71] Color Doppler studies may document focal "peritrophoblastic" flow that demonstrates a low resistance pattern on pulsed Doppler waveform analysis.[71, 72] Color Doppler imaging tends to show a focal area of arterial flow adjacent to the sac that is more intense than other color flashes in the uterus. Because of low diastolic resistance, this area of color flow will appear continuous or nearly continuous during real-time examinations.

These tools also assist both in finding previously unseen, small adnexal masses[71] and in further characterizing such masses (Fig. 32–35). Adnexal masses caused by ectopic pregnancies have a component of trophoblastic tissue. As with trophoblastic tissue surrounding intrauterine pregnancies, extrauterine gestation tends to demonstrate recognizable intense areas of color flow (Fig. 32–36) that have a low resistance pattern of the waveform on duplex Doppler analysis. Unfortunately, the waveform may demonstrate a high resistance pattern even though trophoblastic tissue is present. Nonetheless, these flashes of color flow may draw one's attention to the presence of a small mass that was previously not observed by B-scan imaging alone. Once a mass is seen, the risk for ectopic pregnancy rises dramatically, and if the mass demonstrates color flow, regardless of resistance pattern, the risk for ectopic pregnancy rises further.

Value of Quantitation of hCG

In the patient group with a clinical suspicion of extrauterine gestation, circulating hCG, no sonographically demonstrable intrauterine pregnancy and evidence of either cul-de-sac fluid or an adnexal mass, the potential risk for ectopic pregnancy is sufficiently high (>70%) that laparoscopy would certainly represent a reasonable course of action to further segregate out the falsely suspected case. Of course, patients with documented ectopic pregnancies could even bypass laparoscopy in favor of laparotomy or medical management with cytotoxic drugs. Such patients fall into straightforward management groups.

However, patients who fail to demonstrate either intrauterine pregnancy or adnexal pathology represent a moderately large and particularly difficult management group. Fortunately, additional noninvasive evidence can be obtained in an appropriately short time interval that will further characterize the patient's risk of extrauterine gestation. These women can greatly benefit from quantitation of the level of circulating hCG. The specimen preferably, but not necessarily, should be obtained on the same day as the sonogram.

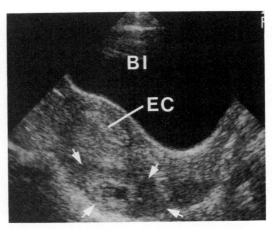

Figure 32–35. Longitudinal sonogram of a patient suspected of harboring an extrauterine pregnancy. There is no evidence of a pregnancy in the endometrial cavity (EC). An ill-defined mass (*arrows*) with a lucent center is identified in the cul-de-sac. The cul-de-sac mass is poorly marginated from the posterior wall of the uterus, unfortunately a not uncommon situation. Color Doppler evaluation may lead to recognition of such masses or greater confidence of the examiner that a mass is truly present.

Recall that the reference standard employed by different laboratories may result in a reported variation of hCG level as great as 50%.

These women have the following differential diagnostic possibilities: (1) they have a normal or abnormal intrauterine pregnancy, but it is too small to be detected sonographically; (2) they have recently spontaneously aborted an abnormal pregnancy but still have measurable levels of circulating hCG; or (3) they do indeed have an ectopic pregnancy that is too small to be detected as an adnexal mass and that has yet to produce visible peritoneal fluid. Although quantitation of the hCG will not unambiguously discriminate between these three possibilities, it can help select the correct management pathway.[20–23]

Evidence indicates that modern sonographic equipment equipped with an endovaginal transducer has the capacity to detect all normal singleton gestational sacs when the hCG level exceeds 1000 mIU/mL (2nd IS).[53, 67, 69] Furthermore, gestational sac size strongly correlates with quantitative hCG levels in normal singleton pregnancies. Ordinarily, abnormal early pregnancies produce low levels of hCG compared with sac size. Therefore, the sac tends to be sonographically visible, although it may lack the usual morphologic features associated with an IUP. This may not be true of all early abnormal gestations. Some produce greater quantities of hCG than normal pregnancies. Therefore, a high hCG level may be present when no sac is visible. The likely culprit in such cases would be pregnancies that would eventually produce trophoblastic disease (true or partial moles).

Patients who have recently spontaneously aborted a pregnancy, either completely or incompletely, are unlikely to have a high level of hCG. Indeed, only 4 of 39 such patients had hCG levels exceeding 1800 IU/L and the history in these 4 patients suggested a very recent passage of tissue (Table 32–4).[21] In contradis-

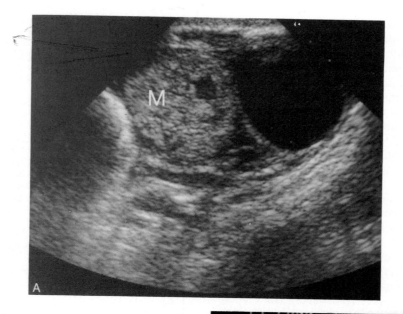

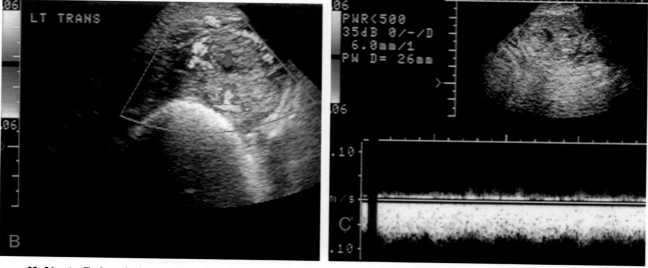

Figure 32–36. *A.* Endovaginal sonogram of a highly suspicious adnexal mass (M). *B.* Color Doppler sonogram shows remarkable "peritrophoblastic" type of flow. *C.* Doppler waveform analysis shows very high diastolic flow.

tinction to these groups, 30 of 68 patients with ectopic pregnancies had hCG levels exceeding 1800 IU/L at the time of initial sonographic evaluation.[22] Thus, if the quantitated hCG is greater than 1800 IU/L (2nd IS), the probability that one is examining a patient with a normal singleton intrauterine pregnancy too early to detect on ultrasound evaluation is remote.

Table 32–4. ABSENT INTRAUTERINE GESTATIONAL SAC CORRELATED WITH SIMULTANEOUS QUANTITATIVE hCG LEVELS (TRANSABDOMINAL SONOGRAPHY)

hCG Level*	Ectopic Pregnancy (n = 68)	Spontaneous Abortion (n = 39)	Intrauterine Pregnancy (n = 19)
>1800 mIU/mL	30	4	0
<1800 mIU/mL	38	35	19

*Based on Second International Standard.

Both patients with a recent spontaneous abortion or an extrauterine gestation could have an "empty" uterus and an hCG greater than 1800 IU/L, but when such a level is documented the diagnosis of ectopic pregnancy is strongly favored. The higher the hCG level in a patient without a visible intrauterine pregnancy, the more likely one is dealing with a patient who harbors an extrauterine gestation.

If the quantitated level of hCG is low, all three differential diagnostic possibilities remain in effect (see Table 32–6), but within 48 hours the referring physician can further segregate the falsely suspected case from this remaining, most troublesome, patient group. A normal intrauterine pregnancy demonstrates an hCG doubling time of approximately 2 days (range, 1.2 to 2.2 days),[24] whereas patients with a recent spontaneous abortion would show a substantial decline in their circulating hCG level during an equivalent time course.[19] By contrast, women with ectopic pregnancies would tend to show a subnormal increase in circulating hCG over a 48-hour span.[16] Unfortunately, ectopic pregnancies occasionally show hCG doubling times similar to a normal pregnancy or declining hCG levels similar to a spontaneous abortion. Early abnormal intrauterine pregnancy may show a variety of patterns of hCG rise or fall but would uncommonly show a normal rise. When doubt remains, and the clinical status of the patient does not mandate immediate invasive testing, serial hCG levels and repeat sonography may be necessary to further assess the patient's status.

Sonography is a pivotal examination in the evaluation of a patient suspected of harboring an extrauterine gestation. In a majority of cases, this diagnosis can be promptly excluded with reasonable certainty by the sonographic demonstration of an intrauterine pregnancy. Although a definitive sonographic diagnosis of the presence of an ectopic pregnancy is more commonly seen with endovaginal transducers (i.e., documentation of living extrauterine embryo or yolk sac), still the majority of ectopic pregnancies cannot be diagnosed with certainty by sonography alone. However, sonography can be employed effectively to assist in determining a patient's risk status. Concomitant measurement of hCG levels can further assist the clinician in risk assessment.

References

1. Estes JW: The practice of medicine in 18th century Massachusetts. N Engl J Med 305:1040, 1981.
2. Dorfman SF: Deaths from ectopic pregnancy, United States: 1979 to 1980. Obstet Gynecol 62:334, 1983.
3. Weinstein L, Morris MB, Dotters D, Christian CD: Ectopic pregnancy: A new surgical epidemic. Obstet Gynecol 61:698, 1983.
4. Lebolt SA, Grimes DA, Cates W: Mortality from abortion and childbirth: Are the populations comparable? JAMA 248:188, 1982.
5. Nagami M, London S, St. Amand P: Factors influencing fertility after ectopic pregnancy. Am J Obstet Gynecol 149:533, 1984.
6. Schoen JA, Nowak RJ: Repeat ectopic pregnancy: A 16-year clinical survey. Obstet Gynecol 45:542, 1975.
7. Grant A: The effect of ectopic pregnancy on fertility. Clin Obstet Gynecol 5:861, 1962.
8. James AE, Fleischer AC, Sacks GA, Greeson T: Ectopic pregnancy: A malpractice paradigm. Radiology 160:411, 1986.
9. Berlin L: Malpractice and radiologists. AJR 135:587, 1980.
10. Stempel LE: Eenie, meenie, minie, mo . . . what do the data really show? Am J Obstet Gynecol 144:745, 1982.
11. Phillips WC, Scott JA, Blaszczynski G: How sensitive is "sensitivity"; how specific is "specificity"? AJR 140:1265, 1983.
12. Breen J: A 21-year survey of 654 ectopic pregnancies. Am J Obstet Gynecol 106:1004, 1970.
13. Tancer ML, Delke I, Veridiano NP: A fifteen-year experience with ectopic pregnancy. Surg Gynecol Obstet 152:179, 1981.
14. Lawless M, Vessey M: Risk of intrauterine contraceptive devices. (Letter) Br Med J 288:1919, 1984.
15. McCausland A: High rate of ectopic pregnancy following laparoscopic tubal coagulation failures, incidence and etiology. Am J Obstet Gynecol 136:97, 1980.
16. Cartwright PS, DiPietro DL: Ectopic pregnancy: Changes in serum human chorionic gonadotropin concentration. Obstet Gynecol 63:76, 1984.
17. Brown TW, Filly RA, Laing FC, et al: Analysis of ultrasonographic criteria in the evaluation for ectopic pregnancy. AJR 131:965, 1978.
18. Bangham DR, Storring PL: Standardization of human chorionic gonadotropin hCG subunits and pregnancy tests. (Letter) Lancet 1:390, 1982.
19. Batzer FR, Weiner S, Corson SL, et al: Landmarks during the first forty-two days of gestation demonstrated by the β-subunit of human chorionic gonadotropin and ultrasound. Am J Obstet Gynecol 146:973, 1983.
20. Nyberg DA, Filly RA, Mahony BS, et al: Early gestation: correlation of hCG levels and sonographic identification. AJR 144:195, 1985.
21. Nyberg DA, Filly RA, Duarte Filho DL, et al: Abnormal pregnancy: Early diagnosis by US and serum chorionic gonadotropin levels. Radiology 158:393, 1986.
22. Nyberg DA, Laing FC, Filly RA, et al: Ectopic pregnancy: Diagnosis by sonography correlated with quantitative hCG levels. J Ultrasound Med 156:150, 1987.
23. Romero R, Kadar N, Jeanty P, et al: A prospective study of the value of the discriminatory zone in the diagnosis of ectopic pregnancy. Obstet Gynecol 66:357, 1985.
24. Batzer R: Guidelines for choosing a pregnancy test. Contemp Obstet Gynecol 30:57, 1985.
25. Romero R, Kadar N, Copel JA, et al: The effect of different human chorionic gonadotropin assay sensitivity on screening for ectopic pregnancy. Am J Obstet Gynecol 153:72, 1985.
26. Olson CM, Holt JA, Alenghat E, et al: Limitations of qualitative serum β-hCG assays in the diagnosis of ectopic pregnancy. J Reprod Med 28:838, 1983.
27. Berry CM, Thompson JD, Hatcher R: The radioreceptor assay for hCG in ectopic pregnancy. Obstet Gynecol 54:43, 1979.
28. Droegemueller W: Ectopic pregnancy. In Danforth DN (ed): Obstetrics and Gynecology, p 407. Philadelphia, Harper & Row, 1982.
29. Mahony BS, Filly RA, Nyberg DA, et al: Sonographic evaluation of ectopic pregnancy. J Ultrasound Med 4:221, 1985.
30. Lawson TL: Ectopic pregnancy: Criteria and accuracy of ultrasonic diagnosis. AJR 131:153, 1978.
31. Pedersen JF: Ultrasonic scanning in suspected ectopic pregnancy. Br J Radiol 53:1, 1980.
32. Maklad NF, Wright CH: Gray scale ultrasonography in the diagnosis of ectopic pregnancy. Radiology 126:221, 1978.
33. Subramanyam BR, Raghavendra BN, Bathazar EJ, et al: Hematosalpinx in tubal pregnancy: Sonographic-pathologic correlation. AJR 141:361, 1983.
34. Schoenbaum S, Rosendorf L, Kappelman N: Gray-scale ultrasound in tubal pregnancy. Radiology 127:757, 1978.
35. Weiner CP: The pseudogestational sac in ectopic pregnancy. Am J Obstet Gynecol 139:959, 1981.
36. Nelson P, Bowie JD, Rosenberg ER: Early intrauterine pregnancy or decidual cast: An anatomic-sonographic approach. J Ultrasound Med 2:543, 1983.
37. Bradley WG, Fiske CE, Filly RA: The double sac sign of early intrauterine pregnancy: Use in exclusion of ectopic pregnancy. Radiology 143:223, 1983.
38. Berger MJ, Taymor ML. Simultaneous intrauterine and tubal pregnancies following ovulation induction. Am J Obstet Gynecol 113:812, 1972.
39. Reece EA, Petrie RH, Sirmans MF: Combined intrauterine and extrauterine gestations: A review. Am J Obstet Gynecol 146:323, 1983.
40. Bello G, Schonholz D, Moshipor J, et al: Combined pregnancy: The Mt. Sinai experience. Obstet Gynecol Surv 41:603, 1986.
41. Sondheimer SJ, Tureck RW, Blasco L, et al: Simultaneous ectopic pregnancy with intrauterine twin gestation after in vitro fertilization and embryo transfer. Fertil Steril 43:313, 1985.
42. Hann LE, Bachman DB, McArdle CR: Coexistent intrauterine and ectopic pregnancy: A re-evaluation. Radiology 152:151, 1984.
43. Yaghoobian J, Pinck RL, Ramanathan K, et al: Sonographic demonstration of simultaneous intrauterine and extrauterine gestation. J Ultrasound Med 5:309, 1986.
44. Dimitry ES, Subak-Sharpe R, Mills M, et al: Nine cases of heterotopic pregnancies in 4 years of in vitro fertilization. Fertil Steril 53:107, 1990.
45. Molloy D, Deambrosis W, Keeping D, et al: Multi-sited (heterotopic) pregnancy after in vitro fertilization and gamete intrafallopian transfer. Fertil Steril 53:1068, 1990.

46. Marks WM, Filly RA, Callen PW, et al: The decidual cast of ectopic pregnancy: A confusing ultrasonographic appearance. Radiology 133:451, 1979.

47. Spirt BA, Ohara KR, Gordon L: Pseudogestational sac in ectopic pregnancy: Sonographic and pathologic correlation. J Clin Ultrasound 9:338, 1981.

48. Laing FC, Filly RA, Marks WM, et al: Ultrasonic demonstration of endometrial fluid collections unassociated with pregnancy. Radiology 137:471, 1980.

49. Mueller CE: Intrauterine pseudogestational sac in ectopic pregnancy. J Clin Ultrasound 7:133, 1979.

50. Abramovich H, Auslender R, Lewin A, et al: Gestational-pseudogestational sac: A new ultrasonic criterion for differential diagnosis. Am J Obstet Gynecol 145:377, 1983.

51. Nyberg DA, Laing FC, Filly RA, et al: Ultrasonographic differentiation of the gestational sac of early intrauterine pregnancy from the pseudogestational sac of ectopic pregnancy. Radiology 146:755, 1983.

52. Jain KA, Hamper UM, Sanders RC: Comparison of transvaginal and transabdominal sonography in detection of early pregnancy and it complications. AJR 151:1139, 1988.

53. Levi CS, Lyons EA, Lindsay DJ: Early diagnosis of nonviable pregnancy with endovaginal US. Radiology 167:383, 1988.

54. Bree RL, Edwards M, Bohm-Velez M, et al: Transvaginal sonography in the evaluation of normal early pregnancy: Correlations with hCG levels. AJR 153:75, 1989.

55. Cadkin AV, McAlpin J: Detection of fetal cardiac activity between 41 and 43 days' gestation. J Ultrasound Med 3:499, 1984.

56. Levi CS, Lyons EA, Zheng XH, et al: Endovaginal US: Demonstration of cardiac activity in embryos of less than 5.0 mm in crown-rump length. Radiology 176:71, 1990.

57. Russel S, Filly RA, Damato N: Sonographic diagnosis of ectopic pregnancy with EV probes: What really has changed? J Ultrasound Med 12:145, 1993.

58. Rempen A: Vaginal sonography in ectopic pregnancy: A prospective evaluation. J Ultrasound Med 7:381, 1988.

59. Nyberg DA, Laing FC, Filly RA: Threatened abortion: Sonographic distinction of normal and abnormal gestation sacs. Radiology 158:397, 1986.

60. Cadkin AV, McAlpin J: The decidua-chorionic sac: A reliable sonographic indicator of intrauterine pregnancy prior to detection of a fetal pole. J Ultrasound Med 3:539, 1984.

61. Nyberg DA, Mack LA, Brooke Jeffrey R Jr, Laing FC: Endovaginal sonographic evaluation of ectopic pregnancy: A prospective study. AJR 149:1181, 1987.

62. Pennel RG, Baltarowich OH, Kurtz AB, et al: Complicated first-trimester pregnancies: Evaluation with endovaginal US versus transabdominal technique. Radiology 165:79, 1987.

63. Filly RA: Ectopic pregnancy: The role of sonography. Radiology 162:661, 1987.

64. Timor-Tritsch IE, Rottem S: Diagnosis and management of ectopic pregnancy using transvaginal sonography. In Fredericks CM, Paulson JD, Holtz G (eds): Ectopic Pregnancy: Pathophysiology and Clinical Management, p 71. Washington, DC, Hemisphere, 1989.

65. Dashefsky SM, Lyons EA, Levi CS, Lindsay DJ: Suspected ectopic pregnancy endovaginal and transvesical US. Radiology 169:181, 1988.

66. Cacciatore B, Stenman UH, Ylostalo P: Comparison of abdominal and vaginal sonography in suspected ectopic pregnancy. Obstet Gynecol 73:770, 1989.

67. Cacciatore B: Can the status of tubal pregnancy be predicted with transvaginal sonography? A prospective comparison of sonographic, surgical, and serum hCG findings. Radiology 177:481, 1990.

68. Kadar N, DeVre G, Romero R: Discriminatory hCG zone: Its use in sonographic evaluation for ectopic pregnancy. Obstet Gynecol 58:156, 1981.

69. Nyberg DA, Mack LA, Laing FC, Jeffrey RB: Early pregnancy complications: Endovaginal sonographic findings correlated with human chorionic gonadotrophin levels. Radiology 167:619, 1988.

70. Fleischer AC, Pennell RG, McKee MS et al: Ectopic pregnancy: Features at transvaginal sonography. Radiology 174:375, 1990.

71. Emerson DS, Cartier MS, Altieri LA, et al: Diagnostic efficacy of endovaginal color Doppler flow imaging in an ectopic pregnancy screening program. Radiology 183:413, 1992.

72. Pellerito JS, Taylor KJW, Quendens-Case C, et al: Ectopic pregnancy: Evaluation with endovaginal color flow imaging. Radiology 183:407, 1992.

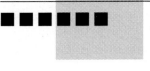

CHAPTER 33

The Role of Magnetic Resonance Imaging in the Evaluation of Gynecologic Disease

MARK J. POPOVICH, M.D.
HEDVIG HRICAK, M.D., Ph.D.

Magnetic resonance imaging (MRI) has become an important modality in the evaluation of the female pelvis. Ultrasonography remains the screening examination of choice in patients with suspected gynecologic disease, given its relative safety and lower cost.[1, 2] However, ultrasonography may be limited by technical considerations (operator dependence, patient's body habitus, low signal-to-noise ratio) and is inadequate in staging pelvic malignancies.[1, 3–5] MRI is considered the next step in the imaging assessment of benign disease and is becoming the primary modality for evaluating gynecologic malignancies.[6–36] The multiplanar imaging capability of MRI, as well as superior soft tissue contrast and large field of view, offer distinct advantages over either ultrasonography or computed tomography (CT) in the assessment of gynecologic abnormalities.

This chapter is an overview of the more common gynecologic entities as studied with MRI. The strengths of MRI in relation to ultrasonography and its role in the clinical workup of specific diseases are emphasized. A comprehensive coverage of MRI of the female pelvis is beyond the scope of this book.

MAJOR CLINICAL INDICATIONS

Although ultrasonography generally remains the initial modality used in evaluating clinically suspected gynecologic disease,[1–3] MRI can offer supplemental diagnostic information in cases of a suboptimal or equivocal ultrasound examination.

The most common indications for the use of MRI in gynecologic disease include the following:

I. Congenital Anomalies
  A. Precise diagnostic classification for obstetric counseling and treatment options
  B. Before surgical intervention
II. Leiomyomas
  A. Precise delineation of number, size, and location
  B. Type of surgery—myomectomy versus hysterectomy
  C. Question of adnexal versus uterine mass on sonography
  D. In selected patients before and after hormonal treatment
III. Adenomyosis
  A. Adenomyosis versus leiomyoma
IV. Adnexal Masses (when ultrasonography is limited)
  A. Detection
  B. Characterization
    1. Benign versus malignant
    2. Specific diagnosis (e.g., teratoma versus endometrioma)
V. Pelvic Malignancies
  A. Staging primary tumors. MRI is the primary imaging modality for cancers of the
    1. Endometrium
    2. Cervix
    3. Vagina
    4. Ovary (the role of MRI is still evolving)
  B. Detection of recurrent disease
  C. Secondary malignancies

TECHNIQUES

In general, both T1- and T2-weighted MR images are necessary to evaluate the female pelvis. T1-weighted images offer excellent contrast between the pelvic organs and adjacent fat, allow optimal depiction of lymph nodes, and are necessary for tissue and fluid characterization (essential for hemorrhagic or fat-containing lesions). T2-weighted sequences are needed to demonstrate the zonal anatomy of the uterus and vagina, as well as to facilitate identification of normal ovaries. In addition, T2-weighted images are usually superior in depicting pathologic conditions of the uterus and ovaries. Intravenous contrast media is routinely used in the evaluation of endometrial and ovarian carcinoma. Currently, in the United States gadolinium-DTPA (Gd-DTPA) is the only contrast material approved for MR imaging.

The direct multiplanar capability of MRI allows a study to be individualized to the particular clinical question. The transverse plane of imaging is routinely acquired in all cases, with additional sequences obtained in either the sagittal or the coronal plane. The sagittal plane optimizes evaluation of the uterus, while the coronal plane is sometimes preferred for studying the ovaries. Unless medically contraindicated, glucagon is routinely administered to reduce bowel peristalsis and improve image quality.

NORMAL MAGNETIC RESONANCE IMAGING APPEARANCE

Uterus

The appearance of the uterus on MRI is influenced by the age and hormonal status of the patient.[10-13] In women of reproductive age, uterine zonal anatomy is appreciated on T2-weighted or contrast-enhanced T1-weighted images, consisting of three distinct layers: the endometrium, the junctional zone, and the myometrium (Figs. 33–1 and 33–2).[11-13] The endometrium demonstrates signal intensity higher than adjacent myometrium, and its thickness varies during the menstrual cycle. The endometrium is at its thinnest at the end of menstruation, while the thickest appearance is seen during the mid-secretory phase.[11-13] During menstruation or after dilatation and curettage, a low signal intensity blood clot may be seen within the high signal intensity endometrium.[37]

The myometrium images with medium signal intensity on T2-weighted or contrast-enhanced T1-weighted images and is of relatively increased intensity in mid-secretory phase.[11-13] The junctional zone is seen as a low signal intensity stripe situated between the myometrium and the endometrium (see Figs. 33–1 and 33–2). Although there is no histologic equivalent to the junctional zone, in vitro studies indicate that it represents inner myometrium.[10, 38-40] The inner myometrium has a lower water content than the outer myometrium, a finding that is believed to account for the different signal intensity of the two zones.[38] Although three uterine zones can be delineated on ultrasound evaluation, these are not directly comparable to the zonal anatomy depicted on MRI.[41]

In premenarchal girls and postmenopausal women,

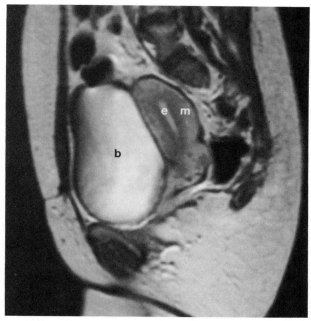

Figure 33–2. Normal uterus on contrast-enhanced T1-weighted sagittal image. The uterine zonal anatomy is discernible, consisting of the endometrium (e) and myometrium (m), separated by the low signal intensity junctional zone. The accumulation of contrast media within the urinary bladder (b) produces high signal intensity on T1-weighted images.

the MRI appearance of the uterus is similar and demonstrates several differences from women of reproductive age (Fig. 33–3). The uterine corpus is shorter in length, the endometrium is thin, and the

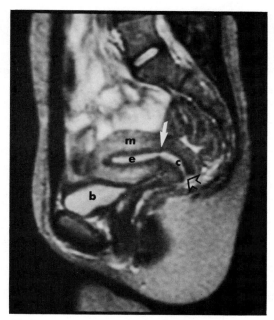

Figure 33–1. Normal uterus. Sagittal T2-weighted image. The zonal anatomy of the uterus is depicted, consisting of the endometrium (e) and myometrium (m), separated by the low signal intensity junctional zone. The cervix (c) extends from the level of the internal os (*white arrow*) to the external os (*open arrow*). b, bladder.

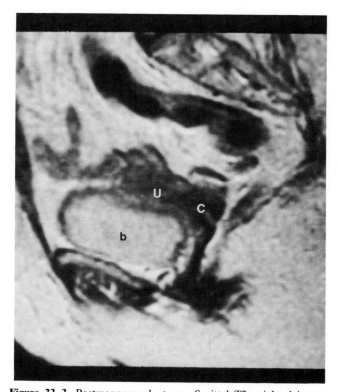

Figure 33–3. Postmenopausal uterus. Sagittal T2-weighted image. The uterus (U) is small, with the cervix (C) accounting for a larger proportion of uterine length. The myometrium is of low signal intensity with indistinct zonal anatomy. b, bladder.

zonal anatomy is often indistinct with comparatively lower signal intensity of the myometrium.[6, 11, 42]

In addition to reproductive status and patient age, exogenous hormonal therapy may affect the appearance of the uterus on MRI. In women taking oral contraceptives, the myometrium is of higher than normal signal intensity.[11, 13] The hypoestrogenic state caused by gonadotropin-releasing hormone analogues (i.e., leuprolide [Lupron]) leads to an MRI appearance of the uterus mimicking that of a postmenopausal woman.[43] In a postmenopausal woman taking estrogen replacement therapy, the uterus appears similar to that of a woman of reproductive age, with clear definition of the three uterine zones.[11]

Intrauterine devices can be safely imaged with MRI, and their presence does not create artifacts that impede image interpretation.[31] All intrauterine devices demonstrate low signal intensity on both T1- and T2-weighted images, although their configuration varies with the type of device.[31] Ultrasonography remains the primary modality for documenting the location of an intrauterine device.

Cervix

Zonal anatomy of the cervix can be appreciated on T2-weighted or contrast-enhanced T1-weighted images (see Fig. 33–1). The normal cervix demonstrates a central area of high signal intensity (endocervical glands and mucus) surrounded by low signal intensity stroma (elastic fibrous tissue).[6–11] Around the periphery of the cervix smooth muscle predominates, resulting in a rim of medium signal intensity similar to that of myometrium.[44, 45]

Vagina

As with the uterus and cervix, vaginal anatomy is most readily appreciated on T2-weighted or contrast-enhanced T1-weighted images (Fig. 33–4). The central high signal intensity of the vaginal mucosa is contrasted to surrounding low signal intensity of the vaginal wall. The MRI appearance of the vagina changes during the menstrual cycle.[29] Additionally, premenarchal or post-

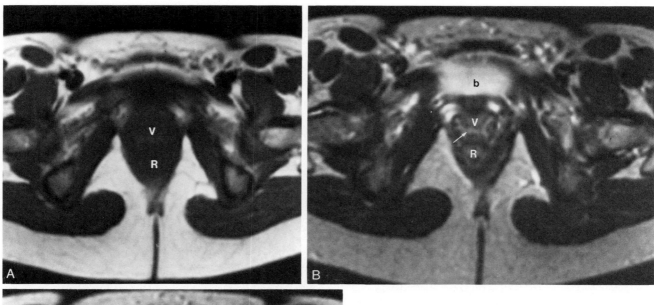

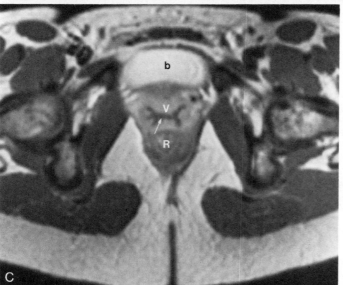

Figure 33–4. Normal vagina. Transaxial T1-weighted (A), T2-weighted (B), and contrast-enhanced T1-weighted (C) images. The vagina (V) is located between the bladder (b) and rectum (R). Although the vagina is of intermediate signal intensity on the T1-weighted image (A), both the T2-weighted (B) and contrast-enhanced T1-weighted (C) images demonstrate vaginal zonal anatomy with differentiation between the wall and the intraepithelial part (arrow).

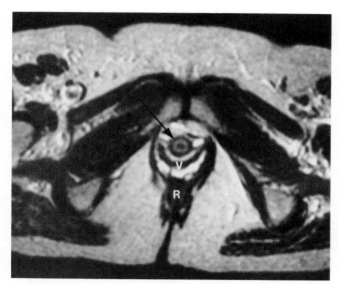

Figure 33–5. Postmenopausal vagina. Transaxial T2-weighted image demonstrates the uniform low signal intensity vagina (V) (lacking the high signal intensity mucosal lining seen in women of reproductive age) located between the urethra (*arrow*) and the rectum (R) posteriorly.

menopausal females demonstrate a thin or absent central high signal intensity stripe (Fig. 33–5). However, the MRI appearance of the vagina in postmenopausal women on estrogen replacement therapy is similar to that of women of reproductive age.[29]

Ovaries

Normal ovaries are of intermediate signal intensity on T1-weighted images and increase in signal intensity on T2-weighted sequences (Fig. 33–6). In women of reproductive age, MRI can identify normal ovaries in 87% to 96% of cases.[25, 46] Contrast administration facilitates detection of the ovaries, since ovarian tissue enhances while small follicular cysts do not.[47]

PATHOLOGIC CONDITIONS

Uterus

CONGENITAL ANOMALIES

Müllerian duct anomalies result from nondevelopment or varying degrees of nonfusion of the müllerian ducts. These occur in 1% to 15% of women.[48] Müllerian duct anomalies are associated with menstrual disorders, infertility, and obstetric complications.[49] Furthermore, renal anomalies (especially agenesis or ectopia) may be present in up to 50% of these patients. The clinical classification of müllerian duct anomalies follow the guidelines proposed by Buttram and Gibbons.[50]

Evaluation of müllerian duct anomalies with physical examination and imaging studies (hysterosalpingography and ultrasonography) is often inconclusive.[51, 52] Before the advent of MRI, laparoscopy or surgery was often necessary for proper diagnosis and classification of these abnormalities. MRI has proven to be an accurate and noninvasive means of evaluating patients with congenital anomalies,[53–60] allowing precise classification and demonstration of associated complications.

Uterine agenesis or hypoplasia results from nondevelopment or rudimentary development of the müllerian ducts. The T2-weighted sagittal images are most useful

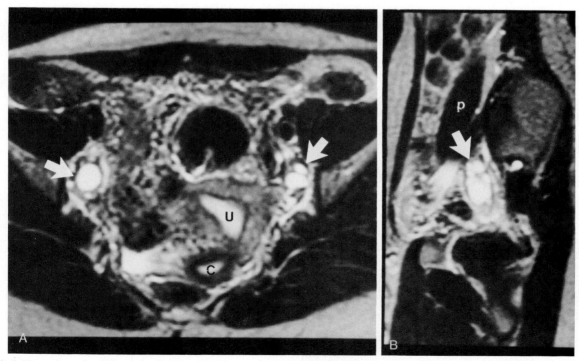

Figure 33–6. Normal ovaries. T2-weighted transaxial (*A*) and sagittal (*B*) images in a woman of reproductive age. Both ovaries (*arrows*) are identified containing several small follicular cysts, which are of high signal intensity. Zonal anatomy of the uterus (U) and cervix (C) are well shown. p, psoas muscle.

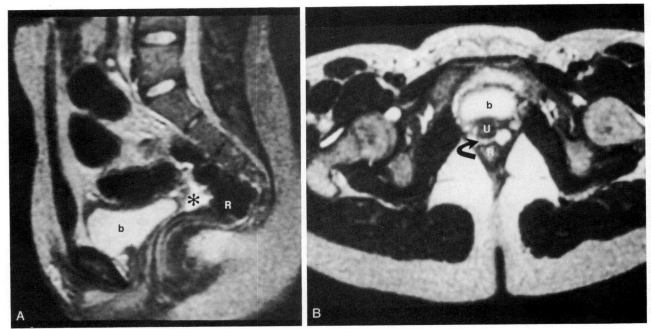

Figure 33–7. Uterine and vaginal agenesis—Mayer-Rokitansky-Küster-Hauser syndrome. T2-weighted sagittal (*A*) and transaxial (*B*) images in an 18-year-old woman with primary amenorrhea. *A*. The sagittal image demonstrates absence of normal uterine or cervical tissue in the expected location (*asterisk*), between the bladder (b) and rectum (R). *B*. The transaxial image demonstrates absence of any vaginal tissue (*arrow*) between the urethra (U) and rectum (R). b, bladder.

for identifying the presence of a uterus. The main advantage of MRI compared with other modalities relates to the ability to differentiate complete from segmental uterine agenesis. A subtype of uterine agenesis, termed the Mayer-Rokitansky-Küster-Hauser syndrome, is accurately displayed on MRI (Fig. 33–7). In these patients, complete absence of the uterus and upper vagina, with varying degrees of development of the lower vagina, is consistently seen on a combination of sagittal and transaxial images.[29, 59] Normal ovaries are usually present. Uterine hypoplasia is diagnosed when the uterus is small in size and the myometrium is of lower than normal signal intensity.

A unicornuate uterus results from nondevelopment or rudimentary development of one müllerian duct. Three subtypes of this anomaly are classified on the basis of the presence of a rudimentary horn and whether it contains endometrium and communicates with the main uterine cavity. The characteristic appearance of the banana-shaped uterine cavity is seen on MRI, with normal dimensions of the endometrium and myometrium (Fig. 33–8). If a rudimentary horn is present, MRI can usually distinguish it from an adnexal mass suspected on ultrasound evaluation as well as determine if there is endometrium contained within it.

The didelphys uterus results from nonfusion of the

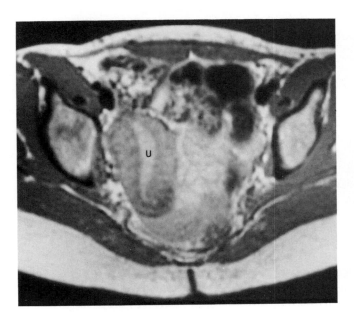

Figure 33–8. Unicornuate uterus. Transaxial proton density image. The uterus (U) has a banana-shaped configuration with normal endometrial and myometrial widths. (From Hricak H, Popovich MJ: The uterus and vagina. In Higgins CB, Hricak H, Helms CA [eds]: Magnetic Resonance Imaging of the Body, 2nd ed, p 831. New York, Raven Press, 1992.)

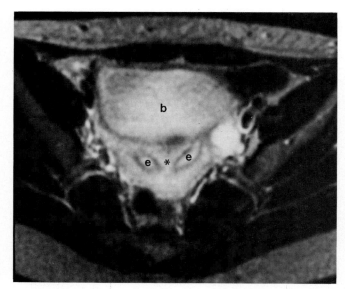

Figure 33–9. Bicornuate uterus. Transaxial T2-weighted image. There are two uterine horns, each containing an endometrial cavity (e). The high signal intensity tissue (*asterisk*) separating the endometrial cavities is composed of myometrium. b, bladder. (From Hricak H, Popovich MJ: The uterus and vagina. In Higgins CB, Hricak H, Helms CA [eds]: Magnetic Resonance Imaging of the Body, 2nd ed, p 832. New York, Raven Press, 1992.)

two müllerian ducts. Two separate normal-sized uteri and cervices are demonstrated on MRI, with a septum extending into the upper vagina. The two uteri are usually widely separated with preservation of the endometrial and myometrial widths.

Partial fusion of the müllerian ducts produces the bicornuate uterus (Fig. 33–9). The resulting septum is composed of myometrium. While the myometrial septum may only project into the uterine cavity, it may extend to the internal os (bicornuate unicollis) or as far as the external os (bicornuate bicollis). MRI often demonstrates an outward fundal concavity as opposed to the normal convexity, with two endometrial cavities separated by myometrium.

Septate uterus is due to incomplete resorption of the final fibrous septum between the two müllerian ducts. The fundal contour is normal (convex), and, in addition, the uterine septum is of low signal intensity on both T1- and T2-weighted images (Fig. 33–10) (in contrast to the medium to high signal intensity myometrium separating the two endometrial cavities in the bicornuate uterus). The differentiation between this entity and the bicornuate uterus is clinically significant, since each is treated with a different surgical procedure.

LEIOMYOMAS

Leiomyomas are the most common uterine tumors. They are found in up to 40% of women in their reproductive years.[42] Although ultrasonography is typically the initial radiologic evaluation of these patients, there is a false-negative rate of up to 20% in detecting these tumors with sonography.[61] Sonographic limitations include uterine orientation (e.g., retroflexed uterus), concurrent uterine or adnexal abnormalities,

and small tumor size.[1, 2, 61, 62] MRI provides more precise information than that available from ultrasonography.[14, 15, 46] MRI is not limited by the location or size of the leiomyomas, with tumors as small as 5 mm being accurately demonstrated.[15, 46]

MRI is indicated when the ultrasound examination is indeterminate or limited.[63] It is useful in patients considered for myomectomy, allowing precise determination of the location and number of leiomyomas.[15, 46, 63, 64] MRI facilitates differentiation of a pedunculated leiomyoma from an adnexal mass. The effects of hormonal therapy on leiomyomas can be monitored.[43, 65, 66] MRI is the only noninvasive means available for differentiating a leiomyoma from adenomyosis,[16, 67, 68] an important clinical distinction since each requires a different surgical procedure.

On T1-weighted images, leiomyomas present as well-circumscribed, rounded lesions with intermediate signal intensity, often indistinguishable from adjacent myometrium. Optimum contrast is achieved on T2-weighted images, where the tumor is of lower signal intensity relative to the myometrium or endometrium (Figs. 33–11 and 33–12).[14, 15, 67, 69] The presence of calcifications usually causes areas of signal void on both T1- and T2-weighted images, but the finding (unlike CT) is not specific. A variety of degenerative processes can alter the characteristic appearance of a leiomyoma (Figs. 33–13 and 33–14). For example, the most common hyaline degeneration produces a "cobblestone" appearance, while rapid growth during pregnancy leading to muscle infarction (red or carneous degeneration) produces a tumor of high signal intensity on T1- and/or T2-weighted sequences.[67]

The vast majority of leiomyomas are found within the uterine corpus (90%), with a small proportion found within the cervix or broad ligament. MRI further allows precise classification by location within the uter-

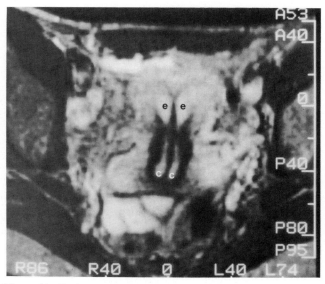

Figure 33–10. Septate uterus. Transaxial T2-weighted image demonstrates a low signal intensity fibrous septum separating the two endometrial cavities (e). The septum extends down to the level of the external cervical os, producing two separate cervical canals (c).

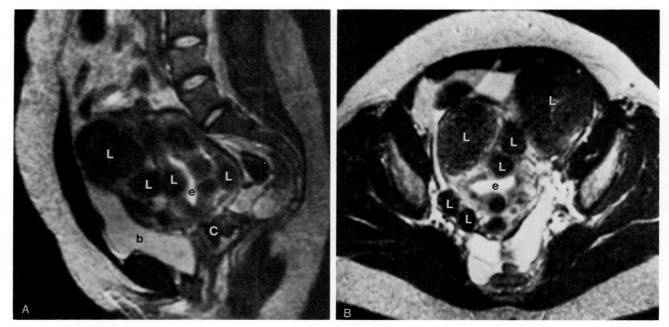

Figure 33–11. Multiple leiomyomas. T2-weighted sagittal (*A*) and transaxial (*B*) images. Multiple rounded, well-defined low signal intensity leiomyomas (L) are demonstrated, contrasting to the higher signal intensity of the myometrium. The endometrial cavity (e) is distorted by the presence of these tumors. c, cervix; b, bladder.

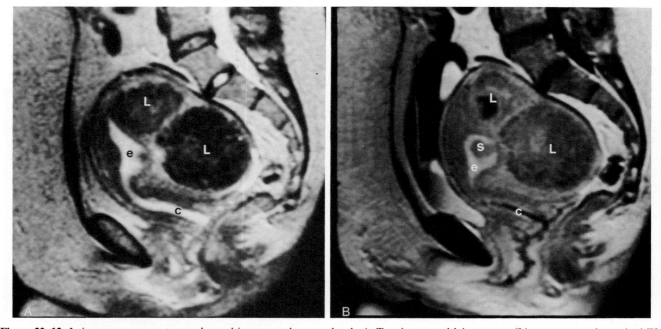

Figure 33–12. Leiomyomas on contrast-enhanced images at the same level. *A.* Two intramural leiomyomas (L) are seen on the sagittal T2-weighted image. *B.* The tumors demonstrate various degrees of enhancement on contrast-enhancement scan. The submucosal leiomyoma (s) protruding into the endometrial cavity (e) is more clearly evident. c, cervix.

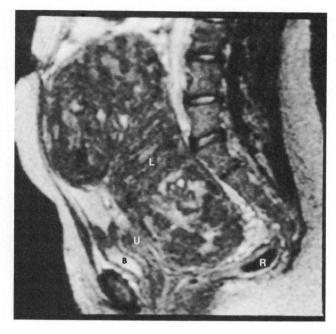

Figure 33–13. Large degenerative leiomyoma. Sagittal T2-weighted image demonstrates a large leiomyoma (L) extending above the level of the umbilicus. The tumor arises from the posterior wall of the uterus (U). The heterogeneous cobblestone appearance of the leiomyoma is consistent with hyaline degeneration. B, bladder; R, rectum.

ine wall.[15, 46, 63, 64] Submucosal leiomyomas protrude into the endometrial cavity (Figs. 33–12, 33–15, and 33–16). Intramural lesions are centered within the myometrium (see Fig. 33–14). Subserosal tumors are largely centered outside the uterus and may be pedunculated (see Figs. 33–13 and 33–17).

ADENOMYOSIS

Adenomyosis is defined as the presence of endometrial tissue (basalis layer) within the myometrium.[42] It is found in 15% to 27% of hysterectomy specimens,[42, 70] with an increased incidence in multiparous women. The symptoms and physical findings of adenomyosis are varied, frequently mimicking those seen with leiomyomas.[42, 70] Before the advent of MRI, the diagnosis could only be made at surgery, since it is not possible to differentiate adenomyosis from leiomyomas clinically or sonographically.

MRI is the examination of choice in the evaluation of suspected adenomyosis. The accuracy of MRI in distinguishing adenomyosis from leiomyomas has been reported as high as 90%.[16, 67] Although MRI can accurately diagnose diffuse adenomyosis, the differentiation of a focal adenomyoma from a leiomyoma may be difficult and the two entities may look alike.[16] Although the distinction between adenomyosis and leiomyomas may not be important in patients opting for hysterectomy, MRI does play a role in cases in which uterine-preserving surgery is contemplated. Leiomyomas can be excised by myomectomy, but adenomyosis can only be treated by hysterectomy.

There are two forms of adenomyosis: diffuse and focal. In diffuse adenomyosis, the uterus demonstrates

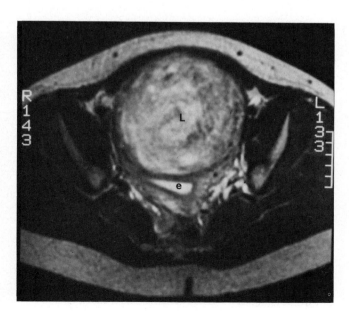

Figure 33–14. Degenerative leiomyoma. Transaxial T2-weighted image demonstrates a leiomyoma (L) of heterogeneous high signal intensity. This tumor is intramural in location. e, endometrial cavity.

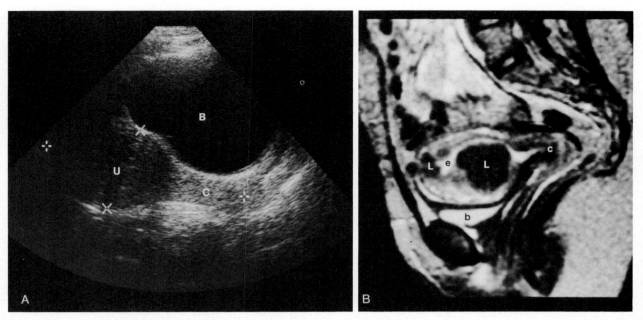

Figure 33–15. Submucosal leiomyoma. *A,* Sagittal transabdominal sonogram reveals a diffusely enlarged uterine body (U). c, cervix; B, bladder. *B.* On the sagittal T2-weighted image there is clear delineation of a large submucosal leiomyoma (L) projecting into the endometrial cavity (e). Several other small leiomyomas are also present in the uterine fundus. b, bladder; c, cervix.

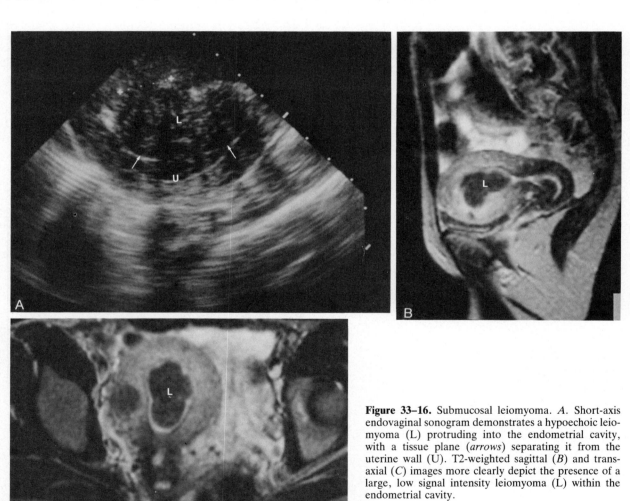

Figure 33–16. Submucosal leiomyoma. *A.* Short-axis endovaginal sonogram demonstrates a hypoechoic leiomyoma (L) protruding into the endometrial cavity, with a tissue plane (*arrows*) separating it from the uterine wall (U). T2-weighted sagittal (*B*) and transaxial (*C*) images more clearly depict the presence of a large, low signal intensity leiomyoma (L) within the endometrial cavity.

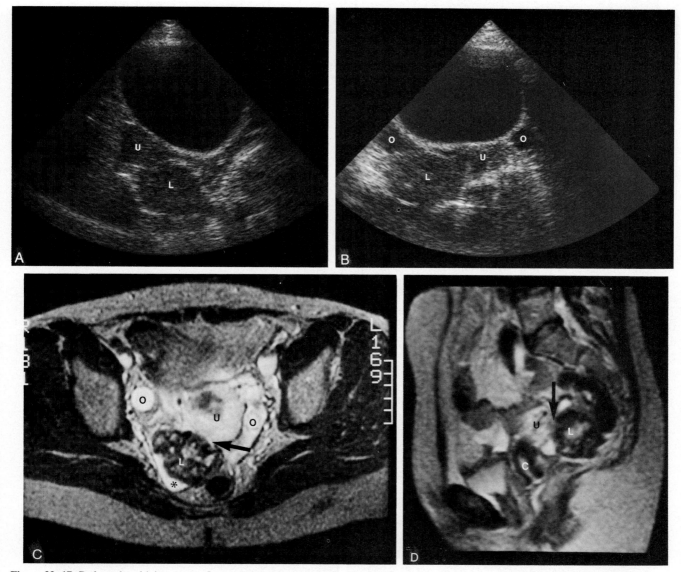

Figure 33–17. Pedunculated leiomyoma. On transabdominal sagittal (*A*) and transverse axial (*B*) sonograms a mass (L) was identified to the right and posterior of the uterus, but it could not be confidently determined if the origin was from the uterus (U) or ovary (O). On T2-weighted transaxial (*C*) and sagittal (*D*) images a connection (*arrow*) between the leiomyoma (L) and uterus (U) is seen. Additionally, the MR images show both ovaries (O) to be separate from the lesion. Asterisk indicates cul-de-sac fluid. C, cervix.

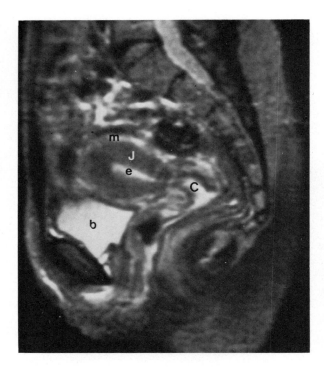

Figure 33–18. Diffuse adenomyosis. Sagittal T2-weighted image. There is widening of the low signal intensity junctional zone (J), separating the myometrium (m) from the endometrium (e). b, bladder; C, cervix.

varying degrees of diffuse enlargement. On T2-weighted images, the low signal intensity junctional zone is thickened either diffusely or segmentally and extends peripherally into the myometrium (Fig. 33–18).[16] Foci of high signal intensity may be seen within the adenomyosis.[16, 68] When present on both T1- and T2-weighted sequences these foci are believed to represent hemorrhage, while if only present on T2-weighted images they are thought to represent endometrial tissue.[68]

Focal adenomyosis (adenomyoma) presents as a mass of low signal intensity on T2-weighted images (Fig. 33–19). Differentiation between an adenomyoma and a leiomyoma depends on the configuration and margin of the lesion.[16, 67, 68] Focal adenomyosis is often oval, compared with the rounded appearance of a

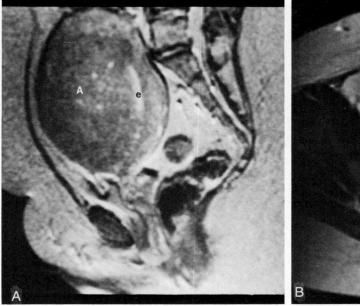

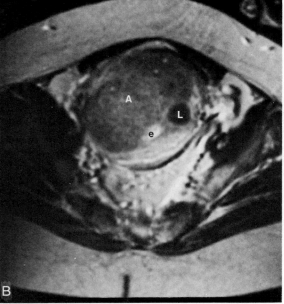

Figure 33–19. Focal adenomyosis (adenomyoma). T2-weighted sagittal (A) and transaxial (B) images in a woman with an enlarged uterus on clinical examination. Focal adenomyosis (A) is characterized by an oval area of low signal intensity, with poorly defined margins. This appearance differs from the more rounded, well-defined low signal intensity appearance of a leiomyoma (L). High signal intensity foci within the adenomyoma represent endometrial tissue. Note the distortion of the endometrial cavity (e) by the adenomyoma.

leiomyoma. An adenomyoma demonstrates an irregular and/or ill-defined margin at its interface with the myometrium, in contrast to the usually sharply defined margin of a leiomyoma. However, sometimes a leiomyoma may have indistinct margins and in this case the two conditions may be difficult to differentiate.[16]

ENDOMETRIAL CARCINOMA

Endometrial carcinoma is the fourth most common female cancer and most commonly presents as postmenopausal bleeding. The disease occurs more frequently in white women and is associated with unopposed estrogen intake, nulliparity, obesity, diabetes, and the Stein-Levanthal syndrome.

These tumors can be either localized or diffuse. Tumor spread initially occurs through the myometrium (involving both corpus and cervix), followed by extrauterine extension and involvement of adjacent organs. If the tumor secondarily obstructs the cervical canal, hematometra or pyometra may occur. The prognosis of endometrial carcinoma depends on a number of factors, including stage, depth of myometrial invasion, lymphadenopathy, and grade.[71-73] Determination of the depth of myometrial invasion is important, since it correlates with the incidence of lymph node metastases.[72-74]

Although surgical staging is the most accurate method of disease assessment,[75, 76] radiographic staging has also been employed. Transabdominal ultrasonography is considered unreliable in staging endometrial carcinoma.[3, 77, 78] The use of endovaginal sonography has shown promise in the evaluation of myometrial invasion,[78, 79] with one report achieving an accuracy of 87%.[79] MRI has been found highly accurate in staging endometrial carcinoma.[18, 19, 80-88] The overall staging accuracy has been reported between 83% and 92%.[19, 81]

The primary strengths of MRI are in the evaluation of depth of myometrial invasion, extension into the cervix, and detection of extrauterine disease.[19, 81, 82, 88]

MRI is not useful in the detection of endometrial carcinoma and histologic diagnosis is required. The signal intensity of endometrial carcinoma is often similar to normal high intensity endometrium on T2-weighted images (Fig. 33–20).[19, 80, 81] Indirect signs of endometrial tumor include widening or lobularity of the endometrial canal.[18, 19, 80-86] After the administration of contrast media there is improved contrast between tumor and normal endometrium, resulting in improved tumor detection. Furthermore, contrast-enhanced images allow differentiation of tumor mass from fluid or necrosis, providing a more accurate assessment of tumor volume and improved staging accuracy (see Fig. 33–20).[47, 87]

The MRI staging classification of endometrial carcinoma follows the surgical International Federation of Gynecologists and Obstetricians (FIGO) staging system,[76] evaluating depth of myometrial invasion and lymph node metastases. Stage I disease is confined to the uterine corpus and subdivided depending on the degree of myometrial invasion—confined to the endometrium (IA), inner half of myometrium invaded (IB), and outer half of myometrium invaded (IC). The most reliable finding on MRI indicating myometrial invasion is disruption of the junctional zone. Tumors are considered confined to the endometrium (stage IA) when the junctional zone is preserved (Figs. 33–20 and 33–21). The differentiation of invasive disease (stage IB from stage IC) is determined by the depth of tumor extension into the myometrium—inner half versus outer half (Fig. 33–22). Tumor extension into the cervix (stage II) or extrauterine disease (stages III and IV) can be accurately assessed with MRI (Fig. 33–23). The ability of MRI to detect involved pelvic lymph nodes is similar to that of CT.

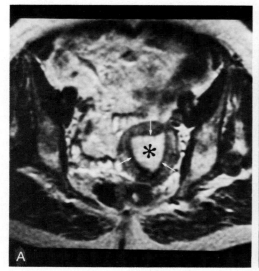 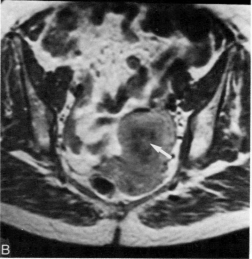

Figure 33–20. Endometrial carcinoma stage IA—tumor confined to the endometrium. Oblique off-axis T2-weighted (*A*) and contrast-enhanced T1-weighted (*B*) images. On the T2-weighted sequence, diffuse high signal intensity within the endometrial cavity (*asterisk*) prevents differentiation of tumor from normal endometrial tissue. Contrast-enhanced images (*B*) allow distinction of enhancing tumor (*large arrow*) from nonenhancing fluid or debris. The junctional zone remains intact (*small arrows*), excluding the presence of myometrial invasion.

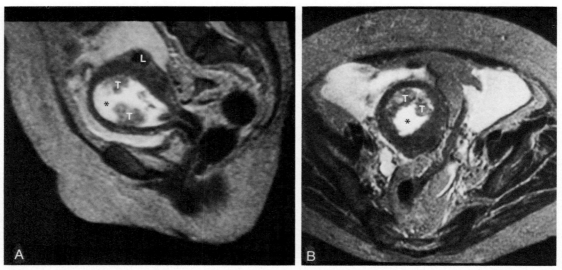

Figure 33–21. Endometrial carcinoma stage IA—tumor confined to the endometrium. T2-weighted sagittal (*A*) and transaxial (*B*) images. Multiple polypoid tumors (T) are present within the distended, fluid-filled endometrial cavity (*asterisk*). L, leiomyoma.

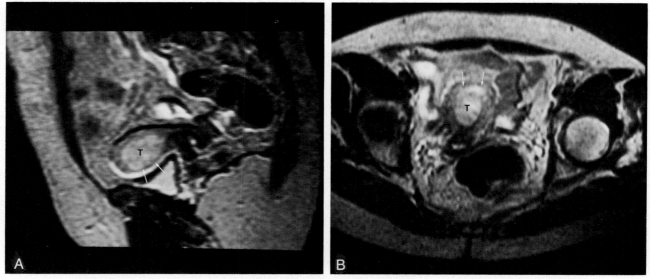

Figure 33–22. Endometrial carcinoma stage IC—tumor invading the outer half of the myometrium. T2-weighted sagittal (*A*) and transaxial (*B*) images. The endometrial tumor (T) distends the uterine cavity and violates the junctional zone, with high signal intensity tumor extending into the outer half of the myometrium (*arrows*).

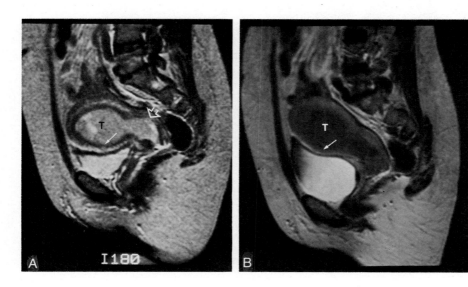

Figure 33–23. Endometrial carcinoma stage II—tumor invading the cervix. Sagittal T2-weighted (*A*) and contrast-enhanced T1-weighted (*B*) images. A large endometrial tumor (T) distends the endometrial cavity and extends into the cervical canal. Violation of the junctional zone and deep invasion of the myometrium is seen anteriorly (*small arrow*). In addition, there is invasion into the cervix (*open arrow*). (With permission from Hricak H, Popovich MJ: The uterus and vagina. In Higgins CB, Hricak H, Helms CA [eds]: Magnetic Resonance Imaging of the Body, 2nd ed, p 852. New York, Raven Press, 1992.)

Cervix

CERVICAL INCOMPETENCE

Cervical incompetence is responsible for approximately 15% of second- and third-trimester abortions. Primary incompetence may be congenital, associated with diethylstilbestrol exposure, or caused by reduced collagen within the cervix. Secondary incompetence usually results from multiple gestations, gynecologic/obstetric trauma, or increased prostaglandin production.[89]

Ultrasonography is currently the modality of choice for diagnosing cervical incompetence during pregnancy. A number of sonographic parameters have been described to indicate cervical incompetence[90]; however, no data are available on this diagnosis in the nonpregnant female. MRI offers the potential to make the diagnosis of cervical incompetence, both in the pregnant and nonpregnant patient.[45]

Four MRI findings have been described as suggestive of cervical incompetence.[45] These include (1) shortening of the endocervical canal (less than 3 cm), (2) widening of the internal cervical os (greater than 4 mm), (3) asymmetric widening of the endocervical canal, and (4) thinning or absence of the low signal intensity cervical stroma. When these findings are present, alone or in combination, cervical incompetence is suspected (Fig. 33–24).

CERVICAL CARCINOMA

Cervical carcinoma is the third most common gynecologic malignancy, but it is the most common malig-

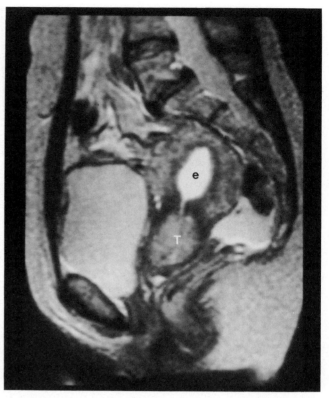

Figure 33–25. Cervical carcinoma stage IB. Sagittal T2-weighted image demonstrates a high signal intensity endocervical tumor (T), causing secondary obstruction of the endometrial cavity (e). The tumor is confined to the cervix, with low signal intensity cervical stroma seen around the periphery of the lesion.

nancy in women younger than 50 years of age. Patients most often present with vaginal bleeding or discharge. Accurate tumor staging is important not only for prognosis but also in determining appropriate therapy. The prognosis is determined by a number of factors, but among the most critical morphologic factors are tumor size, depth of stromal invasion, parametrial extension, and lymph node involvement.[72, 91, 92]

MRI has been shown to be the optimal modality for staging cervical carcinoma, with an overall staging accuracy of between 80% and 90%.[20, 93–96] Correlation with pathologic specimens has shown that MRI accurately determines the size of cervical tumors.[87] The most important staging factor that influences treatment is the presence of parametrial invasion, and the accuracy of MRI in evaluating this parameter has been shown to be approximately 90%.[20, 93, 96–99] MRI also shows promise in monitoring tumor response to preoperative chemotherapy in those patients with invasive cervical carcinoma.[99]

The appearance of cervical carcinoma on T2-weighted images is that of an abnormal area of high signal intensity, contrasted to the normal low signal intensity cervical stroma (Fig. 33–25).[20, 23, 93] MRI tumor staging follows the FIGO staging guidelines.[76] Stage I tumors are confined to the cervix and/or uterine corpus (see Fig. 33–25). These tumors may be restricted to the endocervical canal or have varying degrees of invasion into the low signal intensity cervical stroma. Cervical carcinoma extending beyond the

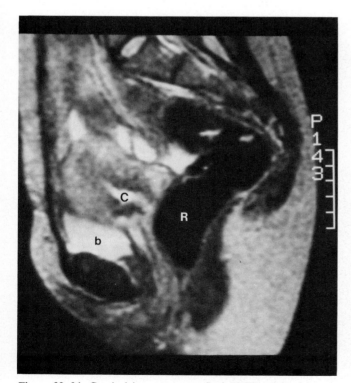

Figure 33–24. Cervical incompetence. Sagittal T2-weighted image. There is shortening of the endocervical canal (C) with asymmetric widening at the level of the internal cervical os. b, bladder; R, rectum.

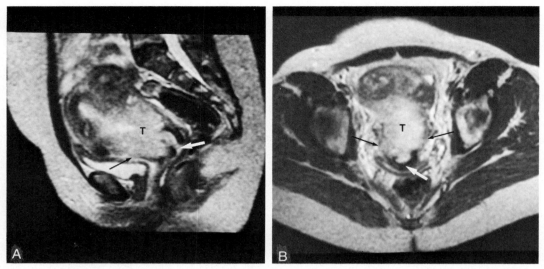

Figure 33–26. Cervical carcinoma stage IIB. T2-weighted sagittal (*A*) and transaxial (*B*) images. The high signal intensity cervical tumor (T) extends into the uterine corpus, while the external cervical os (*white arrow*) remains uninvolved. There is full thickness invasion of the low signal intensity cervical stroma, with bilateral parametrial extension (*black arrows*).

uterus indicates stage II disease, either into the upper vagina (stage IIA) or parametrial invasion (stage IIB) (Figs. 33–26 and 33–27). Stage IIB disease is indicated by complete disruption of the low signal intensity cervical stroma and abnormal tumor mass/signal intensity in the paracervical region.[20, 93, 96] The multiplanar imaging capability of MRI improves evaluation of higher stage tumors, where involvement of the lower vagina (stage IIIA), pelvic sidewall (stage IIIB), and bladder or rectum (stage IVA) can be readily appreciated (Fig. 33–28).[20, 93, 96] Although the use of contrast material does not improve accuracy in evaluating lower stage tumors,[87] contrast-enhanced images are helpful in assessing advanced disease, particularly when the bladder or rectum is involved. The presence of metastatic lymphadenopathy denotes stage IVB disease (Fig. 33–29).

Vagina

VAGINAL MALIGNANCIES

Primary malignancies of the vagina are uncommon, accounting for less than 2% of gynecologic neoplasms.

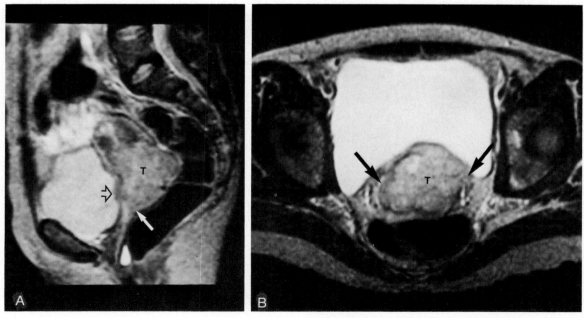

Figure 33–27. Cervical carcinoma stage IVA. T2-weighted sagittal (*A*) and transaxial (*B*) images. The high signal intensity cervical tumor (T) involves the entire cervix as well as extending into the uterine corpus. Additionally, tumor extends into the upper vagina (*white arrow*). There is also full thickness stromal invasion, bilateral parametrial extension (*black arrows*), and direct tumor invasion of the urinary bladder (*open arrow*).

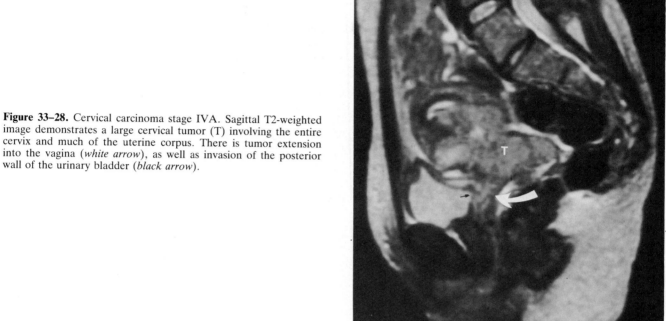

Figure 33–28. Cervical carcinoma stage IVA. Sagittal T2-weighted image demonstrates a large cervical tumor (T) involving the entire cervix and much of the uterine corpus. There is tumor extension into the vagina (*white arrow*), as well as invasion of the posterior wall of the urinary bladder (*black arrow*).

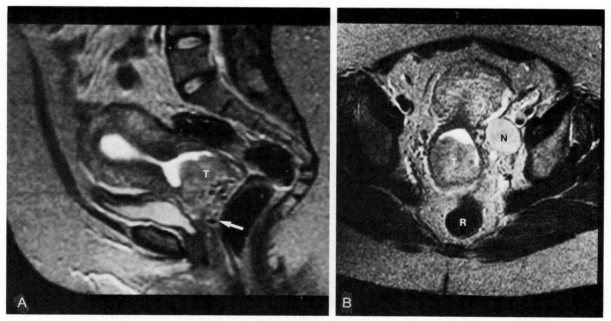

Figure 33–29. Cervical carcinoma stage IVB. T2-weighted sagittal (*A*) and transaxial (*B*) images. The endocervical tumor (T) distends the cervical canal, with extension into the upper vagina (*arrow*). The presence of external iliac lymphadenopathy (N) designates this as stage IVB disease. R, rectum.

There is an increased incidence of clear cell carcinoma in patients with a diethylstilbestrol exposure history.[100] Patients typically present with bleeding, discharge, or pain. Metastatic tumors to the vagina are more common than primary tumors. The most common primary sites of metastasis to the vagina are from the endometrium and cervix, followed by the colon, kidney, and melanoma.[101-103]

The diagnosis of vaginal carcinoma is made primarily by clinical means. Thus, the main role of MRI is not in primary diagnosis but rather in determining the stage and extent of the tumor.[29, 104] Primary tumors of the vagina cannot be differentiated from metastatic tumors on MRI. On T2-weighted images, a medium-to-high signal intensity ill-defined mass represents the vaginal neoplasm (Fig. 33–30).

As in carcinoma of the endometrium and cervix, MRI staging of vaginal carcinoma follows the FIGO staging system.[76] Superficial vaginal tumors (stage I) can be distinguished from extravaginal tumors (stage II) by the presence of tumor extending into the paravaginal tissue. Tumor invasion of the pelvic sidewall muscles is seen in stage III disease. Involvement of the urinary bladder denotes stage IV. Frequently there is formation of a vesicovaginal fistula, the presence of which can be confirmed with the use of intravenous contrast media.

Ovaries

The detection and characterization of ovarian masses is a continuing clinical and radiographic challenge. The sensitivity of MRI in detecting adnexal lesions (87% to 100%) is slightly superior to that of ultrasonography (86% to 92%).[36, 105–107] In the characterization of adnexal masses, MRI also has a higher accuracy than ultrasonography, reported to range from 60% to 95% compared with 53% to 88%, respectively.[36, 107–109] So-

nographic criteria have been described to differentiate a simple benign cyst from other complex masses. These include a well-defined smooth cyst outline, thin wall, anechoic contents, and few or no septations.[110–112] Recently, similar guidelines have been described using MRI to differentiate benign from malignant ovarian lesions.[36] In addition to primary lesion characteristics (similar to those of ultrasonography), additional secondary findings suggestive of malignancy include ascites, adenopathy, pelvic sidewall involvement, or involvement of the peritoneum, mesentery, or omentum. When all of these criteria were used, MRI was found to be 95% accurate in differentiating benign from malignant ovarian lesions.[36]

ENDOMETRIOSIS

Endometriosis is defined as the presence of secretory endometrium in an ectopic location.[113] It is seen most commonly in women between 30 and 40 years of age and affects up to 40% of infertile women.[114] There is an increased incidence in patients with müllerian duct anomalies. The most common sites for endometriosis are the ovaries, which are involved in two thirds of patients, frequently bilaterally. Patients usually complain of dysmenorrhea and other symptoms specifically referable to involved organs. The severity of symptoms does not correlate with the extent of endometriosis.

Foci of endometriosis may enlarge to produce nodules (implants) or cysts. Internal hemorrhage within a nodule of endometriosis produces an endometrial cyst (endometrioma). Dense fibrous adhesions frequently accompany endometriosis, often resulting in fixation of adjacent structures. A rare complication of endometriosis is the development of a malignant neoplasm within an ovarian endometrioma.

Although ultrasonography can identify the presence of an adnexal lesion, it is sometimes unable to provide confident differentiation of an endometrioma from

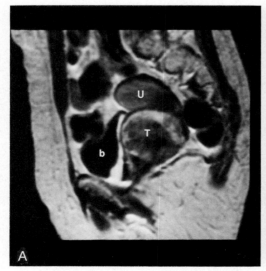
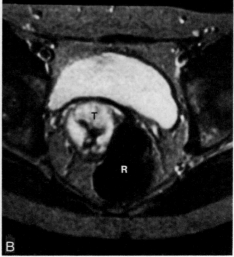

Figure 33–30. Vaginal sarcoma. Sagittal contrast-enhanced T1-weighted (*A*) and transaxial T2-weighted (*B*) images. There is a large tumor mass (T) originating from the vaginal fornix, displacing the uterus (U) superiorly. The mass abuts but does not invade either the bladder (b) or the rectum (R).

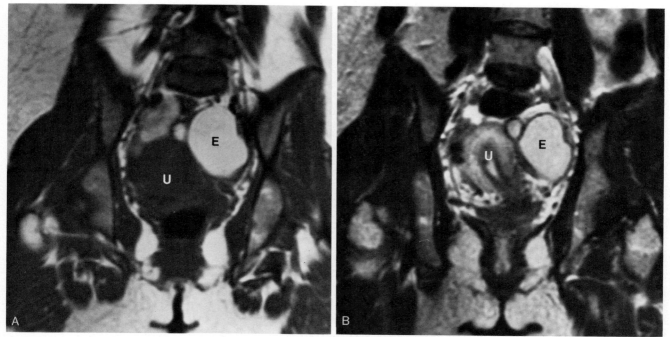

Figure 33–31. Endometrioma. Coronal T1-weighted (*A*) and T2-weighted (*B*) images. On the T1-weighted image, the endometrioma (E) is of high signal intensity consistent with hemorrhage. The endometrioma demonstrates multilocularity and an indistinct interface with the adjacent uterus (U).

other adnexal masses.[115–117] Furthermore, sonography is insensitive in evaluating endometrial implants or adhesions or in detecting diffuse forms of endometriosis.[114] MRI is the most sensitive (approximately 70%) modality for the diagnosis of endometriosis[118, 119] and the most accurate means (96%) of differentiating an endometrioma from other gynecologic masses.[120] Although MRI is useful in demonstrating endometriomas, ovarian adhesions, and some extraperitoneal endometrial implants, extraovarian adhesions and intraperitoneal implants cannot be reliably visualized.[119] As a result, laparoscopy remains the primary means of staging endometriosis.

Endometriosis produces three distinct appearances on MRI, namely, ovarian endometriomas, endometrial implants, and adhesions.

Endometriomas. Endometriomas are typically multiloculated and thin walled, with variable signal intensity depending on the age of the hemorrhage (Figs. 33–31 and 33–32). A number of characteristic MRI appearances have been ascribed to endometriomas.[26, 119–121] Specific findings include (1) presence of a loculus with hemorrhagic fluid (high signal intensity on T1- and T2-weighted images), (2) low signal intensity shading on T2-weighted images,[26] (3) low signal intensity thick fibrous capsule surrounding a cyst loculus on both T1- and T2-weighted images, and (4) indistinct interface with adjacent organs due to adhesions. A hematocrit effect with layering within an endometrioma may also be seen.[121] Although the standard MRI sequences can usually provide the diagnosis of an endometrioma, occasionally the findings may be equivocal, and in these instances utilization of the fat-suppression technique further enhances the characterization of endometriomas on MRI (see Fig. 33–32).[122]

Endometrial Implants. Endometrial implants may be either intraperitoneal or extraperitoneal, although the former are generally more difficult to detect on MRI.[119] Implants typically are small raised lesions with signal characteristics similar to normal endometrium. However, as a result of hormonal stimulation, implants may undergo hemorrhage resulting in foci of high signal intensity on both T1- and T2-weighted images.

Adhesions. The presence of adhesions is suggested on MRI when (1) the tissue plane between an endometrioma and adjacent organs is indistinct or (2) there is fixation and angulation of adjacent bowel loops (see Fig. 33–31).[26, 119]

BENIGN CYSTIC OVARIAN DISEASE

Ultrasonography continues to be the initial modality of choice for evaluating cystic adnexal masses, with MRI reserved for problem solving when further fluid characterization is needed or in cases in which ultrasonography cannot determine if a pelvic mass is of uterine or adnexal origin.

Functional Cysts. Follicular cysts and corpus luteum cysts are thin walled and unilocular. The cyst fluid contents may range from serous to highly proteinaceous to hemorrhagic. Although functional cysts are usually asymptomatic, they may undergo spontaneous rupture or torsion. If these cysts fail to regress with hormonal therapy, surgical removal may be required.

Functional cysts appear on MRI as smooth, well-circumscribed, rounded lesions with a thin, barely perceptible wall (Fig. 33–33). They are typically of homogeneous low signal intensity on T1-weighted images and high signal intensity on T2-weighted images, similar to the intensity of urine.[25, 123] Hemorrhage may

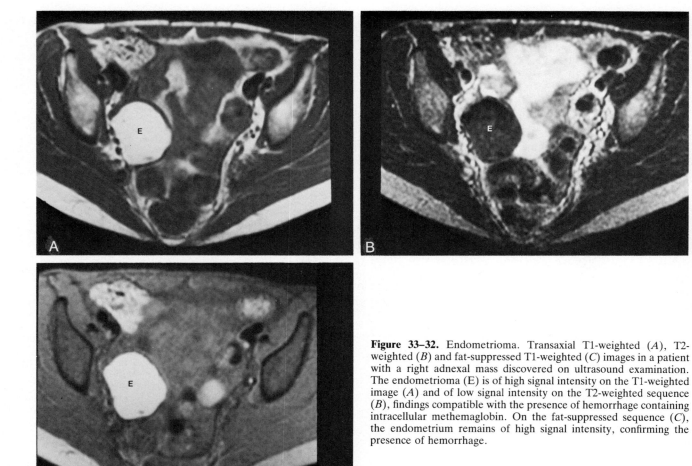

Figure 33–32. Endometrioma. Transaxial T1-weighted (*A*), T2-weighted (*B*) and fat-suppressed T1-weighted (*C*) images in a patient with a right adnexal mass discovered on ultrasound examination. The endometrioma (E) is of high signal intensity on the T1-weighted image (*A*) and of low signal intensity on the T2-weighted sequence (*B*), findings compatible with the presence of hemorrhage containing intracellular methemaglobin. On the fat-suppressed sequence (*C*), the endometrium remains of high signal intensity, confirming the presence of hemorrhage.

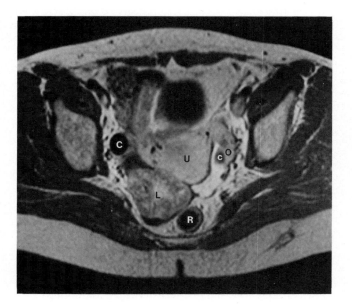

Figure 33–33. Functional ovarian cysts. Transaxial T1-weighted contrast-enhanced image. There are bilateral functional ovarian cysts (c) appearing as smooth, well-circumscribed lesions of homogeneous low signal intensity with an imperceptible wall. The normally enhancing ovarian tissue (O) is seen on the left adjacent to the cyst. U, uterus; L, pedunculated leiomyoma; R, rectum.

occur within a functional cyst, resulting in variable signal intensity on T1- and T2-weighted images depending on the age of the hemorrhage. Fat-suppression T1-weighted spin-echo images are helpful in distinguishing the high signal intensity of hemorrhagic lesions from fat-containing lesions (teratomas).[122] After the administration of contrast media, ovarian tissue enhances surrounding the nonenhancing cyst fluid, resulting in improved conspicuousness of functional cysts (see Fig. 33–33).

Cystadenomas. Cystadenomas are epithelial tumors of the ovary, which can be divided into serous and mucinous subtypes. Serous cystadenomas account for approximately 20% of all benign ovarian neoplasms, with a bilateral rate of 15%. These lesions are typically unilocular cystic masses filled with clear fluid. Mucinous cystadenomas comprise 15% of benign ovarian tumors and are bilateral in about 5% of cases. The appearance of a multiloculated cystic mass is typical, with thick, viscous material being evident on gross inspection. The distinction between these two subtypes of cystadenomas is, however, based on the pathologic examination of the epithelium rather than on the cyst contents.

On MRI, these lesions are typically unilocular or multilocular cystic lesions with thin walls and septa (Fig. 33–34). The cyst fluid may be of variable signal intensity depending on its proteinaceous contents. After the administration of contrast material, enhancement of the cyst wall and any septations may be seen (see Fig. 33–34). Although attempts have been made to differentiate serous from mucinous cystadenomas using criteria including locularity, cystic fluid signal intensity, and septa thickness,[124, 125] the appearance of these lesions may be virtually indistinguishable.

Teratomas. The vast majority of ovarian teratomas are of the cystic, mature (benign) form, which are also known as dermoid cysts. These tumors account for 5% to 25% of all ovarian neoplasms and are the most common ovarian tumor of childhood.[126] Teratomas are bilateral in 10% to 15% of patients. These lesions contain all three germ cell layers, although ectodermal derivatives predominate. A dermoid plug or Rokitansky nodule often arises from the tumor wall and may contain well-differentiated tissue such as bone, teeth, fat, and hair.[126] Complications of cystic teratomas include torsion, rupture, infection, and malignant transformation. Since the treatment of choice for a cystic teratoma is oophorectomy, MRI may play a role in differentiating these lesions from other benign cystic ovarian masses, which may not require surgical excision.

Cystic teratomas are well-defined, heterogeneous masses that usually contain some component of fat seen to be isointense to subcutaneous fat on both T1- and T2-weighted images (Figs. 33–35 through 33–37).[25, 123, 127] The presence of fluid-fluid or fat-fluid levels, as well as a characteristic chemical-shift artifact are other common findings (see Figs. 33–36 and 33–37). Rokitansky nodules are often seen within the dermoid cyst, with their signal intensity depending on the predominant tissue component (fat, calcification, fibrous tissue) (see Figs. 33–35 and 33–36). On occasion, the differentiation between cystic teratomas and hemorrhagic ovarian masses (i.e., endometrioma) on MRI may be difficult, since both may be isointense to subcutaneous fat on T1- and T2-weighted images. In these instances, the use of an additional fat-suppression imaging sequence provides accurate distinction between these two entities (see Fig. 33–37).[122]

MALIGNANT OVARIAN LESIONS

Ovarian Carcinoma. Ovarian cancer represents the most lethal of all gynecologic malignancies. Unfortunately, early detection of ovarian carcinoma remains difficult since the disease is noted for being clinically silent until relatively far advanced. At initial diagnosis,

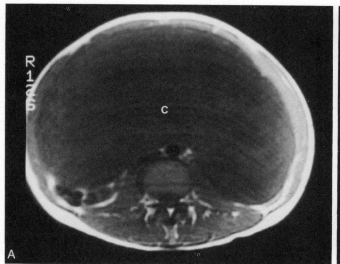
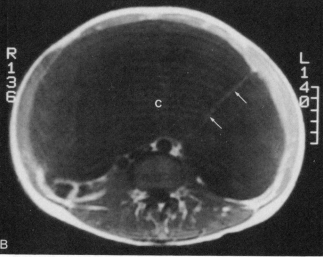

Figure 33–34. Cystadenoma. *A.* A huge cystadenoma (c) fills the entire abdomen and is of homogeneous low signal intensity on the nonenhanced transaxial T1-weighted image. *B.* Following contrast enhancement, only a single, thin septation (*arrows*) is seen, without the presence of a solid component, nodularity, or thick septation or wall. These findings are characteristic of a benign lesion.

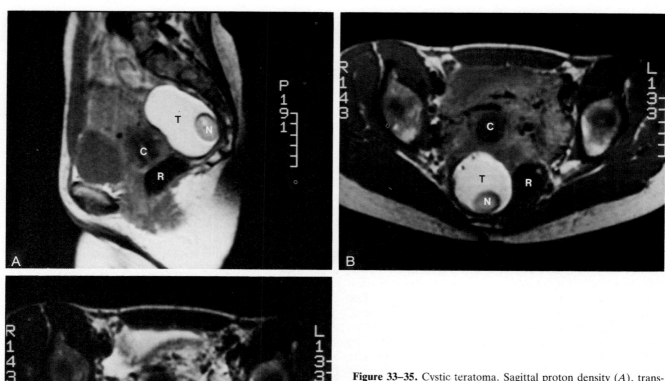

Figure 33–35. Cystic teratoma. Sagittal proton density (*A*), transaxial proton density (*B*), and T2-weighted (*C*) images. The ovarian teratoma (T) is of high signal intensity on all sequences and contains an intermediate signal intensity Rokitansky nodule (N). C, cervix; R, rectum.

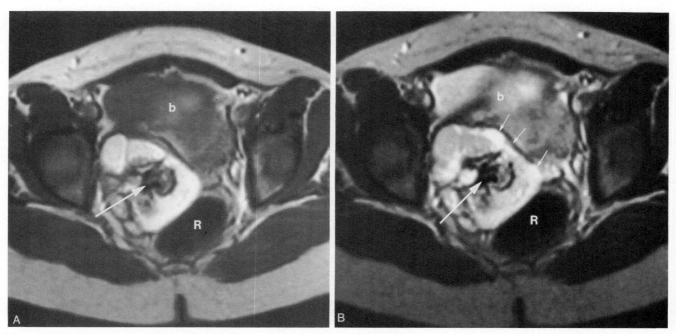

Figure 33–36. Right ovarian teratoma. Transaxial proton density (*A*) and T2-weighted (*B*) images. The teratoma is of heterogeneous signal intensity on both sequences, with areas of high signal intensity compatible with fat. There is a central area of signal void (*large arrow*) representing an area of calcification. Typical chemical shift artifact is seen at the periphery of the lesion (*small arrows*). b, bladder; R, rectum.

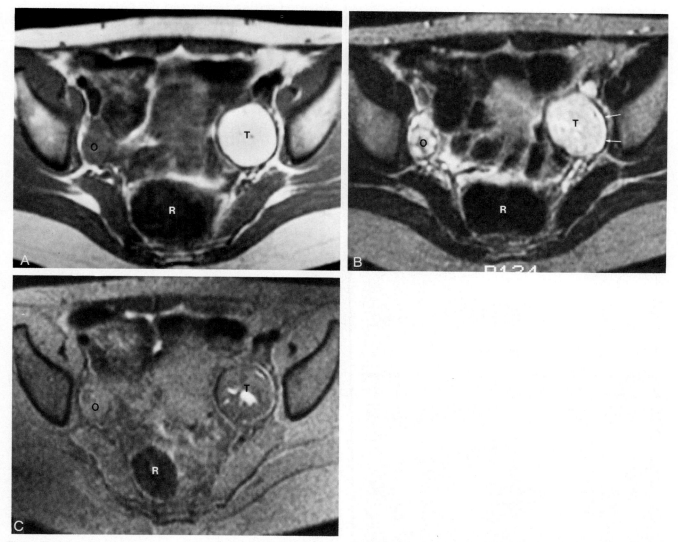

Figure 33–37. Left ovarian teratoma. The teratoma (T) is of high signal intensity on both the transaxial T1-weighted (*A*) and T2-weighted (*B*) images, with typical chemical shift artifact seen (*small arrows*). *C.* On the fat-suppressed T1-weighted image, the majority of the teratoma becomes of low signal intensity, confirming the presence of intratumoral fat. O, normal right ovary; R, rectum.

approximately 75% of patients with ovarian carcinoma have disease beyond the ovary.[128]

Ovarian cancer is classified according to the cell of origin and consists of (1) epithelial (80% to 90%), (2) germ cell (5% to 15%), and (3) stromal (5% to 10%).[128] Among epithelial tumors, the serous cystadenocarcinoma is the most common histologic type, followed by mucinous cystadenocarcinoma.[128] Germ cell tumors include malignant teratoma, dysgerminoma, endodermal sinus tumor, and embryonal carcinoma. The most common stromal tumor is the granulosa cell tumor.[128]

The role of imaging in the evaluation of suspected ovarian cancer remains controversial. The goals of radiologic assessment of suspected adnexal neoplasms include lesion detection, characterization, and staging.

Following initial clinical discovery, patients with a suspected adnexal mass are usually studied by ultrasonography. The role of MRI in ovarian cancer remains to be defined; however, some advantages of MRI compared with ultrasonography have been shown. MRI is superior to ultrasonography in lesion detection and characterization, as well as in evaluation of extraovarian spread of tumor within the pelvis and to the abdomen.[36, 105–109] In limited experience to date, the accuracy of MRI in staging of ovarian carcinoma has been reported to be 75%, which is similar to the reported staging accuracy of CT.[36, 129, 130]

The MRI appearance of ovarian carcinoma includes both solid and mixed solid/cystic masses (Figs. 33–38 through 33–41). These lesions are generally of heterogeneous signal intensity. They tend to have irregular

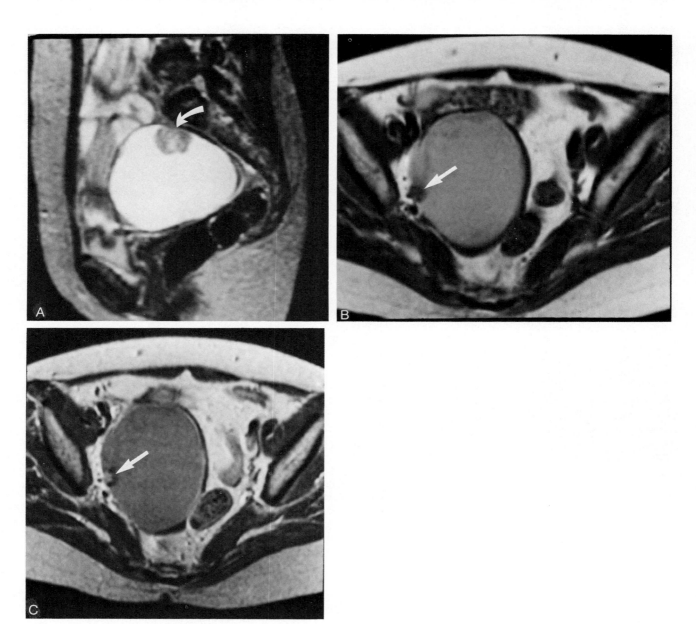

Figure 33–38. Moderately differentiated mucinous cystadenocarcinoma. *A.* Sagittal T2-weighted image demonstrates a homogeneously high signal intensity ovarian lesion containing a medium signal intensity nodule along its superior aspect (*arrow*). *B.* On the transaxial T1-weighted image, a second solid nodule (*arrow*) can be seen along the right lateral aspect of the lesion. *C.* Note enhancement of the nodule following the administration of contrast agent (*arrow*).

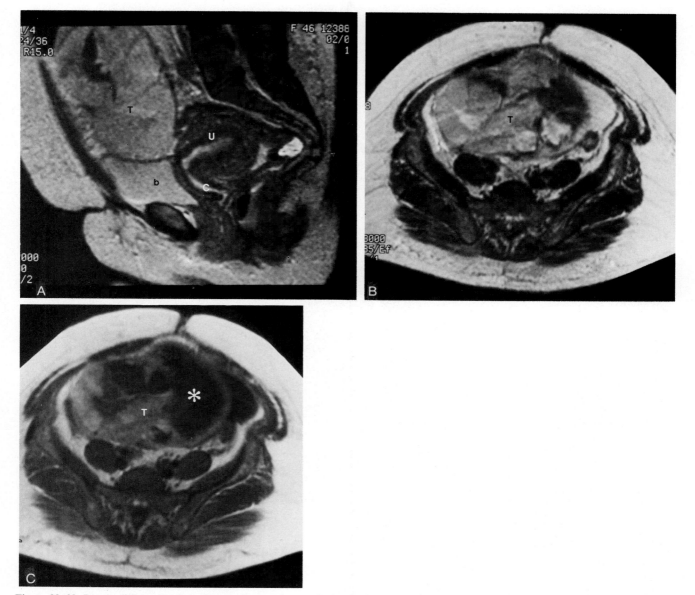

Figure 33–39. Poorly differentiated mucinous adenocarcinoma. Sagittal T2-weighted (*A*), transaxial T2-weighted (*B*), and contrast-enhanced T1-weighted (*C*) images. On the sagittal image, a large ovarian tumor (T) can be seen separate from the uterus (U) and the urinary bladder (b). The contrast-enhanced transaxial image allows differentiation of solid tumor (T) from areas of nonenhancing necrosis (*asterisk*). C, cervix.

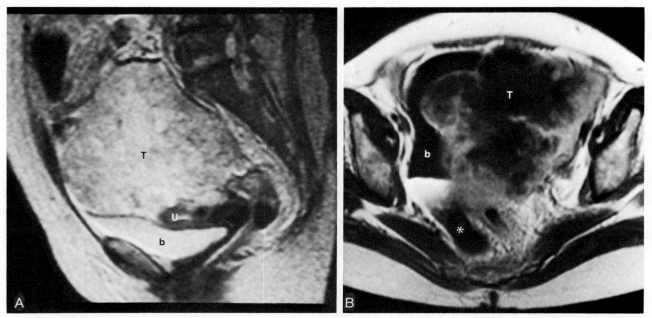

Figure 33–40. Granulosa cell tumor. *A.* The tumor (T) is of high signal intensity on a sagittal T2-weighted image and can be seen superior to both the uterus (U) and the bladder (b). *B.* Following administration of contrast, intratumoral architecture is well appreciated on this transaxial T1-weighted image, with areas of low signal intensity representing nonviable tissue. Asterisk indicates cul-de-sac fluid.

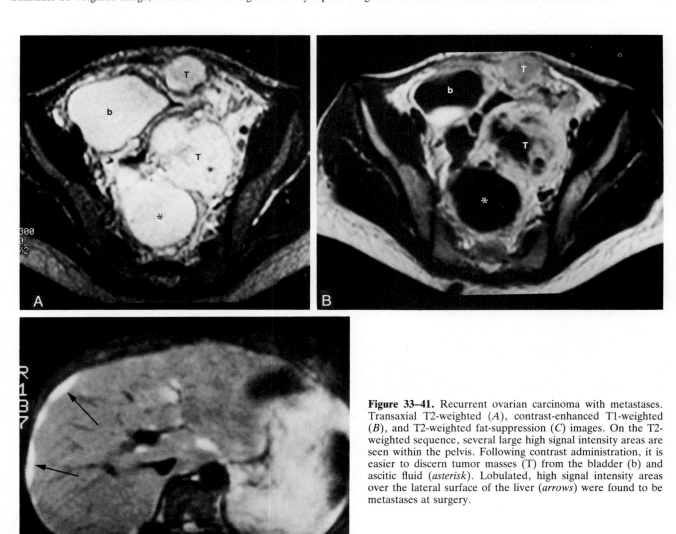

Figure 33–41. Recurrent ovarian carcinoma with metastases. Transaxial T2-weighted (*A*), contrast-enhanced T1-weighted (*B*), and T2-weighted fat-suppression (*C*) images. On the T2-weighted sequence, several large high signal intensity areas are seen within the pelvis. Following contrast administration, it is easier to discern tumor masses (T) from the bladder (b) and ascitic fluid (*asterisk*). Lobulated, high signal intensity areas over the lateral surface of the liver (*arrows*) were found to be metastases at surgery.

margins and often contain thick walls and thick, nodular internal septations. Malignant ovarian masses are usually over 4 cm in size.[36] The presence of a solid, nodular element within an otherwise cystic mass must still be considered suspicious for containing malignancy (see Fig. 33–38). The administration of contrast media improves visualization of intratumoral architecture, more readily demonstrating septations, nodularity, wall thickness, and areas of necrosis,[36, 107] thus facilitating lesion characterization (see Figs. 33–38 through 33–41).

Extraovarian disease within the pelvis involving the uterus, bladder, rectum, or pelvic sidewall may be depicted with MRI. Spread of disease to the abdomen may be manifested by peritoneal implants, omental cake, or mesenteric disease. MRI is currently limited by peristaltic motion artifact and lack of a bowel contrast agent, thus impairing identification of peritoneal implants and mesenteric involvement. Metastatic spread to the liver, either within the parenchyma or on the capsular surface, may also be seen (see Fig. 33–41). The ability of MRI to detect pelvic and retroperitoneal lymphadenopathy is similar to that of CT.[131]

Metastatic Tumors of the Ovary. Approximately 6% of ovarian cancers found during surgery for a pelvic or abdominal mass are metastatic.[132] The most common primary tumors originate from the gastrointestinal tract, breast, and other pelvic organs. Metastases to the ovary are bilateral in 75% of cases. Krukenberg tumor is a specific type of metastasis to the ovary,

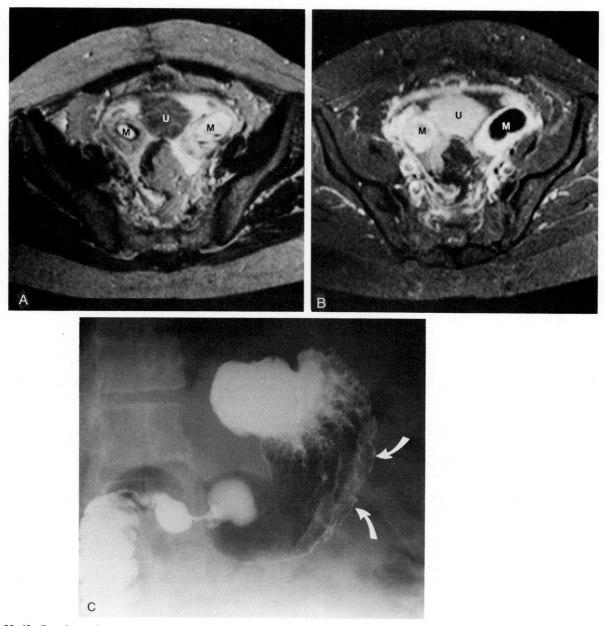

Figure 33–42. Gastric carcinoma metastatic to the ovaries. Transaxial T2-weighted (*A*) and contrast-enhanced T1-weighted fat-suppression (*B*) images demonstrate bilateral, heterogeneous ovarian masses (M) separate from the uterine fundus (U). On a film from an upper gastrointestinal series (*C*) there is diffuse thickening of the folds in the greater curvature of the stomach (*arrows*) caused by the primary adenocarcinoma.

containing signet ring cells. The vast majority arise from a primary gastric carcinoma, but other reported primary sites include breast, intestine, and gallbladder. Krukenberg tumors are large, solid lesions that are usually bilateral and may contain hemorrhage and necrosis.

The MRI appearance of metastases to the ovary is nonspecific and indistinguishable from other ovarian malignancies (Fig. 33–42). However, this diagnosis may be suspected with a known history of malignancy and bilateral ovarian masses. These lesions may be cystic, as can be seen with primary colon carcinoma, or completely solid, as in Krukenberg tumors.

References

1. O'Brien WF, Buck DR, Nash JD: Evaluation of sonography in the initial assessment of the gynecologic patient. Gynecology 149:598, 1984.
2. Fleischer AC, Gordon AN, Entman SS: Transabdominal and transvaginal sonography of pelvic masses. Ultrasound Med Biol 15:529, 1989.
3. Kerr-Wilson RM, Shingleton HM, Orr JN: The use of US and CT scanning in the management of the gynecologic cancer patient. Gynecol Oncol 18:54, 1984.
4. Andreotti RF, Zusmer NR, Sheldon JJ, Ames M: Ultrasound and magnetic resonance imaging of pelvic masses. Surg Gynecol Obstet 166:327, 1988.
5. Lewis E: Imaging techniques in gynecologic cancer. In Rutledge FN, Freedman RS, Gershenson DM (eds): Gynecologic Cancer: Diagnosis and Treatment Strategies, vol 29, pp 397–427. Austin, University of Texas Press, 1987.
6. Hricak H, Alpers C, Crooks LE, Sheldon PE: Magnetic resonance imaging of the female pelvis: Initial experience. AJR 141:1119, 1983.
7. Bryan PJ, Butter HE, LiPuma JP, et al: NMR scanning of the pelvis: Initial experiences with 0.3T system. AJR 141:1111, 1983.
8. Butler H, Bryan PJ, LiPuma JP, et al: Magnetic resonance imaging of the abnormal female pelvis. AJR 143:1259, 1984.
9. Hricak H, Schriock E, Lacey C, et al: Gynecologic masses: Value of MRI. Am J Obstet Gynecol 153:31, 1985.
10. Lee JKT, Gersell DJ, Balfe DM, et al: The uterus: In vitro MR anatomic correlation of normal and abnormal specimens. Radiology 157:175, 1985.
11. Demas BE, Hricak H, Jaffe RB: Uterine MR imaging: Effects of hormonal stimulation. Radiology 159:123, 1986.
12. Haynor D, Mack L, Soules M, et al: Changing appearance of the normal uterus during the menstrual cycle: MR studies. Radiology 161:459, 1986.
13. McCarthy S, Tauber C, Gore J: Female pelvic anatomy: MR assessment of variations during the menstrual cycle and with use of oral contraceptives. Radiology 160:119, 1986.
14. Hamlin DJ, Petersson H, Fitzsimmons J, Morgan LS: MR imaging of uterine leiomyomas and their complications. JCAT 9:902, 1985.
15. Hricak H, Tscholakoff D, Heinrichs L, et al: Uterine leiomyoma correlation by magnetic resonance imaging: Clinical symptoms and histopathology. Radiology 158:385, 1986.
16. Mark AS, Hricak H: Adenomyosis and leiomyoma: Differential diagnosis by means of magnetic resonance imaging. Radiology 163:527, 1987.
17. Bies JR, Ellis JH, Kopecky KK, et al: Assessment of primary gynecologic malignancies: Comparison of 0.15-T resistive MRI with CT. AJR 143:1249, 1984.
18. Worthington JL, Balfe DM, Lee JKT, et al: Uterine neoplasms: MR imaging. Radiology 159:725, 1986.
19. Hricak H, Stern J, Fisher MR: MRI in the evaluation of endometrial carcinoma and its staging. Radiology 162:297, 1987.
20. Hricak H, Lacey CG, Sandles LG, et al: Invasive cervical carcinoma: Comparison of MR imaging and surgical findings. Radiology 166:623, 1988.
21. Hricak H, Demas B, Braga C, et al: Gestational trophoblastic neoplasm of the uterus: MR assessment. Radiology 161:11, 1986.
22. Powell MC, Buckley J, Worthington BS, et al: Magnetic resonance imaging and hydatidiform mole. Br J Radiol 59:561, 1986.
23. Togashi K, Nishimura K, Itoh K, et al: Uterine cervical cancer: Assessment with high-field MR imaging. Radiology 160:431, 1986.
24. Hamlin DJ, Peterson H, Ramey SL, et al: Magnetic resonance imaging of bicornuate uterus with unilateral hematometrosalpinx and ipsilateral renal agenesis. Urol Radiol 8:52, 1986.
25. Dooms GC, Hricak H, Tscholakoff D: Magnetic resonance imaging of adnexal structures: Normal and pathologic. Radiology 158:639, 1986.
26. Nishimura K, Togashi K, Itoh K, et al: Endometrial cysts of the ovary: MR imaging. Radiology 162:315, 1987.
27. Mitchell DG, Gefter WB, Spritzer CE, et al: Polycystic ovaries: MR imaging. Radiology 160:425, 1986.
28. Hamlin DJ, Fitzsimmons JR, Peterson H, et al: Magnetic resonance imaging of the pelvis: Evaluation of ovarian masses at 0.15-T. AJR 145:585, 1985.
29. Hricak H, Chang YCF, Thurnher S: Vagina: Evaluation with MR imaging: I. Normal anatomy and congenital anomalies. Radiology 169:169, 1988.
30. Hricak H: MRI of the female pelvis: A review. AJR 146: 1115, 1986.
31. Mark AS, Hricak H: Magnetic resonance imaging of intrauterine contraceptive devices. Radiology 162:311, 1987.
32. Shapiro I, Lanir A, Sharf M, et al: Magnetic resonance imaging of gynecologic masses. Gynecol Oncol 28:186, 1987.
33. Hricak H: Guidelines for magnetic resonance imaging in obstetrics and gynecology. In American College of Radiology: Clinical Applications of Magnetic Resonance Imaging, pp 31–35. Washington, American College of Radiology, 1989.
34. Hricak H, Carrington BM (eds): MRI of the Pelvis: A Text Atlas, pp 93–248. London, Martin Dunitz Publishers, 1990.
35. Hricak H: Carcinoma of the female reproductive organs: Value of cross-sectional imaging. Cancer 67(suppl 4):1209, 1991.
36. Stevens SK, Hricak H, Stern JL: Detection and characterization of ovarian lesions at 1.5T using gadolinium-DTPA. Radiology 181:481, 1991.
37. Ascher SM, Scoutt LM, McCarthy SM, et al: Uterine changes after dilatation and curettage: MR imaging findings. Radiology 180:433, 1991.
38. McCarthy S, Scott G, Majumdar S, et al: Uterine junctional zone: MR study of water content and relaxation properties. Radiology 171:241, 1989.
39. Scoutt LM, Flynn SD, Luthringer DJ, et al: Junctional zone of the uterus: Correlation of MR imaging and histologic examination of hysterectomy specimens. Radiology 179:403, 1991.
40. Brown HK, Stoll BS, Nicosia SV, et al: Uterine junctional zone: Correlation between histologic findings and MR imaging. Radiology 179:409, 1991.
41. Mitchell DG, Schonholz L, Hilpert PH, et al: Zones of the uterus: Discrepancy between US and MR images. Radiology 174:827, 1990.
42. Hendrickson MR, Kempson RL (eds): Surgical Pathology of the Uterine Corpus, p 452. Philadelphia, WB Saunders, 1980.
43. Andreyko JL, Blumenfeld Z, Marshall LA, et al: Use of an agonistic analog of GnRH (NAFARELIN) to treat leiomyomata: Assessment by magnetic resonance imaging. Am J Obstet Gynecol 158:903, 1988.
44. Danforth DN: The distribution and functional activity of the cervical musculature. Am J Obstet Gynecol 68:1261, 1954.
45. Hricak H, Chang YCF, Cann CE, et al: Cervical incompetence: Preliminary evaluation with MR imaging. Radiology 174:821, 1990.
46. Zawin M, McCarthy S, Scoutt LM, Comite F: High-field MRI and US evaluation of the pelvis in women with leiomyomas. Magn Reson Imaging 8:371, 1990.
47. Hricak H, Hamm B, Wolf K-J: Use of Gd-DTPA in MRI of the female pelvis. Proceedings, Contrast Media in MRI, Berlin, 1990.

48. Sorenson SS: Estimated prevalence of müllerian anomalies. Acta Obstet Gynecol Scan 67:441, 1988.
49. Sorenson SS: Hysteroscopic evaluation and endocrinological aspects of women with müllerian anomalies and oligomenorrhea. Int J Fertil 32:445, 1987.
50. Buttram VC, Gibbons WE: Müllerian anomalies: A proposed classification (an analysis of 144 cases). Fertil Steril 32:40, 1979.
51. Malini S, Valdes C, Malinak R: Sonographic diagnosis and classification of anomalies of the female genital tract. J Ultrasound Med 3:397, 1984.
52. Reuter KL, Daly DC, Cohen SM: Septate versus bicornuate uteri: Errors in imaging diagnosis. Radiology 172:749, 1989.
53. Carrington BM, Hricak H, Nuruddin R, et al: Müllerian duct anomalies: MR imaging evaluation. Radiology 176:715, 1990.
54. Secaf E, Nuruddin R, Hricak H, et al: MR evaluation of ambiguous genitalia. Presented at the 75th Scientific Assembly and Annual Meeting of the Radiological Society of North America, 1989.
55. Togashi K, Nishimujra K, Itoh K, et al: Vaginal agenesis: Classification by MR imaging. Radiology 162:675, 1987.
56. Mintz MC, Thickman DI, Gussman D, et al: MR evaluation of uterine anomalies. AJR 148:287, 1987.
57. Fedele L, Dorta M, Brioschi D, et al: Magnetic resonance evaluation of double uteri. Obstet Gynecol 74:844, 1989.
58. Fedele L, Dorta M, Brioschi D, et al: Magnetic resonance imaging of unicornuate uterus. Acta Obstet Gynecol Scand 69:511, 1990.
59. Fedele L, Dorta M, Brioschi D, et al: Magnetic resonance imaging in Mayer-Rokitansky-Kuster-Hauser syndrome. Obstet Gynecol 76:593, 1990.
60. Shatzkes DR, Haller JO, Velcek FT: Imaging of uterovaginal anomalies in the pediatric patient. Urol Radiol 13:58, 1991.
61. Gross BH, Silver TM, Jaffe MH: Sonographic features of uterine leiomyomas. J Ultrasound Med 2:401, 1983.
62. Baltarowich OH, Kurtz AB, Pennel R, et al: Pitfalls in the sonographic diagnosis of uterine fibroids. AJR 154:725, 1988.
63. Weinreb JC, Barkoff ND, Megibow A, et al: The value of MR imaging in distinguishing leiomyomas from other solid pelvic masses when sonography is indeterminate. AJR 154:295, 1990.
64. Dudiak CM, Turner DA, Patal SK, et al: Uterine leiomyomas in the infertile patient: Preoperative localization with MR imaging versus US and hysterosalpingography. Radiology 167:627, 1988.
65. Zawin M, McCarthy S, Scoutt L, et al: Monitoring therapy with a gonadotropin-releasing hormone analog: Utility of MR imaging. Radiology 175:503, 1990.
66. Lubich LM, Alderman MG, Ros PR: Magnetic resonance imaging of leiomyomata uteri: Assessing therapy with the gonadotropin-releasing hormone agonist leuprolide. Magn Reson Imaging 9:331, 1991.
67. Togashi K, Ozasa H, Konishi I, et al: Enlarged uterus: Differentiation between adenomyosis and leiomyoma with MRI. Radiology 171:531, 1989.
68. Togashi K, Nishimura K, Itoh K, et al: Adenomyosis: Diagnosis with MR imaging. Radiology 166:111, 1988.
69. Hricak H, Tscholakoff D, Heinrichs L, et al: Uterine leiomyomas: Correlation of MR, histopathologic findings and symptoms. Radiology 158:385, 1986.
70. Kilkku P, Erkkola R, Grönroos M: Nonspecificity of symptoms related to adenomyosis: A prospective comparative survey. Acta Obstet Gynecol Scand 63:229, 1984.
71. Berman ML, Ballan SC, Lagasse LK, Watring WG: Prognosis and treatment of endometrial cancer. Am J Obstet Gynecol 136:679, 1980.
72. Hoskins WJ, Perez C, Young RC: Gynecologic tumors. In DeVita VT Jr, Hellman S, Rosenberg SA (eds): Cancer, Principles & Practice of Oncology, 3rd ed, vol 1, pp 1099–1150. Philadelphia, JB Lippincott, 1989.
73. Morrow PC: Melville Cody memorial lecture: Prognostic factors in endometrial carcinoma. In Rutledge FN, Freedman RS, Gershenson DM (ed): Gynecologic Cancer: Diagnosis and Treatment Strategies, pp 293–312. Austin, University of Texas Press, 1987.
74. Chen SS, Lee L: Retroperitoneal lymph node metastases in stage I carcinoma of endometrium: Correlation with risk factors. Gynecol Oncol 16:319, 1983.
75. Boronow RC, Morrow CP, Creasman WT, et al: Surgical staging in endometrial cancer: Clinical pathologic findings of a prospective study. Obstet Gynecol 63:825, 1984.
76. Announcements: FIGO stages, 1988 revision. Gynecol Oncol 35:125, 1989.
77. Thorvinger B, Gudmundsson T, Horvath G, et al: Staging in local endometrial carcinoma: Assessment of magnetic resonance and ultrasound examinations. Acta Radiol 30:252, 1989.
78. Fleischer AC, Dudley BS, Entman SS, et al: Myometrial invasion by endometrial carcinoma: Sonographic assessment. Radiology 162:307, 1987.
79. Cacciatore B, Lehtovirta P, Wahlström T, et al: Contribution of vaginal scanning to sonographic evaluation of endometrial cancer invasion. Acta Oncol 28:585, 1989.
80. Belloni C, Vigano R, del Maschio A, et al: Magnetic resonance imaging in endometrial carcinoma staging. Gynecol Oncol 37:172, 1990.
81. Hricak H, Rubinstein L, Gherman GM, Karstaedt N: MR imaging evaluation of endometrial carcinoma: Results of an NCI cooperative study. Radiology 179:829, 1991.
82. Chen SS, Rumancik WM, Spiegel G: Magnetic resonance imaging in stage I endometrial carcinoma. Obstet Gynecol 75:274, 1990.
83. Javitt MC, Stein HL, Lovecchio JL: MRI in staging of endometrial and cervical carcinoma. Magn Reson Imaging 5:83, 1987.
84. Sironi S, Mellone R, Venzulli A, et al: Assessment of the myometrial infiltration of endometrial carcinoma (FIGO stage I-II): The accuracy of magnetic resonance. Radiol Med (Torino) 77:386, 1989.
85. Yazigi R, Cohen G, Munoz AK, et al: Magnetic resonance imaging Determination of myometrial invasion in endometrial carcinoma. Gynecol Oncol 34:94, 1989.
86. Gordon AN, Fleischer AC, Dudley BS: Preoperative assessment of myometrial invasion of endometrial adenocarcinoma by sonography (US) and magnetic resonance imaging. Gynecol Oncol 34:175, 1989.
87. Hricak H, Hamm B, Semelka RC, et al: Carcinoma of the uterus: Use of gadopentetate dimeglumine in MR imaging. Radiology 181:95, 1991.
88. Sironi S, Taccagni G, Garancini P, et al: Myometrial invasion by endometrial carcinoma: Assessment by MR imaging. AJR 158:565, 1992.
89. Ansari AH, Reynolds RA: Cervical incompetence: A review. J Reprod Med 32:161, 1987.
90. Mahran M. The role of ultrasound in the diagnosis and management of the incompetent cervix. In Kurjak A (ed): Recent Advances in Ultrasound Diagnosis, vol 2, pp 505–514. International Congress series no. 498. Amsterdam, Elsevier, 1980.
91. Morrow PC, Townsend DE: Tumors of the cervix. In Morrow PC, Townsend DE (eds): Synopsis of Gynecologic Oncology 3rd ed, pp 103–158. New York, Churchill Livingstone, 1987.
92. Chung CK, Nahhas WA, Zaino R, et al: Histologic grade and lymph node metastasis in squamous cell carcinoma of the cervix. Gynecol Oncol 12:348, 1981.
93. Kim SH, Choi BI, Lee HP, et al: Uterine cervical carcinoma: Comparison of CT and MR findings. Radiology 175:45, 1990.
94. Cobby M, Browning J, Jones A, et al: Magnetic resonance imaging, computed tomography and endosonography in the local staging of carcinoma of the cervix. Br J Radiol 63:673, 1990.
95. Greco A, Mason P, Leung AWL, et al: Staging of carcinoma of the uterine cervix: MRI—surgical correlation. Clin Radiol 40:401, 1989.
96. Togashi K, Nishimura K, Sago T, et al: Carcinoma of the cervix: Staging with MR imaging. Radiology 171:245, 1989.
97. Lien HH, Blomlie V, Kjorstad K, et al: Clinical stage I carcinoma of the cervix: Value of MR imaging in determining degree of invasiveness. AJR 156:1191, 1991.
98. Sironi S, Belloni C, Taccagni G, et al: Carcinoma of the cervix: Value of MR imaging in detecting parametrial involvement. AJR 156:753, 1991.
99. Sironi S, Belloni C, Taccagni G, DelMaschio A: Invasive cervical carcinoma: MR imaging after preoperative chemotherapy. Radiology 180:719, 1991.
100. Morrow PC, Townsend DE: Vaginal adenosis, adenocarcinoma

and diethylstilbestrol. In Morrow PC, Townsend DE (eds): Synopsis of Gynecologic Oncology, 3rd ed, pp 45–55. New York, Churchill Livingstone, 1987.

101. Rutledge F: Cancer of the vagina. Am J Obstet Gynecol 97:635, 1967.
102. Phillips GL, Prem KA, Adcock LL, et al: Vaginal recurrence of adenocarcinoma of the endometrium. Gynecol Oncol 13:323, 1982.
103. Chen NJ: Vaginal invasion by cervical carcinoma. Acta Med Okayama 38:305, 1984.
104. Chang YCF, Hricak H, Thurnher S, et al: Evaluation of the vagina by magnetic resonance imaging: II. Neoplasm. Radiology 169:569, 1988.
105. Andreotti RF, Zusmer NR, Sheldon JJ, Ames M: Ultrasound and magnetic resonance imaging of pelvic masses. Surg Gynecol Obstet 166:327, 1988.
106. Lewis E: Imaging techniques in gynecologic cancer. In Rutledge FN, Freedman RS, Gershenson DM (eds): Gynecologic Cancer: Diagnosis and Treatment Strategies, vol 29, pp 397–427. Austin, University of Texas Press, 1987.
107. Thurnher S, Hodler J, Baer S, et al: Gadolinium-DOTA enhanced MR imaging of adnexal tumors. JCAT 14:939, 1990.
108. Smith FW, Cherryman GR, Bayliss AP, et al: Comparative study of the accuracy of ultrasound imaging, x-ray computerized tomography and low field MRI diagnosis of ovarian malignancy. Magn Reson Imaging 6:225, 1988.
109. Buy J-N, Ghossain MA, Sciot C, et al: Epithelial tumors of the ovary: CT findings and correlation with US. Radiology 178:811, 1991.
110. Meire HB, Farrant P, Guha T: Distinction of benign from malignant cysts by ultrasound. Br J Obstet Gynaecol 85:893, 1978.
111. Walsh JW, Taylor KJW, Wasson JFM, et al: Gray-scale ultrasound in 204 proved gynecologic masses: Accuracy and specific diagnostic criteria. Radiology 130:391, 1979.
112. Moyle JW, Rochester D, Silder L, et al: Sonography of ovarian tumors: Predictability of tumor type. AJR 141:985, 1983.
113. Clement PB: Endometriosis, lesions of the secondary müllerian system, and pelvic mesothelial proliferations. In Kurman RJ (ed): Blaustein's Pathology of the Female Genital Tract, 3rd ed, pp 516–559. New York, Springer-Verlag, 1987.
114. Friedman H, Vogelzang RL, Mendelson EB, et al: Endometriosis detection by US with laparoscopic correlation. Radiology 157:217, 1985.
115. Fleischer AC, James AE Jr, Millis JB, Julian C: Differential diagnosis of pelvic masses by gray scale sonography. AJR 131:469, 1978.

116. Walsh JW, Taylor KJW, Wasson JFM, et al: Gray-scale ultrasound in 204 proved gynecologic masses: Accuracy and specific diagnostic criteria. Radiology 130:391, 1979.
117. Berland LL, Lawson TL, Albarelli JN, Foley WD: Ultrasonic diagnosis of ovarian and adnexal disease. Semin Ultrasound 1:17, 1980.
118. Zawin M, McCarthy S, Scoutt L, Comite F: Endometriosis: Appearance and detection at MR imaging. Radiology 171:693, 1989.
119. Arrivé L, Hricak H, Martin MC: Pelvic endometriosis: MR imaging. Radiology 171:687, 1989.
120. Togashi K, Nishimura K, Kimura I: Endometrial cysts: Diagnosis with MR imaging. Radiology 180:73, 1991.
121. Nyberg DA, Porter BA, Olds MO, et al: MR imaging of hemorrhagic adnexal masses. JCAT 11:664, 1987.
122. Kier R, Smith RC, McCarthy SM: Value of lipid- and water-suppression MR images in distinguishing between blood and lipid within ovarian masses. AJR 158:321, 1992.
123. Mitchell DG, Mintz MC, Spritzer CE, et al: Adnexal masses: MR imaging observations at 1.5T, with US and CT correlation. Radiology 162:319, 1987.
124. Ghossain MA, Buy J-N, Lignères C, et al: Epithelial tumors of the ovary: Comparison of MR and CT findings. Radiology 181:863, 1991.
125. Mawhinney RR, Powell MC, Worthington BS, Symonds EM: Magnetic resonance imaging of benign ovarian masses. Br J Radiol 61:179, 1988.
126. Talerman A: Germ cell tumors of the ovary. In Kurman RJ (ed): Blaustein's Pathology of the Female Genital Tract, 3rd ed, pp 660–721. New York, Springer-Verlag, 1987.
127. Togashi K, Nishimura K, Itoh K, et al: Ovarian cystic teratomas: MR imaging. Radiology 162:669, 1987.
128. Young RC, Fuks Z, Hoskins WJ: Cancer of the ovary. In DeVita VT, Hellman S, Rosenberg SA (eds): Cancer Principles & Practice of Oncology, 3rd ed, pp 1162–1196. Philadelphia, JB Lippincott, 1989.
129. Amendola MA: The role of CT in the evaluation of ovarian malignancy. CRC Crit Rev Diagn Imaging 24:329, 1985.
130. Kormano M, Grönroos M: Computer-tomographic evaluation of gynecologic tumors. Acta Obstet Gynecol Scand 63:509, 1984.
131. Dooms GC, Hricak H, Crooks LE, Higgins CB: Magnetic resonance imaging of the lymph nodes: Comparison with CT. Radiology 153:719, 1984.
132. Young RH, Scully RE: Metastatic tumors of the ovary. In Kurman RJ (ed): Blaustein's Pathology of the Female Genital Tract, 3rd ed, pp 742–768. New York, Springer-Verlag, 1987.

CHAPTER 34

Artifacts, Pitfalls, and Normal Variants

PETER W. CALLEN, M.D.

When I began my involvement with diagnostic ultrasonography 18 years ago, this chapter would have been considered ludicrous. Virtually all of ultrasonography was considered to be either an artifact or a pitfall. Clinicians did not take this modality seriously, and few critical decisions were ever based on the results of the ultrasound examination alone. With time, improvements in both technology and our understanding of normal and abnormal findings made this a useful clinical diagnostic modality. It did not take long for important clinical decisions to be based solely on the results of the ultrasound examination, which, for example, may be surgery, early delivery of the fetus, or even termination of the pregnancy. This evolution, while welcomed by many, has placed a large responsibility on the sonographer. The phrase "primum non nocere" has never proven more true—first do no harm.

This chapter is not an attempt to explain the physical principles of ultrasound or artifact production. It is also unlikely that such a chapter could ever be all inclusive. I have attempted to find examples of pitfalls, the diagnostic dilemmas that have the potential to lead us to the wrong diagnosis. I have tried to cover both basic potential pitfalls and some of the more esoteric normal variants. There will undoubtedly be some readers who will find some examples that will be so basic as to almost seem insulting. I apologize in advance and will only answer by saying that this chapter is meant to appeal to a wide audience of beginners and "well-seasoned" experts. I also do not attempt to give an overly detailed explanation for each example but try to offer what is theorized at the time.

If I am able to avoid one false-positive diagnosis and prevent unnecessary surgery, termination of a pregnancy, or even 20 weeks of an emotional rollercoaster for the parents, I have fulfilled my goal.

GYNECOLOGY

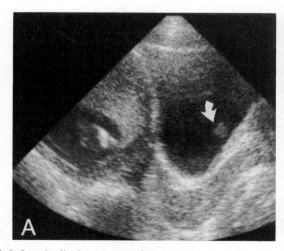 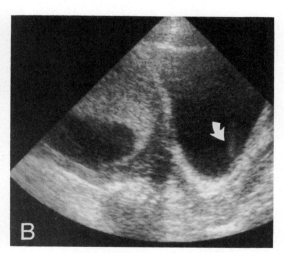

Figure 34–1. Longitudinal sonograms demonstrating the maternal urinary bladder and the gravid uterus. *A.* An apparent soft tissue mass is seen in the urinary bladder (*arrow*). *B.* In fact, this is the stream of urine entering the bladder through the ureteral orifice.

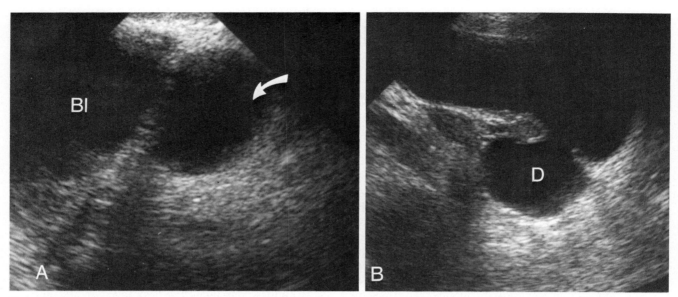

Figure 34–2. *A.* What appears to be a large pelvic cyst is seen in this patient (*arrow*). Bl, bladder. *B.* Although the connection to the bladder was not seen in *A,* this bladder diverticulum (D) is clearly seen in another plane of section.

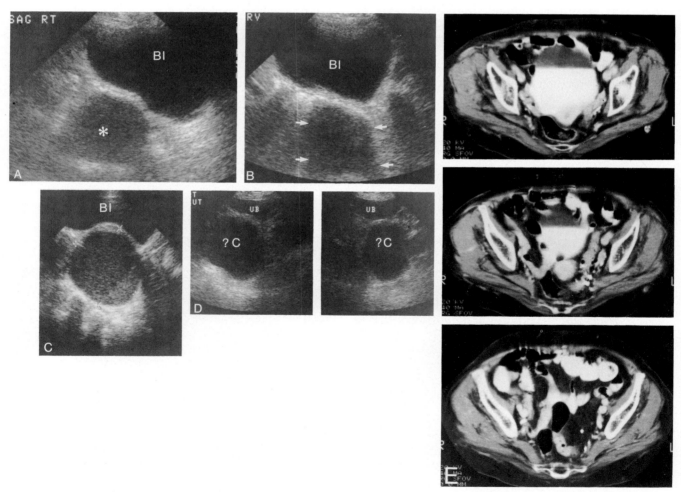

Figure 34–3. Bowel within the pelvis can masquerade as ovarian cysts. *A.* In this patient, bowel gas and its shadowing creates the appearance of a mass (*asterisk*). Bl, bladder. *B.* The strong reflection adjacent to the urinary bladder (Bl) or the "squared" appearance (*arrows*) to the "cyst" should make one suspicious that bowel gas artifact is causing this appearance. *C.* A true ovarian cyst (*cursors*) has borders on nearly every side and has enhanced through sound transmission and internal echoes. Bl, bladder. *D.* In this patient two different planes of section demonstrate what appears to be a large pelvic cyst (?C). In fact, this was due to bowel gas artifact. UB, bladder. *E.* Because this appearance was virtually indistinguishable from a pelvic cyst, a computed tomographic scan was performed immediately after the sonogram, confirming the artifactual nature of this "cyst." The scans were normal without evidence of a pelvic mass.

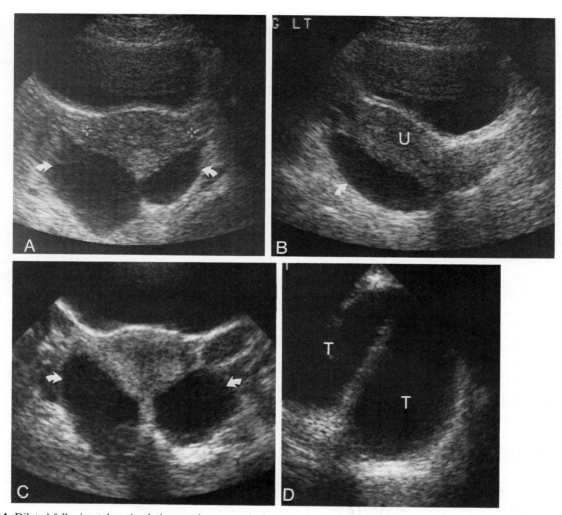

Figure 34–4. Dilated fallopian tubes simulating ovarian cysts. *A.* A transverse sonogram in this patient demonstrates what appear to be two ovarian cysts (*arrows*) posterior to the uterus (*cursors*). *B.* A longitudinal sonogram displays the elongated tubular nature of this fluid collection (*arrow*), which is more compatible with a dilated fallopian tube. U, uterus. *C.* In another patient two large, rounded fluid collections are seen (*arrows*) simulating ovarian cysts. *D.* A longitudinal plane of section through one of these collections demonstrates the tubular (T) retort nature of these dilated fallopian tubes.

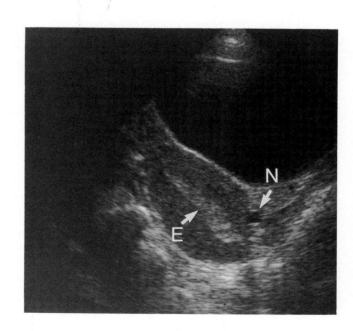

Figure 34–5. Longitudinal scan through the nongravid uterus. A small nabothian cyst (N) is seen in the cervical area. These retention cysts are quite commonly seen and should not be confused with low implanted gestational sacs or other pathology. E, endometrium.

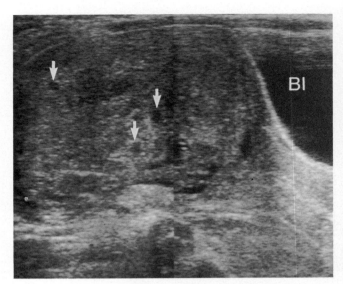

Figure 34–6. In this patient, the uterus is markedly enlarged and lobular with numerous small cystic areas (*arrows*) throughout. Although this has a similar appearance to a hydatidiform mole, in fact, the serum β-hCG was zero and the mass was due to myomatous disease. Bl, bladder.

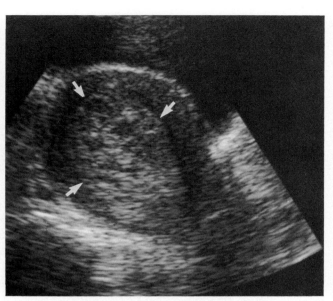

Figure 34–7. A large echogenic mass (*arrows*) is seen filling the uterine cavity in this patient. This has the appearance of a hydatidiform mole; however, no vesicles are seen. This patient had been known to be pregnant although the serum hCG level was zero. This represents a nonviable, missed abortion.

THE GRAVID UTERUS

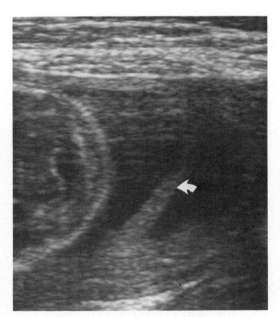

Figure 34–8. Transverse scan through the gravid uterus. A uterine synechia is seen (*arrow*). The fetus was seen to move on either side of the myometrial ridge. This should not be confused with an amniotic band.

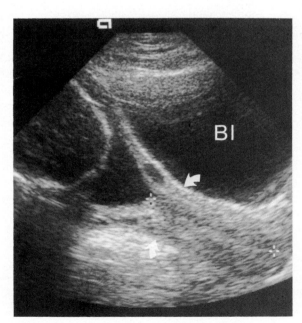

Figure 34–9. Overdistended urinary bladder causing the lower uterine segment to simulate the cervix. In this longitudinal scan the overdistended urinary bladder (Bl) causes apposition of the anterior and posterior lower uterine segment (*arrow*). The cursors are measuring both the cervical canal and lower uterine segment. Any time the cervix measures greater than 4 cm one should make sure an overdistended bladder is not the cause of this appearance.

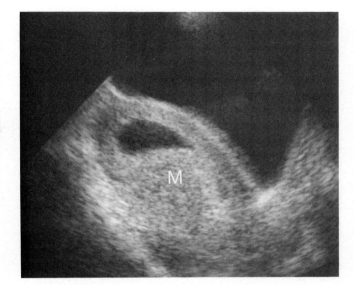

Figure 34–10. A myometrial contraction (M) in the posterior uterine segment is quite common in first-trimester sonograms. This should not be confused with a myoma.

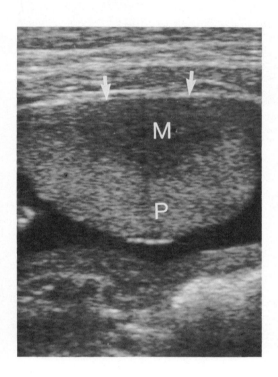

Figure 34–11. A myometrial contraction (M) in this second-trimester pregnancy simulates a myoma. Two features help make this distinction: First, in general, myometrial contractions tend to bulge inwardly without affecting the outer contour of the uterus (*arrows*). Uterine fibroids tend to bulge inward and outward, and myometrial contractions may resolve during the time of scanning. P, placenta.

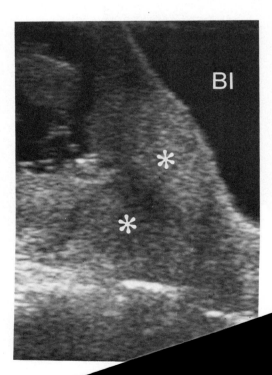

Figure 34–12. Myometrial contractions of the lower uterine segment may often touch one another (*asterisks*). These have been referred to as "kissing contractions." Bl, bladder.

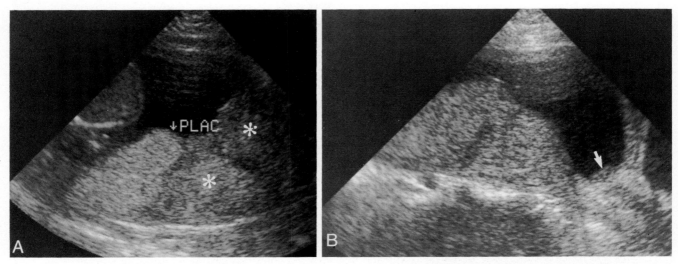

Figure 34–13. *A.* "Kissing contractions" of the lower uterine segment (*asterisks*). The caudal end of the placenta rests at the junction of these contractions. These contractions should not be confused with the cervix and mistakenly called a placenta previa. PLAC, placenta. *B.* With time there was resolution of the anterior contraction so that the cervical area could be identified (*arrow*).

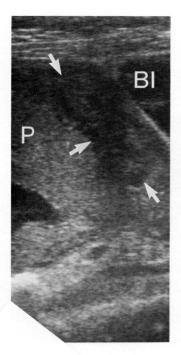

Figure 34–14. A lobular poorly echogenic mass in this patient is a uterine fibroid (*arrows*). This persisted over several examinations. P, placenta; Bl, bladder.

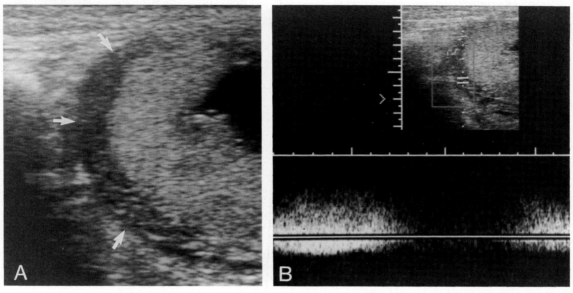

Figure 34–15. *A.* Veins present in the decidua basalis and myometrium contribute to a hypoechoic region beneath the placenta (*arrows*). This should not be misinterpreted as an abruption. *B.* Doppler interrogation of this region will often confirm the venous nature of this area.

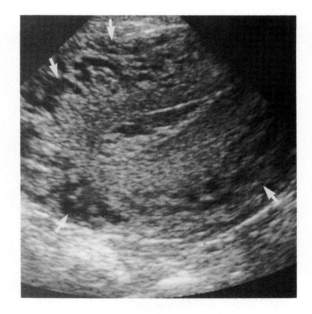

Figure 34–16. Prominent veins (*arrows*) at the periphery of the uterus. These are quite common in the gravid uterus and should not be mistaken as a precursor to an abruption or as trophoblastic disease.

THE FIRST TRIMESTER

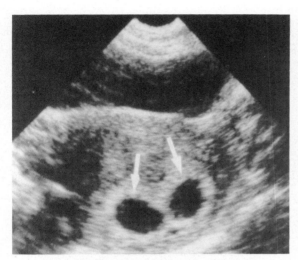

Figure 34–17. Transverse scan over the lower abdomen of an early gravid uterus. Although there appear to be two gestational sacs (*arrows*), in fact, there was only one sac. Moving the transducer slightly over to one side demonstrated the single gestational sac. This effect is believed to be due to the refraction of sound at the interface between the abdominal musculature and fat.

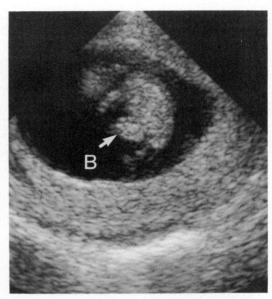

Figure 34–19. Before 12 weeks' gestation the embryonic bowel (B) is extra-abdominal within the umbilical cord. One should be cautious of diagnosing an abdominal wall defect at this stage of gestation.

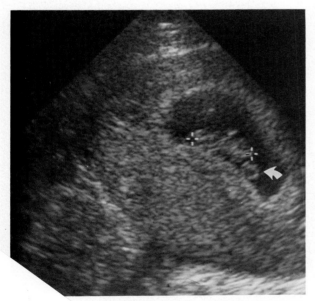

e yolk sac (*arrow*) is commonly identified in first-
This should not be included in the measure-
crown-rump length or mistakenly called a

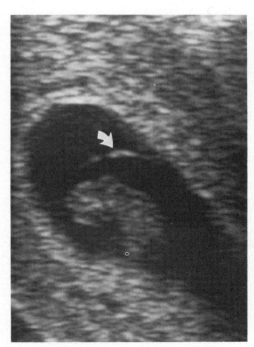

Figure 34–20. The amnion (*arrow*) is frequently identified in first-trimester gestations. It apposes the chorion between 12 and 16 weeks' gestations. It should not be mistaken for the amniotic band syndrome.

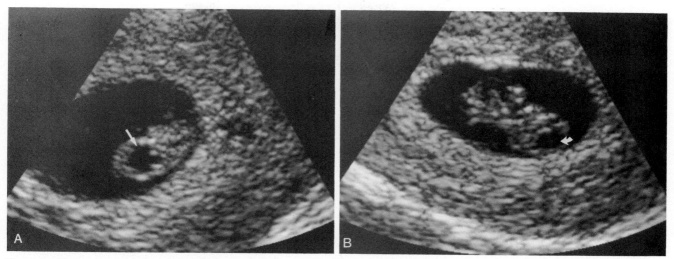

Figure 34–21. *A* and *B*. A prominent fluid-filled intracranial area (*arrow*) can be seen in the cranium of the embryo particularly with endovaginal sonography. This may represent the rhombencephalon and should not be mistaken for either hydrocephalus or holoprosencephaly.

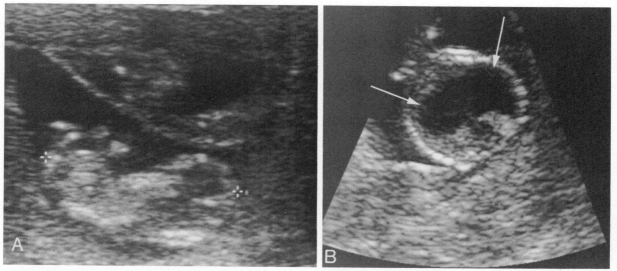

Figure 34–22. *A*. A transabdominal sonogram of the gravid uterus demonstrated what appeared to be a normal embryo. *B*. An endovaginal sonogram of the same patient done at the time of chorionic villus sampling demonstrates a large monoventricular cavity (*arrows*) consistent with holoprosencephaly. Trisomy 13 was detected.

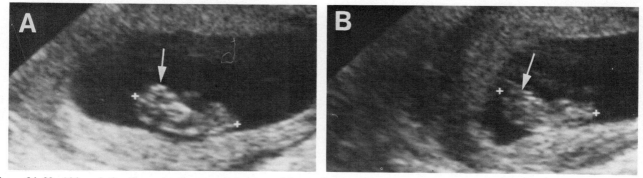

Figure 34–23. Although the diagnosis of anencephaly is certainly possible in the first trimester, the likelihood of a false-negative diagnosis is high. The angiomatous stroma (*A, arrow*) in a case of anencephaly simulates the normal brain (*B, arrow*).

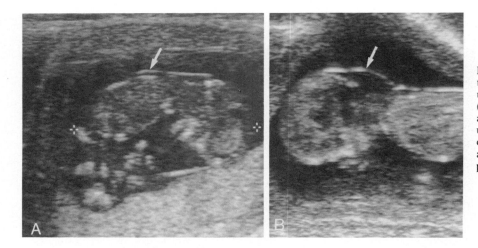

Figure 34–24. *A.* The normal integument of the embryo may be quite sonolucent, particularly in the region of the neck and thorax (*arrow*). *B.* This should not be diagnosed as an early cystic hygroma or lymphangiectasia unless there is prominent rounded protrusion or generalized edema (*arrow*). If there is any question, a follow-up scan should be performed.

THE FETAL NEURAL AXIS

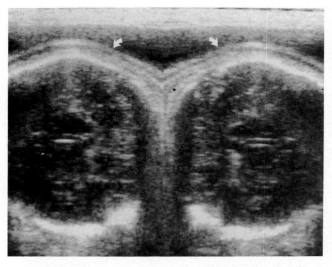

Figure 34–25. This is neither a case of conjoined twins nor hydrops fetalis. These are dual transverse images of the fetal calvarium of a fetus in longitudinal lie and cephalic presentation. The arrows do not point to scalp edema but rather to the maternal urinary bladder. Remember, the head abuts the urinary bladder in fetuses in cephalic presentation.

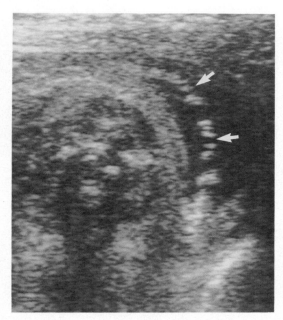

Figure 34–26. Normal fetal hair (*arrows*) may be seen commonly in third-trimester fetuses. This should not be mistaken for a calvarial mass or scalp edema.

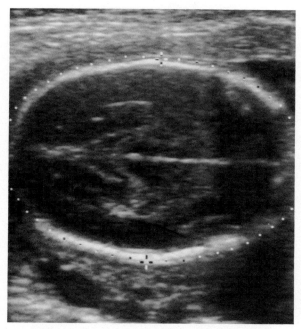

Figure 34–27. Sonogram of the fetal head commonly used for measurement of the biparietal diameter and head circumference. This case has a common variation referred to as dolichocephaly. The importance is that measurement of the biparietal diameter in such fetuses will tend to underestimate gestational age. Dolichocephaly may also be seen in cases of breech presentation, oligohydramnios, and myelomeningoceles.

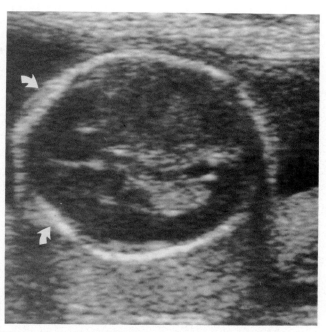

Figure 34–29. Frontal concave scalloping (*arrows*), the so-called lemon sign has been described in patients with a myelomeningocele. This may also be a normal finding, as it was in this case.

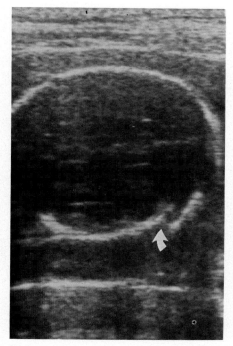

Figure 34–28. Interaction of the sound beam with the curved surface of the calvarium produces troubling appearances. This fetus appears to have overlapping sutures (*arrow*). In fact, this was an artifact related to refraction of the sound beam. The fetal calvarium was normal when the transducer angle was changed.

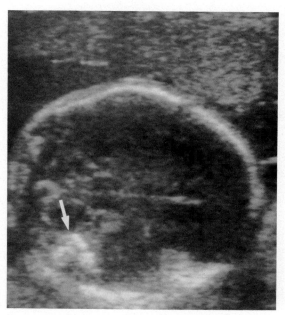

Figure 34–30. In this case a transverse axial plane of section demonstrates an echogenic mass (*arrow*) within the fetal brain. This is due to a slightly obliqued scan in which projection of the petrous ridge at the same level of the normal brain on the opposite side is seen.

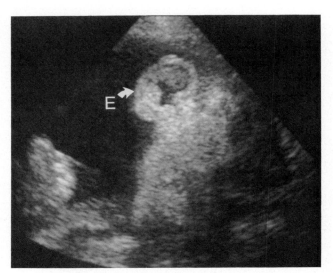

Figure 34–31. Projections from the fetal cranium can often be quite disturbing. In cases of polyhydramnios the fetal ear (E) can be seen perpendicular to the fetal skull and may simulate an encephalocele, which would be quite uncommon in this location.

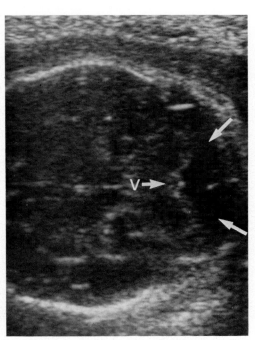

Figure 34–33. The cisterna magna (*arrows*) may be prominent in some persons. Controversy exists regarding the significance of a prominent cisterna magna in the absence of ventricular dilatation. It is my belief that if the cisterna magna is prominent, the cerebellar vermis (v) is normal, the ventricles are normal, and no other malformations are detected, then the overwhelming likelihood is that this is a normal variant.

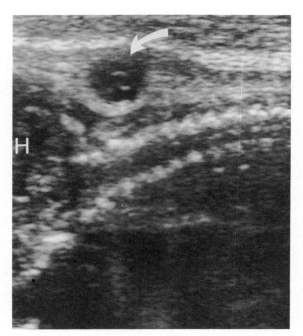

Figure 34–32. Amniotic fluid (*arrow*) is "trapped" between the posterior fetal neck and the myometrium. This may simulate such pathology as a cystic hygroma. Identification of structures within the fluid, such as umbilical cord, as in this case, or displacing the fetus away from the uterine wall will often reveal this to be "artifactual." H, head.

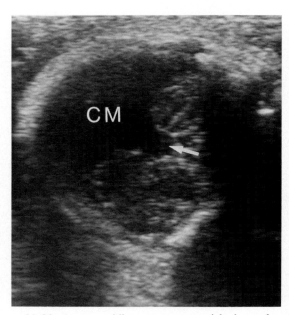

Figure 34–34. A steep oblique transverse axial plane of section through the posterior fossa may contribute to two pitfalls: the cisterna magna (CM) may appear overly prominent, and the normal space (vallecula) between the cerebellar hemispheres (*arrow*) may simulate vermian agenesis.

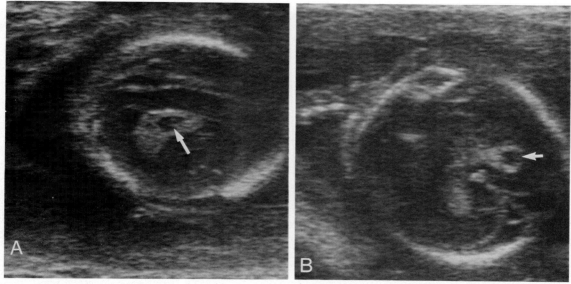

Figure 34–35. *A* and *B*. The choroid plexus cyst (*arrow*) is a normal variant that has been the subject of much controversy during the past several years. Although most cases are simply normal variants that will resolve by 24 to 26 weeks of gestation, some cases may be associated with other anomalies and trisomy 18.

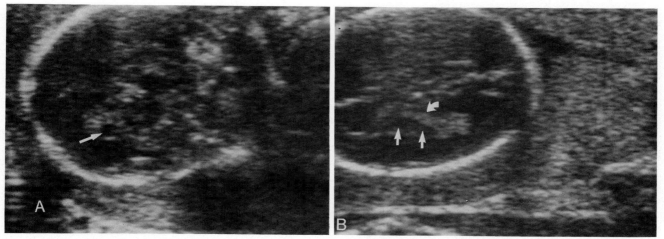

Figure 34–36. *A*. This patient has what appears to be a choroid plexus cyst (*arrow*) on this somewhat obliqued scan of the fetal head. *B*. On a more conventional transverse axial plane of section this "pseudocyst" elongates (*arrows*), proving to indent rather than be within the substance of the choroid plexus. Although the exact etiology of this is uncertain it may represent the corpus striatum.

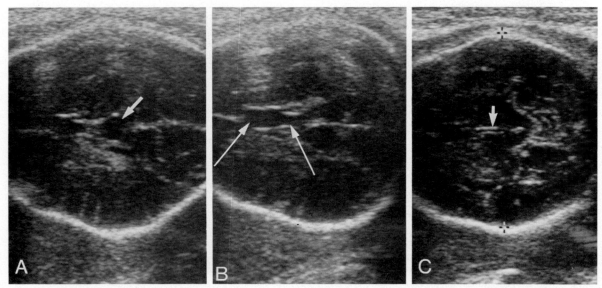

Figure 34–37. The cavum septi pellucidi is normally seen in scans of the second-trimester fetal brain. At times, a prominent but normal posterior continutation referred to as the cavum vergae can be seen. *A* and *B*. Portions of the cavum (*arrows*) may simulate either an arachnoid cyst or dilated third ventricle. *C*. The normal third ventricle (*arrow*) is easily identified in this case.

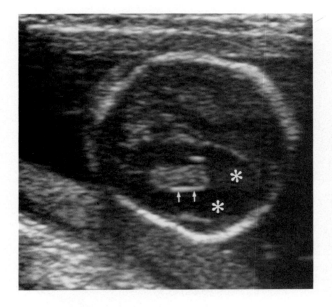

Figure 34–38. The normal fetal brain is quite sonolucent (*asterisks*) and may simulate cerebrospinal fluid. This may incorrectly lead to the diagnosis of hydrocephalus. Identification of the lateral ventricular walls (*arrows*) and the choroid plexus within will help clear up this confusion.

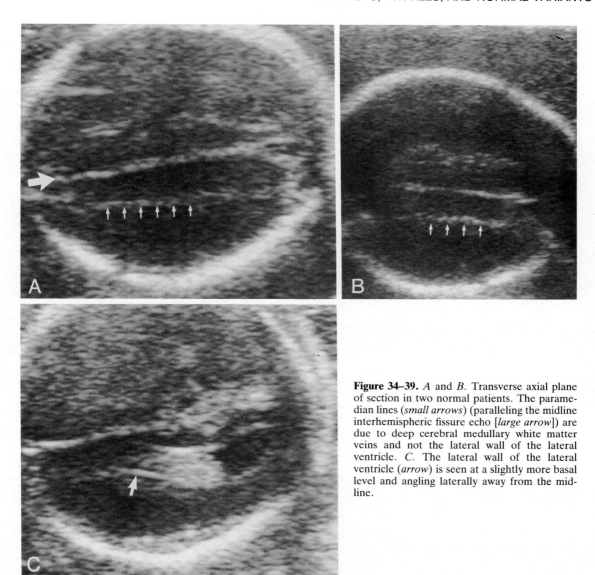

Figure 34–39. *A* and *B*. Transverse axial plane of section in two normal patients. The paramedian lines (*small arrows*) (paralleling the midline interhemispheric fissure echo [*large arrow*]) are due to deep cerebral medullary white matter veins and not the lateral wall of the lateral ventricle. *C*. The lateral wall of the lateral ventricle (*arrow*) is seen at a slightly more basal level and angling laterally away from the midline.

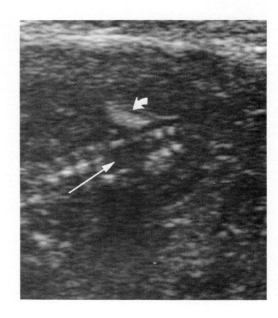

Figure 34–40. Shadowing (*arrow*) from the iliac wing (*curved arrow*) may simulate a gap or fluid-filled cystic space (i.e., myelomeningocele) of the lumbar spine.

THE FETAL THORAX

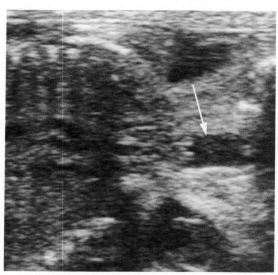

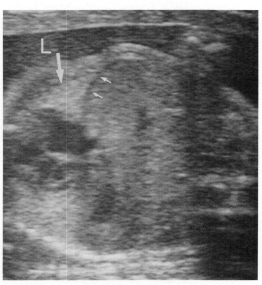

Figure 34–41. The fetal hypopharynx (*arrow*) may be quite prominent. It may be seen to fill and empty with fluid during the examination. This should not be mistaken as representing esophageal obstruction.

Figure 34–42. The echogenicity of the fetal lung (L) may often be misleading. The lung in this oblique coronal scan appears quite echogenic; however, this fetus is neither mature nor has lung pathology. Small arrows indicate diaphragm.

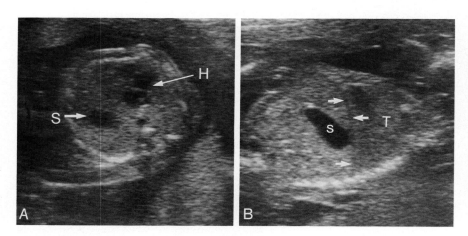

Figure 34–43. *A.* Transverse axial plane of section at the level of the fetal heart (H). The fetal stomach (S) is seen at the same level as the heart, raising the possibility of a diaphragmatic hernia. *B.* This sagittal plane of section from the same patient reminds us that the diaphragms (*arrows*) are curved, and a slightly angled transverse plane of section will portray what appears to be a diaphragmatic hernia, although the stomach (S) is, in fact, below the diaphragm. T, thorax.

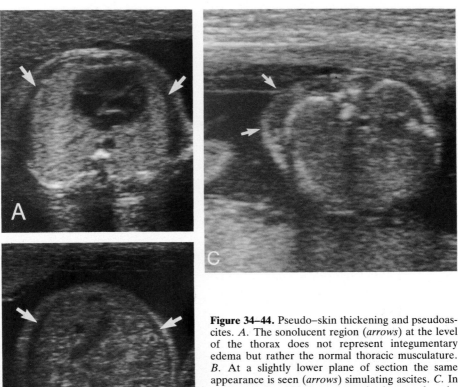

Figure 34–44. Pseudo–skin thickening and pseudoascites. *A.* The sonolucent region (*arrows*) at the level of the thorax does not represent integumentary edema but rather the normal thoracic musculature. *B.* At a slightly lower plane of section the same appearance is seen (*arrows*) simulating ascites. *C.* In another patient this appearance is also noted at the region of the scapula (*arrows*) where it is often most prominent.

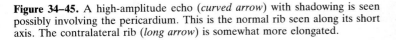

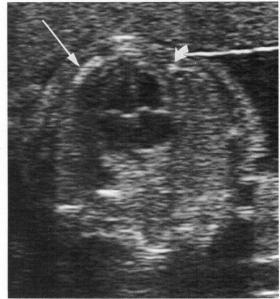

Figure 34–45. A high-amplitude echo (*curved arrow*) with shadowing is seen possibly involving the pericardium. This is the normal rib seen along its short axis. The contralateral rib (*long arrow*) is somewhat more elongated.

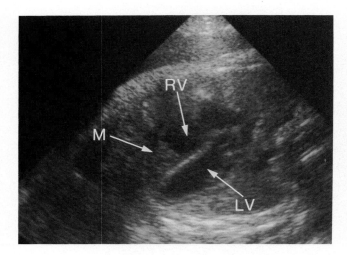

Figure 34–46. Tissue seen within the ventricle is always worrisome for either thrombus or neoplasm. In this patient the normal but prominent moderator band of the right ventricle (M) is seen. RV, right ventricle; LV, left ventricle.

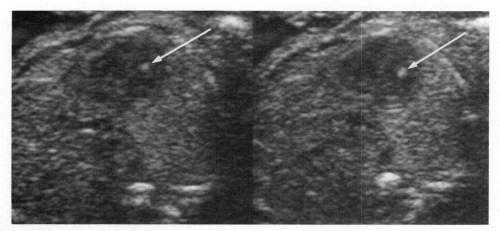

Figure 34–47. A high-amplitude echo (*arrow*) is seen in the ventricle in this patient. This appearance is believed to be due to reflection from the chordae tendineae/papillary muscle.

THE FETAL ABDOMEN

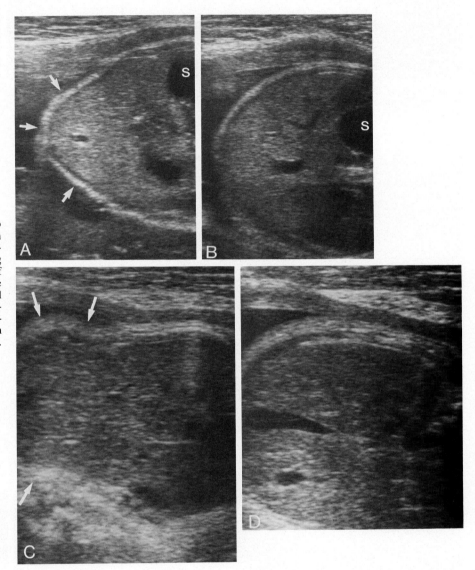

Figure 34–48. Pseudo-omphalocele in two patients. *A* and *C*. Excessive pressure with the linear array transducer causes deformation of the abdominal wall, simulating an abdominal wall defect. Identification of the normal skin covering this protuberance (*arrows*) and less pressure on the maternal abdomen will usually clear up the confusion. *B* and *D*. Same patients demonstrating normal anterior abdominal wall with light pressure on the maternal abdomen. S, stomach.

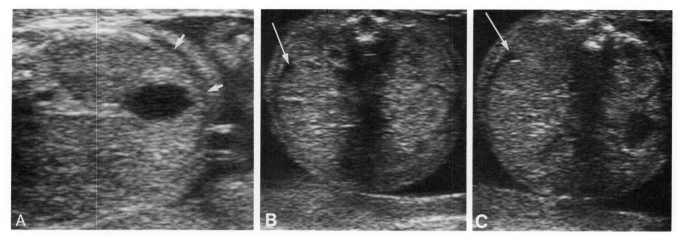

Figure 34–49. *A.* Pseudoascites due to the poorly echogenic appearance of the normal integument (*arrows*). *B* and *C.* A small of amount of real ascites is identified in this patient. Notice that the fluid invaginates between the viscera on the right side (*arrows*).

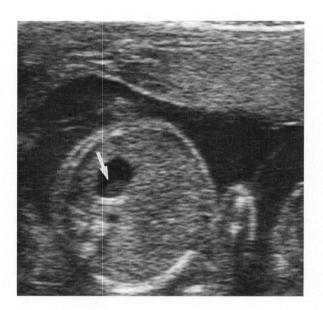

Figure 34–50. Debris within the fetal stomach (*arrow*). Although occasionally the cause may be known (i.e., swallowed blood from an intrauterine transfusion), most often the etiology is unknown. This is almost always an innocuous finding.

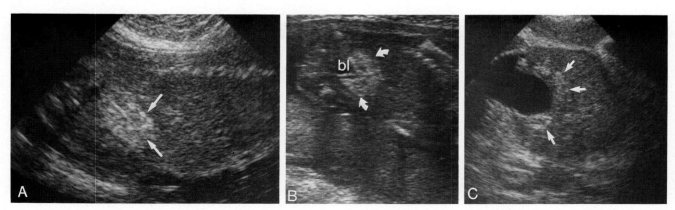

Figure 34–51. Hyperechogenicity within the fetal abdomen (*arrows*). This finding has received recent attention in the literature as a possible clue to the diagnosis of either cystic fibrosis or aneuploidy. The problem is in differentiating normal from abnormal. *A* and *B.* Normal chromosomes and no evidence of cystic fibrosis. bl, bladder. *C.* A case of meconium ileus and cystic fibrosis at birth (*arrows*).

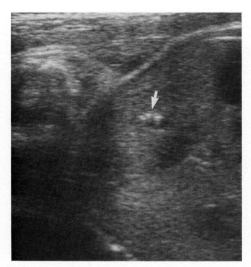

Figure 34–52. Fetal gallstones (*arrows*) seen in a early third-trimester fetus. The fetus was otherwise normal. This finding does not indicate biliary pathology and may resolve before birth.

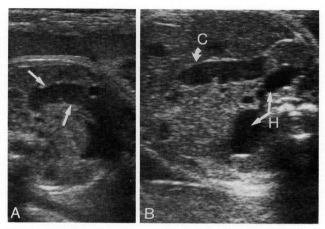

Figure 34–54. The fetal colon may be quite prominent in the third-trimester fetus. *A.* Normal colon in a fetus (*arrows*) in the third trimester. *B.* The colon (C) is prominent but normal in this patient who was evaluated for bilateral ureteropelvic junction obstruction, ultimately repaired. H, hydronephrosis.

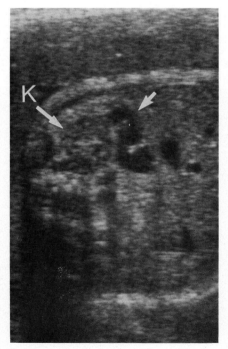

Figure 34–53. The fetal intestine (*arrow*) may simulate other non-intestinal structures such as a dilated ureter. This is especially true in the second trimester when the meconium-filled distal small bowel and colon are quite sonolucent. K, kidney.

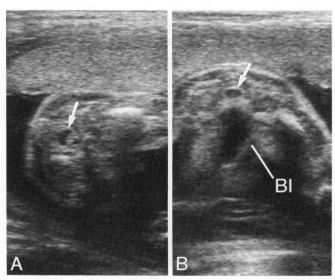

Figure 34–55. *A* and *B*. The normal rectum (*arrows*) can occasionally be seen in the second- and third-trimester fetus. This should not be mistaken for a myelomeningocele or other intrapelvic pathology. Bl, bladder.

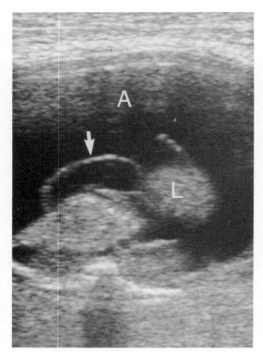

Figure 34–56. In the presence of fetal ascites (A) fluid may enter the lesser sac and result in outlining of the greater omentum (*arrow*). This should not be mistaken for a dilated loop of intestine. L, liver.

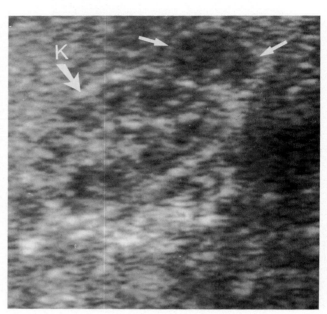

Figure 34–58. The nonfluid filled colon (*arrows*) is seen adjacent to the kidney (K) in this patient. This should not be misinterpreted as a renal mass.

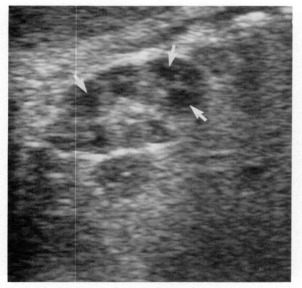

Figure 34–57. The normal fetal renal pyramids may be quite sonolucent (*arrows*) and simulate hydronephrosis. This appearance is normal and should be seen as a normal and expected finding. Failure to identify a dilated medial renal pelvis should reassure the interpreter.

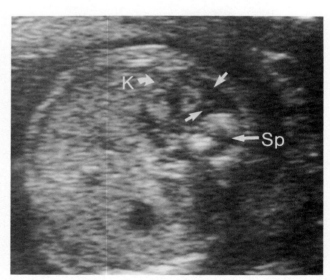

Figure 34–59. The normal poorly echogenic pararenal musculature (quadratus lumborum and psoas) (*arrows*) may simulate fluid around the kidney (K). Sp, spine.

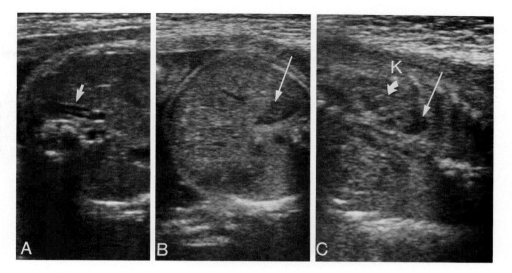

Figure 34–60. *A* through *C.* The normal fetal adrenal gland (*arrow*) may have either a linear appearance or be rounded and should not be mistaken for either the fetal kidney or a renal mass. K, kidney.

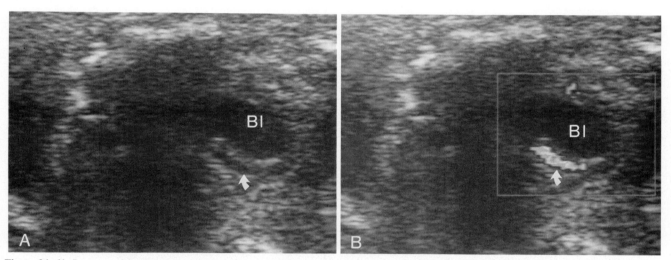

Figure 34–61. In cases of fetal hydroephrosis, evaluation of the urinary bladder size and wall thickness are important steps in identifying the level of obstruction. *A.* In this case the normal umbilical/iliac artery (*arrow*) coursing around the urinary bladder (Bl) may simulate a thickened bladder wall. *B.* Doppler interrogation of this structure will confirm that this is a normal vessel (*arrow*).

Figure 34–62. Dilatation of the intra-abdominal umbilical vein (varix) has been reported to be associated with a poor outcome in some fetuses. *A.* Umbilical vein varix (V). *B.* Doppler flow (*arrow*) will differentiate this from a cystic mass.

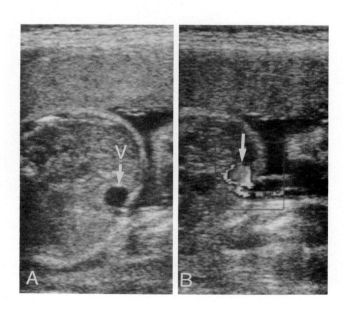

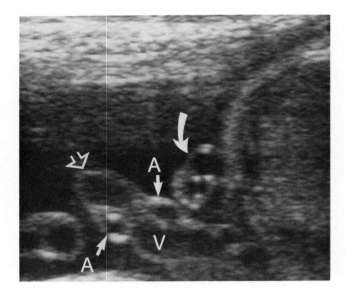

Figure 34–63. A short-axis view of the umbilical cord should always be obtained when attempting to identify the number of vessels. In this case the long-axis view (*open arrow*) appears to show two umbilical arteries (A) and one vein (V). In the short-axis view (*curved arrow*) the correct interpretation of a single umbilical artery in a two-vessel cord can be made.

AMNIOTIC FLUID AND MEMBRANES

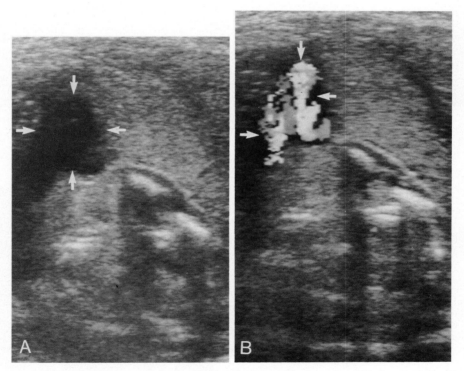

Figure 34–64. When amniotic fluid volume is assessed the "pocket" of fluid should be free of umbilical cord. *A.* In this patient there appears to be a 3-cm pocket of amniotic fluid (*arrows*). *B.* Doppler evaluation of this area revealed that this "pocket" was not amniotic fluid but all umbilical cord (*arrows*).

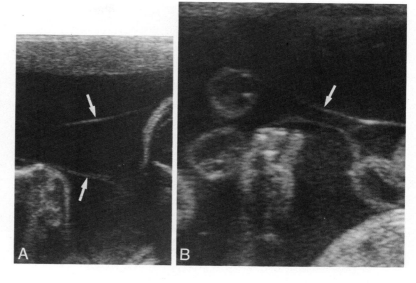

Figure 34–65. Chorioamniotic separation may occur, although rarely after an amniocentesis. *A* and *B*. In both of these patients, chorioamniotic separation has occurred after an amniocentesis. The membranes (*arrows*) are intact, although they "enshroud" the fetus. These patients are likely *not* at risk for deformities owing to the amniotic band syndrome but may be at increased risk for preterm rupture of the membranes and delivery.

THE FETAL SKELETON

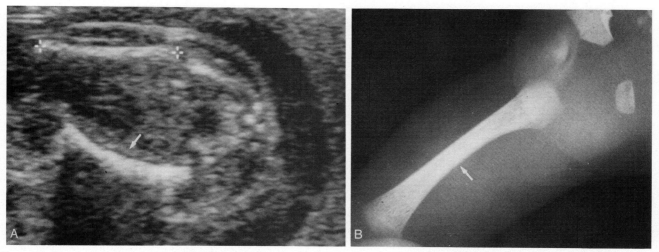

Figure 34–66. *A*. The normal fetal femur has a medial curve to the metadiaphyseal region. This is seen in the femur farthest from the transducer (*arrow*). The femur closest to the transducer (*cursors*) will demonstrate a straight appearance because the lateral aspect is reflecting the sound and the medial aspect is within its shadow. *B*. Radiograph of a normal neonatal femur demonstrating the normal curved appearance of its medial aspect (*arrow*).

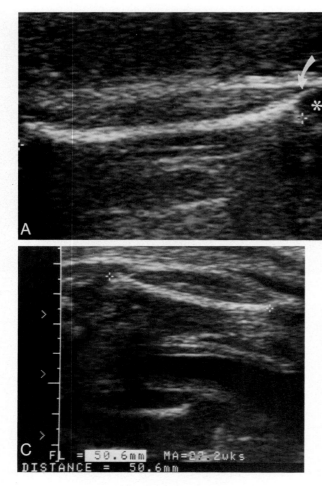

Figure 34–67. Scans of the fetal femur often demonstrate a linear projection from the distal end. *A.* This projection (*arrow*) is a specular reflection from the distal epiphyseal cartilage (*asterisk*). *B.* The measurement of the femur should *not* include this reflection (*arrow*). *C.* The measurement should only include the calcified bone. Inclusion of this reflection would have overestimated the gestational age by as much as 3 weeks.

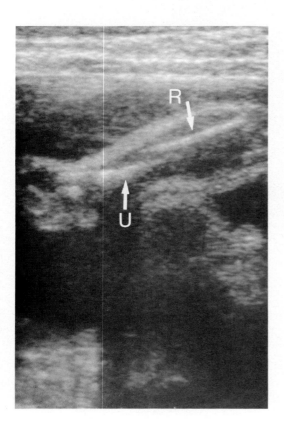

Figure 34–68. Pronation and supination of the forearm may create the appearance that the radius (R) or the ulna (U) is abnormally short (limb reduction abnormality). When both bones are "short" at opposite ends in the same scan one should be suspicious that this is a technical rather than a real abnormality.

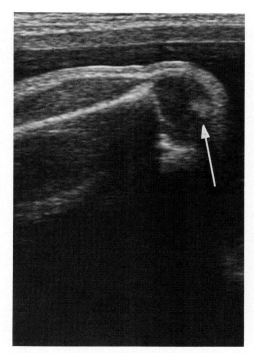

Figure 34–69. The appearance of the epiphyseal ossification centers is helpful in trying to assess gestational age. The synovial tissue is quite echogenic (*arrow*) and may simulate the appearance of one of these centers as in this case. The real epiphyseal center would be slightly more proximal.

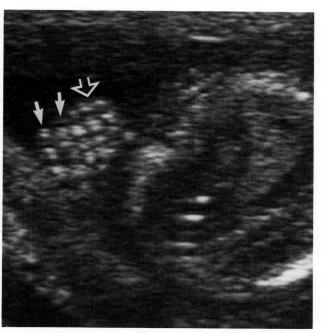

Figure 34–70. In this case, both hands of the fetus are adjacent to one another. The fingers (*arrows*) from one hand and the fingers (*open arrow*) from the other simulate the appearance of polydactyly.

MULTIPLE GESTATIONS

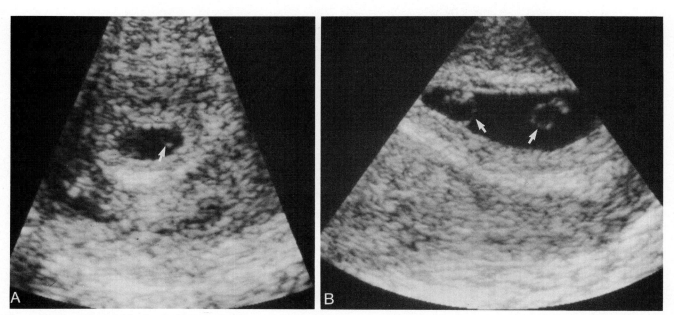

Figure 34–71. Although ideally, multiple-gestation pregnancies should never be missed, it is my experience that when cases are missed it is usually in the first trimester, even with endovaginal scanning. *A.* An endovaginal sonogram done for vaginal bleeding revealed a yolk sac (*arrow*) with cardiac activity noted at the edge of the yolk sac. *B.* Because of continued spotting the patient returned the following week. At this time, two yolk sacs (*arrows*) were identified in this monochorionic pregnancy.

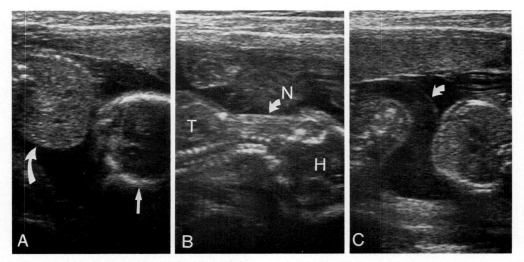

Figure 34–72. The false-negative diagnosis of twins is unusual in the second trimester. If this occurs it likely results from not connecting the fetal head to its body while routine scanning is performed. *A.* In this patient, the fetal head (*straight arrow*) and body (*curved arrow*) are seen in this longitudinal plane of section. Unfortunately, these structures are from different fetuses in this twin pregnancy. *B.* The only way to be absolutely sure of the relation of the head (H) to the body is to demonstrate both structures on the same scan connected to one another through the neck (N). *T,* thorax. *C.* The dividing membrane (*arrow*) is seen on another plane of section clearly dividing the two fetuses.

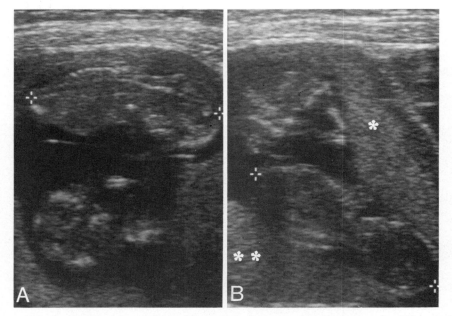

Figure 34–73. Membrane thickness is often quite useful in differentiating between monochorionic twins (thin membrane) and dichorionic twins (thick membrane). This method is not always successful, however. *A.* In this twin pregnancy a scan done at 14 weeks' gestation demonstrates a thin membrane dividing the two gestational sacs. This would imply monochorionicity. *B.* A longitudinal plane of section done at the same time reveals both an anterior (*asterisk*) and a posterior (*double asterisks*) placenta.

ARTIFACTS

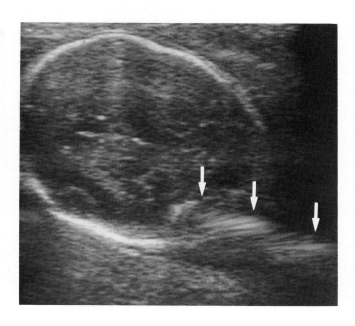

Figure 34–74. Side lobe (gradient) artifact can occur with even the most sophisticated of ultrasound scanning equipment. In this case a side lobe artifact is seen overlying the fetal head (*arrows*). The artifactual nature of these echoes can be confirmed by noting that these echoes are not confined to the head but extend beyond its confines. In addition, changing the scan plane orientation will show the region to be normal.

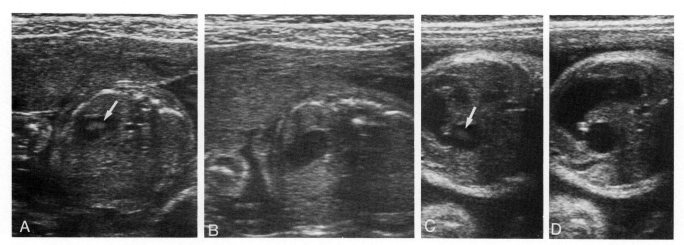

Figure 34–75. *A* and *C.* Two cases of artifact (*arrow*) appear in the fetal stomach. *B* and *D.* If one changes the scanning plane these echoes will disappear from the area of concern.

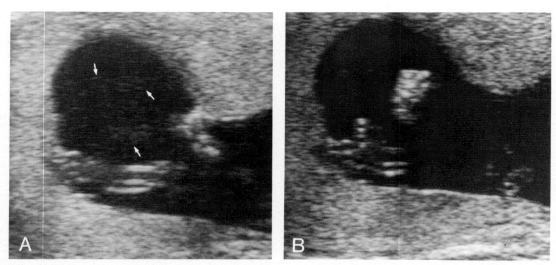

Figure 34–76. The differentiation of real from artifactual echoes is often problematic during sonographic scanning. A common misconception is that by changing to a lower-frequency transducer and decreasing the overall system gain or just reducing the system gain alone will cause the artifactual echoes alone to disappear. Although it is true that artifactual echoes will not be displayed with these maneuvers, it should be remembered that the real echoes will not be displayed either. *A.* In this patient numerous low-level echoes (*arrows*) were seen swirling around in the amniotic fluid during real-time scanning. Although the origin of the echoes is not known, they may represent shed fetal epithelial cells. *B.* When the system gain was decreased, these real echoes virtually disappeared. Although the hard-copy images do not resolve this dilemma, the echoes were quite clearly seen to be moving and real when the sonologist was performing the scan.

The teaching point of this last case of this chapter—and the book as a whole—is that when there is a difficult case or problem, there is no substitute for being in the room and scanning the patient yourself.

■ APPENDIX A

Measurements Frequently Used to Estimate Gestational Age and Fetal Biometry

Table A–1. METHODS FOR DETERMINING MENSTRUAL AGE

Clinical or Sonographic Parameter	Variability Estimate (2 SD)
In vitro fertilization*	±1 day
Ovulation induction*	±3 days
Artificial insemination*	±3 days
Single intercourse record*	±3 days
Basal body temperature record*	±4 days
First-trimester physical examination	±2 weeks
Second-trimester physical examination	±4 weeks
Third-trimester physical examination	±6 weeks
First-trimester sonographic examination (CRL)	±8% of the estimate
Second-trimester sonographic examination (HC, FL)	±8% of the estimate
Third-trimester sonographic examination (HC, FL)	±8% of the estimate

CRL, crown-rump length; HC, head circumference; FL, femur length.
*These are indicators of conceptual age (menstrual age = conceptual age + 14 days).
Adapted from Frank P. Hadlock, M.D., and James D. Bowie, M.D.

Table A–2. VARIABILITY IN PREDICTING MENSTRUAL AGE FROM SONOGRAPHIC MEASUREMENTS (14–20 WEEKS)

Parameter	Variability (2 SD)			
	Hadlock et al.*	Rossavik and Fishburne†	Persson and Weldner‡	Benson and Doubilet§
BPD	0.94 wk	1.02 wk	0.92 wk	1.40 wk
HC	0.84 wk	0.92 wk	ND	1.20 wk
AC	1.04 wk	1.12 wk	ND	2.10 wk
FL	0.96 wk	ND	0.98 wk	1.40 wk
BPD, FL	0.80 wk	ND	0.78 wk	ND
HC, FL	0.76 wk	ND	ND	ND

BPD, biparietal diameter; HC, head circumference; AC, abdominal circumference; FL, femur length; ND, no data.
*Data from Hadlock FP, Harrist RB, Martinez-Poyer J: How accurate is second trimester fetal dating? J Ultrasound Med 10:557, 1992.
†Data from Rossavik IK, Fishburne JI: Conceptional age, menstrual age, and ultrasound age: A second trimester comparison of pregnancies of known conception date with pregnancies dated from the last menstrual period. Obstet Gynecol 73:243, 1989.
‡Data from Persson PH, Weldner BM: Reliability of ultrasound fetometry in estimating gestational age in the second trimester. Acta Obstet Gynecol Scand 65:481, 1986.
§Data from Benson CB, Doubilet PM: Sonographic prediction of gestational age: Accuracy of second and third trimester fetal measurements. AJR 157:1275, 1991.

Table A–3. VARIABILITY IN PREDICTING MENSTRUAL AGE IN THE SECOND HALF OF PREGNANCY (20–42 WEEKS)

Parameter	Variability in Weeks (±2 SD)		
	20–26 Weeks	26–32 Weeks	32–42 Weeks
BPD	2.1 wk	3.8 wk	4.1 wk
Corrected BPD	1.9 wk	3.3 wk	3.8 wk
HC	1.9 wk	3.4 wk	3.8 wk
AC	3.7 wk	3.0 wk	4.5 wk
FL	2.5 wk	3.1 wk	3.5 wk

BPD, biparietal diameter; HC, head circumference; AC, abdominal circumference; FL, femur length.
Adapted from Benson CB, Doubilet PM: Sonographic prediction of gestational age: Accuracy of second and third trimester fetal measurements. AJR 157:1275, 1991.

Table A–4. VARIABILITY ESTIMATES FOR SECONDARY BIOMETRIC PARAMETERS

Parameter	Variability in Weeks (±2 SD)				
	12–18 Weeks	18–24 Weeks	24–30 Weeks	30–36 Weeks	36–42 Weeks
Binocular Distance*	1.8	2.4	3.0	4.0	4.0
Cerebellar diameter†	1.0	1.8	2.0	2.4	3.2
Clavicle length‡	6.5	6.5	6.5	6.5	6.5
Radius length§	1.8	2.2	2.9	3.5	4.1
Ulna length‖	3.6	3.6	3.6	3.6	3.6
Tibia length‖	3.5	3.5	3.5	3.5	3.5
Foot length¶	1.2	1.7	2.2	2.6	3.1

*Data from Jeanty P, Cantraine F, Cousaert E, et al: The binocular distance: A new way to estimate fetal age. J Ultrasound Med 3:241, 1984.
†Data from Hill LM, et al: Transverse cerebellar diameter as a predictor of menstrual age. Obstet Gynecol 75:983, 1990.
‡Data from Yarkoni S, Schmidt W, Jeanty P, et al: Clavicular measurement: A new biometric parameter for fetal evaluation. J Ultrasound Med 4:467, 1985.
§Data from Hill LM, Guzick D, Thomas ML, Fries JK: Fetal radius length: A critical evaluation of race as a factor in gestational age assessment. Am J Obstet Gynecol 161:193, 1989.
‖Data from Jeanty P, Rodesch F, Delbeke D: Estimation of fetal age by long bone measurements. J Ultrasound Med 3:75, 1984.
¶Data from Mercer BM, Sklar S, Shariatmadar A, et al: Fetal foot length as a predictor of gestational age. Am J Obstet Gynecol 15:350, 1987.

Table A–5. GESTATIONAL SAC MEASUREMENT

Mean Predicted Gestational Sac (cm)	Gestational Age (wk)	Mean Predicted Gestational Sac (cm)	Gestational Age (wk)
1.0	5.0	3.6	8.8
1.1	5.2	3.7	8.9
1.2	5.3	3.8	9.0
1.3	5.5	3.9	9.2
1.4	5.6	4.0	9.3
1.5	5.8	4.1	9.5
1.6	5.9	4.2	9.6
1.7	6.0	4.3	9.7
1.8	6.2	4.4	9.9
1.9	6.3	4.5	10.0
2.0	6.5	4.6	10.2
2.1	6.6	4.7	10.3
2.2	6.8	4.8	10.5
2.3	6.9	4.9	10.6
2.4	7.0	5.0	10.7
2.5	7.2	5.1	10.9
2.6	7.3	5.2	11.0
2.7	7.5	5.3	11.2
2.8	7.6	5.4	11.3
2.9	7.8	5.5	11.5
3.0	7.9	5.6	11.6
3.1	8.0	5.7	11.7
3.2	8.2	5.8	11.9
3.3	8.3	5.9	12.0
3.4	8.5	6.0	12.2
3.5	8.6		

From Hellman LM, Kobayashi M, Fillisti L, et al: Growth and development of the human fetus prior to the twentieth week of gestation. Am J Obstet Gynecol 103:789, 1969.

Table A–6. RELATION BETWEEN MEAN SAC DIAMETER, MENSTRUAL AGE, AND HUMAN CHORIONIC GONADOTROPIN

Mean Gestational Sac Diameter (mm)	Predicted Age (wk) Range = 95% CI*	Predicted hCG (mIU/mL) Range = 95% CI†
2	5.0 (4.5–5.5)	1,164 (629–2,188)
3	5.1 (4.6–5.6)	1,377 (771–2,589)
4	5.2 (4.8–5.7)	1,629 (863–3,036)
5	5.4 (4.9–5.8)	1,932 (1,026–3,636)
6	5.5 (5.0–6.0)	2,165 (1,226–4,256)
7	5.6 (5.1–6.1)	2,704 (1,465–4,990)
8	5.7 (5.3–6.2)	3,199 (1,749–5,852)
9	5.9 (5.4–6.3)	3,785 (2,085–6,870)
10	6.0 (5.5–6.5)	4,478 (2,483–8,075)
11	6.1 (5.6–6.6)	5,297 (2,952–9,508)
12	6.2 (5.8–6.7)	6,267 (3,502–11,218)
13	6.4 (5.9–6.8)	7,415 (4,145–13,266)
14	6.5 (6.0–7.0)	8,773 (4,894–15,726)
15	6.6 (6.2–7.1)	10,379 (5,766–18,682)
16	6.7 (6.3–7.2)	12,270 (6,776–22,235)
17	6.9 (6.4–7.3)	14,528 (7,964–26,501)
18	7.0 (6.5–7.5)	17,188 (9,343–31,621)
19	7.1 (6.6–7.6)	20,337 (10,951–37,761)
20	7.3 (6.8–7.7)	24,060 (12,820–45,130)
21	7.4 (6.9–7.8)	28,464 (15,020–53,970)
22	7.5 (7.0–8.0)	33,675 (17,560–64,570)
23	7.6 (7.2–8.1)	39,843 (20,573–77,164)
24	7.8 (7.3–8.2)	47,138 (24,067–93,325)

*Predicted age from mean sac diameter is from Daya S, Woods S, Ward S, et al: Early pregnancy assessment with transvaginal ultrasound scanning. Can Med Assoc J 144:441, 1991.

†Predicted hCG from mean sac diameter is from Nyberg DA, Filly RA, Filho DL, et al: Abnormal pregnancy: Early diagnosis by US and serum gonadotropin levels. Radiology 158:393, 1986 (hCG calibrated against the Second International Standard).

Table A–7. PREDICTED MENSTRUAL AGE (MA) IN WEEKS FROM CROWN-RUMP LENGTH (CRL) MEASUREMENTS (CM)*

CRL	MA	CRL	MA	CRL	MA	CRL	MA	CRL	MA	CRL	MA
0.2	5.7	2.2	8.9	4.2	11.1	6.2	12.6	8.2	14.2	10.2	16.1
0.3	5.9	2.3	9.0	4.3	11.2	6.3	12.7	8.3	14.2	10.3	16.2
0.4	6.1	2.4	9.1	4.4	11.2	6.4	12.8	8.4	14.3	10.4	16.3
0.5	6.2	2.5	9.2	4.5	11.3	6.5	12.8	8.5	14.4	10.5	16.4
0.6	6.4	2.6	9.4	4.6	11.4	6.6	12.9	8.6	14.5	10.6	16.5
0.7	6.6	2.7	9.5	4.7	11.5	6.7	13.0	8.7	14.6	10.7	16.6
0.8	6.7	2.8	9.6	4.8	11.6	6.8	13.1	8.8	14.7	10.8	16.7
0.9	6.9	2.9	9.7	4.9	11.7	6.9	13.1	8.9	14.8	10.9	16.8
1.0	7.2	3.0	9.9	5.0	11.7	7.0	13.2	9.0	14.9	11.0	16.9
1.1	7.2	3.1	10.0	5.1	11.8	7.1	13.3	9.1	15.0	11.1	17.0
1.2	7.4	3.2	10.1	5.2	11.9	7.2	13.4	9.2	15.1	11.2	17.1
1.3	7.5	3.3	10.2	5.3	12.0	7.3	13.4	9.3	15.2	11.3	17.2
1.4	7.7	3.4	10.3	5.4	12.0	7.4	13.5	9.4	15.3	11.4	17.3
1.5	7.9	3.5	10.4	5.5	12.1	7.5	13.6	9.5	15.3	11.5	17.4
1.6	8.0	3.6	10.5	5.6	12.2	7.6	13.7	9.6	15.4	11.6	17.5
1.7	8.1	3.7	10.6	5.7	12.3	7.7	13.8	9.7	15.5	11.7	17.6
1.8	8.3	3.8	10.7	5.8	12.3	7.8	13.8	9.8	15.6	11.8	17.7
1.9	8.4	3.9	10.8	5.9	12.4	7.9	13.9	9.9	15.7	11.9	17.8
2.0	8.6	4.0	10.9	6.0	12.5	8.0	14.0	10.0	15.9	12.0	17.9
2.1	8.7	4.1	11.0	6.1	12.6	8.1	14.1	10.1	16.0	12.1	18.0

*The 95% confidence interval is ± 8% of the predicted age.

From Hadlock FP, Shah YP, Kanon DJ, Lindsey JV: Fetal crown-rump length: Reevaluation of relation to menstrual age (5–18 weeks) with high-resolution real-time US. Radiology 182:501–505, 1992.

Table A–8. PREDICTED MENSTRUAL AGE FOR BIPARIETAL DIAMETER MEASUREMENTS (2.6–9.7 cm)

BPD (cm)	Menstrual Age (wk)	BPD (cm)	Menstrual Age (wk)
2.6	13.9	6.2	25.3
2.7	14.2	6.3	25.7
2.8	14.5	6.4	26.1
2.9	14.7	6.5	26.4
3.0	15.0	6.6	26.8
3.1	15.3	6.7	27.2
3.2	15.6	6.8	27.6
3.3	15.9	6.9	28.0
3.4	16.2	7.0	28.3
3.5	16.5	7.1	28.7
3.6	16.8	7.2	29.1
3.7	17.1	7.3	29.5
3.8	17.4	7.4	29.9
3.9	17.7	7.5	30.4
4.0	18.0	7.6	30.8
4.1	18.3	7.7	31.2
4.2	18.6	7.8	31.6
4.3	18.9	7.9	32.0
4.4	19.2	8.0	32.5
4.5	19.5	8.1	32.9
4.6	19.9	8.3	33.3
4.7	20.2	8.3	33.8
4.8	20.5	8.4	34.2
4.9	20.8	8.5	34.7
5.0	21.2	8.6	35.1
5.1	21.5	8.7	35.6
5.2	21.8	8.8	36.1
5.3	22.2	8.9	36.5
5.4	22.5	9.0	37.0
5.5	22.8	9.1	37.5
5.6	23.2	9.2	38.0
5.7	23.5	9.3	38.5
5.8	23.9	9.4	38.9
5.9	24.2	9.5	39.4
6.0	24.6	9.6	39.9
6.1	25.0	9.7	40.5

Variability Estimates (±2 SD)

12–18 wk	±1.2 wk
18–24 wk	±1.7 wk
24–30 wk	±2.2 wk
30–36 wk	±3.1 wk
36–42 wk	±3.2 wk

Data from Hadlock FP, Deter RL, Harrist RB, et al: Fetal biparietal diameter: A critical reevaluation of the relation to menstrual age by means of realtime ultrasound. J Ultrasound Med 1:97, 1982; and Hadlock FP, Deter LR, Harrist RB, Park SK: Estimating fetal age: Computer-assisted analysis of multiple fetal growth parameters. Radiology 152:497, 1984.

Table A–9. PREDICTED MENSTRUAL AGE FOR HEAD CIRCUMFERENCE MEASUREMENTS (8.5–36.0 cm)

Head Circumference (cm)	Menstrual Age (wk)	Head Circumference (cm)	Menstrual Age (wk)
8.5	13.7	22.5	24.4
9.0	14.0	23.0	24.9
9.5	14.3	23.5	25.4
10.0	14.6	24.0	25.9
10.5	15.0	24.5	26.4
11.0	15.3	25.0	26.9
11.5	15.6	25.5	27.5
12.0	15.9	26.0	28.0
12.5	16.3	26.5	28.6
13.0	16.6	27.0	29.2
13.5	17.0	27.5	29.8
14.0	17.3	28.0	30.3
14.5	17.7	28.5	31.0
15.0	18.1	29.0	31.6
15.5	18.4	29.5	32.2
16.0	18.8	30.0	32.8
16.5	19.2	30.5	33.5
17.0	19.6	31.0	34.2
17.5	20.0	31.5	34.9
18.0	20.4	32.0	35.5
18.5	20.8	32.5	36.3
19.0	21.2	33.0	37.0
19.5	21.6	33.5	37.7
20.0	22.1	34.0	38.5
20.5	22.5	34.5	39.2
21.0	23.0	35.0	40.0
21.5	23.4	35.5	40.8
22.0	23.9	36.0	41.6

Variability Estimates (±2 SD)

12–18 wk	±1.3 wk
18–24 wk	±1.6 wk
24–30 wk	±2.3 wk
30–36 wk	±2.7 wk
34–42 wk	±3.4 wk

From Hadlock FP, Deter RL, Harrist RB, Park SK: Fetal head circumference: Relation to menstrual age. AJR 138:649, 1982.

Table A–10. PERCENTILE VALUES FOR FETAL HEAD CIRCUMFERENCE

Menstrual Weeks	Head Circumference (cm)				
	3rd	*10th*	*50th*	*90th*	*97th*
14	8.8	9.1	9.7	10.3	10.6
15	10.0	10.4	11.0	11.6	12.0
16	11.3	11.7	12.4	13.1	13.5
17	12.6	13.0	13.8	14.6	15.0
18	13.7	14.2	15.1	16.0	16.5
19	14.9	15.5	16.4	17.4	17.9
20	16.1	16.7	17.7	18.7	19.3
21	17.2	17.8	18.9	20.0	20.6
22	18.3	18.9	20.1	21.3	21.9
23	19.4	20.1	21.3	22.5	23.2
24	20.4	21.1	22.4	23.7	24.3
25	21.4	22.2	23.5	24.9	25.6
26	22.4	23.2	24.6	26.0	26.8
27	23.3	24.1	25.6	27.1	27.9
28	24.2	25.1	26.6	28.1	29.0
29	25.0	25.9	27.5	29.1	30.0
30	25.8	26.8	28.4	30.0	31.0
31	26.7	27.6	29.3	31.0	31.9
32	27.4	28.4	30.1	31.8	32.8
33	28.0	29.0	30.8	32.6	33.6
34	28.7	29.7	31.5	33.3	34.3
35	29.3	30.4	32.2	34.1	35.1
36	29.9	30.9	32.8	34.7	35.8
37	30.3	31.4	33.3	35.2	36.3
38	30.8	31.9	33.8	35.8	36.8
39	31.1	32.2	34.2	36.2	37.3
40	31.5	32.6	34.6	36.6	37.7

Adapted from Hadlock FP, Deter RL, Harrist RB, Park SK: Estimating fetal age: Computer-assisted analysis of multiple fetal growth parameters. Radiology 152:497–501, 1984.

Table A–11. PREDICTED MENSTRUAL AGE FOR ABDOMINAL CIRCUMFERENCE MEASUREMENTS (10–36 cm)

Abdominal Circumference (cm)	Menstrual Age (wk)	Abdominal Circumference (cm)	Menstrual Age (wk)
10.0	15.6	23.5	27.7
10.5	16.1	24.0	28.2
11.0	16.5	24.5	28.7
11.5	16.9	25.0	29.2
12.0	17.3	25.5	29.7
12.5	17.8	26.0	30.1
13.0	18.2	26.5	30.6
13.5	18.6	27.0	31.1
14.0	19.1	27.5	31.6
14.5	19.5	28.0	32.1
15.0	20.0	28.5	32.6
15.5	20.4	29.0	33.1
16.0	20.8	29.5	33.6
16.5	21.3	30.0	34.1
17.0	21.7	30.5	34.6
17.5	22.2	31.0	35.1
18.0	22.6	31.5	35.6
18.5	23.1	32.0	36.1
19.0	23.6	32.5	36.6
19.5	24.0	33.0	37.1
20.0	24.5	33.5	37.6
20.5	24.9	34.0	38.1
21.0	25.4	34.5	38.7
21.5	25.9	35.0	39.2
22.0	26.3	35.5	39.7
22.5	26.8	36.0	40.2
23.0	27.3		

Variability Estimates (±2 SD)

12–18 wk	±1.9 wk
18–24 wk	±2.0 wk
24–30 wk	±2.2 wk
30–36 wk	±3.0 wk
36–42 wk	±2.5 wk

From Hadlock FP, Deter RL, Harrist RB, Park SK: Fetal abdominal circumference as a predictor of menstrual age. AJR 139:367, 1982.

Table A–12. PERCENTILE VALUES FOR FETAL ABDOMINAL CIRCUMFERENCE

Menstrual Weeks	Abdominal Circumference (cm)				
	3rd	10th	50th	90th	97th
14	6.4	6.7	7.3	7.9	8.3
15	7.5	7.9	8.6	9.3	9.7
16	8.6	9.1	9.9	10.7	11.2
17	9.7	10.3	11.2	12.1	12.7
18	10.9	11.5	12.5	13.5	14.1
19	11.9	12.6	13.7	14.8	15.5
20	13.1	13.8	15.0	16.3	17.0
21	14.1	14.9	16.2	17.6	18.3
22	15.1	16.0	17.4	18.8	19.7
23	16.1	17.0	18.5	20.0	20.9
24	17.1	18.1	19.7	21.3	22.3
25	18.1	19.1	20.8	22.5	23.5
26	19.1	20.1	21.9	23.7	24.8
27	20.0	21.1	23.0	24.9	26.0
28	20.9	22.0	24.0	26.0	27.1
29	21.8	23.0	25.1	27.2	28.4
30	22.7	23.9	26.1	28.3	29.5
31	23.6	24.9	27.1	29.4	30.6
32	24.5	25.8	28.1	30.4	31.8
33	25.3	26.7	29.1	31.5	32.9
34	26.1	27.5	30.0	32.5	33.9
35	26.9	28.3	30.9	33.5	34.9
36	27.7	29.2	31.8	34.4	35.9
37	28.5	30.0	32.7	35.4	37.0
38	29.2	30.8	33.6	36.4	38.0
39	29.9	31.6	34.4	37.3	38.9
40	30.7	32.4	35.3	38.2	39.9

Adapted from Hadlock FP, Deter RL, Harrist RB, Park SK: Estimating fetal age: Computer-assisted analysis of multiple fetal growth parameters. Radiology 152:497–501, 1984.

Table A–13. A COMPARISON OF ABDOMINAL CIRCUMFERENCE PERCENTILES USING SONOGRAPHY

Percentile Menstrual Weeks	Abdominal Circumference (cm)					
	10th Percentile			90th Percentile		
	Jeanty et al*	Hadlock et al†	Tamura and Sabbagha‡	Jeanty et al*	Hadlock et al†	Tamura and Sabbagha‡
18	10.2	11.5	11.7	13.6	13.5	12.0
20	12.4	13.7	14.2	15.8	16.3	16.7
22	14.6	16.0	14.7	18.0	18.8	19.7
24	16.7	18.1	18.9	20.1	21.3	22.8
26	18.8	20.1	19.8	22.2	23.7	26.7
28	20.8	22.0	23.1	24.2	26.0	27.2
30	22.7	23.9	24.4	26.1	28.3	30.1
32	24.5	25.8	26.7	27.9	30.4	32.4
34	26.2	27.5	28.6	29.6	32.5	33.6
36	27.6	29.2	31.0	31.0	34.4	37.8
38	28.9	30.8	32.8	32.3	36.4	38.5
40	29.9	32.4	33.3	33.3	38.2	41.2

*Adapted from Jeanty P, Cousaert E, Cantraine F: Normal growth of the abdominal perimeter. Am J Perinatol 1:129, 1984.
†Adapted from Tamura RK, Sabbagha RE: Percentile ranks of sonar fetal abdominal circumference measurements. Am J Obstet Gynecol 138:475, 1980.
‡Adapted from Hadlock FP, Deter RL, Harrist RB, Park SK: Estimating fetal age: Computer-assisted analysis of multiple fetal growth parameters. Radiology 152:497, 1984.

Table A–14. PREDICTED MENSTRUAL AGE FOR FEMUR LENGTHS (1.0–7.9 cm)

Femur Length (cm)	Menstrual Age (wk)	Femur Length (cm)	Menstrual Age (wk)
1.0	12.8	4.5	24.5
1.1	13.1	4.6	24.9
1.2	13.4	4.7	25.3
1.3	13.6	4.8	25.7
1.4	13.9	4.9	26.1
1.5	14.2	5.0	26.5
1.6	14.5	5.1	27.0
1.7	14.8	5.2	27.4
1.8	15.1	5.3	27.8
1.9	15.4	5.4	28.2
2.0	15.7	5.5	28.7
2.1	16.0	5.6	29.1
2.2	16.3	5.7	29.6
2.3	16.6	5.8	30.0
2.4	16.9	5.9	30.5
2.5	17.2	6.0	30.9
2.6	17.6	6.1	31.4
2.7	17.9	6.2	31.9
2.8	18.2	6.3	32.3
2.9	18.6	6.4	32.8
3.0	18.9	6.5	33.3
3.1	19.2	6.6	33.8
3.2	19.6	6.7	34.2
3.3	19.9	6.8	34.7
3.4	20.3	6.9	35.2
3.5	20.7	7.0	35.7
3.6	21.0	7.1	36.2
3.7	21.4	7.2	36.7
3.8	21.8	7.3	37.2
3.9	22.1	7.4	37.7
4.0	22.5	7.5	38.3
4.1	22.9	7.6	38.8
4.2	23.3	7.7	39.3
4.3	23.7	7.8	39.8
4.4	24.1	7.9	40.4

Variability Estimates (± 2 SD)

12–18 wk	± 1.0 wk
18–24 wk	± 1.8 wk
24–30 wk	± 2.0 wk
30–36 wk	± 2.4 wk
36–42 wk	± 3.2 wk

From Hadlock FP, Deter RL, Harrist RB, Park SK: Fetal femur length as a predictor of menstrual age: Sonographically measured. AJR 138:875, 1982.

Table A–15. PERCENTILE VALUES FOR FETAL FEMUR LENGTH

Menstrual Weeks	Femur Length (cm)				
	3rd	10th	50th	90th	97th
14	1.2	1.3	1.4	1.5	1.6
15	1.5	1.6	1.7	1.9	1.9
16	1.7	1.8	2.0	2.2	2.3
17	2.1	2.2	2.4	2.6	2.7
18	2.3	2.5	2.7	2.9	3.1
19	2.6	2.7	3.0	3.3	3.4
20	2.8	3.0	3.3	3.6	3.8
21	3.0	3.2	3.5	3.8	4.0
22	3.3	3.5	3.8	4.1	4.3
23	3.5	3.7	4.1	4.5	4.7
24	3.8	4.0	4.4	4.8	5.0
25	4.0	4.2	4.6	5.0	5.2
26	4.2	4.5	4.9	5.3	5.6
27	4.4	4.6	5.1	5.6	5.8
28	4.6	4.9	5.4	5.9	6.2
29	4.8	5.1	5.6	6.1	6.4
30	5.0	5.3	5.8	6.3	6.6
31	5.2	5.5	6.0	6.5	6.8
32	5.3	5.6	6.2	6.8	7.1
33	5.5	5.8	6.4	7.0	7.3
34	5.7	6.0	6.6	7.2	7.5
35	5.9	6.2	6.8	7.4	7.8
36	6.0	6.4	7.0	7.6	8.0
37	6.2	6.6	7.2	7.9	8.2
38	6.4	6.7	7.4	8.1	8.4
39	6.5	6.8	7.5	8.2	8.6
40	6.6	7.0	7.7	8.4	8.8

Adapted from Hadlock FP, Deter RL, Harrist RB, Park SK: Estimating fetal age: Computer-assisted analysis of multiple fetal growth parameters. Radiology 152:497–501, 1984.

Table A–16. LENGTH OF FETAL LONG BONES (mm)

Week No.	Humerus Percentile			Ulna Percentile			Radius Percentile			Femur Percentile			Tibia Percentile			Fibula Percentile		
	5	50	95	5	50	95	5	50	95	5	50	95	5	50	95	5	50	95
11	—	6	—	—	5	—	—	5	—	—	6	—	—	4	—	—	2	—
12	3	9	10	—	8	—	—	7	—	—	9	—	—	7	—	—	5	—
13	5	13	20	3	11	18	—	10	—	6	12	19	4	10	17	—	8	—
14	5	16	20	4	13	17	8	13	12	5	15	19	2	13	19	6	11	10
15	11	18	26	10	16	22	12	15	19	11	19	26	5	16	27	10	14	18
16	12	21	25	8	19	24	9	18	21	13	22	24	7	19	25	6	17	22
17	19	24	29	11	21	32	11	20	29	20	25	29	15	22	29	7	19	31
18	18	27	30	13	24	30	14	22	26	19	28	31	14	24	29	10	22	28
19	22	29	36	20	26	32	20	24	29	23	31	38	19	27	35	18	24	30
20	23	32	36	21	29	32	21	27	28	22	33	39	19	29	35	18	27	30
21	28	34	40	25	31	36	25	29	32	27	36	45	24	32	39	24	29	34
22	28	36	40	24	33	37	24	31	34	29	39	44	25	34	39	21	31	37
23	32	38	45	27	35	43	26	32	39	35	41	48	30	36	43	23	33	44
24	31	41	46	29	37	41	27	34	38	34	44	49	28	39	45	26	35	41
25	35	43	51	34	39	44	31	36	40	38	46	54	31	41	50	33	37	42
26	36	45	49	34	41	44	30	37	41	39	49	53	33	43	49	32	39	43
27	42	46	51	37	43	48	33	39	45	45	51	57	39	45	51	35	41	47
28	41	48	52	37	44	48	33	40	45	45	53	57	38	47	52	36	43	47
29	44	50	56	40	46	51	36	42	47	49	56	62	40	49	57	40	45	50
30	44	52	56	38	47	54	34	43	49	49	58	62	41	51	56	38	47	52
31	47	53	59	39	49	59	34	44	53	53	60	67	46	52	58	40	48	57
32	47	55	59	40	50	58	37	45	51	53	62	67	46	54	59	40	50	56
33	50	56	62	43	52	60	41	46	51	56	64	71	49	56	62	43	51	59
34	50	57	62	44	53	59	39	47	53	57	65	70	47	57	64	46	52	56
35	52	58	65	47	54	61	38	48	57	61	67	73	48	59	69	51	54	57
36	53	60	63	47	55	61	41	48	54	61	69	74	49	60	68	51	55	56
37	57	61	64	49	56	62	45	49	53	64	71	77	52	61	71	55	56	58
38	55	61	66	48	57	63	45	49	53	62	72	79	54	62	69	54	57	59
39	56	62	69	49	57	66	46	50	54	64	74	83	58	64	69	55	58	62
40	56	63	69	50	58	65	46	50	54	66	75	81	58	65	69	54	59	62

From Jeanty P: Fetal limb biometry. (Letter) Radiology 147:602, 1983.

Table A–17. GESTATIONAL AGE FOR CLAVICLE LENGTH

Clavicle Length (mm)	Gestational Age (weeks and days) Percentile		
	5th	50th	95th
11	8 + 3	13 + 6	17 + 2
12	9 + 1	14 + 4	18 + 1
13	10 + 0	14 + 3	19 + 6
14	11 + 6	15 + 2	20 + 5
15	12 + 5	16 + 1	21 + 4
16	12 + 3	18 + 0	21 + 3
17	13 + 2	18 + 5	22 + 2
18	14 + 1	19 + 4	23 + 0
19	16 + 0	19 + 3	24 + 6
20	16 + 6	20 + 2	25 + 5
21	17 + 4	21 + 1	26 + 4
22	17 + 3	22 + 6	26 + 2
23	18 + 2	23 + 5	27 + 1
24	19 + 1	24 + 4	28 + 0
25	21 + 0	24 + 3	29 + 6
26	21 + 5	25 + 1	30 + 5
27	22 + 4	26 + 0	30 + 3
28	22 + 3	27 + 6	31 + 2
29	23 + 2	28 + 5	32 + 1
30	24 + 0	29 + 4	34 + 0
31	25 + 6	29 + 2	34 + 6
32	26 + 5	30 + 1	35 + 4
33	27 + 4	31 + 0	35 + 3
34	27 + 3	32 + 6	36 + 2
35	28 + 1	33 + 5	37 + 1
36	29 + 0	33 + 3	39 + 0
37	30 + 6	34 + 2	39 + 5
38	31 + 5	35 + 1	40 + 4
39	32 + 4	37 + 0	40 + 3
40	32 + 2	37 + 6	41 + 2
41	33 + 1	38 + 4	42 + 0
42	35 + 0	38 + 3	43 + 6
43	35 + 6	39 + 2	44 + 5
44	36 + 5	40 + 1	45 + 4
45	36 + 3	41 + 6	45 + 3

From Yarkoni S, Schmidt W, Jeanty P, et al: Clavicular measurement: A new biometric parameter for fetal evaluation. J Ultrasound Med 4:467, 1985.

Table A–18. COMPARISON OF MEAN POSTPARTUM AND ULTRASONOGRAPHIC FOOT LENGTH WITH STREETER'S PATHOLOGIC DATA (1920)

Gestation Week	Streeter's Data (mm)	Ultrasonographic Foot Length (mm)	Postpartum Foot Length (mm)
11	7	8	
12	9	9	
13	11	10	
14	14	16	
15	17	16	
16	20	21	
17	23	24	
18	27	27	
19	31	28	
20	33	33	33
21	35	35	
22	40	38	
23	42	42	
24	45	44	
25	48	47	48
26	50	51	
27	53	54	52
28	55	58	
29	57	57	57
30	59	61	60
31	61	62	60
32	63	63	66
33	65	67	68
34	68	68	71
35	71	71	72
36	74	74	74
37	77	75	78
38	79	78	78
39	81	78	80
40	83	82	81
41			82
42			82
43			84

From Mercer BM, Sklar S, Shariatmadar A, et al: Fetal foot length as a predictor of gestational age. Am J Obstet Gynecol 156:350, 1987.

Table A–19. PREDICTED MENSTRUAL AGES FOR TRANSVERSE CEREBELLAR DIAMETERS OF 14 TO 56 mm

Cerebellum Diameter (mm)	Menstrual Age (wk)	Cerebellum Diameter (mm)	Menstrual Age (wk)
14	15.2	35	29.4
15	15.8	36	30.0
16	16.5	37	30.6
17	17.2	38	31.2
18	17.9	39	31.8
19	18.6	40	32.3
20	19.3	41	32.8
21	20.0	42	33.4
22	20.7	43	33.9
23	21.4	44	34.4
24	22.1	45	34.8
25	22.8	46	35.3
26	23.5	47	35.7
27	24.2	48	36.1
28	24.9	49	36.5
29	25.5	50	36.8
30	26.2	51	37.2
31	26.9	52	37.5
32	27.5	54	38.0
33	28.1	55	38.3
34	28.8	56	38.5

Variability Estimates (±2 SD)

12–18 wk	±1.0 wk
18–24 wk	±1.8 wk
24–30 wk	±2.0 wk
30–36 wk	±2.4 wk
36–42 wk	±3.2 wk

From Hill LM, Guzick D, Fries J, et al: The transverse cerebellar diameter in estimating gestational age in the large-for-gestational-age fetus. Reprinted with permission from the American College of Obstetricians and Gynecologists (Obstetrics and Gynecology 1990, 75:983).

Table A–20. NOMOGRAM OF THE TRANSVERSE CEREBELLAR DIAMETER ACCORDING TO PERCENTILE DISTRIBUTION

Gestational Age (wk)	Cerebellum Diameter (mm)				
	10	25	50	75	90
15	10	12	14	15	16
16	14	16	16	16	17
17	16	17	17	18	18
18	17	18	18	19	19
19	18	18	19	19	22
20	18	19	20	20	22
21	19	20	22	23	24
22	21	23	23	24	24
23	22	23	24	25	26
24	22	24	25	27	28
25	23	21.5	28	28	29
26	25	28	29	30	32
27	26	28.5	30	31	32
28	27	30	31	32	34
29	29	32	34	36	38
30	31	32	35	37	40
31	32	35	38	39	43
32	33	36	38	40	42
33	32	36	40	43	44
34	33	38	40	41	44
35	31	37	40.5	43	47
36	36	29	43	52	55
37	37	37	45	52	55
38	40	40	48.5	52	55
39	52	52	52	55	55

From Goldstein I, Reece A, Pilu G, et al: Cerebellar measurements with ultrasonography in the evaluation of fetal growth and development. Am J Obstet Gynecol 156:1065, 1987.

Table A–21. PREDICTED BIPARIETAL DIAMETER (BPD) AND WEEKS' GESTATION FROM THE INNER (IOD) AND OUTER (OOD) ORBITAL DISTANCES

BPD (cm)	Gestation (wk)	IOD (cm)	OOD (cm)	BPD (cm)	Gestation (wk)	IOD (cm)	OOD (cm)
1.9	11.6	0.5	1.3	5.8	24.3	1.6	4.1
2.0	11.6	0.5	1.4	5.9	24.3	1.6	4.2
2.1	12.1	0.6	1.5	6.0	24.7	1.6	4.3
2.2	12.6	0.6	1.6	6.1	25.2	1.6	4.3
2.3	12.6	0.6	1.7	6.2	25.2	1.6	4.4
2.4	13.1	0.7	1.7	6.3	25.7	1.7	4.4
2.5	13.6	0.7	1.8	6.4	26.2	1.7	4.5
2.6	13.6	0.7	1.9	6.5	26.2	1.7	4.5
2.7	14.1	0.8	2.0	6.6	26.7	1.7	4.6
2.8	14.6	0.8	2.1	6.7	27.2	1.7	4.6
2.9	14.6	0.8	2.1	6.8	27.6	1.7	4.7
3.0	15.0	0.9	2.2	6.9	28.1	1.7	4.7
3.1	15.5	0.9	2.3	7.0	28.6	1.8	4.8
3.2	15.5	0.9	2.4	7.1	29.1	1.8	4.8
3.3	16.0	1.0	2.5	7.3	29.6	1.8	4.9
3.4	16.5	1.0	2.5	7.4	30.0	1.8	5.0
3.5	16.5	1.0	2.6	7.5	30.6	1.8	5.0
3.6	17.0	1.0	2.7	7.6	31.0	1.8	5.1
3.7	17.5	1.1	2.7	7.7	31.5	1.8	5.1
3.8	17.9	1.1	2.8	7.8	32.0	1.8	5.2
4.0	18.4	1.2	3.0	7.9	32.5	1.9	5.2
4.2	18.9	1.2	3.1	8.0	33.0	1.9	5.3
4.3	19.4	1.2	3.2	8.2	33.5	1.9	5.4
4.4	19.4	1.3	3.2	8.3	34.0	1.9	5.4
4.5	19.9	1.3	3.3	8.4	34.4	1.9	5.4
4.6	20.4	1.3	3.4	8.5	35.0	1.9	5.5
4.7	20.4	1.3	3.4	8.6	35.4	1.9	5.5
4.8	20.9	1.4	3.5	8.8	35.9	1.9	5.6
4.9	21.3	1.4	3.6	8.9	36.4	1.9	5.6
5.0	21.3	1.4	3.6	9.0	36.9	1.9	5.7
5.1	21.8	1.4	3.7	9.1	37.3	1.9	5.7
5.2	22.3	1.4	3.8	9.2	37.8	1.9	5.8
5.3	22.3	1.5	3.8	9.3	38.3	1.9	5.8
5.4	22.8	1.5	3.9	9.4	38.8	1.9	5.8
5.5	23.3	1.5	4.0	9.6	39.3	1.9	5.9
5.6	23.3	1.5	4.0	9.7	39.8	1.9	5.9
5.7	23.8	1.5	4.1				

From Mayden KL, Tortora M, Berkowitz RL, et al: Orbital diameters: A new parameter for prenatal diagnosis and dating. Am J Obstet Gynecol 144:289, 1982.

Table A–22. FETAL THORACIC CIRCUMFERENCE MEASUREMENTS*

Gestational Age (wk)	No.	Predictive Percentiles								
		2.5	5	10	25	50	75	90	95	97.5
16	6	5.9	6.4	7.0	8.0	9.1	10.3	11.3	11.9	12.4
17	22	6.8	7.3	7.9	8.9	10.0	11.2	12.2	12.8	13.3
18	31	7.7	8.2	8.8	9.8	11.0	12.1	13.1	13.7	14.2
19	21	8.6	9.1	9.7	10.7	11.9	13.0	14.0	14.6	15.1
20	20	9.5	10.0	10.6	11.7	12.8	13.9	15.0	15.5	16.0
21	30	10.4	11.0	11.6	12.6	13.7	14.8	15.8	16.4	16.9
22	18	11.3	11.9	12.5	13.5	14.6	15.7	16.7	17.3	17.8
23	21	12.2	12.8	13.4	14.4	15.5	16.6	17.6	18.2	18.8
24	27	13.2	13.7	14.3	15.3	16.4	17.5	18.5	19.1	19.7
25	20	14.1	14.6	15.2	16.2	17.3	18.4	19.4	20.0	20.6
26	25	15.0	15.5	16.1	17.1	18.2	19.3	20.3	21.0	21.5
27	24	15.9	16.4	17.0	18.0	19.1	20.2	21.3	21.9	22.4
28	24	16.8	17.3	17.9	18.9	20.0	21.2	22.2	22.8	23.3
29	24	17.7	18.2	18.8	19.8	21.0	22.1	23.1	23.7	24.2
30	27	18.6	19.1	19.7	20.7	21.9	23.0	24.0	24.6	25.1
31	24	19.5	20.0	20.6	21.6	22.8	23.9	24.9	25.5	26.0
32	28	20.4	20.9	21.5	22.6	23.7	24.8	25.8	26.4	26.9
33	27	21.3	21.8	22.5	23.5	24.6	25.7	26.7	27.3	27.8
34	25	22.2	22.8	23.4	24.4	25.5	26.6	27.6	28.2	28.7
35	20	23.1	23.7	24.3	25.3	26.4	27.5	28.5	29.1	29.6
36	23	24.0	24.6	25.2	26.2	27.3	28.4	29.4	30.0	30.6
37	22	24.9	25.5	26.1	27.1	28.2	29.3	30.3	30.9	31.5
38	21	25.9	26.4	27.0	28.0	29.1	30.2	31.2	31.9	32.4
39	7	26.8	27.3	27.9	28.9	30.0	31.1	32.2	32.8	33.3
40	6	27.7	28.2	28.8	29.8	30.9	32.1	33.1	33.7	34.2

*Measurements in centimeters.
From Chitkara U, Rosenberg J, Chervenak FA, et al: Prenatal sonographic assessment of the fetal thorax: Normal values. Am J Obstet Gynecol 156:1069, 1987.

Measurements Used in Assessing Fetal Weight, Growth, and Body Proportions

Table B–1. PUBLISHED REGRESSION EQUATIONS FOR SONOGRAPHIC ESTIMATION OF FETAL WEIGHT

Reference	Equation [$\log_{10}$ (Birthweight)] =
Hadlock et al.*	$1.3596 - 0.00386 \, (AC)(FL) + 0.0064 \, (HC) + 0.00061 \, (BPD)(AC) + 0.0424 \, (AC) + 0.174 \, (FL)$
Hadlock et al.†	$1.5115 + 0.0436 \, (AC) + 0.1517 \, (FL) - \dfrac{0.321 \, (AC)(FL)}{100} + \dfrac{0.6923 \, (BPD)(HC)}{10000}$
Shepard et al.‡	$-1.7492 + 0.166 \, (BPD) + 0.046 \, (AC) - \dfrac{2.646 \, (AC)(BPD)}{1000}$
Warsof et al.§	$-1.599 + 0.144 \, (BPD) + 0.032 \, (AC) - \dfrac{0.111(BPD)^2 \, (AC)}{1000}$
Roberts et al. ‖	$1.6758 + 0.01707 \, (AC) + 0.042478 \, (BPD) + 0.05216 \, (FL) + 0.01604 \, (HC)$

AC, abdominal circumference; FL, femur length; HC, head circumference; BPD, biparietal diameter.

*Hadlock FP, Harrist RB, Sharman RS, et al: Estimation of fetal weight with the use of head, body, and femur measurements: A prospective study. Am J Obstet Gynecol 151:333, 1985.

†Hadlock FP, Harrist RB, Carpenter RJ, et al: Sonographic estimation of fetal weight. Radiology 150:535, 1984.

‡Shepard MJ, Richards VA, Berkowitz FL, et al: An evaluation of two equations for predicting fetal weight by ultrasound. Am J Obstet Gynecol 142:47, 1982.

§Warsof SL, Gohari P, Berkowitz RL, Hobbins JC: The estimation of fetal weight by computer-assisted analysis. Am J Obstet Gynecol 128:881, 1977.

‖Roberts AB, Lee AJ, James AG: Ultrasonic estimation of fetal weight: A new predictive model incorporating femur length for the low-birthweight fetus. J Clin Ultrasound 13:555, 1985

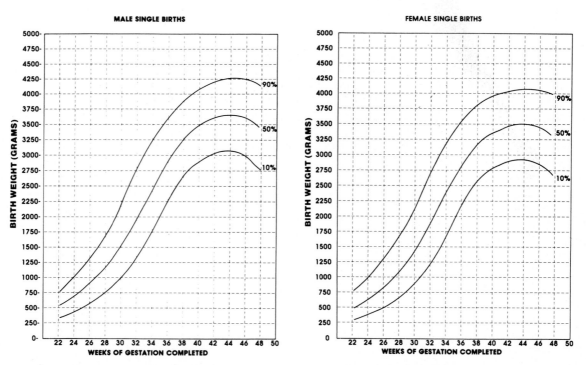

Figure B–1. California birth weight gestational age. (From Williams RL, Creasy RK, Cunningham GC: Fetal growth and perinatal viability in California. Obstet Gynecol 59:624, 1982.)

Table B–2. IN UTERO FETAL SONOGRAPHIC WEIGHT STANDARDS

Menstrual Weeks	Estimated Fetal Weight (g) by Percentile				
	3rd	10th	50th	90th	97th
10	26	29	35	41	44
11	34	37	45	53	56
12	43	48	58	68	73
13	55	61	73	85	91
14	70	77	93	109	116
15	88	97	117	137	146
16	110	121	146	171	183
17	136	150	181	212	226
18	167	185	223	261	279
19	205	227	273	319	341
20	248	275	331	387	414
21	299	331	399	467	499
22	359	398	478	559	598
23	426	471	568	665	710
24	503	556	670	784	838
25	589	652	785	918	981
26	685	758	913	1068	1141
27	791	876	1055	1234	1319
28	908	1004	1210	1416	1513
29	1034	1145	1379	1613	1724
30	1169	1294	1559	1824	1949
31	1313	1453	1751	2049	2189
32	1465	1621	1953	2285	2441
33	1622	1794	2162	2530	2703
34	1783	1973	2377	2781	2971
35	1946	2154	2595	3036	3244
36	2110	2335	2813	3291	3516
37	2271	2513	3028	3543	3785
38	2427	2686	3236	3786	4045
39	2576	2851	3435	4019	4294
40	2714	3004	3619	4234	4524

From Hadlock FP, Harrist RB, Martinez-Poyer J: In utero analysis of fetal growth: A sonographic weight standard. Radiology 181:129–133, 1991.

Table B–3. NOMOGRAM OF ESTIMATED FETAL WEIGHT IN TWIN GESTATIONS

Gestational Age (wk)	Estimated Fetal Weight (g) by Percentile				
	5th	25th	50th	75th	95th
16	132	141	154	189	207
17	173	194	215	239	249
18	214	248	276	289	291
19	223	253	300	333	412
20	232	259	324	378	534
21	275	355	432	482	705
22	319	452	540	586	876
23	347	497	598	684	880
24	376	543	656	783	885
25	549	677	793	916	1118
26	722	812	931	1049	1352
27	755	978	1087	1193	1563
28	789	1145	1244	1337	1774
29	900	1266	1395	1509	1883
30	1011	1387	1546	1682	1992
31	1198	1532	1693	1875	2392
32	1385	1677	1840	2068	2793
33	1491	1771	2032	2334	3000
34	1597	1866	2224	2601	3208
35	1703	2093	2427	2716	3336
36	1809	2321	2631	2832	3465
37	2239	2540	2824	3035	3679
38	2669	2760	3017	3239	3894

From Yarkoni S, Reece EA, Holford T, et al: Estimated fetal weight in the evaluation of growth in twin gestations: A prospective longitudinal study. Obstet Gynecol 69:636, 1987. Reprinted with permission from The American College of Obstetricians and Gynecologists.

Table B–4. ESTIMATES OF FETAL WEIGHT (g) BASED ON ABDOMINAL CIRCUMFERENCE AND FEMUR LENGTH

Femur Length (cm)	Abdominal Circumference (cm)																				
	20.0	20.5	21.0	21.5	22.0	22.5	23.0	23.5	24.0	24.5	25.0	25.5	26.0	26.5	27.0	27.5	28.0	28.5	29.0	29.5	30.0
4.0	663	691	720	751	783	816	851	887	925	964	1006	1048	1093	1139	1188	1239	1291	1346	1403	1463	1525
4.1	680	709	738	769	802	836	871	907	946	986	1027	1070	1115	1162	1211	1262	1315	1371	1429	1489	1551
4.2	697	726	757	788	821	855	891	928	967	1007	1049	1093	1138	1186	1235	1287	1340	1396	1454	1515	1578
4.3	715	745	776	808	841	875	912	949	988	1029	1071	1116	1162	1209	1259	1311	1365	1422	1480	1541	1605
4.4	734	764	795	827	861	896	933	971	1010	1051	1094	1139	1185	1234	1284	1336	1391	1448	1507	1568	1632
4.5	753	783	815	847	882	917	954	993	1033	1074	1118	1163	1210	1259	1309	1362	1417	1474	1534	1596	1660
4.6	772	803	835	868	903	939	976	1015	1056	1098	1142	1187	1235	1284	1335	1388	1444	1501	1561	1623	1688
4.7	792	823	856	889	924	961	999	1038	1079	1122	1166	1212	1260	1310	1361	1415	1471	1529	1589	1652	1717
4.8	812	844	877	911	947	984	1022	1062	1103	1146	1191	1237	1286	1336	1388	1442	1498	1557	1618	1681	1746
4.9	833	865	899	933	969	1007	1046	1086	1128	1171	1216	1263	1312	1363	1415	1470	1527	1585	1647	1710	1776
5.0	855	887	921	956	993	1031	1070	1111	1153	1197	1243	1290	1339	1390	1443	1498	1555	1615	1676	1740	1806
5.1	877	910	944	980	1016	1055	1095	1136	1179	1223	1269	1317	1367	1418	1471	1527	1584	1644	1706	1770	1837
5.2	899	933	967	1004	1041	1080	1120	1162	1205	1250	1296	1344	1395	1447	1500	1556	1614	1674	1737	1801	1868
5.3	922	956	992	1028	1066	1105	1146	1188	1232	1277	1324	1373	1423	1476	1530	1586	1645	1705	1768	1833	1900
5.4	946	981	1016	1053	1091	1131	1172	1215	1259	1305	1352	1401	1452	1505	1560	1617	1675	1736	1799	1865	1933
5.5	971	1005	1041	1079	1118	1158	1199	1242	1287	1333	1381	1431	1482	1535	1591	1648	1707	1768	1832	1897	1966
5.6	995	1031	1067	1105	1144	1185	1227	1271	1316	1362	1411	1461	1513	1566	1622	1679	1739	1801	1864	1931	1999
5.7	1021	1057	1094	1132	1172	1213	1255	1299	1345	1392	1441	1491	1544	1598	1654	1712	1772	1834	1898	1964	2033
5.8	1047	1084	1121	1160	1200	1242	1285	1329	1375	1422	1472	1523	1575	1630	1686	1744	1805	1867	1932	1999	2068
5.9	1074	1111	1149	1188	1229	1271	1314	1359	1406	1454	1503	1555	1608	1663	1719	1778	1839	1902	1966	2034	2103
6.0	1102	1139	1178	1217	1258	1301	1345	1390	1437	1485	1535	1587	1641	1696	1753	1812	1873	1936	2002	2069	2139
6.1	1130	1168	1207	1247	1289	1331	1376	1421	1469	1518	1568	1620	1674	1730	1788	1847	1908	1972	2038	2105	2175
6.2	1160	1198	1237	1278	1319	1363	1408	1454	1501	1551	1602	1654	1709	1765	1823	1882	1944	2008	2074	2142	2212
6.3	1189	1228	1268	1309	1351	1395	1440	1487	1535	1585	1636	1689	1744	1800	1858	1919	1981	2045	2111	2180	2250
6.4	1220	1259	1299	1341	1384	1428	1473	1520	1569	1619	1671	1724	1779	1836	1895	1956	2018	2082	2149	2218	2289
6.5	1251	1291	1332	1373	1417	1461	1507	1555	1604	1655	1707	1760	1816	1873	1932	1993	2056	2121	2188	2256	2328
6.6	1284	1324	1365	1407	1451	1496	1542	1590	1640	1691	1743	1797	1853	1911	1970	2031	2094	2160	2227	2296	2367
6.7	1317	1357	1399	1441	1486	1531	1578	1626	1676	1728	1780	1835	1891	1949	2009	2070	2134	2199	2267	2336	2408
6.8	1351	1391	1433	1477	1521	1567	1615	1663	1713	1765	1819	1873	1930	1988	2048	2110	2174	2240	2307	2377	2449
6.9	1385	1427	1469	1513	1558	1604	1652	1701	1752	1804	1857	1913	1970	2028	2089	2151	2215	2281	2348	2418	2490
7.0	1421	1463	1506	1550	1595	1642	1690	1740	1791	1843	1897	1953	2010	2069	2130	2192	2256	2322	2391	2461	2533
7.1	1458	1500	1543	1588	1633	1681	1729	1779	1830	1883	1938	1994	2051	2110	2171	2234	2299	2365	2433	2504	2576
7.2	1495	1538	1581	1626	1673	1720	1769	1819	1871	1924	1979	2035	2093	2153	2214	2277	2342	2408	2477	2547	2620
7.3	1534	1577	1621	1666	1713	1761	1810	1861	1913	1966	2021	2078	2136	2196	2258	2321	2386	2453	2521	2592	2665
7.4	1573	1616	1661	1707	1754	1802	1852	1903	1955	2009	2065	2122	2180	2240	2302	2365	2431	2498	2566	2637	2710
7.5	1614	1657	1702	1749	1796	1845	1895	1946	1999	2053	2109	2166	2225	2285	2347	2411	2476	2543	2612	2683	2756
7.6	1655	1699	1745	1791	1839	1888	1939	1990	2043	2098	2154	2211	2270	2331	2393	2457	2523	2590	2659	2730	2803
7.7	1698	1742	1788	1835	1883	1933	1983	2035	2089	2144	2200	2258	2317	2378	2440	2504	2570	2638	2707	2778	2851
7.8	1741	1786	1833	1880	1928	1978	2029	2082	2135	2191	2247	2305	2365	2426	2488	2553	2618	2686	2755	2827	2899
7.9	1786	1832	1878	1926	1975	2025	2076	2129	2183	2238	2295	2353	2413	2474	2537	2602	2668	2735	2805	2876	2949
8.0	1832	1878	1925	1973	2022	2073	2124	2177	2232	2287	2344	2403	2463	2524	2587	2652	2718	2785	2855	2926	2999
8.1	1879	1926	1973	2021	2071	2121	2173	2227	2281	2337	2394	2453	2513	2575	2638	2702	2769	2837	2906	2977	3050
8.2	1928	1974	2022	2070	2120	2171	2224	2277	2332	2388	2446	2504	2565	2626	2690	2754	2821	2889	2958	3029	3102
8.3	1978	2024	2072	2121	2171	2223	2275	2329	2384	2440	2498	2557	2617	2679	2743	2807	2874	2942	3011	3082	3155

Abdominal Circumference (cm)

Femur Length (cm)	30.5	31.0	31.5	32.0	32.5	33.0	33.5	34.0	34.5	35.0	35.5	36.0	36.5	37.0	37.5	38.0	38.5	39.0	39.5	40.0
4.0	1590	1658	1729	1802	1879	1959	2042	2129	2220	2314	2413	2515	2622	2734	2850	2972	3098	3230	3367	3511
4.1	1617	1685	1756	1830	1907	1987	2071	2158	2249	2344	2442	2545	2652	2764	2880	3002	3128	3260	3397	3540
4.2	1644	1712	1783	1858	1935	2016	2100	2187	2279	2373	2472	2575	2683	2794	2911	3032	3159	3290	3427	3570
4.3	1671	1740	1812	1886	1964	2045	2129	2217	2308	2404	2503	2606	2713	2825	2942	3063	3189	3321	3458	3600
4.4	1699	1768	1840	1915	1993	2075	2159	2247	2339	2434	2533	2637	2744	2856	2973	3094	3220	3352	3488	3630
4.5	1727	1797	1869	1944	2023	2105	2189	2278	2370	2465	2565	2668	2776	2888	3004	3125	3251	3383	3519	3661
4.6	1756	1826	1898	1974	2053	2135	2220	2309	2401	2497	2596	2700	2807	2919	3036	3157	3283	3414	3550	3692
4.7	1785	1855	1928	2004	2084	2166	2251	2340	2432	2528	2628	2732	2840	2952	3068	3189	3315	3446	3582	3723
4.8	1814	1885	1959	2035	2115	2197	2283	2372	2464	2560	2660	2764	2872	2984	3100	3221	3347	3478	3613	3754
4.9	1845	1916	1990	2066	2146	2229	2315	2404	2497	2593	2693	2797	2905	3017	3133	3254	3380	3510	3645	3786
5.0	1875	1947	2021	2098	2178	2261	2347	2437	2530	2626	2726	2830	2938	3050	3166	3287	3412	3542	3677	3818
5.1	1906	1978	2053	2130	2210	2294	2380	2470	2563	2659	2760	2864	2972	3084	3200	3320	3445	3575	3710	3850
5.2	1938	2010	2085	2163	2243	2327	2413	2503	2597	2693	2794	2898	3006	3117	3234	3354	3479	3608	3743	3882
5.3	1970	2043	2118	2196	2277	2360	2447	2537	2631	2728	2828	2932	3040	3152	3268	3388	3513	3642	3776	3915
5.4	2003	2076	2151	2229	2311	2395	2482	2572	2665	2762	2863	2967	3075	3186	3302	3422	3547	3676	3809	3948
5.5	2036	2109	2185	2264	2345	2429	2516	2607	2700	2797	2898	3002	3110	3221	3337	3457	3581	3710	3843	3981
5.6	2070	2143	2220	2298	2380	2464	2552	2642	2736	2833	2933	3038	3145	3257	3372	3492	3616	3744	3877	4015
5.7	2104	2178	2254	2333	2415	2500	2587	2678	2772	2869	2970	3074	3181	3293	3408	3527	3651	3779	3911	4048
5.8	2139	2213	2290	2369	2451	2536	2624	2714	2808	2905	3006	3110	3218	3329	3444	3563	3686	3814	3946	4082
5.9	2175	2249	2326	2405	2488	2573	2660	2751	2845	2942	3043	3147	3254	3366	3480	3599	3722	3849	3981	4117
6.0	2211	2286	2363	2442	2525	2610	2698	2789	2883	2980	3080	3184	3292	3403	3517	3636	3758	3885	4016	4151
6.1	2248	2323	2400	2480	2562	2647	2736	2827	2921	3018	3118	3222	3329	3440	3554	3673	3795	3921	4052	4186
6.2	2285	2360	2438	2518	2600	2686	2774	2865	2959	3056	3157	3260	3367	3478	3592	3710	3832	3957	4087	4222
6.3	2323	2398	2476	2556	2639	2725	2813	2904	2998	3095	3195	3299	3406	3516	3630	3747	3869	3994	4124	4257
6.4	2362	2437	2515	2595	2678	2764	2852	2943	3037	3134	3235	3338	3445	3555	3668	3785	3906	4031	4160	4293
6.5	2401	2477	2555	2635	2718	2804	2892	2983	3077	3174	3274	3378	3484	3594	3707	3824	3944	4069	4197	4329
6.6	2441	2517	2595	2675	2759	2844	2933	3024	3118	3215	3315	3418	3524	3633	3746	3863	3983	4106	4234	4366
6.7	2481	2557	2636	2716	2800	2885	2974	3065	3159	3256	3355	3458	3564	3673	3786	3902	4021	4144	4271	4402
6.8	2523	2599	2677	2758	2841	2927	3016	3107	3200	3297	3397	3499	3605	3714	3826	3941	4060	4183	4309	4439
6.9	2564	2641	2719	2800	2884	2969	3058	3149	3242	3339	3438	3541	3646	3754	3866	3981	4100	4222	4347	4477
7.0	2607	2683	2762	2843	2927	3012	3101	3192	3285	3381	3481	3583	3688	3796	3907	4022	4140	4261	4386	4514
7.1	2650	2727	2806	2887	2970	3056	3144	3235	3328	3424	3523	3625	3730	3838	3948	4062	4180	4300	4425	4552
7.2	2694	2771	2850	2931	3014	3100	3188	3279	3372	3468	3567	3668	3772	3880	3990	4104	4220	4340	4464	4591
7.3	2739	2816	2895	2976	3059	3145	3233	3323	3416	3512	3610	3712	3816	3922	4032	4145	4261	4381	4503	4629
7.4	2785	2861	2940	3021	3105	3190	3278	3369	3461	3557	3655	3756	3859	3966	4075	4187	4303	4421	4543	4668
7.5	2831	2908	2987	3068	3151	3236	3324	3414	3507	3602	3700	3800	3903	4009	4118	4230	4344	4462	4583	4708
7.6	2878	2955	3034	3115	3198	3283	3371	3461	3553	3648	3745	3845	3948	4053	4161	4272	4387	4504	4624	4747
7.7	2926	3003	3081	3162	3245	3331	3418	3508	3600	3694	3791	3891	3993	4098	4205	4316	4429	4545	4665	4787
7.8	2974	3051	3130	3211	3294	3379	3466	3555	3647	3741	3838	3937	4039	4143	4250	4360	4472	4588	4706	4827
7.9	3024	3100	3179	3260	3343	3427	3514	3604	3695	3789	3885	3984	4085	4188	4295	4404	4515	4630	4748	4868
8.0	3074	3151	3229	3310	3392	3477	3564	3653	3744	3837	3933	4031	4131	4234	4340	4448	4559	4673	4790	4909
8.1	3125	3202	3280	3360	3443	3527	3614	3702	3793	3886	3981	4079	4179	4281	4386	4493	4604	4716	4832	4950
8.2	3177	3253	3332	3412	3494	3578	3664	3752	3843	3935	4030	4127	4226	4328	4432	4539	4648	4760	4875	4992
8.3	3230	3306	3384	3464	3546	3630	3716	3803	3893	3985	4080	4176	4275	4376	4479	4585	4693	4804	4918	5034

From Hadlock FP, Harrist RB, Carpenter RJ, et al: Sonographic estimation of fetal weight. Radiology 150:535, 1984.

733

Table B–5. NORMAL BODY RATIO DATA (14–21 WK)

Menstrual Week	Cephalic Index (SD = 3.7)*	Femur/BPD × 100 (SD = 4.0)†	Femur/HC × 100 (SD = 1.0)†	Femur/AC × 100 (SD = 1.3)†
14	81.5	58.0	15.0	19.0
15	81.0	59.0	15.7	19.3
16	80.5	61.0	16.4	19.8
17	80.1	63.0	16.9	20.3
18	79.7	65.0	17.5	20.8
19	79.4	67.0	18.1	21.0
20	79.1	69.0	18.4	21.3
21	78.8	70.0	18.6	21.5

BPD, biparietal diameter; HC, head circumference; AC, abdominal circumference; SD, standard deviation.

*Data from Gray DL, Songster GS, Parvin CA, Crane JP: Cephalic index: A gestational age-dependent biometric parameter. Obstet Gynecol, 74:600, 1989.

†Data from Hadlock FP, Harrist RB, Martinez-Poyer J: Fetal body ratios in second trimester: A useful tool for identifying chromosomal abnormalities? J Ultrasound Med 11:81, 1992.

Table B–6. NORMAL FETAL BODY RATIOS (22–40 WK)

Menstrual Week	Cephalic Index (SD = 4.4)*	Femur/BPD × 100 (SD = 5.0)†	Femur/HC × 100 (SD = 1.1)‡	Femur/AC × 100 (SD = 1.3)§
22	78.3	77.4	18.6	21.6
23	78.3	77.6	18.8	21.7
24	78.3	77.8	19.0	21.7
25	78.3	78.0	19.2	21.8
26	78.3	78.2	19.4	21.8
27	78.3	78.4	19.6	21.9
28	78.3	78.6	19.8	21.9
29	78.3	78.8	20.0	21.9
30	78.3	79.0	20.3	22.0
31	78.3	79.2	20.5	22.0
32	78.3	79.4	20.7	22.1
33	78.3	79.6	20.9	22.1
34	78.3	79.8	21.1	22.2
35	78.3	80.0	21.4	22.2
36	78.3	80.2	21.6	22.2
37	78.3	80.4	21.8	22.3
38	78.3	80.6	22.0	22.3
39	78.3	80.8	22.2	22.3
40	78.3	81.0	22.4	22.4

BPD, biparietal diameter; HC, head circumference; AC, abdominal circumference; SD, standard deviation.

*Data from Hadlock FP, Deter RL, Carpenter RL, et al: The effect of head shape on the accuracy of BPD in estimating fetal gestational age. AJR 137:83, 1981.

†Data from Hohler CW, Quetel TA: The relationship between fetal femur length and biparietal diameter in the last half of pregnancy. Am J Obstet Gynecol 141:759, 1981.

‡Data from Hadlock FP, Harrist RB, Shah YP, et al: The use of femur length/head circumference relation in obstetrical sonography. J Ultrasound Med 3:439, 1984.

§Data from Hadlock FP, Deter RL, Harrist RB, et al: A date-independent predictor of intrauterine growth retardation: Femur length/abdominal circumference ratio. AJR 141:979, 1983.

Table B–7. COMPARISON OF FETAL PARAMETERS IN
LGA AND AGA FETUSES

Parameter	AGA Group (mean ± SD)	LGA Group (mean ± SD)	P Value
BPD (cm)	9.2 ± 0.4	9.6 ± 0.4	<.0001
HC (cm)	33.7 ± 1.1	35.2 ± 1.3	<.0001
AC (cm)	33.6 ± 1.6	37.4 ± 1.3	<.0001
FL (cm)	7.4 ± 0.4	7.6 ± 0.3	<.0001
HC/AC	1.0 ± 0.05	0.94 ± 0.04	<.0001
FL/AC*	22.0 ± 1.0	20.5 ± 1.0	<.0001

AGA, appropriate for gestational age; LGA, large for gestational age; BPD, biparietal diameter; HC, head circumference; AC, abdominal circumference; FL, femur length.

*FL/AC expressed as FL/AC × 100.

From Hadlock FP, Harrist RB, Fearneyhough TC, et al: Use of femur length/abdominal circumference ratio in detecting the macrosomic fetus. Radiology 154:503–505, 1985.

Table B–8. SENSITIVITY OF INDIVIDUAL SONOGRAPHIC
PARAMETERS FOR DETECTING INTRAUTERINE
GROWTH RETARDATION

Parameter	Sensitivity	
	Hadlock et al. (37.5 ± 2.1 wk)	Brown et al. (37.9 ± 1.9 wk)
Abdominal circumference (AC)	100%	96%
Femur length (FL)	20%	45%
Head circumference/abdominal circumference (HC/AC)	70%	ND
Femur length/abdominal circumference (FL/AC)	63%	57%
Estimated weight percentile	87%	63%
Ponderal index	47%	54%

ND, no data.

Data from Hadlock FP, Deter RL, Harrist RB, et al: A date-independent predictor of intrauterine growth retardation: Femur length/abdominal circumference ratio. AJR 141:979, 1983.

Data from Brown HL, Miller JM, Gabert HA, Kissling G: Ultrasonic recognition of the small-for-gestational-age fetus. Obstet Gynecol 69:693, 1987.

■ APPENDIX C

Frequently Used Measurements for Amniotic Fluid and Fetal Doppler Assessment

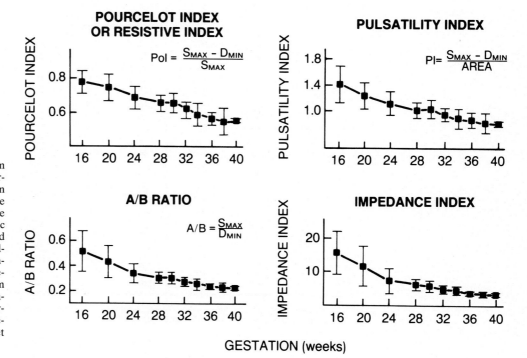

Figure C–1. Doppler waveform analysis of the fetal umbilical artery. With advancing gestation and increasing compliance of the placenta, there is a progressive decrease in the systolic/diastolic ratio, Pourcelot index (PoI), and pulsatility index (PI) of the umbilical artery that is a result of increased placental flow due to decreased resistance. (Modified from Erskine RLA, Ritchie JWK: Umbilical artery blood flow characteristics in normal and growth retarded fetuses. Br J Obstet Gynecol 92:605, 1985.)

POURCELOT INDEX
OR RESISTIVE INDEX

$$PoI = \frac{S_{MAX} - D_{MIN}}{S_{MAX}}$$

PULSATILITY INDEX

$$PI = \frac{S_{MAX} - D_{MIN}}{AREA}$$

A/B RATIO

$$A/B = \frac{S_{MAX}}{D_{MIN}}$$

IMPEDANCE INDEX

GESTATION (weeks)

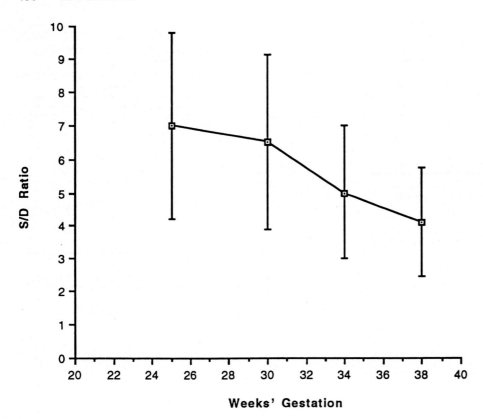

Figure C–2. Middle cerebral artery Doppler systolic/diastolic ratios. (Modified from Woo JSK, Liang ST, et al: Middle cerebral artery Doppler flow velocity. Reprinted with permission from the American College of Obstetricians and Gynecologists [Obstetrics and Gynecology, 1987, 70:613].)

Table C–1. AMNIOTIC FLUID INDEX VALUES IN NORMAL PREGNANCY

Week	Amniotic Fluid Index Percentile Values (mm)				
	3rd	5th	50th	95th	97th
16	73	79	121	185	201
17	77	83	127	194	211
18	80	87	133	202	220
19	83	90	137	207	225
20	86	93	141	212	230
21	88	95	143	214	233
22	89	97	145	216	235
23	90	98	146	218	237
24	90	98	147	219	238
25	89	97	147	221	240
26	89	97	147	223	242
27	85	95	146	226	245
28	86	94	146	228	249
29	84	92	145	231	254
30	82	90	145	234	258
31	79	88	144	238	263
32	77	86	144	242	269
33	74	83	143	245	274
34	72	81	142	248	278
35	70	79	140	249	279
36	68	77	138	249	279
37	66	75	135	244	275
38	65	73	132	239	269
39	64	72	127	226	255
40	63	71	123	214	240
41	63	70	116	194	216
42	63	69	110	175	192

Adapted from Moore TR, Cayle JE: The amniotic fluid index in normal human pregnancy. Am J Obstet Gynecol 162:1168, 1990.

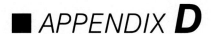

APPENDIX D

Normal Measurements of the Uterus and Ovaries

Table D–1. OVARIAN VOLUME BY DECADE OF LIFE

Decade	Mean Volume (cm³)	Standard Deviation	No. of Ovaries	95% Confidence Interval (cm³)*
1	1.7	1.4	19	0.2–4.9
2	7.8	4.4	83	1.7–18.5
3	10.2	6.2	308	2.6–23.1
4	9.5	5.4	358	2.6–20.7
5	9.0	5.8	206	2.1–20.9
6	6.2	3.6	57	1.6–14.2
7	6.0	3.8	44	1.0–15.0

*Calculated on the basis of cube root values, then transformed back to cubic centimeters.
From Cohen HL, Tice HM, Mandel FS: Ovarian volumes measured by US: Bigger than we think. Radiology 177:189–192, 1990.

Table D–2. OVARIAN VOLUME BY MENSTRUAL STATUS

Group	Mean Volume (cm³)	Standard Deviation	No. of Ovaries	95% Confidence Interval (cm³)*
Premenarchal	3.0	2.3	32	0.2–9.1
Menstruating	9.8	5.8	866	2.5–21.9
Postmenopausal	5.8	3.6	100	1.2–14.1

*Calculated on the basis of cube root values, then transformed back to cubic centimeters.
From Cohen HL, Tice HM, Mandel FS: Ovarian volumes measured by US: Bigger than we think. Radiology 177:189–192, 1990.

Table D–3. NORMAL UTERINE DIAMETERS AND VOLUME*

Age (yr)	No. of Patients	Uterine Diameters (mm) TUL Mean SD	COAP Mean SD	CEAP Mean SD	COAP/CEAP Mean SD	Uterine Volume (cm³) By Chronologic Age Mean SD	By Bone Age Mean SD
2	7	33.1 ± 4.4	7.0 ± 3.4	8.3 ± 2.0	0.84 ± 0.29	1.98 ± 1.58	1.76 ± 0.72
3	8	32.4 ± 4.3	6.4 ± 1.3	7.6 ± 2.2	0.89 ± 0.29	1.63 ± 0.81	1.80 ± 0.74
4	15	32.9 ± 3.3	7.6 ± 1.8	8.6 ± 1.8	0.90 ± 0.22	2.10 ± 0.57	1.97 ± 0.74
5	7	33.1 ± 5.5	8.0 ± 2.8	8.4 ± 1.6	0.95 ± 0.28	2.36 ± 1.39	2.19 ± 1.16
6	9	33.2 ± 4.1	6.7 ± 2.9	7.5 ± 1.8	0.86 ± 0.18	1.80 ± 1.57	1.65 ± 0.93
7	9	32.3 ± 3.9	8.0 ± 2.2	7.7 ± 2.5	1.08 ± 0.26	2.32 ± 1.07	2.81 ± 1.44
8	11	35.8 ± 7.3	9.0 ± 2.8	8.4 ± 1.7	1.05 ± 0.20	3.12 ± 1.52	2.70 ± 1.43
9	11	37.1 ± 4.4	9.7 ± 3.0	8.8 ± 2.0	1.10 ± 0.24	3.70 ± 1.62	2.69 ± 1.83
10	13	40.3 ± 6.4	12.8 ± 5.3	10.7 ± 2.6	1.17 ± 0.31	6.54 ± 3.78	4.66 ± 3.03
11	13	42.2 ± 5.1	12.8 ± 3.1	10.7 ± 2.6	1.22 ± 0.26	6.66 ± 2.87	6.24 ± 3.07
12	6	54.3 ± 8.4	17.3 ± 5.3	14.3 ± 5.2	1.23 ± 0.16	16.18 ± 9.15	8.88 ± 3.65
13	5	53.8 ± 11.4	15.8 ± 4.5	15.0 ± 2.4	1.03 ± 0.15	13.18 ± 5.64	15.55 ± 5.98

*As determined by ultrasonography in 114 girls from age 2 to 13. TUL, total uterine length; COAP, anteroposterior diameter of the corpus; CEAP, anteroposterior diameter of the cervix; SD, standard deviation.
From Orsini LF: Pelvic organs in premenarcheal girls: Real-time ultrasonography. Radiology 153:113–116, 1984.

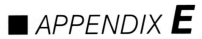

Medications and Reported Associated Malformations

Table E–1. SELECTED MEDICATIONS AND REPORTED ASSOCIATED MALFORMATIONS*

Drug	Malformation
Acetazolamide	Sacrococcygeal teratoma
Amantadine	Cardiac defects
Aminopterin	Neural tube defects, hydrocephalus, limb shortening, cleft lip/palate, clubfoot
p-Aminosalicylic acid	Ear deformity, limb deformity, hypospadias
Amitriptyline	Limb reduction, micrognathia, hypospadias
Amobarbital	Anencephaly, cardiac defects, limb deformity, cleft lip/palate, polydactyly, genitourinary defects, clubfoot
Amphetamine	Cerebral injury in neonates
Aspirin	Intracranial hemorrhage, intrauterine growth retardation
Bromides	Polydactyly, gastrointestinal anomalies, clubfoot
Busulfan	Intrauterine growth retardation, cleft palate, neural tube defects
Captopril†	Second-trimester hypocalvaria
Carbamazepine†	Neural tube defects, cardiac defects
Chlorambucil	Renal agenesis, cardiac defects
Chlordiazepoxide	Microcephaly, duodenal atresia, cardiac defects
Chloroquine	Wilms tumor, hemihypertrophy, tetralogy of Fallot
Chlorothiazide	Fetal bradycardia
Chlorpheniramine	Polydactyly, gastrointestinal defects, hydrocephalus
Chlorpromazine	Microcephaly, syndactyly
Chlorpropamide	Microcephaly, hand anomalies
Clomiphene	Microcephaly, neural tube defects, cleft lip/palate, cardiac defects, syndactyly, clubfoot
Cocaine	Spontaneous abortion, placental abruption, cardiac defects, urinary tract and limb abnormalities, bowel atresias, intrauterine growth retardation
Coumarin derivatives†	Spontaneous abortion, intrauterine growth retardation, neural tube defects [open and closed] (dorsal midline dysplasia), cardiac defects, scoliosis, limb hypoplasia, cleft palate
Cyclophosphamide	Cleft palate, hand abnormalities, cardiac defects, intrauterine growth retardation
Cytarabine	Hand abnormalities (lobster claw deformity), lower limb defects, neural tube defects, cardiac defects
Daunorubicin	Intrauterine growth retardation
Diphenhydramine	Cleft lip/palate, genitourinary defects, clubfoot, cardiac defects
Disulfiram	Clubfoot, VACTERL syndrome, phocomelia
Ethanol (alcohol)†	Intrauterine growth retardation, microphthalmia, micrognathia, microcephaly, hypoplastic maxilla, cardiac defects, genitourinary defects, radioulnar synostosis, Klippel-Feil anomaly, diaphragmatic hernia
Ethoheptazine	Umbilical hernia, hip dislocation
Ethosuximide	Cleft lip/palate, hydrocephalus, patent ductus arteriosus, spontaneous hemorrhage in the neonate
Etretinate†	Neural tube defects, facial dysmorphia, multiple synostoses, syndactylies, limb reduction
Fluorouracil	Radial aplasia, pulmonary hypoplasia, esophageal and duodenal atresia, cloacal malformation
Fluphenazine	Ocular hypertelorism, cleft lip/palate, imperforate anus
Griseofulvin	Conjoined twins
Haloperidol	Limb reduction, aortic valve defect
Heroin	Intrauterine growth retardation, multiple and varied congenital malformations
Ibuprofen	Oligohydramnios, premature closure of patent ductus arteriosus
Imipramine	Diaphragmatic hernia, cleft palate, exencephaly, renal cystic dysplasia
Indomethacin	Oligohydramnios, premature closure of patent ductus arteriosus, phocomelia, penile agenesis
Isoetharine	Clubfoot
Levothyroxine	Cardiac defects, polydactyly
Lithium†	Cardiac defects (Ebstein anomaly, ventricular septal defect, coarctation, mitral atresia), neural tube defects

Table E–1. SELECTED MEDICATIONS AND REPORTED ASSOCIATED MALFORMATIONS* *Continued*

Drug	Malformation
Lysergic acid diethylamide	Intrauterine growth retardation, limb reduction, neural tube defects, cardiac defects
Marijuana	Intrauterine growth retardation, facial anomalies
Mechlorethamine	Intrauterine growth retardation, oligodactyly, malformed kidneys
Meclizine	Eye and ear defects, hypoplastic heart, respiratory defects
Melphalan	Intrauterine growth retardation
Meprobamate	Cardiac defects, omphalocele, joint abnormalities
Mercaptopurine	Cleft palate, microphthalmia, intrauterine growth retardation
Methimazole	Patent urachus
Methotrexate	Intrauterine growth retardation, hypertelorism, dextroposition of the heart, absent digits, absence of frontal bone
Methotrimeprazine	Hydrocephalus, cardiac defects
Metronidazole	Spontaneous abortion and limb, cardiac, urinary, and facial abnormalities
Minoxidil	Omphalocele, clinodactyly, cardiac defects (ventricular septal defects and transposition)
Norethindrone	Neural tube defects, hydrocephalus
Norethynodrel	Cardiac defects
Nortriptyline	Limb reduction
Oxazepam	Neural tube defects, intrauterine growth retardation
Paramethadione†	Spontaneous abortions, intrauterine growth retardation, cardiac defects
Penicillamine	Hydrocephalus, flexion deformities, perforated bowel
Phenacetin	Craniosynostosis, anal atresia, musculoskeletal and urinary tract defects
Phensuximide	Ambiguous genitalia
Phenylephrine	Eye and ear abnormalities, syndactyly, clubfoot, musculoskeletal defects
Phenylpropanolamine	Eye and ear abnormalities, polydactyly
Phenytoin†	Microcephaly, hypertelorism, cleft lip/palate, hypoplasia of distal phalanges, short neck, broad nasal ridge
Procarbazine	Intrauterine growth retardation, cardiac defects, oligodactyly, malformed kidneys
Prochlorperazine	Cleft palate/micrognathia, cardiac defects, skeletal defects
Propoxyphene	Limb abnormalities, omphalocele, micrognathia, clubfoot, microcephaly
Quinacrine	Renal agenesis, neural tube defects
Quinine	Neural tube defects, hydrocephalus, limb defects, facial defects, cardiac defects, urogenital abnormalities, vertebral abnormality, gastrointestinal anomaly
Retinoic acid†	Hydrocephalus, neural tube defects, microphthalmia, microcephaly, cardiac defects, limb abnormalities, cleft palate
Sodium iodide†	Ablation of fetal thyroid gland
Sulfasalazine	Cleft lip/palate, hydrocephalus, cardiac defects, urinary tract abnormalities
Sulfonamides	Limb hypoplasia, urinary tract abnormalities
Thioguanine	Absent digits
Tolbutamide	Syndactyly, cardiac defects
Trimethadione†	Intrauterine growth retardation, microcephaly, cleft lip/palate, cardiac defects, malformed hand, clubfoot, ambiguous genitalia, esophageal atresia, tracheoesophageal fistula
Valproic acid†	Neural tube defects, cardiac defects, facial dysmorphism, hypertelorism, protruding eyes, micrognathia, hydrocephalus, cleft lip/palate, microcephaly, limb reduction, scoliosis, renal hypoplasia, duodenal atresia, hand deformity

*Many of the listed associations are based on case reports that have appeared in the medical literature. It is likely that in many cases the reported association was coincidental to, rather than resultant from, the medication. In all cases of suspected teratogenetic effects a reproductive geneticist or teratologist should be consulted.

†Proven teratogens.

Modified from Briggs GG, Freeman RK, Yaffe SJ: Drugs in Pregnancy and Lactation. Baltimore, Williams & Wilkins, 1990.

Index

Note: Page numbers in *italics* refer to illustrations; page numbers followed by t refer to tables.

ISBN 0-7216-6712-0